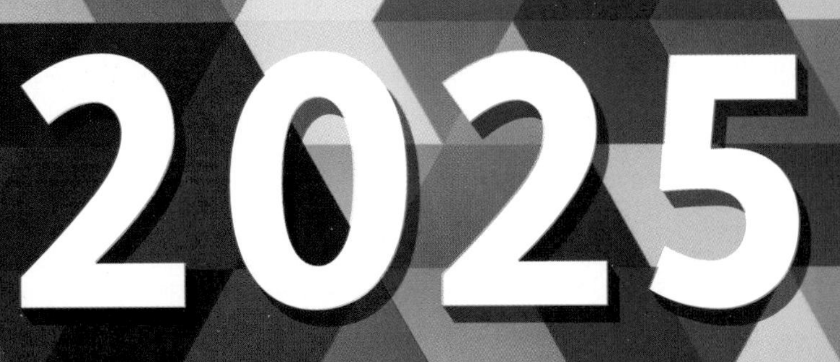
2025

BUCK'S 2025 ICD-10-PCS

Jackie L. Koesterman, CPC
Coding and Reimbursement Specialist
JDK Medical Coding EDU
Grand Forks, North Dakota

INCLUDES NETTER'S ANATOMY ART

T0308345

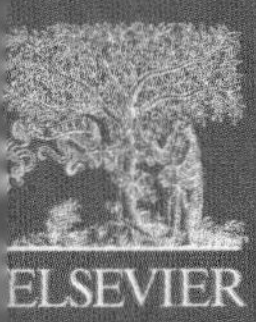
ELSEVIER

Elsevier
3251 Riverport Lane
St. Louis, Missouri 63043

BUCK'S 2025 ICD-10-PCS ISBN: 978-0-443-24884-9

Copyright © 2025 Elsevier Inc. All rights reserved, including those for text and data mining, AI training, and similar technologies.

Publisher's note: Elsevier takes a neutral position with respect to territorial disputes or jurisdictional claims in its published content, including in maps and institutional affiliations.

Some material was previously published.

No part of this publication may be reproduced or transmitted in any form or by any means, electronic or mechanical, including photocopying, recording, or any information storage and retrieval system, without permission in writing from the publisher. Details on how to seek permission, further information about the Publisher's permissions policies and our arrangements with organizations such as the Copyright Clearance Center and the Copyright Licensing Agency, can be found at our website: www.elsevier.com/permissions.

This book and the individual contributions contained in it are protected under copyright by the Publisher (other than as may be noted herein).

Notice

Practitioners and researchers must always rely on their own experience and knowledge in evaluating and using any information, methods, compounds or experiments described herein. Because of rapid advances in the medical sciences, in particular, independent verification of diagnoses and drug dosages should be made. To the fullest extent of the law, no responsibility is assumed by Elsevier, authors, editors or contributors for any injury and/or damage to persons or property as a matter of products liability, negligence or otherwise, or from any use or operation of any methods, products, instructions, or ideas contained in the material herein.

Previous editions copyrighted 2024, 2023, 2022, 2021, 2020, 2019, 2018, 2017, 2016, 2015, 2014, 2013, 2010.

International Standard Book Number: 978-0-443-24884-9

Content Strategist: Luke Held
Content Development Manager: Danielle Frazier
Senior Content Development Specialist: Joshua S. Rapplean
Publishing Services Manager: Deepthi Unni
Project Manager: Nayagi Anandan
Senior Book Designer: Maggie Reid

Printed in Canada

Last digit is the print number: 9 8 7 6 5 4 3 2 1

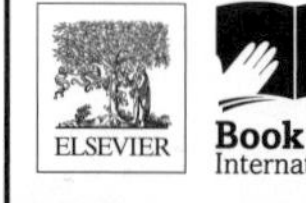
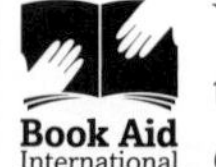
Working together to grow libraries in developing countries

www.elsevier.com • www.bookaid.org

DEDICATION

To all who require of themselves the highest level of accuracy, integrity, and professionalism. You enhance our profession and are a tremendous asset to health care. May this manual be of assistance to you.

With Greatest Admiration.

Carol J. Buck, MS

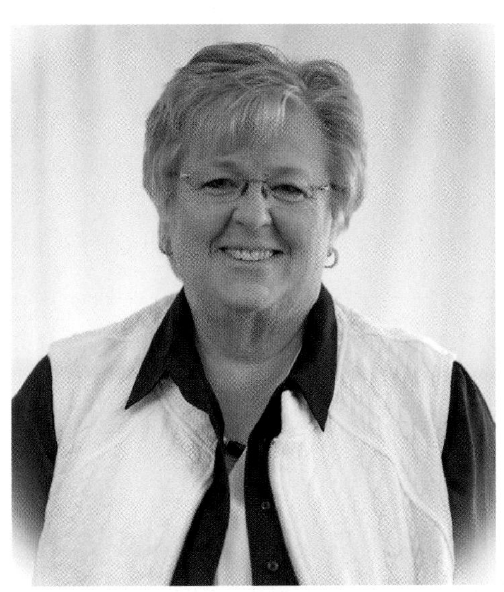

DEVELOPMENT OF THIS EDITION

Lead Technical Collaborator

Jackie L. Koesterman, CPC
Coding and Reimbursement Specialist
JDK Medical Coding EDU
Grand Forks, North Dakota

Query Team

Robin Linker, CHCA, CHCAS, CPC-I, COC, CCS-P, CPC-P, MCS-P, CHC
AAPC Approved Instructor
CEO, Robin Linker & Education Associates, Inc.; and
Association of Health Care Auditors and Educators
Aurora, Colorado

CONTENTS

ICD-10-PCS SYMBOLS AND CONVENTIONS vii

GUIDE TO THE 2025 UPDATES viii

INTRODUCTION 1

ICD-10-PCS Official Guidelines for Coding and Reporting 1

Anatomy Illustrations 9

TABLES 41

Ø Medical and Surgical 41

ØØ Central Nervous System and Cranial Nerves 42

Ø1 Peripheral Nervous System 59

Ø2 Heart and Great Vessels 7Ø

Ø3 Upper Arteries 89

Ø4 Lower Arteries 1Ø8

Ø5 Upper Veins 129

Ø6 Lower Veins 146

Ø7 Lymphatic and Hemic Systems 163

Ø8 Eye 175

Ø9 Ear, Nose, Sinus 192

ØB Respiratory System 21Ø

ØC Mouth and Throat 227

ØD Gastrointestinal System 242

ØF Hepatobiliary System and Pancreas 268

ØG Endocrine System 284

ØH Skin and Breast 292

ØJ Subcutaneous Tissue and Fascia 31Ø

ØK Muscles 329

ØL Tendons 345

ØM Bursae and Ligaments 36Ø

ØN Head and Facial Bones 375

ØP Upper Bones 39Ø

ØQ Lower Bones 4Ø7

ØR Upper Joints 423

ØS Lower Joints 44Ø

ØT Urinary System 457

ØU Female Reproductive System 473
ØV Male Reproductive System 49Ø
ØW Anatomical Regions, General 5Ø5
ØX Anatomical Regions, Upper Extremities 517
ØY Anatomical Regions, Lower Extremities 526
1 Obstetrics 535
2 Placement 54Ø
3 Administration 549
4 Measurement and Monitoring 567
5 Extracorporeal or Systemic Assistance and Performance 573
6 Extracorporeal or Systemic Therapies 576
7 Osteopathic 58Ø
8 Other Procedures 582
9 Chiropractic 585
B Imaging 587
C Nuclear Medicine 645
D Radiation Therapy 666
F Physical Rehabilitation and Diagnostic Audiology 69Ø
G Mental Health 7Ø8
H Substance Abuse Treatment 712
X New Technology 716
INDEX 739
APPENDIX A – Definitions 863
APPENDIX B – Body Part Key 91Ø
APPENDIX C – Device Key 939
APPENDIX D – Substance Key 951
APPENDIX E – Device Aggregation Table 952
APPENDIX F – Procedure Combinations Table on codingupdates.com

SYMBOLS AND CONVENTIONS

Annotated

Throughout the manual, revisions, additions, and deleted codes or words are indicated by the following symbols:

New and revised content from the previous edition are indicated by green font.

~~deleted~~ Deletions from the previous edition are struck through.

ICD-10-PCS Table Symbols

Throughout the manual information is indicated by the following symbols:

♀♂ **Sex conflict:** *Definitions of Medicare Code Edits* (MCE) detects inconsistencies between a patient's sex and any diagnosis or procedure on the patient's record. For example, a male patient with cervical cancer (diagnosis) or a female patient with a prostatectomy (procedure). In both instances, the indicated diagnosis or the procedure conflicts with the stated sex of the patient. Therefore, the patient's diagnosis, procedure, or sex is presumed to be incorrect.

Non-covered: There are some procedures for which Medicare does not provide reimbursement. There are also procedures that would normally not be reimbursed by Medicare but due to the presence of certain diagnoses are reimbursed.

Limited Coverage: For certain procedures whose medical complexity and serious nature incur extraordinary associated costs, Medicare limits coverage to a portion of the cost.

DRG Non-OR A **non-operating room procedure that does affect MS-DRG assignment** is indicated by a purple highlight.

Non-OR A **non-operating room procedure that does not affect MS-DRG assignment** is indicated by a yellow highlight.

Combination: Certain combinations of procedures are treated differently than their constituent codes.

Hospital-Acquired Condition: Some procedures are always associated with Hospital Acquired Conditions (HAC) according to the MS-DRG.

Coding Clinic: American Hospital Association's *Coding Clinic*® citations provide reference information to official ICD-10-PCS coding advice.

OGCR The ***Official Guidelines for Coding and Reporting*** symbol includes the placement of a portion of a guideline as that guideline pertains to the code by which it is located. The complete OGCR are located in the Introduction.

[ ] Brackets below the tables enclose the alphanumeric options for Non-covered, Limited Coverage, DRG Non-OR, Non-OR, and HAC.

Note: The final FY2025 MS-DRG and Medicare Code Edits were unavailable at the time of printing. Proposed new DRG Non-OR procedures were available and have been included below the appropriate tables with "(proposed)" appearing behind the codes. Please check codingupdates.com for final FY2025 MS-DRG and MCE information.

GUIDE TO THE 2025 UPDATES

The ICD-1Ø-PCS codes that have changed are shown in the lists below.
If you would like to see this information in table format, please visit codingupdates.com for a complete listing.

2025 ICD-10-PCS New, Revised, and Deleted Codes

NEW CODES

ØØ5Ø3Z4
ØØKØXZ1
Ø413Ø9R
Ø413ØAR
Ø413ØJR
Ø413ØKR
Ø413ØZR
Ø41349R
Ø4134AR
Ø4134JR
Ø4134KR
Ø4134ZR
Ø414Ø9R
Ø414ØAR
Ø414ØJR
Ø414ØKR
Ø414ØZR
Ø41449R
Ø4144AR
Ø4144JR
Ø4144KR
Ø4144ZR
Ø47K342
Ø47K352
Ø47K362
Ø47K372
Ø47L342
Ø47L352
Ø47L362
Ø47L372
Ø47M342
Ø47M352
Ø47M362
Ø47M372
Ø47N342
Ø47N352
Ø47N362
Ø47N372
Ø47P342
Ø47P352
Ø47P362
Ø47P372
Ø47Q342
Ø47Q352
Ø47Q362
Ø47Q372
Ø47R342
Ø47R352
Ø47R362
Ø47R372
Ø47S342
Ø47S362
Ø47S372
Ø47T342
Ø47T352
Ø47T362
Ø47T372
Ø47U342
Ø47U352
Ø47U362
Ø47U372
Ø71
Ø71ØØZ3
Ø71ØØZ4
Ø71ØØZ7
Ø71ØØZK
Ø71ØØZL
Ø71Ø4Z3
Ø71Ø4Z4
Ø71Ø4Z7
Ø71Ø4ZK
Ø71Ø4ZL
Ø711ØZ3
Ø711ØZ4
Ø711ØZ7
Ø711ØZK
Ø711ØZL
Ø7114Z3
Ø7114Z4
Ø7114Z7
Ø7114ZK
Ø7114ZL
Ø712ØZ3
Ø712ØZ4
Ø712ØZ7
Ø712ØZK
Ø712ØZL
Ø7124Z3
Ø7124Z4
Ø7124Z7
Ø7124ZK
Ø7124ZL
Ø713ØZ3
Ø713ØZ4
Ø713ØZ7
Ø713ØZK
Ø713ØZL
Ø7134Z3
Ø7134Z4
Ø7134Z7
Ø7134ZK
Ø7134ZL
Ø714ØZ3
Ø714ØZ4
Ø714ØZ7
Ø714ØZK
Ø714ØZL
Ø7144Z3
Ø7144Z4
Ø7144Z7
Ø7144ZK
Ø7144ZL
Ø715ØZ3
Ø715ØZ4
Ø715ØZ7
Ø715ØZK
Ø715ØZL
Ø7154Z3
Ø7154Z4
Ø7154Z7
Ø7154ZK
Ø7154ZL
Ø716ØZ3
Ø716ØZ4
Ø716ØZ7
Ø716ØZK
Ø716ØZL
Ø7164Z3
Ø7164Z4
Ø7164Z7
Ø7164ZK
Ø7164ZL
Ø717ØZ3
Ø717ØZ4
Ø717ØZ7
Ø717ØZK
Ø717ØZL
Ø7174Z3
Ø7174Z4
Ø7174Z7
Ø7174ZK
Ø7174ZL
Ø718ØZ3
Ø718ØZ4
Ø718ØZ7
Ø718ØZK
Ø718ØZL
Ø7184Z3
Ø7184Z4
Ø7184Z7
Ø7184ZK
Ø7184ZL
Ø719ØZ3
Ø719ØZ4
Ø719ØZ7
Ø719ØZK
Ø719ØZL
Ø7194Z3
Ø7194Z4
Ø7194Z7
Ø7194ZK
Ø7194ZL
Ø71BØZ3
Ø71BØZ4
Ø71BØZ7
Ø71BØZK
Ø71BØZL
Ø71B4Z3
Ø71B4Z4
Ø71B4Z7
Ø71B4ZK
Ø71B4ZL
Ø71CØZ3
Ø71CØZ4
Ø71CØZ7
Ø71CØZK
Ø71CØZL
Ø71C4Z3
Ø71C4Z4
Ø71C4Z7
Ø71C4ZK
Ø71C4ZL
Ø71DØZ3
Ø71DØZ4
Ø71DØZ7
Ø71DØZK
Ø71DØZL
Ø71D4Z3
Ø71D4Z4
Ø71D4Z7
Ø71D4ZK
Ø71D4ZL
Ø71FØZ3
Ø71FØZ4
Ø71FØZ7
Ø71FØZK
Ø71FØZL
Ø71F4Z3
Ø71F4Z4
Ø71F4Z7
Ø71F4ZK
Ø71F4ZL
Ø71GØZ3
Ø71GØZ4
Ø71GØZ7
Ø71GØZK
Ø71GØZL
Ø71G4Z3
Ø71G4Z4
Ø71G4Z7
Ø71G4ZK
Ø71G4ZL
Ø71HØZ3
Ø71HØZ4
Ø71HØZ7
Ø71HØZK
Ø71HØZL
Ø71H4Z3
Ø71H4Z4
Ø71H4Z7
Ø71H4ZK
Ø71H4ZL
Ø71JØZ3
Ø71JØZ4
Ø71JØZ7
Ø71JØZK
Ø71JØZL
Ø71J4Z3
Ø71J4Z4
Ø71J4Z7
Ø71J4ZK
Ø71J4ZL
Ø71KØZ3
Ø71KØZ4
Ø71KØZ7
Ø71KØZK
Ø71KØZL
Ø71K4Z3
Ø71K4Z4
Ø71K4Z7
Ø71K4ZK
Ø71K4ZL
Ø71LØZ3
Ø71LØZ4
Ø71LØZ7
Ø71LØZK
Ø71LØZL
Ø71L4Z3
Ø71L4Z4
Ø71L4Z7
Ø71L4ZK
Ø71L4ZL
ØFP48ØZ
ØFPG8ØZ
ØFW48ØZ
ØFWG8ØZ
ØHRTØ7B
ØHRUØ7B
ØHRVØ7B
ØNPBØ5Z
ØNPB35Z
ØNPB45Z
ØNPBX5Z
ØNPWØ5Z
ØNPW35Z
ØNPW45Z
ØNPWX5Z
ØNWBØ5Z
ØNWB35Z
ØNWB45Z
ØNWBX5Z
ØNWWØ5Z
ØNWW35Z
ØNWW45Z
ØNWWX5Z
5AØ5AØL
8EØ23FZ
XØ5133A
X27P3TA
X27Q3TA
X27R3TA
X27S3TA
X27T3TA
X27U3TA
X28
X28F3VA
X2R5ØWA
X2R6ØWA
X2R7ØWA
X2R8ØWA
X2RJ3RA
X2VE3SA
XHRØXGA
XHR1XGA
XHR2XGA
XHR3XGA
XHR4XGA
XHR5XGA
XHR6XGA
XHR7XGA
XRGAØEA
XRGBØEA
XRGCØEA
XRGDØEA
XRGJØCA
XRGKØCA
XRGLØCA
XRGMØCA
XRH6ØFA
XRH63FA
XRH64FA
XRH7ØFA
XRH73FA
XRH74FA
XRH8ØFA
XRH83FA
XRH84FA
XRHAØFA
XRHA3FA
XRHA4FA
XRHBØFA
XRHB3FA
XRHB4FA
XRHCØFA
XRHC3FA
XRHC4FA
XRHDØFA
XRHD3FA
XRHD4FA
XWØ136A
XWØ333A
XWØ334A
XWØ335A
XWØ338A
XWØ339A
XWØ33BA
XWØ33CA
XWØ33DA
XWØ33FA
XWØ433A
XWØ434A
XWØ435A

NEW CODES (continued)

XWØ438A
XWØ439A
XWØ43BA
XWØ43CA
XWØ43FA
XWØJ3HA
XWØJ3JA
XWØJ3KA
XWØJ3LA
XWØK3HA
XWØK3JA
XWØK3KA
XWØK3LA
XWØL3HA
XWØL3JA
XWØL3KA
XWØL3LA
XWØM3HA
XWØM3JA
XWØM3KA
XWØM3LA
XWØUØGA
XWØV3WA
XW1337A
XW1437A
XX25XØA
XXA
XXA536A
XXEØX1A
XXE5X2A
XXE5X4A

REVISED CODES

DELETED CODES

X27H385
X27H395
X27H3B5
X27H3C5
X27J385
X27J395
X27J3B5
X27J3C5
X27K385
X27K395
X27K3B5
X27K3C5
X27L385
X27L395
X27L3B5
X27L3C5
X27M385
X27M395
X27M3B5
X27M3C5
X27N385
X27N395
X27N3B5
X27N3C5
X27P385
X27P395
X27P3B5
X27P3C5
X27Q385
X27Q395
X27Q3B5
X27Q3C5
X27R385
X27R395
X27R3B5
X27R3C5
X27S385
X27S395
X27S3B5
X27S3C5
X27T385
X27T395
X27T3B5
X27T3C5
X27U385
X27U395
X27U3B5
X27U3C5
XWØ33K5
XWØ33N5
XWØ33U5
XWØ43K5
XWØ43N5
XWØ43U5
XWØ97M5
XWØDXJ5
XWØDXL5
XWØDXR5
XWØDXT5
XWØDXV5
XXE5XM5

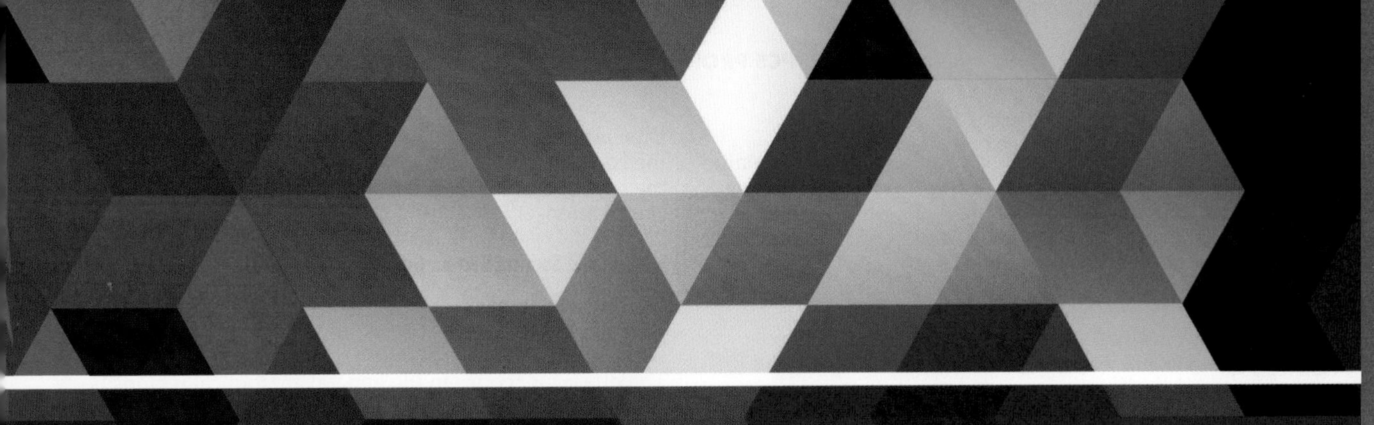

OGCR

Introduction

ICD-10-PCS Official Guidelines for Coding and Reporting

2025

The Centers for Medicare and Medicaid Services (CMS) and the National Center for Health Statistics (NCHS), two departments within the U.S. Federal Government's Department of Health and Human Services (DHHS) provide the following guidelines for coding and reporting using the International Classification of Diseases, 10th Revision, Procedure Coding System (ICD-10-PCS). These guidelines should be used as a companion document to the official version of the ICD-10-PCS as published on the CMS website. The ICD-10-PCS is a procedure classification published by the United States for classifying procedures performed in hospital inpatient health care settings.

These guidelines have been approved by the four organizations that make up the Cooperating Parties for the ICD-10-PCS: the American Hospital Association (AHA), the American Health Information Management Association (AHIMA), CMS, and NCHS.

These guidelines are a set of rules that have been developed to accompany and complement the official conventions and instructions provided within the ICD-10-PCS itself. They are intended to provide direction that is applicable in most circumstances. However, there may be unique circumstances where exceptions are applied. The instructions and conventions of the classification take precedence over guidelines. These guidelines are based on the coding and sequencing instructions in the Tables, Index and Definitions of ICD-10-PCS, but provide additional instruction. Adherence to these guidelines when assigning ICD-10-PCS procedure codes is required under the Health Insurance Portability and Accountability Act (HIPAA). The procedure codes have been adopted under HIPAA for hospital inpatient healthcare settings. A joint effort between the healthcare provider and the coder is essential to achieve complete and accurate documentation, code assignment, and reporting of diagnoses and procedures. These guidelines have been developed to assist both the healthcare provider and the coder in identifying those procedures that are to be reported. The importance of consistent, complete documentation in the medical record cannot be overemphasized. Without such documentation accurate coding cannot be achieved.

Table of Contents

A. Conventions
B. Medical and Surgical Section Guidelines
    2. Body System
    3. Root Operation
    4. Body Part
    5. Approach
    6. Device
C. Obstetrics Section Guidelines
D. Radiation Therapy Guidelines
E. New Technology Section Guidelines
F. Selection of Principal Procedure

Conventions

A1

ICD-10-PCS codes are composed of seven characters. Each character is an axis of classification that specifies information about the procedure performed. Within a defined code range, a character specifies the same type of information in that axis of classification.

Example: The fifth axis of classification specifies the approach in sections 0 through 4 and 7 through 9 of the system.

A2

One of 34 possible values can be assigned to each axis of classification in the seven-character code: they are the numbers 0 through 9 and the alphabet (except I and O because they are easily confused with the numbers 1 and 0). The number of unique values used in an axis of classification differs as needed.

Example: Where the fifth axis of classification specifies the approach, seven different approach values are currently used to specify the approach.

A3

The valid values for an axis of classification can be added to as needed.

Example: If a significantly distinct type of device is used in a new procedure, a new device value can be added to the system.

A4
As with words in their context, the meaning of any single value is a combination of its axis of classification and any preceding values on which it may be dependent.
Example: The meaning of a body part value in the Medical and Surgical section is always dependent on the body system value. The body part value Ø in the Central Nervous body system specifies Brain and the body part value Ø in the Peripheral Nervous body system specifies Cervical Plexus.

A5
As the system is expanded to become increasingly detailed, over time more values will depend on preceding values for their meaning.
Example: In the Lower Joints body system, the device value 3 in the root operation Insertion specifies Infusion Device and the device value 3 in the root operation Replacement specifies Ceramic Synthetic Substitute.

A6
The purpose of the alphabetic index is to locate the appropriate table that contains all information necessary to construct a procedure code. The PCS Tables should always be consulted to find the most appropriate valid code.

A7
It is not required to consult the index first before proceeding to the tables to complete the code. A valid code may be chosen directly from the tables.

A8
All seven characters must be specified to be a valid code. If the documentation is incomplete for coding purposes, the physician should be queried for the necessary information.

A9
Within a PCS table, valid codes include all combinations of choices in characters 4 through 7 contained in the same row of the table. In the example below, ØJHT3VZ is a valid code, and ØJHW3VZ is *not* a valid code.

A1Ø
"And," when used in a code description, means "and/or," except when used to describe a combination of multiple body parts for which separate values exist for each body part (e.g., Skin and Subcutaneous Tissue used as a qualifier, where there are separate body part values for "Skin" and "Subcutaneous Tissue").
Example: Lower Arm and Wrist Muscle means lower arm and/or wrist muscle.

A11
Many of the terms used to construct PCS codes are defined within the system. It is the coder's responsibility to determine what the documentation in the medical record equates to in the PCS definitions. The physician is not expected to use the terms used in PCS code descriptions, nor is the coder required to query the physician when the correlation between the documentation and the defined PCS terms is clear.
Example: When the physician documents "partial resection" the coder can independently correlate "partial resection" to the root operation Excision without querying the physician for clarification.

Medical and Surgical Section Guidelines (section Ø)

B2. Body System

General guidelines

B2.1a
The procedure codes in the general anatomical regions body systems expressed concern with the coding options based on 1) the Index entry and Device Key for Brachytherapy seeds that instructs to use Radioactive Element and 2) published coding advice for the GammaTile™ collagen implant for which a new code was created effective XXXX that describes Insertion with radioactive element and for which a corresponding Index entry exists. Anatomical Regions, General, Anatomical Regions, Upper Extremities and Anatomical Regions, Lower Extremities can be used when the procedure is performed on an anatomical region rather than a specific body part or on the rare occasion when no information is available to support assignment of a code to a specific body part.
Examples: Chest tube drainage of the pleural cavity is coded to the root operation Drainage found in the body system Anatomical Regions, General. Suture repair of the abdominal wall is coded to the root operation Repair in the body system Anatomical Regions, General.
Amputation of the foot is coded to the root operation Detachment in the body system Anatomical Regions, Lower Extremities.

B2.1b
Where the general body part values "upper" and "lower" are provided as an option in the Upper Arteries, Lower Arteries, Upper Veins, Lower Veins, Muscles and Tendons body systems, "upper" or "lower" specifies body parts located above or below the diaphragm respectively.
Example: Vein body parts above the diaphragm are found in the Upper Veins body system; vein body parts below the diaphragm are found in the Lower Veins body system.

B3. Root Operation

General guidelines

B3.1a
In order to determine the appropriate root operation, the full definition of the root operation as contained in the PCS Tables must be applied.

B3.1b
Components of a procedure specified in the root operation definition or explanation as integral to that root operation are not coded separately. Procedural steps necessary to reach the operative site and close the operative site, including anastomosis of a tubular body part, are also not coded separately.

SECTION: Ø **MEDICAL AND SURGICAL**
BODY SYSTEM: J **SUBCUTANEOUS TISSUE AND FASCIA**
OPERATION: H **INSERTION:** Putting in a nonbiological appliance that monitors, assists, performs, or prevents a physiological function but does not physically take the place of a body part

Body Part	Approach	Device	Qualifier
S Subcutaneous Tissue and Fascia, Head and Neck V Subcutaneous Tissue and Fascia, Upper Extremity W Subcutaneous Tissue and Fascia, Lower Extremity	Ø Open 3 Percutaneous	1 Radioactive Element 3 Infusion Device Y Other Device	Z No Qualifier
T Subcutaneous Tissue and Fascia, Trunk	Ø Open 3 Percutaneous	1 Radioactive Element 3 Infusion Device V Infusion Pump Y Other Device	Z No Qualifier

Examples: Resection of a joint as part of a joint replacement procedure is included in the root operation definition of Replacement and is not coded separately. Laparotomy performed to reach the site of an open liver biopsy is not coded separately. In a resection of sigmoid colon with anastomosis of descending colon to rectum, the anastomosis is not coded separately.

Multiple procedures
B3.2
During the same operative episode, multiple procedures are coded if:

a. The same root operation is performed on different body parts as defined by distinct values of the body part character. *Examples:* Diagnostic excision of liver and pancreas are coded separately.
b. The same root operation is repeated in multiple body parts, and those body parts are separate and distinct body parts classified to a single ICD-10-PCS body part value. *Examples:* Excision of the sartorius muscle and excision of the gracilis muscle are both included in the upper leg muscle body part value, and multiple procedures are coded. Extraction of multiple toenails are coded separately.
c. Multiple root operations with distinct objectives are performed on the same body part. *Example:* Destruction of sigmoid lesion and bypass of sigmoid colon are coded separately.
d. The intended root operation is attempted using one approach, but is converted to a different approach. *Example:* Laparoscopic cholecystectomy converted to an open cholecystectomy is coded as percutaneous endoscopic Inspection and open Resection.

Discontinued or incomplete procedures
B3.3
If the intended procedure is discontinued or otherwise not completed, code the procedure to the root operation performed. If a procedure is discontinued before any other root operation is performed, code the root operation Inspection of the body part or anatomical region inspected. *Example:* A planned aortic valve replacement procedure is discontinued after the initial thoracotomy and before any incision is made in the heart muscle, when the patient becomes hemodynamically unstable. This procedure is coded as an open Inspection of the mediastinum.

Biopsy procedures
B3.4a
Biopsy procedures are coded using the root operations Excision, Extraction, or Drainage and the qualifier Diagnostic. *Examples:* Fine needle aspiration biopsy of fluid in the lung is coded to the root operation Drainage with the qualifier Diagnostic. Biopsy of bone marrow is coded to the root operation Extraction with the qualifier Diagnostic. Lymph node sampling for biopsy is coded to the root operation Excision with the qualifier Diagnostic.

Biopsy followed by more definitive treatment
B3.4b
If a diagnostic Excision, Extraction, or Drainage procedure (biopsy) is followed by a more definitive procedure, such as Destruction, Excision or Resection at the same procedure site, both the biopsy and the more definitive treatment are coded. *Example:* Biopsy of breast followed by partial mastectomy at the same procedure site, both the biopsy and the partial mastectomy procedure are coded.

Overlapping body layers
B3.5
If root operations such as, Excision, Extraction, Repair or Inspection are performed on overlapping layers of the musculoskeletal system, the body part specifying the deepest layer is coded.
Example: Excisional debridement that includes skin and subcutaneous tissue and muscle is coded to the muscle body part.

Bypass procedures
B3.6a
Bypass procedures are coded by identifying the body part bypassed "from" and the body part bypassed "to." The fourth character body part specifies the body part bypassed from, and the qualifier specifies the body part bypassed to.
Example: Bypass from stomach to jejunum, stomach is the body part and jejunum is the qualifier.

B3.6b
Coronary artery bypass procedures are coded differently than other bypass procedures as described in the previous guideline. Rather than identifying the body part bypassed from, the body part identifies the number of coronary arteries bypassed to, and the qualifier specifies the vessel bypassed from.
Example: Aortocoronary artery bypass of the left anterior descending coronary artery and the obtuse marginal coronary artery is classified in the body part axis of classification as two coronary arteries, and the qualifier specifies the aorta as the body part bypassed from.

B3.6c
If multiple coronary arteries are bypassed, a separate procedure is coded for each coronary artery that uses a different device and/or qualifier.
Example: Aortocoronary artery bypass and internal mammary coronary artery bypass are coded separately.

Control vs. more specific root operations
B3.7
The root operation Control is defined as, "Stopping, or attempting to stop, postprocedural or other acute bleeding." Control is the root operation coded when the procedure performed to achieve hemostasis, beyond what would be considered integral to a procedure, utilizes techniques (e.g. cautery, application of substances or pressure, suturing or ligation or clipping of bleeding points at the site) that are not described by a more specific root operation, such as Bypass, Detachment, Excision, Extraction, Reposition, Replacement, or Resection. If a more specific root operation definition applies to the procedure performed, then the more specific root operation is coded instead of Control.
Example: Silver nitrate cautery to treat acute nasal bleeding is coded to the root operation Control.
Example: Liquid embolization of the right internal iliac artery to treat acute hematoma by stopping blood flow is coded to the root operation Occlusion.
Example: Suctioning of residual blood to achieve hemostasis during a transbronchial cryobiopsy is considered integral to the cryobiopsy procedure and is not coded separately.

Excision vs. Resection
B3.8
PCS contains specific body parts for anatomical subdivisions of a body part, such as lobes of the lungs or liver and regions of the intestine. Resection of the specific body part is coded whenever all of the body part is cut out or off, rather than coding Excision of a less specific body part.
Example: Left upper lung lobectomy is coded to Resection of Upper Lung Lobe, Left rather than Excision of Lung, Left.

Excision for graft
B3.9
If an autograft is obtained from a different procedure site in order to complete the objective of the procedure, a separate procedure is coded, except when the seventh character qualifier value in the ICD-10-PCS table fully specifies the site from which the autograft was obtained.
Examples: Coronary bypass with excision of saphenous vein graft, excision of saphenous vein is coded separately.
Replacement of breast with autologous deep inferior epigastric artery perforator (DIEP) flap, excision of the DIEP flap is not coded separately. The seventh character qualifier value Deep Inferior Epigastric Artery Perforator Flap in the Replacement table fully specifies the site of the autograft harvest.

Fusion procedures of the spine
B3.1Øa
The body part coded for a spinal vertebral joint(s) rendered immobile by a spinal fusion procedure is classified by the level of the spine (e.g., thoracic). There are distinct body part values for a single vertebral joint and for multiple vertebral joints at each spinal level.
Example: Body part values specify Lumbar Vertebral Joint, Lumbar Vertebral Joints, 2 or More and Lumbosacral Vertebral Joint.
B3.1Øb
If multiple vertebral joints are fused, a separate procedure is coded for each vertebral joint that uses a different device and/or qualifier.
Example: Fusion of lumbar vertebral joint, posterior approach, anterior column and fusion of lumbar vertebral joint, posterior approach, posterior column are coded separately.
B3.1Øc
Combinations of devices and materials are often used on a vertebral joint to render the joint immobile. When combinations of devices are used on the same vertebral joint, the device value coded for the procedure is as follows:

- If an interbody fusion device is used to render the joint immobile (containing bone graft or bone graft sustitute), the procedure is coded with the device value Interbody Fusion Device
- If bone graft is the *only* device used to render the joint immobile, the procedure is coded with the device value Nonautologous Tissue Substitute or Autologous Tissue Substitute
- If a mixture of autologous and nonautologous bone graft (with or without biological or synthetic extenders or binders) is used to render the joint immobile, code the procedure with the device value Autologous Tissue Substitute

Examples: Fusion of a vertebral joint using a cage style interbody fusion device containing morsellized bone graft is coded to the device Interbody Fusion Device. Fusion of a vertebral joint using a bone dowel interbody fusion device made of cadaver bone and packed with a mixture of local morsellized bone and demineralized bone matrix is coded to the device Interbody Fusion Device.
Fusion of a vertebral joint using both autologous bone graft and bone bank bone graft is coded to the device Autologous Tissue Substitute.

Inspection procedures
B3.11a
Inspection of a body part(s) performed in order to achieve the objective of a procedure is not coded separately.
Example: Fiberoptic bronchoscopy performed for irrigation of bronchus, only the irrigation procedure is coded.
B3.11b
If multiple tubular body parts are inspected, the most distal body part (the body part furthest from the starting point of the inspection) is coded. If multiple non-tubular body parts in a region are inspected, the body part that specifies the entire area inspected is coded.
Examples: Cystoureteroscopy with inspection of bladder and ureters is coded to the ureter body part value. Exploratory laparotomy with general inspection of abdominal contents is coded to the peritoneal cavity body part value.
B3.11c
When both an Inspection procedure and another procedure are performed on the same body part during the same episode, if the Inspection procedure is performed using a different approach than the other procedure, the Inspection procedure is coded separately.
Example: Endoscopic Inspection of the duodenum is coded separately when open.
Excision of the duodenum is performed during the same procedural episode.

Occlusion vs. Restriction for vessel embolization procedures
B3.12
If the objective of an embolization procedure is to completely close a vessel, the root operation Occlusion is coded. If the objective of an embolization procedure is to narrow the lumen of a vessel, the root operation Restriction is coded.
Examples: Tumor embolization is coded to the root operation Occlusion, because the objective of the procedure is to cut off the blood supply to the vessel.
Embolization of a cerebral aneurysm is coded to the root operation Restriction, because the objective of the procedure is not to close off the vessel entirely, but to narrow the lumen of the vessel at the site of the aneurysm where it is abnormally wide.

Release procedures
B3.13
In the root operation Release, the body part value coded is the body part being freed and not the tissue being manipulated or cut to free the body part.
Example: Lysis of intestinal adhesions is coded to the specific intestine body part value.

Release vs. Division
B3.14
If the sole objective of the procedure is freeing a body part without cutting the body part, the root operation is Release. If the sole objective of the procedure is separating or transecting a body part, the root operation is Division.
Examples: Freeing a nerve root from surrounding scar tissue to relieve pain is coded to the root operation Release. Severing a nerve root to relieve pain is coded to the root operation Division.

Reposition for fracture treatment
B3.15
Reduction of a displaced fracture is coded to the root operation Reposition and the application of a cast or splint in conjunction with the Reposition procedure is not coded separately. Treatment of a nondisplaced fracture is coded to the procedure performed.
Examples: Casting of a nondisplaced fracture is coded to the root operation Immobilization in the Placement section.
Putting a pin in a nondisplaced fracture is coded to the root operation Insertion.

Transplantation vs. Administration
B3.16
Putting in a mature and functioning living body part taken from another individual or animal is coded to the root operation Transplantation. Putting in autologous or nonautologous cells is coded to the Administration section.
Example: Putting in autologous or nonautologous bone marrow, pancreatic islet cells or stem cells is coded to the Administration section.

Transfer procedures using multiple tissue layers
B3.17
The root operation Transfer contains qualifiers that can be used to specify when a transfer flap is composed of more than one tissue layer, such as a musculocutaneous flap. For procedures involving transfer of multiple tissue layers including skin, subcutaneous tissue, fascia or muscle, the procedure is coded to the body part value that describes the deepest tissue layer in the flap, and the qualifier can be used to describe the other tissue layer(s) in the transfer flap.
Example: A musculocutaneous flap transfer is coded to the appropriate body part value in the body system Muscles, and the qualifier is used to describe the additional tissue layer(s) in the transfer flap.

Excision/Resection followed by replacement
B3.18
If an excision or resection of a body part is followed by a replacement procedure, code both procedures to identify each distinct objective, except when the excision or resection is considered integral and preparatory for the replacement procedure.
Examples: Mastectomy followed by reconstruction, both resection and replacement of the breast are coded to fully capture the distinct objectives of the procedures performed. Maxillectomy with obturator reconstruction, both excision and replacement of the maxilla are coded to fully capture the distinct objectives of the procedures performed. Excisional debridement of tendon with skin graft, both the excision of the tendon and the replacement of the skin with a graft are coded to fully capture the distinct objectives of the procedures performed. Esophagectomy followed by reconstruction with colonic interposition, both the resection and the transfer of the large intestine to function as the esophagus are coded to fully capture the distinct objectives of the procedures performed.
Examples: Resection of a joint as part of a joint replacement procedure is considered integral and preparatory for the replacement of the joint and the resection is not coded separately. Resection of a valve as part of a valve replacement procedure is considered integral and preparatory for the valve replacement and the resection is not coded separately.

Detachment procedures of extremities
B3.19
The root operation Detachment contains qualifiers that can be used to specify the level where the extremity was amputated. These qualifiers are dependent on the body part value in the "upper extremities" and "lower extremities" body systems. For procedures involving the detachment of all or part of the upper or lower extremities, the procedure is coded to the body part value that describes the site of the detachment.
Example: An amputation at the proximal portion of the shaft of the tibia and fibula is coded to the Lower leg body part value in the body system Anatomical Regions, Lower Extremities, and the qualifier High is used to specify the level where the extremity was detached.

The following definitions were developed for the Detachment qualifiers

Body Part	Qualifier	Definition
Upper arm and upper leg	1	High: Amputation at the proximal portion of the shaft of the humerus or femur
	2	Mid: Amputation at the middle portion of the shaft of the humerus or femur
	3	Low: Amputation at the distal portion of the shaft of the humerus or femur
Lower arm and lower leg	1	High: Amputation at the proximal portion of the shaft of the radius/ulna or tibia/fibula
	2	Mid: Amputation at the middle portion of the shaft of the radius/ulna or tibia/fibula
	3	Low: Amputation at the distal portion of the shaft of the radius/ulna or tibia/fibula
Hand and Foot	Ø	Complete*
	4	Complete 1st Ray
	5	Complete 2nd Ray
	6	Complete 3rd Ray
	7	Complete 4th Ray
	8	Complete 5th Ray
	9	Partial 1st Ray
	B	Partial 2nd Ray
	C	Partial 3rd Ray
	D	Partial 4th Ray
	F	Partial 5th Ray
Thumb, finger, or toe	Ø	Complete: Amputation at the metacarpophalangeal/metatarsal-phalangeal joint
	1	High: Amputation anywhere along the proximal phalanx
	2	Mid: Amputation through the proximal interphalangeal joint or anywhere along the middle phalanx
	3	Low: Amputation through the distal interphalangeal joint or anywhere along the distal phalanx

*When coding amputation of Hand and Foot, the following definitions are followed:
Complete: Amputation through the carpometacarpal joint of the hand, or through the tarsal-metatarsal joint of the foot.
Partial: Amputation anywhere along the shaft or head of the metacarpal bone of the hand, or of the metatarsal bone of the foot.

GUIDELINES (ICD-10-PCS)

B4. Body Part

General guidelines

B4.1a

If a procedure is performed on a portion of a body part that does not have a separate body part value, code the body part value corresponding to the whole body part.

Example: A procedure performed on the alveolar process of the mandible is coded to the mandible body part.

B4.1b

If the prefix "peri" is combined with a body part to identify the site of the procedure, and the site of the procedure is not further specified, then the procedure is coded to the body part named. This guideline applies only when a more specific body part value is not available.

Examples: A procedure site identified as perirenal is coded to the kidney body part when the site of the procedure is not further specified. A procedure site described in the documentation as peri-urethral, and the documentation also indicates that it is the vulvar tissue and not the urethral tissue that is the site of the procedure, then the procedure is coded to the vulva body part.

A procedure site documented as involving the periosteum is coded to the corresponding bone body part.

B4.1c

If a procedure is performed on a continuous section of an arterial or venous single vascular body part, code the body part value corresponding to the anatomically most proximal (closest to the heart) portion of the arterial or venous body part.

Example: A procedure performed on a continuous section of artery from the femoral artery to the external iliac artery with the point of entry at the femoral artery is coded to the external iliac body part. A procedure performed on a continuous section of artery from the femoral artery to the external iliac artery with the point of entry at the external iliac artery is also coded to the external iliac artery body part.

Branches of body parts

B4.2

Where a specific branch of a body part does not have its own body part value in PCS, the body part is typically coded to the closest proximal branch that has a specific body part value. In the cardiovascular body systems, if a general body part is available in the correct root operation table, and coding to a proximal branch would require assigning a code in a different body system, the procedure is coded using the general body part value.

Example: A procedure performed on the mandibular branch of the trigeminal nerve is coded to the trigeminal nerve body part value.

Bilateral body part values

B4.3

Bilateral body part values are available for a limited number of body parts. If the identical procedure is performed on contralateral body parts, and a bilateral body part value exists for that body part, a single procedure is coded using the bilateral body part value. If no bilateral body part value exists, each procedure is coded separately using the appropriate body part value.

Examples: The identical procedure performed on both fallopian tubes is coded once using the body part value Fallopian Tube, Bilateral. The identical procedure performed on both knee joints is coded twice using the body part values Knee Joint, Right and Knee Joint, Left.

Coronary arteries

B4.4

The coronary arteries are classified as a single body part that is further specified by number of arteries treated. One procedure code specifying multiple arteries is used when the same procedure is performed, including the same device and qualifier values.

Examples: Angioplasty of two distinct coronary arteries with placement of two stents is coded as Dilation of Coronary Artery, Two Arteries with Two Intraluminal Devices.

Angioplasty of two distinct coronary arteries, one with stent placed and one without, is coded separately as Dilation of Coronary Artery, One Artery with Intraluminal Device, and Dilation of Coronary Artery, One Artery with no device.

Tendons, ligaments, bursae and fascia near a joint

B4.5

Procedures performed on tendons, ligaments, bursae and fascia supporting a joint are coded to the body part in the respective body system that is the focus of the procedure. Procedures performed on joint structures themselves are coded to the body part in the joint body systems.

Examples: Repair of the anterior cruciate ligament of the knee is coded to the knee bursae and ligament body part in the bursae and ligaments body system. Knee arthroscopy with shaving of articular cartilage is coded to the knee joint body part in the Lower Joints body system.

Skin, subcutaneous tissue and fascia overlying a joint

B4.6

If a procedure is performed on the skin, subcutaneous tissue or fascia overlying a joint, the procedure is coded to the following body part:

- Shoulder is coded to Upper Arm
- Elbow is coded to Lower Arm
- Wrist is coded to Lower Arm
- Hip is coded to Upper Leg
- Knee is coded to Lower Leg
- Ankle is coded to Foot

Fingers and toes

B4.7

If a body system does not contain a separate body part value for fingers, procedures performed on the fingers are coded to the body part value for the hand. If a body system does not contain a separate body part value for toes, procedures performed on the toes are coded to the body part value for the foot.

Example: Excision of finger muscle is coded to one of the hand muscle body part values in the Muscles body system.

Upper and lower intestinal tract

B4.8

In the Gastrointestinal body system, the general body part values Upper Intestinal Tract and Lower Intestinal Tract are provided as an option for the root operations such as Change, Inspection, Removal and Revision. Upper Intestinal Tract includes the portion of the gastrointestinal tract from the esophagus down to and including the duodenum, and Lower Intestinal Tract includes the portion of the gastrointestinal tract from the jejunum down to and including the rectum and anus.

Example: In the root operation Change table, change of a device in the jejunum is coded using the body part Lower Intestinal Tract.

B5. Approach

Open approach with percutaneous endoscopic assistance

B5.2a

Procedures performed using the open approach with percutaneous endoscopic assistance are coded to the approach Open.

Example: Laparoscopic-assisted sigmoidectomy is coded to the approach Open.

Percutaneous endoscopic approach with hand-assistance or extension of incision
B5.2b
Procedures performed using the percutaneous endoscopic approach with hand-assistance, or with an incision or extension of an incision to assist in the removal of all or a portion of a body part, or to anastomose a tubular body part with or without the temporary exteriorization of a body structure, are coded to the approach value Percutaneous Endoscopic.
Examples: Hand-assisted laparoscopic sigmoid colon resection with exteriorization of a segment of the colon for removal of specimen with return of colon back into abdominal cavity is coded to the approach value percutaneous endoscopic.
Laparoscopic sigmoid colectomy with extension of stapling port for removal of specimen and direct anastomosis is coded to the approach value percutaneous endoscopic.
Laparoscopic nephrectomy with midline incision for removing the resected kidney is coded to the approach value percutaneous endoscopic.
Robotic-assisted laparoscopic prostatectomy with extension of incision for removal of the resected prostate is coded to the approach value percutaneous endoscopic.

External approach
B5.3a
Procedures performed within an orifice on structures that are visible without the aid of any instrumentation are coded to the approach External.
Example: Resection of tonsils is coded to the approach External.

B5.3b
Procedures performed indirectly by the application of external force through the intervening body layers are coded to the approach External.
Example: Closed reduction of fracture is coded to the approach External.

Percutaneous procedure via device
B5.4
Procedures performed percutaneously via a device placed for the procedure are coded to the approach Percutaneous.
Example: Fragmentation of kidney stone performed via percutaneous nephrostomy is coded to the approach Percutaneous.

B6. Device
General guidelines
B6.1a
A device is coded only if a device remains after the procedure is completed. If no device remains, the device value No Device is coded. In limited root operations, the classification provides the qualifier values Temporary and Intraoperative, for specific procedures involving clinically significant devices, where the purpose of the device is to be utilized for a brief duration during the procedure or current inpatient stay. If a device that is intended to remain after the procedure is completed requires removal before the end of the operative episode in which it was inserted, both the insertion and removal of the device should be coded.

B6.1b
Materials such as sutures, ligatures, radiological markers and temporary post-operative wound drains are considered integral to the performance of a procedure and are not coded as devices.

B6.1c
Procedures performed on a device only and not on a body part are specified in the root operations Change, Irrigation, Removal and Revision, and are coded to the procedure performed.
Example: Irrigation of percutaneous nephrostomy tube is coded to the root operation Irrigation of indwelling device in the Administration section.

Drainage device
B6.2
A separate procedure to put in a drainage device is coded to the root operation Drainage with the device value Drainage Device.

Obstetric Section Guidelines (section 1)

C. Obstetrics Section
Products of conception
C1
Procedures performed on the products of conception are coded to the Obstetrics section. Procedures performed on the pregnant female other than the products of conception are coded to the appropriate root operation in the Medical and Surgical section.
Example: Amniocentesis is coded to the products of conception body part in the Obstetrics section. Repair of obstetric urethral laceration is coded to the urethra body part in the Medical and Surgical section.

Procedures following delivery or abortion
C2
Procedures performed following a delivery or abortion for curettage of the endometrium or evacuation of retained products of conception are all coded in the Obstetrics section, to the root operation Extraction and the body part Products of Conception, Retained. Diagnostic or therapeutic dilation and curettage performed during times other than the postpartum or post-abortion period are all coded in the Medical and Surgical section, to the root operation Extraction and the body part Endometrium.

Radiation Therapy Section Guidelines (section D)

D. Radiation Therapy Section
Brachytherapy
D1.a
Brachytherapy is coded to the modality Brachytherapy in the Radiation Therapy section. When a radioactive brachytherapy source is left in the body at the end of the procedure, it is coded separately to the root operation Insertion with the device value Radioactive Element.
Example: Brachytherapy with implantation of a low dose rate brachytherapy source left in the body at the end of the procedure is coded to the applicable treatment site in section D, Radiation Therapy, with the modality Brachytherapy, the modality qualifier value Low Dose Rate, and the applicable isotope value and qualifier value. The implantation of the brachytherapy source is coded separately to the device value Radioactive Element in the appropriate Insertion table of the Medical and Surgical section. The Radiation Therapy section code identifies the specific modality and isotope of the brachytherapy, and the root operation Insertion code identifies the implantation of the brachytherapy source that remains in the body at the end of the procedure.
Exception: Implantation of Cesium-131 brachytherapy seeds embedded in a collagen matrix to the treatment site after resection of brain tumor is coded to the root operation Insertion with the device value Radioactive Element, Cesium-131 Collagen Implant. The procedure is coded to the root operation Insertion only, because the device value identifies both the implantation of the radioactive element and a specific brachytherapy isotope that is not included in the Radiation Therapy section tables.

D1.b
A separate procedure to place a temporary applicator for delivering the brachytherapy is coded to the root operation Insertion and the device value Other Device.
Examples: Intrauterine brachytherapy applicator placed as a separate procedure from the brachytherapy procedure is coded to Insertion of Other Device, and the brachytherapy is coded separately using the modality Brachytherapy in the Radiation Therapy section.
Intrauterine brachytherapy applicator placed concomitantly with delivery of the brachytherapy dose is coded with a single code using the modality Brachytherapy in the Radiation Therapy section.

New Technology Section Guidelines (section X)

E. New Technology Section

General guidelines

E1.a

Section X codes fully represent the specific procedure described in the code title, and do not require additional codes from other sections of ICD-10-PCS. When section X contains a code title which fully describes a specific new technology procedure, and is the only procedure performed, only the section X code is reported for the procedure. There is no need to report an additional code in another section of ICD-10-PCS.

Example: XW043A6 Introduction of Cefiderocol Anti-infective into Central Vein, Percutaneous Approach, New Technology Group 6, can be coded to indicate that Cefiderocol Anti-infective was administered via a central vein. A separate code from table 3E0 in the Administration section of ICD-10-PCS is not coded in addition to this code.

E1.b

When multiple procedures are performed, New Technology section X codes are coded following the multiple procedures guideline.

Examples: Dual filter cerebral embolic filtration used during transcatheter aortic valve replacement (TAVR), X2A5312 Cerebral Embolic Filtration, Dual Filter in Innominate Artery and Left Common Carotid Artery, Percutaneous Approach, New Technology Group 2, is coded for the cerebral embolic filtration, along with an ICD-10-PCS code for the TAVR procedure.

An extracorporeal flow reversal circuit for embolic neuroprotection placed during a transcarotid arterial revascularization procedure, a code from table X2A, Assistance of the Cardiovascular System is coded for the use of the extracoporeal flow reversal circuit, along with an ICD-10-PCS code for the transcarotid arterial revascularization procedure.

F. Selection of Principal Procedure

The following instructions should be applied in the selection of principal procedure and clarification on the importance of the relation to the principal diagnosis when more than one procedure is performed:

1. Procedure performed for definitive treatment of both principal diagnosis and secondary diagnosis
   a. Sequence procedure performed for definitive treatment most related to principal diagnosis as principal procedure.
2. Procedure performed for definitive treatment and diagnostic procedures performed for both principal diagnosis and secondary diagnosis
   a. Sequence procedure performed for definitive treatment most related to principal diagnosis as principal procedure
3. A diagnostic procedure was performed for the principal diagnosis and a procedure is performed for definitive treatment of a secondary diagnosis.
   a. Sequence diagnostic procedure as principal procedure, since the procedure most related to the principal diagnosis takes precedence.
4. No procedures performed that are related to principal diagnosis; procedures performed for definitive treatment and diagnostic procedures were performed for secondary diagnosis
   a. Sequence procedure performed for definitive treatment of secondary diagnosis as principal procedure, since there are no procedures (definitive or nondefinitive treatment) related to principal diagnosis.

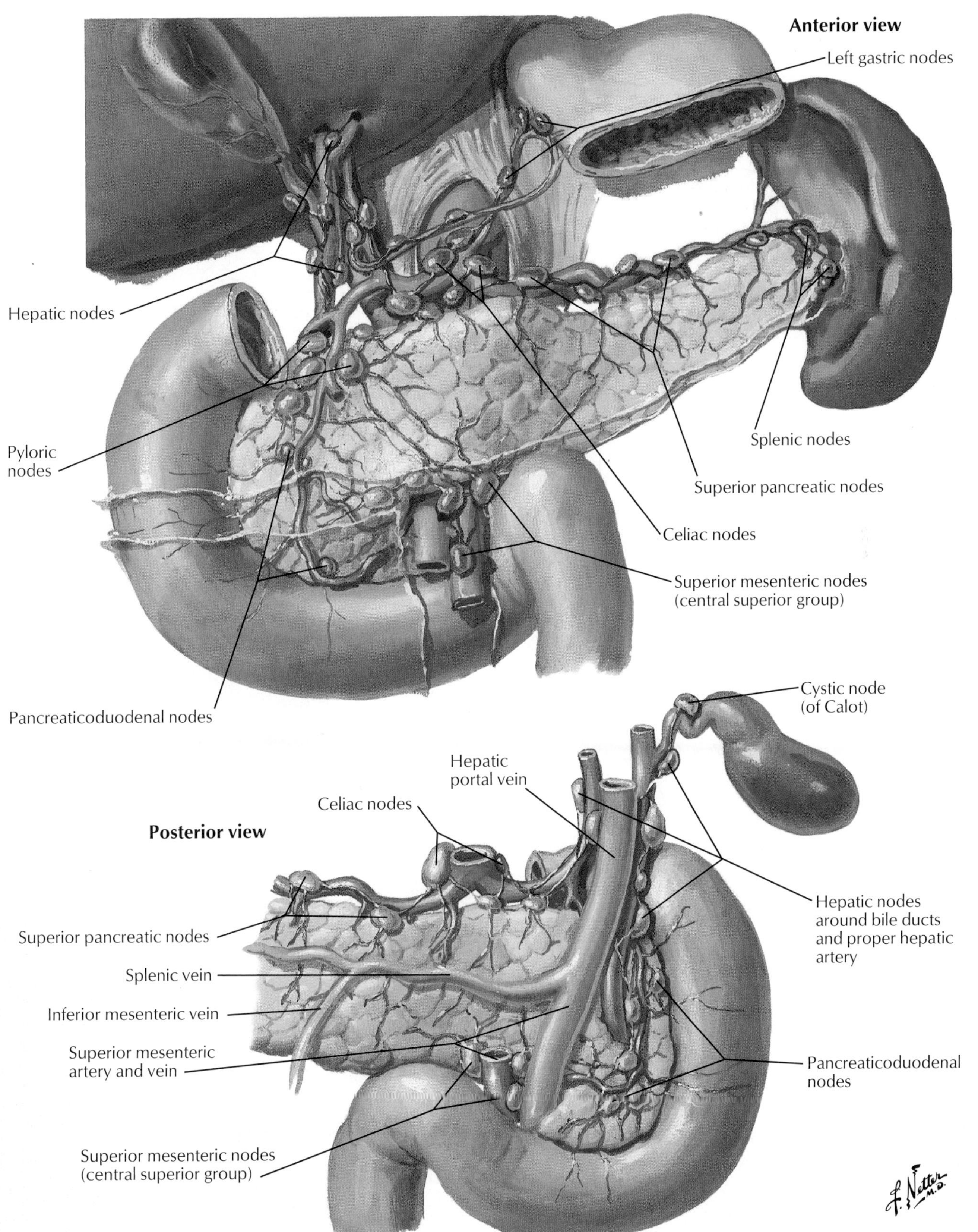
Anterior view
Left gastric nodes
Hepatic nodes
Pyloric nodes
Splenic nodes
Superior pancreatic nodes
Celiac nodes
Superior mesenteric nodes (central superior group)
Pancreaticoduodenal nodes
Cystic node (of Calot)
Hepatic portal vein
Celiac nodes
Posterior view
Hepatic nodes around bile ducts and proper hepatic artery
Superior pancreatic nodes
Splenic vein
Inferior mesenteric vein
Superior mesenteric artery and vein
Pancreaticoduodenal nodes
Superior mesenteric nodes (central superior group)
F. Netter M.D.

Plate 1 Lymph Vessels and Nodes of Pancreas. (Copyright 2024 Elsevier Inc. All rights reserved. www.netterimages.com. Image ID: 4420)

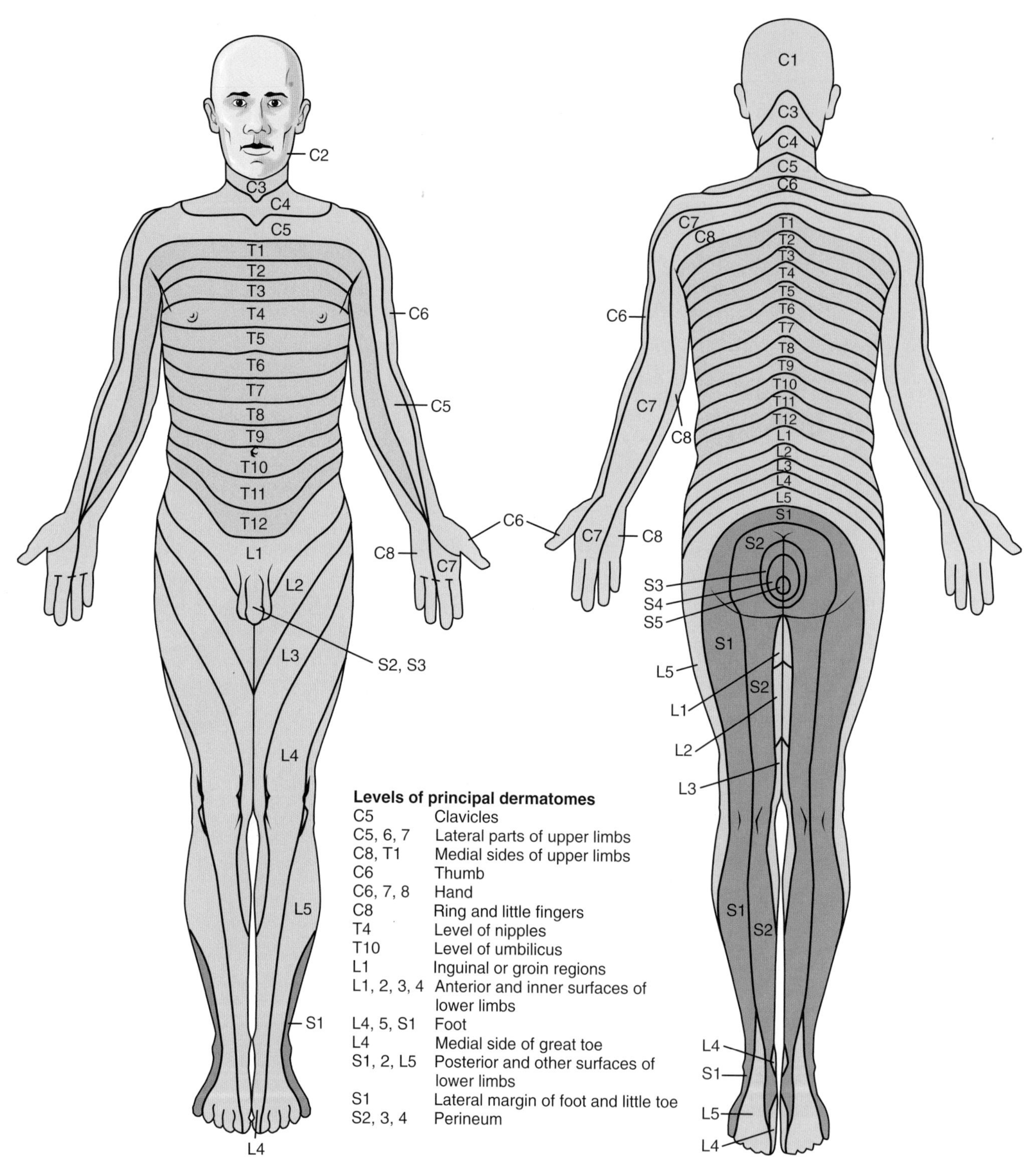
C2
C3
C4
C5
T1
T2
T3
T4
T5
T6
T7
T8
T9
T10
T11
T12
L1
L2
L3
L4
L5
S1
L4
C6
C5
C8
C7
C6
S2, S3
C1
C3
C4
C5
C6
C7
C8
C6
C7
C8
C7
C8
S2
S3
S4
S5
S1
L5
L1
L2
L3
S2
S1
S2
L4
S1
L5
L4
Levels of principal dermatomes
C5 Clavicles
C5, 6, 7 Lateral parts of upper limbs
C8, T1 Medial sides of upper limbs
C6 Thumb
C6, 7, 8 Hand
C8 Ring and little fingers
T4 Level of nipples
T10 Level of umbilicus
L1 Inguinal or groin regions
L1, 2, 3, 4 Anterior and inner surfaces of lower limbs
L4, 5, S1 Foot
L4 Medial side of great toe
S1, 2, L5 Posterior and other surfaces of lower limbs
S1 Lateral margin of foot and little toe
S2, 3, 4 Perineum

Plate 2 Schematic demarcation of Dermatomes. (Miller MD, Hart JA, MacKnight JM: Essential Orthopaedics, ed 2, Philadelphia, 2020, Elsevier.)

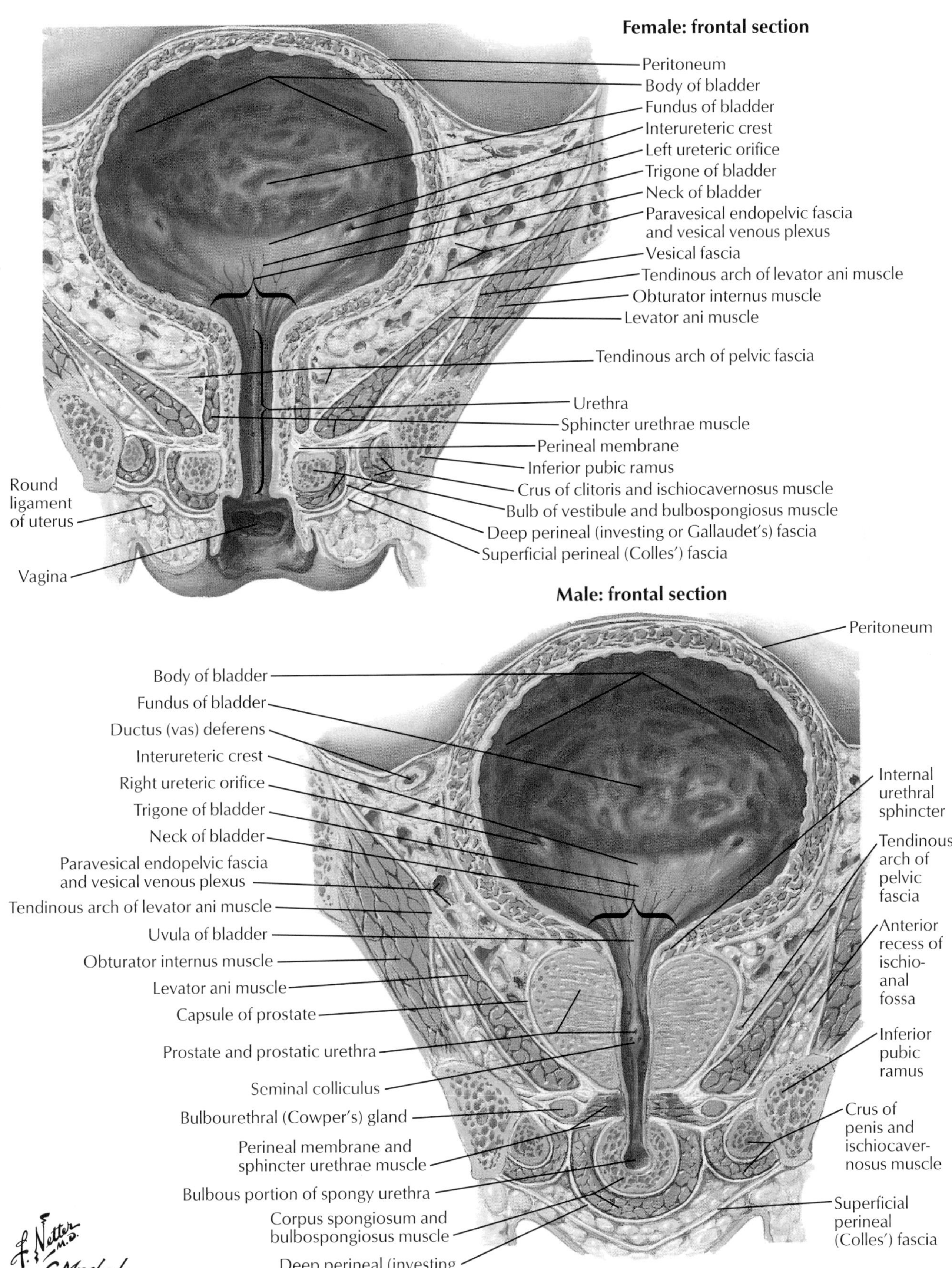
Female: frontal section
Peritoneum
Body of bladder
Fundus of bladder
Interureteric crest
Left ureteric orifice
Trigone of bladder
Neck of bladder
Paravesical endopelvic fascia and vesical venous plexus
Vesical fascia
Tendinous arch of levator ani muscle
Obturator internus muscle
Levator ani muscle
Tendinous arch of pelvic fascia
Urethra
Sphincter urethrae muscle
Perineal membrane
Inferior pubic ramus
Crus of clitoris and ischiocavernosus muscle
Bulb of vestibule and bulbospongiosus muscle
Deep perineal (investing or Gallaudet's) fascia
Superficial perineal (Colles') fascia
Round ligament of uterus
Vagina
Male: frontal section
Peritoneum
Body of bladder
Fundus of bladder
Ductus (vas) deferens
Interureteric crest
Right ureteric orifice
Trigone of bladder
Neck of bladder
Paravesical endopelvic fascia and vesical venous plexus
Tendinous arch of levator ani muscle
Uvula of bladder
Obturator internus muscle
Levator ani muscle
Capsule of prostate
Prostate and prostatic urethra
Seminal colliculus
Bulbourethral (Cowper's) gland
Perineal membrane and sphincter urethrae muscle
Bulbous portion of spongy urethra
Corpus spongiosum and bulbospongiosus muscle
Deep perineal (investing or Gallaudet's) fascia
Internal urethral sphincter
Tendinous arch of pelvic fascia
Anterior recess of ischio-anal fossa
Inferior pubic ramus
Crus of penis and ischiocavernosus muscle
Superficial perineal (Colles') fascia
F. Netter M.D.
C. Machado M.D.

ANATOMY ILLUSTRATIONS

Plate 3 Urinary Bladder: Female and Male. (Copyright 2024 Elsevier Inc. All rights reserved. www.netterimages.com. Image ID: 4714)

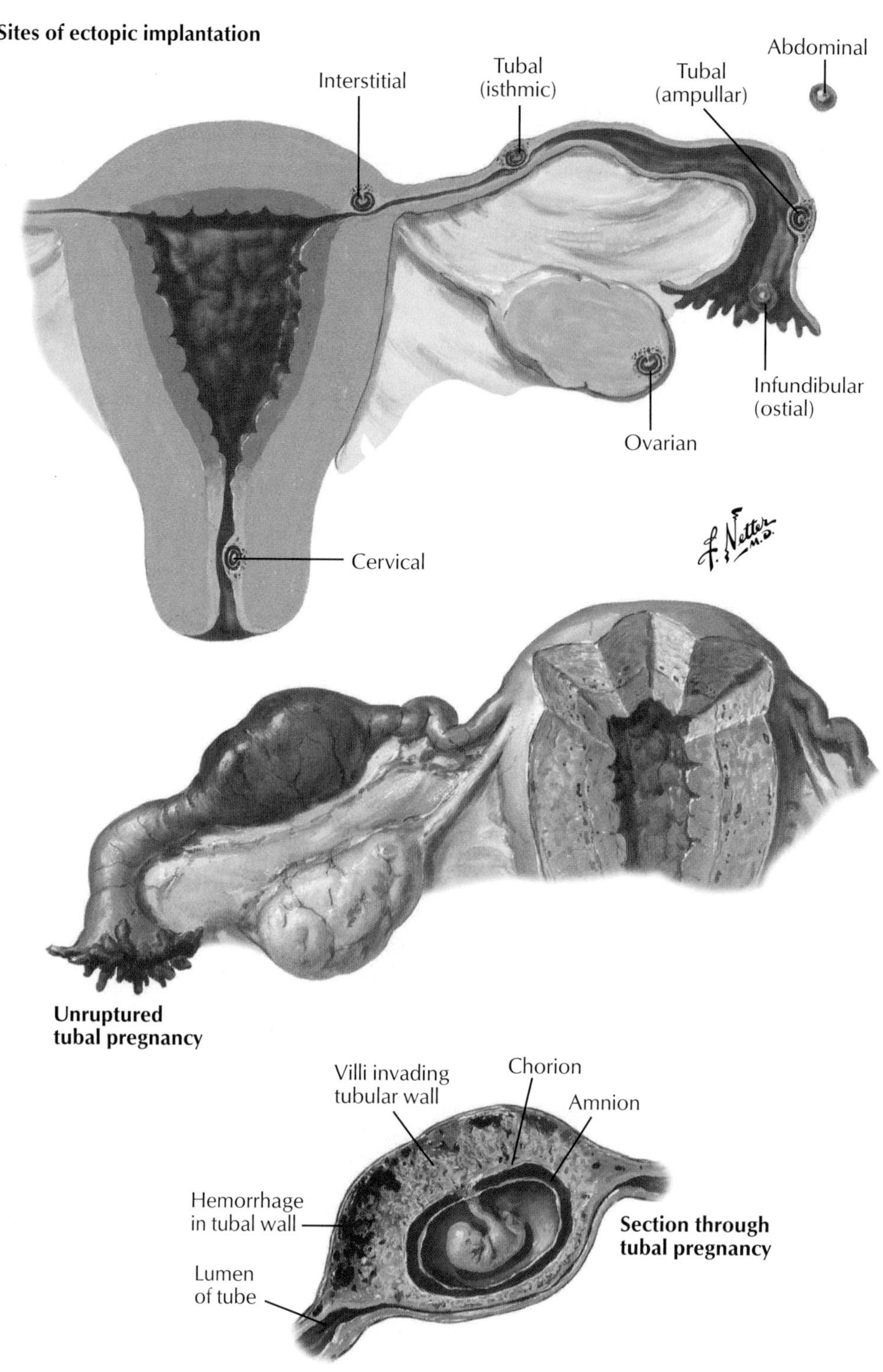
Sites of ectopic implantation
Interstitial
Tubal
(isthmic)
Tubal
(ampullar)
Abdominal
Infundibular
(ostial)
Ovarian
Cervical
Unruptured
tubal pregnancy
Villi invading
tubular wall
Chorion
Amnion
Hemorrhage
in tubal wall
Lumen
of tube
Section through
tubal pregnancy

Plate 4 Ectopic Pregnancy. (Copyright 2024 Elsevier Inc. All rights reserved. www.netterimages.com. Image ID: 5148)

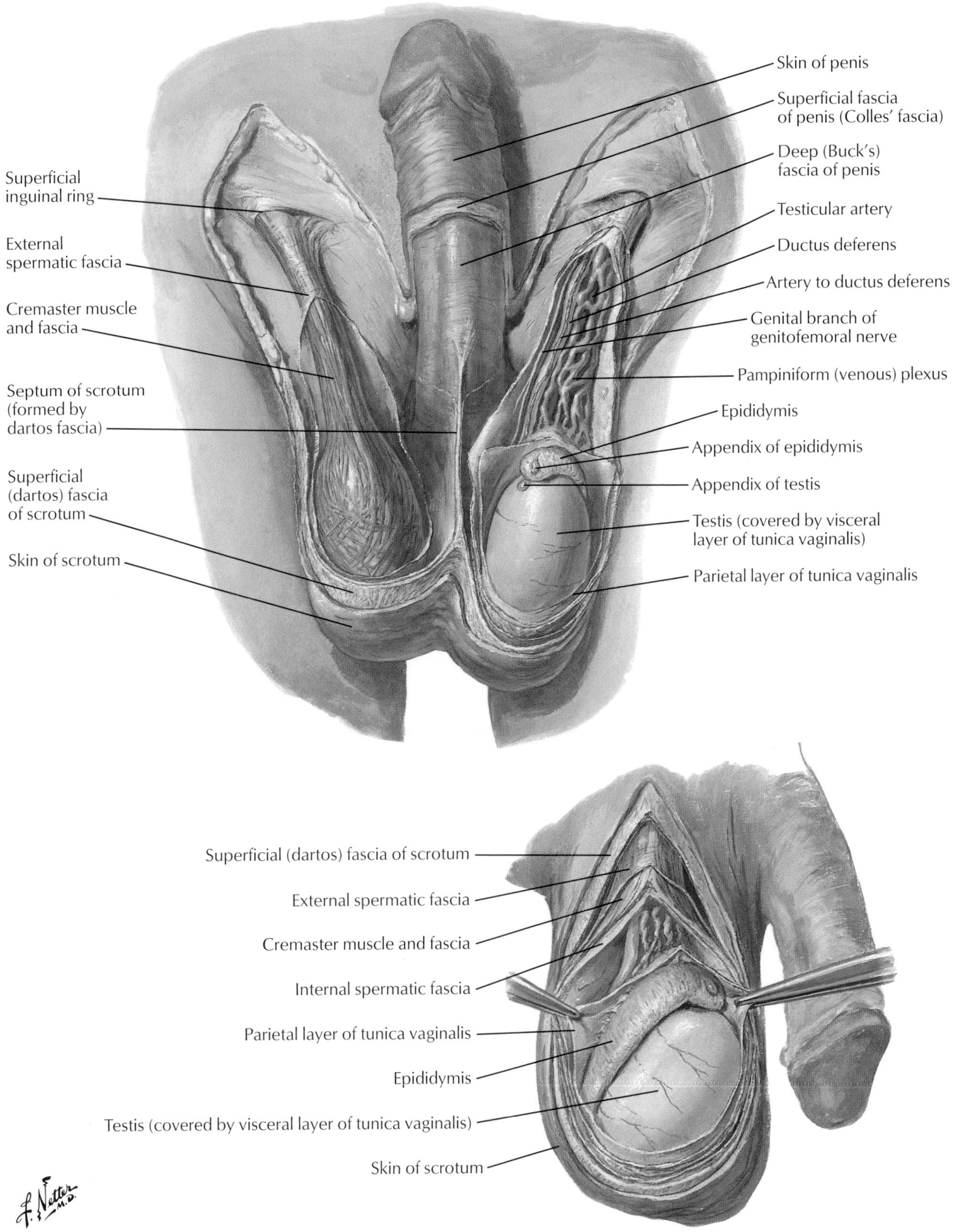
Skin of penis
Superficial fascia of penis (Colles' fascia)
Deep (Buck's) fascia of penis
Testicular artery
Ductus deferens
Artery to ductus deferens
Genital branch of genitofemoral nerve
Pampiniform (venous) plexus
Epididymis
Appendix of epididymis
Appendix of testis
Testis (covered by visceral layer of tunica vaginalis)
Parietal layer of tunica vaginalis
Superficial inguinal ring
External spermatic fascia
Cremaster muscle and fascia
Septum of scrotum (formed by dartos fascia)
Superficial (dartos) fascia of scrotum
Skin of scrotum
Superficial (dartos) fascia of scrotum
External spermatic fascia
Cremaster muscle and fascia
Internal spermatic fascia
Parietal layer of tunica vaginalis
Epididymis
Testis (covered by visceral layer of tunica vaginalis)
Skin of scrotum

Plate 5 Scrotum and Contents. (Copyright 2024 Elsevier Inc. All rights reserved. www.netterimages.com. Image ID: 4686.)

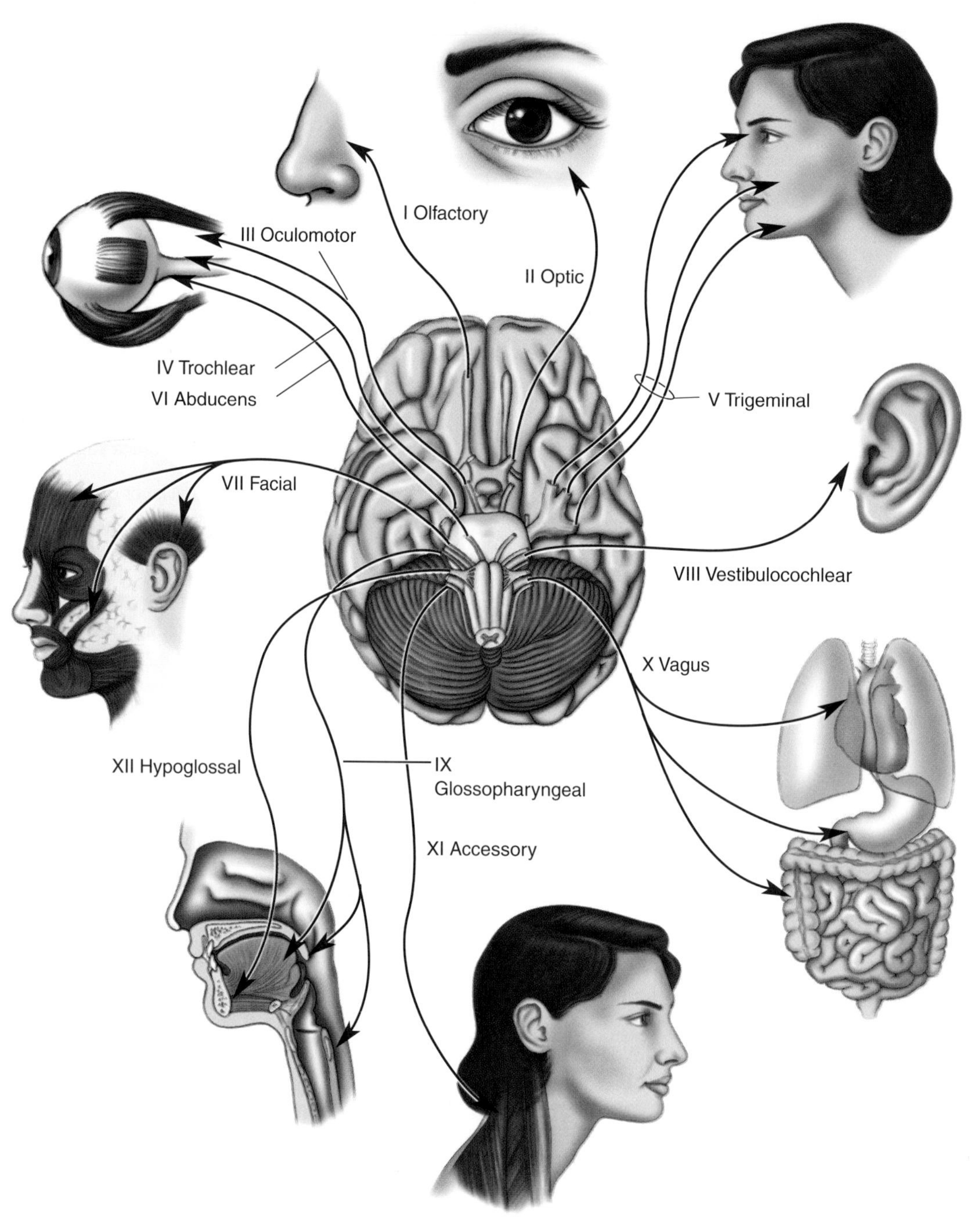
I Olfactory
III Oculomotor
II Optic
IV Trochlear
VI Abducens
V Trigeminal
VII Facial
VIII Vestibulocochlear
X Vagus
XII Hypoglossal
IX
Glossopharyngeal
XI Accessory

Plate 6 Cranial Nerves (12 pairs) are known by their numbers (Roman numerals) and names. (Herlihy BL: The Human Body in Health and Illness, ed 6, St. Louis, 2018, Elsevier.)

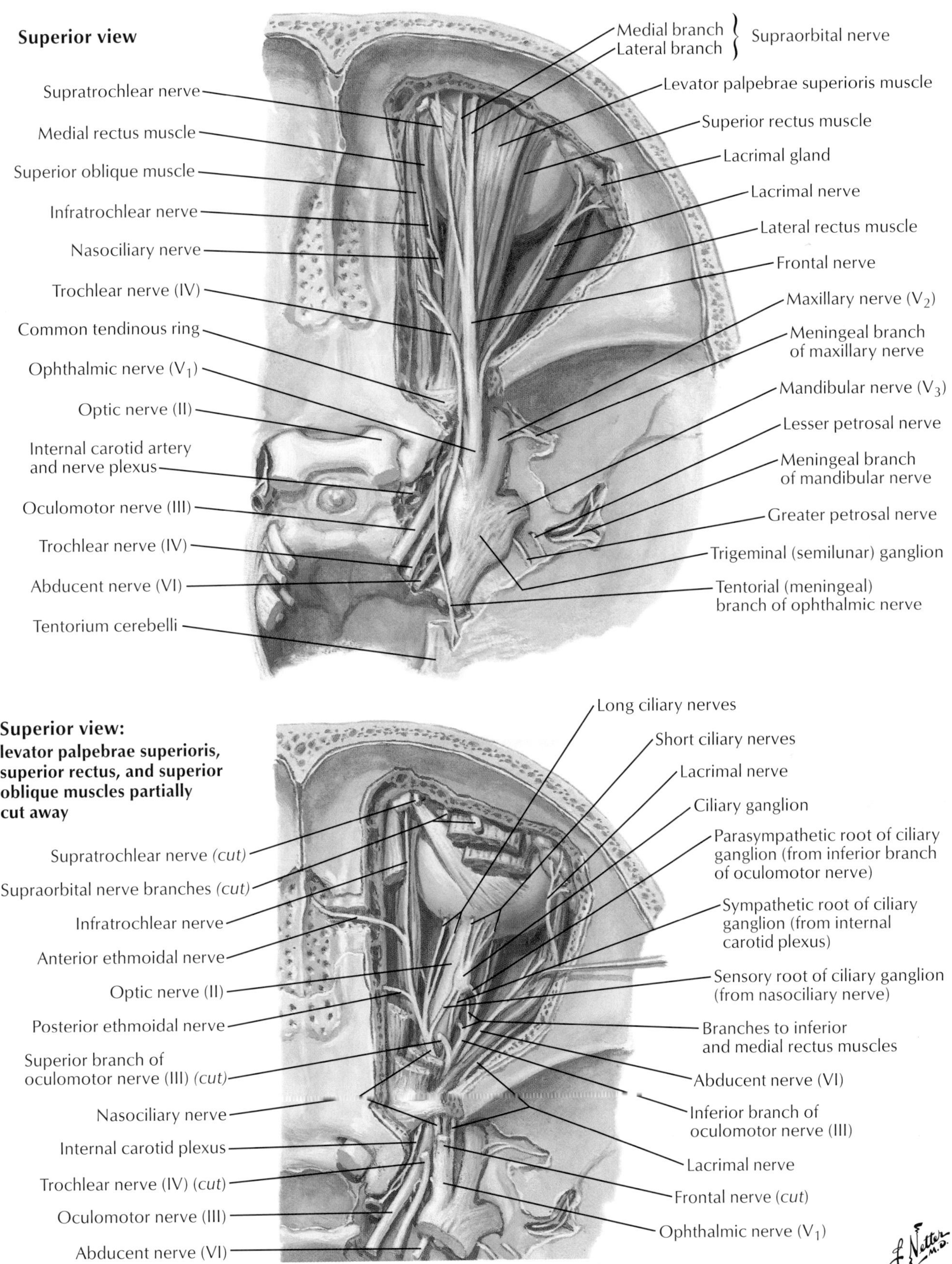

Superior view
Medial branch
Lateral branch
Supraorbital nerve
Supratrochlear nerve
Levator palpebrae superioris muscle
Medial rectus muscle
Superior rectus muscle
Superior oblique muscle
Lacrimal gland
Infratrochlear nerve
Lacrimal nerve
Nasociliary nerve
Lateral rectus muscle
Frontal nerve
Trochlear nerve (IV)
Maxillary nerve (V_2)
Common tendinous ring
Meningeal branch of maxillary nerve
Ophthalmic nerve (V_1)
Mandibular nerve (V_3)
Optic nerve (II)
Lesser petrosal nerve
Internal carotid artery and nerve plexus
Meningeal branch of mandibular nerve
Oculomotor nerve (III)
Greater petrosal nerve
Trochlear nerve (IV)
Trigeminal (semilunar) ganglion
Abducent nerve (VI)
Tentorial (meningeal) branch of ophthalmic nerve
Tentorium cerebelli
Long ciliary nerves
Superior view: levator palpebrae superioris, superior rectus, and superior oblique muscles partially cut away
Short ciliary nerves
Lacrimal nerve
Ciliary ganglion
Supratrochlear nerve (cut)
Parasympathetic root of ciliary ganglion (from inferior branch of oculomotor nerve)
Supraorbital nerve branches (cut)
Infratrochlear nerve
Sympathetic root of ciliary ganglion (from internal carotid plexus)
Anterior ethmoidal nerve
Sensory root of ciliary ganglion (from nasociliary nerve)
Optic nerve (II)
Posterior ethmoidal nerve
Branches to inferior and medial rectus muscles
Superior branch of oculomotor nerve (III) (cut)
Abducent nerve (VI)
Nasociliary nerve
Inferior branch of oculomotor nerve (III)
Internal carotid plexus
Lacrimal nerve
Trochlear nerve (IV) (cut)
Frontal nerve (cut)
Oculomotor nerve (III)
Ophthalmic nerve (V_1)
Abducent nerve (VI)
F. Netter M.D.

ANATOMY ILLUSTRATIONS

Plate 7 Nerves of Orbit. (Copyright 2024 Elsevier Inc. All rights reserved. www.netterimages.com. Image ID: 4615.)

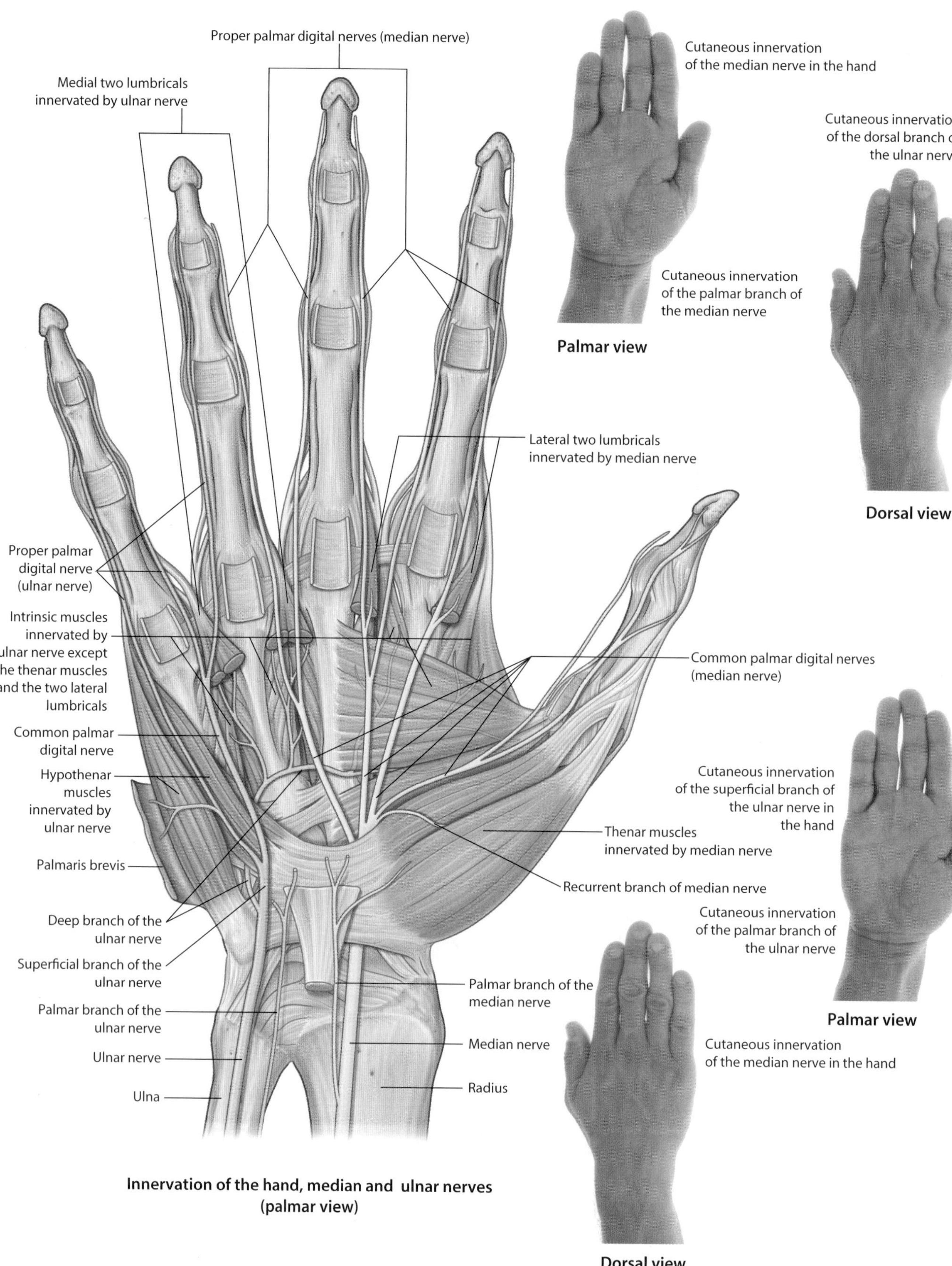
Proper palmar digital nerves (median nerve)
Medial two lumbricals innervated by ulnar nerve
Lateral two lumbricals innervated by median nerve
Proper palmar digital nerve (ulnar nerve)
Intrinsic muscles innervated by ulnar nerve except the thenar muscles and the two lateral lumbricals
Common palmar digital nerves (median nerve)
Common palmar digital nerve
Hypothenar muscles innervated by ulnar nerve
Thenar muscles innervated by median nerve
Palmaris brevis
Recurrent branch of median nerve
Deep branch of the ulnar nerve
Superficial branch of the ulnar nerve
Palmar branch of the median nerve
Palmar branch of the ulnar nerve
Median nerve
Ulnar nerve
Radius
Ulna
Innervation of the hand, median and ulnar nerves (palmar view)
Cutaneous innervation of the median nerve in the hand
Cutaneous innervation of the palmar branch of the median nerve
Palmar view
Cutaneous innervation of the dorsal branch of the ulnar nerve
Dorsal view
Cutaneous innervation of the superficial branch of the ulnar nerve in the hand
Cutaneous innervation of the palmar branch of the ulnar nerve
Palmar view
Cutaneous innervation of the median nerve in the hand
Dorsal view

Plate 8 Innervation of the Hand: Median and Ulnar Nerves. (From Drake RL, Vogl AW, Mitchell AWM, Tibbitts RM, Richardson PE: Gray's Atlas of Anatomy, ed 2, Philadelphia, 2015, Churchill Livingstone.)

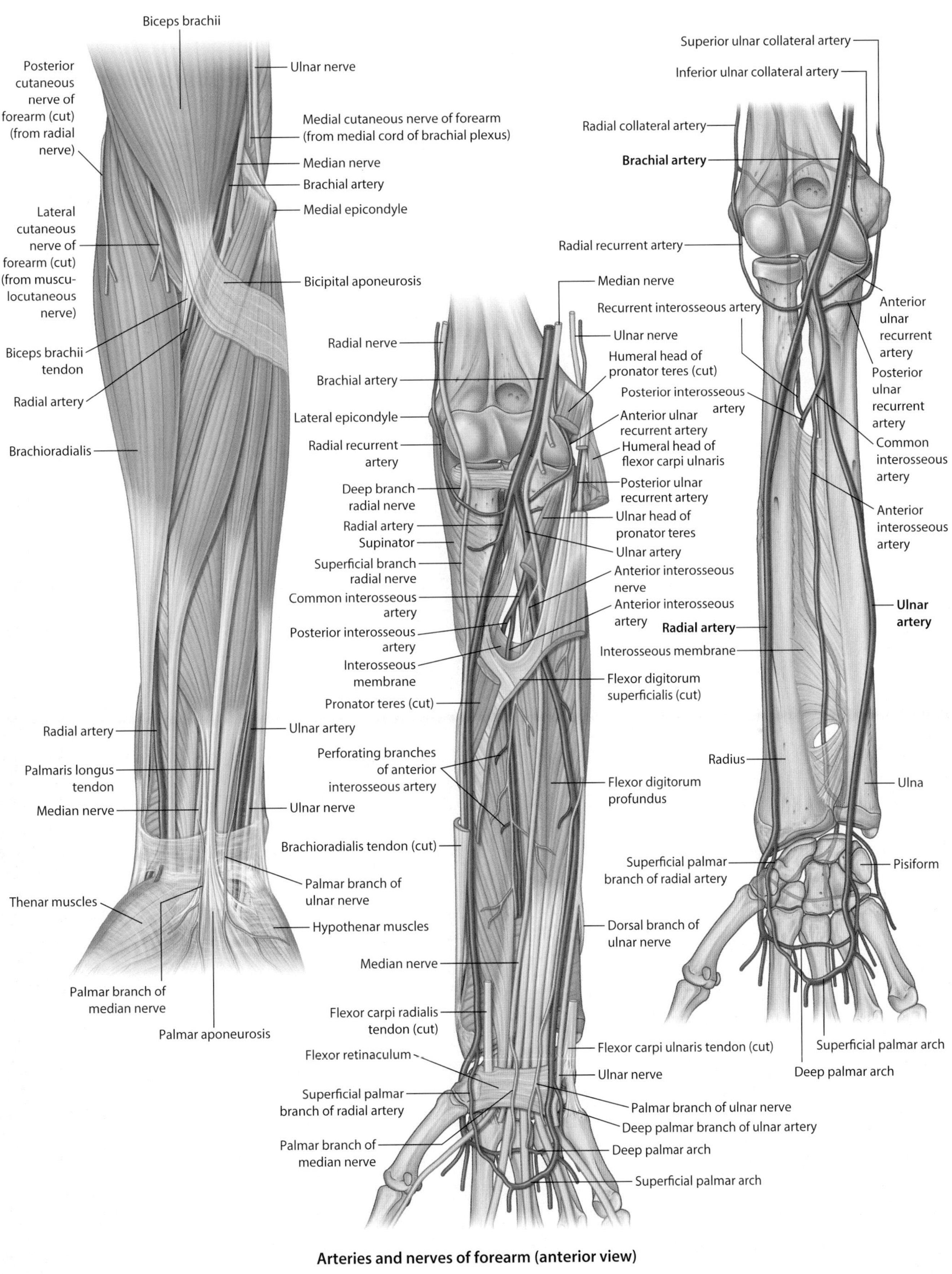
Biceps brachii
Posterior cutaneous nerve of forearm (cut) (from radial nerve)
Ulnar nerve
Medial cutaneous nerve of forearm (from medial cord of brachial plexus)
Median nerve
Brachial artery
Medial epicondyle
Lateral cutaneous nerve of forearm (cut) (from musculocutaneous nerve)
Bicipital aponeurosis
Biceps brachii tendon
Radial artery
Brachioradialis
Radial artery
Ulnar artery
Palmaris longus tendon
Median nerve
Ulnar nerve
Thenar muscles
Palmar branch of ulnar nerve
Hypothenar muscles
Palmar branch of median nerve
Palmar aponeurosis
Median nerve
Recurrent interosseous artery
Radial nerve
Ulnar nerve
Humeral head of pronator teres (cut)
Brachial artery
Posterior interosseous artery
Lateral epicondyle
Anterior ulnar recurrent artery
Radial recurrent artery
Humeral head of flexor carpi ulnaris
Deep branch radial nerve
Posterior ulnar recurrent artery
Radial artery
Ulnar head of pronator teres
Supinator
Ulnar artery
Superficial branch radial nerve
Anterior interosseous nerve
Common interosseous artery
Anterior interosseous artery
Posterior interosseous artery
Interosseous membrane
Flexor digitorum superficialis (cut)
Pronator teres (cut)
Perforating branches of anterior interosseous artery
Flexor digitorum profundus
Brachioradialis tendon (cut)
Dorsal branch of ulnar nerve
Median nerve
Flexor carpi radialis tendon (cut)
Flexor retinaculum
Flexor carpi ulnaris tendon (cut)
Ulnar nerve
Superficial palmar branch of radial artery
Palmar branch of ulnar nerve
Deep palmar branch of ulnar artery
Palmar branch of median nerve
Deep palmar arch
Superficial palmar arch
Superior ulnar collateral artery
Inferior ulnar collateral artery
Radial collateral artery
Brachial artery
Radial recurrent artery
Anterior ulnar recurrent artery
Posterior ulnar recurrent artery
Common interosseous artery
Anterior interosseous artery
Ulnar artery
Radial artery
Interosseous membrane
Radius
Ulna
Superficial palmar branch of radial artery
Pisiform
Superficial palmar arch
Deep palmar arch

Arteries and nerves of forearm (anterior view)

Plate 9 Arteries and Nerves of the Forearm (Anterior View). (From Drake RL, Vogl AW, Mitchell AWM, Tibbitts RM, Richardson PE: Gray's Atlas of Anatomy, ed 2, Philadelphia, 2015, Churchill Livingstone.)

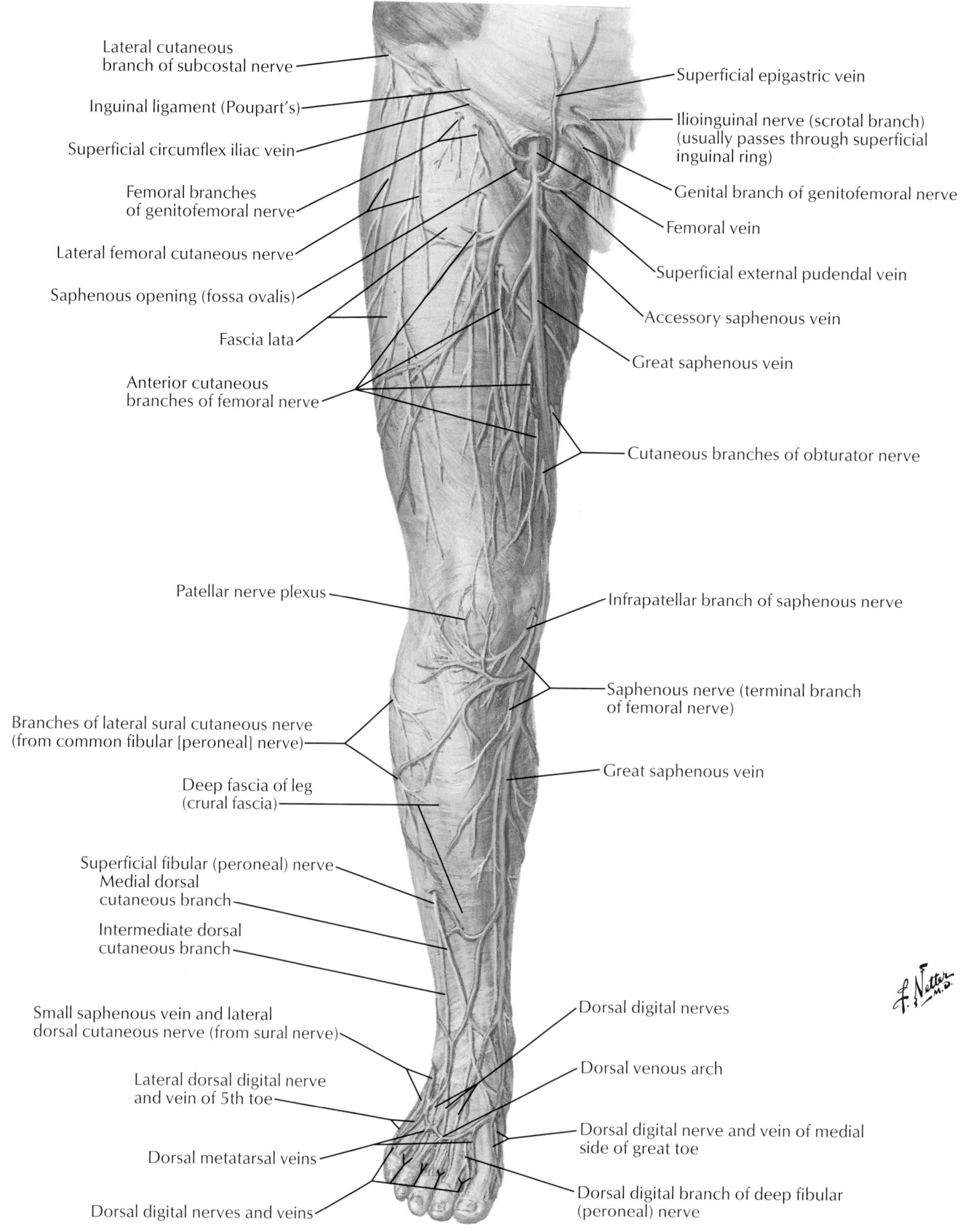
Lateral cutaneous
branch of subcostal nerve
Inguinal ligament (Poupart's)
Superficial circumflex iliac vein
Femoral branches
of genitofemoral nerve
Lateral femoral cutaneous nerve
Saphenous opening (fossa ovalis)
Fascia lata
Anterior cutaneous
branches of femoral nerve
Superficial epigastric vein
Ilioinguinal nerve (scrotal branch)
(usually passes through superficial
inguinal ring)
Genital branch of genitofemoral nerve
Femoral vein
Superficial external pudendal vein
Accessory saphenous vein
Great saphenous vein
Cutaneous branches of obturator nerve
Patellar nerve plexus
Infrapatellar branch of saphenous nerve
Saphenous nerve (terminal branch
of femoral nerve)
Branches of lateral sural cutaneous nerve
(from common fibular [peroneal] nerve)
Great saphenous vein
Deep fascia of leg
(crural fascia)
Superficial fibular (peroneal) nerve
Medial dorsal
cutaneous branch
Intermediate dorsal
cutaneous branch
Small saphenous vein and lateral
dorsal cutaneous nerve (from sural nerve)
Lateral dorsal digital nerve
and vein of 5th toe
Dorsal metatarsal veins
Dorsal digital nerves and veins
Dorsal digital nerves
Dorsal venous arch
Dorsal digital nerve and vein of medial
side of great toe
Dorsal digital branch of deep fibular
(peroneal) nerve
F. Netter M.D.

Plate 10 Superficial Nerves and Veins of Lower Limb: Anterior View. (Copyright 2024 Elsevier Inc. All rights reserved. www.netterimages.com. Image ID: 4846.)

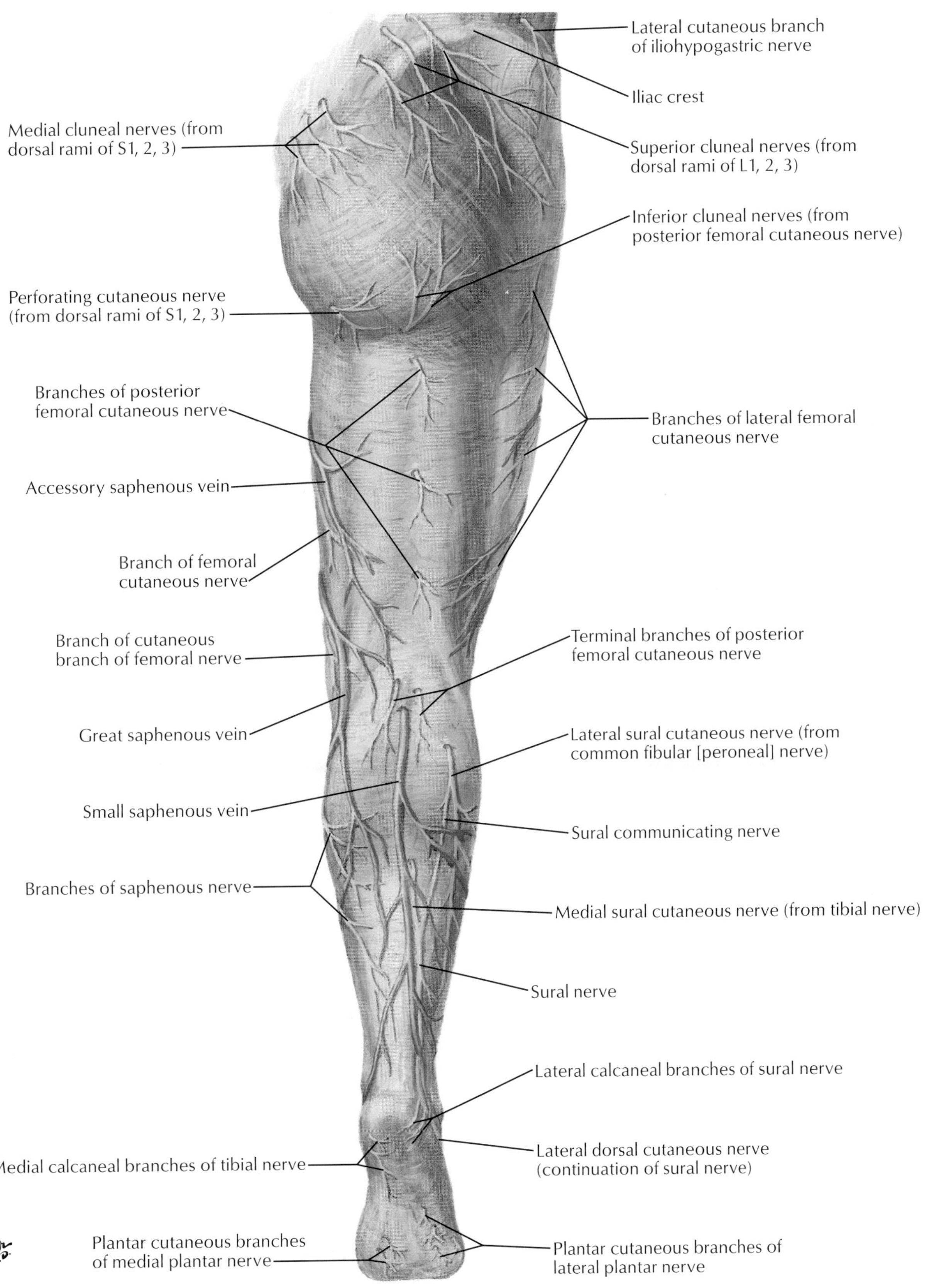
Lateral cutaneous branch of iliohypogastric nerve
Iliac crest
Medial cluneal nerves (from dorsal rami of S1, 2, 3)
Superior cluneal nerves (from dorsal rami of L1, 2, 3)
Inferior cluneal nerves (from posterior femoral cutaneous nerve)
Perforating cutaneous nerve (from dorsal rami of S1, 2, 3)
Branches of posterior femoral cutaneous nerve
Branches of lateral femoral cutaneous nerve
Accessory saphenous vein
Branch of femoral cutaneous nerve
Branch of cutaneous branch of femoral nerve
Terminal branches of posterior femoral cutaneous nerve
Great saphenous vein
Lateral sural cutaneous nerve (from common fibular [peroneal] nerve)
Small saphenous vein
Sural communicating nerve
Branches of saphenous nerve
Medial sural cutaneous nerve (from tibial nerve)
Sural nerve
Lateral calcaneal branches of sural nerve
Medial calcaneal branches of tibial nerve
Lateral dorsal cutaneous nerve (continuation of sural nerve)
Plantar cutaneous branches of medial plantar nerve
Plantar cutaneous branches of lateral plantar nerve

Plate 11 Superficial Nerves and Veins of Lower Limb: Posterior View. (Copyright 2024 Elsevier Inc. All rights reserved. www.netterimages.com. Image ID: 4669.)

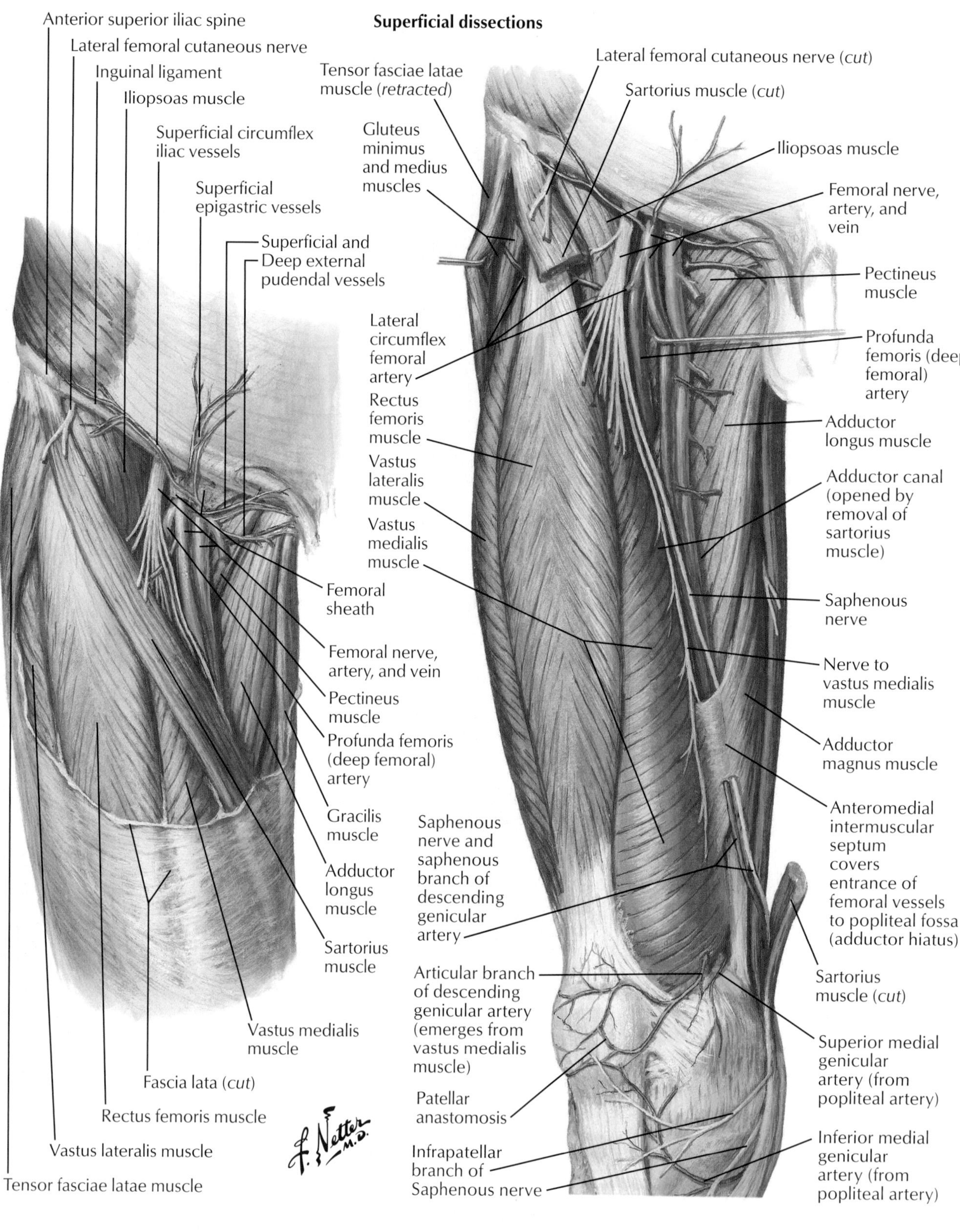
Superficial dissections
Anterior superior iliac spine
Lateral femoral cutaneous nerve
Inguinal ligament
Iliopsoas muscle
Superficial circumflex iliac vessels
Superficial epigastric vessels
Superficial and
Deep external pudendal vessels
Femoral sheath
Femoral nerve, artery, and vein
Pectineus muscle
Profunda femoris (deep femoral) artery
Gracilis muscle
Adductor longus muscle
Sartorius muscle
Vastus medialis muscle
Fascia lata (*cut*)
Rectus femoris muscle
Vastus lateralis muscle
Tensor fasciae latae muscle
Tensor fasciae latae muscle (*retracted*)
Gluteus minimus and medius muscles
Lateral circumflex femoral artery
Rectus femoris muscle
Vastus lateralis muscle
Vastus medialis muscle
Saphenous nerve and saphenous branch of descending genicular artery
Articular branch of descending genicular artery (emerges from vastus medialis muscle)
Patellar anastomosis
Infrapatellar branch of Saphenous nerve
Lateral femoral cutaneous nerve (*cut*)
Sartorius muscle (*cut*)
Iliopsoas muscle
Femoral nerve, artery, and vein
Pectineus muscle
Profunda femoris (deep femoral) artery
Adductor longus muscle
Adductor canal (opened by removal of sartorius muscle)
Saphenous nerve
Nerve to vastus medialis muscle
Adductor magnus muscle
Anteromedial intermuscular septum covers entrance of femoral vessels to popliteal fossa (adductor hiatus)
Sartorius muscle (*cut*)
Superior medial genicular artery (from popliteal artery)
Inferior medial genicular artery (from popliteal artery)
F. Netter M.D.

Plate 12 Arteries and Nerves of Thigh: Anterior Views. (Copyright 2024 Elsevier Inc. All rights reserved. www.netterimages.com. Image ID: 4475.)

Deep dissection

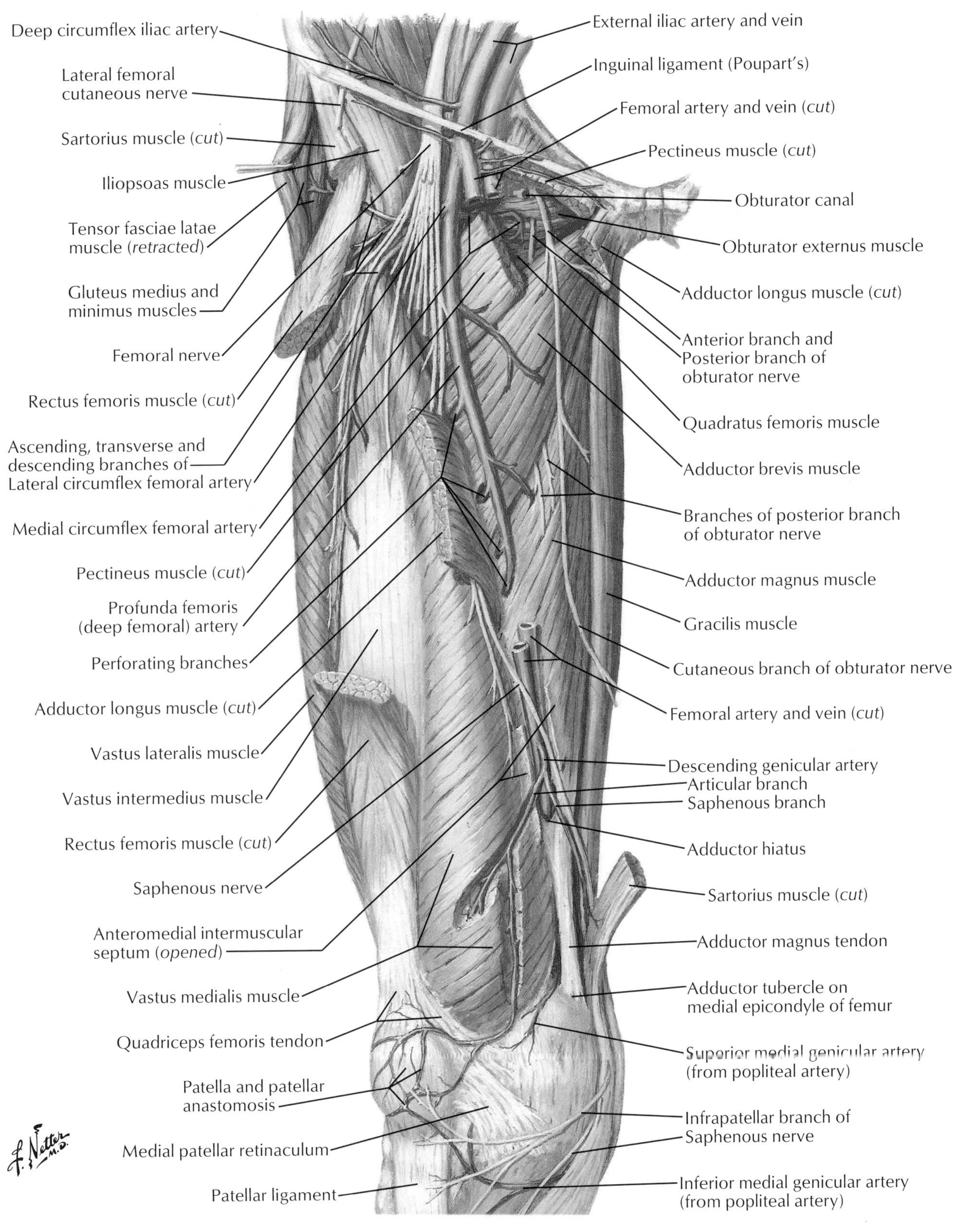

Deep circumflex iliac artery
Lateral femoral cutaneous nerve
Sartorius muscle (*cut*)
Iliopsoas muscle
Tensor fasciae latae muscle (*retracted*)
Gluteus medius and minimus muscles
Femoral nerve
Rectus femoris muscle (*cut*)
Ascending, transverse and descending branches of Lateral circumflex femoral artery
Medial circumflex femoral artery
Pectineus muscle (*cut*)
Profunda femoris (deep femoral) artery
Perforating branches
Adductor longus muscle (*cut*)
Vastus lateralis muscle
Vastus intermedius muscle
Rectus femoris muscle (*cut*)
Saphenous nerve
Anteromedial intermuscular septum (*opened*)
Vastus medialis muscle
Quadriceps femoris tendon
Patella and patellar anastomosis
Medial patellar retinaculum
Patellar ligament
External iliac artery and vein
Inguinal ligament (Poupart's)
Femoral artery and vein (*cut*)
Pectineus muscle (*cut*)
Obturator canal
Obturator externus muscle
Adductor longus muscle (*cut*)
Anterior branch and
Posterior branch of obturator nerve
Quadratus femoris muscle
Adductor brevis muscle
Branches of posterior branch of obturator nerve
Adductor magnus muscle
Gracilis muscle
Cutaneous branch of obturator nerve
Femoral artery and vein (*cut*)
Descending genicular artery
Articular branch
Saphenous branch
Adductor hiatus
Sartorius muscle (*cut*)
Adductor magnus tendon
Adductor tubercle on medial epicondyle of femur
Superior medial genicular artery (from popliteal artery)
Infrapatellar branch of
Saphenous nerve
Inferior medial genicular artery (from popliteal artery)
F. Netter M.D.

Plate 13 Arteries and Nerves of Thigh: Posterior View. (Copyright 2024 Elsevier Inc. All rights reserved. www.netterimages.com. Image ID: 49316.)

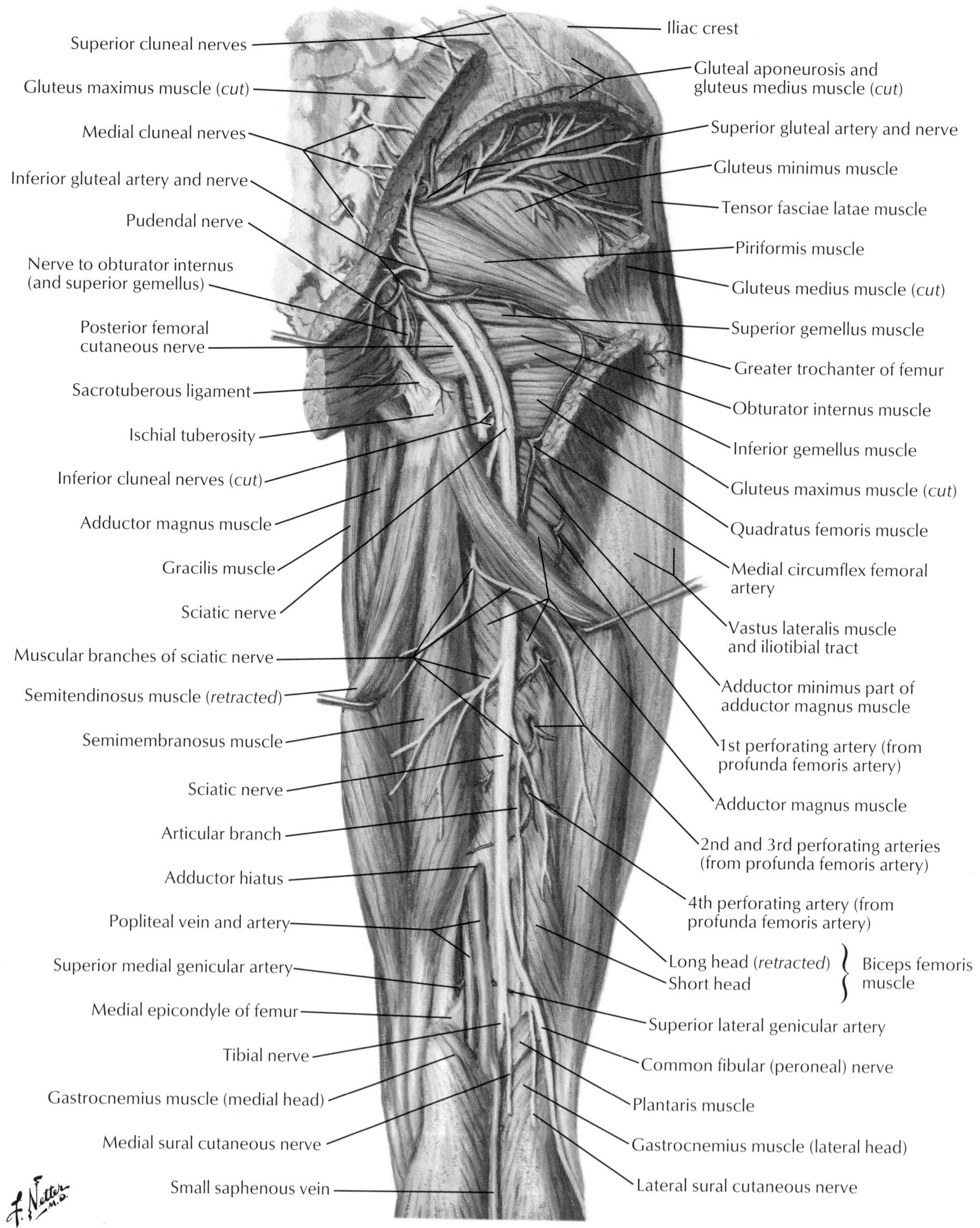
Deep dissection
Superior cluneal nerves
Gluteus maximus muscle (cut)
Medial cluneal nerves
Inferior gluteal artery and nerve
Pudendal nerve
Nerve to obturator internus (and superior gemellus)
Posterior femoral cutaneous nerve
Sacrotuberous ligament
Ischial tuberosity
Inferior cluneal nerves (cut)
Adductor magnus muscle
Gracilis muscle
Sciatic nerve
Muscular branches of sciatic nerve
Semitendinosus muscle (retracted)
Semimembranosus muscle
Sciatic nerve
Articular branch
Adductor hiatus
Popliteal vein and artery
Superior medial genicular artery
Medial epicondyle of femur
Tibial nerve
Gastrocnemius muscle (medial head)
Medial sural cutaneous nerve
Small saphenous vein
Iliac crest
Gluteal aponeurosis and gluteus medius muscle (cut)
Superior gluteal artery and nerve
Gluteus minimus muscle
Tensor fasciae latae muscle
Piriformis muscle
Gluteus medius muscle (cut)
Superior gemellus muscle
Greater trochanter of femur
Obturator internus muscle
Inferior gemellus muscle
Gluteus maximus muscle (cut)
Quadratus femoris muscle
Medial circumflex femoral artery
Vastus lateralis muscle and iliotibial tract
Adductor minimus part of adductor magnus muscle
1st perforating artery (from profunda femoris artery)
Adductor magnus muscle
2nd and 3rd perforating arteries (from profunda femoris artery)
4th perforating artery (from profunda femoris artery)
Long head (retracted)
Short head
Biceps femoris muscle
Superior lateral genicular artery
Common fibular (peroneal) nerve
Plantaris muscle
Gastrocnemius muscle (lateral head)
Lateral sural cutaneous nerve
F. Netter M.D.

Plate 14 Arteries and Nerves of Thigh: Posterior View. (Copyright 2024 Elsevier Inc. All rights reserved. www.netterimages.com. Image ID: 49317.)

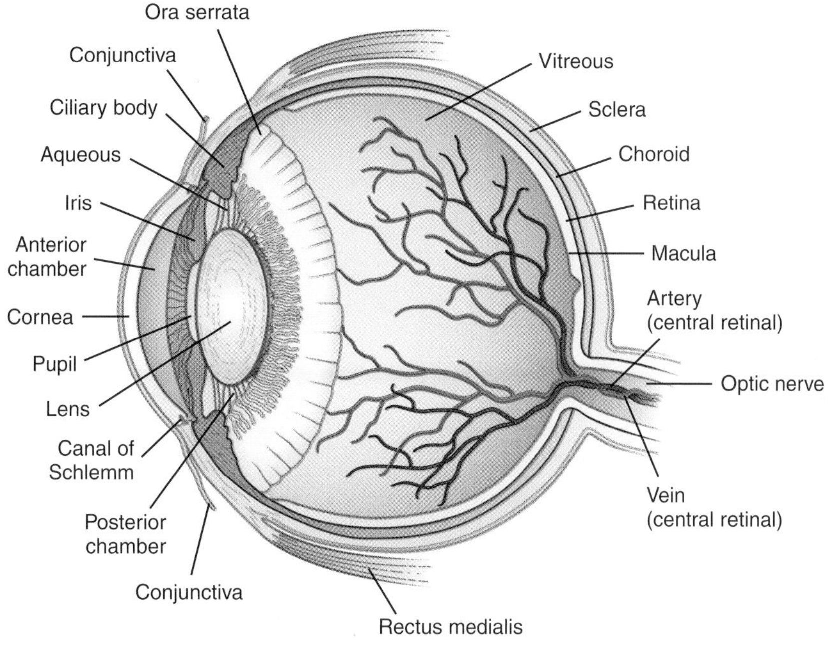
Ora serrata
Conjunctiva
Ciliary body
Aqueous
Iris
Anterior chamber
Cornea
Pupil
Lens
Canal of Schlemm
Posterior chamber
Conjunctiva
Rectus medialis
Vitreous
Sclera
Choroid
Retina
Macula
Artery (central retinal)
Optic nerve
Vein (central retinal)

Plate 15 Anatomy of the eye. (Dehn RW, Asprey DP: Essential Clinical Procedures, ed 3, Philadelphia, 2013, Saunders.)

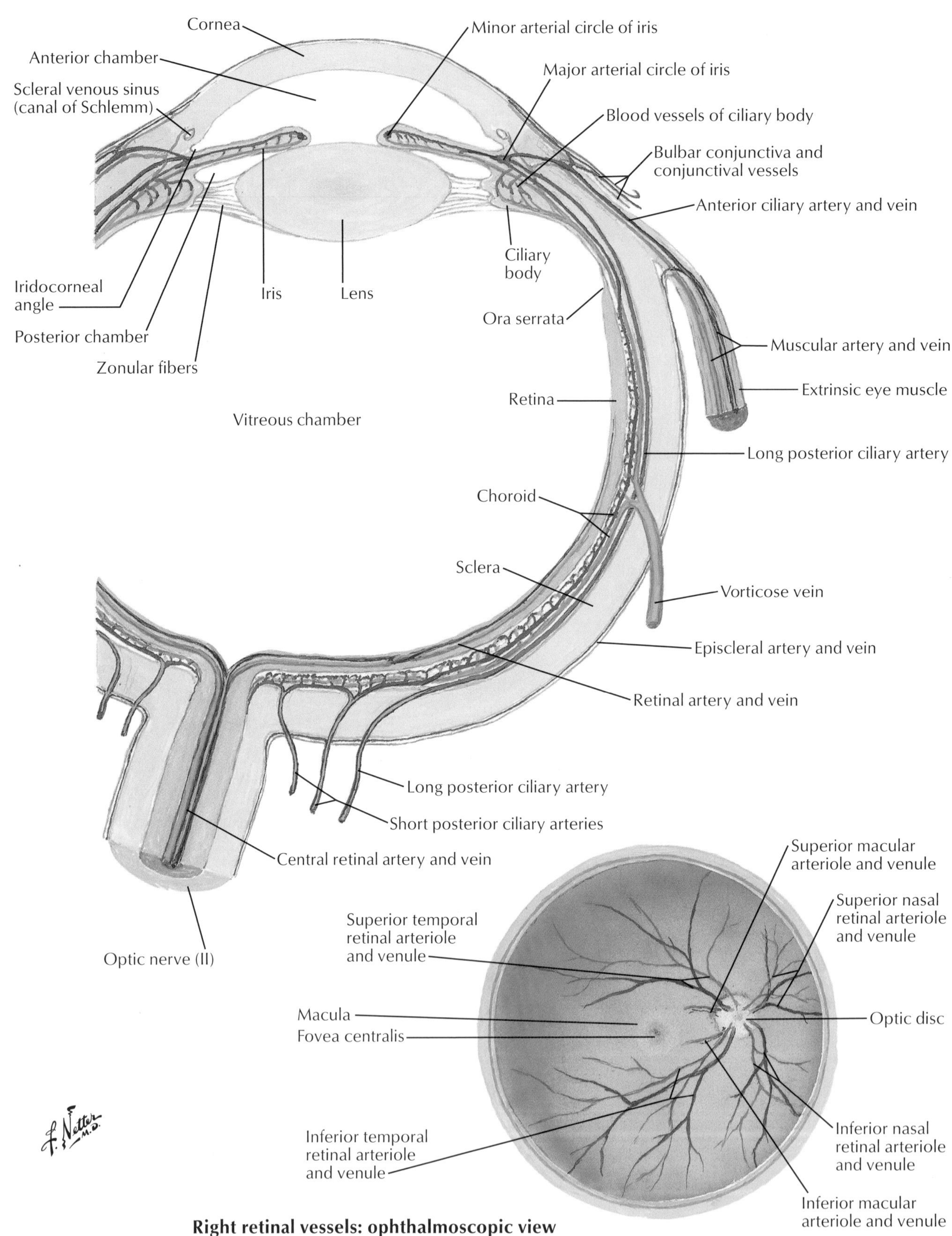
Cornea
Anterior chamber
Scleral venous sinus
(canal of Schlemm)
Minor arterial circle of iris
Major arterial circle of iris
Blood vessels of ciliary body
Bulbar conjunctiva and
conjunctival vessels
Anterior ciliary artery and vein
Iridocorneal
angle
Posterior chamber
Zonular fibers
Iris
Lens
Ciliary
body
Ora serrata
Muscular artery and vein
Extrinsic eye muscle
Retina
Vitreous chamber
Long posterior ciliary artery
Choroid
Sclera
Vorticose vein
Episcleral artery and vein
Retinal artery and vein
Long posterior ciliary artery
Short posterior ciliary arteries
Central retinal artery and vein
Optic nerve (II)
Superior macular
arteriole and venule
Superior nasal
retinal arteriole
and venule
Superior temporal
retinal arteriole
and venule
Macula
Fovea centralis
Optic disc
Inferior temporal
retinal arteriole
and venule
Inferior nasal
retinal arteriole
and venule
Inferior macular
arteriole and venule
Right retinal vessels: ophthalmoscopic view

Plate 16 Intrinsic Arteries and Veins of Eye. (Copyright 2024 Elsevier Inc. All rights reserved. www.netterimages.com. Image ID: 49107.)

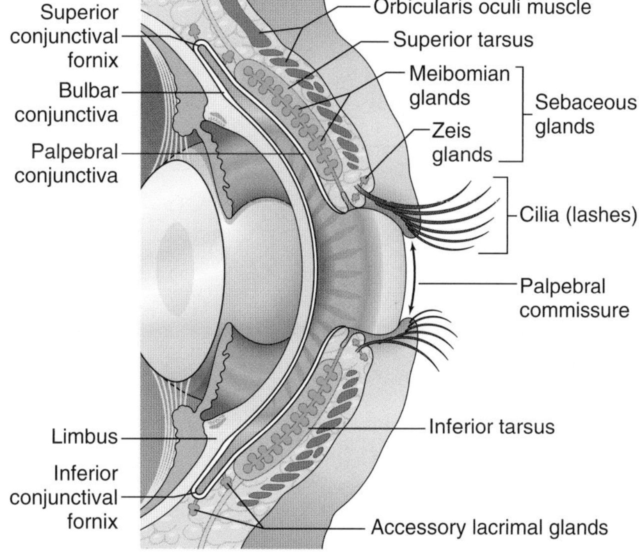
Superior conjunctival fornix
Bulbar conjunctiva
Palpebral conjunctiva
Limbus
Inferior conjunctival fornix
Orbicularis oculi muscle
Superior tarsus
Meibomian glands
Zeis glands
Sebaceous glands
Cilia (lashes)
Palpebral commissure
Inferior tarsus
Accessory lacrimal glands

Plate 17 Anatomy of the conjunctiva and eyelids. (Kumar V, Abbas AK, Aster JC: Robbins and Cotran Pathologic Basis of Disease, ed 9, Philadelphia, 2015, Saunders.)

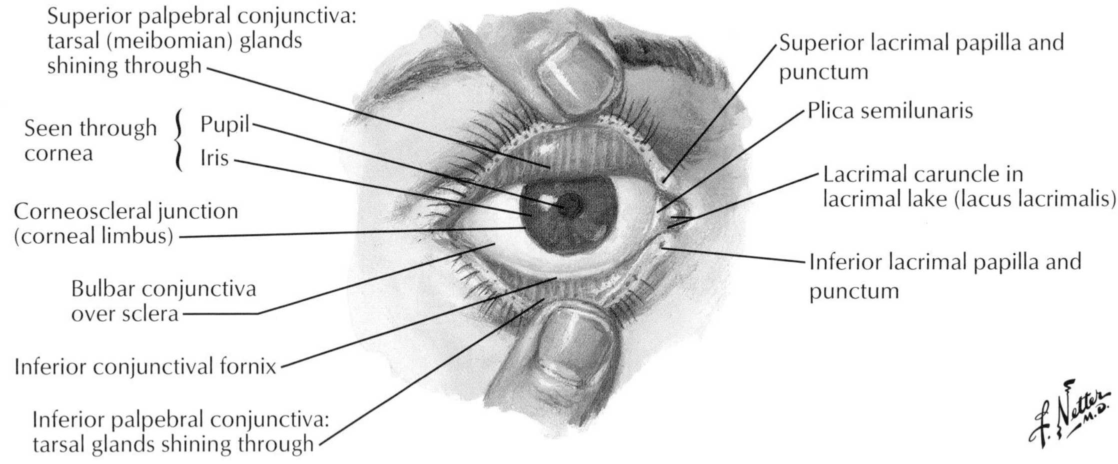
Superior palpebral conjunctiva: tarsal (meibomian) glands shining through
Seen through cornea
Pupil
Iris
Corneoscleral junction (corneal limbus)
Bulbar conjunctiva over sclera
Inferior conjunctival fornix
Inferior palpebral conjunctiva: tarsal glands shining through
Superior lacrimal papilla and punctum
Plica semilunaris
Lacrimal caruncle in lacrimal lake (lacus lacrimalis)
Inferior lacrimal papilla and punctum
F. Netter M.D.

Plate 18 Eyelid. (Copyright 2024 Elsevier Inc. All rights reserved. www.netterimages.com. Image ID: 4557.)

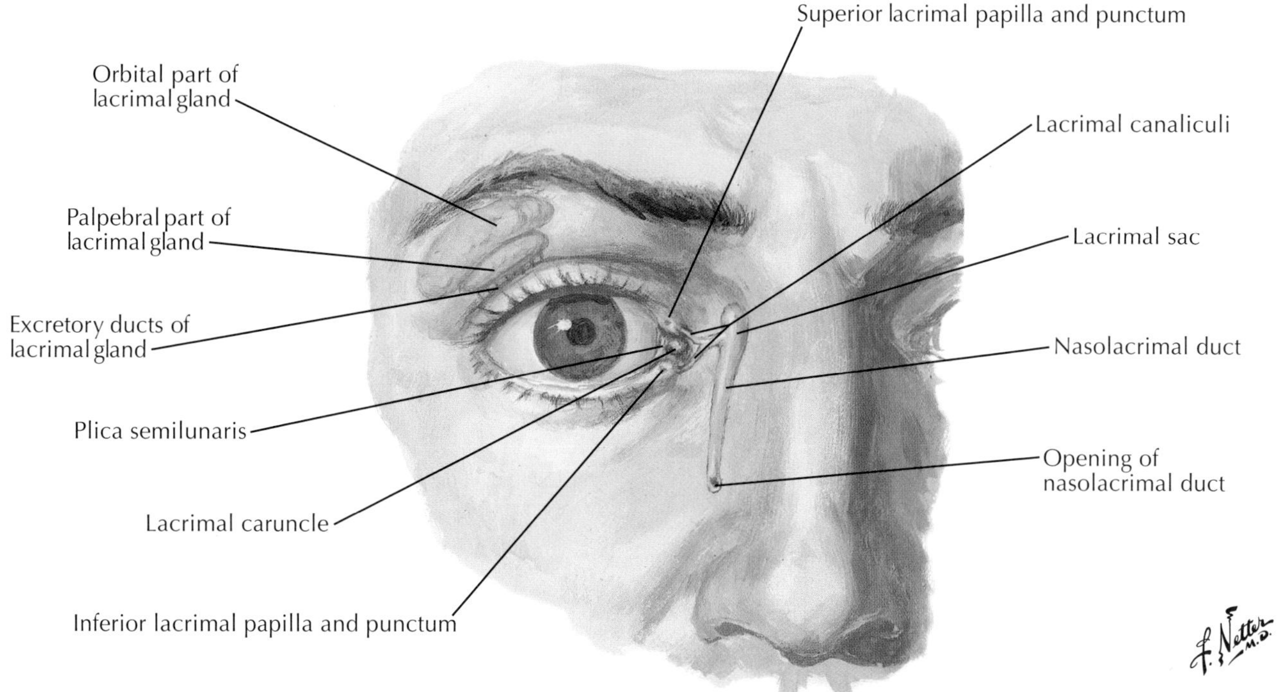
Superior lacrimal papilla and punctum
Orbital part of lacrimal gland
Lacrimal canaliculi
Palpebral part of lacrimal gland
Lacrimal sac
Excretory ducts of lacrimal gland
Nasolacrimal duct
Plica semilunaris
Opening of nasolacrimal duct
Lacrimal caruncle
Inferior lacrimal papilla and punctum

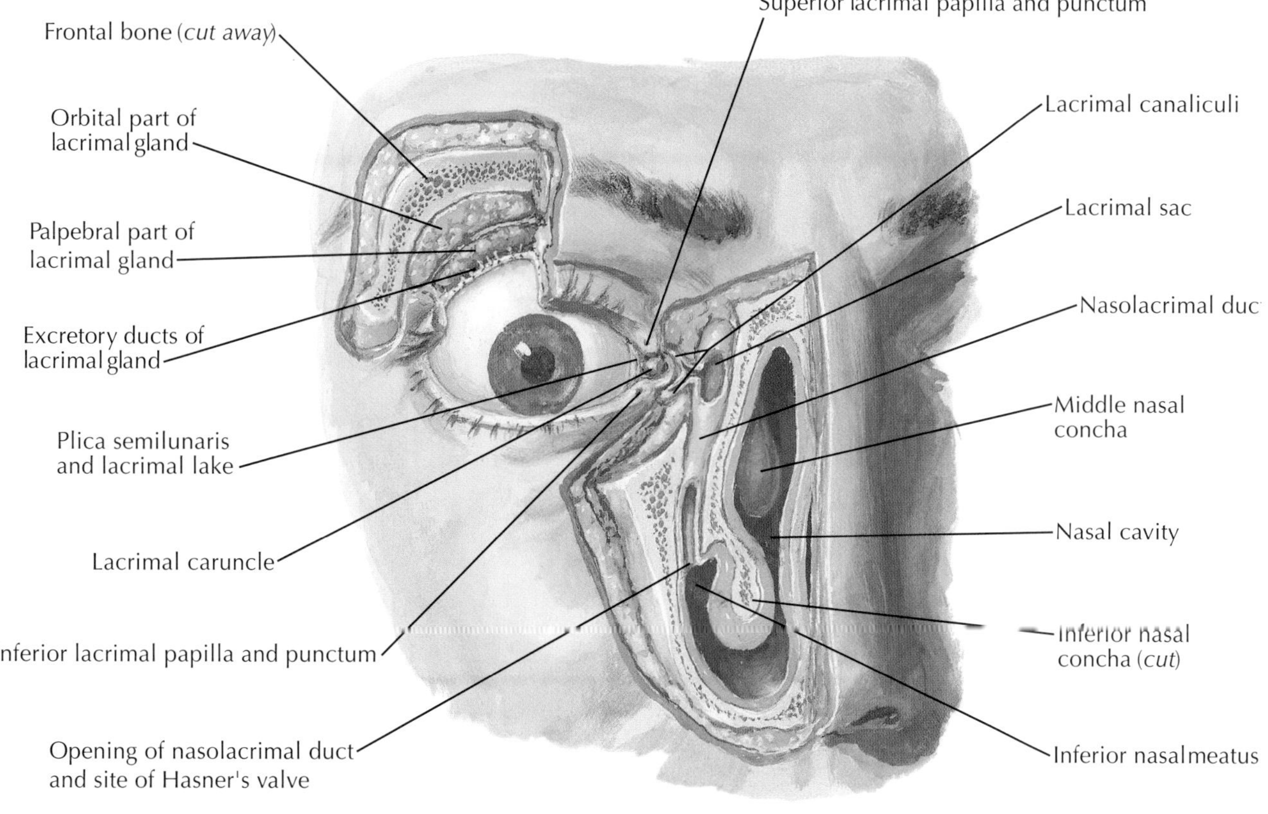
Superior lacrimal papilla and punctum
Frontal bone (*cut away*)
Lacrimal canaliculi
Orbital part of lacrimal gland
Lacrimal sac
Palpebral part of lacrimal gland
Nasolacrimal duc
Excretory ducts of lacrimal gland
Middle nasal concha
Plica semilunaris and lacrimal lake
Nasal cavity
Lacrimal caruncle
Inferior nasal concha (*cut*)
Inferior lacrimal papilla and punctum
Opening of nasolacrimal duct and site of Hasner's valve
Inferior nasalmeatus

Plate 19 Lacrimal Apparatus. (Copyright 2024 Elsevier Inc. All rights reserved. www.netterimages.com. Image ID: 49103.)

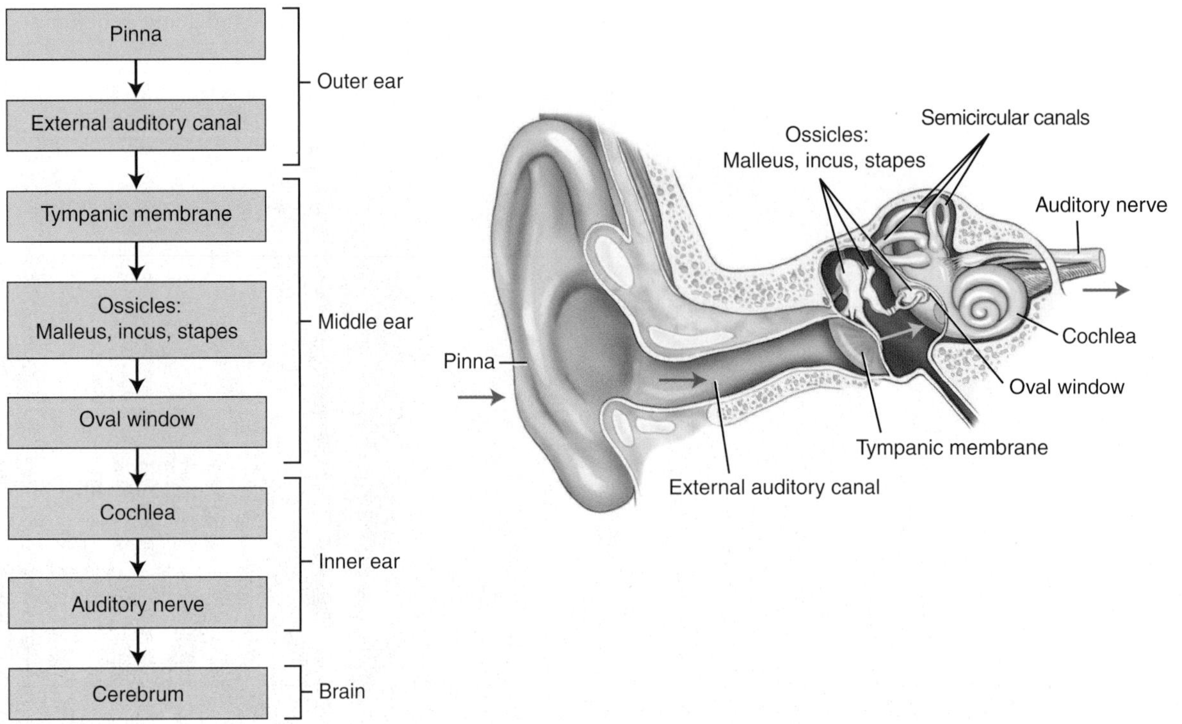
Pinna
External auditory canal
Outer ear
Tympanic membrane
Ossicles:
Malleus, incus, stapes
Middle ear
Oval window
Cochlea
Inner ear
Auditory nerve
Cerebrum
Brain
Semicircular canals
Ossicles:
Malleus, incus, stapes
Auditory nerve
Cochlea
Oval window
Pinna
Tympanic membrane
External auditory canal

Plate 20 Pathway of Sound. (LaFleur Brooks D, LaFleur Brooks M: Basic Medical Language, ed 4, St. Louis, 2013, Mosby.)

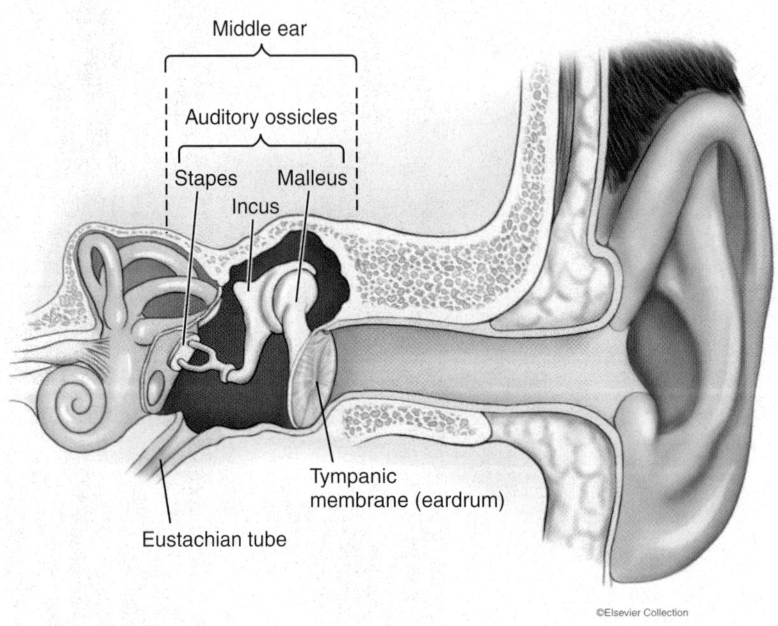
Middle ear
Auditory ossicles
Stapes
Malleus
Incus
Tympanic
membrane (eardrum)
Eustachian tube
©Elsevier Collection

Plate 21 Middle ear structures. (©Elsevier Collection.)

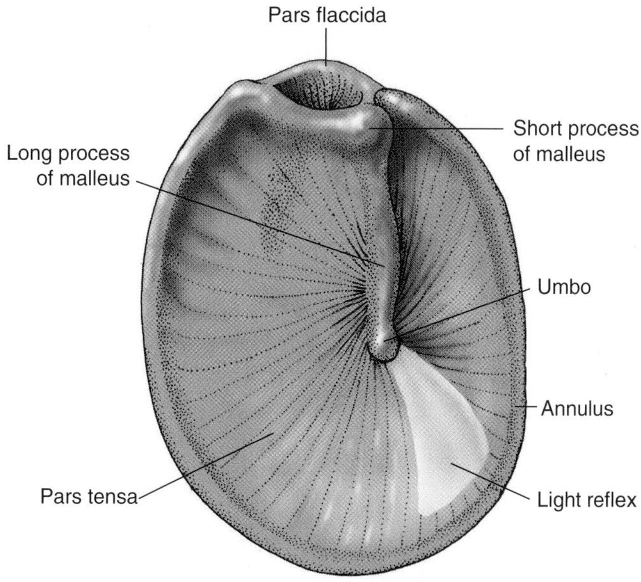
RIGHT TYMPANIC MEMBRANE
Pars flaccida
Short process of malleus
Long process of malleus
Umbo
Annulus
Pars tensa
Light reflex

Plate 22 Structural landmarks of tympanic membrane. (Ignatavicius DD, Workman ML: Medical-Surgical Nursing: Patient-Centered Collaborative Care, ed 7, St. Louis, 2013, Saunders.)

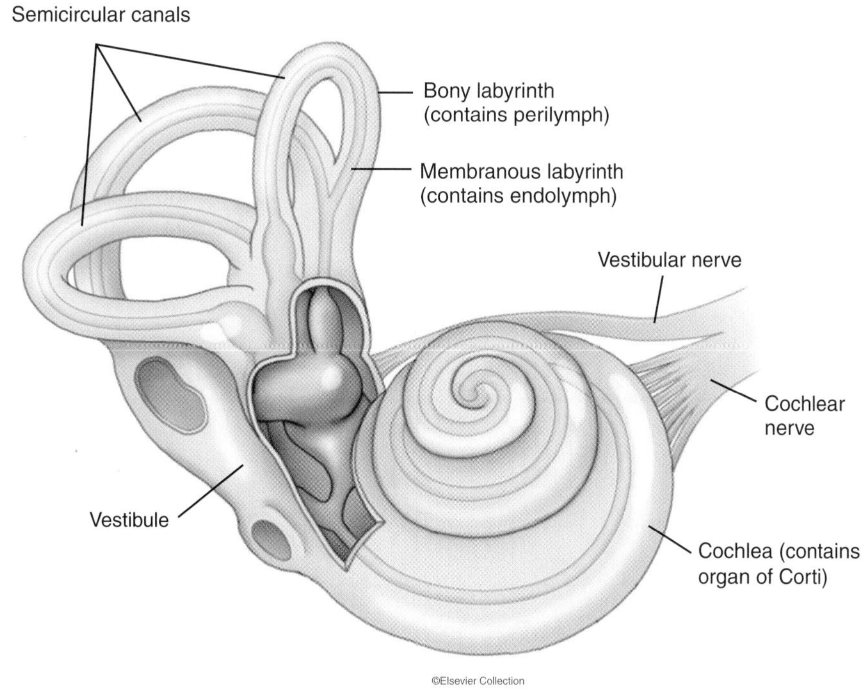
Semicircular canals
Bony labyrinth (contains perilymph)
Membranous labyrinth (contains endolymph)
Vestibular nerve
Cochlear nerve
Vestibule
Cochlea (contains organ of Corti)
©Elsevier Collection

Plate 23 Inner ear structures. (©Elsevier Collection.)

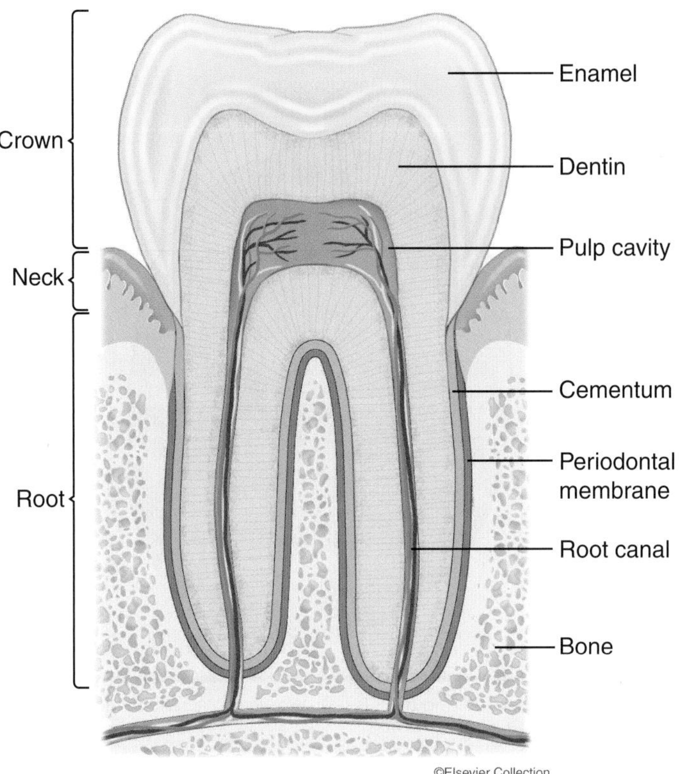
Crown
Neck
Root
Enamel
Dentin
Pulp cavity
Cementum
Periodontal membrane
Root canal
Bone
©Elsevier Collection

Plate 24 The Tooth. (©Elsevier Collection).

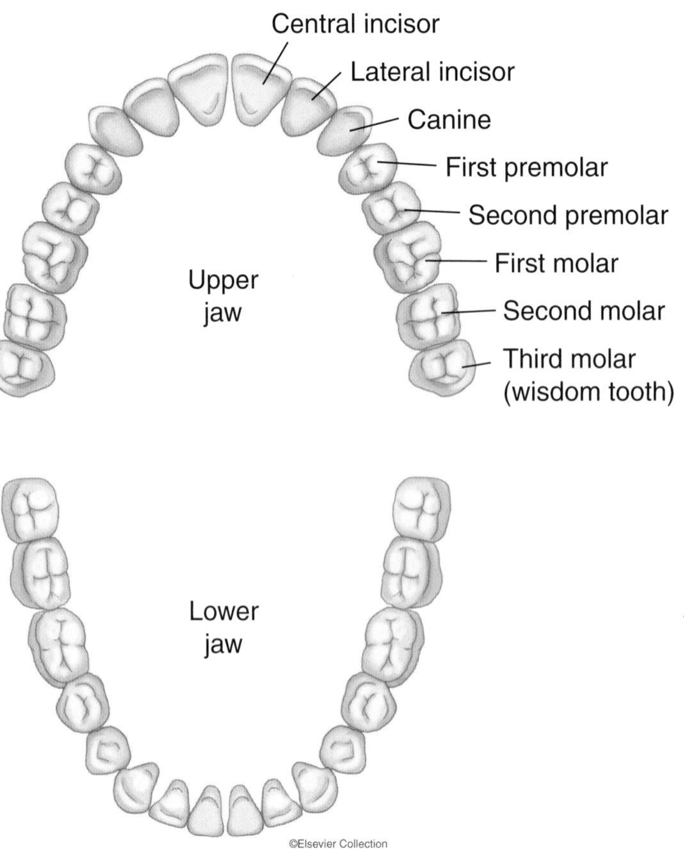
Central incisor
Lateral incisor
Canine
First premolar
Second premolar
First molar
Second molar
Third molar (wisdom tooth)
Upper jaw
Lower jaw
©Elsevier Collection

Plate 25 Adult Teeth. (©Elsevier Collection).

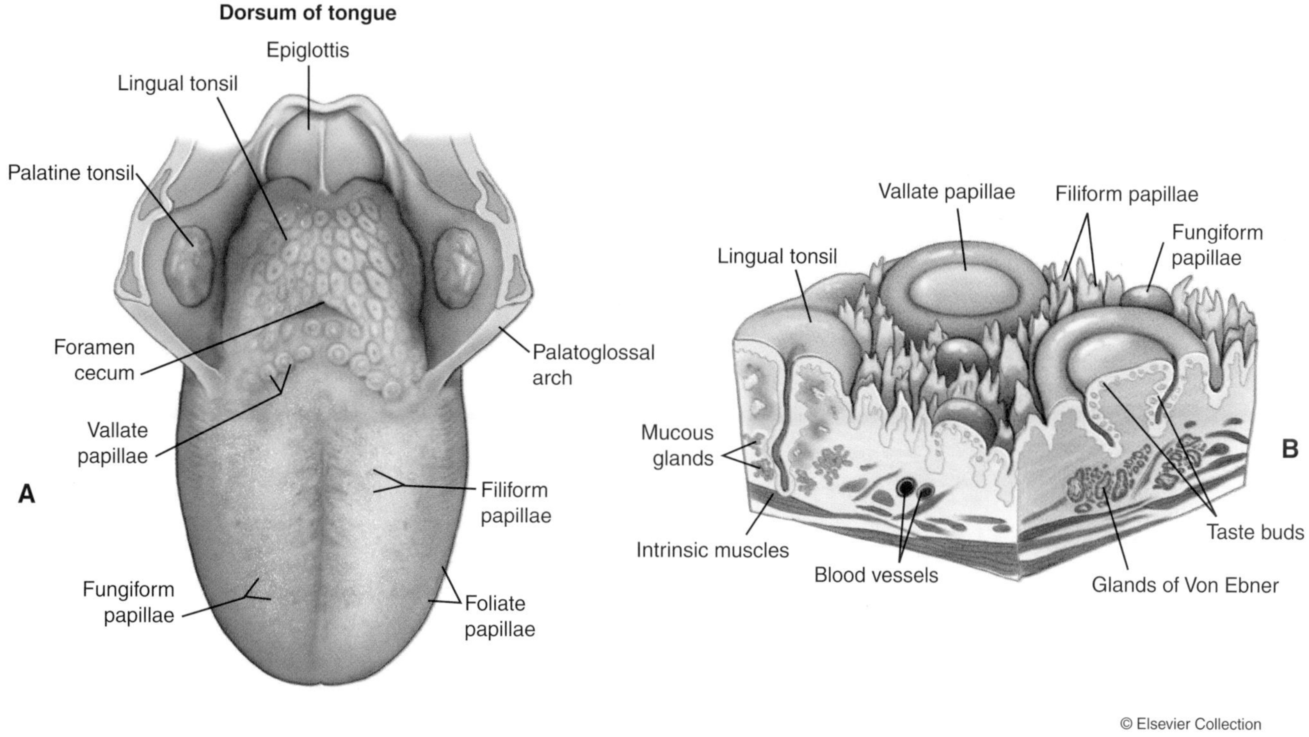

Dorsum of tongue
Epiglottis
Lingual tonsil
Palatine tonsil
Foramen cecum
Palatoglossal arch
Vallate papillae
A
Filiform papillae
Fungiform papillae
Foliate papillae
Vallate papillae
Filiform papillae
Fungiform papillae
Lingual tonsil
Mucous glands
B
Intrinsic muscles
Taste buds
Blood vessels
Glands of Von Ebner

© Elsevier Collection

Plate 26 A, Dorsal view of tongue showing the roughened large lingual tonsils on the posterior of the tongue and the foliate papillae on the side. B, Section of dorsal of the tongue showing a cutaway through lingual papillae and showing von Ebner's glands at the base of the vallate papilla. (Brand RW, Isselhard DE: Anatomy of Orofacial Structures: A Comprehensive Approach, ed 8, St. Louis, 2019, Elsevier.)

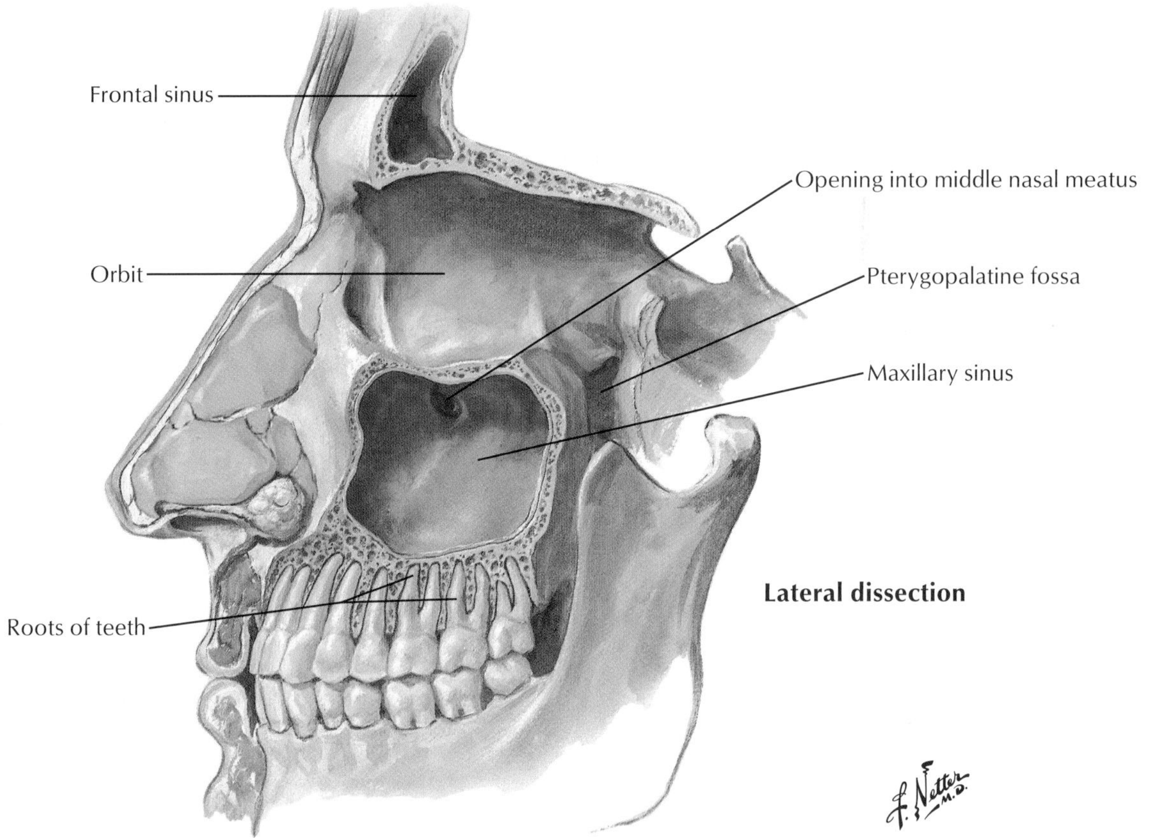
Frontal sinus
Opening into middle nasal meatus
Orbit
Pterygopalatine fossa
Maxillary sinus
Lateral dissection
Roots of teeth

Plate 27 Paranasal Sinuses. (Copyright 2024 Elsevier Inc. All rights reserved. www.netterimages.com. Image ID: 8427.)

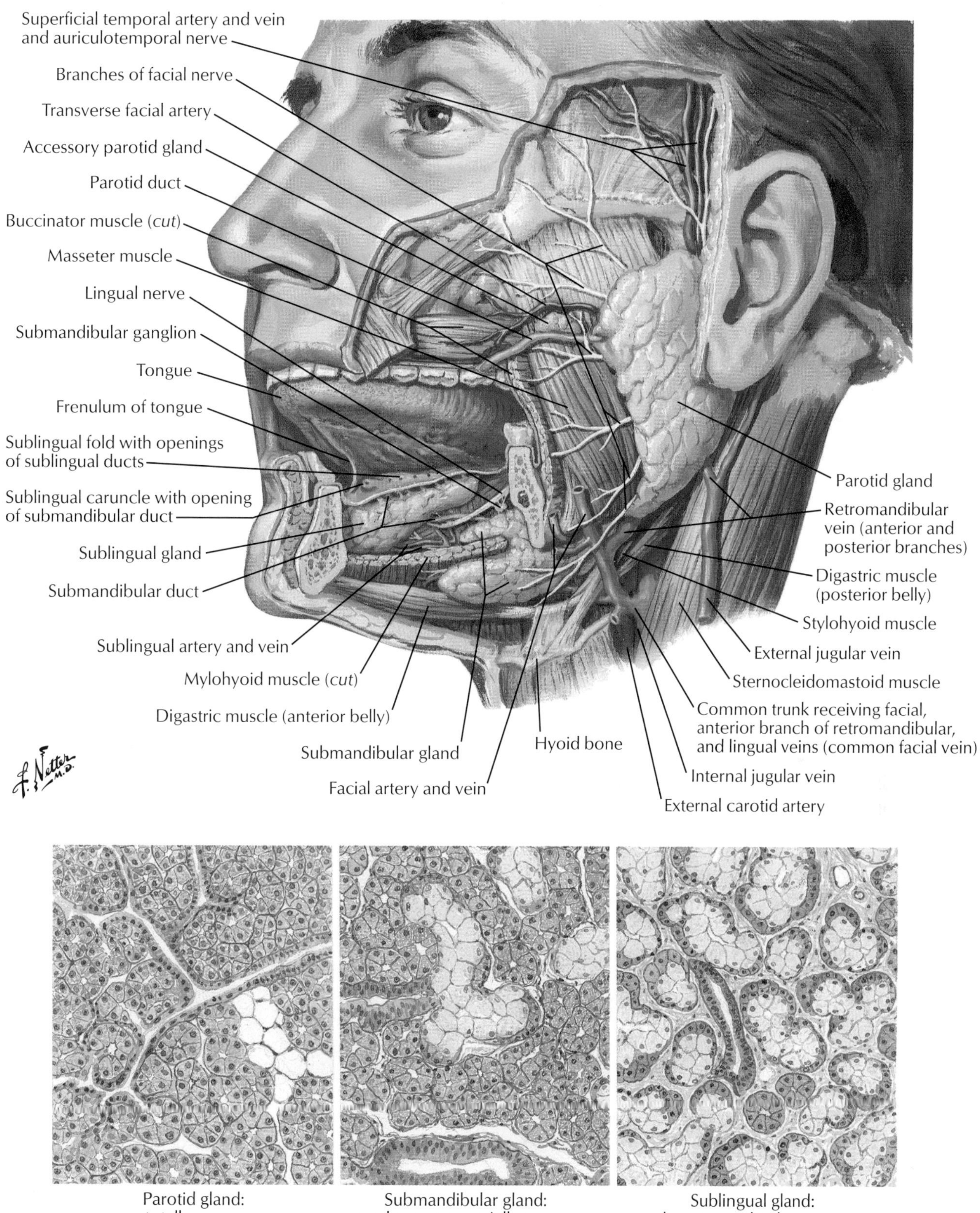
Superficial temporal artery and vein and auriculotemporal nerve
Branches of facial nerve
Transverse facial artery
Accessory parotid gland
Parotid duct
Buccinator muscle (cut)
Masseter muscle
Lingual nerve
Submandibular ganglion
Tongue
Frenulum of tongue
Sublingual fold with openings of sublingual ducts
Sublingual caruncle with opening of submandibular duct
Sublingual gland
Submandibular duct
Sublingual artery and vein
Mylohyoid muscle (cut)
Digastric muscle (anterior belly)
Submandibular gland
Facial artery and vein
Hyoid bone
Parotid gland
Retromandibular vein (anterior and posterior branches)
Digastric muscle (posterior belly)
Stylohyoid muscle
External jugular vein
Sternocleidomastoid muscle
Common trunk receiving facial, anterior branch of retromandibular, and lingual veins (common facial vein)
Internal jugular vein
External carotid artery
Parotid gland: totally serous
Submandibular gland: mostly serous, partially mucous
Sublingual gland: almost completely mucous

Plate 28 Salivary Glands. (Copyright 2024 Elsevier Inc. All rights reserved. www.netterimages.com. Image ID: 4396.)

Coronary Arteries: Arteriographic Views

Right coronary artery: left anterior oblique view

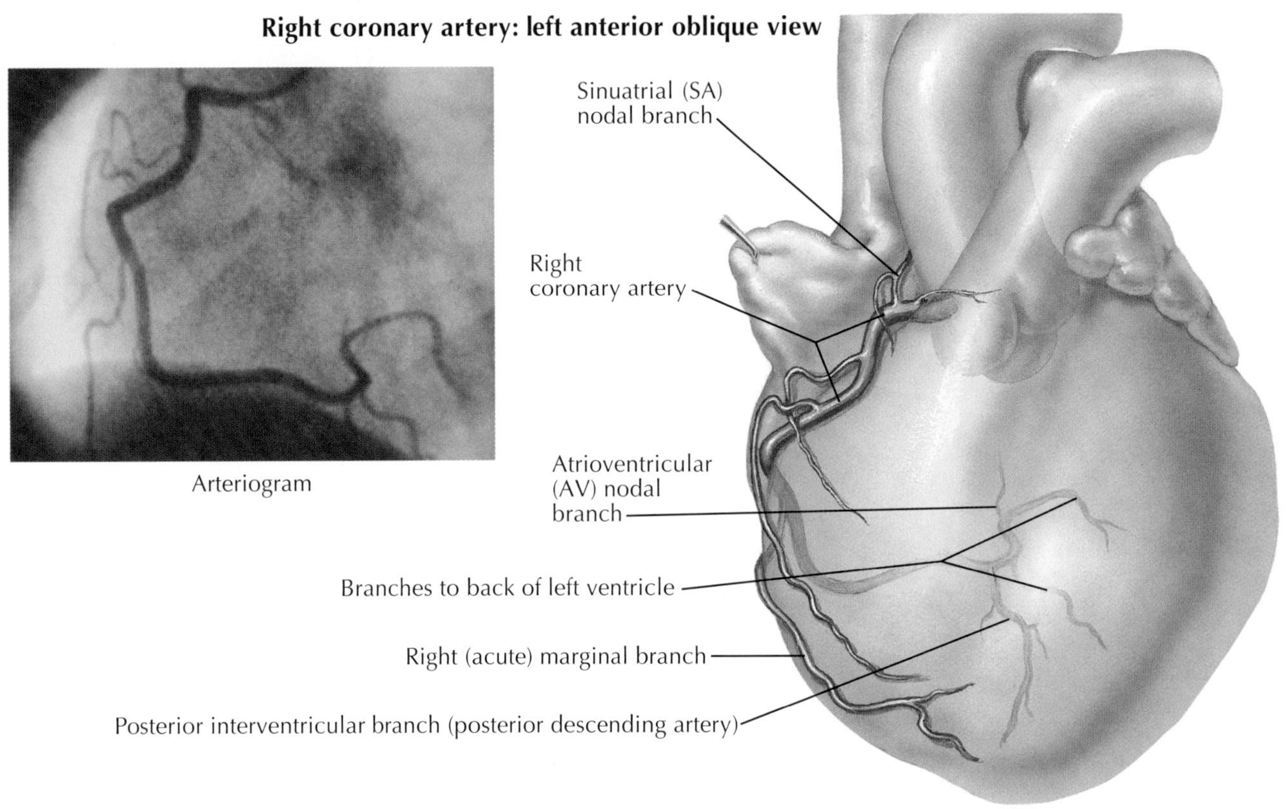
Arteriogram
Sinuatrial (SA) nodal branch
Right coronary artery
Atrioventricular (AV) nodal branch
Branches to back of left ventricle
Right (acute) marginal branch
Posterior interventricular branch (posterior descending artery)

Right coronary artery: right anterior oblique view

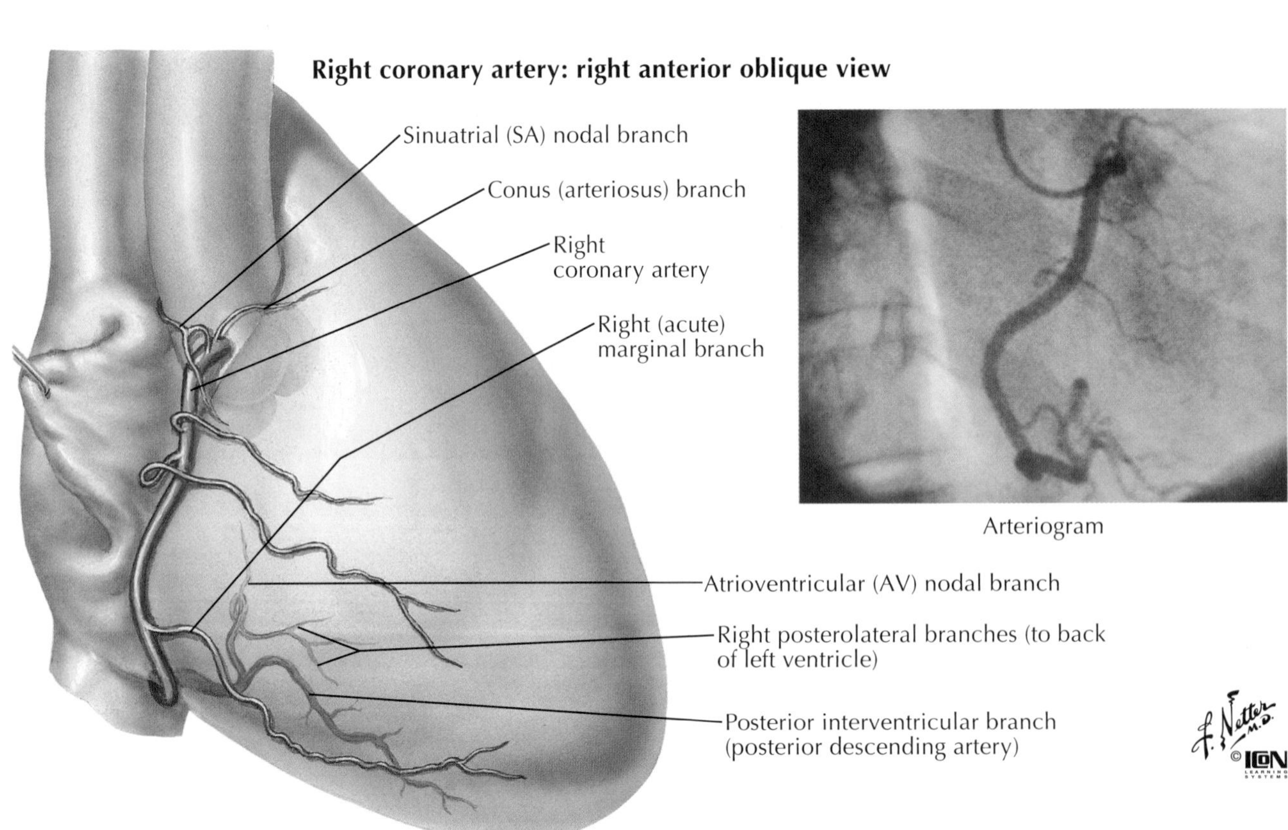
Sinuatrial (SA) nodal branch
Conus (arteriosus) branch
Right coronary artery
Right (acute) marginal branch
Arteriogram
Atrioventricular (AV) nodal branch
Right posterolateral branches (to back of left ventricle)
Posterior interventricular branch (posterior descending artery)
F. Netter M.D.
© ICON LEARNING SYSTEMS

Plate 29 Coronary Arteries: Arteriographic Views. (Copyright 2024 Elsevier Inc. All rights reserved. www.netterimages.com. Image ID: 4725.)

Left coronary artery: left anterior oblique view

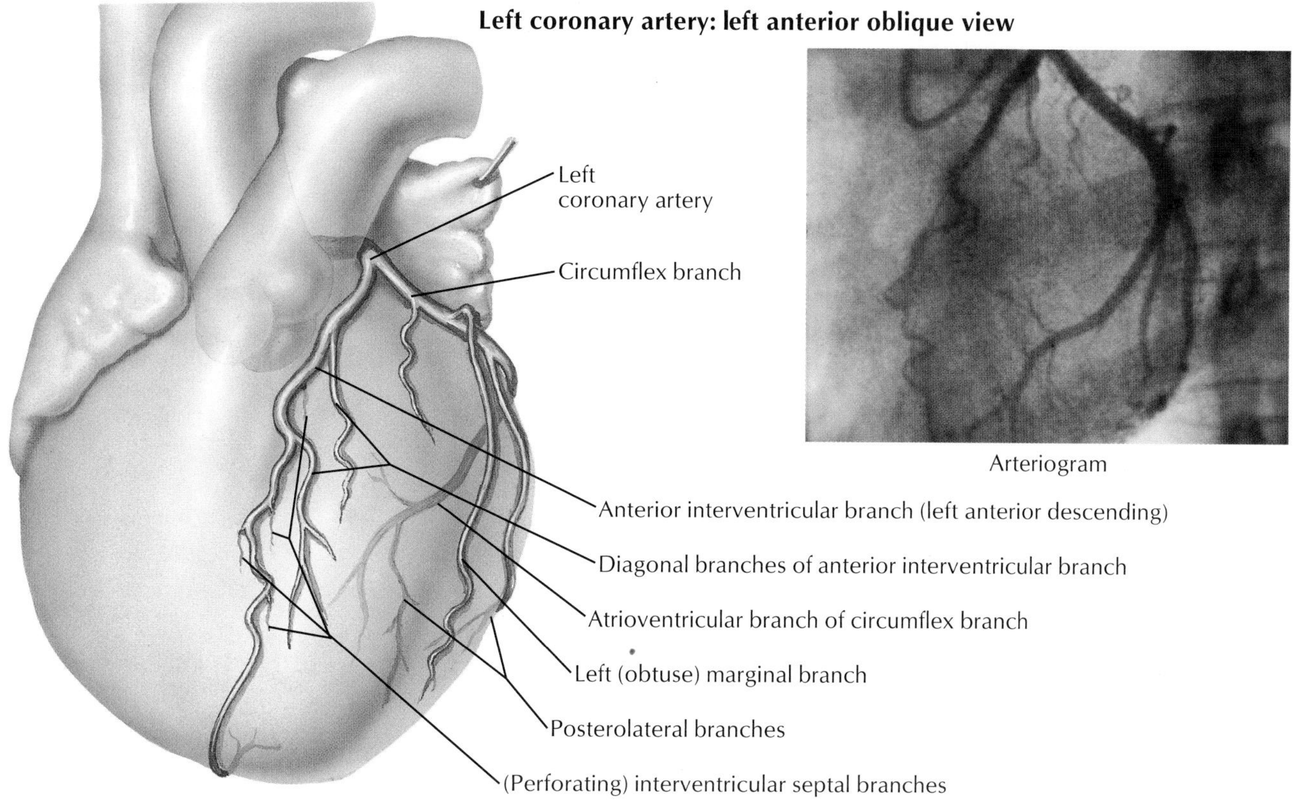

Left coronary artery
Circumflex branch
Arteriogram
Anterior interventricular branch (left anterior descending)
Diagonal branches of anterior interventricular branch
Atrioventricular branch of circumflex branch
Left (obtuse) marginal branch
Posterolateral branches
(Perforating) interventricular septal branches

Left coronary artery: right anterior oblique view

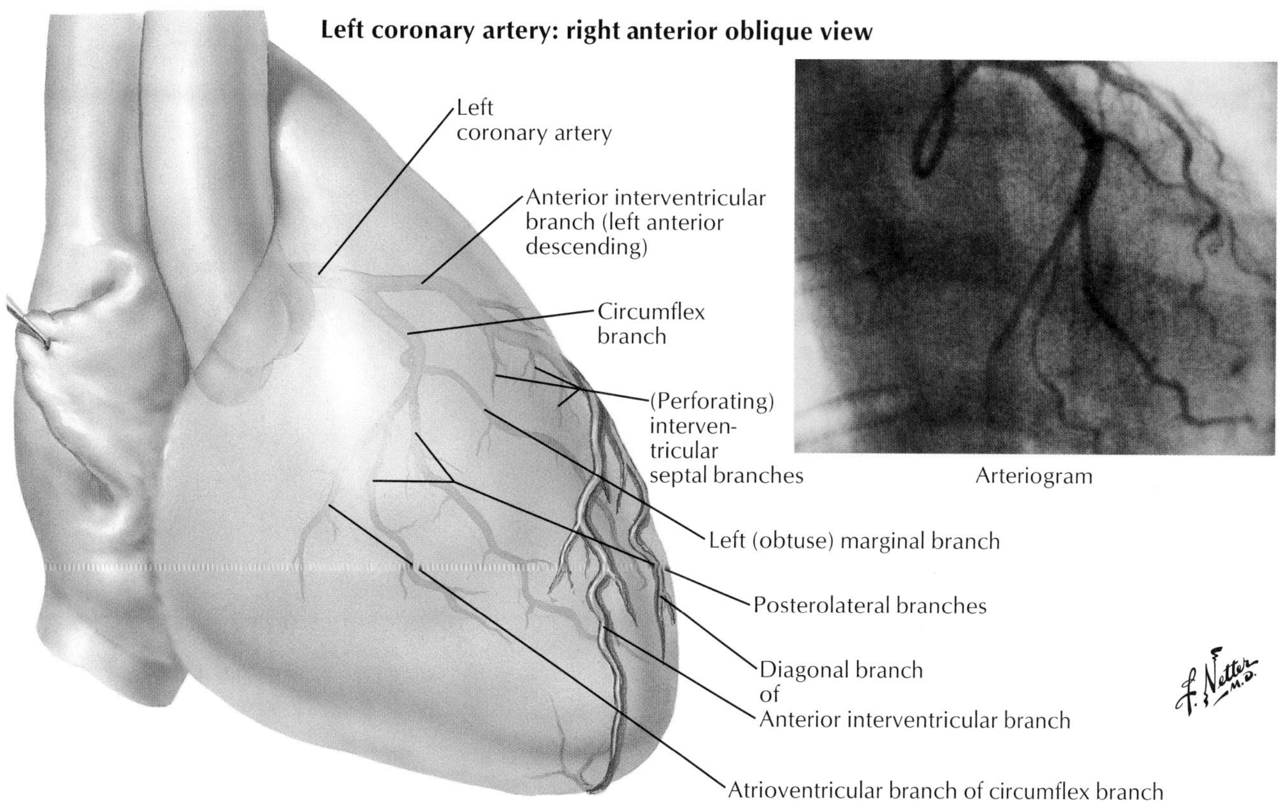

Left coronary artery
Anterior interventricular branch (left anterior descending)
Circumflex branch
(Perforating) interventricular septal branches
Arteriogram
Left (obtuse) marginal branch
Posterolateral branches
Diagonal branch of Anterior interventricular branch
Atrioventricular branch of circumflex branch

Plate 30 Coronary Arteries: Arteriographic Views. (Copyright 2024 Elsevier Inc. All rights reserved. www.netterimages.com. Image ID: 4542.)

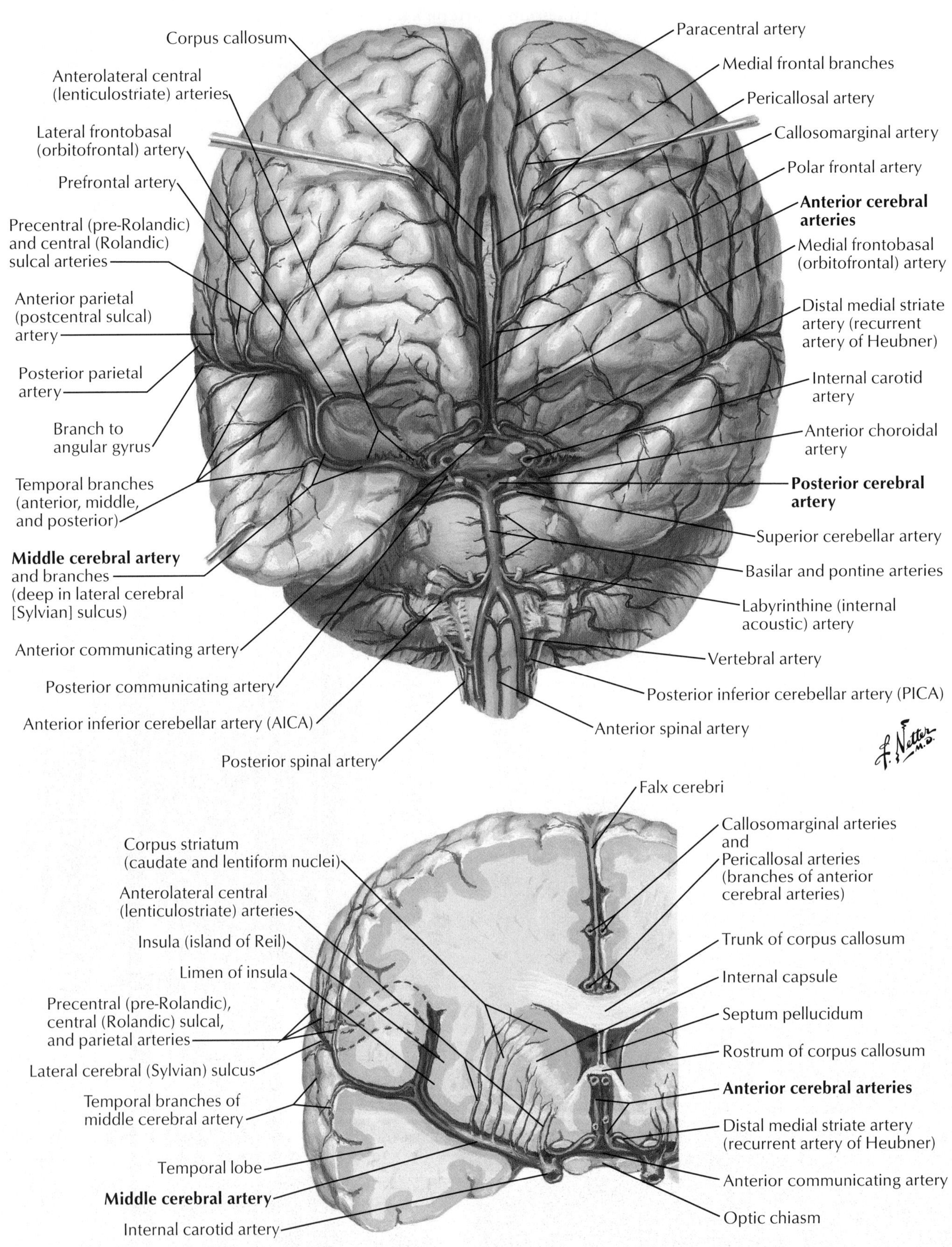
Corpus callosum
Anterolateral central (lenticulostriate) arteries
Lateral frontobasal (orbitofrontal) artery
Prefrontal artery
Precentral (pre-Rolandic) and central (Rolandic) sulcal arteries
Anterior parietal (postcentral sulcal) artery
Posterior parietal artery
Branch to angular gyrus
Temporal branches (anterior, middle, and posterior)
Middle cerebral artery and branches (deep in lateral cerebral [Sylvian] sulcus)
Anterior communicating artery
Posterior communicating artery
Anterior inferior cerebellar artery (AICA)
Posterior spinal artery
Paracentral artery
Medial frontal branches
Pericallosal artery
Callosomarginal artery
Polar frontal artery
Anterior cerebral arteries
Medial frontobasal (orbitofrontal) artery
Distal medial striate artery (recurrent artery of Heubner)
Internal carotid artery
Anterior choroidal artery
Posterior cerebral artery
Superior cerebellar artery
Basilar and pontine arteries
Labyrinthine (internal acoustic) artery
Vertebral artery
Posterior inferior cerebellar artery (PICA)
Anterior spinal artery
F. Netter M.D.
Falx cerebri
Corpus striatum (caudate and lentiform nuclei)
Anterolateral central (lenticulostriate) arteries
Insula (island of Reil)
Limen of insula
Precentral (pre-Rolandic), central (Rolandic) sulcal, and parietal arteries
Lateral cerebral (Sylvian) sulcus
Temporal branches of middle cerebral artery
Temporal lobe
Middle cerebral artery
Internal carotid artery
Callosomarginal arteries and Pericallosal arteries (branches of anterior cerebral arteries)
Trunk of corpus callosum
Internal capsule
Septum pellucidum
Rostrum of corpus callosum
Anterior cerebral arteries
Distal medial striate artery (recurrent artery of Heubner)
Anterior communicating artery
Optic chiasm

Plate 31 Arteries of Brain: Frontal View and Section. (Copyright 2024 Elsevier Inc. All rights reserved. www.netterimages.com. Image ID: 4588.)

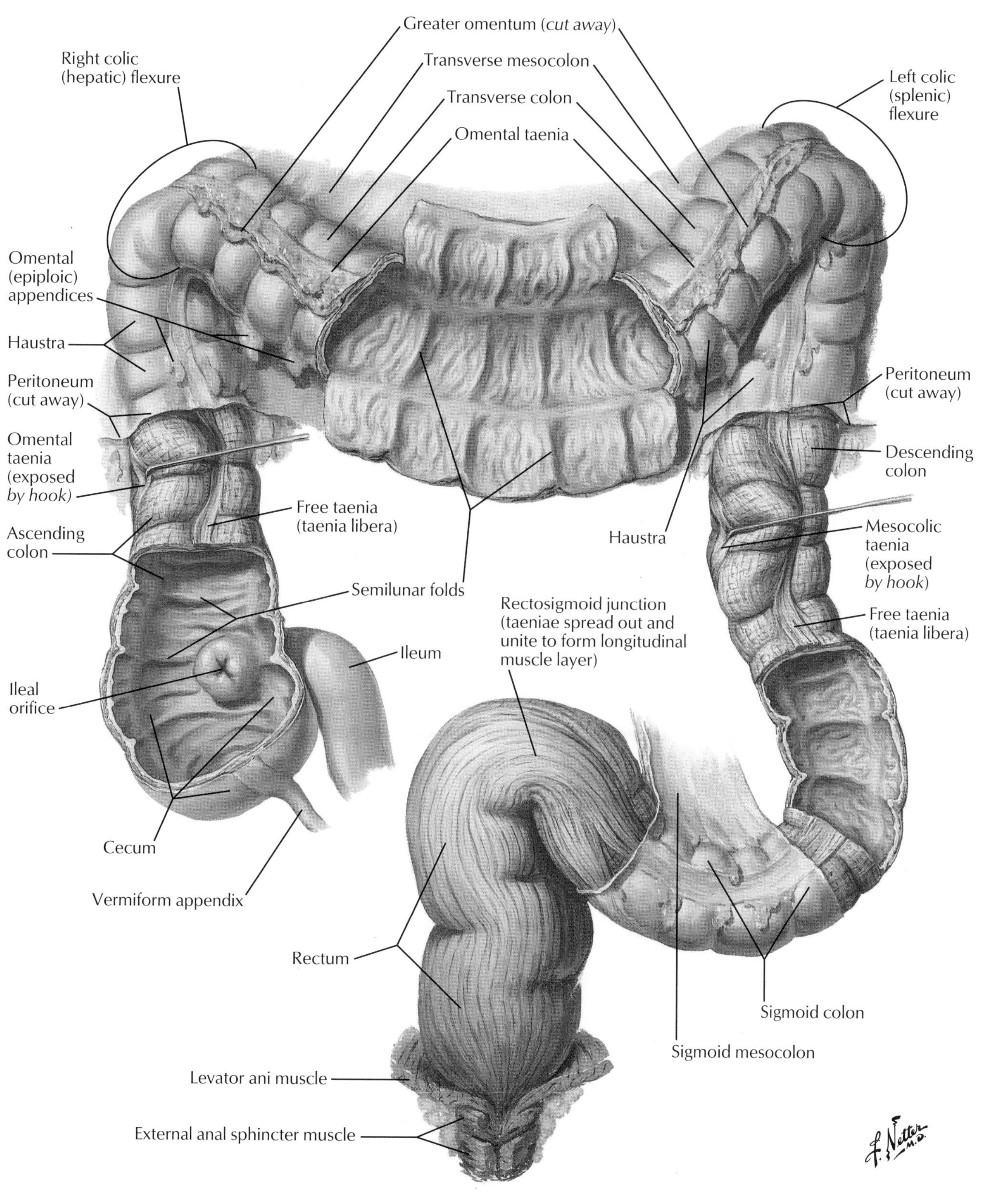
Greater omentum (*cut away*)
Right colic (hepatic) flexure
Transverse mesocolon
Transverse colon
Omental taenia
Left colic (splenic) flexure
Omental (epiploic) appendices
Haustra
Peritoneum (cut away)
Omental taenia (exposed *by hook)*
Ascending colon
Free taenia (taenia libera)
Semilunar folds
Haustra
Peritoneum (cut away)
Descending colon
Mesocolic taenia (exposed *by hook)*
Free taenia (taenia libera)
Rectosigmoid junction (taeniae spread out and unite to form longitudinal muscle layer)
Ileum
Ileal orifice
Cecum
Vermiform appendix
Rectum
Sigmoid colon
Sigmoid mesocolon
Levator ani muscle
External anal sphincter muscle

Plate 32 Mucosa and Musculature of Large Intestine. (Copyright 2024 Elsevier Inc. All rights reserved. www.netterimages.com. Image ID: 4778.)

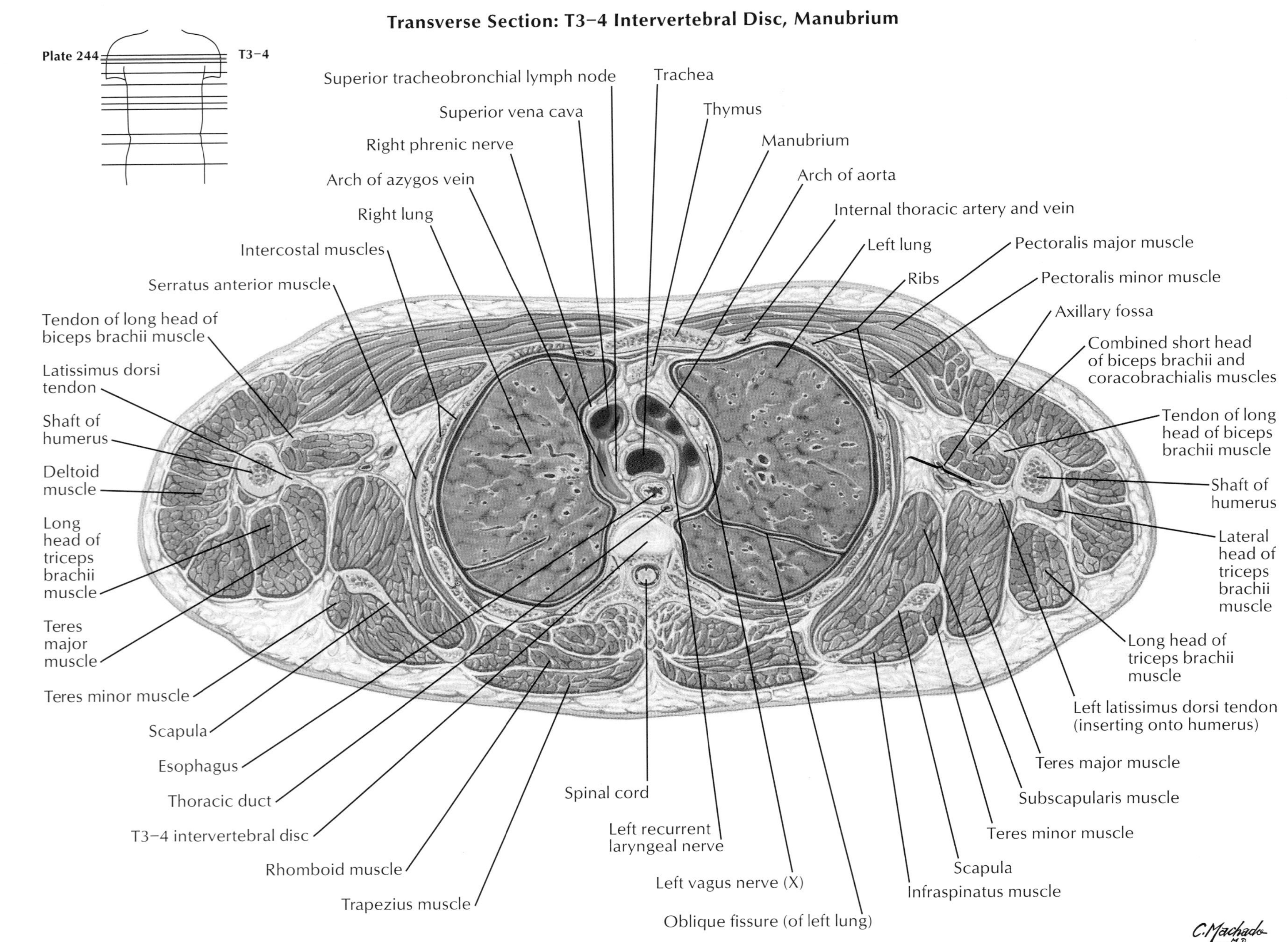
Transverse Section: T3–4 Intervertebral Disc, Manubrium
Plate 244
T3–4
Superior tracheobronchial lymph node
Trachea
Superior vena cava
Thymus
Right phrenic nerve
Manubrium
Arch of azygos vein
Arch of aorta
Right lung
Internal thoracic artery and vein
Intercostal muscles
Left lung
Pectoralis major muscle
Serratus anterior muscle
Ribs
Pectoralis minor muscle
Axillary fossa
Tendon of long head of biceps brachii muscle
Combined short head of biceps brachii and coracobrachialis muscles
Latissimus dorsi tendon
Tendon of long head of biceps brachii muscle
Shaft of humerus
Shaft of humerus
Deltoid muscle
Lateral head of triceps brachii muscle
Long head of triceps brachii muscle
Teres major muscle
Long head of triceps brachii muscle
Teres minor muscle
Left latissimus dorsi tendon (inserting onto humerus)
Scapula
Esophagus
Teres major muscle
Thoracic duct
Spinal cord
Subscapularis muscle
T3–4 intervertebral disc
Left recurrent laryngeal nerve
Teres minor muscle
Rhomboid muscle
Scapula
Left vagus nerve (X)
Infraspinatus muscle
Trapezius muscle
Oblique fissure (of left lung)
C. Machado M.D.

Plate 33 Cross Section of Thorax at T3-4 Disc Level. (Copyright 2024 Elsevier Inc. All rights reserved. www.netterimages.com. Image ID: 4880.)

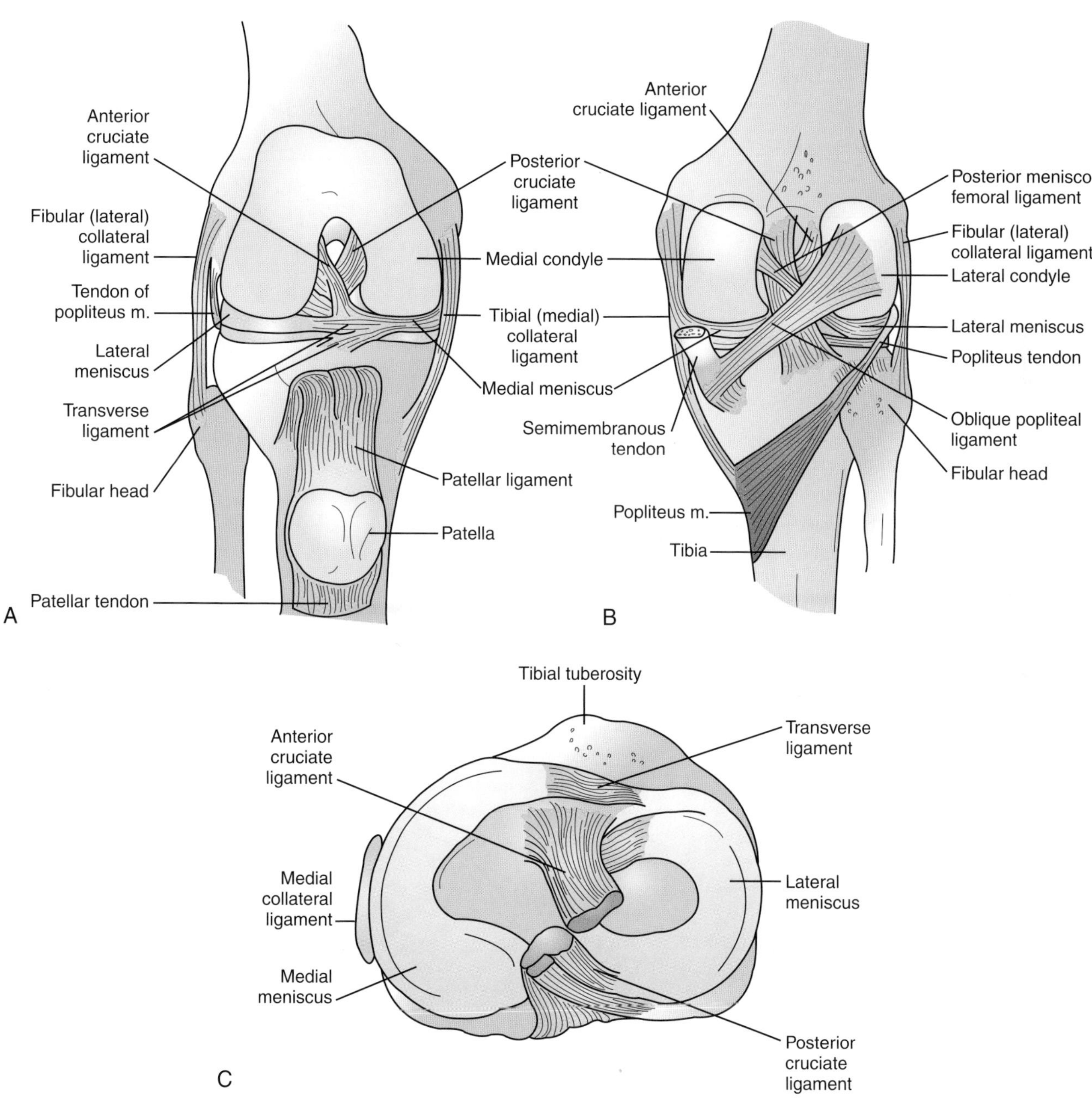

Anterior cruciate ligament
Fibular (lateral) collateral ligament
Tendon of popliteus m.
Lateral meniscus
Transverse ligament
Fibular head
Patellar tendon
A
Posterior cruciate ligament
Medial condyle
Tibial (medial) collateral ligament
Medial meniscus
Patellar ligament
Patella
Anterior cruciate ligament
Posterior menisco-femoral ligament
Fibular (lateral) collateral ligament
Lateral condyle
Lateral meniscus
Popliteus tendon
Oblique popliteal ligament
Fibular head
Semimembranous tendon
Popliteus m.
Tibia
B
Tibial tuberosity
Anterior cruciate ligament
Transverse ligament
Medial collateral ligament
Lateral meniscus
Medial meniscus
Posterior cruciate ligament
C

Plate 34 Knee joint opened; anterior, posterior, and proximal views. A, Anterior view of the knee joint, opened by folding the patella and patellar ligament inferiorly. On the lateral side is the fibular collateral ligament, separated by the popliteal tendon from the lateral meniscus. On the medial side, the tibial collateral ligament is attached to the medial meniscus. The anterior and posterior cruciate ligaments are seen between the femoral condyles. B, Posterior view of the opened knee joint with a more complete view of the posterior cruciate ligament. C, The femur is removed, showing the proximal (articular) end of the right tibia. On the medial side is the gently curved medial meniscus; on the lateral side is the more tightly curved lateral meniscus. The anterior end of the medial meniscus is anchored to the surface of the tibia by the transverse ligament. The cut ends of the anterior and posterior cruciate ligaments are shown, as well as the meniscofemoral ligament. (Fritz S: Mosby's Essential Sciences for Therapeutic Massage: Anatomy, Physiology, Biomechanics, and Pathology, ed 5, St. Louis, 2017, Elsevier.)

Paramedian (sagittal) dissection

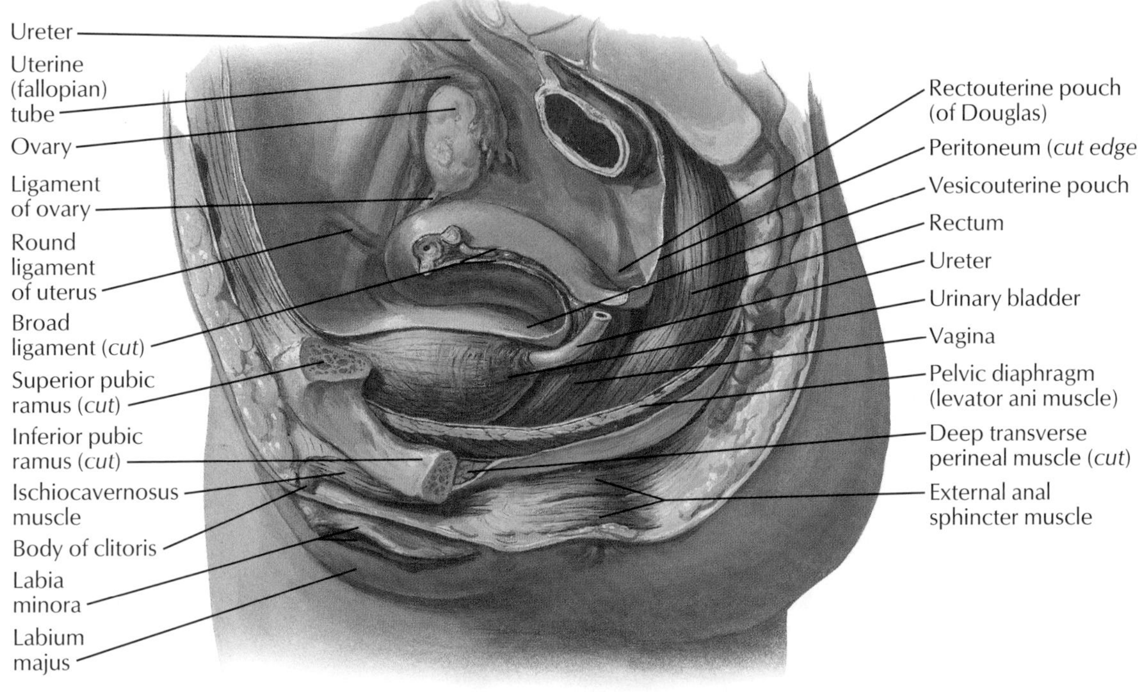
Ureter
Uterine (fallopian) tube
Ovary
Ligament of ovary
Round ligament of uterus
Broad ligament (*cut*)
Superior pubic ramus (*cut*)
Inferior pubic ramus (*cut*)
Ischiocavernosus muscle
Body of clitoris
Labia minora
Labium majus
Rectouterine pouch (of Douglas)
Peritoneum (*cut edge*)
Vesicouterine pouch
Rectum
Ureter
Urinary bladder
Vagina
Pelvic diaphragm (levator ani muscle)
Deep transverse perineal muscle (*cut*)
External anal sphincter muscle

Median (sagittal) section

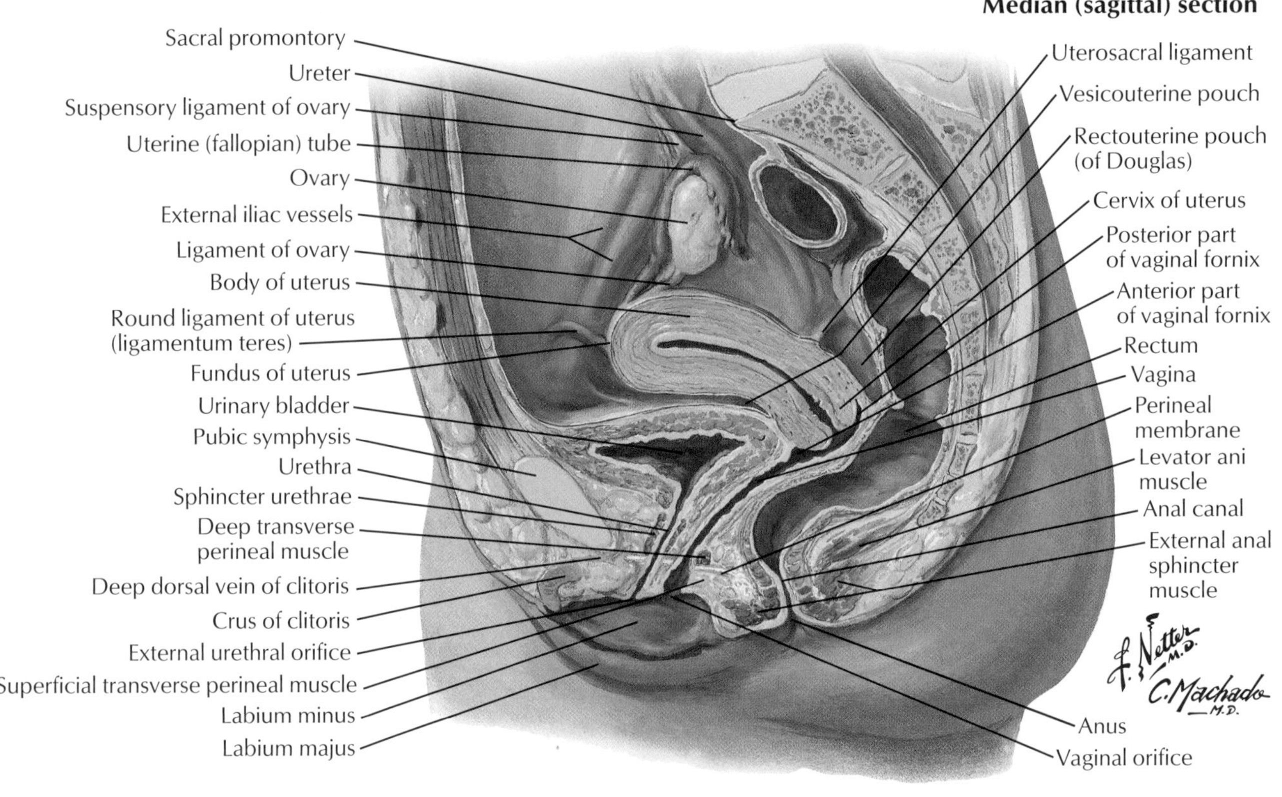
Sacral promontory
Ureter
Suspensory ligament of ovary
Uterine (fallopian) tube
Ovary
External iliac vessels
Ligament of ovary
Body of uterus
Round ligament of uterus (ligamentum teres)
Fundus of uterus
Urinary bladder
Pubic symphysis
Urethra
Sphincter urethrae
Deep transverse perineal muscle
Deep dorsal vein of clitoris
Crus of clitoris
External urethral orifice
Superficial transverse perineal muscle
Labium minus
Labium majus
Uterosacral ligament
Vesicouterine pouch
Rectouterine pouch (of Douglas)
Cervix of uterus
Posterior part of vaginal fornix
Anterior part of vaginal fornix
Rectum
Vagina
Perineal membrane
Levator ani muscle
Anal canal
External anal sphincter muscle
Anus
Vaginal orifice
F. Netter M.D.
C. Machado M.D.

Plate 35 Pelvic Viscera and Perineum: Female. (Copyright 2024 Elsevier Inc. All rights reserved. www.netterimages.com. Image ID: 4463.)

TABLES

Medical and Surgical

00. Central Nervous System and Cranial Nerves....42
- 001. Bypass....43
- 002. Change....43
- 005. Destruction....44
- 007. Dilation....45
- 008. Division....45
- 009. Drainage....46
- 00B. Excision....48
- 00C. Extirpation....49
- 00D. Extraction....50
- 00F. Fragmentation....50
- 00H. Insertion....51
- 00J. Inspection....51
- 00K. Map....52
- 00N. Release....52
- 00P. Removal....53
- 00Q. Repair....54
- 00R. Replacement....55
- 00S. Reposition....55
- 00T. Resection....56
- 00U. Supplement....56
- 00W. Revision....57
- 00X. Transfer....58

SECTION: Ø MEDICAL AND SURGICAL
BODY SYSTEM: Ø CENTRAL NERVOUS SYSTEM AND CRANIAL NERVES
OPERATION: 1 BYPASS: Altering the route of passage of the contents of a tubular body part

Body Part	Approach	Device	Qualifier
6 Cerebral Ventricle	Ø Open 3 Percutaneous 4 Percutaneous Endoscopic	7 Autologous Tissue Substitute J Synthetic Substitute K Nonautologous Tissue Substitute	Ø Nasopharynx 1 Mastoid Sinus 2 Atrium 3 Blood Vessel 4 Pleural Cavity 5 Intestine 6 Peritoneal Cavity 7 Urinary Tract 8 Bone Marrow A Subgaleal Space B Cerebral Cisterns
6 Cerebral Ventricle	Ø Open 3 Percutaneous 4 Percutaneous Endoscopic	Z No Device	B Cerebral Cisterns
U Spinal Canal	Ø Open 3 Percutaneous 4 Percutaneous Endoscopic	7 Autologous Tissue Substitute J Synthetic Substitute K Nonautologous Tissue Substitute	2 Atrium 4 Pleural Cavity 6 Peritoneal Cavity 7 Urinary Tract 9 Fallopian Tube

Coding Clinic: 2021, Q2, P19; 2013, Q2, P37 – ØØ163J6
Coding Clinic: 2018, Q4, P86 – ØØ1UØJ2
Coding Clinic: 2019, Q4, P22 – ØØ163JA

SECTION: Ø MEDICAL AND SURGICAL
BODY SYSTEM: Ø CENTRAL NERVOUS SYSTEM AND CRANIAL NERVES
OPERATION: 2 CHANGE: Taking out or off a device from a body part and putting back an identical or similar device in or on the same body part without cutting or puncturing the skin or a mucous membrane

Body Part	Approach	Device	Qualifier
Ø Brain E Cranial Nerve U Spinal Canal	X External	Ø Drainage Device Y Other Device	Z No Qualifier

Non-OR All Values

SECTION: Ø MEDICAL AND SURGICAL

BODY SYSTEM: Ø CENTRAL NERVOUS SYSTEM AND CRANIAL NERVES

OPERATION: 5 DESTRUCTION: Physical eradication of all or a portion of a body part by the direct use of energy, force, or a destructive agent

Body Part	Approach	Device	Qualifier
Ø Brain	Ø Open 4 Percutaneous Endoscopic	Z No Device	3 Laser Interstitial Thermal Therapy Z No Qualifier
Ø Brain	3 Percutaneous	Z No Device Therapy	3 Laser Interstitial Thermal 4 Stereoelectroencephalographic Radiofrequency Ablation Z No Qualifier
~~Ø Brain~~ ~~W Cervical Spinal Cord~~ ~~X Thoracic Spinal Cord~~ ~~Y Lumbar Spinal Cord~~	~~Ø Open~~ ~~3 Percutaneous~~ ~~4 Percutaneous Endoscopic~~	~~Z No Device~~	~~3 Laser Interstitial Thermal~~ ~~Z No Qualifier~~
1 Cerebral Meninges 2 Dura Mater 6 Cerebral Ventricle 7 Cerebral Hemisphere 8 Basal Ganglia 9 Thalamus A Hypothalamus B Pons C Cerebellum D Medulla Oblongata F Olfactory Nerve G Optic Nerve H Oculomotor Nerve J Trochlear Nerve K Trigeminal Nerve L Abducens Nerve M Facial Nerve N Acoustic Nerve P Glossopharyngeal Nerve Q Vagus Nerve R Accessory Nerve S Hypoglossal Nerve T Spinal Meninges	Ø Open 3 Percutaneous 4 Percutaneous Endoscopic	Z No Device	Z No Qualifier
W Cervical Spinal Cord X Thoracic Spinal Cord Y Lumbar Spinal Cord	Ø Open 3 Percutaneous 4 Percutaneous Endoscopic	Z No Device	3 Laser Interstitial Thermal Therapy Z No Qualifier

Non-OR ØØ5[ØFGHJKLMNPQRSWXY][Ø34]ZZ

Coding Clinic: 2Ø21, Q2, P18 – ØØ5[WX]ØZZ
Coding Clinic: 2Ø21, Q3, P17 – ØØ5CØZZ
Coding Clinic: 2Ø22, Q1, P5Ø – ØØ5K3ZZ

SECTION: Ø MEDICAL AND SURGICAL
BODY SYSTEM: Ø CENTRAL NERVOUS SYSTEM AND CRANIAL NERVES
OPERATION: 7 DILATION: Expanding an orifice or the lumen of a tubular body part

Body Part	Approach	Device	Qualifier
6 Cerebral Ventricle	Ø Open 3 Percutaneous 4 Percutaneous Endoscopic	Z No Device	Z No Qualifier

Coding Clinic: 2017, Q4, P4Ø – ØØ764ZZ

SECTION: Ø MEDICAL AND SURGICAL
BODY SYSTEM: Ø CENTRAL NERVOUS SYSTEM AND CRANIAL NERVES
OPERATION: 8 DIVISION: Cutting into a body part, without draining fluids and/or gases from the body part, in order to separate or transect a body part

Body Part	Approach	Device	Qualifier
Ø Brain 7 Cerebral Hemisphere 8 Basal Ganglia F Olfactory Nerve G Optic Nerve H Oculomotor Nerve J Trochlear Nerve K Trigeminal Nerve L Abducens Nerve M Facial Nerve N Acoustic Nerve P Glossopharyngeal Nerve Q Vagus Nerve R Accessory Nerve S Hypoglossal Nerve W Cervical Spinal Cord X Thoracic Spinal Cord Y Lumbar Spinal Cord	Ø Open 3 Percutaneous 4 Percutaneous Endoscopic	Z No Device	Z No Qualifier

SECTION: Ø MEDICAL AND SURGICAL
BODY SYSTEM: Ø CENTRAL NERVOUS SYSTEM AND CRANIAL NERVES
OPERATION: 9 DRAINAGE: *(on multiple pages)*
Taking or letting out fluids and/or gases from a body part

Body Part	Approach	Device	Qualifier
Ø Brain 1 Cerebral Meninges 2 Dura Mater 3 Epidural Space, Intracranial 4 Subdural Space, Intracranial 5 Subarachnoid Space, Intracranial 6 Cerebral Ventricle 7 Cerebral Hemisphere 8 Basal Ganglia 9 Thalamus A Hypothalamus B Pons C Cerebellum D Medulla Oblongata F Olfactory Nerve G Optic Nerve H Oculomotor Nerve J Trochlear Nerve K Trigeminal Nerve L Abducens Nerve M Facial Nerve N Acoustic Nerve P Glossopharyngeal Nerve Q Vagus Nerve R Accessory Nerve S Hypoglossal Nerve T Spinal Meninges U Spinal Canal W Cervical Spinal Cord X Thoracic Spinal Cord Y Lumbar Spinal Cord	Ø Open 3 Percutaneous 4 Percutaneous Endoscopic	Ø Drainage Device	Z No Qualifier

DRG Non-OR ØØ9[3TWXY]3ØZ
Non-OR ØØ9U[34]ØZ

Coding Clinic: 2015, Q2, P3Ø – ØØ9WØØZ
Coding Clinic: 2018, Q4, P85 – ØØ9UØØZ

SECTION: Ø MEDICAL AND SURGICAL
BODY SYSTEM: Ø CENTRAL NERVOUS SYSTEM AND CRANIAL NERVES
OPERATION: 9 DRAINAGE: *(continued)*
Taking or letting out fluids and/or gases from a body part

Body Part	Approach	Device	Qualifier
Ø Brain 1 Cerebral Meninges 2 Dura Mater 3 Epidural Space, Intracranial 4 Subdural Space, Intracranial 5 Subarachnoid Space, Intracranial 6 Cerebral Ventricle 7 Cerebral Hemisphere 8 Basal Ganglia 9 Thalamus A Hypothalamus B Pons C Cerebellum D Medulla Oblongata F Olfactory Nerve G Optic Nerve H Oculomotor Nerve J Trochlear Nerve K Trigeminal Nerve L Abducens Nerve M Facial Nerve N Acoustic Nerve P Glossopharyngeal Nerve Q Vagus Nerve R Accessory Nerve S Hypoglossal Nerve T Spinal Meninges U Spinal Canal W Cervical Spinal Cord X Thoracic Spinal Cord Y Lumbar Spinal Cord	Ø Open 3 Percutaneous 4 Percutaneous Endoscopic	Z No Device	X Diagnostic Z No Qualifier

DRG Non-OR ØØ933ZZ
Non-OR ØØ9[Ø123456789ABCDFGHJKLMNPQRSU][34]ZX
Non-OR ØØ9U[34]ZZ
Non-OR ØØ9[TWXY]3[XZ]

Coding Clinic: 2Ø15, Q3, P12-13 – ØØ9[46]3ØZ

SECTION: Ø MEDICAL AND SURGICAL
BODY SYSTEM: Ø CENTRAL NERVOUS SYSTEM AND CRANIAL NERVES
OPERATION: B EXCISION: Cutting out or off, without replacement, a portion of a body part

Body Part	Approach	Device	Qualifier
Ø Brain 1 Cerebral Meninges 2 Dura Mater 6 Cerebral Ventricle 7 Cerebral Hemisphere 8 Basal Ganglia 9 Thalamus A Hypothalamus B Pons C Cerebellum D Medulla Oblongata F Olfactory Nerve G Optic Nerve H Oculomotor Nerve J Trochlear Nerve K Trigeminal Nerve L Abducens Nerve M Facial Nerve N Acoustic Nerve P Glossopharyngeal Nerve Q Vagus Nerve R Accessory Nerve S Hypoglossal Nerve T Spinal Meninges W Cervical Spinal Cord X Thoracic Spinal Cord Y Lumbar Spinal Cord	Ø Open 3 Percutaneous 4 Percutaneous Endoscopic	Z No Device	X Diagnostic Z No Qualifier

Non-OR ØØB[Ø126789ABCDFGHJKLMNPQRS][34]ZX

Coding Clinic: 2Ø15, Q1, P13 – ØØBØØZZ
Coding Clinic: 2Ø16, Q2, P13 – ØØB[MRS]ØZZ
Coding Clinic: 2Ø16, Q2, P18 – ØØB7ØZZ
Coding Clinic: 2Ø21, Q3, P17 – ØØBCØZZ

New/Revised Text in Green ~~deleted~~ Deleted ♀ Females Only ♂ Males Only Coding Clinic
Non-covered Limited Coverage Combination (See Appendix E) DRG Non-OR Non-OR Hospital-Acquired Condition

SECTION: Ø MEDICAL AND SURGICAL
BODY SYSTEM: Ø CENTRAL NERVOUS SYSTEM AND CRANIAL NERVES
OPERATION: C EXTIRPATION: Taking or cutting out solid matter from a body part

Body Part	Approach	Device	Qualifier
Ø Brain 1 Cerebral Meninges 2 Dura Mater 3 Epidural Space, Intracranial 4 Subdural Space, Intracranial 5 Subarachnoid Space, Intracranial 6 Cerebral Ventricle 7 Cerebral Hemisphere 8 Basal Ganglia 9 Thalamus A Hypothalamus B Pons C Cerebellum D Medulla Oblongata F Olfactory Nerve G Optic Nerve H Oculomotor Nerve J Trochlear Nerve K Trigeminal Nerve L Abducens Nerve M Facial Nerve N Acoustic Nerve P Glossopharyngeal Nerve Q Vagus Nerve R Accessory Nerve S Hypoglossal Nerve T Spinal Meninges U Spinal Canal W Cervical Spinal Cord X Thoracic Spinal Cord Y Lumbar Spinal Cord	Ø Open 3 Percutaneous 4 Percutaneous Endoscopic	Z No Device	Z No Qualifier

Coding Clinic: 2Ø15, Q1, P12 – ØØCØØZZ
Coding Clinic: 2Ø19, Q3, P4; 2Ø16, Q2, P29; 2Ø15, Q3, P11 – ØØC4ØZZ
Coding Clinic: 2Ø15, Q3, P13 – ØØC74ZZ
Coding Clinic: 2Ø16, Q4, P28 – ØØCØØZZ
Coding Clinic: 2Ø17, Q4, P48 – ØØCUØZZ
Coding Clinic: 2Ø19, Q2, P37 – ØØCØ4ZZ

SECTION: Ø MEDICAL AND SURGICAL
BODY SYSTEM: Ø CENTRAL NERVOUS SYSTEM AND CRANIAL NERVES
OPERATION: D EXTRACTION: Pulling or stripping out or off all or a portion of a body part by the use of force

Body Part	Approach	Device	Qualifier
Ø Brain 1 Cerebral Meninges 2 Dura Mater 7 Cerebral Hemisphere C Cerebellum F Olfactory Nerve G Optic Nerve H Oculomotor Nerve J Trochlear Nerve K Trigeminal Nerve L Abducens Nerve M Facial Nerve N Acoustic Nerve P Glossopharyngeal Nerve Q Vagus Nerve R Accessory Nerve S Hypoglossal Nerve T Spinal Meninges	Ø Open 3 Percutaneous 4 Percutaneous Endoscopic	Z No Device	Z No Qualifier

Non-OR ØØDC[Ø34]ZZ

Coding Clinic: 2Ø15, Q3, P14 – ØØD2ØZZ
Coding Clinic: 2Ø21, Q4, P4Ø – ØØD[Ø7]ØZZ

SECTION: Ø MEDICAL AND SURGICAL
BODY SYSTEM: Ø CENTRAL NERVOUS SYSTEM AND CRANIAL NERVES
OPERATION: F FRAGMENTATION: Breaking solid matter in a body part into pieces

Body Part	Approach	Device	Qualifier
3 Epidural Space, Intracranial 4 Subdural Space, Intracranial 5 Subarachnoid Space, Intracranial 6 Cerebral Ventricle U Spinal Canal	Ø Open 3 Percutaneous 4 Percutaneous Endoscopic X External	Z No Device	Z No Qualifier

ØØF[3456]XZZ
Non-OR ØØF[3456]XZZ

SECTION: Ø MEDICAL AND SURGICAL
BODY SYSTEM: Ø CENTRAL NERVOUS SYSTEM AND CRANIAL NERVES
OPERATION: H INSERTION: Putting in a nonbiological appliance that monitors, assists, performs, or prevents a physiological function but does not physically take the place of a body part

Body Part	Approach	Device	Qualifier
Ø Brain ⊞	Ø Open	1 Radioactive Element 2 Monitoring Device 3 Infusion Device 4 Radioactive Element, Cesium-131 Collagen Implant 5 Radioactive Element, Palladium-1Ø3 CollagenImplant M Neurostimulator Lead Y Other Device	Z No Qualifier
Ø Brain ⊞	3 Percutaneous 4 Percutaneous Endoscopic	1 Radioactive Element 2 Monitoring Device 3 Infusion Device M Neurostimulator Lead Y Other Device	Z No Qualifier
6 Cerebral Ventricle ⊞ E Cranial Nerve ⊞ U Spinal Canal ⊞ V Spinal Cord ⊞	Ø Open 3 Percutaneous 4 Percutaneous Endoscopic	1 Radioactive Element 2 Monitoring Device 3 Infusion Device M Neurostimulator Lead Y Other Device	Z No Qualifier

⊞ ØØHØ[Ø34]MZ
⊞ ØØH[6EUV][Ø34]MZ
DRG Non-OR ØØH[O3][Ø3][24]Z
DRG Non-OR ØØH[6UV]32Z
Non-OR ØØH[UV][Ø34]3Z

Coding Clinic: 2Ø2Ø, Q2, P15 – ØØH633Z
Coding Clinic: 2Ø2Ø, Q2, P17 – ØØHUØ3Z

SECTION: Ø MEDICAL AND SURGICAL
BODY SYSTEM: Ø CENTRAL NERVOUS SYSTEM AND CRANIAL NERVES
OPERATION: J INSPECTION: Visually and/or manually exploring a body part

Body Part	Approach	Device	Qualifier
Ø Brain E Cranial Nerve U Spinal Canal V Spinal Cord	Ø Open 3 Percutaneous 4 Percutaneous Endoscopic	Z No Device	Z No Qualifier

Non-OR ØØJE3ZZ
Non-OR ØØJ[EUV][Ø3][2Y]Z

Coding Clinic: 2Ø17, Q1, P5Ø – ØØJU3ZZ
Coding Clinic: 2Ø19, Q2, P37 – ØØJØØZZ
Coding Clinic: 2Ø21, Q2, P18 – ØØJØ4ZZ

SECTION: Ø MEDICAL AND SURGICAL
BODY SYSTEM: Ø CENTRAL NERVOUS SYSTEM AND CRANIAL NERVES
OPERATION: K MAP: Locating the route of passage of electrical impulses and/or locating functional areas in a body part

Body Part	Approach	Device	Qualifier
Ø Brain	Ø Open 3 Percutaneous 4 Percutaneous Endoscopic	Z No Device	Z No Qualifier
Ø Brain	X External	Z No Device	1 Connectomic Analysis
~~Ø Brain~~ 7 Cerebral Hemisphere 8 Basal Ganglia 9 Thalamus A Hypothalamus B Pons C Cerebellum D Medulla Oblongata	Ø Open 3 Percutaneous 4 Percutaneous Endoscopic	Z No Device	Z No Qualifier

SECTION: Ø MEDICAL AND SURGICAL
BODY SYSTEM: Ø CENTRAL NERVOUS SYSTEM AND CRANIAL NERVES
OPERATION: N RELEASE: Freeing a body part from an abnormal physical constraint by cutting or by the use of force

Body Part	Approach	Device	Qualifier
Ø Brain 1 Cerebral Meninges 2 Dura Mater 6 Cerebral Ventricle 7 Cerebral Hemisphere 8 Basal Ganglia 9 Thalamus A Hypothalamus B Pons C Cerebellum D Medulla Oblongata F Olfactory Nerve G Optic Nerve H Oculomotor Nerve J Trochlear Nerve K Trigeminal Nerve L Abducens Nerve M Facial Nerve N Acoustic Nerve P Glossopharyngeal Nerve Q Vagus Nerve R Accessory Nerve S Hypoglossal Nerve T Spinal Meninges W Cervical Spinal Cord X Thoracic Spinal Cord Y Lumbar Spinal Cord	Ø Open 3 Percutaneous 4 Percutaneous Endoscopic	Z No Device	Z No Qualifier

Coding Clinic: 2017, Q2, P24; 2015, Q2, P22 – ØØNWØZZ
Coding Clinic: 2016, Q2, P29 – ØØNØØZZ
Coding Clinic: 2017, Q3, P1Ø – ØØNCØZZ
Coding Clinic: 2018, Q4, P1Ø – ØØNM4ZZ
Coding Clinic: 2019, Q1, P29 – ØØNYØZZ
Coding Clinic: 2019, Q2, P2Ø – ØØNW3ZZ

SECTION: Ø MEDICAL AND SURGICAL
BODY SYSTEM: Ø CENTRAL NERVOUS SYSTEM AND CRANIAL NERVES
OPERATION: P REMOVAL: Taking out or off a device from a body part

Body Part	Approach	Device	Qualifier
Ø Brain V Spinal Cord	Ø Open 3 Percutaneous 4 Percutaneous Endoscopic	Ø Drainage Device 2 Monitoring Device 3 Infusion Device 7 Autologous Tissue Substitute J Synthetic Substitute K Nonautologous Tissue Substitute M Neurostimulator Lead Y Other Device	Z No Qualifier
Ø Brain V Spinal Cord	X External	Ø Drainage Device 2 Monitoring Device 3 Infusion Device M Neurostimulator Lead	Z No Qualifier
6 Cerebral Ventricle U Spinal Canal	Ø Open 3 Percutaneous 4 Percutaneous Endoscopic	Ø Drainage Device 2 Monitoring Device 3 Infusion Device J Synthetic Substitute M Neurostimulator Lead Y Other Device	Z No Qualifier
6 Cerebral Ventricle U Spinal Canal	X External	Ø Drainage Device 2 Monitoring Device 3 Infusion Device M Neurostimulator Lead	Z No Qualifier
E Cranial Nerve	Ø Open 3 Percutaneous 4 Percutaneous Endoscopic	Ø Drainage Device 2 Monitoring Device 3 Infusion Device 7 Autologous Tissue Substitute M Neurostimulator Lead Y Other Device	Z No Qualifier
E Cranial Nerve	X External	Ø Drainage Device 2 Monitoring Device 3 Infusion Device M Neurostimulator Lead	Z No Qualifier

Non-OR ØØP[ØV]X[Ø23M]Z
Non-OR ØØP6X[Ø3]Z
Non-OR ØØPEX[Ø23]Z
Non-OR ØØPUX[Ø23M]Z
Non-OR ØØP[Ø6EUV][3X][Ø23M]Z

SECTION: 0 MEDICAL AND SURGICAL
BODY SYSTEM: 0 CENTRAL NERVOUS SYSTEM AND CRANIAL NERVES
OPERATION: Q REPAIR: Restoring, to the extent possible, a body part to its normal anatomic structure and function

Body Part	Approach	Device	Qualifier
0 Brain 1 Cerebral Meninges 2 Dura Mater 6 Cerebral Ventricle 7 Cerebral Hemisphere 8 Basal Ganglia 9 Thalamus A Hypothalamus B Pons C Cerebellum D Medulla Oblongata F Olfactory Nerve G Optic Nerve H Oculomotor Nerve J Trochlear Nerve K Trigeminal Nerve L Abducens Nerve M Facial Nerve N Acoustic Nerve P Glossopharyngeal Nerve Q Vagus Nerve R Accessory Nerve S Hypoglossal Nerve T Spinal Meninges W Cervical Spinal Cord X Thoracic Spinal Cord Y Lumbar Spinal Cord	0 Open 3 Percutaneous 4 Percutaneous Endoscopic	Z No Device	Z No Qualifier

Coding Clinic: 2013, Q3, P25 – 00Q20ZZ

SECTION: Ø MEDICAL AND SURGICAL
BODY SYSTEM: Ø CENTRAL NERVOUS SYSTEM AND CRANIAL NERVES
OPERATION: R REPLACEMENT: Putting in or on biological or synthetic material that physically takes the place and/or function of all or a portion of a body part

Body Part	Approach	Device	Qualifier
1 Cerebral Meninges 2 Dura Mater 6 Cerebral Ventricle F Olfactory Nerve G Optic Nerve H Oculomotor Nerve J Trochlear Nerve K Trigeminal Nerve L Abducens Nerve M Facial Nerve N Acoustic Nerve P Glossopharyngeal Nerve Q Vagus Nerve R Accessory Nerve S Hypoglossal Nerve T Spinal Meninges	Ø Open 4 Percutaneous Endoscopic	7 Autologous Tissue Substitute J Synthetic Substitute K Nonautologous Tissue Substitute	Z No Qualifier

SECTION: Ø MEDICAL AND SURGICAL
BODY SYSTEM: Ø CENTRAL NERVOUS SYSTEM AND CRANIAL NERVES
OPERATION: S REPOSITION: Moving to its normal location, or other suitable location, all or a portion of a body part

Body Part	Approach	Device	Qualifier
F Olfactory Nerve G Optic Nerve H Oculomotor Nerve J Trochlear Nerve K Trigeminal Nerve L Abducens Nerve M Facial Nerve N Acoustic Nerve P Glossopharyngeal Nerve Q Vagus Nerve R Accessory Nerve S Hypoglossal Nerve W Cervical Spinal Cord X Thoracic Spinal Cord Y Lumbar Spinal Cord	Ø Open 3 Percutaneous 4 Percutaneous Endoscopic	Z No Device	Z No Qualifier

SECTION: Ø MEDICAL AND SURGICAL
BODY SYSTEM: Ø CENTRAL NERVOUS SYSTEM AND CRANIAL NERVES
OPERATION: T RESECTION: Cutting out or off, without replacement, all of a body part

Body Part	Approach	Device	Qualifier
7 Cerebral Hemisphere	Ø Open 3 Percutaneous 4 Percutaneous Endoscopic	Z No Device	Z No Qualifier

SECTION: Ø MEDICAL AND SURGICAL
BODY SYSTEM: Ø CENTRAL NERVOUS SYSTEM AND CRANIAL NERVES
OPERATION: U SUPPLEMENT: Putting in or on biological or synthetic material that physically reinforces and/or augments the function of a portion of a body part

Body Part	Approach	Device	Qualifier
1 Cerebral Meninges 2 Dura Mater 6 Cerebral Ventricle F Olfactory Nerve G Optic Nerve H Oculomotor Nerve J Trochlear Nerve K Trigeminal Nerve L Abducens Nerve M Facial Nerve N Acoustic Nerve P Glossopharyngeal Nerve Q Vagus Nerve R Accessory Nerve S Hypoglossal Nerve T Spinal Meninges	Ø Open 3 Percutaneous 4 Percutaneous Endoscopic	7 Autologous Tissue Substitute J Synthetic Substitute K Nonautologous Tissue Substitute	Z No Qualifier

Coding Clinic: 2Ø18, Q1, P9; 2Ø17, Q3, P11 – ØØU2ØKZ
Coding Clinic: 2Ø21, Q3, P17 – ØØU2ØKZ

SECTION: Ø MEDICAL AND SURGICAL
BODY SYSTEM: Ø CENTRAL NERVOUS SYSTEM AND CRANIAL NERVES
OPERATION: W REVISION: Correcting, to the extent possible, a portion of a malfunctioning device or the position of a displaced device

Body Part	Approach	Device	Qualifier
Ø Brain V Spinal Cord	Ø Open 3 Percutaneous 4 Percutaneous Endoscopic	Ø Drainage Device 2 Monitoring Device 3 Infusion Device 7 Autologous Tissue Substitute J Synthetic Substitute K Nonautologous Tissue Substitute M Neurostimulator Lead Y Other Device	Z No Qualifier
Ø Brain V Spinal Cord	X External	Ø Drainage Device 2 Monitoring Device 3 Infusion Device 7 Autologous Tissue Substitute J Synthetic Substitute K Nonautologous Tissue Substitute M Neurostimulator Lead	Z No Qualifier
6 Cerebral Ventricle U Spinal Canal	Ø Open 3 Percutaneous 4 Percutaneous Endoscopic	Ø Drainage Device 2 Monitoring Device 3 Infusion Device J Synthetic Substitute M Neurostimulator Lead Y Other Device	Z No Qualifier
6 Cerebral Ventricle U Spinal Canal	X External	Ø Drainage Device 2 Monitoring Device 3 Infusion Device J Synthetic Substitute M Neurostimulator Lead	Z No Qualifier
E Cranial Nerve	Ø Open 3 Percutaneous 4 Percutaneous Endoscopic	Ø Drainage Device 2 Monitoring Device 3 Infusion Device 7 Autologous Tissue Substitute M Neurostimulator Lead Y Other Device	Z No Qualifier
E Cranial Nerve	X External	Ø Drainage Device 2 Monitoring Device 3 Infusion Device 7 Autologous Tissue Substitute M Neurostimulator Lead	Z No Qualifier

Non-OR ØØW[ØV]X[Ø237JKM]Z
Non-OR ØØW[6U]X[Ø23JM]Z
Non-OR ØØWEX[Ø237M]Z

SECTION: Ø MEDICAL AND SURGICAL
BODY SYSTEM: Ø CENTRAL NERVOUS SYSTEM AND CRANIAL NERVES
OPERATION: X TRANSFER: Moving, without taking out, all or a portion of a body part to another location to take over the function of all or a portion of a body part

Body Part	Approach	Device	Qualifier
F Olfactory Nerve G Optic Nerve H Oculomotor Nerve J Trochlear Nerve K Trigeminal Nerve L Abducens Nerve M Facial Nerve N Acoustic Nerve P Glossopharyngeal Nerve Q Vagus Nerve R Accessory Nerve S Hypoglossal Nerve	Ø Open 4 Percutaneous Endoscopic	Z No Device	F Olfactory Nerve G Optic Nerve H Oculomotor Nerve J Trochlear Nerve K Trigeminal Nerve L Abducens Nerve M Facial Nerve N Acoustic Nerve P Glossopharyngeal Nerve Q Vagus Nerve R Accessory Nerve S Hypoglossal Nerve

Ø1. Peripheral Nervous System 59
Ø12. Change 6Ø
Ø15. Destruction 6Ø
Ø18. Division 61
Ø19. Drainage 62
Ø1B. Excision 63
Ø1C. Extirpation 64
Ø1D. Extraction 65
Ø1H. Insertion 65
Ø1J. Inspection 65
Ø1N. Release 66
Ø1P. Removal 66
Ø1Q. Repair 67
Ø1R. Replacement 67
Ø1S. Reposition 68
Ø1U. Supplement 68
Ø1W. Revision 69
Ø1X. Transfer 69

SECTION: Ø MEDICAL AND SURGICAL
BODY SYSTEM: 1 PERIPHERAL NERVOUS SYSTEM
OPERATION: 2 CHANGE: Taking out or off a device from a body part and putting back an identical or similar device in or on the same body part without cutting or puncturing the skin or a mucous membrane

Body Part	Approach	Device	Qualifier
Y Peripheral Nerve	X External	Ø Drainage Device Y Other Device	Z No Qualifier

Non-OR Ø12YX[ØY]Z

SECTION: Ø MEDICAL AND SURGICAL
BODY SYSTEM: 1 PERIPHERAL NERVOUS SYSTEM
OPERATION: 5 DESTRUCTION: Physical eradication of all or a portion of a body part by the direct use of energy, force, or a destructive agent

Body Part	Approach	Device	Qualifier
Ø Cervical Plexus 1 Cervical Nerve 2 Phrenic Nerve 3 Brachial Plexus 4 Ulnar Nerve 5 Median Nerve 6 Radial Nerve 8 Thoracic Nerve 9 Lumbar Plexus A Lumbosacral Plexus B Lumbar Nerve C Pudendal Nerve D Femoral Nerve F Sciatic Nerve G Tibial Nerve H Peroneal Nerve K Head and Neck Sympathetic Nerve L Thoracic Sympathetic Nerve M Abdominal Sympathetic Nerve N Lumbar Sympathetic Nerve P Sacral Sympathetic Nerve Q Sacral Plexus R Sacral Nerve	Ø Open 3 Percutaneous 4 Percutaneous Endoscopic	Z No Device	Z No Qualifier

Non-OR Ø15[Ø234569ACDFGHQ][Ø34]ZZ
Non-OR Ø15[18BR]3ZZ

SECTION: Ø MEDICAL AND SURGICAL
BODY SYSTEM: 1 PERIPHERAL NERVOUS SYSTEM
OPERATION: 8 DIVISION: Cutting into a body part, without draining fluids and/or gases from the body part, in order to separate or transect a body part

Body Part	Approach	Device	Qualifier
Ø Cervical Plexus 1 Cervical Nerve 2 Phrenic Nerve 3 Brachial Plexus 4 Ulnar Nerve 5 Median Nerve 6 Radial Nerve 8 Thoracic Nerve 9 Lumbar Plexus A Lumbosacral Plexus B Lumbar Nerve C Pudendal Nerve D Femoral Nerve F Sciatic Nerve G Tibial Nerve H Peroneal Nerve K Head and Neck Sympathetic Nerve L Thoracic Sympathetic Nerve M Abdominal Sympathetic Nerve N Lumbar Sympathetic Nerve P Sacral Sympathetic Nerve Q Sacral Plexus R Sacral Nerve	Ø Open 3 Percutaneous 4 Percutaneous Endoscopic	Z No Device	Z No Qualifier

SECTION: Ø MEDICAL AND SURGICAL
BODY SYSTEM: 1 PERIPHERAL NERVOUS SYSTEM
OPERATION: 9 DRAINAGE: Taking or letting out fluids and/or gases from a body part

Body Part	Approach	Device	Qualifier
Ø Cervical Plexus 1 Cervical Nerve 2 Phrenic Nerve 3 Brachial Plexus 4 Ulnar Nerve 5 Median Nerve 6 Radial Nerve 8 Thoracic Nerve 9 Lumbar Plexus A Lumbosacral Plexus B Lumbar Nerve C Pudendal Nerve D Femoral Nerve F Sciatic Nerve G Tibial Nerve H Peroneal Nerve K Head and Neck Sympathetic Nerve L Thoracic Sympathetic Nerve M Abdominal Sympathetic Nerve N Lumbar Sympathetic Nerve P Sacral Sympathetic Nerve Q Sacral Plexus R Sacral Nerve	Ø Open 3 Percutaneous 4 Percutaneous Endoscopic	Ø Drainage Device	Z No Qualifier
Ø Cervical Plexus 1 Cervical Nerve 2 Phrenic Nerve 3 Brachial Plexus 4 Ulnar Nerve 5 Median Nerve 6 Radial Nerve 8 Thoracic Nerve 9 Lumbar Plexus A Lumbosacral Plexus B Lumbar Nerve C Pudendal Nerve D Femoral Nerve F Sciatic Nerve G Tibial Nerve H Peroneal Nerve K Head and Neck Sympathetic Nerve L Thoracic Sympathetic Nerve M Abdominal Sympathetic Nerve N Lumbar Sympathetic Nerve P Sacral Sympathetic Nerve Q Sacral Plexus R Sacral Nerve	Ø Open 3 Percutaneous 4 Percutaneous Endoscopic	Z No Device	X Diagnostic Z No Qualifier

Non-OR Ø19[Ø12345689ABCDFGHKLMNPQR]3ØZ
Non-OR Ø19[Ø12345689ABCDFGHKLMNPQR]3ZZ
Non-OR Ø19[Ø12345689ABCDFGHQR][34]ZX

SECTION: Ø MEDICAL AND SURGICAL
BODY SYSTEM: 1 PERIPHERAL NERVOUS SYSTEM
OPERATION: B EXCISION: Cutting out or off, without replacement, a portion of a body part

Body Part	Approach	Device	Qualifier
Ø Cervical Plexus 1 Cervical Nerve 2 Phrenic Nerve 3 Brachial Plexus ⊞ 4 Ulnar Nerve 5 Median Nerve 6 Radial Nerve 8 Thoracic Nerve 9 Lumbar Plexus A Lumbosacral Plexus B Lumbar Nerve C Pudendal Nerve D Femoral Nerve F Sciatic Nerve G Tibial Nerve H Peroneal Nerve K Head and Neck Sympathetic Nerve L Thoracic Sympathetic Nerve ⊞ M Abdominal Sympathetic Nerve N Lumbar Sympathetic Nerve P Sacral Sympathetic Nerve Q Sacral Plexus R Sacral Nerve	Ø Open 3 Percutaneous 4 Percutaneous Endoscopic	Z No Device	X Diagnostic Z No Qualifier

⊞ Ø1B[3L]ØZZ

Non-OR Ø1B[Ø12345689ABCDFGHQR][34]ZX

Coding Clinic: 2Ø17, Q2, P19 – Ø1BLØZZ

SECTION: Ø MEDICAL AND SURGICAL
BODY SYSTEM: 1 PERIPHERAL NERVOUS SYSTEM
OPERATION: C EXTIRPATION: Taking or cutting out solid matter from a body part

Body Part	Approach	Device	Qualifier
Ø Cervical Plexus 1 Cervical Nerve 2 Phrenic Nerve 3 Brachial Plexus 4 Ulnar Nerve 5 Median Nerve 6 Radial Nerve 8 Thoracic Nerve 9 Lumbar Plexus A Lumbosacral Plexus B Lumbar Nerve C Pudendal Nerve D Femoral Nerve F Sciatic Nerve G Tibial Nerve H Peroneal Nerve K Head and Neck Sympathetic Nerve L Thoracic Sympathetic Nerve M Abdominal Sympathetic Nerve N Lumbar Sympathetic Nerve P Sacral Sympathetic Nerve Q Sacral Plexus R Sacral Nerve	Ø Open 3 Percutaneous 4 Percutaneous Endoscopic	Z No Device	Z No Qualifier

SECTION: Ø MEDICAL AND SURGICAL
BODY SYSTEM: 1 PERIPHERAL NERVOUS SYSTEM
OPERATION: D EXTRACTION: Pulling or stripping out or off all or a portion of a body part by the use of force

Body Part	Approach	Device	Qualifier
Ø Cervical Plexus 1 Cervical Nerve 2 Phrenic Nerve 3 Brachial Plexus 4 Ulnar Nerve 5 Median Nerve 6 Radial Nerve 8 Thoracic Nerve 9 Lumbar Plexus A Lumbosacral Plexus B Lumbar Nerve C Pudendal Nerve D Femoral Nerve F Sciatic Nerve G Tibial Nerve H Peroneal Nerve K Head and Neck Sympathetic Nerve L Thoracic Sympathetic Nerve M Abdominal Sympathetic Nerve N Lumbar Sympathetic Nerve P Sacral Sympathetic Nerve Q Sacral Plexus R Sacral Nerve	Ø Open 3 Percutaneous 4 Percutaneous Endoscopic	Z No Device	Z No Qualifier

SECTION: Ø MEDICAL AND SURGICAL
BODY SYSTEM: 1 PERIPHERAL NERVOUS SYSTEM
OPERATION: H INSERTION: Putting in a nonbiological appliance that monitors, assists, performs, or prevents a physiological function but does not physically take the place of a body part

Body Part	Approach	Device	Qualifier
Y Peripheral Nerve ⊞	Ø Open 3 Percutaneous 4 Percutaneous Endoscopic	1 Radioactive Element 2 Monitoring Device M Neurostimulator Lead Y Other Device	Z No Qualifier

⊞ Ø1HY[Ø34][1M]Z

SECTION: Ø MEDICAL AND SURGICAL
BODY SYSTEM: 1 PERIPHERAL NERVOUS SYSTEM
OPERATION: J INSPECTION: Visually and/or manually exploring a body part

Body Part	Approach	Device	Qualifier
Y Peripheral Nerve	Ø Open 3 Percutaneous 4 Percutaneous Endoscopic	Z No Device	Z No Qualifier

Non-OR Ø1JY3ZZ

SECTION: Ø MEDICAL AND SURGICAL
BODY SYSTEM: 1 PERIPHERAL NERVOUS SYSTEM
OPERATION: N RELEASE: Freeing a body part from an abnormal physical constraint by cutting or by the use of force

Body Part	Approach	Device	Qualifier
Ø Cervical Plexus 1 Cervical Nerve 2 Phrenic Nerve 3 Brachial Plexus 4 Ulnar Nerve 5 Median Nerve 6 Radial Nerve 8 Thoracic Nerve 9 Lumbar Plexus A Lumbosacral Plexus B Lumbar Nerve C Pudendal Nerve D Femoral Nerve F Sciatic Nerve G Tibial Nerve H Peroneal Nerve K Head and Neck Sympathetic Nerve L Thoracic Sympathetic Nerve M Abdominal Sympathetic Nerve N Lumbar Sympathetic Nerve P Sacral Sympathetic Nerve Q Sacral Plexus R Sacral Nerve	Ø Open 3 Percutaneous 4 Percutaneous Endoscopic	Z No Device	Z No Qualifier

Coding Clinic: 2Ø16, Q2, P16; 2Ø15, Q2, P34 – Ø1NBØZZ
Coding Clinic: 2Ø16, Q2, P17 – Ø1N1ØZZ
Coding Clinic: 2Ø16, Q2, P23 – Ø1N3ØZZ
Coding Clinic: 2Ø19, Q1, P29; 2Ø18, Q2, P23 – Ø1NBØZZ
Coding Clinic: 2Ø19, Q1, P29 – Ø1NRØZZ

SECTION: Ø MEDICAL AND SURGICAL
BODY SYSTEM: 1 PERIPHERAL NERVOUS SYSTEM
OPERATION: P REMOVAL: Taking out or off a device from a body part

Body Part	Approach	Device	Qualifier
Y Peripheral Nerve	Ø Open 3 Percutaneous 4 Percutaneous Endoscopic	Ø Drainage Device 2 Monitoring Device 7 Autologous Tissue Substitute M Neurostimulator Lead Y Other Device	Z No Qualifier
Y Peripheral Nerve	X External	Ø Drainage Device 2 Monitoring Device M Neurostimulator Lead	Z No Qualifier

Non-OR Ø1PY[3X][Ø2M]Z

SECTION: Ø MEDICAL AND SURGICAL
BODY SYSTEM: 1 PERIPHERAL NERVOUS SYSTEM
OPERATION: Q REPAIR: Restoring, to the extent possible, a body part to its normal anatomic structure and function

Body Part	Approach	Device	Qualifier
Ø Cervical Plexus 1 Cervical Nerve 2 Phrenic Nerve 3 Brachial Plexus 4 Ulnar Nerve 5 Median Nerve 6 Radial Nerve 8 Thoracic Nerve 9 Lumbar Plexus A Lumbosacral Plexus B Lumbar Nerve C Pudendal Nerve D Femoral Nerve F Sciatic Nerve G Tibial Nerve H Peroneal Nerve K Head and Neck Sympathetic Nerve L Thoracic Sympathetic Nerve M Abdominal Sympathetic Nerve N Lumbar Sympathetic Nerve P Sacral Sympathetic Nerve Q Sacral Plexus R Sacral Nerve	Ø Open 3 Percutaneous 4 Percutaneous Endoscopic	Z No Device	Z No Qualifier

SECTION: Ø MEDICAL AND SURGICAL
BODY SYSTEM: 1 PERIPHERAL NERVOUS SYSTEM
OPERATION: R REPLACEMENT: Putting in or on biological or synthetic material that physically takes the place and/or function of all or a portion of a body part

Body Part	Approach	Device	Qualifier
1 Cervical Nerve 2 Phrenic Nerve 4 Ulnar Nerve 5 Median Nerve 6 Radial Nerve 8 Thoracic Nerve B Lumbar Nerve C Pudendal Nerve D Femoral Nerve F Sciatic Nerve G Tibial Nerve H Peroneal Nerve R Sacral Nerve	Ø Open 4 Percutaneous Endoscopic	7 Autologous Tissue Substitute J Synthetic Substitute K Nonautologous Tissue Substitute	Z No Qualifier

SECTION: Ø MEDICAL AND SURGICAL
BODY SYSTEM: 1 PERIPHERAL NERVOUS SYSTEM
OPERATION: S REPOSITION: Moving to its normal location, or other suitable location, all or a portion of a body part

Body Part	Approach	Device	Qualifier
Ø Cervical Plexus 1 Cervical Nerve 2 Phrenic Nerve 3 Brachial Plexus 4 Ulnar Nerve 5 Median Nerve 6 Radial Nerve 8 Thoracic Nerve 9 Lumbar Plexus A Lumbosacral Plexus B Lumbar Nerve C Pudendal Nerve D Femoral Nerve F Sciatic Nerve G Tibial Nerve H Peroneal Nerve Q Sacral Plexus R Sacral Nerve	Ø Open 3 Percutaneous 4 Percutaneous Endoscopic	Z No Device	Z No Qualifier

Coding Clinic: 2Ø21, Q3, P2Ø – Ø1S[3456]ØZZ

SECTION: Ø MEDICAL AND SURGICAL
BODY SYSTEM: 1 PERIPHERAL NERVOUS SYSTEM
OPERATION: U SUPPLEMENT: Putting in or on biological or synthetic material that physically reinforces and/or augments the function of a portion of a body part

Body Part	Approach	Device	Qualifier
1 Cervical Nerve 2 Phrenic Nerve 4 Ulnar Nerve 5 Median Nerve 6 Radial Nerve 8 Thoracic Nerve B Lumbar Nerve C Pudendal Nerve D Femoral Nerve F Sciatic Nerve G Tibial Nerve H Peroneal Nerve R Sacral Nerve	Ø Open 3 Percutaneous 4 Percutaneous Endoscopic	7 Autologous Tissue Substitute J Synthetic Substitute K Nonautologous Tissue Substitute	Z No Qualifier

Coding Clinic: 2Ø17, Q4, P62 – Ø1U5ØKZ
Coding Clinic: 2Ø19, Q3, P33 – Ø1U8ØKZ

SECTION: Ø MEDICAL AND SURGICAL
BODY SYSTEM: 1 PERIPHERAL NERVOUS SYSTEM
OPERATION: W REVISION: Correcting, to the extent possible, a portion of a malfunctioning device or the position of a displaced device

Body Part	Approach	Device	Qualifier
Y Peripheral Nerve	Ø Open 3 Percutaneous 4 Percutaneous Endoscopic	Ø Drainage Device 2 Monitoring Device 7 Autologous Tissue Substitute M Neurostimulator Lead Y Other Device	Z No Qualifier
Y Peripheral Nerve	X External	Ø Drainage Device 2 Monitoring Device 7 Autologous Tissue Substitute M Neurostimulator Lead	Z No Qualifier

Non-OR Ø1WY[ØX][Ø27M]Z

SECTION: Ø MEDICAL AND SURGICAL
BODY SYSTEM: 1 PERIPHERAL NERVOUS SYSTEM
OPERATION: X TRANSFER: Moving, without taking out, all or a portion of a body part to another location to take over the function of all or a portion of a body part

Body Part	Approach	Device	Qualifier
1 Cervical Nerve 2 Phrenic Nerve	Ø Open 4 Percutaneous Endoscopic	Z No Device	1 Cervical Nerve 2 Phrenic Nerve
4 Ulnar Nerve 5 Median Nerve 6 Radial Nerve	Ø Open 4 Percutaneous Endoscopic	Z No Device	4 Ulnar Nerve 5 Median Nerve 6 Radial Nerve
8 Thoracic Nerve	Ø Open 4 Percutaneous Endoscopic	Z No Device	8 Thoracic Nerve
B Lumbar Nerve C Pudendal Nerve	Ø Open 4 Percutaneous Endoscopic	Z No Device	B Lumbar Nerve C Pudendal Nerve
D Femoral Nerve F Sciatic Nerve G Tibial Nerve H Peroneal Nerve	Ø Open 4 Percutaneous Endoscopic	Z No Device	D Femoral Nerve F Sciatic Nerve G Tibial Nerve H Peroneal Nerve

Ø2. Heart and Great Vessels 70
Ø21. Bypass 71
Ø24. Creation 73
Ø25. Destruction 74
Ø27. Dilation 75
Ø28. Division 76
Ø2B. Excision 76
Ø2C. Extirpation 77
Ø2F. Fragmentation 77
Ø2H. Insertion 78
Ø2J. Inspection 79
Ø2K. Map 79
Ø2L. Occlusion 8Ø
Ø2N. Release 8Ø
Ø2P. Removal 81
Ø2Q. Repair 82
Ø2R. Replacement 83
Ø2S. Reposition 84
Ø2T. Resection 84
Ø2U. Supplement 85
Ø2V. Restriction 86
Ø2W. Revision 87
Ø2Y. Transplantation 88

SECTION: Ø MEDICAL AND SURGICAL
BODY SYSTEM: 2 HEART AND GREAT VESSELS
OPERATION: 1 BYPASS: *(on multiple pages)*
Altering the route of passage of the contents of a tubular body part

Body Part	Approach	Device	Qualifier
Ø Coronary Artery, One Artery 1 Coronary Artery, Two Arteries 2 Coronary Artery, Three Arteries 3 Coronary Artery, Four or More Arteries	Ø Open	8 Zooplastic Tissue 9 Autologous Venous Tissue A Autologous Arterial Tissue J Synthetic Substitute K Nonautologous Tissue Substitute	3 Coronary Artery 8 Internal Mammary, Right 9 Internal Mammary, Left C Thoracic Artery F Abdominal Artery W Aorta
Ø Coronary Artery, One Artery 1 Coronary Artery, Two Arteries 2 Coronary Artery, Three Arteries 3 Coronary Artery, Four or More Arteries	Ø Open	Z No Device	3 Coronary Artery 8 Internal Mammary, Right 9 Internal Mammary, Left C Thoracic Artery F Abdominal Artery
Ø Coronary Artery, One Artery 1 Coronary Artery, Two Arteries 2 Coronary Artery, Three Arteries 3 Coronary Artery, Four or More Arteries	3 Percutaneous	4 Drug-eluting Intraluminal Device D Intraluminal Device	4 Coronary Vein
Ø Coronary Artery, One Artery 1 Coronary Artery, Two Arteries 2 Coronary Artery, Three Arteries 3 Coronary Artery, Four or More Arteries	4 Percutaneous Endoscopic	4 Drug-eluting Intraluminal Device D Intraluminal Device	4 Coronary Vein
Ø Coronary Artery, One Artery 1 Coronary Artery, Two Arteries 2 Coronary Artery, Three Arteries 3 Coronary Artery, Four or More Arteries	4 Percutaneous Endoscopic	8 Zooplastic Tissue 9 Autologous Venous Tissue A Autologous Arterial Tissue J Synthetic Substitute K Nonautologous Tissue Substitute	3 Coronary Artery 8 Internal Mammary, Right 9 Internal Mammary, Left C Thoracic Artery F Abdominal Artery W Aorta
Ø Coronary Artery, One Artery 1 Coronary Artery, Two Arteries 2 Coronary Artery, Three Arteries 3 Coronary Artery, Four or More Arteries	4 Percutaneous Endoscopic	Z No Device	3 Coronary Artery 8 Internal Mammary, Right 9 Internal Mammary, Left C Thoracic Artery F Abdominal Artery
6 Atrium, Right	Ø Open 4 Percutaneous Endoscopic	8 Zooplastic Tissue 9 Autologous Venous Tissue A Autologous Arterial Tissue J Synthetic Substitute K Nonautologous Tissue Substitute	P Pulmonary Trunk Q Pulmonary Artery, Right R Pulmonary Artery, Left
6 Atrium, Right	Ø Open 4 Percutaneous Endoscopic	Z No Device	7 Atrium, Left P Pulmonary Trunk Q Pulmonary Artery, Right R Pulmonary Artery, Left
6 Atrium, Right	3 Percutaneous	Z No Device	7 Atrium, Left

Non-OR Ø21[Ø123]4[4D]4
Non-OR Ø21[Ø123]3[4D]4
Ø21[Ø123]Ø[89AJK][389CFW] when reported with Secondary Diagnosis J98.5
Ø21[Ø123]ØZ[389CF] when reported with Secondary Diagnosis J98.5
Ø21[Ø123]4[89AJK][389CFW] when reported with Secondary Diagnosis J98.5
Ø21[Ø123]4Z[389CF] when reported with Secondary Diagnosis J98.5

Coding Clinic: 2015, Q4, P23 P25, Q3, P17 – Ø21KØKP
Coding Clinic: 2016, Q1, P28 – Ø21ØØZ9, Ø212Ø9W
Coding Clinic: 2016, Q4, P81-82, 1Ø2, 1Ø8-1Ø9 – Ø21
Coding Clinic: 2016, Q4, P83 – Ø21ØØAW, Ø211Ø9W
Coding Clinic: 2016, Q4, P84 – Ø21ØØZ9
Coding Clinic: 2016, Q4, P1Ø8 – Ø217ØZU
Coding Clinic: 2016, Q4, P1Ø2 – Ø21WØJQ
Coding Clinic: 2016, Q4, P1Ø3 – Ø21QØJA
Coding Clinic: 2016, Q4, P1Ø7 – Ø21KØKP
Coding Clinic: 2016, Q4, P144 – Ø21VØ9S
Coding Clinic: 2016, Q4, P145 – Ø21VØ8S
Coding Clinic: 2017, Q1, P19 – Ø21KØJP
Coding Clinic: 2017, Q4, P56 – Ø2163Z7
Coding Clinic: 2021, Q3, P22 – Ø21ØØA3

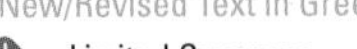
New/Revised Text in Green ~~deleted~~ Deleted ♀ Females Only ♂ Males Only **Coding Clinic**
Non-covered Limited Coverage Combination (See Appendix E) DRG Non-OR Non-OR Hospital-Acquired Condition

SECTION: Ø MEDICAL AND SURGICAL
BODY SYSTEM: 2 HEART AND GREAT VESSELS
OPERATION: 1 BYPASS: *(continued)*
Altering the route of passage of the contents of a tubular body part

Body Part	Approach	Device	Qualifier
7 Atrium, Left ⊞ V Superior Vena Cava	Ø Open 4 Percutaneous Endoscopic	8 Zooplastic Tissue 9 Autologous Venous Tissue A Autologous Arterial Tissue J Synthetic Substitute K Nonautologous Tissue Substitute Z No Device	P Pulmonary Trunk Q Pulmonary Artery, Right R Pulmonary Artery, Left S Pulmonary Vein, Right T Pulmonary Vein, Left U Pulmonary Vein, Confluence
7 Atrium, Left	3 Percutaneous	J Synthetic Substitute	6 Atrium, Right
K Ventricle, Right L Ventricle, Left	Ø Open 4 Percutaneous Endoscopic	8 Zooplastic Tissue 9 Autologous Venous Tissue A Autologous Arterial Tissue J Synthetic Substitute K Nonautologous Tissue Substitute	P Pulmonary Trunk Q Pulmonary Artery, Right R Pulmonary Artery, Left
K Ventricle, Right L Ventricle, Left	Ø Open 4 Percutaneous Endoscopic	Z No Device	5 Coronary Circulation 8 Internal Mammary, Right 9 Internal Mammary, Left C Thoracic Artery F Abdominal Artery P Pulmonary Trunk Q Pulmonary Artery, Right R Pulmonary Artery, Left W Aorta
P Pulmonary Trunk Q Pulmonary Artery, Right R Pulmonary Artery, Left	Ø Open 4 Percutaneous Endoscopic	8 Zooplastic Tissue 9 Autologous Venous Tissue A Autologous Arterial Tissue J Synthetic Substitute K Nonautologous Tissue Substitute Z No Device	A Innominate Artery B Subclavian D Carotid
V Superior Vena Cava	Ø Open 4 Percutaneous Endoscopic	8 Zooplastic Tissue 9 Autologous Venous Tissue A Autologous Arterial Tissue J Synthetic Substitute K Nonautologous Tissue Substitute Z No Device	P Pulmonary Trunk Q Pulmonary Artery, Right R Pulmonary Artery, Left S Pulmonary Vein, Right T Pulmonary Vein, Left U Pulmonary Vein, Confluence
W Thoracic Aorta, Descending	Ø Open	8 Zooplastic Tissue 9 Autologous Venous Tissue A Autologous Arterial Tissue J Synthetic Substitute K Nonautologous Tissue Substitute	A Innominate Artery B Subclavian D Carotid F Abdominal Artery G Axillary Artery H Brachial Artery P Pulmonary Trunk Q Pulmonary Artery, Right R Pulmonary Artery, Left V Lower Extremity Artery
W Thoracic Aorta, Descending	Ø Open	Z No Device	A Innominate Artery B Subclavian D Carotid P Pulmonary Trunk Q Pulmonary Artery, Right R Pulmonary Artery, Left

Ø217ØZ[PQR]

Coding Clinic: 2Ø18, Q4, P46 – Ø21WØJV
Coding Clinic: 2Ø19, Q3, P31 – Ø21XØJ[B,D]
Coding Clinic: 2Ø19, Q4, P23 – Ø21XØJA
Coding Clinic: 2Ø2Ø, Q1, P25 – Ø21KØJP

SECTION: Ø MEDICAL AND SURGICAL
BODY SYSTEM: 2 HEART AND GREAT VESSELS
OPERATION: 1 BYPASS: *(continued)*
Altering the route of passage of the contents of a tubular body part

Body Part	Approach	Device	Qualifier
W Thoracic Aorta, Descending	4 Percutaneous Endoscopic	8 Zooplastic Tissue 9 Autologous Venous Tissue A Autologous Arterial Tissue J Synthetic Substitute K Nonautologous Tissue Substitute Z No Device	A Innominate Artery B Subclavian D Carotid P Pulmonary Trunk Q Pulmonary Artery, Right R Pulmonary Artery, Left
X Thoracic Aorta, Ascending/Arch	Ø Open 4 Percutaneous Endoscopic	8 Zooplastic Tissue 9 Autologous Venous Tissue A Autologous Arterial Tissue J Synthetic Substitute K Nonautologous Tissue Substitute Z No Device	A Innominate Artery B Subclavian D Carotid P Pulmonary Trunk Q Pulmonary Artery, Right R Pulmonary Artery, Left

SECTION: Ø MEDICAL AND SURGICAL
BODY SYSTEM: 2 HEART AND GREAT VESSELS
OPERATION: 4 CREATION: Putting in or on biological or synthetic material to form a new body part that to the extent possible replicates the anatomic structure or function of an absent body part

Body Part	Approach	Device	Qualifier
F Aortic Valve	Ø Open	7 Autologous Tissue Substitute 8 Zooplastic Tissue J Synthetic Substitute K Nonautologous Tissue Substitute	J Truncal Valve
G Mitral Valve J Tricuspid Valve	Ø Open	7 Autologous Tissue Substitute 8 Zooplastic Tissue J Synthetic Substitute K Nonautologous Tissue Substitute	2 Common Atrioventricular Valve

Coding Clinic: 2Ø16, Q4, P1Ø1-1Ø2, 1Ø6 – Ø24
Coding Clinic: 2Ø16, Q4, P1Ø5 – ØØ2[GJ]Ø[JK]2
Coding Clinic: 2Ø16, Q4, P1Ø7 – Ø24FØ[8J]J

Ø: M/S 2: HEART AND GREAT VESSELS 1: BYPASS 4: CREATION

SECTION: Ø MEDICAL AND SURGICAL
BODY SYSTEM: 2 HEART AND GREAT VESSELS
OPERATION: 5 DESTRUCTION: Physical eradication of all or a portion of a body part by the direct use of energy, force, or a destructive agent

Body Part	Approach	Device	Qualifier
4 Coronary Vein 5 Atrial Septum 6 Atrium, Right ~~7 Atrium, Left~~ ~~8 Conduction Mechanism~~ 9 Chordae Tendineae D Papillary Muscle F Aortic Valve G Mitral Valve H Pulmonary Valve J Tricuspid Valve K Ventricle, Right L Ventricle, Left M Ventricular Septum N Pericardium P Pulmonary Trunk Q Pulmonary Artery, Right R Pulmonary Artery, Left S Pulmonary Vein, Right T Pulmonary Vein, Left V Superior Vena Cava W Thoracic Aorta, Descending X Thoracic Aorta, Ascending/Arch	Ø Open 3 Percutaneous 4 Percutaneous Endoscopic	Z No Device	Z No Qualifier
7 Atrium, Left	Ø Open 3 Percutaneous 4 Percutaneous Endoscopic	Z No Device	K Left Atrial Appendage Z No Qualifier
8 Conduction Mechanism	Ø Open 4 Percutaneous Endoscopic	Z No Device	Z No Qualifier
8 Conduction Mechanism	3 Percutaneous	Z No Device	F Irreversible Electroporation Z No Qualifier

DRG Non-OR Ø257[Ø34]ZK

Coding Clinic: 2Ø13, Q2, P39 – Ø25S3ZZ, Ø25T3ZZ
Coding Clinic: 2Ø16, Q2, P18 – Ø25NØZZ
Coding Clinic: 2Ø2Ø, Q1, P33; 2Ø16, Q3, P43 – Ø2583ZZ
Coding Clinic: 2Ø16, Q3, P44 – Ø258ØZZ
Coding Clinic: 2Ø16, Q3, P44 – Ø257ØZK
Coding Clinic: 2Ø16, Q4, P81 – Ø25
Coding Clinic: 2Ø2Ø, Q1, P32 – Ø2584ZZ

SECTION: Ø MEDICAL AND SURGICAL
BODY SYSTEM: 2 HEART AND GREAT VESSELS
OPERATION: 7 DILATION: Expanding an orifice or the lumen of a tubular body part

Body Part	Approach	Device	Qualifier
Ø Coronary Artery, One Artery 1 Coronary Artery, Two Arteries 2 Coronary Artery, Three Arteries 3 Coronary Artery, Four or More Arteries	Ø Open 3 Percutaneous 4 Percutaneous Endoscopic	4 Drug-eluting Intraluminal Device 5 Intraluminal Device, Drug-eluting, Two 6 Intraluminal Device, Drug-eluting, Three 7 Intraluminal Device, Drug-eluting, Four or More D Intraluminal Device E Intraluminal Device, Two F Intraluminal Device, Three G Intraluminal Device, Four or More T Radioactive Intraluminal Device Z No Device	6 Bifurcation Z No Qualifier
F Aortic Valve G Mitral Valve H Pulmonary Valve J Tricuspid Valve K Ventricle, Right L Ventricle, Left P Pulmonary Trunk Q Pulmonary Artery, Right S Pulmonary Vein, Right T Pulmonary Vein, Left V Superior Vena Cava W Thoracic Aorta, Descending X Thoracic Aorta, Ascending/Arch	Ø Open 3 Percutaneous 4 Percutaneous Endoscopic	4 Drug-eluting Intraluminal Device D Intraluminal Device Z No Device	Z No Qualifier
R Pulmonary Artery, Left	Ø Open 3 Percutaneous 4 Percutaneous Endoscopic	4 Drug-eluting Intraluminal Device D Intraluminal Device Z No Device	T Ductus Arteriosus Z No Qualifier

Coding Clinic: 2Ø15, Q2, P3-5 – Ø27234Z, Ø27Ø3[4D]Z, Ø27Ø346, Ø27134Z
Coding Clinic: 2Ø15, Q3, P1Ø, P17 – Ø27Ø3ZZ, Ø27QØDZ
Coding Clinic: 2Ø19, Q4, P4Ø; 2Ø15, Q4, P14 – Ø27Ø34Z
Coding Clinic: 2Ø16, Q1, P17 – Ø27HØZZ
Coding Clinic: 2Ø16, Q4, P81-82 – Ø27
Coding Clinic: 2Ø16, Q4, P85 – Ø27Ø3EZ, Ø27136Z
Coding Clinic: 2Ø16, Q4, P86 – Ø27Ø37Z
Coding Clinic: 2Ø16, Q4, P87 – Ø271356
Coding Clinic: 2Ø16, Q4, P88 – Ø27Ø346, Ø27Ø3ZZ
Coding Clinic: 2Ø17, Q4, P33 – Ø27LØZZ

SECTION: Ø MEDICAL AND SURGICAL
BODY SYSTEM: 2 HEART AND GREAT VESSELS
OPERATION: 8 DIVISION: Cutting into a body part, without draining fluids and/or gases from the body part, in order to separate or transect a body part

Body Part	Approach	Device	Qualifier
8 Conduction Mechanism 9 Chordae Tendineae D Papillary Muscle	Ø Open 3 Percutaneous 4 Percutaneous Endoscopic	Z No Device	Z No Qualifier

SECTION: Ø MEDICAL AND SURGICAL
BODY SYSTEM: 2 HEART AND GREAT VESSELS
OPERATION: B EXCISION: Cutting out or off, without replacement, a portion of a body part

Body Part	Approach	Device	Qualifier
4 Coronary Vein 5 Atrial Septum 6 Atrium, Right 8 Conduction Mechanism 9 Chordae Tendineae D Papillary Muscle F Aortic Valve G Mitral Valve H Pulmonary Valve J Tricuspid Valve K Ventricle, Right L Ventricle, Left M Ventricular Septum N Pericardium P Pulmonary Trunk Q Pulmonary Artery, Right R Pulmonary Artery, Left S Pulmonary Vein, Right T Pulmonary Vein, Left V Superior Vena Cava W Thoracic Aorta, Descending X Thoracic Aorta, Ascending/Arch	Ø Open 3 Percutaneous 4 Percutaneous Endoscopic	Z No Device	X Diagnostic Z No Qualifier
7 Atrium, Left	Ø Open 3 Percutaneous 4 Percutaneous Endoscopic	Z No Device	K Left Atrial Appendage X Diagnostic Z No Qualifier

Ø2B[KL][Ø34]ZZ
Ø2BKØZZ
DRG Non-OR Ø2B7[Ø34]ZK
Non-OR Ø2B[45689DFGHJKLM][Ø34]ZX
Non-OR Ø2B7[Ø34]ZX

Coding Clinic: 2Ø15, Q2, P24 – Ø2BGØZZ
Coding Clinic: 2Ø16, Q4, P81 – Ø2B
Coding Clinic: 2Ø19, Q2, P21 – Ø2BNØZZ
Coding Clinic: 2Ø19, Q3, P32 – Ø2BK3ZX

SECTION: Ø MEDICAL AND SURGICAL
BODY SYSTEM: 2 HEART AND GREAT VESSELS
OPERATION: C EXTIRPATION: Taking or cutting out solid matter from a body part

Body Part	Approach	Device	Qualifier
Ø Coronary Artery, One Artery 1 Coronary Artery, Two Arteries 2 Coronary Artery, Three Arteries 3 Coronary Artery, Four or More Arteries	Ø Open 4 Percutaneous Endoscopic	Z No Device	6 Bifurcation Z No Qualifier
Ø Coronary Artery, One Artery 1 Coronary Artery, Two Arteries 2 Coronary Artery, Three Arteries 3 Coronary Artery, Four or More Arteries	3 Percutaneous	Z No Device	6 Bifurcation 7 Orbital Atherectomy Technique Z No Qualifier
4 Coronary Vein 5 Atrial Septum 6 Atrium, Right 7 Atrium, Left 8 Conduction Mechanism 9 Chordae Tendineae D Papillary Muscle F Aortic Valve G Mitral Valve H Pulmonary Valve J Tricuspid Valve K Ventricle, Right L Ventricle, Left M Ventricular Septum N Pericardium P Pulmonary Trunk Q Pulmonary Artery, Right R Pulmonary Artery, Left S Pulmonary Vein, Right T Pulmonary Vein, Left V Superior Vena Cava W Thoracic Aorta, Descending X Thoracic Aorta, Ascending/Arch	Ø Open 3 Percutaneous 4 Percutaneous Endoscopic	Z No Device	Z No Qualifier

Coding Clinic: 2Ø16, Q2, P25 – Ø2CGØZZ **Coding Clinic: 2Ø16, Q4, P81-82, 87 – Ø2C**

SECTION: Ø MEDICAL AND SURGICAL
BODY SYSTEM: 2 HEART AND GREAT VESSELS
OPERATION: F FRAGMENTATION: Breaking solid matter in a body part into pieces

Body Part	Approach	Device	Qualifier
Ø Coronary Artery, One Artery 1 Coronary Artery, Two Arteries 2 Coronary Artery, Three Arteries 3 Coronary Artery, Four or More Arteries	3 Percutaneous	Z No Device	Z No Qualifier
N Pericardium	Ø Open 3 Percutaneous 4 Percutaneous Endoscopic X External	Z No Device	Z No Qualifier
P Pulmonary Trunk Q Pulmonary Artery, Right R Pulmonary Artery, Left S Pulmonary Vein, Right T Pulmonary Vein, Left	3 Percutaneous	Z No Device	Ø Ultrasonic Z No Qualifier

Ø2FNXZZ

Non-OR Ø2FNXZZ

SECTION: Ø MEDICAL AND SURGICAL
BODY SYSTEM: 2 HEART AND GREAT VESSELS
OPERATION: H INSERTION: *(on multiple pages)*

Putting in a nonbiological appliance that monitors, assists, performs, or prevents a physiological function but does not physically take the place of a body part

Body Part	Approach	Device	Qualifier
Ø Coronary Artery, One Artery 1 Coronary Artery, Two Arteries 2 Coronary Artery, Three Arteries 3 Coronary Artery, Four or More Arteries	Ø Open 3 Percutaneous 4 Percutaneous Endoscopic	D Intraluminal Device Y Other Device	Z No Qualifier
4 Coronary Vein 6 Atrium, Right 7 Atrium, Left K Ventricle, Right L Ventricle, Left	Ø Open 3 Percutaneous 4 Percutaneous Endoscopic	Ø Monitoring Device, Pressure Sensor 2 Monitoring Device 3 Infusion Device D Intraluminal Device J Cardiac Lead, Pacemaker K Cardiac Lead, Defibrillator M Cardiac Lead N Intracardiac Pacemaker Y Other Device	Z No Qualifier
A Heart	Ø Open 3 Percutaneous 4 Percutaneous Endoscopic	Q Implantable Heart Assist System Y Other Device	Z No Qualifier
A Heart	Ø Open 3 Percutaneous 4 Percutaneous Endoscopic	R Short-term External Heart Assist System	J Intraoperative S Biventricular Z No Qualifier
N Pericardium	Ø Open 3 Percutaneous 4 Percutaneous Endoscopic	Ø Monitoring Device, Pressure Sensor 2 Monitoring Device J Cardiac Lead, Pacemaker K Cardiac Lead, Defibrillator M Cardiac Lead Y Other Device	Z No Qualifier

Ø2HA[34]QZ
Ø2H4[Ø4]KZ
Ø2H43[K]Z
Ø2H[67][Ø34]KZ
Ø2HK[Ø34][Ø2K]Z
Ø2HL[Ø34][KM]Z
Ø2HA[Ø4]R[SZ]
Ø2HA3RS
Ø2HN[Ø34][K]Z
DRG Non-OR Ø2H[467][Ø34][JM]Z
DRG Non-OR Ø2H[67]3JZ
DRG Non-OR Ø2H[KLN][Ø34][JM]Z
DRG Non-OR Ø2HK3[2JM]Z
DRG Non-OR Ø2H[467KL]3DZ
DRG Non-OR Ø2H[PQRSTVW]3DZ
Non-OR Ø2H[467KL]3[23M]Z
Non-OR Ø2HK33Z
Ø2H43[JKM]Z when reported with Secondary Diagnosis K68.11, T81.4XXA, T82.6XXA, or T82.7XXA
Ø2H[6K]33Z when reported with Secondary Diagnosis J95.811
Ø2H[67]3[JM]Z when reported with Secondary Diagnosis K68.11, T81.4XXA, T82.6XXA, or T82.7XXA
Ø2H[KL]3JZ when reported with Secondary Diagnosis K68.11, T81.4XXA, T82.6XXA, or T82.7XXA
Ø2HN[Ø34][JM]Z when reported with Secondary Diagnosis K68.11, T81.4XXA, T82.6XXA, or T82.7XXA

Coding Clinic: 2Ø13, Q3, P18 – Ø2HV33Z
Coding Clinic: 2Ø15, Q2, P32-33 – Ø2HK3DZ, Ø2HV33Z
Coding Clinic: 2Ø15, Q3, P35 – Ø2HP32Z
Coding Clinic: 2Ø17, Q4, P63; 2Ø15, Q4, P14, P28-32 – Ø2HV33Z
Coding Clinic: 2Ø16, Q2, P15 – Ø2H633Z
Coding Clinic: 2Ø17, Q1, P1Ø; 2Ø16, Q4, P81, 95, 137 – Ø2H
Coding Clinic: 2Ø17, Q1, P11-12; 2Ø16, Q4, P139 – Ø2HA3RS
Coding Clinic: 2Ø17, Q2, P25 – Ø2H633Z
Coding Clinic: 2Ø17, Q4, P44-45 – Ø2HA3E[JZ]
Coding Clinic: 2Ø17, Q4, P1Ø5 – Ø2H73DZ
Coding Clinic: 2Ø18, Q2, P19 – Ø2H63KZ
Coding Clinic: 2Ø19, Q1, P24 – Ø2HAØQZ
Coding Clinic: 2Ø19, Q3, P2Ø – Ø2HLØDZ
Coding Clinic: 2Ø19, Q3, P23 – Ø2HL3JZ
Coding Clinic: 2Ø19, Q4, P24 – Ø2H13DZ
Coding Clinic: 2Ø22, Q2, P25 – Ø2HK3JZ
Coding Clinic: 2Ø24, Q1, P3Ø – Ø2HA3RZ
Coding Clinic: 2Ø24, Q2, P3Ø – Ø2HL3YZ

SECTION: Ø MEDICAL AND SURGICAL
BODY SYSTEM: 2 HEART AND GREAT VESSELS
OPERATION: H INSERTION: *(continued)*

Putting in a nonbiological appliance that monitors, assists, performs, or prevents a physiological function but does not physically take the place of a body part

Body Part	Approach	Device	Qualifier
P Pulmonary Trunk Q Pulmonary Artery, Right R Pulmonary Artery, Left S Pulmonary Vein, Right T Pulmonary Vein, Left V Superior Vena Cava	Ø Open 3 Percutaneous 4 Percutaneous Endoscopic	Ø Monitoring Device, Pressure Sensor 2 Monitoring Device 3 Infusion Device D Intraluminal Device Y Other Device	Z No Qualifier
W Thoracic Aorta, Descending	Ø Open 4 Percutaneous Endoscopic	Ø Monitoring Device, Pressure Sensor 2 Monitoring Device 3 Infusion Device D Intraluminal Device Y Other Device	Z No Qualifier
W Thoracic Aorta,	3 Percutaneous	Ø Monitoring Device, Pressure Sensor 2 Monitoring Device 3 Infusion Device D Intraluminal Device R Short-term External Heart Assist System Y Other Device	Z No Qualifier
X Thoracic Aorta, Ascending/Arch	Ø Open 3 Percutaneous 4 Percutaneous Endoscopic	Ø Monitoring Device, Pressure Sensor 2 Monitoring Device 3 Infusion Device D Intraluminal Device	Z No Qualifier

Non-OR Ø2HP[Ø34][Ø23]Z
Non-OR Ø2H[QR][Ø34][23]Z
Non-OR Ø2H[STV][Ø34]3Z
Non-OR Ø2H[STVW]32Z
Non-OR Ø2HW[Ø34][Ø3]Z

Ø2H[STV][34]3Z when reported with Secondary Diagnosis J95.811

SECTION: Ø MEDICAL AND SURGICAL
BODY SYSTEM: 2 HEART AND GREAT VESSELS
OPERATION: J INSPECTION: Visually and/or manually exploring a body part

Body Part	Approach	Device	Qualifier
A Heart Y Great Vessel	Ø Open 3 Percutaneous 4 Percutaneous Endoscopic	Z No Device	Z No Qualifier

Non-OR Ø2J[AY]3ZZ

Coding Clinic: 2Ø15, Q3, P9 – Ø2JA3ZZ

SECTION: Ø MEDICAL AND SURGICAL
BODY SYSTEM: 2 HEART AND GREAT VESSELS
OPERATION: K MAP: Locating the route of passage of electrical impulses and/or locating functional areas in a body part

Body Part	Approach	Device	Qualifier
8 Conduction Mechanism	Ø Open 3 Percutaneous 4 Percutaneous Endoscopic	Z No Device	Z No Qualifier

DRG Non-OR Ø2K8[Ø34]ZZ

SECTION: Ø MEDICAL AND SURGICAL
BODY SYSTEM: 2 HEART AND GREAT VESSELS
OPERATION: L OCCLUSION: Completely closing an orifice or the lumen of a tubular body part

Body Part	Approach	Device	Qualifier
7 Atrium, Left	Ø Open 3 Percutaneous 4 Percutaneous Endoscopic	C Extraluminal Device D Intraluminal Device Z No Device	K Left Atrial Appendage
H Pulmonary Valve P Pulmonary Trunk Q Pulmonary Artery, Right S Pulmonary Vein, Right T Pulmonary Vein, Left V Superior Vena Cava	Ø Open 3 Percutaneous 4 Percutaneous Endoscopic	C Extraluminal Device D Intraluminal Device Z No Device	Z No Qualifier
R Pulmonary Artery, Left	Ø Open 3 Percutaneous 4 Percutaneous Endoscopic	C Extraluminal Device D Intraluminal Device Z No Device	T Ductus Arteriosus Z No Qualifier
W Thoracic Aorta, Descending	Ø Open 3 Percutaneous	D Intraluminal Device	J Temporary

DRG Non-OR Ø2L7[Ø34][CDZ]K

Coding Clinic: 2Ø15, Q4, P24 – Ø2LRØZT

Coding Clinic: 2Ø16, Q2, P26 – Ø2LS3DZ
Coding Clinic: 2Ø16, Q4, P1Ø2, 1Ø4 – Ø2L
Coding Clinic: 2Ø17, Q4, P34 – Ø2L[QS]3DZ

SECTION: Ø MEDICAL AND SURGICAL
BODY SYSTEM: 2 HEART AND GREAT VESSELS
OPERATION: N RELEASE: Freeing a body part from an abnormal physical constraint by cutting or by the use of force

Body Part	Approach	Device	Qualifier
Ø Coronary Artery, One Artery 1 Coronary Artery, Two Arteries 2 Coronary Artery, Three Arteries 3 Coronary Artery, Four or More Arteries 4 Coronary Vein 5 Atrial Septum 6 Atrium, Right 7 Atrium, Left 8 Conduction Mechanism 9 Chordae Tendineae D Papillary Muscle F Aortic Valve G Mitral Valve H Pulmonary Valve J Tricuspid Valve K Ventricle, Right L Ventricle, Left M Ventricular Septum N Pericardium P Pulmonary Trunk Q Pulmonary Artery, Right R Pulmonary Artery, Left S Pulmonary Vein, Right T Pulmonary Vein, Left V Superior Vena Cava W Thoracic Aorta, Descending X Thoracic Aorta, Ascending/Arch	Ø Open 3 Percutaneous 4 Percutaneous Endoscopic	Z No Device	Z No Qualifier

Coding Clinic: 2Ø16, Q4, P81 – Ø2N

Coding Clinic: 2Ø19, Q2, P14, 21 – Ø2NØØZZ

SECTION: Ø MEDICAL AND SURGICAL
BODY SYSTEM: 2 HEART AND GREAT VESSELS
OPERATION: P REMOVAL: Taking out or off a device from a body part

Body Part	Approach	Device	Qualifier
A Heart	Ø Open 3 Percutaneous 4 Percutaneous Endoscopic	2 Monitoring Device 3 Infusion Device 7 Autologous Tissue Substitute 8 Zooplastic Tissue C Extraluminal Device D Intraluminal Device J Synthetic Substitute K Nonautologous Tissue Substitute M Cardiac Lead N Intracardiac Pacemaker Q Implantable Heart Assist System Y Other Device	Z No Qualifier
A Heart	Ø Open 3 Percutaneous 4 Percutaneous Endoscopic	R Short-term External Heart Assist System	S Biventricular Z No Qualifier
A Heart	X External	2 Monitoring Device 3 Infusion Device D Intraluminal Device M Cardiac Lead	Z No Qualifier
W Thoracic Aorta, Descending	3 Percutaneous	R Short-term External Heart Assist System	Z No Qualifier
Y Great Vessel	Ø Open 3 Percutaneous 4 Percutaneous Endoscopic	2 Monitoring Device 3 Infusion Device 7 Autologous Tissue Substitute 8 Zooplastic Tissue C Extraluminal Device D Intraluminal Device J Synthetic Substitute K Nonautologous Tissue Substitute Y Other Device	Z No Qualifier
Y Great Vessel	X External	2 Monitoring Device 3 Infusion Device D Intraluminal Device	Z No Qualifier

Ø2PA[Ø34]RZ
Ø2PAXMZ
DRG Non-OR Ø2PAXMZ
Non-OR Ø2PAX[23DM]Z
Non-OR Ø2PA3[23D]Z
Non-OR Ø2PY3[23D]Z
Non-OR Ø2PYX[23D]Z
Ø2PA[Ø34]MZ when reported with Secondary Diagnosis K68.11, T81.4XXA, T82.6XXA, or T82.7XXA
Ø2PAXMZ when reported with Secondary Diagnosis K68.11, T81.4XXA, T82.6XXA, or T82.7XXA

Coding Clinic: 2015, Q3, P33 – Ø2PA3MZ
Coding Clinic: 2016, Q2, P15; 2015, Q4, P32 – Ø2PY33Z
Coding Clinic: 2016, Q3, P19 – Ø2PYX3Z
Coding Clinic: 2016, Q4, P95 – Ø2P
Coding Clinic: 2016, Q4, P97 – Ø2PA3NZ
Coding Clinic: 2018, Q4, P54; 2017, Q1, P11-21; 2016, Q4, P139 – Ø2PA3RZ
Coding Clinic: 2017, Q1, P14 – Ø2PAØRZ
Coding Clinic: 2017, Q2, P25 – Ø2PY33Z
Coding Clinic: 2017, Q4, P45, 105 – Ø2PA[DQ]Z
Coding Clinic: 2018, Q4, P85 – Ø2PY3JZ
Coding Clinic: 2019, Q1, P24 – Ø2PAØQZ
Coding Clinic: 2022, Q2, P25 – Ø2PA3MZ

SECTION: Ø MEDICAL AND SURGICAL
BODY SYSTEM: 2 HEART AND GREAT VESSELS
OPERATION: Q REPAIR: Restoring, to the extent possible, a body part to its normal anatomic structure and function

Body Part	Approach	Device	Qualifier
Ø Coronary Artery, One Artery 1 Coronary Artery, Two Arteries 2 Coronary Artery, Three Arteries 3 Coronary Artery, Four or More Arteries 4 Coronary Vein 5 Atrial Septum 6 Atrium, Right 7 Atrium, Left 8 Conduction Mechanism 9 Chordae Tendineae A Heart B Heart, Right C Heart, Left D Papillary Muscle H Pulmonary Valve K Ventricle, Right L Ventricle, Left M Ventricular Septum N Pericardium P Pulmonary Trunk Q Pulmonary Artery, Right R Pulmonary Artery, Left S Pulmonary Vein, Right T Pulmonary Vein, Left V Superior Vena Cava W Thoracic Aorta, Descending X Thoracic Aorta, Ascending/Arch	Ø Open 3 Percutaneous 4 Percutaneous Endoscopic	Z No Device	Z No Qualifier
F Aortic Valve	Ø Open 3 Percutaneous 4 Percutaneous Endoscopic	Z No Device	J Truncal Valve Z No Qualifier
G Mitral Valve	Ø Open 3 Percutaneous 4 Percutaneous Endoscopic	Z No Device	E Atrioventricular Valve, Left Z No Qualifier
J Tricuspid Valve	Ø Open 3 Percutaneous 4 Percutaneous Endoscopic	Z No Device	G Atrioventricular Valve, Right Z No Qualifier

Non-OR Ø2Q[WX][Ø34]ZZ

Coding Clinic: 2Ø15, Q3, P16 – Ø2QWØZZ
Coding Clinic: 2Ø15, Q4, P24 – Ø2Q5ØZZ
Coding Clinic: 2Ø16, Q4, P81, 83, 1Ø2 – Ø2Q
Coding Clinic: 2Ø16, Q4, P1Ø6 – Ø2QGØZE, Ø2QJØZG
Coding Clinic: 2Ø16, Q4, P1Ø7 – Ø2QFØZJ
Coding Clinic: 2Ø17, Q18, P1Ø – Ø2Q[ST]ØZZ
Coding Clinic: 2Ø21, Q3, P27 – Ø2Q[6V]ØZZ
Coding Clinic: 2Ø22, Q1, P4Ø-41 – Ø2QAØZZ
Coding Clinic: 2Ø23, Q3, P28 – Ø2QW3ZZ

SECTION: Ø MEDICAL AND SURGICAL
BODY SYSTEM: 2 HEART AND GREAT VESSELS
OPERATION: R REPLACEMENT: *(on multiple pages)*

Putting in or on biological or synthetic material that physically takes the place and/or function of all or a portion of a body part

Body Part	Approach	Device	Qualifier
5 Atrial Septum 6 Atrium, Right 7 Atrium, Left 9 Chordae Tendineae D Papillary Muscle K Ventricle, Right L Ventricle, Left M Ventricular Septum N Pericardium P Pulmonary Trunk Q Pulmonary Artery, Right R Pulmonary Artery, Left S Pulmonary Vein, Right T Pulmonary Vein, Left V Superior Vena Cava W Thoracic Aorta, Descending X Thoracic Aorta, Ascending/Arch	Ø Open 4 Percutaneous Endoscopic	7 Autologous Tissue Substitute 8 Zooplastic Tissue J Synthetic Substitute K Nonautologous Tissue Substitute	Z No Qualifier
A Heart	Ø Open	L Biologic with Synthetic Substitute, Autoregulated M Synthetic Substitute, Pneumatic	Z No Qualifier
F Aortic Valve	Ø Open 4 Percutaneous Endoscopic	7 Autologous Tissue Substitute J Synthetic Substitute K Nonautologous Tissue Substitute	Z No Qualifier
F Aortic Valve	Ø Open 4 Percutaneous Endoscopic	8 Zooplastic Tissue	N Rapid Deployment Technique Z No Qualifier
F Aortic Valve	3 Percutaneous	7 Autologous Tissue Substitute J Synthetic Substitute K Nonautologous Tissue Substitute	H Transapical Z No Qualifier
F Aortic Valve	3 Percutaneous	8 Zooplastic Tissue	H Transapical N Rapid Deployment Technique Z No Qualifier
G Mitral Valve J Tricuspid Valve	Ø Open 5 Percutaneous 6 Endoscopic	7 Autologous Tissue Substitute 8 Zooplastic Tissue J Synthetic Substitute K Nonautologous TissueSubstitute	Z No Qualifier
G Mitral Valve J Tricuspid Valve	3 Percutaneous	7 Autologous Tissue Substitute 8 Zooplastic Tissue J Synthetic Substitute K Nonautologous Tissue Substitute	H Transapical Z No Qualifier
H Pulmonary Valve	Ø Open 4 Percutaneous Endoscopic	7 Autologous Tissue Substitute 8 Zooplastic Tissue J Synthetic Substitute K Nonautologous Tissue Substitute	Z No Qualifier

Non-OR Ø2RF[Ø34]8N

Ø2R[KL]ØJZ when combined with ZØØ.6

Ø2R[KL]ØJZ

Coding Clinic: 2Ø16, Q3, P32 – Ø2RJ48Z

Coding Clinic: 2Ø16, Q4, P81 – Ø2R
Coding Clinic: 2Ø17, Q1, P13 – Ø2R[KL]ØJZ
Coding Clinic: 2Ø17, Q4, P56 – Ø2RJ3JZ
Coding Clinic: 2Ø19, Q1, P31 – Ø2RF38Z
Coding Clinic: 2Ø24, Q2, P19, 31 – Ø2R[FX]Ø[8J]Z

SECTION: Ø MEDICAL AND SURGICAL
BODY SYSTEM: 2 HEART AND GREAT VESSELS
OPERATION: R REPLACEMENT: *(continued)*
Putting in or on biological or synthetic material that physically takes the place and/or function of all or a portion of a body part

Body Part	Approach	Device	Qualifier
H Pulmonary Valve	3 Percutaneous	7 Autologous Tissue Substitute 8 Zooplastic Tissue J Synthetic Substitute K Nonautologous Tissue Substitute	H Transapical Z No Qualifier
H Pulmonary Valve	3 Percutaneous	8 Zooplastic Tissue	H Transapical L In Existing Conduit M Native Site Z No Qualifier

Coding Clinic: 2Ø19, Q3, P24 – Ø2RGØ8Z, Ø2RXØJZ
Coding Clinic: 2Ø19, Q4, P24 – Ø2RF3JZ
Coding Clinic: 2Ø2Ø, Q1, P26 – Ø2RXØJZ

SECTION: Ø MEDICAL AND SURGICAL
BODY SYSTEM: 2 HEART AND GREAT VESSELS
OPERATION: S REPOSITION: Moving to its normal location, or other suitable location, all or a portion of a body part

Body Part	Approach	Device	Qualifier
Ø Coronary Artery, One Artery 1 Coronary Artery, Two Arteries P Pulmonary Trunk Q Pulmonary Artery, Right R Pulmonary Artery, Left S Pulmonary Vein, Right T Pulmonary Vein, Left V Superior Vena Cava W Thoracic Aorta, Descending X Thoracic Aorta, Ascending/Arch	Ø Open	Z No Device	Z No Qualifier

Coding Clinic: 2Ø15, Q4, P24 – Ø2S[PW]ØZZ
Coding Clinic: 2Ø16, Q4, P81, 83, 1Ø2 – Ø2S
Coding Clinic: 2Ø16, Q4, P1Ø3-1Ø4 – Ø2S[1PX]ØZZ

SECTION: Ø MEDICAL AND SURGICAL
BODY SYSTEM: 2 HEART AND GREAT VESSELS
OPERATION: T RESECTION: Cutting out or off, without replacement, all of a body part

Body Part	Approach	Device	Qualifier
5 Atrial Septum 8 Conduction Mechanism 9 Chordae Tendineae D Papillary Muscle H Pulmonary Valve M Ventricular Septum N Pericardium	Ø Open 3 Percutaneous 4 Percutaneous Endoscopic	Z No Device	Z No Qualifier

SECTION: Ø MEDICAL AND SURGICAL

BODY SYSTEM: 2 HEART AND GREAT VESSELS

OPERATION: U SUPPLEMENT: Putting in or on biological or synthetic material that physically reinforces and/or augments the function of a portion of a body part

Body Part	Approach	Device	Qualifier
Ø Coronary Artery, One Artery 1 Coronary Artery, Two Arteries 2 Coronary Artery, Three Arteries 3 Coronary Artery, Four or More Arteries 5 Atrial Septum 6 Atrium, Right 7 Atrium, Left 9 Chordae Tendineae A Heart D Papillary Muscle H Pulmonary Valve K Ventricle, Right L Ventricle, Left M Ventricular Septum N Pericardium P Pulmonary Trunk Q Pulmonary Artery, Right R Pulmonary Artery, Left S Pulmonary Vein, Right T Pulmonary Vein, Left V Superior Vena Cava W Thoracic Aorta, Descending X Thoracic Aorta, Ascending/Arch	Ø Open 3 Percutaneous 4 Percutaneous Endoscopic	7 Autologous Tissue Substitute 8 Zooplastic Tissue J Synthetic Substitute K Nonautologous Tissue Substitute	Z No Qualifier
F Aortic Valve	Ø Open 3 Percutaneous 4 Percutaneous Endoscopic	7 Autologous Tissue Substitute 8 Zooplastic Tissue J Synthetic Substitute K Nonautologous Tissue Substitute	J Truncal Valve Z No Qualifier
G Mitral Valve	Ø Open 3 Percutaneous 4 Percutaneous Endoscopic	7 Autologous Tissue Substitute 8 Zooplastic Tissue J Synthetic Substitute K Nonautologous Tissue Substitute	E Atrioventricular Valve, Left Z No Qualifier
G Mitral Valve	Ø Open 4 Percutaneous Endoscopic	7 Autologous Tissue Substitute 8 Zooplastic Tissue J Synthetic Substitute K Nonautologous Tissue Substitute	E Atrioventricular Valve, Left Z No Qualifier
G Mitral Valve	3 Percutaneous	7 Autologous Tissue Substitute 8 Zooplastic Tissue K Nonautologous Tissue Substitute	E Atrioventricular Valve, Left Z No Qualifier
G Mitral Valve	3 Percutaneous	J Synthetic Substitute	E Atrioventricular Valve, Left H Transapical Z No Qualifier
J Tricuspid Valve	Ø Open 3 Percutaneous 4 Percutaneous Endoscopic	7 Autologous Tissue Substitute 8 Zooplastic Tissue J Synthetic Substitute K Nonautologous Tissue Substitute	G Atrioventricular Valve, Right Z No Qualifier

DRG Non-OR Ø2U7[34]JZ

Coding Clinic: 2015, Q2, P24 – Ø2UGØJZ
Coding Clinic: 2015, Q3, P17 – Ø2U[QR]ØKZ
Coding Clinic: 2015, Q4, P23-25 – Ø2UFØ8Z, Ø2UMØJZ, Ø2UMØ8Z, Ø2UWØ7Z
Coding Clinic: 2016, Q2, P24 – Ø2U[PR]Ø7Z
Coding Clinic: 2016, Q2, P27 – Ø2UWØJZ
Coding Clinic: 2016, Q4, P81, 1Ø2 – Ø2U
Coding Clinic: 2016, Q4, P1Ø6 – Ø2UGØJE, Ø2UJØKG
Coding Clinic: 2016, Q4, P1Ø7 – Ø2UMØ8Z, Ø2UFØKJ
Coding Clinic: 2017, Q1, P2Ø – Ø2UXØKZ
Coding Clinic: 2017, Q3, P7 - Ø2U[67]Ø7Z
Coding Clinic: 2017, Q4, P36 - Ø2UGØ8Z
Coding Clinic: 2019, Q4, P26 – Ø2UØ3JZ
Coding Clinic: 2020, Q1, P25 – Ø2UPØ8Z
Coding Clinic: 2023, Q2, P21; 2021, Q3, P28 – Ø2UG3JZ
Coding Clinic: 2022, Q1, P38 – Ø2U73JZ, Ø2UAØ8Z

SECTION: Ø MEDICAL AND SURGICAL
BODY SYSTEM: 2 HEART AND GREAT VESSELS
OPERATION: V RESTRICTION: Partially closing an orifice or the lumen of a tubular body part

Body Part	Approach	Device	Qualifier
A Heart	Ø Open 3 Percutaneous 4 Percutaneous Endoscopic	C Extraluminal Device Z No Device	Z No Qualifier
G Mitral Valve	Ø Open 3 Percutaneous 4 Percutaneous Endoscopic	Z No Device	Z No Qualifier
L Ventricle, Left P Pulmonary Trunk Q Pulmonary Artery, Right S Pulmonary Vein, Right T Pulmonary Vein, Left V Superior Vena Cava	Ø Open 3 Percutaneous 4 Percutaneous Endoscopic	C Extraluminal Device D Intraluminal Device Z No Device	Z No Qualifier
R Pulmonary Artery, Left	Ø Open 3 Percutaneous 4 Percutaneous Endoscopic	C Extraluminal Device D Intraluminal Device Z No Device	T Ductus Arteriosus Z No Qualifier
W Thoracic Aorta, Descending X Thoracic Aorta, Ascending/Arch	Ø Open 3 Percutaneous 4 Percutaneous Endoscopic	C Extraluminal Device D Intraluminal Device E Intraluminal Device, Branched or Fenestrated, One or Two Arteries F Intraluminal Device, Branched or Fenestrated, Three or More Arteries Z No Device	Z No Qualifier

Coding Clinic: 2Ø16, Q4, P81, 89 – Ø2V
Coding Clinic: 2Ø16, Q4, P93 – Ø2VW3DZ
Coding Clinic: 2Ø17, Q4, P36 – Ø2VGØZZ
Coding Clinic: 2Ø2Ø, Q1, P26 – Ø2VWØDZ
Coding Clinic: 2Ø21, Q4, P45 – Ø2VL3DZ

SECTION: Ø MEDICAL AND SURGICAL
BODY SYSTEM: 2 HEART AND GREAT VESSELS
OPERATION: W REVISION: *(on multiple pages)*

Correcting, to the extent possible, a portion of a malfunctioning device or the position of a displaced device

Body Part	Approach	Device	Qualifier
5 Atrial Septum M Ventricular Septum	Ø Open 4 Percutaneous Endoscopic	J Synthetic Substitute	Z No Qualifier
A Heart	Ø Open 3 Percutaneous 4 Percutaneous Endoscopic	2 Monitoring Device 3 Infusion Device 7 Autologous Tissue Substitute 8 Zooplastic Tissue C Extraluminal Device D Intraluminal Device J Synthetic Substitute K Nonautologous Tissue Substitute M Cardiac Lead N Intracardiac Pacemaker Q Implantable Heart Assist System Y Other Device	Z No Qualifier
A Heart	Ø Open 3 Percutaneous 4 Percutaneous Endoscopic	R Short-term External Heart Assist System	S Biventricular Z No Qualifier
A Heart	X External	2 Monitoring Device 3 Infusion Device 7 Autologous Tissue Substitute 8 Zooplastic Tissue C Extraluminal Device D Intraluminal Device J Synthetic Substitute K Nonautologous Tissue Substitute M Cardiac Lead N Intracardiac Pacemaker Q Implantable Heart Assist System	Z No Qualifier
A Heart	X External	R Short-term External Heart Assist System	S Biventricular Z No Qualifier
F Aortic Valve G Mitral Valve H Pulmonary Valve J Tricuspid Valve	Ø Open 3 Percutaneous 4 Percutaneous Endoscopic	7 Autologous Tissue Substitute 8 Zooplastic Tissue J Synthetic Substitute K Nonautologous Tissue Substitute	Z No Qualifier

Ø2WA[Ø34][QR]Z
Non-OR Ø2WAX[2378CDJKMQ]Z
Non-OR Ø2WAXRZ
Non-OR Ø2WA3[23D]Z
Ø2WA[Ø34]MZ when reported with Secondary Diagnosis K68.11, T81.4XXA, T82.6XXA, or T82.7XXA
Ø2WA[34]QZ

Coding Clinic: 2015, Q3, P32 – Ø2WA3MZ
Coding Clinic: 2016, Q4, P95 – Ø2W
Coding Clinic: 2016, Q4, P96 – Ø2WA3NZ
Coding Clinic: 2018, Q1, P17 – Ø2WAXRZ

SECTION: Ø MEDICAL AND SURGICAL
BODY SYSTEM: 2 HEART AND GREAT VESSELS
OPERATION: W REVISION: *(continued)*
Correcting, to the extent possible, a portion of a malfunctioning device or the position of a displaced device

Body Part	Approach	Device	Qualifier
W Thoracic Aorta, Descending	3 Percutaneous	R Short-term External Heart Assist System	Z No Qualifier
Y Great Vessel	Ø Open 3 Percutaneous 4 Percutaneous Endoscopic	2 Monitoring Device 3 Infusion Device 7 Autologous Tissue Substitute 8 Zooplastic Tissue C Extraluminal Device D Intraluminal Device J Synthetic Substitute K Nonautologous Tissue Substitute Y Other Device	Z No Qualifier
Y Great Vessel	X External	2 Monitoring Device 3 Infusion Device 7 Autologous Tissue Substitute 8 Zooplastic Tissue C Extraluminal Device D Intraluminal Device J Synthetic Substitute K Nonautologous Tissue Substitute	Z No Qualifier

Non-OR Ø2WY[3X][2378CDJK]Z

SECTION: Ø MEDICAL AND SURGICAL
BODY SYSTEM: 2 HEART AND GREAT VESSELS
OPERATION: Y TRANSPLANTATION: Putting in or on all or a portion of a living body part taken from another individual or animal to physically take the place and/or function of all or a portion of a similar body part

Body Part	Approach	Device	Qualifier
A Heart	Ø Open	Z No Device	Ø Allogeneic 1 Syngeneic 2 Zooplastic

Ø2YAØZ[Ø12]

Coding Clinic: 2Ø13, Q3, P19 – Ø2YAØZØ

Ø3. Upper Arteries 89
Ø31. Bypass....9Ø
Ø35. Destruction....92
Ø37. Dilation....93
Ø39. Drainage 94
Ø3B. Excision 96
Ø3C. Extirpation....97
Ø3F. Fragmentation....98
Ø3H. Insertion....99
Ø3J. Inspection 1ØØ
Ø3L. Occlusion 1ØØ
Ø3N. Release 1Ø1
Ø3P. Removal 1Ø1
Ø3Q. Repair 1Ø2
Ø3R. Replacement 1Ø3
Ø3S. Reposition....1Ø4
Ø3U. Supplement....1Ø5
Ø3V. Restriction....1Ø6
Ø3W. Revision....1Ø7

SECTION: Ø MEDICAL AND SURGICAL
BODY SYSTEM: 3 UPPER ARTERIES
OPERATION: 1 BYPASS: *(on multiple pages)*
Altering the route of passage of the contents of a tubular body part

Body Part	Approach	Device	Qualifier
2 Innominate Artery	Ø Open	9 Autologous Venous Tissue A Autologous Arterial Tissue J Synthetic Substitute K Nonautologous Tissue Substitute Z No Device	Ø Upper Arm Artery, Right 1 Upper Arm Artery, Left 2 Upper Arm Artery, Bilateral 3 Lower Arm Artery, Right 4 Lower Arm Artery, Left 5 Lower Arm Artery, Bilateral 6 Upper Leg Artery, Right 7 Upper Leg Artery, Left 8 Upper Leg Artery, Bilateral 9 Lower Leg Artery, Right B Lower Leg Artery, Left C Lower Leg Artery, Bilateral D Upper Arm Vein F Lower Arm Vein J Extracranial Artery, Right K Extracranial Artery, Left W Lower Extremity Vein
3 Subclavian Artery, Right 4 Subclavian Artery, Left	Ø Open	9 Autologous Venous Tissue A Autologous Arterial Tissue J Synthetic Substitute K Nonautologous Tissue Substitute Z No Device	Ø Upper Arm Artery, Right 1 Upper Arm Artery, Left 2 Upper Arm Artery, Bilateral 3 Lower Arm Artery, Right 4 Lower Arm Artery, Left 5 Lower Arm Artery, Bilateral 6 Upper Leg Artery, Right 7 Upper Leg Artery, Left 8 Upper Leg Artery, Bilateral 9 Lower Leg Artery, Right B Lower Leg Artery, Left C Lower Leg Artery, Bilateral D Upper Arm Vein F Lower Arm Vein J Extracranial Artery, Right K Extracranial Artery, Left M Pulmonary Artery, Right N Pulmonary Artery, Left W Lower Extremity Vein
5 Axillary Artery, Right 6 Axillary Artery, Left	Ø Open	9 Autologous Venous Tissue A Autologous Arterial Tissue J Synthetic Substitute K Nonautologous Tissue Substitute Z No Device	Ø Upper Arm Artery, Right 1 Upper Arm Artery, Left 2 Upper Arm Artery, Bilateral 3 Lower Arm Artery, Right 4 Lower Arm Artery, Left 5 Lower Arm Artery, Bilateral 6 Upper Leg Artery, Right 7 Upper Leg Artery, Left 8 Upper Leg Artery, Bilateral 9 Lower Leg Artery, Right B Lower Leg Artery, Left C Lower Leg Artery, Bilateral D Upper Arm Vein F Lower Arm Vein J Extracranial Artery, Right K Extracranial Artery, Left T Abdominal Artery V Superior Vena Cava W Lower Extremity Vein

Coding Clinic: 2Ø16, Q3, P38 – Ø318ØJD

SECTION: Ø MEDICAL AND SURGICAL
BODY SYSTEM: 3 UPPER ARTERIES
OPERATION: 1 BYPASS: *(continued)*
Altering the route of passage of the contents of a tubular body part

Body Part	Approach	Device	Qualifier
7 Brachial Artery, Right	Ø Open	9 Autologous Venous Tissue A Autologous Arterial Tissue J Synthetic Substitute K Nonautologous Tissue Substitute Z No Device	Ø Upper Arm Artery, Right 3 Lower Arm Artery, Right D Upper Arm Vein F Lower Arm Vein V Superior Vena Cava W Lower Extremity Vein
7 Brachial Artery, Right	3 Percutaneous	Z No Device	F Lower Arm Vein
8 Brachial Artery, Left	Ø Open	9 Autologous Venous Tissue A Autologous Arterial Tissue J Synthetic Substitute K Nonautologous Tissue Substitute Z No Device	1 Upper Arm Artery, Left 4 Lower Arm Artery, Left D Upper Arm Vein F Lower Arm Vein V Superior Vena Cava W Lower Extremity Vein
8 Brachial Artery, Left	3 Percutaneous	Z No Device	F Lower Arm Vein
9 Ulnar Artery, Right B Radial Artery, Right	Ø Open	9 Autologous Venous Tissue A Autologous Arterial Tissue J Synthetic Substitute K Nonautologous Tissue Substitute Z No Device	3 Lower Arm Artery, Right F Lower Arm Vein
9 Ulnar Artery, Right B Radial Artery, Right	3 Percutaneous	Z No Device	F Lower Arm Vein
A Ulnar Artery, Left C Radial Artery, Left	Ø Open	9 Autologous Venous Tissue A Autologous Arterial Tissue J Synthetic Substitute K Nonautologous Tissue Substitute Z No Device	4 Lower Arm Artery, Left F Lower Arm Vein
A Ulnar Artery, Left C Radial Artery, Left	3 Percutaneous	Z No Device	F Lower Arm Vein
G Intracranial Artery S Temporal Artery, Right T Temporal Artery, Left	Ø Open	9 Autologous Venous Tissue A Autologous Arterial Tissue J Synthetic Substitute K Nonautologous Tissue Substitute Z No Device	G Intracranial Artery
H Common Carotid Artery, Right J Common Carotid Artery, Left	Ø Open	9 Autologous Venous Tissue A Autologous Arterial Tissue J Synthetic Substitute K Nonautologous Tissue Substitute Z No Device	G Intracranial Artery J Extracranial Artery, Right K Extracranial Artery, Left Y Upper Artery
K Internal Carotid Artery, Right L Internal Carotid Artery, Left M External Carotid Artery, Right N External Carotid Artery, Left	Ø Open	9 Autologous Venous Tissue A Autologous Arterial Tissue J Synthetic Substitute K Nonautologous Tissue Substitute Z No Device	J Extracranial Artery, Right K Extracranial Artery, Left

Non-OR Ø31[789ABCGHJ]Ø[9AJKZ][Ø134DFGJK]
Coding Clinic: 2Ø13, Q1, P228 – Ø31CØZF
Coding Clinic: 2Ø17, Q2, P22 – Ø31JØZK
Coding Clinic: 2Ø17, Q4, P65 – Ø31JØJJ
Coding Clinic: 2Ø21, Q3, P15 – Ø317ØKF.

SECTION: Ø MEDICAL AND SURGICAL
BODY SYSTEM: 3 UPPER ARTERIES
OPERATION: 5 DESTRUCTION: Physical eradication of all or a portion of a body part by the direct use of energy, force, or a destructive agent

Body Part	Approach	Device	Qualifier
Ø Internal Mammary Artery, Right 1 Internal Mammary Artery, Left 2 Innominate Artery 3 Subclavian Artery, Right 4 Subclavian Artery, Left 5 Axillary Artery, Right 6 Axillary Artery, Left 7 Brachial Artery, Right 8 Brachial Artery, Left 9 Ulnar Artery, Right A Ulnar Artery, Left B Radial Artery, Right C Radial Artery, Left D Hand Artery, Right F Hand Artery, Left G Intracranial Artery H Common Carotid Artery, Right J Common Carotid Artery, Left K Internal Carotid Artery, Right L Internal Carotid Artery, Left M External Carotid Artery, Right N External Carotid Artery, Left P Vertebral Artery, Right Q Vertebral Artery, Left R Face Artery S Temporal Artery, Right T Temporal Artery, Left U Thyroid Artery, Right V Thyroid Artery, Left Y Upper Artery	Ø Open 3 Percutaneous 4 Percutaneous Endoscopic	Z No Device	Z No Qualifier

SECTION: Ø MEDICAL AND SURGICAL
BODY SYSTEM: 3 UPPER ARTERIES
OPERATION: 7 DILATION: Expanding an orifice or the lumen of a tubular body part

Body Part	Approach	Device	Qualifier
Ø Internal Mammary Artery, Right 1 Internal Mammary Artery, Left 2 Innominate Artery 3 Subclavian Artery, Right 4 Subclavian Artery, Left 5 Axillary Artery, Right 6 Axillary Artery, Left 7 Brachial Artery, Right 8 Brachial Artery, Left 9 Ulnar Artery, Right A Ulnar Artery, Left B Radial Artery, Right C Radial Artery, Left	Ø Open 3 Percutaneous 4 Percutaneous Endoscopic	4 Intraluminal Device, Drug-eluting 5 Intraluminal Device, Drug-eluting, Two 6 Intraluminal Device, Drug-eluting, Three 7 Intraluminal Device, Drug-eluting, Four or More E Intraluminal Device, Two F Intraluminal Device, Three G Intraluminal Device, Four or More	Z No Qualifier
Ø Internal Mammary Artery, Right 1 Internal Mammary Artery, Left 2 Innominate Artery 3 Subclavian Artery, Right 4 Subclavian Artery, Left 5 Axillary Artery, Right 6 Axillary Artery, Left 7 Brachial Artery, Right 8 Brachial Artery, Left 9 Ulnar Artery, Right A Ulnar Artery, Left B Radial Artery, Right C Radial Artery, Left	Ø Open 3 Percutaneous 4 Percutaneous Endoscopic	D Intraluminal Device Z No Device	1 Drug-Coated Balloon Z No Qualifier
D Hand Artery, Right F Hand Artery, Left G Intracranial Artery H Common Carotid Artery, Right J Common Carotid Artery, Left K Internal Carotid Artery, Right L Internal Carotid Artery, Left M External Carotid Artery, Right N External Carotid Artery, Left P Vertebral Artery, Right Q Vertebral Artery, Left R Face Artery S Temporal Artery, Right T Temporal Artery, Left U Thyroid Artery, Right V Thyroid Artery, Left Y Upper Artery	Ø Open 3 Percutaneous 4 Percutaneous Endoscopic	4 Intraluminal Device, Drug-eluting 5 Intraluminal Device, Drug-eluting, Two 6 Intraluminal Device, Drug-eluting, Three 7 Intraluminal Device, Drug-eluting, Four or More D Intraluminal Device E Intraluminal Device, Two F Intraluminal Device, Three G Intraluminal Device, Four or More Z No Device	Z No Qualifier

Ø37G[34]Z[6Z]

Coding Clinic: 2Ø16, Q4, P87 – Ø37
Coding Clinic: 2Ø19, Q3, P3Ø – Ø37K3DZ

SECTION: Ø MEDICAL AND SURGICAL
BODY SYSTEM: 3 UPPER ARTERIES
OPERATION: 9 DRAINAGE: *(on multiple pages)*
Taking or letting out fluids and/or gases from a body part

Body Part	Approach	Device	Qualifier
Ø Internal Mammary Artery, Right 1 Internal Mammary Artery, Left 2 Innominate Artery 3 Subclavian Artery, Right 4 Subclavian Artery, Left 5 Axillary Artery, Right 6 Axillary Artery, Left 7 Brachial Artery, Right 8 Brachial Artery, Left 9 Ulnar Artery, Right A Ulnar Artery, Left B Radial Artery, Right C Radial Artery, Left D Hand Artery, Right F Hand Artery, Left G Intracranial Artery H Common Carotid Artery, Right J Common Carotid Artery, Left K Internal Carotid Artery, Right L Internal Carotid Artery, Left M External Carotid Artery, Right N External Carotid Artery, Left P Vertebral Artery, Right Q Vertebral Artery, Left R Face Artery S Temporal Artery, Right T Temporal Artery, Left U Thyroid Artery, Right V Thyroid Artery, Left Y Upper Artery	Ø Open 3 Percutaneous 4 Percutaneous Endoscopic	Ø Drainage Device	Z No Qualifier

Non-OR Ø39[Ø123456789ABCDFGHJKLMNPQRSTUVY][Ø34]ØZ

SECTION: Ø MEDICAL AND SURGICAL
BODY SYSTEM: 3 UPPER ARTERIES
OPERATION: 9 DRAINAGE: *(continued)*

Taking or letting out fluids and/or gases from a body part

Body Part	Approach	Device	Qualifier
Ø Internal Mammary Artery, Right 1 Internal Mammary Artery, Left 2 Innominate Artery 3 Subclavian Artery, Right 4 Subclavian Artery, Left 5 Axillary Artery, Right 6 Axillary Artery, Left 7 Brachial Artery, Right 8 Brachial Artery, Left 9 Ulnar Artery, Right A Ulnar Artery, Left B Radial Artery, Right C Radial Artery, Left D Hand Artery, Right F Hand Artery, Left G Intracranial Artery H Common Carotid Artery, Right J Common Carotid Artery, Left K Internal Carotid Artery, Right L Internal Carotid Artery, Left M External Carotid Artery, Right N External Carotid Artery, Left P Vertebral Artery, Right Q Vertebral Artery, Left R Face Artery S Temporal Artery, Right T Temporal Artery, Left U Thyroid Artery, Right V Thyroid Artery, Left Y Upper Artery	Ø Open 3 Percutaneous 4 Percutaneous Endoscopic	Z No Device	X Diagnostic Z No Qualifier

Non-OR Ø39[Ø123456789ABCDFGHJKLMNPQRSTUVY][Ø34]Z[3XZ]

Ø: M/S 3: UPPER ARTERIES 9: DRAINAGE

SECTION: Ø MEDICAL AND SURGICAL
BODY SYSTEM: 3 UPPER ARTERIES
OPERATION: B EXCISION: Cutting out or off, without replacement, a portion of a body part

Body Part	Approach	Device	Qualifier
Ø Internal Mammary Artery, Right 1 Internal Mammary Artery, Left 2 Innominate Artery 3 Subclavian Artery, Right 4 Subclavian Artery, Left 5 Axillary Artery, Right 6 Axillary Artery, Left 7 Brachial Artery, Right 8 Brachial Artery, Left 9 Ulnar Artery, Right A Ulnar Artery, Left B Radial Artery, Right C Radial Artery, Left D Hand Artery, Right F Hand Artery, Left G Intracranial Artery H Common Carotid Artery, Right J Common Carotid Artery, Left K Internal Carotid Artery, Right L Internal Carotid Artery, Left M External Carotid Artery, Right N External Carotid Artery, Left P Vertebral Artery, Right Q Vertebral Artery, Left R Face Artery S Temporal Artery, Right T Temporal Artery, Left U Thyroid Artery, Right V Thyroid Artery, Left Y Upper Artery	Ø Open 3 Percutaneous 4 Percutaneous Endoscopic	Z No Device	X Diagnostic Z No Qualifier

Coding Clinic: 2Ø16, Q2, P13 – Ø3BNØZZ

SECTION: Ø MEDICAL AND SURGICAL
BODY SYSTEM: 3 UPPER ARTERIES
OPERATION: C EXTIRPATION: Taking or cutting out solid matter from a body part

Body Part	Approach	Device	Qualifier
Ø Internal Mammary Artery, Right 1 Internal Mammary Artery, Left 2 Innominate Artery 3 Subclavian Artery, Right 4 Subclavian Artery, Left 5 Axillary Artery, Right 6 Axillary Artery, Left 7 Brachial Artery, Right 8 Brachial Artery, Left 9 Ulnar Artery, Right A Ulnar Artery, Left B Radial Artery, Right C Radial Artery, Left D Hand Artery, Right F Hand Artery, Left R Face Artery S Temporal Artery, Right T Temporal Artery, Left U Thyroid Artery, Right V Thyroid Artery, Left Y Upper Artery	Ø Open 3 Percutaneous 4 Percutaneous Endoscopic	Z No Device	Z No Qualifier
G Intracranial Artery H Common Carotid Artery, Right J Common Carotid Artery, Left K Internal Carotid Artery, Right L Internal Carotid Artery, Left M External Carotid Artery, Right N External Carotid Artery, Left P Vertebral Artery, Right Q Vertebral Artery, Left	Ø Open 4 Percutaneous Endoscopic	Z No Device	Z No Qualifier
G Intracranial Artery H Common Carotid Artery, Right J Common Carotid Artery, Left K Internal Carotid Artery, Right L Internal Carotid Artery, Left M External Carotid Artery, Right N External Carotid Artery, Left P Vertebral Artery, Right Q Vertebral Artery, Left	3 Percutaneous	Z No Device	7 Stent Retriever Z No Qualifier

Coding Clinic: 2Ø16, Q2, P12 – Ø3CKØZZ
Coding Clinic: 2Ø16, Q4, P87 – Ø3C
Coding Clinic: 2Ø17, Q4, P65 – Ø3CNØZZ
Coding Clinic: 2Ø21, Q2, P13 – Ø3CLØZZ
Coding Clinic: 2Ø22, Q1, P43 – Ø3CG3ZZ
Coding Clinic: 2Ø23, Q3, P24 – Ø3C73ZZ

SECTION: Ø MEDICAL AND SURGICAL
BODY SYSTEM: 3 UPPER ARTERIES
OPERATION: F FRAGMENTATION: Breaking solid matter in a body part into pieces

Body Part	Approach	Device	Qualifier
2 Innominate Artery 3 Subclavian Artery, Right 4 Subclavian Artery, Left 5 Axillary Artery, Right 6 Axillary Artery, Left 7 Brachial Artery, Right 8 Brachial Artery, Left 9 Ulnar Artery, Right A Ulnar Artery, Left B Radial Artery, Right C Radial Artery, Left G Intracranial Artery Y Upper Artery	3 Percutaneous	Z No Device	Ø Ultrasonic Z No Qualifier

SECTION: Ø MEDICAL AND SURGICAL
BODY SYSTEM: 3 UPPER ARTERIES
OPERATION: H INSERTION: Putting in a nonbiological appliance that monitors, assists, performs, or prevents a physiological function but does not physically take the place of a body part

Body Part	Approach	Device	Qualifier
Ø Internal Mammary Artery, Right 1 Internal Mammary Artery, Left 2 Innominate Artery 3 Subclavian Artery, Right 4 Subclavian Artery, Left 5 Axillary Artery, Right 6 Axillary Artery, Left 7 Brachial Artery, Right 8 Brachial Artery, Left 9 Ulnar Artery, Right A Ulnar Artery, Left B Radial Artery, Right C Radial Artery, Left D Hand Artery, Right F Hand Artery, Left G Intracranial Artery H Common Carotid Artery, Right J Common Carotid Artery, Left M External Carotid Artery, Right N External Carotid Artery, Left P Vertebral Artery, Right Q Vertebral Artery, Left R Face Artery S Temporal Artery, Right T Temporal Artery, Left U Thyroid Artery, Right V Thyroid Artery, Left	Ø Open 3 Percutaneous 4 Percutaneous Endoscopic	3 Infusion Device D Intraluminal Device	Z No Qualifier
K Internal Carotid Artery, Right L Internal Carotid Artery, Left	Ø Open 3 Percutaneous 4 Percutaneous Endoscopic	3 Infusion Device D Intraluminal Device M Stimulator Lead	Z No Qualifier
Y Upper Artery	Ø Open 3 Percutaneous 4 Percutaneous Endoscopic	2 Monitoring Device 3 Infusion Device D Intraluminal Device Y Other Device	Z No Qualifier

Non-OR Ø3H[Ø123456789ABCDFGHJMNPQRSTUV][Ø34]3Z
Non-OR Ø3H[KL][Ø34]3Z
Non-OR Ø3HY[Ø34]3Z
Non-OR Ø3HY32Z

Coding Clinic: 2Ø16, Q2, P32 – Ø3HY32Z
Coding Clinic: 2Ø2Ø, Q1, P27 – ØHRU7Z
Coding Clinic: 2Ø24, Q2, P19 – Ø3H[4J]DZ

SECTION: Ø MEDICAL AND SURGICAL
BODY SYSTEM: 3 UPPER ARTERIES
OPERATION: J INSPECTION: Visually and/or manually exploring a body part

Body Part	Approach	Device	Qualifier
Y Upper Artery	Ø Open 3 Percutaneous 4 Percutaneous Endoscopic X External	Z No Device	Z No Qualifier

Non-OR Ø3JY[34X]ZZ

Coding Clinic: 2Ø15, Q1, P29 – Ø3JYØZZ
Coding Clinic: 2Ø21, Q1, P17 – Ø3JY3ZZ

SECTION: Ø MEDICAL AND SURGICAL
BODY SYSTEM: 3 UPPER ARTERIES
OPERATION: L OCCLUSION: Completely closing an orifice or the lumen of a tubular body part

Body Part	Approach	Device	Qualifier
Ø Internal Mammary Artery, Right 1 Internal Mammary Artery, Left 2 Innominate Artery 3 Subclavian Artery, Right 4 Subclavian Artery, Left 5 Axillary Artery, Right 6 Axillary Artery, Left 7 Brachial Artery, Right 8 Brachial Artery, Left 9 Ulnar Artery, Right A Ulnar Artery, Left B Radial Artery, Right C Radial Artery, Left D Hand Artery, Right F Hand Artery, Left R Face Artery S Temporal Artery, Right T Temporal Artery, Left U Thyroid Artery, Right V Thyroid Artery, Left Y Upper Artery	Ø Open 3 Percutaneous 4 Percutaneous Endoscopic	C Extraluminal Device D Intraluminal Device Z No Device	Z No Qualifier
G Intracranial Artery H Common Carotid Artery, Right J Common Carotid Artery, Left K Internal Carotid Artery, Right L Internal Carotid Artery, Left M External Carotid Artery, Right N External Carotid Artery, Left P Vertebral Artery, Right Q Vertebral Artery, Left	Ø Open 3 Percutaneous 4 Percutaneous Endoscopic	B Intraluminal Device, Bioactive C Extraluminal Device D Intraluminal Device Z No Device	Z No Qualifier

Coding Clinic: 2Ø16, Q2, P3Ø – Ø3LGØCZ
Coding Clinic: 2Ø21, Q2, P13 – Ø3LLØZZ

SECTION: Ø MEDICAL AND SURGICAL
BODY SYSTEM: 3 UPPER ARTERIES
OPERATION: N RELEASE: Freeing a body part from an abnormal physical constraint by cutting or by the use of force

Body Part	Approach	Device	Qualifier
Ø Internal Mammary Artery, Right 1 Internal Mammary Artery, Left 2 Innominate Artery 3 Subclavian Artery, Right 4 Subclavian Artery, Left 5 Axillary Artery, Right 6 Axillary Artery, Left 7 Brachial Artery, Right 8 Brachial Artery, Left 9 Ulnar Artery, Right A Ulnar Artery, Left B Radial Artery, Right C Radial Artery, Left D Hand Artery, Right F Hand Artery, Left G Intracranial Artery H Common Carotid Artery, Right J Common Carotid Artery, Left K Internal Carotid Artery, Right L Internal Carotid Artery, Left M External Carotid Artery, Right N External Carotid Artery, Left P Vertebral Artery, Right Q Vertebral Artery, Left R Face Artery S Temporal Artery, Right T Temporal Artery, Left U Thyroid Artery, Right V Thyroid Artery, Left Y Upper Artery	Ø Open 3 Percutaneous 4 Percutaneous Endoscopic	Z No Device	Z No Qualifier

SECTION: Ø MEDICAL AND SURGICAL
BODY SYSTEM: 3 UPPER ARTERIES
OPERATION: P REMOVAL: Taking out or off a device from a body part

Body Part	Approach	Device	Qualifier
Y Upper Artery	Ø Open 3 Percutaneous 4 Percutaneous Endoscopic	Ø Drainage Device 2 Monitoring Device 3 Infusion Device 7 Autologous Tissue Substitute C Extraluminal Device D Intraluminal Device J Synthetic Substitute K Nonautologous Tissue Substitute M Stimulator Lead Y Other Device	Z No Qualifier
Y Upper Artery	X External	Ø Drainage Device 2 Monitoring Device 3 Infusion Device D Intraluminal Device M Stimulator Lead	Z No Qualifier

Non-OR Ø3PY3[Ø23D]Z

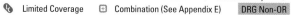

Non-OR Ø3PYX[Ø23DM]Z

SECTION: Ø MEDICAL AND SURGICAL
BODY SYSTEM: 3 UPPER ARTERIES
OPERATION: Q REPAIR: Restoring, to the extent possible, a body part to its normal anatomic structure and function

Body Part	Approach	Device	Qualifier
Ø Internal Mammary Artery, Right 1 Internal Mammary Artery, Left 2 Innominate Artery 3 Subclavian Artery, Right 4 Subclavian Artery, Left 5 Axillary Artery, Right 6 Axillary Artery, Left 7 Brachial Artery, Right 8 Brachial Artery, Left 9 Ulnar Artery, Right A Ulnar Artery, Left B Radial Artery, Right C Radial Artery, Left D Hand Artery, Right F Hand Artery, Left G Intracranial Artery H Common Carotid Artery, Right J Common Carotid Artery, Left K Internal Carotid Artery, Right L Internal Carotid Artery, Left M External Carotid Artery, Right N External Carotid Artery, Left P Vertebral Artery, Right Q Vertebral Artery, Left R Face Artery S Temporal Artery, Right T Temporal Artery, Left U Thyroid Artery, Right V Thyroid Artery, Left Y Upper Artery	Ø Open 3 Percutaneous 4 Percutaneous Endoscopic	Z No Device	Z No Qualifier

Coding Clinic: 2Ø17, Q1, P32 – Ø3QHØZZ

SECTION: Ø MEDICAL AND SURGICAL
BODY SYSTEM: 3 UPPER ARTERIES
OPERATION: R REPLACEMENT: Putting in or on biological or synthetic material that physically takes the place and/or function of all or a portion of a body part

Body Part	Approach	Device	Qualifier
Ø Internal Mammary Artery, Right 1 Internal Mammary Artery, Left 2 Innominate Artery 3 Subclavian Artery, Right 4 Subclavian Artery, Left 5 Axillary Artery, Right 6 Axillary Artery, Left 7 Brachial Artery, Right 8 Brachial Artery, Left 9 Ulnar Artery, Right A Ulnar Artery, Left B Radial Artery, Right C Radial Artery, Left D Hand Artery, Right F Hand Artery, Left G Intracranial Artery H Common Carotid Artery, Right J Common Carotid Artery, Left K Internal Carotid Artery, Right L Internal Carotid Artery, Left M External Carotid Artery, Right N External Carotid Artery, Left P Vertebral Artery, Right Q Vertebral Artery, Left R Face Artery S Temporal Artery, Right T Temporal Artery, Left U Thyroid Artery, Right V Thyroid Artery, Left Y Upper Artery	Ø Open 4 Percutaneous Endoscopic	7 Autologous Tissue Substitute J Synthetic Substitute K Nonautologous Tissue Substitute	Z No Qualifier

SECTION: Ø MEDICAL AND SURGICAL
BODY SYSTEM: 3 UPPER ARTERIES
OPERATION: S REPOSITION: Moving to its normal location, or other suitable location, all or a portion of a body part

Body Part	Approach	Device	Qualifier
Ø Internal Mammary Artery, Right 1 Internal Mammary Artery, Left 2 Innominate Artery 3 Subclavian Artery, Right 4 Subclavian Artery, Left 5 Axillary Artery, Right 6 Axillary Artery, Left 7 Brachial Artery, Right 8 Brachial Artery, Left 9 Ulnar Artery, Right A Ulnar Artery, Left B Radial Artery, Right C Radial Artery, Left D Hand Artery, Right F Hand Artery, Left G Intracranial Artery H Common Carotid Artery, Right J Common Carotid Artery, Left K Internal Carotid Artery, Right L Internal Carotid Artery, Left M External Carotid Artery, Right N External Carotid Artery, Left P Vertebral Artery, Right Q Vertebral Artery, Left R Face Artery S Temporal Artery, Right T Temporal Artery, Left U Thyroid Artery, Right V Thyroid Artery, Left Y Upper Artery	Ø Open 3 Percutaneous 4 Percutaneous Endoscopic	Z No Device	Z No Qualifier

Coding Clinic: 2Ø15, Q3, P28 – Ø3SSØZZ

SECTION: Ø MEDICAL AND SURGICAL
BODY SYSTEM: 3 UPPER ARTERIES
OPERATION: U SUPPLEMENT: Putting in or on biological or synthetic material that physically reinforces and/or augments the function of a portion of a body part

Body Part	Approach	Device	Qualifier
Ø Internal Mammary Artery, Right 1 Internal Mammary Artery, Left 2 Innominate Artery 3 Subclavian Artery, Right 4 Subclavian Artery, Left 5 Axillary Artery, Right 6 Axillary Artery, Left 7 Brachial Artery, Right 8 Brachial Artery, Left 9 Ulnar Artery, Right A Ulnar Artery, Left B Radial Artery, Right C Radial Artery, Left D Hand Artery, Right F Hand Artery, Left G Intracranial Artery H Common Carotid Artery, Right J Common Carotid Artery, Left K Internal Carotid Artery, Right L Internal Carotid Artery, Left M External Carotid Artery, Right N External Carotid Artery, Left P Vertebral Artery, Right Q Vertebral Artery, Left R Face Artery S Temporal Artery, Right T Temporal Artery, Left U Thyroid Artery, Right V Thyroid Artery, Left Y Upper Artery	Ø Open 3 Percutaneous 4 Percutaneous Endoscopic	7 Autologous Tissue Substitute J Synthetic Substitute K Nonautologous Tissue Substitute	Z No Qualifier

Coding Clinic: 2Ø16, Q2, P12 – Ø3UKØJZ

SECTION: Ø MEDICAL AND SURGICAL
BODY SYSTEM: 3 UPPER ARTERIES
OPERATION: V RESTRICTION: Partially closing an orifice or the lumen of a tubular body part

Body Part	Approach	Device	Qualifier
Ø Internal Mammary Artery, Right 1 Internal Mammary Artery, Left 2 Innominate Artery 3 Subclavian Artery, Right 4 Subclavian Artery, Left 5 Axillary Artery, Right 6 Axillary Artery, Left 7 Brachial Artery, Right 8 Brachial Artery, Left 9 Ulnar Artery, Right A Ulnar Artery, Left B Radial Artery, Right C Radial Artery, Left D Hand Artery, Right F Hand Artery, Left R Face Artery S Temporal Artery, Right T Temporal Artery, Left U Thyroid Artery, Right V Thyroid Artery, Left Y Upper Artery	Ø Open 3 Percutaneous 4 Percutaneous Endoscopic	C Extraluminal Device D Intraluminal Device Z No Device	Z No Qualifier
G Intracranial Artery H Common Carotid Artery, Right J Common Carotid Artery, Left K Internal Carotid Artery, Right L Internal Carotid Artery, Left M External Carotid Artery, Right N External Carotid Artery, Left P Vertebral Artery, Right Q Vertebral Artery, Left	Ø Open 3 Percutaneous 4 Percutaneous Endoscopic	B Intraluminal Device, Bioactive C Extraluminal Device D Intraluminal Device H Intraluminal Device, Flow Diverter Z No Device	Z No Qualifier

Coding Clinic: 2Ø16, Q1, P2Ø – Ø3VG3DZ
Coding Clinic: 2Ø16, Q4, P26 – Ø3VM3DZ
Coding Clinic: 2Ø19, Q1, P22 – Ø3VGØCZ
Coding Clinic: 2Ø23, Q1, P35 – Ø3VK3[DH]Z
Coding Clinic: 2Ø23, Q3, P27 – Ø3VG3HZ

SECTION: Ø MEDICAL AND SURGICAL
BODY SYSTEM: 3 UPPER ARTERIES
OPERATION: W REVISION: Correcting, to the extent possible, a portion of a malfunctioning device or the position of a displaced device

Body Part	Approach	Device	Qualifier
Y Upper Artery	Ø Open 3 Percutaneous 4 Percutaneous Endoscopic	Ø Drainage Device 2 Monitoring Device 3 Infusion Device 7 Autologous Tissue Substitute C Extraluminal Device D Intraluminal Device J Synthetic Substitute K Nonautologous Tissue Substitute M Stimulator Lead Y Other Device	Z No Qualifier
Y Upper Artery	X External	Ø Drainage Device 2 Monitoring Device 3 Infusion Device 7 Autologous Tissue Substitute C Extraluminal Device D Intraluminal Device J Synthetic Substitute K Nonautologous Tissue Substitute M Stimulator Lead	Z No Qualifier

Non-OR Ø3WY3[Ø23D]Z
Non-OR Ø3WYX[Ø237CDJKM]Z

Coding Clinic: 2Ø15, Q1, P33 – ØØWY3DZ
Coding Clinic: 2Ø16, Q3, P4Ø – Ø3WYØJZ

Ø4. Lower Arteries 108
Ø41. Bypass....................109
Ø45. Destruction....................11Ø
Ø47. Dilation....................111
Ø49. Drainage 114
Ø4B. Excision 116
Ø4C. Extirpation 117
Ø4F. Fragmentation....................118
Ø4H. Insertion....................119
Ø4J. Inspection 12Ø
Ø4L. Occlusion 121
Ø4N. Release 122
Ø4P. Removal 123
Ø4Q. Repair 123
Ø4R. Replacement 124
Ø4S. Reposition....................125
Ø4U. Supplement....................126
Ø4V. Restriction....................127
Ø4W. Revision....................128

SECTION: Ø MEDICAL AND SURGICAL
BODY SYSTEM: 4 LOWER ARTERIES
OPERATION: 1 BYPASS: *(on multiple pages)*

Altering the route of passage of the contents of a tubular body part

Body Part	Approach	Device	Qualifier
Ø Abdominal Aorta C Common Iliac Artery, Right D Common Iliac Artery, Left	Ø Open 4 Percutaneous Endoscopic	9 Autologous Venous Tissue A Autologous Arterial Tissue J Synthetic Substitute K Nonautologous Tissue Substitute Z No Device	Ø Abdominal Aorta 1 Celiac Artery 2 Mesenteric Artery 3 Renal Artery, Right 4 Renal Artery, Left 5 Renal Artery, Bilateral 6 Common Iliac Artery, Right 7 Common Iliac Artery, Left 8 Common Iliac Arteries, Bilateral 9 Internal Iliac Artery, Right B Internal Iliac Artery, Left C Internal Iliac Arteries, Bilateral D External Iliac Artery, Right F External Iliac Artery, Left G External Iliac Arteries, Bilateral H Femoral Artery, Right J Femoral Artery, Left K Femoral Arteries, Bilateral Q Lower Extremity Artery R Lower Artery
3 Hepatic Artery 4 Splenic Artery	Ø Open 4 Percutaneous Endoscopic	9 Autologous Venous Tissue A Autologous Arterial Tissue J Synthetic Substitute K Nonautologous Tissue Substitute Z No Device	3 Renal Artery, Right 4 Renal Artery, Left 5 Renal Artery, Bilateral R Lower Artery
E Internal Iliac Artery, Right F Internal Iliac Artery, Left H External Iliac Artery, Right J External Iliac Artery, Left	Ø Open 4 Percutaneous Endoscopic	9 Autologous Venous Tissue A Autologous Arterial Tissue J Synthetic Substitute K Nonautologous Tissue Substitute Z No Device	9 Internal Iliac Artery, Right B Internal Iliac Artery, Left C Internal Iliac Arteries, Bilateral D External Iliac Artery, Right F External Iliac Artery, Left G External Iliac Arteries, Bilateral H Femoral Artery, Right J Femoral Artery, Left K Femoral Arteries, Bilateral P Foot Artery Q Lower Extremity Artery
K Femoral Artery, Right L Femoral Artery, Left	Ø Open 4 Percutaneous Endoscopic	9 Autologous Venous Tissue A Autologous Arterial Tissue J Synthetic Substitute K Nonautologous Tissue Substitute Z No Device	H Femoral Artery, Right J Femoral Artery, Left K Femoral Arteries, Bilateral L Popliteal Artery M Peroneal Artery N Posterior Tibial Artery P Foot Artery Q Lower Extremity Artery S Lower Extremity Vein
K Femoral Artery, Right L Femoral Artery, Left	3 Percutaneous	J Synthetic Substitute	Q Lower Extremity Artery S Lower Extremity Vein
M Popliteal Artery, Right N Popliteal Artery, Left	Ø Open 4 Percutaneous Endoscopic	9 Autologous Venous Tissue A Autologous Arterial Tissue J Synthetic Substitute K Nonautologous Tissue Substitute Z No Device	L Popliteal Artery M Peroneal Artery P Foot Artery Q Lower Extremity Artery S Lower Extremity Vein

Coding Clinic: 2Ø15, Q3, P28 – Ø41ØØZ3, Ø414ØZ4
Coding Clinic: 2Ø16, Q2, P19 – Ø41KØJN
Coding Clinic: 2Ø17, Q3, P6 – Ø41KØ9N, Ø41KØJN
Coding Clinic: 2Ø17, Q3, P16 – Ø41CØJ[25]
Coding Clinic: 2Ø17, Q4, P47 – Ø41[34]ØZ[34]
Coding Clinic: 2Ø22, Q3, P6 – Ø41ØØJH

SECTION: Ø MEDICAL AND SURGICAL
BODY SYSTEM: 4 LOWER ARTERIES
OPERATION: 1 BYPASS: *(continued)*
Altering the route of passage of the contents of a tubular body part

Body Part	Approach	Device	Qualifier
M Popliteal Artery, Right N Popliteal Artery, Left	3 Percutaneous	J Synthetic Substitute	Q Lower Extremity Artery S Lower Extremity Vein
P Anterior Tibial Artery, Right Q Anterior Tibial Artery, Left R Posterior Tibial Artery, Right S Posterior Tibial Artery, Left	Ø Open 3 Percutaneous 4 Percutaneous Endoscopic	J Synthetic Substitute	Q Lower Extremity Artery S Lower Extremity Vein
T Peroneal Artery, Right U Peroneal Artery, Left V Foot Artery, Right W Foot Artery, Left	Ø Open 4 Percutaneous Endoscopic	9 Autologous Venous Tissue A Autologous Arterial Tissue J Synthetic Substitute K Nonautologous Tissue Substitute Z No Device	P Foot Artery Q Lower Extremity Artery S Lower Extremity Vein
T Peroneal Artery, Right U Peroneal Artery, Left V Foot Artery, Right W Foot Artery, Left	3 Percutaneous	J Synthetic Substitute	Q Lower Extremity Artery S Lower Extremity Vein

Coding Clinic: 2Ø17, Q1, P33 – Ø41MØ9P

SECTION: Ø MEDICAL AND SURGICAL
BODY SYSTEM: 4 LOWER ARTERIES
OPERATION: 5 DESTRUCTION: Physical eradication of all or a portion of a body part by the direct use of energy, force, or a destructive agent

Body Part	Approach	Device	Qualifier
Ø Abdominal Aorta 1 Celiac Artery 2 Gastric Artery 3 Hepatic Artery 4 Splenic Artery 5 Superior Mesenteric Artery 6 Colic Artery, Right 7 Colic Artery, Left 8 Colic Artery, Middle 9 Renal Artery, Right A Renal Artery, Left B Inferior Mesenteric Artery C Common Iliac Artery, Right D Common Iliac Artery, Left E Internal Iliac Artery, Right F Internal Iliac Artery, Left H External Iliac Artery, Right J External Iliac Artery, Left K Femoral Artery, Right L Femoral Artery, Left M Popliteal Artery, Right N Popliteal Artery, Left P Anterior Tibial Artery, Right Q Anterior Tibial Artery, Left R Posterior Tibial Artery, Right S Posterior Tibial Artery, Left T Peroneal Artery, Right U Peroneal Artery, Left V Foot Artery, Right W Foot Artery, Left Y Lower Artery	Ø Open 3 Percutaneous 4 Percutaneous Endoscopic	Z No Device	Z No Qualifier

SECTION: Ø MEDICAL AND SURGICAL
BODY SYSTEM: 4 LOWER ARTERIES
OPERATION: 7 DILATION: *(on multiple pages)*
Expanding an orifice or the lumen of a tubular body part

Body Part	Approach	Device	Qualifier
Ø Abdominal Aorta 1 Celiac Artery 2 Gastric Artery 3 Hepatic Artery 4 Splenic Artery 5 Superior Mesenteric Artery 6 Colic Artery, Right 7 Colic Artery, Left 8 Colic Artery, Middle 9 Renal Artery, Right A Renal Artery, Left B Inferior Mesenteric Artery C Common Iliac Artery, Right D Common Iliac Artery, Left E Internal Iliac Artery, Right F Internal Iliac Artery, Left H External Iliac Artery, Right J External Iliac Artery, Left ~~K Femoral Carotid Artery, Right~~ ~~L Femoral Carotid Artery, Left~~ ~~M Popliteal Carotid Artery, Right~~ ~~N Popliteal Carotid Artery, Left~~ ~~P Anterior Tibial Artery, Right~~ ~~Q Anterior Tibial Artery, Left~~ ~~R Posterior Tibial Artery, Right~~ ~~S Posterior Tibial Artery, Left~~ ~~T Peroneal Artery, Right~~ ~~U Peroneal Artery, Left~~ V Foot Artery, Right W Foot Artery, Left Y Lower Artery	Ø Open 3 Percutaneous 4 Percutaneous Endoscopic	4 Intraluminal Device, Drug-eluting D Intraluminal Device Z No Device	1 Drug-Coated Balloon Z No Qualifier

Non-OR Ø47[59A]4DZ

Coding Clinic: 2Ø16, Q3, P39 – Ø47C3DZ
Coding Clinic: 2Ø16, Q4, P87 – Ø47

SECTION: Ø MEDICAL AND SURGICAL
BODY SYSTEM: 4 LOWER ARTERIES
OPERATION: 7 DILATION: *(continued)*
Expanding an orifice or the lumen of a tubular body part

Body Part	Approach	Device	Qualifier
Ø Abdominal Aorta 1 Celiac Artery 2 Gastric Artery 3 Hepatic Artery 4 Splenic Artery 5 Superior Mesenteric Artery 6 Colic Artery, Right 7 Colic Artery, Left 8 Colic Artery, Middle 9 Renal Artery, Right A Renal Artery, Left B Inferior Mesenteric Artery C Common Iliac Artery, Right D Common Iliac Artery, Left E Internal Iliac Artery, Right F Internal Iliac Artery, Left H External Iliac Artery, Right J External Iliac Artery, Left ~~K Femoral Carotid Artery, Right~~ ~~L Femoral Carotid Artery, Left~~ ~~M Popliteal Carotid Artery, Right~~ ~~N Popliteal Carotid Artery, Left~~ ~~P Anterior Tibial Artery, Right~~ ~~Q Anterior Tibial Artery, Left~~ ~~R Posterior Tibial Artery, Right~~ ~~S Posterior Tibial Artery, Left~~ ~~T Peroneal Artery, Right~~ ~~U Peroneal Artery, Left~~ V Foot Artery, Right W Foot Artery, Left Y Lower Artery	Ø Open 3 Percutaneous 4 Percutaneous Endoscopic	5 Intraluminal Device, Drug-eluting, Two 6 Intraluminal Device, Drug-eluting, Three 7 Intraluminal Device, Drug-eluting, Four or More E Intraluminal Device, Two F Intraluminal Device, Three G Intraluminal Device, Four or More	Z No Qualifier
K Femoral Artery, Right L Femoral Artery, Left M Popliteal Artery, Right N Popliteal Artery, Left P Anterior Tibial Artery, Right Q Anterior Tibial Artery, Left R Posterior Tibial Artery, Right S Posterior Tibial Artery, Left T Peroneal Artery, Right U Peroneal Artery, Left	Ø Open 4 Percutaneous Endoscopic	4 Intraluminal Device, Drug-eluting D Intraluminal Device Z No Device	1 Drug-Coated Balloon Z No Qualifier
K Femoral Artery, Right L Femoral Artery, Left M Popliteal Artery, Right N Popliteal Artery, Left P Anterior Tibial Artery, Right Q Anterior Tibial Artery, Left R Posterior Tibial Artery, Right S Posterior Tibial Artery, Left T Peroneal Artery, Right U Peroneal Artery, Left	Ø Open 4 Percutaneous Endoscopic	5 Intraluminal Device, Drug-eluting, Two 6 Intraluminal Device, Drug-eluting, Three 7 Intraluminal Device, Drug-eluting, Four or More E Intraluminal Device, Two F Intraluminal Device, Three G Intraluminal Device, Four or More	Z No Qualifier

New/Revised Text in Green ~~deleted~~ Deleted ♀ Females Only ♂ Males Only Coding Clinic
Non-covered Limited Coverage ⊞ Combination (See Appendix E) DRG Non-OR Non-OR Hospital-Acquired Condition

SECTION: Ø MEDICAL AND SURGICAL
BODY SYSTEM: 4 LOWER ARTERIES
OPERATION: 7 DILATION: *(continued)*
Expanding an orifice or the lumen of a tubular body part

Body Part	Approach	Device	Qualifier
K Femoral Artery, Right L Femoral Artery, Left M Popliteal Artery, Right N Popliteal Artery, Left P Anterior Tibial Artery, Right Q Anterior Tibial Artery, Left R Posterior Tibial Artery, Right S Posterior Tibial Artery, Left T Peroneal Artery, Right U Peroneal Artery, Left	3 Percutaneous	4 Intraluminal Device, Drug-eluting	1 Drug-Coated Balloon 2 Sustained Release Z No Qualifier
K Femoral Artery, Right L Femoral Artery, Left M Popliteal Artery, Right N Popliteal Artery, Left P Anterior Tibial Artery, Right Q Anterior Tibial Artery, Left R Posterior Tibial Artery, Right S Posterior Tibial Artery, Left T Peroneal Artery, Right U Peroneal Artery, Left	3 Percutaneous	5 Intraluminal Device, Drug-eluting, Two 6 Intraluminal Device, Drug-eluting, Three 7 Intraluminal Device, Drug-eluting, Four or More	2 Sustained Release Z No Qualifier
K Femoral Artery, Right L Femoral Artery, Left M Popliteal Artery, Right N Popliteal Artery, Left P Anterior Tibial Artery, Right Q Anterior Tibial Artery, Left R Posterior Tibial Artery, Right S Posterior Tibial Artery, Left T Peroneal Artery, Right U Peroneal Artery, Left	3 Percutaneous	D Intraluminal Device Z No Device	1 Drug-Coated Balloon Z No Qualifier
K Femoral Artery, Right L Femoral Artery, Left M Popliteal Artery, Right N Popliteal Artery, Left P Anterior Tibial Artery, Right Q Anterior Tibial Artery, Left R Posterior Tibial Artery, Right S Posterior Tibial Artery, Left T Peroneal Artery, Right U Peroneal Artery, Left	3 Percutaneous	E Intraluminal Device, Two F Intraluminal Device, Three G Intraluminal Device, Four or More	Z No Qualifier

Coding Clinic: 2Ø15, Q4, P7 – Ø47K3D1
Coding Clinic: 2Ø15, Q4, P15 – Ø47K3D1, Ø47L3Z1
Coding Clinic: 2Ø16, Q4, P89 – Ø47K3Z6

SECTION: Ø MEDICAL AND SURGICAL
BODY SYSTEM: 4 LOWER ARTERIES
OPERATION: 9 DRAINAGE: *(on multiple pages)*
Taking or letting out fluids and/or gases from a body part

Body Part	Approach	Device	Qualifier
Ø Abdominal Aorta 1 Celiac Artery 2 Gastric Artery 3 Hepatic Artery 4 Splenic Artery 5 Superior Mesenteric Artery 6 Colic Artery, Right 7 Colic Artery, Left 8 Colic Artery, Middle 9 Renal Artery, Right A Renal Artery, Left B Inferior Mesenteric Artery C Common Iliac Artery, Right D Common Iliac Artery, Left E Internal Iliac Artery, Right F Internal Iliac Artery, Left H External Iliac Artery, Right J External Iliac Artery, Left K Femoral Artery, Right L Femoral Artery, Left M Popliteal Artery, Right N Popliteal Artery, Left P Anterior Tibial Artery, Right Q Anterior Tibial Artery, Left R Posterior Tibial Artery, Right S Posterior Tibial Artery, Left T Peroneal Artery, Right U Peroneal Artery, Left V Foot Artery, Right W Foot Artery, Left Y Lower Artery	Ø Open 3 Percutaneous 4 Percutaneous Endoscopic	Ø Drainage Device	Z No Qualifier

Non-OR Ø49[Ø123456789ABCDEFHJKLMNPQRSTUVWY][Ø34]ØZ

SECTION: Ø MEDICAL AND SURGICAL

BODY SYSTEM: 4 LOWER ARTERIES

OPERATION: 9 DRAINAGE: *(continued)*

Taking or letting out fluids and/or gases from a body part

Body Part	Approach	Device	Qualifier
Ø Abdominal Aorta 1 Celiac Artery 2 Gastric Artery 3 Hepatic Artery 4 Splenic Artery 5 Superior Mesenteric Artery 6 Colic Artery, Right 7 Colic Artery, Left 8 Colic Artery, Middle 9 Renal Artery, Right A Renal Artery, Left B Inferior Mesenteric Artery C Common Iliac Artery, Right D Common Iliac Artery, Left E Internal Iliac Artery, Right F Internal Iliac Artery, Left H External Iliac Artery, Right J External Iliac Artery, Left K Femoral Artery, Right L Femoral Artery, Left M Popliteal Artery, Right N Popliteal Artery, Left P Anterior Tibial Artery, Right Q Anterior Tibial Artery, Left R Posterior Tibial Artery, Right S Posterior Tibial Artery, Left T Peroneal Artery, Right U Peroneal Artery, Left V Foot Artery, Right W Foot Artery, Left Y Lower Artery	Ø Open 3 Percutaneous 4 Percutaneous Endoscopic	Z No Device	X Diagnostic Z No Qualifier

Non-OR Ø49[Ø123456789ABCDEFHJKLMNPQRSTUVWY][Ø34]Z[XZ]

SECTION: Ø MEDICAL AND SURGICAL
BODY SYSTEM: 4 LOWER ARTERIES
OPERATION: B EXCISION: Cutting out or off, without replacement, a portion of a body part

Body Part	Approach	Device	Qualifier
Ø Abdominal Aorta 1 Celiac Artery 2 Gastric Artery 3 Hepatic Artery 4 Splenic Artery 5 Superior Mesenteric Artery 6 Colic Artery, Right 7 Colic Artery, Left 8 Colic Artery, Middle 9 Renal Artery, Right A Renal Artery, Left B Inferior Mesenteric Artery C Common Iliac Artery, Right D Common Iliac Artery, Left E Internal Iliac Artery, Right F Internal Iliac Artery, Left H External Iliac Artery, Right J External Iliac Artery, Left K Femoral Artery, Right L Femoral Artery, Left M Popliteal Artery, Right N Popliteal Artery, Left P Anterior Tibial Artery, Right Q Anterior Tibial Artery, Left R Posterior Tibial Artery, Right S Posterior Tibial Artery, Left T Peroneal Artery, Right U Peroneal Artery, Left V Foot Artery, Right W Foot Artery, Left Y Lower Artery	Ø Open 3 Percutaneous 4 Percutaneous Endoscopic	Z No Device	X Diagnostic Z No Qualifier

SECTION: Ø MEDICAL AND SURGICAL
BODY SYSTEM: 4 LOWER ARTERIES
OPERATION: C EXTIRPATION: Taking or cutting out solid matter from a body part

Body Part	Approach	Device	Qualifier
Ø Abdominal Aorta 1 Celiac Artery 2 Gastric Artery 3 Hepatic Artery 4 Splenic Artery 5 Superior Mesenteric Artery 6 Colic Artery, Right 7 Colic Artery, Left 8 Colic Artery, Middle 9 Renal Artery, Right A Renal Artery, Left B Inferior Mesenteric Artery C Common Iliac Artery, Right D Common Iliac Artery, Left E Internal Iliac Artery, Right F Internal Iliac Artery, Left H External Iliac Artery, Right J External Iliac Artery, Left K Femoral Artery, Right L Femoral Artery, Left M Popliteal Artery, Right N Popliteal Artery, Left P Anterior Tibial Artery, Right Q Anterior Tibial Artery, Left R Posterior Tibial Artery, Right S Posterior Tibial Artery, Left T Peroneal Artery, Right U Peroneal Artery, Left V Foot Artery, Right W Foot Artery, Left Y Lower Artery	Ø Open 3 Percutaneous 4 Percutaneous Endoscopic	Z No Device	Z No Qualifier

Coding Clinic: 2015, Q1, P36 – Ø4CL3ZZ
Coding Clinic: 2021, Q1, P15; 2016, Q1, P31 – Ø4CJØZZ
Coding Clinic: 2016, Q4, P89 – Ø4CK3Z6
Coding Clinic: 2021, Q1, P16 – Ø4CHØZZ

SECTION: Ø MEDICAL AND SURGICAL
BODY SYSTEM: 4 LOWER ARTERIES
OPERATION: F FRAGMENTATION: Breaking solid matter in a body part into pieces

Body Part	Approach	Device	Qualifier
C Common Iliac Artery, Right D Common Iliac Artery, Left E Internal Iliac Artery, Right F Internal Iliac Artery, Left H External Iliac Artery, Right J External Iliac Artery, Left K Femoral Artery, Right L Femoral Artery, Left M Popliteal Artery, Right N Popliteal Artery, Left P Anterior Tibial Artery, Right Q Anterior Tibial Artery, Left R Posterior Tibial Artery, Right S Posterior Tibial Artery, Left T Peroneal Artery, Right U Peroneal Artery, Left Y Lower Artery	3 Percutaneous	Z No Device	Ø Ultrasonic Z No Qualifier

SECTION: Ø MEDICAL AND SURGICAL
BODY SYSTEM: 4 LOWER ARTERIES
OPERATION: H INSERTION: Putting in a nonbiological appliance that monitors, assists, performs, or prevents a physiological function but does not physically take the place of a body part

Body Part	Approach	Device	Qualifier
Ø Abdominal Aorta	Ø Open 3 Percutaneous 4 Percutaneous Endoscopic	2 Monitoring Device 3 Infusion Device D Intraluminal Device	Z No Qualifier
1 Celiac Artery 2 Gastric Artery 3 Hepatic Artery 4 Splenic Artery 5 Superior Mesenteric Artery 6 Colic Artery, Right 7 Colic Artery, Left 8 Colic Artery, Middle 9 Renal Artery, Right A Renal Artery, Left B Inferior Mesenteric Artery C Common Iliac Artery, Right D Common Iliac Artery, Left E Internal Iliac Artery, Right F Internal Iliac Artery, Left H External Iliac Artery, Right J External Iliac Artery, Left K Femoral Artery, Right L Femoral Artery, Left M Popliteal Artery, Right N Popliteal Artery, Left P Anterior Tibial Artery, Right Q Anterior Tibial Artery, Left R Posterior Tibial Artery, Right S Posterior Tibial Artery, Left T Peroneal Artery, Right U Peroneal Artery, Left V Foot Artery, Right W Foot Artery, Left	Ø Open 3 Percutaneous 4 Percutaneous Endoscopic	3 Infusion Device D Intraluminal Device	Z No Qualifier
Y Lower Artery	Ø Open 3 Percutaneous 4 Percutaneous Endoscopic	2 Monitoring Device 3 Infusion Device D Intraluminal Device Y Other Device	Z No Qualifier

DRG Non-OR Ø4HY32Z
Non-OR Ø4HØ[Ø34][23]Z
Non-OR Ø4H[123456789ABCDEFHJKLMNPQRSTUVW][Ø34]3Z
Non-OR Ø4HY[Ø34]3Z

Coding Clinic: 2Ø17, Q1, P21 – Ø4HY32Z
Coding Clinic: 2Ø19, Q1, P23 – Ø4H1[59A]3DZ
Coding Clinic: 2Ø19, Q3, P21 – Ø4HY33Z
Coding Clinic: 2Ø22, Q3, P2Ø – Ø4HØ3DZ

SECTION: Ø MEDICAL AND SURGICAL
BODY SYSTEM: 4 LOWER ARTERIES
OPERATION: J INSPECTION: Visually and/or manually exploring a body part

Body Part	Approach	Device	Qualifier
Y Lower Artery	Ø Open 3 Percutaneous 4 Percutaneous Endoscopic X External	Z No Device	Z No Qualifier

Non-OR Ø4JY[34X]ZZ

Coding Clinic: 2Ø22, Q4, P56 – Ø4JY3ZZ

SECTION: Ø MEDICAL AND SURGICAL
BODY SYSTEM: 4 LOWER ARTERIES
OPERATION: L OCCLUSION: Completely closing an orifice or the lumen of a tubular body part

Body Part	Approach	Device	Qualifier
Ø Abdominal Aorta	4 Percutaneous Endoscopic	C Extraluminal Device D Intraluminal Device Z No Device	Z No Qualifier
Ø Abdominal Aorta	Ø Open 3 Percutaneous	C Extraluminal Device Z No Device	Z No Qualifier
Ø Abdominal Aorta	Ø Open 3 Percutaneous	D Intraluminal Device	J Temporary Z No Qualifier
1 Celiac Artery 2 Gastric Artery 3 Hepatic Artery 4 Splenic Artery 5 Superior Mesenteric Artery 6 Colic Artery, Right 7 Colic Artery, Left 8 Colic Artery, Middle 9 Renal Artery, Right A Renal Artery, Left B Inferior Mesenteric Artery C Common Iliac Artery, Right D Common Iliac Artery, Left H External Iliac Artery, Right J External Iliac Artery, Left K Femoral Artery, Right L Femoral Artery, Left M Popliteal Artery, Right N Popliteal Artery, Left P Anterior Tibial Artery, Right Q Anterior Tibial Artery, Left R Posterior Tibial Artery, Right S Posterior Tibial Artery, Left T Peroneal Artery, Right U Peroneal Artery, Left V Foot Artery, Right W Foot Artery, Left Y Lower Artery	Ø Open 3 Percutaneous 4 Percutaneous Endoscopic	C Extraluminal Device D Intraluminal Device Z No Device	Z No Qualifier
E Internal Iliac Artery, Right	Ø Open 3 Percutaneous 4 Percutaneous Endoscopic	C Extraluminal Device D Intraluminal Device Z No Device	T Uterine Artery, Right ♀ V Prostatic Artery, Right ♂ Z No Qualifier
F Internal Iliac Artery, Left	Ø Open 3 Percutaneous 4 Percutaneous Endoscopic	C Extraluminal Device D Intraluminal Device Z No Device	U Uterine Artery, Left ♀ W Prostatic Artery, Left ♂ Z No Qualifier

Non-OR Ø4L23DZ
Non-OR Ø4L[EF][CDZ]V

Coding Clinic: 2Ø15, Q2, P27 – Ø4LE3DT
Coding Clinic: 2Ø18, Q2, P18 – Ø4L[HJ]ØCZ
Coding Clinic: 2Ø22, Q4, P56 – Ø4LE3DV

SECTION: Ø MEDICAL AND SURGICAL
BODY SYSTEM: 4 LOWER ARTERIES
OPERATION: N RELEASE: Freeing a body part from an abnormal physical constraint by cutting or by the use of force

Body Part	Approach	Device	Qualifier
Ø Abdominal Aorta 1 Celiac Artery 2 Gastric Artery 3 Hepatic Artery 4 Splenic Artery 5 Superior Mesenteric Artery 6 Colic Artery, Right 7 Colic Artery, Left 8 Colic Artery, Middle 9 Renal Artery, Right A Renal Artery, Left B Inferior Mesenteric Artery C Common Iliac Artery, Right D Common Iliac Artery, Left E Internal Iliac Artery, Right F Internal Iliac Artery, Left H External Iliac Artery, Right J External Iliac Artery, Left K Femoral Artery, Right L Femoral Artery, Left M Popliteal Artery, Right N Popliteal Artery, Left P Anterior Tibial Artery, Right Q Anterior Tibial Artery, Left R Posterior Tibial Artery, Right S Posterior Tibial Artery, Left T Peroneal Artery, Right U Peroneal Artery, Left V Foot Artery, Right W Foot Artery, Left Y Lower Artery	Ø Open 3 Percutaneous 4 Percutaneous Endoscopic	Z No Device	Z No Qualifier

Coding Clinic: 2Ø15, Q2, P28 – Ø4N1ØZZ

SECTION: Ø MEDICAL AND SURGICAL
BODY SYSTEM: 4 LOWER ARTERIES
OPERATION: P REMOVAL: Taking out or off a device from a body part

Body Part	Approach	Device	Qualifier
Y Lower Artery	Ø Open 3 Percutaneous 4 Percutaneous Endoscopic	Ø Drainage Device 2 Monitoring Device 3 Infusion Device 7 Autologous Tissue Substitute C Extraluminal Device D Intraluminal Device J Synthetic Substitute K Nonautologous Tissue Substitute Y Other Device	Z No Qualifier
Y Lower Artery	X External	Ø Drainage Device 1 Radioactive Element 2 Monitoring Device 3 Infusion Device D Intraluminal Device	Z No Qualifier

Non-OR Ø4PYX[Ø123D]Z

Coding Clinic: 2019, Q3, P21 – Ø4PY33Z

SECTION: Ø MEDICAL AND SURGICAL
BODY SYSTEM: 4 LOWER ARTERIES
OPERATION: Q REPAIR: Restoring, to the extent possible, a body part to its normal anatomic structure and function

Body Part	Approach	Device	Qualifier
Ø Abdominal Aorta 1 Celiac Artery 2 Gastric Artery 3 Hepatic Artery 4 Splenic Artery 5 Superior Mesenteric Artery 6 Colic Artery, Right 7 Colic Artery, Left 8 Colic Artery, Middle 9 Renal Artery, Right A Renal Artery, Left B Inferior Mesenteric Artery C Common Iliac Artery, Right D Common Iliac Artery, Left E Internal Iliac Artery, Right F Internal Iliac Artery, Left H External Iliac Artery, Right J External Iliac Artery, Left K Femoral Artery, Right L Femoral Artery, Left M Popliteal Artery, Right N Popliteal Artery, Left P Anterior Tibial Artery, Right Q Anterior Tibial Artery, Left R Posterior Tibial Artery, Right S Posterior Tibial Artery, Left T Peroneal Artery, Right U Peroneal Artery, Left V Foot Artery, Right W Foot Artery, Left Y Lower Artery	Ø Open 3 Percutaneous 4 Percutaneous Endoscopic	Z No Device	Z No Qualifier

Coding Clinic: 2023, Q3, P28 – Ø4QØ3ZZ

SECTION: Ø MEDICAL AND SURGICAL
BODY SYSTEM: 4 LOWER ARTERIES
OPERATION: R REPLACEMENT: Putting in or on biological or synthetic material that physically takes the place and/or function of all or a portion of a body part

Body Part	Approach	Device	Qualifier
Ø Abdominal Aorta 1 Celiac Artery 2 Gastric Artery 3 Hepatic Artery 4 Splenic Artery 5 Superior Mesenteric Artery 6 Colic Artery, Right 7 Colic Artery, Left 8 Colic Artery, Middle 9 Renal Artery, Right A Renal Artery, Left B Inferior Mesenteric Artery C Common Iliac Artery, Right D Common Iliac Artery, Left E Internal Iliac Artery, Right F Internal Iliac Artery, Left H External Iliac Artery, Right J External Iliac Artery, Left K Femoral Artery, Right L Femoral Artery, Left M Popliteal Artery, Right N Popliteal Artery, Left P Anterior Tibial Artery, Right Q Anterior Tibial Artery, Left R Posterior Tibial Artery, Right S Posterior Tibial Artery, Left T Peroneal Artery, Right U Peroneal Artery, Left V Foot Artery, Right W Foot Artery, Left Y Lower Artery	Ø Open 4 Percutaneous Endoscopic	7 Autologous Tissue Substitute J Synthetic Substitute K Nonautologous Tissue Substitute	Z No Qualifier

Coding Clinic: 2Ø15, Q2, P28 – Ø4R1ØJZ
Coding Clinic: 2Ø22, Q3, P5 – Ø4R[ØD]ØJZ

SECTION: Ø MEDICAL AND SURGICAL
BODY SYSTEM: 4 LOWER ARTERIES
OPERATION: S REPOSITION: Moving to its normal location, or other suitable location, all or a portion of a body part

Body Part	Approach	Device	Qualifier
Ø Abdominal Aorta 1 Celiac Artery 2 Gastric Artery 3 Hepatic Artery 4 Splenic Artery 5 Superior Mesenteric Artery 6 Colic Artery, Right 7 Colic Artery, Left 8 Colic Artery, Middle 9 Renal Artery, Right A Renal Artery, Left B Inferior Mesenteric Artery C Common Iliac Artery, Right D Common Iliac Artery, Left E Internal Iliac Artery, Right F Internal Iliac Artery, Left H External Iliac Artery, Right J External Iliac Artery, Left K Femoral Artery, Right L Femoral Artery, Left M Popliteal Artery, Right N Popliteal Artery, Left P Anterior Tibial Artery, Right Q Anterior Tibial Artery, Left R Posterior Tibial Artery, Right S Posterior Tibial Artery, Left T Peroneal Artery, Right U Peroneal Artery, Left V Foot Artery, Right W Foot Artery, Left Y Lower Artery	Ø Open 3 Percutaneous 4 Percutaneous Endoscopic	Z No Device	Z No Qualifier

SECTION: Ø MEDICAL AND SURGICAL
BODY SYSTEM: 4 LOWER ARTERIES
OPERATION: U SUPPLEMENT: Putting in or on biological or synthetic material that physically reinforces and/or augments the function of a portion of a body part

Body Part	Approach	Device	Qualifier
Ø Abdominal Aorta 1 Celiac Artery 2 Gastric Artery 3 Hepatic Artery 4 Splenic Artery 5 Superior Mesenteric Artery 6 Colic Artery, Right 7 Colic Artery, Left 8 Colic Artery, Middle 9 Renal Artery, Right A Renal Artery, Left B Inferior Mesenteric Artery C Common Iliac Artery, Right D Common Iliac Artery, Left E Internal Iliac Artery, Right F Internal Iliac Artery, Left H External Iliac Artery, Right J External Iliac Artery, Left K Femoral Artery, Right L Femoral Artery, Left M Popliteal Artery, Right N Popliteal Artery, Left P Anterior Tibial Artery, Right Q Anterior Tibial Artery, Left R Posterior Tibial Artery, Right S Posterior Tibial Artery, Left T Peroneal Artery, Right U Peroneal Artery, Left V Foot Artery, Right W Foot Artery, Left Y Lower Artery	Ø Open 3 Percutaneous 4 Percutaneous Endoscopic	7 Autologous Tissue Substitute J Synthetic Substitute K Nonautologous Tissue Substitute	Z No Qualifier

Coding Clinic: 2Ø16, Q1, P31 – Ø4UJØKZ
Coding Clinic: 2Ø16, Q2, P19 – Ø4URØ7Z
Coding Clinic: 2Ø23, Q3, P26 – Ø4UL3JZ

SECTION: Ø MEDICAL AND SURGICAL
BODY SYSTEM: 4 LOWER ARTERIES
OPERATION: V RESTRICTION: Partially closing an orifice or the lumen of a tubular body part

Body Part	Approach	Device	Qualifier
Ø Abdominal Aorta	Ø Open 3 Percutaneous 4 Percutaneous Endoscopic	C Extraluminal Device E Intraluminal Device, Branched or Fenestrated, One or Two Arteries F Intraluminal Device, Branched or Fenestrated, Three or More Arteries Z No Device	Z No Qualifier
Ø Abdominal Aorta	Ø Open 3 Percutaneous 4 Percutaneous Endoscopic	D Intraluminal Device	J Temporary Z No Qualifier
1 Celiac Artery 2 Gastric Artery 3 Hepatic Artery 4 Splenic Artery 5 Superior Mesenteric Artery 6 Colic Artery, Right 7 Colic Artery, Left 8 Colic Artery, Middle 9 Renal Artery, Right A Renal Artery, Left B Inferior Mesenteric Artery E Internal Iliac Artery, Right F Internal Iliac Artery, Left H External Iliac Artery, Right J External Iliac Artery, Left K Femoral Artery, Right L Femoral Artery, Left M Popliteal Artery, Right N Popliteal Artery, Left P Anterior Tibial Artery, Right Q Anterior Tibial Artery, Left R Posterior Tibial Artery, Right S Posterior Tibial Artery, Left T Peroneal Artery, Right U Peroneal Artery, Left V Foot Artery, Right W Foot Artery, Left Y Lower Artery	Ø Open 3 Percutaneous 4 Percutaneous Endoscopic	C Extraluminal Device D Intraluminal Device Z No Device	Z No Qualifier
C Common Iliac Artery, Right D Common Iliac Artery, Left	Ø Open 3 Percutaneous 4 Percutaneous Endoscopic	C Extraluminal Device D Intraluminal Device E Intraluminal Device, Branched or Fenestrated, One or Two Arteries F Intraluminal Device, Branched or Fenestrated, Three or More Arteries Z No Device	Z No Qualifier

Non-OR Ø4V[CDY][Ø34][Ø23F]Z

Coding Clinic: 2Ø16, Q3, P39 – Ø4VØ3DZ
Coding Clinic: 2Ø16, Q4, P87, 89-9Ø – Ø4V
Coding Clinic: 2Ø16, Q4, P91 – Ø4VØ3E6
Coding Clinic: 2Ø16, Q4, P93-94 – Ø4VØ3F6
Coding Clinic: 2Ø16, Q4, P94 – Ø4V[CD]3EZ
Coding Clinic: 2Ø19, Q1, P22 – Ø4VØØDZ
Coding Clinic: 2Ø21, Q3, P23 – Ø4V43DZ

SECTION: Ø MEDICAL AND SURGICAL
BODY SYSTEM: 4 LOWER ARTERIES
OPERATION: W REVISION: Correcting, to the extent possible, a portion of a malfunctioning device or the position of a displaced device

Body Part	Approach	Device	Qualifier
Y Lower Artery	Ø Open 3 Percutaneous 4 Percutaneous Endoscopic	Ø Drainage Device 2 Monitoring Device 3 Infusion Device 7 Autologous Tissue Substitute C Extraluminal Device D Intraluminal Device J Synthetic Substitute K Nonautologous Tissue Substitute Y Other Device	Z No Qualifier
Y Lower Artery	X External	Ø Drainage Device 2 Monitoring Device 3 Infusion Device 7 Autologous Tissue Substitute C Extraluminal Device D Intraluminal Device J Synthetic Substitute K Nonautologous Tissue Substitute	Z No Qualifier

DRG Non-OR Ø4WY3[Ø23D]Z *(proposed)*
Non-OR Ø4WYX[Ø237CDJK]Z

Coding Clinic: 2Ø15, Q1, P37 – Ø4WYØ7Z
Coding Clinic: 2Ø19, Q2, P15 – Ø4WYØJZ

Ø5. Upper Veins 129
Ø51. Bypass....130
Ø55. Destruction....131
Ø57. Dilation....132
Ø59. Drainage....133
Ø5B. Excision....134
Ø5C. Extirpation....135
Ø5D. Extraction....136
Ø5F. Fragmentation....136
Ø5H. Insertion....137
Ø5J. Inspection....138
Ø5L. Occlusion....138
Ø5N. Release....139
Ø5P. Removal....139
Ø5Q. Repair....140
Ø5R. Replacement....141
Ø5S. Reposition....142
Ø5U. Supplement....143
Ø5V. Restriction....144
Ø5W. Revision....145

SECTION: Ø MEDICAL AND SURGICAL
BODY SYSTEM: 5 UPPER VEINS
OPERATION: 1 BYPASS: Altering the route of passage of the contents of a tubular body part

Body Part	Approach	Device	Qualifier
Ø Azygos Vein 1 Hemiazygos Vein 3 Innominate Vein, Right 4 Innominate Vein, Left 5 Subclavian Vein, Right 6 Subclavian Vein, Left 7 Axillary Vein, Right 8 Axillary Vein, Left 9 Brachial Vein, Right A Brachial Vein, Left B Basilic Vein, Right C Basilic Vein, Left D Cephalic Vein, Right F Cephalic Vein, Left G Hand Vein, Right H Hand Vein, Left L Intracranial Vein M Internal Jugular Vein, Right N Internal Jugular Vein, Left P External Jugular Vein, Right Q External Jugular Vein, Left R Vertebral Vein, Right S Vertebral Vein, Left T Face Vein, Right V Face Vein, Left	Ø Open 4 Percutaneous Endoscopic	7 Autologous Tissue Substitute 9 Autologous Venous Tissue A Autologous Arterial Tissue J Synthetic Substitute K Nonautologous Tissue Substitute Z No Device	Y Upper Vein

Coding Clinic: 202Ø, Q1, P29 – Ø51Q49Y

SECTION: Ø MEDICAL AND SURGICAL

BODY SYSTEM: 5 UPPER VEINS

OPERATION: 5 DESTRUCTION: Physical eradication of all or a portion of a body part by the direct use of energy, force, or a destructive agent

Body Part	Approach	Device	Qualifier
Ø Azygos Vein 1 Hemiazygos Vein 3 Innominate Vein, Right 4 Innominate Vein, Left 5 Subclavian Vein, Right 6 Subclavian Vein, Left 7 Axillary Vein, Right 8 Axillary Vein, Left 9 Brachial Vein, Right A Brachial Vein, Left B Basilic Vein, Right C Basilic Vein, Left D Cephalic Vein, Right F Cephalic Vein, Left G Hand Vein, Right H Hand Vein, Left L Intracranial Vein M Internal Jugular Vein, Right N Internal Jugular Vein, Left P External Jugular Vein, Right Q External Jugular Vein, Left R Vertebral Vein, Right S Vertebral Vein, Left T Face Vein, Right V Face Vein, Left Y Upper Vein	Ø Open 3 Percutaneous 4 Percutaneous Endoscopic	Z No Device	Z No Qualifier

SECTION: Ø MEDICAL AND SURGICAL
BODY SYSTEM: 5 UPPER VEINS
OPERATION: 7 DILATION: Expanding an orifice or the lumen of a tubular body part

Body Part	Approach	Device	Qualifier
Ø Azygos Vein 1 Hemiazygos Vein G Hand Vein, Right H Hand Vein, Left L Intracranial Vein M Internal Jugular Vein, Right N Internal Jugular Vein, Left P External Jugular Vein, Right Q External Jugular Vein, Left R Vertebral Vein, Right S Vertebral Vein, Left T Face Vein, Right V Face Vein, Left Y Upper Vein	Ø Open 3 Percutaneous 4 Percutaneous Endoscopic	D Intraluminal Device Z No Device	Z No Qualifier
3 Innominate Vein, Right 4 Innominate Vein, Left 5 Subclavian Vein, Right 6 Subclavian Vein, Left 7 Axillary Vein, Right 8 Axillary Vein, Left 9 Brachial Vein, Right A Brachial Vein, Left B Basilic Vein, Right C Basilic Vein, Left D Cephalic Vein, Right F Cephalic Vein, Left	Ø Open 3 Percutaneous 4 Percutaneous Endoscopic	D Intraluminal Device Z No Device	1 Drug-Coated Balloon Z No Qualifier

Ø57L[34]ZZ

SECTION: Ø MEDICAL AND SURGICAL
BODY SYSTEM: 5 UPPER VEINS
OPERATION: 9 DRAINAGE: Taking or letting out fluids and/or gases from a body part

Body Part	Approach	Device	Qualifier
Ø Azygos Vein 1 Hemiazygos Vein 3 Innominate Vein, Right 4 Innominate Vein, Left 5 Subclavian Vein, Right 6 Subclavian Vein, Left 7 Axillary Vein, Right 8 Axillary Vein, Left 9 Brachial Vein, Right A Brachial Vein, Left B Basilic Vein, Right C Basilic Vein, Left D Cephalic Vein, Right F Cephalic Vein, Left G Hand Vein, Right H Hand Vein, Left L Intracranial Vein M Internal Jugular Vein, Right N Internal Jugular Vein, Left P External Jugular Vein, Right Q External Jugular Vein, Left R Vertebral Vein, Right S Vertebral Vein, Left T Face Vein, Right V Face Vein, Left Y Upper Vein	Ø Open 3 Percutaneous 4 Percutaneous Endoscopic	Ø Drainage Device	Z No Qualifier
Ø Azygos Vein 1 Hemiazygos Vein 3 Innominate Vein, Right 4 Innominate Vein, Left 5 Subclavian Vein, Right 6 Subclavian Vein, Left 7 Axillary Vein, Right 8 Axillary Vein, Left 9 Brachial Vein, Right A Brachial Vein, Left B Basilic Vein, Right C Basilic Vein, Left D Cephalic Vein, Right F Cephalic Vein, Left G Hand Vein, Right H Hand Vein, Left L Intracranial Vein M Internal Jugular Vein, Right N Internal Jugular Vein, Left P External Jugular Vein, Right Q External Jugular Vein, Left R Vertebral Vein, Right S Vertebral Vein, Left T Face Vein, Right V Face Vein, Left Y Upper Vein	Ø Open 3 Percutaneous 4 Percutaneous Endoscopic	Z No Device	X Diagnostic Z No Qualifier

Non-OR Ø59[Ø13456789ABCDFGHLMNPQRSTVY][Ø34]ØZ
Non-OR Ø59[Ø13456789ABCDFGHLMNPQRSTVY][Ø34]Z[XZ]

SECTION: Ø MEDICAL AND SURGICAL
BODY SYSTEM: 5 UPPER VEINS
OPERATION: B EXCISION: Cutting out or off, without replacement, a portion of a body part

Body Part	Approach	Device	Qualifier
Ø Azygos Vein 1 Hemiazygos Vein 3 Innominate Vein, Right 4 Innominate Vein, Left 5 Subclavian Vein, Right 6 Subclavian Vein, Left 7 Axillary Vein, Right 8 Axillary Vein, Left 9 Brachial Vein, Right A Brachial Vein, Left B Basilic Vein, Right C Basilic Vein, Left D Cephalic Vein, Right F Cephalic Vein, Left G Hand Vein, Right H Hand Vein, Left L Intracranial Vein M Internal Jugular Vein, Right N Internal Jugular Vein, Left P External Jugular Vein, Right Q External Jugular Vein, Left R Vertebral Vein, Right S Vertebral Vein, Left T Face Vein, Right V Face Vein, Left Y Upper Vein	Ø Open 3 Percutaneous 4 Percutaneous Endoscopic	Z No Device	X Diagnostic Z No Qualifier

Coding Clinic: 2Ø16, Q2, P13-14 – Ø5B[NQ]ØZZ
Coding Clinic: 2Ø21, Q2, P16; 2Ø2Ø, Q1, P24 – Ø5BLØZZ

SECTION: Ø MEDICAL AND SURGICAL
BODY SYSTEM: 5 UPPER VEINS
OPERATION: C EXTIRPATION: Taking or cutting out solid matter from a body part

Body Part	Approach	Device	Qualifier
Ø Azygos Vein 1 Hemiazygos Vein 3 Innominate Vein, Right 4 Innominate Vein, Left 5 Subclavian Vein, Right 6 Subclavian Vein, Left 7 Axillary Vein, Right 8 Axillary Vein, Left 9 Brachial Vein, Right A Brachial Vein, Left B Basilic Vein, Right C Basilic Vein, Left D Cephalic Vein, Right F Cephalic Vein, Left G Hand Vein, Right H Hand Vein, Left L Intracranial Vein M Internal Jugular Vein, Right N Internal Jugular Vein, Left P External Jugular Vein, Right Q External Jugular Vein, Left R Vertebral Vein, Right S Vertebral Vein, Left T Face Vein, Right V Face Vein, Left Y Upper Vein	Ø Open 3 Percutaneous 4 Percutaneous Endoscopic	Z No Device	Z No Qualifier

Coding Clinic: 2023, Q3, P24 – Ø5CY3ZZ

SECTION: Ø MEDICAL AND SURGICAL
BODY SYSTEM: 5 UPPER VEINS
OPERATION: D **EXTRACTION:** Pulling or stripping out or off all or a portion of a body part by the use of force

Body Part	Approach	Device	Qualifier
9 Brachial Vein, Right A Brachial Vein, Left B Basilic Vein, Right C Basilic Vein, Left D Cephalic Vein, Right F Cephalic Vein, Left G Hand Vein, Right H Hand Vein, Left Y Upper Vein	Ø Open 3 Percutaneous	Z No Device	Z No Qualifier

SECTION: Ø MEDICAL AND SURGICAL
BODY SYSTEM: 5 UPPER VEINS
OPERATION: F **FRAGMENTATION:** Breaking solid matter in a body part into pieces

Body Part	Approach	Device	Qualifier
3 Innominate Vein, Right 4 Innominate Vein, Left 5 Subclavian Vein, Right 6 Subclavian Vein, Left 7 Axillary Vein, Right 8 Axillary Vein, Left 9 Brachial Vein, Right A Brachial Vein, Left B Basilic Vein, Right C Basilic Vein, Left D Cephalic Vein, Right F Cephalic Vein, Left Y Upper Vein	3 Percutaneous	Z No Device	Ø Ultrasonic Z No Qualifier

SECTION: Ø MEDICAL AND SURGICAL
BODY SYSTEM: 5 UPPER VEINS
OPERATION: H INSERTION: Putting in a nonbiological appliance that monitors, assists, performs, or prevents a physiological function but does not physically take the place of a body part

Body Part	Approach	Device	Qualifier
Ø Azygos Vein	Ø Open 3 Percutaneous 4 Percutaneous Endoscopic	2 Monitoring Device 3 Infusion Device D Intraluminal Device M Neurostimulator Lead	Z No Qualifier
1 Hemiazygos Vein 5 Subclavian Vein, Right 6 Subclavian Vein, Left 7 Axillary Vein, Right 8 Axillary Vein, Left 9 Brachial Vein, Right A Brachial Vein, Left B Basilic Vein, Right C Basilic Vein, Left D Cephalic Vein, Right F Cephalic Vein, Left G Hand Vein, Right H Hand Vein, Left L Intracranial Vein M Internal Jugular Vein, Right N Internal Jugular Vein, Left P External Jugular Vein, Right Q External Jugular Vein, Left R Vertebral Vein, Right S Vertebral Vein, Left T Face Vein, Right V Face Vein, Left	Ø Open 3 Percutaneous 4 Percutaneous Endoscopic	3 Infusion Device D Intraluminal Device	Z No Qualifier
3 Innominate Vein, Right 4 Innominate Vein, Left	Ø Open 3 Percutaneous 4 Percutaneous Endoscopic	3 Infusion Device D Intraluminal Device M Neurostimulator Lead	Z No Qualifier
Y Upper Vein	Ø Open 3 Percutaneous 4 Percutaneous Endoscopic	2 Monitoring Device 3 Infusion Device D Intraluminal Device Y Other Device	Z No Qualifier

Ø5HØ[Ø34]MZ
Ø5H[34][Ø34]MZ
Non-OR Ø5HØ[Ø34]3Z
Non-OR Ø5H[13789ABCDFGHLRSTV][Ø34]3Z
Non-OR Ø5H[56MNPQ][Ø34]3Z
Non-OR Ø5H[34][Ø34]3Z
Non-OR Ø5HY[Ø34]3Z
Non-OR Ø5HY32Z
Ø5HØ[34]3Z when reported with Secondary Diagnosis J95.811
Ø5H[156][34]3Z when reported with Secondary Diagnosis J95.811
Ø5H[34][34]3Z when reported with Secondary Diagnosis J95.811
Ø5H[MNPQ]33Z when reported with Secondary Diagnosis J95.811

Coding Clinic: 2016, Q4, P98 – Ø5H, Ø5HØ32Z
Coding Clinic: 2016, Q4, P99 – Ø5H43MZ

SECTION: Ø MEDICAL AND SURGICAL
BODY SYSTEM: 5 UPPER VEINS
OPERATION: J INSPECTION: Visually and/or manually exploring a body part

Body Part	Approach	Device	Qualifier
Y Upper Vein	Ø Open 3 Percutaneous 4 Percutaneous Endoscopic X External	Z No Device	Z No Qualifier

Non-OR Ø5JY[3X]ZZ

SECTION: Ø MEDICAL AND SURGICAL
BODY SYSTEM: 5 UPPER VEINS
OPERATION: L OCCLUSION: Completely closing an orifice or the lumen of a tubular body part

Body Part	Approach	Device	Qualifier
Ø Azygos Vein 1 Hemiazygos Vein 3 Innominate Vein, Right 4 Innominate Vein, Left 5 Subclavian Vein, Right 6 Subclavian Vein, Left 7 Axillary Vein, Right 8 Axillary Vein, Left 9 Brachial Vein, Right A Brachial Vein, Left B Basilic Vein, Right C Basilic Vein, Left D Cephalic Vein, Right F Cephalic Vein, Left G Hand Vein, Right H Hand Vein, Left L Intracranial Vein M Internal Jugular Vein, Right N Internal Jugular Vein, Left P External Jugular Vein, Right Q External Jugular Vein, Left R Vertebral Vein, Right S Vertebral Vein, Left T Face Vein, Right V Face Vein, Left Y Upper Vein	Ø Open 3 Percutaneous 4 Percutaneous Endoscopic	C Extraluminal Device D Intraluminal Device Z No Device	Z No Qualifier

SECTION: Ø MEDICAL AND SURGICAL
BODY SYSTEM: 5 UPPER VEINS
OPERATION: N RELEASE: Freeing a body part from an abnormal physical constraint

Body Part	Approach	Device	Qualifier
Ø Azygos Vein 1 Hemiazygos Vein 3 Innominate Vein, Right 4 Innominate Vein, Left 5 Subclavian Vein, Right 6 Subclavian Vein, Left 7 Axillary Vein, Right 8 Axillary Vein, Left 9 Brachial Vein, Right A Brachial Vein, Left B Basilic Vein, Right C Basilic Vein, Left D Cephalic Vein, Right F Cephalic Vein, Left G Hand Vein, Right H Hand Vein, Left L Intracranial Vein M Internal Jugular Vein, Right N Internal Jugular Vein, Left P External Jugular Vein, Right Q External Jugular Vein, Left R Vertebral Vein, Right S Vertebral Vein, Left T Face Vein, Right V Face Vein, Left Y Upper Vein	Ø Open 3 Percutaneous 4 Percutaneous Endoscopic	Z No Device	Z No Qualifier

SECTION: Ø MEDICAL AND SURGICAL
BODY SYSTEM: 5 UPPER VEINS
OPERATION: P REMOVAL: Taking out or off a device from a body part

Body Part	Approach	Device	Qualifier
Ø Azygos Vein	Ø Open 3 Percutaneous 4 Percutaneous Endoscopic X External	2 Monitoring Device M Neurostimulator Lead	Z No Qualifier
3 Innominate Vein, Right 4 Innominate Vein, Left	Ø Open 3 Percutaneous 4 Percutaneous Endoscopic X External	M Neurostimulator Lead	Z No Qualifier
Y Upper Vein	Ø Open 3 Percutaneous 4 Percutaneous Endoscopic	Ø Drainage Device 2 Monitoring Device 3 Infusion Device 7 Autologous Tissue Substitute C Extraluminal Device D Intraluminal Device J Synthetic Substitute K Nonautologous Tissue Substitute Y Other Device	Z No Qualifier
Y Upper Vein	X External	Ø Drainage Device 2 Monitoring Device 3 Infusion Device D Intraluminal Device	Z No Qualifier

Non-OR Ø5PØ[Ø3X]2Z
Non-OR Ø5PY3[Ø23D]Z
Non-OR Ø5PYX[Ø23D]Z

Coding Clinic: 2016, Q4, P98 – Ø5P

SECTION: Ø MEDICAL AND SURGICAL
BODY SYSTEM: 5 UPPER VEINS
OPERATION: Q REPAIR: Restoring, to the extent possible, a body part to its normal anatomic structure and function

Body Part	Approach	Device	Qualifier
Ø Azygos Vein 1 Hemiazygos Vein 3 Innominate Vein, Right 4 Innominate Vein, Left 5 Subclavian Vein, Right 6 Subclavian Vein, Left 7 Axillary Vein, Right 8 Axillary Vein, Left 9 Brachial Vein, Right A Brachial Vein, Left B Basilic Vein, Right C Basilic Vein, Left D Cephalic Vein, Right F Cephalic Vein, Left G Hand Vein, Right H Hand Vein, Left L Intracranial Vein M Internal Jugular Vein, Right N Internal Jugular Vein, Left P External Jugular Vein, Right Q External Jugular Vein, Left R Vertebral Vein, Right S Vertebral Vein, Left T Face Vein, Right V Face Vein, Left Y Upper Vein	Ø Open 3 Percutaneous 4 Percutaneous Endoscopic	Z No Device	Z No Qualifier

Coding Clinic: 2Ø17, Q3, P16 – Ø5Q4ØZZ

SECTION: Ø MEDICAL AND SURGICAL
BODY SYSTEM: 5 UPPER VEINS
OPERATION: R REPLACEMENT: Putting in or on biological or synthetic material that physically takes the place and/or function of all or a portion of a body part

Body Part	Approach	Device	Qualifier
Ø Azygos Vein 1 Hemiazygos Vein 3 Innominate Vein, Right 4 Innominate Vein, Left 5 Subclavian Vein, Right 6 Subclavian Vein, Left 7 Axillary Vein, Right 8 Axillary Vein, Left 9 Brachial Vein, Right A Brachial Vein, Left B Basilic Vein, Right C Basilic Vein, Left D Cephalic Vein, Right F Cephalic Vein, Left G Hand Vein, Right H Hand Vein, Left L Intracranial Vein M Internal Jugular Vein, Right N Internal Jugular Vein, Left P External Jugular Vein, Right Q External Jugular Vein, Left R Vertebral Vein, Right S Vertebral Vein, Left T Face Vein, Right V Face Vein, Left Y Upper Vein	Ø Open 4 Percutaneous Endoscopic	7 Autologous Tissue Substitute J Synthetic Substitute K Nonautologous Tissue Substitute	Z No Qualifier

SECTION: Ø **MEDICAL AND SURGICAL**
BODY SYSTEM: 5 **UPPER VEINS**
OPERATION: S **REPOSITION:** Moving to its normal location, or other suitable location, all or a portion of a body part

Body Part	Approach	Device	Qualifier
Ø Azygos Vein 1 Hemiazygos Vein 3 Innominate Vein, Right 4 Innominate Vein, Left 5 Subclavian Vein, Right 6 Subclavian Vein, Left 7 Axillary Vein, Right 8 Axillary Vein, Left 9 Brachial Vein, Right A Brachial Vein, Left B Basilic Vein, Right C Basilic Vein, Left D Cephalic Vein, Right F Cephalic Vein, Left G Hand Vein, Right H Hand Vein, Left L Intracranial Vein M Internal Jugular Vein, Right N Internal Jugular Vein, Left P External Jugular Vein, Right Q External Jugular Vein, Left R Vertebral Vein, Right S Vertebral Vein, Left T Face Vein, Right V Face Vein, Left Y Upper Vein	Ø Open 3 Percutaneous 4 Percutaneous Endoscopic	Z No Device	Z No Qualifier

Ø5U

SECTION: Ø **MEDICAL AND SURGICAL**

BODY SYSTEM: 5 **UPPER VEINS**

OPERATION: U **SUPPLEMENT:** Putting in or on biological or synthetic material that physically reinforces and/or augments the function of a portion of a body part

Body Part	Approach	Device	Qualifier
Ø Azygos Vein 1 Hemiazygos Vein 3 Innominate Vein, Right 4 Innominate Vein, Left 5 Subclavian Vein, Right 6 Subclavian Vein, Left 7 Axillary Vein, Right 8 Axillary Vein, Left 9 Brachial Vein, Right A Brachial Vein, Left B Basilic Vein, Right C Basilic Vein, Left D Cephalic Vein, Right F Cephalic Vein, Left G Hand Vein, Right H Hand Vein, Left L Intracranial Vein M Internal Jugular Vein, Right N Internal Jugular Vein, Left P External Jugular Vein, Right Q External Jugular Vein, Left R Vertebral Vein, Right S Vertebral Vein, Left T Face Vein, Right V Face Vein, Left Y Upper Vein	Ø Open 3 Percutaneous 4 Percutaneous Endoscopic	7 Autologous Tissue Substitute J Synthetic Substitute K Nonautologous Tissue Substitute	Z No Qualifier

SECTION: Ø MEDICAL AND SURGICAL
BODY SYSTEM: 5 UPPER VEINS
OPERATION: V RESTRICTION: Partially closing an orifice or the lumen of a tubular body part

Body Part	Approach	Device	Qualifier
Ø Azygos Vein 1 Hemiazygos Vein 3 Innominate Vein, Right 4 Innominate Vein, Left 5 Subclavian Vein, Right 6 Subclavian Vein, Left 7 Axillary Vein, Right 8 Axillary Vein, Left 9 Brachial Vein, Right A Brachial Vein, Left B Basilic Vein, Right C Basilic Vein, Left D Cephalic Vein, Right F Cephalic Vein, Left G Hand Vein, Right H Hand Vein, Left L Intracranial Vein M Internal Jugular Vein, Right N Internal Jugular Vein, Left P External Jugular Vein, Right Q External Jugular Vein, Left R Vertebral Vein, Right S Vertebral Vein, Left T Face Vein, Right V Face Vein, Left Y Upper Vein	Ø Open 3 Percutaneous 4 Percutaneous Endoscopic	C Extraluminal Device D Intraluminal Device Z No Device	Z No Qualifier

SECTION: Ø MEDICAL AND SURGICAL
BODY SYSTEM: 5 UPPER VEINS
OPERATION: W REVISION: Correcting, to the extent possible, a portion of a malfunctioning device or the position of a displaced device

Body Part	Approach	Device	Qualifier
Ø Azygos Vein	Ø Open 3 Percutaneous 4 Percutaneous Endoscopic X External	2 Monitoring Device M Neurostimulator Lead	Z No Qualifier
3 Innominate Vein, Right 4 Innominate Vein, Left	Ø Open 3 Percutaneous 4 Percutaneous Endoscopic X External	M Neurostimulator Lead	Z No Qualifier
Y Upper Vein	Ø Open 3 Percutaneous 4 Percutaneous Endoscopic	Ø Drainage Device 2 Monitoring Device 3 Infusion Device 7 Autologous Tissue Substitute C Extraluminal Device D Intraluminal Device J Synthetic Substitute K Nonautologous Tissue Substitute Y Other Device	Z No Qualifier
Y Upper Vein	X External	Ø Drainage Device 2 Monitoring Device 3 Infusion Device 7 Autologous Tissue Substitute C Extraluminal Device D Intraluminal Device J Synthetic Substitute K Nonautologous Tissue Substitute	Z No Qualifier

Non-OR Ø5WY3[Ø23D]Z
Non-OR Ø5WØXMZ
Non-OR Ø5W[34]XMZ
Non-OR Ø5WYX[Ø237CDJK]Z

Coding Clinic: 2Ø16, Q4, P98 – Ø5W

Ø6. Lower Veins 146
Ø61. Bypass 147
Ø65. Destruction 148
Ø67. Dilation 149
Ø69. Drainage 15Ø
Ø6B. Excision 151
Ø6C. Extirpation 152
Ø6D. Extraction 153
Ø6F. Fragmentation 153
Ø6H. Insertion 154
Ø6J. Inspection 155
Ø6L. Occlusion 155
Ø6N. Release 156
Ø6P. Removal 156
Ø6Q. Repair 157
Ø6R. Replacement 158
Ø6S. Reposition 159
Ø6U. Supplement 16Ø
Ø6V. Restriction 161
Ø6W. Revision 162

SECTION: Ø MEDICAL AND SURGICAL
BODY SYSTEM: 6 LOWER VEINS
OPERATION: 1 BYPASS: Altering the route of passage of the contents of a tubular body part

Body Part	Approach	Device	Qualifier
Ø Inferior Vena Cava	Ø Open 4 Percutaneous Endoscopic	7 Autologous Tissue Substitute 9 Autologous Venous Tissue A Autologous Arterial Tissue J Synthetic Substitute K Nonautologous Tissue Substitute Z No Device	5 Superior Mesenteric Vein 6 Inferior Mesenteric Vein P Pulmonary Trunk Q Pulmonary Artery, Right R Pulmonary Artery, Left Y Lower Vein
1 Splenic Vein	Ø Open 4 Percutaneous Endoscopic	7 Autologous Tissue Substitute 9 Autologous Venous Tissue A Autologous Arterial Tissue J Synthetic Substitute K Nonautologous Tissue Substitute Z No Device	9 Renal Vein, Right B Renal Vein, Left Y Lower Vein
2 Gastric Vein 3 Esophageal Vein 4 Hepatic Vein 5 Superior Mesenteric Vein 6 Inferior Mesenteric Vein 7 Colic Vein 9 Renal Vein, Right B Renal Vein, Left C Common Iliac Vein, Right D Common Iliac Vein, Left F External Iliac Vein, Right G External Iliac Vein, Left H Hypogastric Vein, Right J Hypogastric Vein, Left M Femoral Vein, Right N Femoral Vein, Left P Saphenous Vein, Right Q Saphenous Vein, Left T Foot Vein, Right V Foot Vein, Left	Ø Open 4 Percutaneous Endoscopic	7 Autologous Tissue Substitute 9 Autologous Venous Tissue A Autologous Arterial Tissue J Synthetic Substitute K Nonautologous Tissue Substitute Z No Device	Y Lower Vein
8 Portal Vein	Ø Open	7 Autologous Tissue Substitute 9 Autologous Venous Tissue A Autologous Arterial Tissue J Synthetic Substitute K Nonautologous Tissue Substitute Z No Device	9 Renal Vein, Right B Renal Vein, Left Y Lower Vein
8 Portal Vein	3 Percutaneous	J Synthetic Substitute	4 Hepatic Vein Y Lower Vein
8 Portal Vein	4 Percutaneous Endoscopic	7 Autologous Tissue Substitute 9 Autologous Venous Tissue A Autologous Arterial Tissue K Nonautologous Tissue Substitute Z No Device	9 Renal Vein, Right B Renal Vein, Left Y Lower Vein
8 Portal Vein	4 Percutaneous Endoscopic	J Synthetic Substitute	4 Hepatic Vein 9 Renal Vein, Right B Renal Vein, Left Y Lower Vein

Coding Clinic: 2017, Q4, P38 – Ø61ØØJP

SECTION: Ø MEDICAL AND SURGICAL
BODY SYSTEM: 6 LOWER VEINS
OPERATION: 5 DESTRUCTION: Physical eradication of all or a portion of a body part by the direct use of energy, force, or a destructive agent

Body Part	Approach	Device	Qualifier
Ø Inferior Vena Cava 1 Splenic Vein 2 Gastric Vein 3 Esophageal Vein 4 Hepatic Vein 5 Superior Mesenteric Vein 6 Inferior Mesenteric Vein 7 Colic Vein 8 Portal Vein 9 Renal Vein, Right B Renal Vein, Left C Common Iliac Vein, Right D Common Iliac Vein, Left F External Iliac Vein, Right G External Iliac Vein, Left H Hypogastric Vein, Right J Hypogastric Vein, Left M Femoral Vein, Right N Femoral Vein, Left P Saphenous Vein, Right Q Saphenous Vein, Left T Foot Vein, Right V Foot Vein, Left	Ø Open 3 Percutaneous 4 Percutaneous Endoscopic	Z No Device	Z No Qualifier
Y Lower Vein	Ø Open 3 Percutaneous 4 Percutaneous Endoscopic	Z No Device	C Hemorrhoidal Plexus Z No Qualifier

SECTION: Ø MEDICAL AND SURGICAL
BODY SYSTEM: 6 LOWER VEINS
OPERATION: 7 DILATION: Expanding an orifice or the lumen of a tubular body part

Body Part	Approach	Device	Qualifier
Ø Inferior Vena Cava 1 Splenic Vein 2 Gastric Vein 3 Esophageal Vein 4 Hepatic Vein 5 Superior Mesenteric Vein 6 Inferior Mesenteric Vein 7 Colic Vein 8 Portal Vein 9 Renal Vein, Right B Renal Vein, Left C Common Iliac Vein, Right D Common Iliac Vein, Left F External Iliac Vein, Right G External Iliac Vein, Left H Hypogastric Vein, Right J Hypogastric Vein, Left M Femoral Vein, Right N Femoral Vein, Left P Saphenous Vein, Right Q Saphenous Vein, Left T Foot Vein, Right V Foot Vein, Left Y Lower Vein	Ø Open 3 Percutaneous 4 Percutaneous Endoscopic	D Intraluminal Device Z No Device	Z No Qualifier

SECTION: Ø MEDICAL AND SURGICAL
BODY SYSTEM: 6 LOWER VEINS
OPERATION: 9 DRAINAGE: Taking or letting out fluids and/or gases from a body part

Body Part	Approach	Device	Qualifier
Ø Inferior Vena Cava 1 Splenic Vein 2 Gastric Vein 3 Esophageal Vein 4 Hepatic Vein 5 Superior Mesenteric Vein 6 Inferior Mesenteric Vein 7 Colic Vein 8 Portal Vein 9 Renal Vein, Right B Renal Vein, Left C Common Iliac Vein, Right D Common Iliac Vein, Left F External Iliac Vein, Right G External Iliac Vein, Left H Hypogastric Vein, Right J Hypogastric Vein, Left M Femoral Vein, Right N Femoral Vein, Left P Saphenous Vein, Right Q Saphenous Vein, Left T Foot Vein, Right V Foot Vein, Left Y Lower Vein	Ø Open 3 Percutaneous 4 Percutaneous Endoscopic	Ø Drainage Device	Z No Qualifier
Ø Inferior Vena Cava 1 Splenic Vein 2 Gastric Vein 3 Esophageal Vein 4 Hepatic Vein 5 Superior Mesenteric Vein 6 Inferior Mesenteric Vein 7 Colic Vein 8 Portal Vein 9 Renal Vein, Right B Renal Vein, Left C Common Iliac Vein, Right D Common Iliac Vein, Left F External Iliac Vein, Right G External Iliac Vein, Left H Hypogastric Vein, Right J Hypogastric Vein, Left M Femoral Vein, Right N Femoral Vein, Left P Saphenous Vein, Right Q Saphenous Vein, Left T Foot Vein, Right V Foot Vein, Left Y Lower Vein	Ø Open 3 Percutaneous 4 Percutaneous Endoscopic	Z No Device	X Diagnostic Z No Qualifier

Non-OR Ø6933ØZ
Non-OR Ø69[Ø12456789BCDFGHJMNPQTVY][Ø34]ØZ
Non-OR Ø6933ZZ
Non-OR Ø69[Ø123456789BCDFGHJMNPQRSTVY][Ø34]Z[XZ]

SECTION: Ø MEDICAL AND SURGICAL
BODY SYSTEM: 6 LOWER VEINS
OPERATION: B EXCISION: Cutting out or off, without replacement, a portion of a body part

Body Part	Approach	Device	Qualifier
Ø Inferior Vena Cava 1 Splenic Vein 2 Gastric Vein 3 Esophageal Vein 4 Hepatic Vein 5 Superior Mesenteric Vein 6 Inferior Mesenteric Vein 7 Colic Vein 8 Portal Vein 9 Renal Vein, Right B Renal Vein, Left C Common Iliac Vein, Right D Common Iliac Vein, Left F External Iliac Vein, Right G External Iliac Vein, Left H Hypogastric Vein, Right J Hypogastric Vein, Left M Femoral Vein, Right N Femoral Vein, Left P Saphenous Vein, Right Q Saphenous Vein, Left T Foot Vein, Right V Foot Vein, Left	Ø Open 3 Percutaneous 4 Percutaneous Endoscopic	Z No Device	X Diagnostic Z No Qualifier
Y Lower Vein	Ø Open 3 Percutaneous 4 Percutaneous Endoscopic	Z No Device	C Hemorrhoidal Plexus X Diagnostic Z No Qualifier

Coding Clinic: 2Ø16, Q1, P28 – Ø6BQ4ZZ
Coding Clinic: 2Ø16, Q2, P19 – Ø6B9ØZZ
Coding Clinic: 2Ø17, Q1, P32 – Ø6BPØZZ
Coding Clinic: 2Ø2Ø, Q1, P29; 2Ø17, Q1, P33 – Ø6BQØZZ
Coding Clinic: 2Ø17, Q3, P6 – Ø6BPØZZ

SECTION: Ø MEDICAL AND SURGICAL
BODY SYSTEM: 6 LOWER VEINS
OPERATION: C EXTIRPATION: Taking or cutting out solid matter from a body part

Body Part	Approach	Device	Qualifier
Ø Inferior Vena Cava 1 Splenic Vein 2 Gastric Vein 3 Esophageal Vein 4 Hepatic Vein 5 Superior Mesenteric Vein 6 Inferior Mesenteric Vein 7 Colic Vein 8 Portal Vein 9 Renal Vein, Right B Renal Vein, Left C Common Iliac Vein, Right D Common Iliac Vein, Left F External Iliac Vein, Right G External Iliac Vein, Left H Hypogastric Vein, Right J Hypogastric Vein, Left M Femoral Vein, Right N Femoral Vein, Left P Saphenous Vein, Right Q Saphenous Vein, Left T Foot Vein, Right V Foot Vein, Left Y Lower Vein	Ø Open 3 Percutaneous 4 Percutaneous Endoscopic	Z No Device	Z No Qualifier

SECTION: Ø MEDICAL AND SURGICAL
BODY SYSTEM: 6 LOWER VEINS
OPERATION: D EXTRACTION: Pulling or stripping out or off all or a portion of a body part by the use of force

Body Part	Approach	Device	Qualifier
M Femoral Vein, Right N Femoral Vein, Left P Saphenous Vein, Right Q Saphenous Vein, Left T Foot Vein, Right V Foot Vein, Left Y Lower Vein	Ø Open 3 Percutaneous 4 Percutaneous Endoscopic	Z No Device	Z No Qualifier

SECTION: Ø MEDICAL AND SURGICAL
BODY SYSTEM: 6 LOWER VEINS
OPERATION: F FRAGMENTATION: Breaking solid matter in a body part into pieces

Body Part	Approach	Device	Qualifier
C Common Iliac Vein, Right D Common Iliac Vein, Left F External Iliac Vein, Right G External Iliac Vein, Left H Hypogastric Vein, Right J Hypogastric Vein, Left M Femoral Vein, Right N Femoral Vein, Left P Saphenous Vein, Right Q Saphenous Vein, Left Y Lower Vein	3 Percutaneous	Z No Device	Ø Ultrasonic Z No Qualifier

SECTION: Ø MEDICAL AND SURGICAL
BODY SYSTEM: 6 LOWER VEINS
OPERATION: H INSERTION: Putting in a nonbiological appliance that monitors, assists, performs, or prevents a physiological function but does not physically take the place of a body part

Body Part	Approach	Device	Qualifier
Ø Inferior Vena Cava	Ø Open 3 Percutaneous	3 Infusion Device	T Via Unbilical Vein Z No Qualifier
Ø Inferior Vena Cava	Ø Open 3 Percutaneous	D Intraluminal Device	Z No Qualifier
Ø Inferior Vena Cava	4 Percutaneous Endoscopic	3 Infusion Device D Intraluminal Device	Z No Qualifier
1 Splenic Vein 2 Gastric Vein 3 Esophageal Vein 4 Hepatic Vein 5 Superior Mesenteric Vein 6 Inferior Mesenteric Vein 7 Colic Vein 8 Portal Vein 9 Renal Vein, Right B Renal Vein, Left C Common Iliac Vein, Right D Common Iliac Vein, Left F External Iliac Vein, Right G External Iliac Vein, Left H Hypogastric Vein, Right J Hypogastric Vein, Left M Femoral Vein, Right N Femoral Vein, Left P Saphenous Vein, Right Q Saphenous Vein, Left T Foot Vein, Right V Foot Vein, Left	Ø Open 3 Percutaneous 4 Percutaneous Endoscopic	3 Infusion Device D Intraluminal Device	Z No Qualifier
Y Lower Vein	Ø Open 3 Percutaneous 4 Percutaneous Endoscopic	2 Monitoring Device 3 Infusion Device D Intraluminal Device Y Other Device	Z No Qualifier

Non-OR Ø6HØ[Ø3]3[DTZ]
Non-OR Ø6HØ43Z
Non-OR Ø6H[123456789BCDFGHJPQTV][Ø34]3Z
Non-OR Ø6H[MN][Ø34]3Z
Non-OR Ø6HY32Z
Non-OR Ø6HY[Ø34]3Z

Coding Clinic: 2Ø13, Q3, P19 – Ø6HØ33Z
Coding Clinic: 2Ø17, Q1, P31 – Ø6HØ33T, Ø6HY33Z
Coding Clinic: 2Ø21, Q3, P19 – Ø6HY33Z

SECTION: Ø MEDICAL AND SURGICAL
BODY SYSTEM: 6 LOWER VEINS
OPERATION: J INSPECTION: Visually and/or manually exploring a body part

Body Part	Approach	Device	Qualifier
Y Lower Vein	Ø Open 3 Percutaneous 4 Percutaneous Endoscopic X External	Z No Device	Z No Qualifier

Non-OR Ø6JY[3X]ZZ

SECTION: Ø MEDICAL AND SURGICAL
BODY SYSTEM: 6 LOWER VEINS
OPERATION: L OCCLUSION: Completely closing an orifice or the lumen of a tubular body part

Body Part	Approach	Device	Qualifier
Ø Inferior Vena Cava 1 Splenic Vein 4 Hepatic Vein 5 Superior Mesenteric Vein 6 Inferior Mesenteric Vein 7 Colic Vein 8 Portal Vein 9 Renal Vein, Right B Renal Vein, Left C Common Iliac Vein, Right D Common Iliac Vein, Left F External Iliac Vein, Right G External Iliac Vein, Left H Hypogastric Vein, Right J Hypogastric Vein, Left M Femoral Vein, Right N Femoral Vein, Left P Saphenous Vein, Right Q Saphenous Vein, Left T Foot Vein, Right V Foot Vein, Left	Ø Open 3 Percutaneous 4 Percutaneous Endoscopic	C Extraluminal Device D Intraluminal Device Z No Device	Z No Qualifier
2 Gastric Vein 3 Esophageal Vein	Ø Open 3 Percutaneous 4 Percutaneous Endoscopic 7 Via Natural or Artificial Opening 8 Via Natural or Artificial Opening Endoscopic	C Extraluminal Device D Intraluminal Device Z No Device	Z No Qualifier
Y Lower Vein	Ø Open 3 Percutaneous 4 Percutaneous Endoscopic 7 Via Natural or Artificial Opening 8 Via Natural or Artificial Opening Endoscopic	C Extraluminal Device D Intraluminal Device Z No Device	C Hemorrhoidal Plexus Z No Qualifier

Non-OR Ø6L3[34][CDZ]Z

Coding Clinic: 2017, Q4, P57 – ØØ6L38CZ
Coding Clinic: 2018, Q2, P19 – Ø6LFØCZ
Coding Clinic: 2021, Q4, P5Ø – Ø6L84CZ

Ø: M/S 6: LOWER VEINS J: INSPECTION L: OCCLUSION

SECTION: Ø MEDICAL AND SURGICAL
BODY SYSTEM: 6 LOWER VEINS
OPERATION: N RELEASE: Freeing a body part from an abnormal physical constraint by cutting or by the use of force

Body Part	Approach	Device	Qualifier
Ø Inferior Vena Cava 1 Splenic Vein 2 Gastric Vein 3 Esophageal Vein 4 Hepatic Vein 5 Superior Mesenteric Vein 6 Inferior Mesenteric Vein 7 Colic Vein 8 Portal Vein 9 Renal Vein, Right B Renal Vein, Left C Common Iliac Vein, Right D Common Iliac Vein, Left F External Iliac Vein, Right G External Iliac Vein, Left H Hypogastric Vein, Right J Hypogastric Vein, Left M Femoral Vein, Right N Femoral Vein, Left P Saphenous Vein, Right Q Saphenous Vein, Left T Foot Vein, Right V Foot Vein, Left Y Lower Vein	Ø Open 3 Percutaneous 4 Percutaneous Endoscopic	Z No Device	Z No Qualifier

SECTION: Ø MEDICAL AND SURGICAL
BODY SYSTEM: 6 LOWER VEINS
OPERATION: P REMOVAL: Taking out or off a device from a body part

Body Part	Approach	Device	Qualifier
Y Lower Vein	Ø Open 3 Percutaneous 4 Percutaneous Endoscopic	Ø Drainage Device 2 Monitoring Device 3 Infusion Device 7 Autologous Tissue Substitute C Extraluminal Device D Intraluminal Device J Synthetic Substitute K Nonautologous Tissue Substitute Y Other Device	Z No Qualifier
Y Lower Vein	X External	Ø Drainage Device 2 Monitoring Device 3 Infusion Device D Intraluminal Device	Z No Qualifier

Non-OR Ø6PY3[Ø23D]Z
Non-OR Ø6PYX[Ø23D]Z

Coding Clinic: 2021, Q3, P19 – Ø6PY33Z

SECTION: Ø MEDICAL AND SURGICAL
BODY SYSTEM: 6 LOWER VEINS
OPERATION: Q REPAIR: Restoring, to the extent possible, a body part to its normal anatomic structure and function

Body Part	Approach	Device	Qualifier
Ø Inferior Vena Cava 1 Splenic Vein 2 Gastric Vein 3 Esophageal Vein 4 Hepatic Vein 5 Superior Mesenteric Vein 6 Inferior Mesenteric Vein 7 Colic Vein 8 Portal Vein 9 Renal Vein, Right B Renal Vein, Left C Common Iliac Vein, Right D Common Iliac Vein, Left F External Iliac Vein, Right G External Iliac Vein, Left H Hypogastric Vein, Right J Hypogastric Vein, Left M Femoral Vein, Right N Femoral Vein, Left P Saphenous Vein, Right Q Saphenous Vein, Left T Foot Vein, Right V Foot Vein, Left Y Lower Vein	Ø Open 3 Percutaneous 4 Percutaneous Endoscopic	Z No Device	Z No Qualifier

SECTION: Ø MEDICAL AND SURGICAL
BODY SYSTEM: 6 LOWER VEINS
OPERATION: R REPLACEMENT: Putting in or on biological or synthetic material that physically takes the place and/or function of all or a portion of a body part

Body Part	Approach	Device	Qualifier
Ø Inferior Vena Cava 1 Splenic Vein 2 Gastric Vein 3 Esophageal Vein 4 Hepatic Vein 5 Superior Mesenteric Vein 6 Inferior Mesenteric Vein 7 Colic Vein 8 Portal Vein 9 Renal Vein, Right B Renal Vein, Left C Common Iliac Vein, Right D Common Iliac Vein, Left F External Iliac Vein, Right G External Iliac Vein, Left H Hypogastric Vein, Right J Hypogastric Vein, Left M Femoral Vein, Right N Femoral Vein, Left P Saphenous Vein, Right Q Saphenous Vein, Left T Foot Vein, Right V Foot Vein, Left Y Lower Vein	Ø Open 4 Percutaneous Endoscopic	7 Autologous Tissue Substitute J Synthetic Substitute K Nonautologous Tissue Substitute	Z No Qualifier

SECTION: Ø MEDICAL AND SURGICAL
BODY SYSTEM: 6 LOWER VEINS
OPERATION: S REPOSITION: Moving to its normal location, or other suitable location, all or a portion of a body part

Body Part	Approach	Device	Qualifier
Ø Inferior Vena Cava 1 Splenic Vein 2 Gastric Vein 3 Esophageal Vein 4 Hepatic Vein 5 Superior Mesenteric Vein 6 Inferior Mesenteric Vein 7 Colic Vein 8 Portal Vein 9 Renal Vein, Right B Renal Vein, Left C Common Iliac Vein, Right D Common Iliac Vein, Left F External Iliac Vein, Right G External Iliac Vein, Left H Hypogastric Vein, Right J Hypogastric Vein, Left M Femoral Vein, Right N Femoral Vein, Left P Saphenous Vein, Right Q Saphenous Vein, Left T Foot Vein, Right V Foot Vein, Left Y Lower Vein	Ø Open 3 Percutaneous 4 Percutaneous Endoscopic	Z No Device	Z No Qualifier

SECTION: Ø MEDICAL AND SURGICAL

BODY SYSTEM: 6 LOWER VEINS

OPERATION: U SUPPLEMENT: Putting in or on biological or synthetic material that physically reinforces and/or augments the function of a portion of a body part

Body Part	Approach	Device	Qualifier
Ø Inferior Vena Cava 1 Splenic Vein 2 Gastric Vein 3 Esophageal Vein 4 Hepatic Vein 5 Superior Mesenteric Vein 6 Inferior Mesenteric Vein 7 Colic Vein 8 Portal Vein 9 Renal Vein, Right B Renal Vein, Left C Common Iliac Vein, Right D Common Iliac Vein, Left F External Iliac Vein, Right G External Iliac Vein, Left H Hypogastric Vein, Right J Hypogastric Vein, Left M Femoral Vein, Right N Femoral Vein, Left P Saphenous Vein, Right Q Saphenous Vein, Left T Foot Vein, Right V Foot Vein, Left Y Lower Vein	Ø Open 3 Percutaneous 4 Percutaneous Endoscopic	7 Autologous Tissue Substitute J Synthetic Substitute K Nonautologous Tissue Substitute	Z No Qualifier

SECTION: Ø MEDICAL AND SURGICAL
BODY SYSTEM: 6 LOWER VEINS
OPERATION: V RESTRICTION: Partially closing an orifice or the lumen of a tubular body part

Body Part	Approach	Device	Qualifier
Ø Inferior Vena Cava 1 Splenic Vein 2 Gastric Vein 3 Esophageal Vein 4 Hepatic Vein 5 Superior Mesenteric Vein 6 Inferior Mesenteric Vein 7 Colic Vein 8 Portal Vein 9 Renal Vein, Right B Renal Vein, Left C Common Iliac Vein, Right D Common Iliac Vein, Left F External Iliac Vein, Right G External Iliac Vein, Left H Hypogastric Vein, Right J Hypogastric Vein, Left M Femoral Vein, Right N Femoral Vein, Left P Saphenous Vein, Right Q Saphenous Vein, Left T Foot Vein, Right V Foot Vein, Left Y Lower Vein	Ø Open 3 Percutaneous 4 Percutaneous Endoscopic	C Extraluminal Device D Intraluminal Device Z No Device	Z No Qualifier

SECTION: Ø MEDICAL AND SURGICAL
BODY SYSTEM: 6 LOWER VEINS
OPERATION: W REVISION: Correcting, to the extent possible, a portion of a malfunctioning device or the position of a displaced device

Body Part	Approach	Device	Qualifier
Y Lower Vein	Ø Open 3 Percutaneous 4 Percutaneous Endoscopic	Ø Drainage Device 2 Monitoring Device 3 Infusion Device 7 Autologous Tissue Substitute C Extraluminal Device D Intraluminal Device J Synthetic Substitute K Nonautologous Tissue Substitute Y Other Device	Z No Qualifier
Y Lower Vein	X External	Ø Drainage Device 2 Monitoring Device 3 Infusion Device 7 Autologous Tissue Substitute C Extraluminal Device D Intraluminal Device J Synthetic Substitute K Nonautologous Tissue Substitute	Z No Qualifier

Non-OR Ø6WY[3X][Ø237CDJK]Z

Coding Clinic: 2Ø18, Q1, P11 – Ø6WY3DZ

Ø7. Lymphatic and Hemic Systems 163
Ø71. Bypass 164
Ø72. Change 164
Ø75. Destruction 165
Ø79. Drainage 166
Ø7B. Excision 167
Ø7C. Extirpation 167
Ø7D. Extraction 168
Ø7H. Insertion 168
Ø7J. Inspection 169
Ø7L. Occlusion 169
Ø7N. Release 17Ø
Ø7P. Removal 17Ø
Ø7Q. Repair 171
Ø7S. Reposition 171
Ø7T. Resection 172
Ø7U. Supplement 173
Ø7V. Restriction 173
Ø7W. Revision 174
Ø7Y. Transplantation 174

SECTION: Ø MEDICAL AND SURGICAL
BODY SYSTEM: 7 LYMPHATIC AND HEMIC SYSTEMS
OPERATION: 1 BYPASS: Altering the route of passage of the contents of a tubular body part

Body Part	Approach	Device	Qualifier
Ø Lymphatic, Head 1 Lymphatic, Right Neck 2 Lymphatic, Left Neck 3 Lymphatic, Right Upper Extremity 4 Lymphatic, Left Upper Extremity 5 Lymphatic, Right Axillary 6 Lymphatic, Left Axillary 7 Lymphatic, Thorax 8 Lymphatic, Internal Mammary, Right 9 Lymphatic, Internal Mammary, Left B Lymphatic, Mesenteric C Lymphatic, Pelvis D Lymphatic, Aortic F Lymphatic, Right Lower Extremity G Lymphatic, Left Lower Extremity H Lymphatic, Right Inguinal J Lymphatic, Left Inguinal K Thoracic Duct L Cistema Chyli	Ø Open 4 Percutaneous Endoscopic	Z No Device	3 Peripheral Vein 4 Central Vein 7 Lymphatic K Thoracic Duct L Cisterna Chyli

SECTION: Ø MEDICAL AND SURGICAL
BODY SYSTEM: 7 LYMPHATIC AND HEMIC SYSTEMS
OPERATION: 2 CHANGE: Taking out or off a device from a body part and putting back an identical or similar device in or on the same body part without cutting or puncturing the skin or a mucous membrane

Body Part	Approach	Device	Qualifier
K Thoracic Duct L Cisterna Chyli M Thymus N Lymphatic P Spleen T Bone Marrow	X External	Ø Drainage Device Y Other Device	Z No Qualifier

Non-OR All Values

~~Coding Clinic: 2Ø16, Q1, P3Ø – Ø7T5ØZZ~~

SECTION: Ø MEDICAL AND SURGICAL
BODY SYSTEM: 7 LYMPHATIC AND HEMIC SYSTEMS
OPERATION: 5 DESTRUCTION: Physical eradication of all or a portion of a body part by the direct use of energy, force, or a destructive agent

Body Part	Approach	Device	Qualifier
Ø Lymphatic, Head 1 Lymphatic, Right Neck 2 Lymphatic, Left Neck 3 Lymphatic, Right Upper Extremity 4 Lymphatic, Left Upper Extremity 5 Lymphatic, Right Axillary 6 Lymphatic, Left Axillary 7 Lymphatic, Thorax 8 Lymphatic, Internal Mammary, Right 9 Lymphatic, Internal Mammary, Left B Lymphatic, Mesenteric C Lymphatic, Pelvis D Lymphatic, Aortic F Lymphatic, Right Lower Extremity G Lymphatic, Left Lower Extremity H Lymphatic, Right Inguinal J Lymphatic, Left Inguinal K Thoracic Duct L Cisterna Chyli M Thymus P Spleen	Ø Open 3 Percutaneous 4 Percutaneous Endoscopic	Z No Device	Z No Qualifier

SECTION: Ø MEDICAL AND SURGICAL
BODY SYSTEM: 7 LYMPHATIC AND HEMIC SYSTEMS
OPERATION: 9 DRAINAGE: Taking or letting out fluids and/or gases from a body part

Body Part	Approach	Device	Qualifier
Ø Lymphatic, Head 1 Lymphatic, Right Neck 2 Lymphatic, Left Neck 3 Lymphatic, Right Upper Extremity 4 Lymphatic, Left Upper Extremity 5 Lymphatic, Right Axillary 6 Lymphatic, Left Axillary 7 Lymphatic, Thorax 8 Lymphatic, Internal Mammary, Right 9 Lymphatic, Internal Mammary, Left B Lymphatic, Mesenteric C Lymphatic, Pelvis D Lymphatic, Aortic F Lymphatic, Right Lower Extremity G Lymphatic, Left Lower Extremity H Lymphatic, Right Inguinal J Lymphatic, Left Inguinal K Thoracic Duct L Cisterna Chyli	Ø Open 3 Percutaneous 4 Percutaneous Endoscopic 8 Via Natural or Artificial Opening Endoscopic	Ø Drainage Device	Z No Qualifier
Ø Lymphatic, Head 1 Lymphatic, Right Neck 2 Lymphatic, Left Neck 3 Lymphatic, Right Upper Extremity 4 Lymphatic, Left Upper Extremity 5 Lymphatic, Right Axillary 6 Lymphatic, Left Axillary 7 Lymphatic, Thorax 8 Lymphatic, Internal Mammary, Right 9 Lymphatic, Internal Mammary, Left B Lymphatic, Mesenteric C Lymphatic, Pelvis D Lymphatic, Aortic F Lymphatic, Right Lower Extremity G Lymphatic, Left Lower Extremity H Lymphatic, Right Inguinal J Lymphatic, Left Inguinal K Thoracic Duct L Cisterna Chyli	Ø Open 3 Percutaneous 4 Percutaneous Endoscopic 8 Via Natural or Artificial Opening Endoscopic	Z No Device	X Diagnostic Z No Qualifier
M Thymus P Spleen T Bone Marrow	Ø Open 3 Percutaneous 4 Percutaneous Endoscopic	Ø Drainage Device	Z No Qualifier
M Thymus P Spleen T Bone Marrow	Ø Open 3 Percutaneous 4 Percutaneous Endoscopic	Z No Device	X Diagnostic Z No Qualifier

Non-OR Ø79[123456789BCDEFGHJKL]3ØZ
Non-OR Ø79P[34]ØZ
Non-OR Ø79T[Ø34]ØZ
Non-OR Ø79[123456789BCDEFGHJKL]3ZZ
Non-OR Ø79P[34]Z[XZ]
Non-OR Ø79T[Ø34]Z[XZ]

Coding Clinic: 2021, Q4, P48 – Ø79T3ZX

SECTION: Ø MEDICAL AND SURGICAL
BODY SYSTEM: 7 LYMPHATIC AND HEMIC SYSTEMS
OPERATION: B EXCISION: Cutting out or off, without replacement, a portion of a body part

Body Part	Approach	Device	Qualifier
Ø Lymphatic, Head 1 Lymphatic, Right Neck 2 Lymphatic, Left Neck 3 Lymphatic, Right Upper Extremity 4 Lymphatic, Left Upper Extremity 5 Lymphatic, Right Axillary 6 Lymphatic, Left Axillary 7 Lymphatic, Thorax 8 Lymphatic, Internal Mammary, Right 9 Lymphatic, Internal Mammary, Left B Lymphatic, Mesenteric C Lymphatic, Pelvis D Lymphatic, Aortic F Lymphatic, Right Lower Extremity G Lymphatic, Left Lower Extremity H Lymphatic, Right Inguinal ⊞ J Lymphatic, Left Inguinal ⊞ K Thoracic Duct L Cisterna Chyli M Thymus P Spleen	Ø Open 3 Percutaneous 4 Percutaneous Endoscopic	Z No Device	X Diagnostic Z No Qualifier

⊞ Ø7B[HJ][Ø4]ZZ
Non-OR Ø7BP[34]ZX

Coding Clinic: 2019, Q1, P7 – Ø7B[D]ØZZ
Coding Clinic: 2022, Q1, P15 – Ø7B6ØZX

SECTION: Ø MEDICAL AND SURGICAL
BODY SYSTEM: 7 LYMPHATIC AND HEMIC SYSTEMS
OPERATION: C EXTIRPATION: Taking or cutting out solid matter from a body part

Body Part	Approach	Device	Qualifier
Ø Lymphatic, Head 1 Lymphatic, Right Neck 2 Lymphatic, Left Neck 3 Lymphatic, Right Upper Extremity 4 Lymphatic, Left Upper Extremity 5 Lymphatic, Right Axillary 6 Lymphatic, Left Axillary 7 Lymphatic, Thorax 8 Lymphatic, Internal Mammary, Right 9 Lymphatic, Internal Mammary, Left B Lymphatic, Mesenteric C Lymphatic, Pelvis D Lymphatic, Aortic F Lymphatic, Right Lower Extremity G Lymphatic, Left Lower Extremity H Lymphatic, Right Inguinal J Lymphatic, Left Inguinal K Thoracic Duct L Cisterna Chyli M Thymus P Spleen	Ø Open 3 Percutaneous 4 Percutaneous Endoscopic	Z No Device	Z No Qualifier

Non-OR Ø7CP[34]ZZ

SECTION: Ø MEDICAL AND SURGICAL
BODY SYSTEM: 7 LYMPHATIC AND HEMIC SYSTEMS
OPERATION: D EXTRACTION: Pulling or stripping out or off all or a portion of a body part by the use of force

Body Part	Approach	Device	Qualifier
Ø Lymphatic, Head 1 Lymphatic, Right Neck 2 Lymphatic, Left Neck 3 Lymphatic, Right Upper Extremity 4 Lymphatic, Left Upper Extremity 5 Lymphatic, Right Axillary 6 Lymphatic, Left Axillary 7 Lymphatic, Thorax 8 Lymphatic, Internal Mammary, Right 9 Lymphatic, Internal Mammary, Left B Lymphatic, Mesenteric C Lymphatic, Pelvis D Lymphatic, Aortic F Lymphatic, Right Lower Extremity G Lymphatic, Left Lower Extremity H Lymphatic, Right Inguinal J Lymphatic, Left Inguinal K Thoracic Duct L Cisterna Chyli	3 Percutaneous 4 Percutaneous Endoscopic 8 Via Natural or Artificial Opening Endoscopic	Z No Device	X Diagnostic
M Thymus P Spleen	3 Percutaneous 4 Percutaneous Endoscopic	Z No Device	X Diagnostic
Q Bone Marrow, Sternum R Bone Marrow, Iliac S Bone Marrow, Vertebral T Bone Marrow	Ø Open 3 Percutaneous	Z No Device	X Diagnostic Z No Qualifier

Non-OR Ø7D[QRS][Ø3]Z[XZ]

Coding Clinic: 2Ø21, Q4, P48 – Ø7DT3ZX

SECTION: Ø MEDICAL AND SURGICAL
BODY SYSTEM: 7 LYMPHATIC AND HEMIC SYSTEMS
OPERATION: H INSERTION: Putting in a nonbiological appliance that monitors, assists, performs, or prevents a physiological function but does not physically take the place of a body part

Body Part	Approach	Device	Qualifier
K Thoracic Duct L Cisterna Chyli M Thymus N Lymphatic P Spleen T Bone Marrow	Ø Open 3 Percutaneous 4 Percutaneous Endoscopic	1 Radioactive Element 3 Infusion Device Y Other Device	Z No Qualifier

DRG Non-OR Ø7H[KLMNP][Ø34]3Z

SECTION: Ø MEDICAL AND SURGICAL
BODY SYSTEM: 7 LYMPHATIC AND HEMIC SYSTEMS
OPERATION: J INSPECTION: Visually and/or manually exploring a body part

Body Part	Approach	Device	Qualifier
K Thoracic Duct L Cisterna Chyli M Thymus T Bone Marrow	Ø Open 3 Percutaneous 4 Percutaneous Endoscopic	Z No Device	Z No Qualifier
N Lymphatic	Ø Open 3 Percutaneous 4 Percutaneous Endoscopic 8 Via Natural or Artificial Opening Endoscopic X External	Z No Device	Z No Qualifier
P Spleen	Ø Open 3 Percutaneous 4 Percutaneous Endoscopic X External	Z No Device	Z No Qualifier

Non-OR Ø7J[KLM]3ZZ
Non-OR Ø7JN[3X]ZZ
Non-OR Ø7JP[34X]ZZ
Non-OR Ø7JT[Ø34]ZZ

SECTION: Ø MEDICAL AND SURGICAL
BODY SYSTEM: 7 LYMPHATIC AND HEMIC SYSTEMS
OPERATION: L OCCLUSION: Completely closing an orifice or the lumen of a tubular body part

Body Part	Approach	Device	Qualifier
Ø Lymphatic, Head 1 Lymphatic, Right Neck 2 Lymphatic, Left Neck 3 Lymphatic, Right Upper Extremity 4 Lymphatic, Left Upper Extremity 5 Lymphatic, Right Axillary 6 Lymphatic, Left Axillary 7 Lymphatic, Thorax 8 Lymphatic, Internal Mammary, Right 9 Lymphatic, Internal Mammary, Left B Lymphatic, Mesenteric C Lymphatic, Pelvis D Lymphatic, Aortic F Lymphatic, Right Lower Extremity G Lymphatic, Left Lower Extremity H Lymphatic, Right Inguinal J Lymphatic, Left Inguinal K Thoracic Duct L Cisterna Chyli	Ø Open 3 Percutaneous 4 Percutaneous Endoscopic	C Extraluminal Device D Intraluminal Device Z No Device	Z No Qualifier

SECTION: Ø MEDICAL AND SURGICAL
BODY SYSTEM: 7 LYMPHATIC AND HEMIC SYSTEMS
OPERATION: N RELEASE: Freeing a body part from an abnormal physical constraint by cutting or by the use of force

Body Part	Approach	Device	Qualifier
Ø Lymphatic, Head 1 Lymphatic, Right Neck 2 Lymphatic, Left Neck 3 Lymphatic, Right Upper Extremity 4 Lymphatic, Left Upper Extremity 5 Lymphatic, Right Axillary 6 Lymphatic, Left Axillary 7 Lymphatic, Thorax 8 Lymphatic, Internal Mammary, Right 9 Lymphatic, Internal Mammary, Left B Lymphatic, Mesenteric C Lymphatic, Pelvis D Lymphatic, Aortic F Lymphatic, Right Lower Extremity G Lymphatic, Left Lower Extremity H Lymphatic, Right Inguinal J Lymphatic, Left Inguinal K Thoracic Duct L Cisterna Chyli M Thymus P Spleen	Ø Open 3 Percutaneous 4 Percutaneous Endoscopic	Z No Device	Z No Qualifier

SECTION: Ø MEDICAL AND SURGICAL
BODY SYSTEM: 7 LYMPHATIC AND HEMIC SYSTEMS
OPERATION: P REMOVAL: Taking out or off a device from a body part

Body Part	Approach	Device	Qualifier
K Thoracic Duct L Cisterna Chyli N Lymphatic	Ø Open 3 Percutaneous 4 Percutaneous Endoscopic	Ø Drainage Device 3 Infusion Device 7 Autologous Tissue Substitute C Extraluminal Device D Intraluminal Device J Synthetic Substitute K Nonautologous Tissue Substitute Y Other Device	Z No Qualifier
K Thoracic Duct L Cisterna Chyli N Lymphatic	X External	Ø Drainage Device 3 Infusion Device D Intraluminal Device	Z No Qualifier
M Thymus P Spleen	Ø Open 3 Percutaneous 4 Percutaneous Endoscopic	Ø Drainage Device 3 Infusion Device Y Other Device	Z No Qualifier
M Thymus P Spleen	X External	Ø Drainage Device 3 Infusion Device	Z No Qualifier
T Bone Marrow	Ø Open 3 Percutaneous 4 Percutaneous Endoscopic X External	Ø Drainage Device	Z No Qualifier

Non-OR Ø7P[KLN]X[Ø3D]Z Non-OR Ø7P[MP]X[Ø3]Z Non-OR Ø7PT[Ø34X]ØZ

New/Revised Text in Green ~~deleted~~ Deleted ♀ Females Only ♂ Males Only Coding Clinic
Non-covered Limited Coverage Combination (See Appendix E) DRG Non-OR Non-OR Hospital-Acquired Condition

SECTION: Ø MEDICAL AND SURGICAL
BODY SYSTEM: 7 LYMPHATIC AND HEMIC SYSTEMS
OPERATION: Q REPAIR: Restoring, to the extent possible, a body part to its normal anatomic structure and function

Body Part	Approach	Device	Qualifier
Ø Lymphatic, Head 1 Lymphatic, Right Neck 2 Lymphatic, Left Neck 3 Lymphatic, Right Upper Extremity 4 Lymphatic, Left Upper Extremity 5 Lymphatic, Right Axillary 6 Lymphatic, Left Axillary 7 Lymphatic, Thorax 8 Lymphatic, Internal Mammary, Right 9 Lymphatic, Internal Mammary, Left B Lymphatic, Mesenteric C Lymphatic, Pelvis D Lymphatic, Aortic F Lymphatic, Right Lower Extremity G Lymphatic, Left Lower Extremity H Lymphatic, Right Inguinal J Lymphatic, Left Inguinal K Thoracic Duct L Cisterna Chyli	Ø Open 3 Percutaneous 4 Percutaneous Endoscopic 8 Via Natural or Artificial Opening Endoscopic	Z No Device	Z No Qualifier
M Thymus P Spleen	Ø Open 3 Percutaneous 4 Percutaneous Endoscopic	Z No Device	Z No Qualifier

Coding Clinic: 2Ø17, Q1, P34 – Ø7Q6ØZZ

SECTION: Ø MEDICAL AND SURGICAL
BODY SYSTEM: 7 LYMPHATIC AND HEMIC SYSTEMS
OPERATION: S REPOSITION: Moving to its normal location, or other suitable location, all or a portion of a body part

Body Part	Approach	Device	Qualifier
M Thymus P Spleen	Ø Open	Z No Device	Z No Qualifier

SECTION: Ø MEDICAL AND SURGICAL
BODY SYSTEM: 7 LYMPHATIC AND HEMIC SYSTEMS
OPERATION: T RESECTION: Cutting out or off, without replacement, all of a body part

Body Part	Approach	Device	Qualifier
Ø Lymphatic, Head 1 Lymphatic, Right Neck 2 Lymphatic, Left Neck 3 Lymphatic, Right Upper Extremity 4 Lymphatic, Left Upper Extremity 5 Lymphatic, Right Axillary ⊞ 6 Lymphatic, Left Axillary ⊞ 7 Lymphatic, Thorax ⊞ 8 Lymphatic, Internal Mammary, Right ⊞ 9 Lymphatic, Internal Mammary, Left ⊞ B Lymphatic, Mesenteric C Lymphatic, Pelvis D Lymphatic, Aortic F Lymphatic, Right Lower Extremity G Lymphatic, Left Lower Extremity H Lymphatic, Right Inguinal J Lymphatic, Left Inguinal K Thoracic Duct L Cisterna Chyli M Thymus ~~P Spleen~~	Ø Open 4 Percutaneous Endoscopic	Z No Device	Z No Qualifier
P Spleen	Ø Open	Z No Device	Z No Qualifier
P Spleen	4 Percutaneous Endoscopic	Z No Device	G Hand-Assisted Z No Qualifier

⊞ Ø7T[56789]ØZZ

Coding Clinic: 2Ø15, Q4, P13 – Ø7TPØZZ
Coding Clinic: 2Ø16, Q1, P3Ø – Ø7T5ØZZ
Coding Clinic: 2Ø16, Q2, P13 – Ø7T2ØZZ

SECTION: Ø MEDICAL AND SURGICAL
BODY SYSTEM: 7 LYMPHATIC AND HEMIC SYSTEMS
OPERATION: U SUPPLEMENT: Putting in or on biological or synthetic material that physically reinforces and/or augments the function of a portion of a body part

Body Part	Approach	Device	Qualifier
Ø Lymphatic, Head 1 Lymphatic, Right Neck 2 Lymphatic, Left Neck 3 Lymphatic, Right Upper Extremity 4 Lymphatic, Left Upper Extremity 5 Lymphatic, Right Axillary 6 Lymphatic, Left Axillary 7 Lymphatic, Thorax 8 Lymphatic, Internal Mammary, Right 9 Lymphatic, Internal Mammary, Left B Lymphatic, Mesenteric C Lymphatic, Pelvis D Lymphatic, Aortic F Lymphatic, Right Lower Extremity G Lymphatic, Left Lower Extremity H Lymphatic, Right Inguinal J Lymphatic, Left Inguinal K Thoracic Duct L Cisterna Chyli	Ø Open 4 Percutaneous Endoscopic	7 Autologous Tissue Substitute J Synthetic Substitute K Nonautologous Tissue Substitute	Z No Qualifier

SECTION: Ø MEDICAL AND SURGICAL
BODY SYSTEM: 7 LYMPHATIC AND HEMIC SYSTEMS
OPERATION: V RESTRICTION: Partially closing an orifice or the lumen of a tubular body part

Body Part	Approach	Device	Qualifier
Ø Lymphatic, Head 1 Lymphatic, Right Neck 2 Lymphatic, Left Neck 3 Lymphatic, Right Upper Extremity 4 Lymphatic, Left Upper Extremity 5 Lymphatic, Right Axillary 6 Lymphatic, Left Axillary 7 Lymphatic, Thorax 8 Lymphatic, Internal Mammary, Right 9 Lymphatic, Internal Mammary, Left B Lymphatic, Mesenteric C Lymphatic, Pelvis D Lymphatic, Aortic F Lymphatic, Right Lower Extremity G Lymphatic, Left Lower Extremity H Lymphatic, Right Inguinal J Lymphatic, Left Inguinal K Thoracic Duct L Cisterna Chyli	Ø Open 3 Percutaneous 4 Percutaneous Endoscopic	C Extraluminal Device D Intraluminal Device Z No Device	Z No Qualifier

SECTION: Ø MEDICAL AND SURGICAL
BODY SYSTEM: 7 LYMPHATIC AND HEMIC SYSTEMS
OPERATION: W **REVISION:** Correcting, to the extent possible, a portion of a malfunctioning device or the position of a displaced device

Body Part	Approach	Device	Qualifier
K Thoracic Duct L Cisterna Chyli N Lymphatic	Ø Open 3 Percutaneous 4 Percutaneous Endoscopic	Ø Drainage Device 3 Infusion Device 7 Autologous Tissue Substitute C Extraluminal Device D Intraluminal Device J Synthetic Substitute K Nonautologous Tissue Substitute Y Other Device	Z No Qualifier
K Thoracic Duct L Cisterna Chyli N Lymphatic	X External	Ø Drainage Device 3 Infusion Device 7 Autologous Tissue Substitute C Extraluminal Device D Intraluminal Device J Synthetic Substitute K Nonautologous Tissue Substitute	Z No Qualifier
M Thymus P Spleen	Ø Open 3 Percutaneous 4 Percutaneous Endoscopic	Ø Drainage Device 3 Infusion Device Y Other Device	Z No Qualifier
M Thymus P Spleen	X External	Ø Drainage Device 3 Infusion Device	Z No Qualifier
T Bone Marrow	Ø Open 3 Percutaneous 4 Percutaneous Endoscopic X External	Ø Drainage Device	Z No Qualifier

Non-OR Ø7W[KLN]X[Ø37CDJK]Z
Non-OR Ø7W[MP]X[Ø3]Z
Non-OR Ø7WT[Ø34X]ØZ

SECTION: Ø MEDICAL AND SURGICAL
BODY SYSTEM: 7 LYMPHATIC AND HEMIC SYSTEMS
OPERATION: Y **TRANSPLANTATION:** Putting in or on all or a portion of a living body part taken from another individual or animal to physically take the place and/or function of all or a portion of a similar body part

Body Part	Approach	Device	Qualifier
M Thymus P Spleen	Ø Open	Z No Device	Ø Allogeneic 1 Syngeneic 2 Zooplastic

Coding Clinic: 2Ø19, Q3, P29 – Ø7YMØZØ

Ø8. Eye 175
Ø8Ø. Alteration 176
Ø81. Bypass 176
Ø82. Change 176
Ø85. Destruction 177
Ø87. Dilation 177
Ø89. Drainage 178
Ø8B. Excision 18Ø
Ø8C. Extirpation 181
Ø8D. Extraction 181
Ø8F. Fragmentation 182
Ø8H. Insertion 182
Ø8J. Inspection 182
Ø8L. Occlusion 183
Ø8M. Reattachment 183
Ø8N. Release 184
Ø8P. Removal 185
Ø8Q. Repair 186
Ø8R. Replacement 187
Ø8S. Reposition 188
Ø8T. Resection 189
Ø8U. Supplement 19Ø
Ø8V. Restriction 19Ø
Ø8W. Revision 191
Ø8X. Transfer 191

SECTION: Ø MEDICAL AND SURGICAL
BODY SYSTEM: 8 EYE
OPERATION: Ø ALTERATION: Modifying the anatomic structure of a body part without affecting the function of the body part

Body Part	Approach	Device	Qualifier
N Upper Eyelid, Right P Upper Eyelid, Left Q Lower Eyelid, Right R Lower Eyelid, Left	Ø Open 3 Percutaneous X External	7 Autologous Tissue Substitute J Synthetic Substitute K Nonautologous Tissue Substitute Z No Device	Z No Qualifier

Non-OR All Values

SECTION: Ø MEDICAL AND SURGICAL
BODY SYSTEM: 8 EYE
OPERATION: 1 BYPASS: Altering the route of passage of the contents of a tubular body part

Body Part	Approach	Device	Qualifier
2 Anterior Chamber, Right 3 Anterior Chamber, Left	3 Percutaneous	J Synthetic Substitute K Nonautologous Tissue Substitute Z No Device	4 Sclera
X Lacrimal Duct, Right Y Lacrimal Duct, Left	Ø Open 3 Percutaneous	J Synthetic Substitute K Nonautologous Tissue Substitute Z No Device	3 Nasal Cavity

Coding Clinic: 2Ø19, Q1, P28 – Ø8133J4

SECTION: Ø MEDICAL AND SURGICAL
BODY SYSTEM: 8 EYE
OPERATION: 2 CHANGE: Taking out or off a device from a body part and putting back an identical or similar device in or on the same body part without cutting or puncturing the skin or a mucous membrane

Body Part	Approach	Device	Qualifier
Ø Eye, Right 1 Eye, Left	X External	Ø Drainage Device Y Other Device	Z No Qualifier

Non-OR All Values

SECTION: Ø MEDICAL AND SURGICAL
BODY SYSTEM: 8 EYE
OPERATION: 5 DESTRUCTION: Physical eradication of all or a portion of a body part by the direct use of energy, force, or a destructive agent

Body Part	Approach	Device	Qualifier
Ø Eye, Right 1 Eye, Left 6 Sclera, Right 7 Sclera, Left 8 Cornea, Right 9 Cornea, Left S Conjunctiva, Right T Conjunctiva, Left	X External	Z No Device	Z No Qualifier
2 Anterior Chamber, Right 3 Anterior Chamber, Left 4 Vitreous, Right 5 Vitreous, Left C Iris, Right D Iris, Left E Retina, Right F Retina, Left G Retinal Vessel, Right H Retinal Vessel, Left J Lens, Right K Lens, Left	3 Percutaneous	Z No Device	Z No Qualifier
A Choroid, Right B Choroid, Left L Extraocular Muscle, Right M Extraocular Muscle, Left V Lacrimal Gland, Right W Lacrimal Gland, Left	Ø Open 3 Percutaneous	Z No Device	Z No Qualifier
N Upper Eyelid, Right P Upper Eyelid, Left Q Lower Eyelid, Right R Lower Eyelid, Left	Ø Open 3 Percutaneous X External	Z No Device	Z No Qualifier
X Lacrimal Duct, Right Y Lacrimal Duct, Left	Ø Open 3 Percutaneous 7 Via Natural or Artificial Opening 8 Via Natural or Artificial Opening Endoscopic	Z No Device	Z No Qualifier

SECTION: Ø MEDICAL AND SURGICAL
BODY SYSTEM: 8 EYE
OPERATION: 7 DILATION: Expanding an orifice or the lumen of a tubular body part

Body Part	Approach	Device	Qualifier
X Lacrimal Duct, Right Y Lacrimal Duct, Left	Ø Open 3 Percutaneous 7 Via Natural or Artificial Opening 8 Via Natural or Artificial Opening Endoscopic	D Intraluminal Device Z No Device	Z No Qualifier

SECTION: Ø MEDICAL AND SURGICAL
BODY SYSTEM: 8 EYE
OPERATION: 9 DRAINAGE: *(on multiple pages)*
Taking or letting out fluids and/or gases from a body part

Body Part	Approach	Device	Qualifier
Ø Eye, Right 1 Eye, Left 6 Sclera, Right 7 Sclera, Left 8 Cornea, Right 9 Cornea, Left S Conjunctiva, Right T Conjunctiva, Left	X External	Ø Drainage Device	Z No Qualifier
Ø Eye, Right 1 Eye, Left 6 Sclera, Right 7 Sclera, Left 8 Cornea, Right 9 Cornea, Left S Conjunctiva, Right T Conjunctiva, Left	X External	Z No Device	X Diagnostic Z No Qualifier
2 Anterior Chamber, Right 3 Anterior Chamber, Left 4 Vitreous, Right 5 Vitreous, Left C Iris, Right D Iris, Left E Retina, Right F Retina, Left G Retinal Vessel, Right H Retinal Vessel, Left J Lens, Right K Lens, Left	3 Percutaneous	Ø Drainage Device	Z No Qualifier
2 Anterior Chamber, Right 3 Anterior Chamber, Left 4 Vitreous, Right 5 Vitreous, Left C Iris, Right D Iris, Left E Retina, Right F Retina, Left G Retinal Vessel, Right H Retinal Vessel, Left J Lens, Right K Lens, Left	3 Percutaneous	Z No Device	X Diagnostic Z No Qualifier
A Choroid, Right B Choroid, Left L Extraocular Muscle, Right M Extraocular Muscle, Left V Lacrimal Gland, Right W Lacrimal Gland, Left	Ø Open 3 Percutaneous	Ø Drainage Device	Z No Qualifier

DRG Non-OR Ø89[Ø16789ST]XZ[XZ] *(proposed)*

Coding Clinic: 2Ø16, Q2, P21 – Ø8923ZZ

SECTION: Ø MEDICAL AND SURGICAL
BODY SYSTEM: 8 EYE
OPERATION: 9 DRAINAGE: *(continued)*
Taking or letting out fluids and/or gases from a body part

Body Part	Approach	Device	Qualifier
A Choroid, Right B Choroid, Left L Extraocular Muscle, Right M Extraocular Muscle, Left V Lacrimal Gland, Right W Lacrimal Gland, Left	Ø Open 3 Percutaneous	Z No Device	X Diagnostic Z No Qualifier
N Upper Eyelid, Right P Upper Eyelid, Left Q Lower Eyelid, Right R Lower Eyelid, Left	Ø Open 3 Percutaneous X External	Ø Drainage Device	Z No Qualifier
N Upper Eyelid, Right P Upper Eyelid, Left Q Lower Eyelid, Right R Lower Eyelid, Left	Ø Open 3 Percutaneous X External	Z No Device	X Diagnostic Z No Qualifier
X Lacrimal Duct, Right Y Lacrimal Duct, Left	Ø Open 3 Percutaneous 7 Via Natural or Artificial Opening 8 Via Natural or Artificial Opening Endoscopic	Ø Drainage Device	Z No Qualifier
X Lacrimal Duct, Right Y Lacrimal Duct, Left	Ø Open 3 Percutaneous 7 Via Natural or Artificial Opening 8 Via Natural or Artificial Opening Endoscopic	Z No Device	X Diagnostic Z No Qualifier

DRG Non-OR Ø89[NPQR]XZX *(proposed)*
Non-OR Ø89[NPQR][Ø3X]ØZ
Non-OR Ø89[NPQR][Ø3X]ZZ

SECTION: Ø MEDICAL AND SURGICAL

BODY SYSTEM: 8 EYE

OPERATION: B EXCISION: Cutting out or off, without replacement, a portion of a body part

Body Part	Approach	Device	Qualifier
Ø Eye, Right 1 Eye, Left N Upper Eyelid, Right P Upper Eyelid, Left Q Lower Eyelid, Right R Lower Eyelid, Left	Ø Open 3 Percutaneous X External	Z No Device	X Diagnostic Z No Qualifier
4 Vitreous, Right 5 Vitreous, Left C Iris, Right D Iris, Left E Retina, Right F Retina, Left J Lens, Right K Lens, Left	3 Percutaneous	Z No Device	X Diagnostic Z No Qualifier
6 Sclera, Right 7 Sclera, Left 8 Cornea, Right 9 Cornea, Left S Conjunctiva, Right T Conjunctiva, Left	X External	Z No Device	X Diagnostic Z No Qualifier
A Choroid, Right B Choroid, Left L Extraocular Muscle, Right M Extraocular Muscle, Left V Lacrimal Gland, Right W Lacrimal Gland, Left	Ø Open 3 Percutaneous	Z No Device	X Diagnostic Z No Qualifier
X Lacrimal Duct, Right Y Lacrimal Duct, Left	Ø Open 3 Percutaneous 7 Via Natural or Artificial Opening 8 Via Natural or Artificial Opening Endoscopic	Z No Device	X Diagnostic Z No Qualifier

SECTION: Ø MEDICAL AND SURGICAL
BODY SYSTEM: 8 EYE
OPERATION: C EXTIRPATION: Taking or cutting out solid matter from a body part

Body Part	Approach	Device	Qualifier
Ø Eye, Right 1 Eye, Left 6 Sclera, Right 7 Sclera, Left 8 Cornea, Right 9 Cornea, Left S Conjunctiva, Right T Conjunctiva, Left	X External	Z No Device	Z No Qualifier
2 Anterior Chamber, Right 3 Anterior Chamber, Left 4 Vitreous, Right 5 Vitreous, Left C Iris, Right D Iris, Left E Retina, Right F Retina, Left G Retinal Vessel, Right H Retinal Vessel, Left J Lens, Right K Lens, Left	3 Percutaneous X External	Z No Device	Z No Qualifier
A Choroid, Right B Choroid, Left L Extraocular Muscle, Right M Extraocular Muscle, Left N Upper Eyelid, Right P Upper Eyelid, Left Q Lower Eyelid, Right R Lower Eyelid, Left V Lacrimal Gland, Right W Lacrimal Gland, Left	Ø Open 3 Percutaneous X External	Z No Device	Z No Qualifier
X Lacrimal Duct, Right Y Lacrimal Duct, Left	Ø Open 3 Percutaneous 7 Via Natural or Artificial Opening 8 Via Natural or Artificial Opening Endoscopic	Z No Device	Z No Qualifier

Non-OR Ø8C[23]XZZ
Non-OR Ø8C[67]XZZ
Non-OR Ø8C[NPQR][Ø3X]ZZ

SECTION: Ø MEDICAL AND SURGICAL
BODY SYSTEM: 8 EYE
OPERATION: D EXTRACTION: Pulling or stripping out or off all or a portion of a body part by the use of force

Body Part	Approach	Device	Qualifier
8 Cornea, Right 9 Cornea, Left	X External	Z No Device	X Diagnostic Z No Qualifier
J Lens, Right K Lens, Left	3 Percutaneous	Z No Device	Z No Qualifier

SECTION: Ø MEDICAL AND SURGICAL
BODY SYSTEM: 8 EYE
OPERATION: F **FRAGMENTATION:** Breaking solid matter in a body part into pieces

Body Part	Approach	Device	Qualifier
4 Vitreous, Right 5 Vitreous, Left	3 Percutaneous X External	Z No Device	Z No Qualifier

Ø8F[45]XZZ
Non-OR Ø8F[45]XZZ

SECTION: Ø MEDICAL AND SURGICAL
BODY SYSTEM: 8 EYE
OPERATION: H **INSERTION:** Putting in a nonbiological appliance that monitors, assists, performs, or prevents a physiological function but does not physically take the place of a body part

Body Part	Approach	Device	Qualifier
Ø Eye, Right 1 Eye, Left	Ø Open	5 Epiretinal Visual Prosthesis Y Other Device	Z No Qualifier
Ø Eye, Right 1 Eye, Left	3 Percutaneous	1 Radioactive Element 3 Infusion Device Y Other Device	Z No Qualifier
Ø Eye, Right 1 Eye, Left	7 Via Natural or Artificial Opening 8 Via Natural or Artificial Opening Endoscopic	Y Other Device	Z No Qualifier
Ø Eye, Right 1 Eye, Left	X External	1 Radioactive Element 3 Infusion Device	Z No Qualifier

SECTION: Ø MEDICAL AND SURGICAL
BODY SYSTEM: 8 EYE
OPERATION: J **INSPECTION:** Visually and/or manually exploring a body part

Body Part	Approach	Device	Qualifier
Ø Eye, Right 1 Eye, Left J Lens, Right K Lens, Left	X External	Z No Device	Z No Qualifier
L Extraocular Muscle, Right M Extraocular Muscle, Left	Ø Open X External	Z No Device	Z No Qualifier

Non-OR Ø8J[Ø1JK]XZZ
Non-OR Ø8J[LM]XZZ

Coding Clinic: 2015, Q1, P36 – Ø8JØXZZ

SECTION: Ø MEDICAL AND SURGICAL
BODY SYSTEM: 8 EYE
OPERATION: L **OCCLUSION:** Completely closing an orifice or the lumen of a tubular body part

Body Part	Approach	Device	Qualifier
X Lacrimal Duct, Right Y Lacrimal Duct, Left	Ø Open 3 Percutaneous	C Extraluminal Device D Intraluminal Device Z No Device	Z No Qualifier
X Lacrimal Duct, Right Y Lacrimal Duct, Left	7 Via Natural or Artificial Opening 8 Via Natural or Artificial Opening Endoscopic	D Intraluminal Device Z No Device	Z No Qualifier

SECTION: Ø MEDICAL AND SURGICAL
BODY SYSTEM: 8 EYE
OPERATION: M **REATTACHMENT:** Putting back in or on all or a portion of a separated body part to its normal location or other suitable location

Body Part	Approach	Device	Qualifier
N Upper Eyelid, Right P Upper Eyelid, Left Q Lower Eyelid, Right R Lower Eyelid, Left	X External	Z No Device	Z No Qualifier

SECTION: Ø MEDICAL AND SURGICAL
BODY SYSTEM: 8 EYE
OPERATION: N RELEASE: Freeing a body part from an abnormal physical constraint by cutting or by the use of force

Body Part	Approach	Device	Qualifier
Ø Eye, Right 1 Eye, Left 6 Sclera, Right 7 Sclera, Left 8 Cornea, Right 9 Cornea, Left S Conjunctiva, Right T Conjunctiva, Left	X External	Z No Device	Z No Qualifier
2 Anterior Chamber, Right 3 Anterior Chamber, Left 4 Vitreous, Right 5 Vitreous, Left C Iris, Right D Iris, Left E Retina, Right F Retina, Left G Retinal Vessel, Right H Retinal Vessel, Left J Lens, Right K Lens, Left	3 Percutaneous	Z No Device	Z No Qualifier
A Choroid, Right B Choroid, Left L Extraocular Muscle, Right M Extraocular Muscle, Left V Lacrimal Gland, Right W Lacrimal Gland, Left	Ø Open 3 Percutaneous	Z No Device	Z No Qualifier
N Upper Eyelid, Right P Upper Eyelid, Left Q Lower Eyelid, Right R Lower Eyelid, Left	Ø Open 3 Percutaneous X External	Z No Device	Z No Qualifier
X Lacrimal Duct, Right Y Lacrimal Duct, Left	Ø Open 3 Percutaneous 7 Via Natural or Artificial Opening 8 Via Natural or Artificial Opening Endoscopic	Z No Device	Z No Qualifier

Coding Clinic: 2Ø15, Q2, P25 – Ø8NC3ZZ

SECTION: Ø MEDICAL AND SURGICAL
BODY SYSTEM: 8 EYE
OPERATION: P REMOVAL: Taking out or off a device from a body part

Body Part	Approach	Device	Qualifier
Ø Eye, Right 1 Eye, Left	Ø Open 3 Percutaneous 7 Via Natural or Artificial Opening 8 Via Natural or Artificial Opening Endoscopic	Ø Drainage Device 1 Radioactive Element 3 Infusion Device 7 Autologous Tissue Substitute C Extraluminal Device D Intraluminal Device J Synthetic Substitute K Nonautologous Tissue Substitute Y Other Device	Z No Qualifier
Ø Eye, Right 1 Eye, Left	X External	Ø Drainage Device 1 Radioactive Element 3 Infusion Device 7 Autologous Tissue Substitute C Extraluminal Device D Intraluminal Device J Synthetic Substitute K Nonautologous Tissue Substitute	Z No Qualifier
J Lens, Right K Lens, Left	3 Percutaneous	J Synthetic Substitute Y Other Device	Z No Qualifier
L Extraocular Muscle, Right M Extraocular Muscle, Left	Ø Open 3 Percutaneous	Ø Drainage Device 7 Autologous Tissue Substitute J Synthetic Substitute K Nonautologous Tissue Substitute Y Other Device	Z No Qualifier

Non-OR Ø8P[Ø1][78][Ø3D]Z
Non-OR Ø8PØX[Ø3CD]Z
Non-OR Ø8P1X[Ø13CD]Z

SECTION: Ø MEDICAL AND SURGICAL
BODY SYSTEM: 8 EYE
OPERATION: Q REPAIR: Restoring, to the extent possible, a body part to its normal anatomic structure and function

Body Part	Approach	Device	Qualifier
Ø Eye, Right 1 Eye, Left 6 Sclera, Right 7 Sclera, Left 8 Cornea, Right 9 Cornea, Left S Conjunctiva, Right T Conjunctiva, Left	X External	Z No Device	Z No Qualifier
2 Anterior Chamber, Right 3 Anterior Chamber, Left 4 Vitreous, Right 5 Vitreous, Left C Iris, Right D Iris, Left E Retina, Right F Retina, Left G Retinal Vessel, Right H Retinal Vessel, Left J Lens, Right K Lens, Left	3 Percutaneous	Z No Device	Z No Qualifier
A Choroid, Right B Choroid, Left L Extraocular Muscle, Right M Extraocular Muscle, Left V Lacrimal Gland, Right W Lacrimal Gland, Left	Ø Open 3 Percutaneous	Z No Device	Z No Qualifier
N Upper Eyelid, Right P Upper Eyelid, Left Q Lower Eyelid, Right R Lower Eyelid, Left	Ø Open 3 Percutaneous X External	Z No Device	Z No Qualifier
X Lacrimal Duct, Right Y Lacrimal Duct, Left	Ø Open 3 Percutaneous 7 Via Natural or Artificial Opening 8 Via Natural or Artificial Opening Endoscopic	Z No Device	Z No Qualifier

Ø8Q[89]XZZ
Non-OR Ø8Q[NPQR][Ø3X]ZZ

SECTION: Ø MEDICAL AND SURGICAL
BODY SYSTEM: 8 EYE
OPERATION: R REPLACEMENT: Putting in or on biological or synthetic material that physically takes the place and/or function of all or a portion of a body part

Body Part	Approach	Device	Qualifier
Ø Eye, Right 1 Eye, Left A Choroid, Right B Choroid, Left	Ø Open 3 Percutaneous	7 Autologous Tissue Substitute J Synthetic Substitute K Nonautologous Tissue Substitute	Z No Qualifier
4 Vitreous, Right 5 Vitreous, Left C Iris, Right D Iris, Left G Retinal Vessel, Right H Retinal Vessel, Left	3 Percutaneous	7 Autologous Tissue Substitute J Synthetic Substitute K Nonautologous Tissue Substitute	Z No Qualifier
6 Sclera, Right 7 Sclera, Left S Conjunctiva, Right T Conjunctiva, Left	X External	7 Autologous Tissue Substitute J Synthetic Substitute K Nonautologous Tissue Substitute	Z No Qualifier
8 Cornea, Right 9 Cornea, Left	3 Percutaneous X External	7 Autologous Tissue Substitute J Synthetic Substitute K Nonautologous Tissue Substitute	Z No Qualifier
J Lens, Right K Lens, Left	3 Percutaneous	Ø Synthetic Substitute, Intraocular Telescope 7 Autologous Tissue Substitute J Synthetic Substitute K Nonautologous Tissue Substitute	Z No Qualifier
N Upper Eyelid, Right P Upper Eyelid, Left Q Lower Eyelid, Right R Lower Eyelid, Left	Ø Open 3 Percutaneous X External	7 Autologous Tissue Substitute J Synthetic Substitute K Nonautologous Tissue Substitute	Z No Qualifier
X Lacrimal Duct, Right Y Lacrimal Duct, Left	Ø Open 3 Percutaneous 7 Via Natural or Artificial Opening 8 Via Natural or Artificial Opening Endoscopic	7 Autologous Tissue Substitute J Synthetic Substitute K Nonautologous Tissue Substitute	Z No Qualifier

Coding Clinic: 2Ø15, Q2, P25-26 – Ø8R8XKZ

SECTION: Ø MEDICAL AND SURGICAL
BODY SYSTEM: 8 EYE
OPERATION: S REPOSITION: Moving to its normal location, or other suitable location, all or a portion of a body part

Body Part	Approach	Device	Qualifier
C Iris, Right D Iris, Left G Retinal Vessel, Right H Retinal Vessel, Left J Lens, Right K Lens, Left	3 Percutaneous	Z No Device	Z No Qualifier
L Extraocular Muscle, Right M Extraocular Muscle, Left V Lacrimal Gland, Right W Lacrimal Gland, Left	Ø Open 3 Percutaneous	Z No Device	Z No Qualifier
N Upper Eyelid, Right P Upper Eyelid, Left Q Lower Eyelid, Right R Lower Eyelid, Left	Ø Open 3 Percutaneous X External	Z No Device	Z No Qualifier
X Lacrimal Duct, Right Y Lacrimal Duct, Left	Ø Open 3 Percutaneous 7 Via Natural or Artificial Opening 8 Via Natural or Artificial Opening Endoscopic	Z No Device	Z No Qualifier

SECTION: Ø MEDICAL AND SURGICAL
BODY SYSTEM: 8 EYE
OPERATION: T RESECTION: Cutting out or off, without replacement, all of a body part

Body Part	Approach	Device	Qualifier
Ø Eye, Right 1 Eye, Left 8 Cornea, Right 9 Cornea, Left	X External	Z No Device	Z No Qualifier
4 Vitreous, Right 5 Vitreous, Left C Iris, Right D Iris, Left J Lens, Right K Lens, Left	3 Percutaneous	Z No Device	Z No Qualifier
L Extraocular Muscle, Right M Extraocular Muscle, Left V Lacrimal Gland, Right W Lacrimal Gland, Left	Ø Open 3 Percutaneous	Z No Device	Z No Qualifier
N Upper Eyelid, Right P Upper Eyelid, Left Q Lower Eyelid, Right R Lower Eyelid, Left	Ø Open X External	Z No Device	Z No Qualifier
X Lacrimal Duct, Right Y Lacrimal Duct, Left	Ø Open 3 Percutaneous 7 Via Natural or Artificial Opening 8 Via Natural or Artificial Opening Endoscopic	Z No Device	Z No Qualifier

Coding Clinic: 2Ø15, Q2, P13 – Ø8T1XZZ, Ø8T[MR]ØZZ

SECTION: Ø MEDICAL AND SURGICAL
BODY SYSTEM: 8 EYE
OPERATION: U **SUPPLEMENT:** Putting in or on biological or synthetic material that physically reinforces and/or augments the function of a portion of a body part

Body Part	Approach	Device	Qualifier
Ø Eye, Right 1 Eye, Left C Iris, Right D Iris, Left E Retina, Right F Retina, Left G Retinal Vessel, Right H Retinal Vessel, Left L Extraocular Muscle, Right M Extraocular Muscle, Left	Ø Open 3 Percutaneous	7 Autologous Tissue Substitute J Synthetic Substitute K Nonautologous Tissue Substitute	Z No Qualifier
8 Cornea, Right 9 Cornea, Left N Upper Eyelid, Right P Upper Eyelid, Left Q Lower Eyelid, Right R Lower Eyelid, Left	Ø Open 3 Percutaneous X External	7 Autologous Tissue Substitute J Synthetic Substitute K Nonautologous Tissue Substitute	Z No Qualifier
X Lacrimal Duct, Right Y Lacrimal Duct, Left	Ø Open 3 Percutaneous 7 Via Natural or Artificial Opening 8 Via Natural or Artificial Opening Endoscopic	7 Autologous Tissue Substitute J Synthetic Substitute K Nonautologous Tissue Substitute	Z No Qualifier

Ø8U[89][Ø3X]KZ

SECTION: Ø MEDICAL AND SURGICAL
BODY SYSTEM: 8 EYE
OPERATION: V **RESTRICTION:** Partially closing an orifice or the lumen of a tubular body part

Body Part	Approach	Device	Qualifier
X Lacrimal Duct, Right Y Lacrimal Duct, Left	Ø Open 3 Percutaneous	C Extraluminal Device D Intraluminal Device Z No Device	Z No Qualifier
X Lacrimal Duct, Right Y Lacrimal Duct, Left	7 Via Natural or Artificial Opening 8 Via Natural or Artificial Opening Endoscopic	D Intraluminal Device Z No Device	Z No Qualifier

SECTION: Ø MEDICAL AND SURGICAL
BODY SYSTEM: 8 EYE
OPERATION: W REVISION: Correcting, to the extent possible, a portion of a malfunctioning device or the positon of a displaced device

Body Part	Approach	Device	Qualifier
Ø Eye, Right 1 Eye, Left	Ø Open 3 Percutaneous 7 Via Natural or Artificial Opening 8 Via Natural or Artificial Opening Endoscopic	Ø Drainage Device 3 Infusion Device 7 Autologous Tissue Substitute C Extraluminal Device D Intraluminal Device J Synthetic Substitute K Nonautologous Tissue Substitute Y Other Device	Z No Qualifier
Ø Eye, Right 1 Eye, Left	X External	Ø Drainage Device 3 Infusion Device 7 Autologous Tissue Substitute C Extraluminal Device D Intraluminal Device J Synthetic Substitute K Nonautologous Tissue Substitute	Z No Qualifier
J Lens, Right K Lens, Left	3 Percutaneous	J Synthetic Substitute Y Other Device	Z No Qualifier
J Lens, Right K Lens, Left	X External	J Synthetic Substitute	Z No Qualifier
L Extraocular Muscle, Right M Extraocular Muscle, Left	Ø Open 3 Percutaneous	Ø Drainage Device 7 Autologous Tissue Substitute J Synthetic Substitute K Nonautologous Tissue Substitute Y Other Device	Z No Qualifier

Non-OR Ø8W[Ø1]X[Ø37CDJK]Z
Non-OR Ø8W[JK]XJZ

SECTION: Ø MEDICAL AND SURGICAL
BODY SYSTEM: 8 EYE
OPERATION: X TRANSFER: Moving, without taking out, all or a portion of a body part to another location to take over the function of all or a portion of a body part

Body Part	Approach	Device	Qualifier
L Extraocular Muscle, Right M Extraocular Muscle, Left	Ø Open 3 Percutaneous	Z No Device	Z No Qualifier

Ø9. Ear, Nose, Sinus 192
Ø9Ø. Alteration 193
Ø91. Bypass 193
Ø92. Change 193
Ø93. Control 193
Ø95. Destruction 194
Ø97. Dilation 195
Ø98. Division 195
Ø99. Drainage 196
Ø9B. Excision 198
Ø9C. Extirpation 199
Ø9D. Extraction 2ØØ
Ø9H. Insertion 2ØØ
Ø9J. Inspection 2Ø1
Ø9M. Reattachment 2Ø1
Ø9N. Release 2Ø2
Ø9P. Removal 2Ø3
Ø9Q. Repair 2Ø4
Ø9R. Replacement 2Ø5
Ø9S. Reposition 2Ø6
Ø9T. Resection 2Ø7
Ø9U. Supplement 2Ø8
Ø9W. Revision 2Ø9

SECTION: Ø MEDICAL AND SURGICAL
BODY SYSTEM: 9 EAR, NOSE, SINUS
OPERATION: Ø ALTERATION: Modifying the anatomic structure of a body part without affecting the function of the body part

Body Part	Approach	Device	Qualifier
Ø External Ear, Right 1 External Ear, Left 2 External Ear, Bilateral K Nasal Mucosa and Soft Tissue	Ø Open 3 Percutaneous 4 Percutaneous Endoscopic X External	7 Autologous Tissue Substitute J Synthetic Substitute K Nonautologous Tissue Substitute Z No Device	Z No Qualifier

SECTION: Ø MEDICAL AND SURGICAL
BODY SYSTEM: 9 EAR, NOSE, SINUS
OPERATION: 1 BYPASS: Altering the route of passage of the contents of a tubular body part

Body Part	Approach	Device	Qualifier
D Inner Ear, Right E Inner Ear, Left	Ø Open	7 Autologous Tissue Substitute J Synthetic Substitute K Nonautologous Tissue Substitute Z No Device	Ø Endolymphatic

SECTION: Ø MEDICAL AND SURGICAL
BODY SYSTEM: 9 EAR, NOSE, SINUS
OPERATION: 2 CHANGE: Taking out or off a device from a body part and putting back an identical or similar device in or on the same body part without cutting or puncturing the skin or a mucous membrane

Body Part	Approach	Device	Qualifier
H Ear, Right J Ear, Left K Nasal Mucosa and Soft Tissue Y Sinus	X External	Ø Drainage Device Y Other Device	Z No Qualifier

Non-OR All Values

SECTION: Ø MEDICAL AND SURGICAL
BODY SYSTEM: 9 EAR, NOSE, SINUS
OPERATION: 3 CONTROL: Stopping, or attempting to stop, postprocedural or other acute bleeding

Body Part	Approach	Device	Qualifier
K Nasal Mucosa and Soft Tissue	7 Via Natural or Artificial Opening 8 Via Natural or Artificial Opening Endoscopic	Z No Device	Z No Qualifier

Coding Clinic: 2Ø18, Q4, P38 – Ø93K8ZZ

SECTION: Ø MEDICAL AND SURGICAL
BODY SYSTEM: 9 EAR, NOSE, SINUS
OPERATION: 5 DESTRUCTION: Physical eradication of all or a portion of a body part by the direct use of energy, force, or a destructive agent

Body Part	Approach	Device	Qualifier
Ø External Ear, Right 1 External Ear, Left	Ø Open 3 Percutaneous 4 Percutaneous Endoscopic X External	Z No Device	Z No Qualifier
3 External Auditory Canal, Right 4 External Auditory Canal, Left	Ø Open 3 Percutaneous 4 Percutaneous Endoscopic 7 Via Natural or Artificial Opening 8 Via Natural or Artificial Opening Endoscopic X External	Z No Device	Z No Qualifier
5 Middle Ear, Right 6 Middle Ear, Left 9 Auditory Ossicle, Right A Auditory Ossicle, Left D Inner Ear, Right E Inner Ear, Left	Ø Open 8 Via Natural or Artificial Opening Endoscopic	Z No Device	Z No Qualifier
7 Tympanic Membrane, Right 8 Tympanic Membrane, Left F Eustachian Tube, Right G Eustachian Tube, Left L Nasal Turbinate N Nasopharynx	Ø Open 3 Percutaneous 4 Percutaneous Endoscopic 7 Via Natural or Artificial Opening 8 Via Natural or Artificial Opening Endoscopic	Z No Device	Z No Qualifier
B Mastoid Sinus, Right C Mastoid Sinus, Left M Nasal Septum P Accessory Sinus Q Maxillary Sinus, Right R Maxillary Sinus, Left S Frontal Sinus, Right T Frontal Sinus, Left U Ethmoid Sinus, Right V Ethmoid Sinus, Left W Sphenoid Sinus, Right X Sphenoid Sinus, Left	Ø Open 3 Percutaneous 4 Percutaneous Endoscopic 8 Via Natural or Artificial Opening Endoscopic	Z No Device	Z No Qualifier
K Nasal Mucosa and Soft Tissue	Ø Open 3 Percutaneous 4 Percutaneous Endoscopic 8 Via Natural or Artificial Opening Endoscopic X External	Z No Device	Z No Qualifier

Non-OR Ø95[Ø1][Ø34X]ZZ
Non-OR Ø95[34][Ø3478X]ZZ
Non-OR Ø95[FG][Ø3478]ZZ
Non-OR Ø95M[Ø34]ZZ
Non-OR Ø95K[Ø34X]ZZ

SECTION: Ø MEDICAL AND SURGICAL
BODY SYSTEM: 9 EAR, NOSE, SINUS
OPERATION: 7 DILATION: Expanding an orifice or the lumen of a tubular body part

Body Part	Approach	Device	Qualifier
F Eustachian Tube, Right G Eustachian Tube, Left	Ø Open 7 Via Natural or Artificial Opening 8 Via Natural or Artificial Opening Endoscopic	D Intraluminal Device Z No Device	Z No Qualifier
F Eustachian Tube, Right G Eustachian Tube, Left	3 Percutaneous 4 Percutaneous Endoscopic	Z No Device	Z No Qualifier
N Nasopharynx	Ø Open 7 Via Natural or Artificial Opening 8 Via Natural or Artificial Opening Endoscopic	Z No Device	Z No Qualifier

Non-OR All Values

SECTION: Ø MEDICAL AND SURGICAL
BODY SYSTEM: 9 EAR, NOSE, SINUS
OPERATION: 8 DIVISION: Cutting into a body part, without draining fluids and/or gases from the body part, in order to separate or transect a body part

Body Part	Approach	Device	Qualifier
L Nasal Turbinate	Ø Open 3 Percutaneous 4 Percutaneous Endoscopic 7 Via Natural or Artificial Opening 8 Via Natural or Artificial Opening Endoscopic	Z No Device	Z No Qualifier

SECTION: Ø MEDICAL AND SURGICAL
BODY SYSTEM: 9 EAR, NOSE, SINUS
OPERATION: 9 DRAINAGE: *(on multiple pages)*
Taking or letting out fluids and/or gases from a body part

Body Part	Approach	Device	Qualifier
Ø External Ear, Right 1 External Ear, Left	Ø Open 3 Percutaneous 4 Percutaneous Endoscopic X External	Ø Drainage Device	Z No Qualifier
Ø External Ear, Right 1 External Ear, Left	Ø Open 3 Percutaneous 4 Percutaneous Endoscopic X External	Z No Device	X Diagnostic Z No Qualifier
3 External Auditory Canal, Right 4 External Auditory Canal, Left K Nasal Mucosa and Soft Tissue	Ø Open 3 Percutaneous 4 Percutaneous Endoscopic 7 Via Natural or Artificial Opening 8 Via Natural or Artificial Opening Endoscopic X External	Ø Drainage Device	Z No Qualifier
3 External Auditory Canal, Right 4 External Auditory Canal, Left K Nasal Mucosa and Soft Tissue	Ø Open 3 Percutaneous 4 Percutaneous Endoscopic 7 Via Natural or Artificial Opening 8 Via Natural or Artificial Opening Endoscopic X External	Z No Device	X Diagnostic Z No Qualifier
5 Middle Ear, Right 6 Middle Ear, Left 9 Auditory Ossicle, Right A Auditory Ossicle, Left D Inner Ear, Right E Inner Ear, Left	Ø Open 7 Via Natural or Artificial Opening 8 Via Natural or Artificial Opening Endoscopic	Ø Drainage Device	Z No Qualifier
5 Middle Ear, Right 6 Middle Ear, Left 9 Auditory Ossicle, Right A Auditory Ossicle, Left D Inner Ear, Right E Inner Ear, Left	Ø Open 7 Via Natural or Artificial Opening 8 Via Natural or Artificial Opening Endoscopic	Z No Device	X Diagnostic Z No Qualifier

Non-OR Ø99[Ø1][Ø34X]ØZ
Non-OR Ø99[Ø1][Ø34X]Z[XZ]
Non-OR Ø99[34][Ø3478X]ØZ
Non-OR Ø99K[Ø34X]ØZ
Non-OR Ø99[34][Ø3478X]Z[XZ]
Non-OR Ø99K[Ø34X]Z[XZ]
Non-OR Ø99[56]ØZZ

SECTION: Ø MEDICAL AND SURGICAL
BODY SYSTEM: 9 EAR, NOSE, SINUS
OPERATION: 9 DRAINAGE: *(continued)*
Taking or letting out fluids and/or gases from a body part

Body Part	Approach	Device	Qualifier
7 Tympanic Membrane, Right 8 Tympanic Membrane, Left B Mastoid Sinus, Right C Mastoid Sinus, Left F Eustachian Tube, Right G Eustachian Tube, Left L Nasal Turbinate M Nasal Septum N Nasopharynx P Accessory Sinus Q Maxillary Sinus, Right R Maxillary Sinus, Left S Frontal Sinus, Right T Frontal Sinus, Left U Ethmoid Sinus, Right V Ethmoid Sinus, Left W Sphenoid Sinus, Right X Sphenoid Sinus, Left	Ø Open 3 Percutaneous 4 Percutaneous Endoscopic 7 Via Natural or Artificial Opening 8 Via Natural or Artificial Opening Endoscopic	Ø Drainage Device	Z No Qualifier
7 Tympanic Membrane, Right 8 Tympanic Membrane, Left B Mastoid Sinus, Right C Mastoid Sinus, Left F Eustachian Tube, Right G Eustachian Tube, Left L Nasal Turbinate M Nasal Septum N Nasopharynx P Accessory Sinus Q Maxillary Sinus, Right R Maxillary Sinus, Left S Frontal Sinus, Right T Frontal Sinus, Left U Ethmoid Sinus, Right V Ethmoid Sinus, Left W Sphenoid Sinus, Right X Sphenoid Sinus, Left	Ø Open 3 Percutaneous 4 Percutaneous Endoscopic 7 Via Natural or Artificial Opening 8 Via Natural or Artificial Opening Endoscopic	Z No Device	X Diagnostic Z No Qualifier

Non-OR Ø99[FGL][Ø3478]ØZ
Non-OR Ø99N3ØZ
Non-OR Ø99[78FG][Ø3478]ZZ
Non-OR Ø99L[Ø3478]Z[XZ]
Non-OR Ø99N[Ø3478]ZX
Non-OR Ø99N3ZZ
Non-OR Ø99[BC]3ØZ
Non-OR Ø99M[Ø34]ØZ
Non-OR Ø99[PQRSTUVWX][34]ØZ
Non-OR Ø99[BC]3ZZ
Non-OR Ø99M[Ø34]Z[XZ]
Non-OR Ø99[PQRSTUVWX][34]Z[XZ]

SECTION: Ø MEDICAL AND SURGICAL
BODY SYSTEM: 9 EAR, NOSE, SINUS
OPERATION: B EXCISION: Cutting out or off, without replacement, a portion of a body part

Body Part	Approach	Device	Qualifier
Ø External Ear, Right 1 External Ear, Left	Ø Open 3 Percutaneous 4 Percutaneous Endoscopic X External	Z No Device	X Diagnostic Z No Qualifier
3 External Auditory Canal, Right 4 External Auditory Canal, Left	Ø Open 3 Percutaneous 4 Percutaneous Endoscopic 7 Via Natural or Artificial Opening 8 Via Natural or Artificial Opening Endoscopic X External	Z No Device	X Diagnostic Z No Qualifier
5 Middle Ear, Right 6 Middle Ear, Left 9 Auditory Ossicle, Right A Auditory Ossicle, Left D Inner Ear, Right E Inner Ear, Left	Ø Open 8 Via Natural or Artificial Opening Endoscopic	Z No Device	X Diagnostic Z No Qualifier
7 Tympanic Membrane, Right 8 Tympanic Membrane, Left F Eustachian Tube, Right G Eustachian Tube, Left L Nasal Turbinate N Nasopharynx	Ø Open 3 Percutaneous 4 Percutaneous Endoscopic 7 Via Natural or Artificial Opening 8 Via Natural or Artificial Opening Endoscopic	Z No Device	X Diagnostic Z No Qualifier
B Mastoid Sinus, Right C Mastoid Sinus, Left M Nasal Septum P Accessory Sinus Q Maxillary Sinus, Right R Maxillary Sinus, Left S Frontal Sinus, Right T Frontal Sinus, Left U Ethmoid Sinus, Right V Ethmoid Sinus, Left W Sphenoid Sinus, Right X Sphenoid Sinus, Left	Ø Open 3 Percutaneous 4 Percutaneous Endoscopic 8 Via Natural or Artificial Opening Endoscopic	Z No Device	X Diagnostic Z No Qualifier
K Nasal Mucosa and Soft Tissue	Ø Open 3 Percutaneous 4 Percutaneous Endoscopic 8 Via Natural or Artificial Opening Endoscopic X External	Z No Device	X Diagnostic Z No Qualifier

Non-OR Ø9B[Ø1][Ø34X]Z[XZ]
Non-OR Ø9B[34][Ø3478X]Z[XZ]
Non-OR Ø9B[FG][Ø3478]Z[XZ]
Non-OR Ø9B[LN][Ø3478]ZX
Non-OR Ø9BM[Ø34]ZX
Non-OR Ø9B[PQRSTUVWX][34]ZX
Non-OR Ø9BK[Ø34X]Z[XZ]

SECTION: Ø MEDICAL AND SURGICAL
BODY SYSTEM: 9 EAR, NOSE, SINUS
OPERATION: C EXTIRPATION: Taking or cutting out solid matter from a body part

Body Part	Approach	Device	Qualifier
Ø External Ear, Right 1 External Ear, Left	Ø Open 3 Percutaneous 4 Percutaneous Endoscopic X External	Z No Device	Z No Qualifier
3 External Auditory Canal, Right 4 External Auditory Canal, Left	Ø Open 3 Percutaneous 4 Percutaneous Endoscopic 7 Via Natural or Artificial Opening 8 Via Natural or Artificial Opening Endoscopic X External	Z No Device	Z No Qualifier
5 Middle Ear, Right 6 Middle Ear, Left 9 Auditory Ossicle, Right A Auditory Ossicle, Left D Inner Ear, Right E Inner Ear, Left	Ø Open 8 Via Natural or Artificial Opening Endoscopic	Z No Device	Z No Qualifier
7 Tympanic Membrane, Right 8 Tympanic Membrane, Left F Eustachian Tube, Right G Eustachian Tube, Left L Nasal Turbinate N Nasopharynx	Ø Open 3 Percutaneous 4 Percutaneous Endoscopic 7 Via Natural or Artificial Opening 8 Via Natural or Artificial Opening Endoscopic	Z No Device	Z No Qualifier
B Mastoid Sinus, Right C Mastoid Sinus, Left M Nasal Septum P Accessory Sinus Q Maxillary Sinus, Right R Maxillary Sinus, Left S Frontal Sinus, Right T Frontal Sinus, Left U Ethmoid Sinus, Right V Ethmoid Sinus, Left W Sphenoid Sinus, Right X Sphenoid Sinus, Left	Ø Open 3 Percutaneous 4 Percutaneous Endoscopic 8 Via Natural or Artificial Opening Endoscopic	Z No Device	Z No Qualifier
K Nasal Mucosa and Soft Tissue	Ø Open 3 Percutaneous 4 Percutaneous Endoscopic 8 Via Natural or Artificial Opening Endoscopic X External	Z No Device	Z No Qualifier

Non-OR Ø9C[Ø1][Ø34X]ZZ
Non-OR Ø9C[34][Ø3478X]ZZ
Non-OR Ø9C[78FGL][Ø3478]ZZ
Non-OR Ø9CM[Ø34]ZZ
Non-OR Ø9BK[Ø34X]ZZ

SECTION: Ø MEDICAL AND SURGICAL
BODY SYSTEM: 9 EAR, NOSE, SINUS
OPERATION: D EXTRACTION: Pulling or stripping out or off all or a portion of a body part by the use of force

Body Part	Approach	Device	Qualifier
7 Tympanic Membrane, Right 8 Tympanic Membrane, Left L Nasal Turbinate	Ø Open 3 Percutaneous 4 Percutaneous Endoscopic 7 Via Natural or Artificial Opening 8 Via Natural or Artificial Opening Endoscopic	Z No Device	Z No Qualifier
9 Auditory Ossicle, Right A Auditory Ossicle, Left	Ø Open	Z No Device	Z No Qualifier
B Mastoid Sinus, Right C Mastoid Sinus, Left M Nasal Septum P Accessory Sinus Q Maxillary Sinus, Right R Maxillary Sinus, Left S Frontal Sinus, Right T Frontal Sinus, Left U Ethmoid Sinus, Right V Ethmoid Sinus, Left W Sphenoid Sinus, Right X Sphenoid Sinus, Left	Ø Open 3 Percutaneous 4 Percutaneous Endoscopic	Z No Device	Z No Qualifier

SECTION: Ø MEDICAL AND SURGICAL
BODY SYSTEM: 9 EAR, NOSE, SINUS
OPERATION: H INSERTION: Putting in a nonbiological appliance that monitors, assists, performs, or prevents a physiological function but does not physically take the place of a body part

Body Part	Approach	Device	Qualifier
D Inner Ear, Right E Inner Ear, Left	Ø Open 3 Percutaneous 4 Percutaneous Endoscopic	1 Radioactive Element 4 Hearing Device, Bone Conduction 5 Hearing Device, Single Channel Cochlear Prosthesis 6 Hearing Device, Multiple Channel Cochlear Prosthesis S Hearing Device	Z No Qualifier
H Ear, Right J Ear, Left K Nasal Mucosa and Soft Tissue Y Sinus	Ø Open 3 Percutaneous 4 Percutaneous Endoscopic 7 Via Natural or Artificial Opening 8 Via Natural or Artificial Opening Endoscopic	1 Radioactive Element Y Other Device	Z No Qualifier
N Nasopharynx	7 Via Natural or Artificial Opening 8 Via Natural or Artificial Opening Endoscopic	1 Radioactive Element B Intraluminal Device, Airway	Z No Qualifier

Non-OR Ø9HN[78]BZ
Coding Clinic: 2022, Q2, P18 – Ø9HK7YZ

SECTION: Ø MEDICAL AND SURGICAL
BODY SYSTEM: 9 EAR, NOSE, SINUS
OPERATION: J INSPECTION: Visually and/or manually exploring a body part

Body Part	Approach	Device	Qualifier
7 Tympanic Membrane, Right 8 Tympanic Membrane, Left H Ear, Right J Ear, Left	Ø Open 3 Percutaneous 4 Percutaneous Endoscopic 7 Via Natural or Artificial Opening 8 Via Natural or Artificial Opening Endoscopic X External	Z No Device	Z No Qualifier
D Inner Ear, Right E Inner Ear, Left K Nasal Mucosa and Soft Tissue Y Sinus	Ø Open 3 Percutaneous 4 Percutaneous Endoscopic 8 Via Natural or Artificial Opening Endoscopic X External	Z No Device	Z No Qualifier

Non-OR Ø9J[78][378X]ZZ
Non-OR Ø9J[HJ][Ø3478X]ZZ
Non-OR Ø9J[DE][3X]ZZ
Non-OR Ø9J[KY][Ø34X]ZZ

SECTION: Ø MEDICAL AND SURGICAL
BODY SYSTEM: 9 EAR, NOSE, SINUS
OPERATION: M REATTACHMENT: Putting back in or on all or a portion of a separated body part to its normal location or other suitable location

Body Part	Approach	Device	Qualifier
Ø External Ear, Right 1 External Ear, Left K Nasal Mucosa and Soft Tissue	X External	Z No Device	Z No Qualifier

SECTION: Ø MEDICAL AND SURGICAL
BODY SYSTEM: 9 EAR, NOSE, SINUS
OPERATION: N RELEASE: Freeing a body part from an abnormal physical constraint

Body Part	Approach	Device	Qualifier
Ø External Ear, Right 1 External Ear, Left	Ø Open 3 Percutaneous 4 Percutaneous Endoscopic X External	Z No Device	Z No Qualifier
3 External Auditory Canal, Right 4 External Auditory Canal, Left	Ø Open 3 Percutaneous 4 Percutaneous Endoscopic 7 Via Natural or Artificial Opening 8 Via Natural or Artificial Opening Endoscopic X External	Z No Device	Z No Qualifier
5 Middle Ear, Right 6 Middle Ear, Left 9 Auditory Ossicle, Right A Auditory Ossicle, Left D Inner Ear, Right E Inner Ear, Left	Ø Open 8 Via Natural or Artificial Opening Endoscopic	Z No Device	Z No Qualifier
7 Tympanic Membrane, Right 8 Tympanic Membrane, Left F Eustachian Tube, Right G Eustachian Tube, Left L Nasal Turbinate N Nasopharynx	Ø Open 3 Percutaneous 4 Percutaneous Endoscopic 7 Via Natural or Artificial Opening 8 Via Natural or Artificial Opening Endoscopic	Z No Device	Z No Qualifier
B Mastoid Sinus, Right C Mastoid Sinus, Left M Nasal Septum P Accessory Sinus Q Maxillary Sinus, Right R Maxillary Sinus, Left S Frontal Sinus, Right T Frontal Sinus, Left U Ethmoid Sinus, Right V Ethmoid Sinus, Left W Sphenoid Sinus, Right X Sphenoid Sinus, Left	Ø Open 3 Percutaneous 4 Percutaneous Endoscopic 8 Via Natural or Artificial Opening Endoscopic	Z No Device	Z No Qualifier
K Nasal Mucosa and Soft Tissue	Ø Open 3 Percutaneous 4 Percutaneous Endoscopic 8 Via Natural or Artificial Opening Endoscopic X External	Z No Device	Z No Qualifier

Non-OR Ø9N[FGL][Ø3478]ZZ
Non-OR Ø9NM[Ø34]ZZ
Non-OR Ø9NK[Ø34X]ZZ

SECTION: Ø MEDICAL AND SURGICAL
BODY SYSTEM: 9 EAR, NOSE, SINUS
OPERATION: P REMOVAL: Taking out or off a device from a body part

Body Part	Approach	Device	Qualifier
7 Tympanic Membrane, Right 8 Tympanic Membrane, Left	Ø Open 7 Via Natural or Artificial Opening 8 Via Natural or Artificial Opening Endoscopic X External	Ø Drainage Device	Z No Qualifier
D Inner Ear, Right E Inner Ear, Left	Ø Open 7 Via Natural or Artificial Opening 8 Via Natural or Artificial Opening Endoscopic	S Hearing Device	Z No Qualifier
H Ear, Right J Ear, Left K Nasal Mucosa and Soft Tissue	Ø Open 3 Percutaneous 4 Percutaneous Endoscopic 7 Via Natural or Artificial Opening 8 Via Natural or Artificial Opening Endoscopic	Ø Drainage Device 7 Autologous Tissue Substitute D Intraluminal Device J Synthetic Substitute K Nonautologous Tissue Substitute Y Other Device	Z No Qualifier
H Ear, Right J Ear, Left K Nasal Mucosa and Soft Tissue	X External	Ø Drainage Device 7 Autologous Tissue Substitute D Intraluminal Device J Synthetic Substitute K Nonautologous Tissue Substitute	Z No Qualifier
Y Sinus	Ø Open 3 Percutaneous 4 Percutaneous Endoscopic	Ø Drainage Device Y Other Device	Z No Qualifier
Y Sinus	7 Via Natural or Artificial Opening 8 Via Natural or Artificial Opening Endoscopic	Y Other Device	Z No Qualifier
Y Sinus	X External	Ø Drainage Device	Z No Qualifier

Non-OR Ø9P[78][Ø78X]ØZ
Non-OR Ø9P[HJ][34][ØJK]Z
Non-OR Ø9P[HJ][78][ØD]Z
Non-OR Ø9P[HJ]X[Ø7DJK]Z
Non-OR Ø9PK[Ø3478][Ø7DJK]Z
Non-OR Ø9PYXØZ
Non-OR Ø9PKX[Ø7DJK]Z

SECTION: Ø MEDICAL AND SURGICAL
BODY SYSTEM: 9 EAR, NOSE, SINUS
OPERATION: Q REPAIR: Restoring, to the extent possible, a body part to its normal anatomic structure and function

Body Part	Approach	Device	Qualifier
Ø External Ear, Right 1 External Ear, Left 2 External Ear, Bilateral	Ø Open 3 Percutaneous 4 Percutaneous Endoscopic X External	Z No Device	Z No Qualifier
3 External Auditory Canal, Right 4 External Auditory Canal, Left F Eustachian Tube, Right G Eustachian Tube, Left	Ø Open 3 Percutaneous 4 Percutaneous Endoscopic 7 Via Natural or Artificial Opening 8 Via Natural or Artificial Opening Endoscopic X External	Z No Device	Z No Qualifier
5 Middle Ear, Right 6 Middle Ear, Left 9 Auditory Ossicle, Right A Auditory Ossicle, Left D Inner Ear, Right E Inner Ear, Left	Ø Open 8 Via Natural or Artificial Opening Endoscopic	Z No Device	Z No Qualifier
7 Tympanic Membrane, Right 8 Tympanic Membrane, Left L Nasal Turbinate N Nasopharynx	Ø Open 3 Percutaneous 4 Percutaneous Endoscopic 7 Via Natural or Artificial Opening 8 Via Natural or Artificial Opening Endoscopic	Z No Device	Z No Qualifier
B Mastoid Sinus, Right C Mastoid Sinus, Left M Nasal Septum P Accessory Sinus Q Maxillary Sinus, Right R Maxillary Sinus, Left S Frontal Sinus, Right T Frontal Sinus, Left U Ethmoid Sinus, Right V Ethmoid Sinus, Left W Sphenoid Sinus, Right X Sphenoid Sinus, Left	Ø Open 3 Percutaneous 4 Percutaneous Endoscopic 8 Via Natural or Artificial Opening Endoscopic	Z No Device	Z No Qualifier
K Nasal Mucosa and Soft Tissue	Ø Open 3 Percutaneous 4 Percutaneous Endoscopic 8 Via Natural or Artificial Opening Endoscopic X External	Z No Device	Z No Qualifier

Non-OR Ø9Q[Ø12]XZZ
Non-OR Ø9Q[34]XZZ
Non-OR Ø9Q[FG][Ø3478X]ZZ

SECTION: Ø MEDICAL AND SURGICAL
BODY SYSTEM: 9 EAR, NOSE, SINUS
OPERATION: R REPLACEMENT: Putting in or on biological or synthetic material that physically takes the place and/or function of all or a portion of a body part

Body Part	Approach	Device	Qualifier
Ø External Ear, Right 1 External Ear, Left 2 External Ear, Bilateral K Nasal Mucosa and Soft Tissue	Ø Open X External	7 Autologous Tissue Substitute J Synthetic Substitute K Nonautologous Tissue Substitute	Z No Qualifier
5 Middle Ear, Right 6 Middle Ear, Left 9 Auditory Ossicle, Right A Auditory Ossicle, Left D Inner Ear, Right E Inner Ear, Left	Ø Open	7 Autologous Tissue Substitute J Synthetic Substitute K Nonautologous Tissue Substitute	Z No Qualifier
7 Tympanic Membrane, Right 8 Tympanic Membrane, Left N Nasopharynx	Ø Open 7 Via Natural or Artificial Opening 8 Via Natural or Artificial Opening Endoscopic	7 Autologous Tissue Substitute J Synthetic Substitute K Nonautologous Tissue Substitute	Z No Qualifier
L Nasal Turbinate	Ø Open 3 Percutaneous 4 Percutaneous Endoscopic 7 Via Natural or Artificial Opening 8 Via Natural or Artificial Opening Endoscopic	7 Autologous Tissue Substitute J Synthetic Substitute K Nonautologous Tissue Substitute	Z No Qualifier
M Nasal Septum	Ø Open 3 Percutaneous 4 Percutaneous Endoscopic	7 Autologous Tissue Substitute J Synthetic Substitute K Nonautologous Tissue Substitute	Z No Qualifier

SECTION: Ø MEDICAL AND SURGICAL
BODY SYSTEM: 9 EAR, NOSE, SINUS
OPERATION: S REPOSITION: Moving to its normal location, or other suitable location, all or a portion of a body part

Body Part	Approach	Device	Qualifier
Ø External Ear, Right 1 External Ear, Left 2 External Ear, Bilateral K Nasal Mucosa and Soft Tissue	Ø Open 4 Percutaneous Endoscopic X External	Z No Device	Z No Qualifier
7 Tympanic Membrane, Right 8 Tympanic Membrane, Left F Eustachian Tube, Right G Eustachian Tube, Left L Nasal Turbinate	Ø Open 4 Percutaneous Endoscopic 7 Via Natural or Artificial Opening 8 Via Natural or Artificial Opening Endoscopic	Z No Device	Z No Qualifier
9 Auditory Ossicle, Right A Auditory Ossicle, Left M Nasal Septum	Ø Open 4 Percutaneous Endoscopic	Z No Device	Z No Qualifier

Non-OR Ø9S[FG][Ø478]ZZ

SECTION: Ø MEDICAL AND SURGICAL
BODY SYSTEM: 9 EAR, NOSE, SINUS
OPERATION: T RESECTION: Cutting out or off, without replacement, all of a body part

Body Part	Approach	Device	Qualifier
Ø External Ear, Right 1 External Ear, Left	Ø Open 4 Percutaneous Endoscopic X External	Z No Device	Z No Qualifier
5 Middle Ear, Right 6 Middle Ear, Left 9 Auditory Ossicle, Right A Auditory Ossicle, Left D Inner Ear, Right E Inner Ear, Left	Ø Open 8 Via Natural or Artificial Opening Endoscopic	Z No Device	Z No Qualifier
7 Tympanic Membrane, Right 8 Tympanic Membrane, Left F Eustachian Tube, Right G Eustachian Tube, Left L Nasal Turbinate N Nasopharynx	Ø Open 4 Percutaneous Endoscopic 7 Via Natural or Artificial Opening 8 Via Natural or Artificial Opening Endoscopic	Z No Device	Z No Qualifier
B Mastoid Sinus, Right C Mastoid Sinus, Left M Nasal Septum P Accessory Sinus Q Maxillary Sinus, Right R Maxillary Sinus, Left S Frontal Sinus, Right T Frontal Sinus, Left U Ethmoid Sinus, Right V Ethmoid Sinus, Left W Sphenoid Sinus, Right X Sphenoid Sinus, Left	Ø Open 4 Percutaneous Endoscopic 8 Via Natural or Artificial Opening Endoscopic	Z No Device	Z No Qualifier
K Nasal Mucosa and Soft Tissue	Ø Open 4 Percutaneous Endoscopic 8 Via Natural or Artificial Opening Endoscopic X External	Z No Device	Z No Qualifier

Non-OR Ø9T[FG][Ø478]ZZ

SECTION: Ø MEDICAL AND SURGICAL
BODY SYSTEM: 9 EAR, NOSE, SINUS
OPERATION: U SUPPLEMENT: Putting in or on biological or synthetic material that physically reinforces and/or augments the function of a portion of a body part

Body Part	Approach	Device	Qualifier
Ø External Ear, Right 1 External Ear, Left 2 External Ear, Bilateral	Ø Open X External	7 Autologous Tissue Substitute J Synthetic Substitute K Nonautologous Tissue Substitute	Z No Qualifier
5 Middle Ear, Right 6 Middle Ear, Left 9 Auditory Ossicle, Right A Auditory Ossicle, Left D Inner Ear, Right E Inner Ear, Left	Ø Open 8 Via Natural or Artificial Opening Endoscopic	7 Autologous Tissue Substitute J Synthetic Substitute K Nonautologous Tissue Substitute	Z No Qualifier
7 Tympanic Membrane, Right 8 Tympanic Membrane, Left N Nasopharynx	Ø Open 7 Via Natural or Artificial Opening 8 Via Natural or Artificial Opening Endoscopic	7 Autologous Tissue Substitute J Synthetic Substitute K Nonautologous Tissue Substitute	Z No Qualifier
B Mastoid Sinus, Right C Mastoid Sinus, Left L Nasal Turbinate P Accessory Sinus Q Maxillary Sinus, Right R Maxillary Sinus, Left S Frontal Sinus, Right T Frontal Sinus, Left U Ethmoid Sinus, Right V Ethmoid Sinus, Left W Sphenoid Sinus, Right X Sphenoid Sinus, Left	Ø Open 3 Percutaneous 4 Percutaneous Endoscopic 7 Via Natural or Artificial Opening 8 Via Natural or Artificial Opening Endoscopic	7 Autologous Tissue Substitute J Synthetic Substitute K Nonautologous Tissue Substitute	Z No Qualifier
K Nasal Mucosa and Soft Tissue	Ø Open 8 Via Natural or Artificial Opening Endoscopic X External	7 Autologous Tissue Substitute J Synthetic Substitute K Nonautologous Tissue Substitute	Z No Qualifier
L Nasal Turbinate	Ø Open 3 Percutaneous 4 Percutaneous Endoscopic 7 Via Natural or Artificial Opening 8 Via Natural or Artificial Opening Endoscopic	7 Autologous Tissue Substitute J Synthetic Substitute K Nonautologous Tissue Substitute	Z No Qualifier
M Nasal Septum	Ø Open 3 Percutaneous 4 Percutaneous Endoscopic 8 Via Natural or Artificial Opening Endoscopic	7 Autologous Tissue Substitute J Synthetic Substitute K Nonautologous Tissue Substitute	Z No Qualifier

SECTION: Ø MEDICAL AND SURGICAL
BODY SYSTEM: 9 EAR, NOSE, SINUS
OPERATION: W REVISION: Correcting, to the extent possible, a portion of a malfunctioning device or the position of a displaced device

Body Part	Approach	Device	Qualifier
7 Tympanic Membrane, Right 8 Tympanic Membrane, Left 9 Auditory Ossicle, Right A Auditory Ossicle, Left	Ø Open 7 Via Natural or Artificial Opening 8 Via Natural or Artificial Opening Endoscopic	7 Autologous Tissue Substitute J Synthetic Substitute K Nonautologous Tissue Substitute	Z No Qualifier
D Inner Ear, Right E Inner Ear, Left	Ø Open 7 Via Natural or Artificial Opening 8 Via Natural or Artificial Opening Endoscopic	S Hearing Device	Z No Qualifier
H Ear, Right J Ear, Left K Nasal Mucosa and Soft Tissue	Ø Open 3 Percutaneous 4 Percutaneous Endoscopic 7 Via Natural or Artificial Opening 8 Via Natural or Artificial Opening Endoscopic	Ø Drainage Device 7 Autologous Tissue Substitute D Intraluminal Device J Synthetic Substitute K Nonautologous Tissue Substitute Y Other Device	Z No Qualifier
H Ear, Right J Ear, Left K Nasal Mucosa and Soft Tissue	X External	Ø Drainage Device 7 Autologous Tissue Substitute D Intraluminal Device J Synthetic Substitute K Nonautologous Tissue Substitute	Z No Qualifier
Y Sinus	Ø Open 3 Percutaneous 4 Percutaneous Endoscopic	Ø Drainage Device Y Other Device	Z No Qualifier
Y Sinus	7 Via Natural or Artificial Opening 8 Via Natural or Artificial Opening Endoscopic	Y Other Device	Z No Qualifier
Y Sinus	X External	Ø Drainage Device	Z No Qualifier

Non-OR Ø9W[HJ][34][JK]Z
Non-OR Ø9W[HJ][78]DZ
Non-OR Ø9W[HJ]X[Ø7DJK]Z
Non-OR Ø9WK[Ø3478][Ø7DJK]Z
Non-OR Ø9WYXØZ
Non-OR Ø9QKX[Ø7DJK]Z

ØB. Respiratory System ... 210
ØB1. Bypass ... 211
ØB2. Change ... 211
ØB5. Destruction ... 212
ØB7. Dilation ... 213
ØB9. Drainage ... 213
ØBB. Excision ... 215
ØBC. Extirpation ... 216
ØBD. Extraction ... 216
ØBF. Fragmentation ... 217
ØBH. Insertion ... 217
ØBJ. Inspection ... 218
ØBL. Occlusion ... 219
ØBM. Reattachment ... 219
ØBN. Release ... 220
ØBP. Removal ... 220
ØBQ. Repair ... 222
ØBR. Replacement ... 222
ØBS. Reposition ... 223
ØBT. Resection ... 223
ØBU. Supplement ... 224
ØBV. Restriction ... 224
ØBW. Revision ... 225
ØBY. Transplantation ... 226

SECTION: Ø MEDICAL AND SURGICAL
BODY SYSTEM: B RESPIRATORY SYSTEM
OPERATION: 1 BYPASS: Altering the route of passage of the contents of a tubular body part

Body Part	Approach	Device	Qualifier
1 Trachea	Ø Open	D Intraluminal Device	6 Esophagus
1 Trachea	Ø Open	F Tracheostomy Device Z No Device	4 Cutaneous
1 Trachea	3 Percutaneous 4 Percutaneous Endoscopic	F Tracheostomy Device Z No Device	4 Cutaneous

DRG Non-OR ØB113[FZ]4
Non-OR ØB11ØD6

SECTION: Ø MEDICAL AND SURGICAL
BODY SYSTEM: B RESPIRATORY SYSTEM
OPERATION: 2 CHANGE: Taking out or off a device from a body part and putting back an identical or similar device in or on the same body part without cutting or puncturing the skin or a mucous membrane

Body Part	Approach	Device	Qualifier
Ø Tracheobronchial Tree K Lung, Right L Lung, Left Q Pleura T Diaphragm	X External	Ø Drainage Device Y Other Device	Z No Qualifier
1 Trachea	X External	Ø Drainage Device E Intraluminal Device, Endotracheal Airway F Tracheostomy Device Y Other Device	Z No Qualifier

Non-OR All Values

SECTION: Ø MEDICAL AND SURGICAL
BODY SYSTEM: B RESPIRATORY SYSTEM
OPERATION: 5 DESTRUCTION: Physical eradication of all or a portion of a body part by the direct use of energy, force, or a destructive agent

Body Part	Approach	Device	Qualifier
1 Trachea 2 Carina 3 Main Bronchus, Right 4 Upper Lobe Bronchus, Right 5 Middle Lobe Bronchus, Right 6 Lower Lobe Bronchus, Right 7 Main Bronchus, Left 8 Upper Lobe Bronchus, Left 9 Lingula Bronchus B Lower Lobe Bronchus, Left	Ø Open 3 Percutaneous 4 Percutaneous Endoscopic 7 Via Natural or Artificial Opening 8 Via Natural or Artificial Opening Endoscopic	Z No Device	Z No Qualifier
C Upper Lung Lobe, Right D Middle Lung Lobe, Right F Lower Lung Lobe, Right G Upper Lung Lobe, Left H Lung Lingula J Lower Lung Lobe, Left K Lung, Right L Lung, Left M Lungs, Bilateral	Ø Open 3 Percutaneous 4 Percutaneous Endoscopic	Z No Device	3 Laser Interstitial Thermal Therapy Z No Qualifier
C Upper Lung Lobe, Right D Middle Lung Lobe, Right F Lower Lung Lobe, Right G Upper Lung Lobe, Left H Lung Lingula J Lower Lung Lobe, Left K Lung, Right L Lung, Left M Lungs, Bilateral	7 Via Natural or Artificial Opening 8 Via Natural or Artificial Opening Endoscopic	Z No Device	Z No Qualifier
N Pleura, Right P Pleura, Left T Diaphragm	Ø Open 3 Percutaneous 4 Percutaneous Endoscopic	Z No Device	Z No Qualifier

Non-OR ØB5[3456789B]4ZZ
Non-OR ØB5[CDFGHJKLM]8ZZ
Non-OR ØB5[CDFGHJKLM][Ø34]Z3

Coding Clinic: 2Ø16, Q2, P18 – ØB5[PS]ØZZ

SECTION: Ø MEDICAL AND SURGICAL
BODY SYSTEM: B RESPIRATORY SYSTEM
OPERATION: 7 DILATION: Expanding an orifice or the lumen of a tubular body part

Body Part	Approach	Device	Qualifier
1 Trachea 2 Carina 3 Main Bronchus, Right 4 Upper Lobe Bronchus, Right 5 Middle Lobe Bronchus, Right 6 Lower Lobe Bronchus, Right 7 Main Bronchus, Left 8 Upper Lobe Bronchus, Left 9 Lingula Bronchus B Lower Lobe Bronchus, Left	Ø Open 3 Percutaneous 4 Percutaneous Endoscopic 7 Via Natural or Artificial Opening 8 Via Natural or Artificial Opening Endoscopic	D Intraluminal Device Z No Device	Z No Qualifier

Non-OR ØB5[3456789B][Ø3478][DZ]Z

SECTION: Ø MEDICAL AND SURGICAL
BODY SYSTEM: B RESPIRATORY SYSTEM
OPERATION: 9 DRAINAGE: *(on multiple pages)*
Taking or letting out fluids and/or gases from a body part

Body Part	Approach	Device	Qualifier
1 Trachea 2 Carina 3 Main Bronchus, Right 4 Upper Lobe Bronchus, Right 5 Middle Lobe Bronchus, Right 6 Lower Lobe Bronchus, Right 7 Main Bronchus, Left 8 Upper Lobe Bronchus, Left 9 Lingula Bronchus B Lower Lobe Bronchus, Left C Upper Lung Lobe, Right D Middle Lung Lobe, Right F Lower Lung Lobe, Right G Upper Lung Lobe, Left H Lung Lingula J Lower Lung Lobe, Left K Lung, Right L Lung, Left M Lungs, Bilateral	Ø Open 3 Percutaneous 4 Percutaneous Endoscopic 7 Via Natural or Artificial Opening 8 Via Natural or Artificial Opening Endoscopic	Ø Drainage Device	Z No Qualifier

Coding Clinic: 2016, Q1, P26 – ØB948ZX, ØB9B8ZX
Coding Clinic: 2016, Q1, P27 – ØB988ZX
Coding Clinic: 2017, Q1, P51 – ØB9[BJ]8ZX
Coding Clinic: 2017, Q3, P15 – ØB9M8ZZ

SECTION: Ø MEDICAL AND SURGICAL
BODY SYSTEM: B RESPIRATORY SYSTEM
OPERATION: 9 DRAINAGE: *(continued)*
Taking or letting out fluids and/or gases from a body part

Body Part	Approach	Device	Qualifier
1 Trachea 2 Carina 3 Main Bronchus, Right 4 Upper Lobe Bronchus, Right 5 Middle Lobe Bronchus, Right 6 Lower Lobe Bronchus, Right 7 Main Bronchus, Left 8 Upper Lobe Bronchus, Left 9 Lingula Bronchus B Lower Lobe Bronchus, Left C Upper Lung Lobe, Right D Middle Lung Lobe, Right F Lower Lung Lobe, Right G Upper Lung Lobe, Left H Lung Lingula J Lower Lung Lobe, Left K Lung, Right L Lung, Left M Lungs, Bilateral	Ø Open 3 Percutaneous 4 Percutaneous Endoscopic 7 Via Natural or Artificial Opening 8 Via Natural or Artificial Opening Endoscopic	Z No Device	X Diagnostic Z No Qualifier
N Pleura, Right P Pleura, Left	Ø Open 3 Percutaneous 4 Percutaneous Endoscopic 8 Via Natural or Artificial Opening Endoscopic	Ø Drainage Device	Z No Qualifier
N Pleura, Right P Pleura, Left	Ø Open 3 Percutaneous 4 Percutaneous Endoscopic 8 Via Natural or Artificial Opening Endoscopic	Z No Device	X Diagnostic Z No Qualifier
T Diaphragm	Ø Open 3 Percutaneous 4 Percutaneous Endoscopic	Ø Drainage	Z No Qualifier
T Diaphragm	Ø Open 3 Percutaneous 4 Percutaneous Endoscopic	Z No Device	X Diagnostic Z No Qualifier

DRG Non-OR ØB9[123456789B][78]ØZ *(proposed)*
DRG Non-OR ØB9[123456789B][78]ZZ *(proposed)*
Non-OR ØB9[123456789B][3478]ZX
Non-OR ØB9[CDFGHJKLM][347]ZX
Non-OR ØB9[NP][Ø3]ØZ
Non-OR ØB9[NP][Ø3]Z[XZ]
Non-OR ØB9[NP]4ZX
Non-OR ØB9T3ZZ

SECTION: Ø MEDICAL AND SURGICAL
BODY SYSTEM: B RESPIRATORY SYSTEM
OPERATION: B EXCISION: Cutting out or off, without replacement, a portion of a body part

Body Part	Approach	Device	Qualifier
1 Trachea 2 Carina 3 Main Bronchus, Right 4 Upper Lobe Bronchus, Right 5 Middle Lobe Bronchus, Right 6 Lower Lobe Bronchus, Right 7 Main Bronchus, Left 8 Upper Lobe Bronchus, Left 9 Lingula Bronchus B Lower Lobe Bronchus, Left C Upper Lung Lobe, Right D Middle Lung Lobe, Right F Lower Lung Lobe, Right G Upper Lung Lobe, Left H Lung Lingula J Lower Lung Lobe, Left K Lung, Right L Lung, Left M Lungs, Bilateral	Ø Open 3 Percutaneous 4 Percutaneous Endoscopic 7 Via Natural or Artificial Opening 8 Via Natural or Artificial Opening Endoscopic	Z No Device	X Diagnostic Z No Qualifier
N Pleura, Right P Pleura, Left	Ø Open 3 Percutaneous 4 Percutaneous Endoscopic 8 Via Natural or Artificial Opening Endoscopic	Z No Device	X Diagnostic Z No Qualifier
T Diaphragm	Ø Open 3 Percutaneous 4 Percutaneous Endoscopic	Z No Device	X Diagnostic Z No Qualifier

Non-OR ØBB[123456789B][3478]ZX
Non-OR ØBB[3456789BM][48]ZZ
Non-OR ØBB[CDFGHJKLM]3ZX
Non-OR ØBB[CDFGHJKL]8ZZ
Non-OR ØBB[NP][Ø3]ZX

Coding Clinic: 2Ø15, Q1, P16 – ØBB1ØZZ
Coding Clinic: 2Ø16, Q1, P26 – ØBB48ZX, ØBBC8ZX
Coding Clinic: 2Ø16, Q1, P27 – ØBB88ZX
Coding Clinic: 2Ø22, Q2, P19 – ØBBG8ZX

SECTION: Ø MEDICAL AND SURGICAL
BODY SYSTEM: B RESPIRATORY SYSTEM
OPERATION: C EXTIRPATION: Taking or cutting out solid matter from a body part

Body Part	Approach	Device	Qualifier
1 Trachea 2 Carina 3 Main Bronchus, Right 4 Upper Lobe Bronchus, Right 5 Middle Lobe Bronchus, Right 6 Lower Lobe Bronchus, Right 7 Main Bronchus, Left 8 Upper Lobe Bronchus, Left 9 Lingula Bronchus B Lower Lobe Bronchus, Left C Upper Lung Lobe, Right D Middle Lung Lobe, Right F Lower Lung Lobe, Right G Upper Lung Lobe, Left H Lung Lingula J Lower Lung Lobe, Left K Lung, Right L Lung, Left M Lungs, Bilateral	Ø Open 3 Percutaneous 4 Percutaneous Endoscopic 7 Via Natural or Artificial Opening 8 Via Natural or Artificial Opening Endoscopic	Z No Device	Z No Qualifier
N Pleura, Right P Pleura, Left T Diaphragm	Ø Open 3 Percutaneous 4 Percutaneous Endoscopic	Z No Device	Z No Qualifier

Non-OR ØBC[123456789B][78]ZZ
Non-OR ØBC[NP][Ø34]ZZ

Coding Clinic: 2Ø17, Q3, P15 – ØBC58ZZ

SECTION: Ø MEDICAL AND SURGICAL
BODY SYSTEM: B RESPIRATORY SYSTEM
OPERATION: D EXTRACTION: Pulling or stripping out or off all or a portion of a body part by the use of force

Body Part	Approach	Device	Qualifier
1 Trachea 2 Carina 3 Main Bronchus, Right 4 Upper Lobe Bronchus, Right 5 Middle Lobe Bronchus, Right 6 Lower Lobe Bronchus, Right 7 Main Bronchus, Left 8 Upper Lobe Bronchus, Left 9 Lingula Bronchus B Lower Lobe Bronchus, Left C Upper Lung Lobe, Right D Middle Lung Lobe, Right F Lower Lung Lobe, Right G Upper Lung Lobe, Left H Lung Lingula J Lower Lung Lobe, Left K Lung, Right L Lung, Left M Lungs, Bilateral	4 Percutaneous Endoscopic 8 Via Natural or Artificial Opening Endoscopic	Z No Device	X Diagnostic
N Pleura, Right P Pleura, Left	Ø Open 3 Percutaneous 4 Percutaneous Endoscopic	Z No Device	X Diagnostic Z No Qualifier

SECTION: Ø MEDICAL AND SURGICAL
BODY SYSTEM: B RESPIRATORY SYSTEM
OPERATION: F FRAGMENTATION: Breaking solid matter in a body part into pieces

Body Part	Approach	Device	Qualifier
1 Trachea 2 Carina 3 Main Bronchus, Right 4 Upper Lobe Bronchus, Right 5 Middle Lobe Bronchus, Right 6 Lower Lobe Bronchus, Right 7 Main Bronchus, Left 8 Upper Lobe Bronchus, Left 9 Lingula Bronchus B Lower Lobe Bronchus, Left	Ø Open 3 Percutaneous 4 Percutaneous Endoscopic 7 Via Natural or Artificial Opening 8 Via Natural or Artificial Opening Endoscopic X External	Z No Device	Z No Qualifier

ØBF[123456789B]XZZ
Non-OR ØBF[123456789B]XZZ

SECTION: Ø MEDICAL AND SURGICAL
BODY SYSTEM: B RESPIRATORY SYSTEM
OPERATION: H INSERTION: *(on multiple pages)*

Putting in a nonbiological appliance that monitors, assists, performs, or prevents a physiological function but does not physically take the place of a body part

Body Part	Approach	Device	Qualifier
Ø Tracheobronchial Tree	Ø Open 3 Percutaneous 4 Percutaneous Endoscopic 7 Via Natural or Artificial Opening 8 Via Natural or Artificial Opening Endoscopic	1 Radioactive Element 2 Monitoring Device 3 Infusion Device D Intraluminal Device Y Other Device	Z No Qualifier
1 Trachea	Ø Open	2 Monitoring Device D Intraluminal Device Y Other Device	Z No Qualifier
1 Trachea	3 Percutaneous	D Intraluminal Device E Intraluminal Device, Endotracheal Airway Y Other Device	Z No Qualifier
1 Trachea	4 Percutaneous Endoscopic	D Intraluminal Device Y Other Device	Z No Qualifier
1 Trachea	7 Via Natural or Artificial Opening 8 Via Natural or Artificial Opening Endoscopic	2 Monitoring Device D Intraluminal Device E Intraluminal Device, Endotracheal Airway Y Other Device	Z No Qualifier

Non-OR ØBHØ[78][23D]Z
Non-OR ØBH13EZ

Coding Clinic: 2019, Q3, P34 – ØBHB8GZ
Coding Clinic: 2022, Q3, P23 – ØBH17EZ

SECTION: Ø MEDICAL AND SURGICAL
BODY SYSTEM: B RESPIRATORY SYSTEM
OPERATION: H INSERTION: *(continued)*

Putting in a nonbiological appliance that monitors, assists, performs, or prevents a physiological function but does not physically take the place of a body part

Body Part	Approach	Device	Qualifier
3 Main Bronchus, Right 4 Upper Lobe Bronchus, Right 5 Middle Lobe Bronchus, Right 6 Lower Lobe Bronchus, Right 7 Main Bronchus, Left 8 Upper Lobe Bronchus, Left 9 Lingula Bronchus B Lower Lobe Bronchus, Left	Ø Open 3 Percutaneous 4 Percutaneous Endoscopic 7 Via Natural or Artificial Opening 8 Via Natural or Artificial Opening Endoscopic	G Endobronchial Device, Endobronchial Valve	Z No Qualifier
K Lung, Right L Lung, Left	Ø Open 3 Percutaneous 4 Percutaneous Endoscopic 7 Via Natural or Artificial Opening 8 Via Natural or Artificial Opening Endoscopic	1 Radioactive Element 2 Monitoring Device 3 Infusion Device Y Other Device	Z No Qualifier
Q Pleura	Ø Open 3 Percutaneous 4 Percutaneous Endoscopic 7 Via Natural or Artificial Opening 8 Via Natural or Artificial Opening Endoscopic	Y Other Device	Z No Qualifier
T Diaphragm	Ø Open 3 Percutaneous 4 Percutaneous Endoscopic	2 Monitoring Device M Diaphragmatic Pacemaker Lead Y Other Device	Z No Qualifier
T Diaphragm	7 Via Natural or Artificial Opening 8 Via Natural or Artificial Opening Endoscopic	Y Other Device	Z No Qualifier

Non-OR ØBH1[78]2Z
Non-OR ØBH1[78]EZ
Non-OR ØBH[3456789B]8GZ
Non-OR ØBH[KL][78][23]Z
DRG Non-OR ØBH[3456789B]8GZ

SECTION: Ø MEDICAL AND SURGICAL
BODY SYSTEM: B RESPIRATORY SYSTEM
OPERATION: J INSPECTION: Visually and/or manually exploring a body part

Body Part	Approach	Device	Qualifier
Ø Tracheobronchial Tree 1 Trachea K Lung, Right L Lung, Left Q Pleura T Diaphragm	Ø Open 3 Percutaneous 4 Percutaneous Endoscopic 7 Via Natural or Artificial Opening 8 Via Natural or Artificial Opening Endoscopic X External	Z No Device	Z No Qualifier

Non-OR ØBJ[ØKL][378X]ZZ
Non-OR ØBJ1[3478X]ZZ
Non-OR ØBJ[QT][378X]ZZ

Coding Clinic: 2Ø15, Q2, P31 – ØBJQ4ZZ

New/Revised Text in Green ~~deleted~~ Deleted ♀ Females Only ♂ Males Only Coding Clinic
Non-covered Limited Coverage Combination (See Appendix E) DRG Non-OR Non-OR Hospital-Acquired Condition

SECTION: Ø MEDICAL AND SURGICAL
BODY SYSTEM: B RESPIRATORY SYSTEM
OPERATION: L OCCLUSION: Completely closing an orifice or the lumen of a tubular body part

Body Part	Approach	Device	Qualifier
1 Trachea 2 Carina 3 Main Bronchus, Right 4 Upper Lobe Bronchus, Right 5 Middle Lobe Bronchus, Right 6 Lower Lobe Bronchus, Right 7 Main Bronchus, Left 8 Upper Lobe Bronchus, Left 9 Lingula Bronchus B Lower Lobe Bronchus, Left	Ø Open 3 Percutaneous 4 Percutaneous Endoscopic	C Extraluminal Device D Intraluminal Device Z No Device	Z No Qualifier
1 Trachea 2 Carina 3 Main Bronchus, Right 4 Upper Lobe Bronchus, Right 5 Middle Lobe Bronchus, Right 6 Lower Lobe Bronchus, Right 7 Main Bronchus, Left 8 Upper Lobe Bronchus, Left 9 Lingula Bronchus B Lower Lobe Bronchus, Left	7 Via Natural or Artificial Opening 8 Via Natural or Artificial Opening Endoscopic	D Intraluminal Device Z No Device	Z No Qualifier

SECTION: Ø MEDICAL AND SURGICAL
BODY SYSTEM: B RESPIRATORY SYSTEM
OPERATION: M REATTACHMENT: Putting back in or on all or a portion of a separated body part to its normal location or other suitable location

Body Part	Approach	Device	Qualifier
1 Trachea 2 Carina 3 Main Bronchus, Right 4 Upper Lobe Bronchus, Right 5 Middle Lobe Bronchus, Right 6 Lower Lobe Bronchus, Right 7 Main Bronchus, Left 8 Upper Lobe Bronchus, Left 9 Lingula Bronchus B Lower Lobe Bronchus, Left C Upper Lung Lobe, Right D Middle Lung Lobe, Right F Lower Lung Lobe, Right G Upper Lung Lobe, Left H Lung Lingula J Lower Lung Lobe, Left K Lung, Right L Lung, Left T Diaphragm	Ø Open	Z No Device	Z No Qualifier

SECTION: Ø MEDICAL AND SURGICAL
BODY SYSTEM: B RESPIRATORY SYSTEM
OPERATION: N RELEASE: Freeing a body part from an abnormal physical constraint by cutting or by the use of force

Body Part	Approach	Device	Qualifier
1 Trachea 2 Carina 3 Main Bronchus, Right 4 Upper Lobe Bronchus, Right 5 Middle Lobe Bronchus, Right 6 Lower Lobe Bronchus, Right 7 Main Bronchus, Left 8 Upper Lobe Bronchus, Left 9 Lingula Bronchus B Lower Lobe Bronchus, Left C Upper Lung Lobe, Right D Middle Lung Lobe, Right F Lower Lung Lobe, Right G Upper Lung Lobe, Left H Lung Lingula J Lower Lung Lobe, Left K Lung, Right L Lung, Left M Lungs, Bilateral	Ø Open 3 Percutaneous 4 Percutaneous Endoscopic 7 Via Natural or Artificial Opening 8 Via Natural or Artificial Opening Endoscopic	Z No Device	Z No Qualifier
N Pleura, Right P Pleura, Left T Diaphragm	Ø Open 3 Percutaneous 4 Percutaneous Endoscopic	Z No Device	Z No Qualifier

Coding Clinic: 2Ø15, Q3, P15 – ØBN1ØZZ
Coding Clinic: 2Ø19, Q2, P21 – ØBNNØZZ

SECTION: Ø MEDICAL AND SURGICAL
BODY SYSTEM: B RESPIRATORY SYSTEM
OPERATION: P REMOVAL: *(on multiple pages)* Taking out or off a device from a body part

Body Part	Approach	Device	Qualifier
Ø Tracheobronchial Tree	Ø Open 3 Percutaneous 4 Percutaneous Endoscopic 7 Via Natural or Artificial Opening 8 Via Natural or Artificial Opening Endoscopic	Ø Drainage Device 1 Radioactive Element 2 Monitoring Device 3 Infusion Device 7 Autologous Tissue Substitute C Extraluminal Device D Intraluminal Device J Synthetic Substitute K Nonautologous Tissue Substitute Y Other Device	Z No Qualifier
Ø Tracheobronchial Tree	X External	Ø Drainage Device 1 Radioactive Element 2 Monitoring Device 3 Infusion Device D Intraluminal Device	Z No Qualifier

Non-OR ØBPØ[78][Ø23D]Z   Non-OR ØBPØX[Ø123D]Z   Non-OR ØBP1[Ø34]FZ

SECTION: Ø MEDICAL AND SURGICAL
BODY SYSTEM: B RESPIRATORY SYSTEM
OPERATION: P REMOVAL: *(continued)*
Taking out or off a device from a body part

Body Part	Approach	Device	Qualifier
1 Trachea	Ø Open 3 Percutaneous 4 Percutaneous Endoscopic 7 Via Natural or Artificial Opening 8 Via Natural or Artificial Opening Endoscopic	Ø Drainage Device 2 Monitoring Device 7 Autologous Tissue Substitute C Extraluminal Device D Intraluminal Device F Tracheostomy Device J Synthetic Substitute K Nonautologous Tissue Substitute	Z No Qualifier
1 Trachea	X External	Ø Drainage Device 2 Monitoring Device D Intraluminal Device F Tracheostomy Device	Z No Qualifier
K Lung, Right L Lung, Left	Ø Open 3 Percutaneous 4 Percutaneous Endoscopic 7 Via Natural or Artificial Opening 8 Via Natural or Artificial Opening Endoscopic	Ø Drainage Device 1 Radioactive Element 2 Monitoring Device 3 Infusion Device Y Other Device	Z No Qualifier
K Lung, Right L Lung, Left	X External	Ø Drainage Device 1 Radioactive Element 2 Monitoring Device 3 Infusion Device	Z No Qualifier
Q Pleura	Ø Open 3 Percutaneous 4 Percutaneous Endoscopic 7 Via Natural or Artificial Opening 8 Via Natural or Artificial Opening Endoscopic	Ø Drainage Device 1 Radioactive Element 2 Monitoring Device Y Other Device	Z No Qualifier
Q Pleura	X External	Ø Drainage Device 1 Radioactive Element 2 Monitoring Device	Z No Qualifier
T Diaphragm	Ø Open 3 Percutaneous 4 Percutaneous Endoscopic 7 Via Natural or Artificial Opening 8 Via Natural or Artificial Opening Endoscopic	Ø Drainage Device 2 Monitoring Device 7 Autologous Tissue Substitute J Synthetic Substitute K Nonautologous Tissue Substitute M Diaphragmatic Pacemaker Lead Y Other Device	Z No Qualifier
T Diaphragm	X External	Ø Drainage Device 2 Monitoring Device M Diaphragmatic Pacemaker Lead	Z No Qualifier

Non-OR ØBP1[78][Ø2DF]Z
Non-OR ØBP1X[Ø2DF]Z
Non-OR ØBP[KL][78][Ø23]Z
Non-OR ØBP[KL]X[Ø123]Z
Non-OR ØBPQ[Ø3478X][Ø12]Z
Non-OR ØBPQX[Ø12]Z
Non-OR ØBPT[78][Ø2]Z
Non-OR ØBPTX[Ø2M]Z

SECTION: Ø MEDICAL AND SURGICAL
BODY SYSTEM: B RESPIRATORY SYSTEM
OPERATION: Q REPAIR: Restoring, to the extent possible, a body part to its normal anatomic structure and function

Body Part	Approach	Device	Qualifier
1 Trachea 2 Carina 3 Main Bronchus, Right 4 Upper Lobe Bronchus, Right 5 Middle Lobe Bronchus, Right 6 Lower Lobe Bronchus, Right 7 Main Bronchus, Left 8 Upper Lobe Bronchus, Left 9 Lingula Bronchus B Lower Lobe Bronchus, Left C Upper Lung Lobe, Right D Middle Lung Lobe, Right F Lower Lung Lobe, Right G Upper Lung Lobe, Left H Lung Lingula J Lower Lung Lobe, Left K Lung, Right L Lung, Left M Lungs, Bilateral	Ø Open 3 Percutaneous 4 Percutaneous Endoscopic 7 Via Natural or Artificial Opening 8 Via Natural or Artificial Opening Endoscopic	Z No Device	Z No Qualifier
N Pleura, Right P Pleura, Left T Diaphragm	Ø Open 3 Percutaneous 4 Percutaneous Endoscopic	Z No Device	Z No Qualifier

Coding Clinic: 2Ø16, Q2, P23 – ØBQ[RS]ØZZ

SECTION: Ø MEDICAL AND SURGICAL
BODY SYSTEM: B RESPIRATORY SYSTEM
OPERATION: R REPLACEMENT: Putting in or on biological or synthetic material that physically takes the place and/or function of all or a portion of a body part

Body Part	Approach	Device	Qualifier
1 Trachea 2 Carina 3 Main Bronchus, Right 4 Upper Lobe Bronchus, Right 5 Middle Lobe Bronchus, Right 6 Lower Lobe Bronchus, Right 7 Main Bronchus, Left 8 Upper Lobe Bronchus, Left 9 Lingula Bronchus B Lower Lobe Bronchus, Left T Diaphragm	Ø Open 4 Percutaneous Endoscopic	7 Autologous Tissue Substitute J Synthetic Substitute K Nonautologous Tissue Substitute	Z No Qualifier

SECTION: Ø MEDICAL AND SURGICAL
BODY SYSTEM: B RESPIRATORY SYSTEM
OPERATION: S REPOSITION: Moving to its normal location, or other suitable location, all or a portion of a body part

Body Part	Approach	Device	Qualifier
1 Trachea 2 Carina 3 Main Bronchus, Right 4 Upper Lobe Bronchus, Right 5 Middle Lobe Bronchus, Right 6 Lower Lobe Bronchus, Right 7 Main Bronchus, Left 8 Upper Lobe Bronchus, Left 9 Lingula Bronchus B Lower Lobe Bronchus, Left C Upper Lung Lobe, Right D Middle Lung Lobe, Right F Lower Lung Lobe, Right G Upper Lung Lobe, Left H Lung Lingula J Lower Lung Lobe, Left K Lung, Right L Lung, Left T Diaphragm	Ø Open	Z No Device	Z No Qualifier

SECTION: Ø MEDICAL AND SURGICAL
BODY SYSTEM: B RESPIRATORY SYSTEM
OPERATION: T RESECTION: Cutting out or off, without replacement, all of a body part

Body Part	Approach	Device	Qualifier
1 Trachea 2 Carina 3 Main Bronchus, Right 4 Upper Lobe Bronchus, Right 5 Middle Lobe Bronchus, Right 6 Lower Lobe Bronchus, Right 7 Main Bronchus, Left 8 Upper Lobe Bronchus, Left 9 Lingula Bronchus B Lower Lobe Bronchus, Left C Upper Lung Lobe, Right D Middle Lung Lobe, Right F Lower Lung Lobe, Right G Upper Lung Lobe, Left H Lung Lingula J Lower Lung Lobe, Left K Lung, Right L Lung, Left M Lungs, Bilateral T Diaphragm	Ø Open 4 Percutaneous Endoscopic	Z No Device	Z No Qualifier

SECTION: Ø MEDICAL AND SURGICAL
BODY SYSTEM: B RESPIRATORY SYSTEM
OPERATION: U SUPPLEMENT: Putting in or on biological or synthetic material that physically reinforces and/or augments the function of a portion of a body part

Body Part	Approach	Device	Qualifier
1 Trachea 2 Carina 3 Main Bronchus, Right 4 Upper Lobe Bronchus, Right 5 Middle Lobe Bronchus, Right 6 Lower Lobe Bronchus, Right 7 Main Bronchus, Left 8 Upper Lobe Bronchus, Left 9 Lingula Bronchus B Lower Lobe Bronchus, Left	Ø Open 4 Percutaneous Endoscopic 8 Via Natural or Artificial Opening Endoscopic	7 Autologous Tissue Substitute J Synthetic Substitute K Nonautologous Tissue Substitute	Z No Qualifier
T Diaphragm	Ø Open 4 Percutaneous Endoscopic	7 Autologous Tissue Substitute J Synthetic Substitute K Nonautologous Tissue Substitute	Z No Qualifier

Coding Clinic: 2Ø15, Q1, P28 – ØBU3Ø7Z

SECTION: Ø MEDICAL AND SURGICAL
BODY SYSTEM: B RESPIRATORY SYSTEM
OPERATION: V RESTRICTION: Partially closing an orifice or the lumen of a tubular body part

Body Part	Approach	Device	Qualifier
1 Trachea 2 Carina 3 Main Bronchus, Right 4 Upper Lobe Bronchus, Right 5 Middle Lobe Bronchus, Right 6 Lower Lobe Bronchus, Right 7 Main Bronchus, Left 8 Upper Lobe Bronchus, Left 9 Lingula Bronchus B Lower Lobe Bronchus, Left	Ø Open 3 Percutaneous 4 Percutaneous Endoscopic	C Extraluminal Device D Intraluminal Device Z No Device	Z No Qualifier
1 Trachea 2 Carina 3 Main Bronchus, Right 4 Upper Lobe Bronchus, Right 5 Middle Lobe Bronchus, Right 6 Lower Lobe Bronchus, Right 7 Main Bronchus, Left 8 Upper Lobe Bronchus, Left 9 Lingula Bronchus B Lower Lobe Bronchus, Left	7 Via Natural or Artificial Opening 8 Via Natural or Artificial Opening Endoscopic	D Intraluminal Device Z No Device	Z No Qualifier

SECTION: Ø MEDICAL AND SURGICAL
BODY SYSTEM: B RESPIRATORY SYSTEM
OPERATION: W REVISION: *(on multiple pages)*

Correcting, to the extent possible, a portion of a malfunctioning device or the position of a displaced device

Body Part	Approach	Device	Qualifier
Ø Tracheobronchial Tree	Ø Open 3 Percutaneous 4 Percutaneous Endoscopic 7 Via Natural or Artificial Opening 8 Via Natural or Artificial Opening Endoscopic	Ø Drainage Device 2 Monitoring Device 3 Infusion Device 7 Autologous Tissue Substitute C Extraluminal Device D Intraluminal Device J Synthetic Substitute K Nonautologous Tissue Substitute Y Other Device	Z No Qualifier
Ø Tracheobronchial Tree	X External	Ø Drainage Device 2 Monitoring Device 3 Infusion Device 7 Autologous Tissue Substitute C Extraluminal Device D Intraluminal Device J Synthetic Substitute K Nonautologous Tissue Substitute	Z No Qualifier
1 Trachea	Ø Open 3 Percutaneous 4 Percutaneous Endoscopic 7 Via Natural or Artificial Opening 8 Via Natural or Artificial Opening Endoscopic X External	Ø Drainage Device 2 Monitoring Device 7 Autologous Tissue Substitute C Extraluminal Device D Intraluminal Device F Tracheostomy Device J Synthetic Substitute K Nonautologous Tissue Substitute	Z No Qualifier
K Lung, Right L Lung, Left	Ø Open 3 Percutaneous 4 Percutaneous Endoscopic 7 Via Natural or Artificial Opening 8 Via Natural or Artificial Opening Endoscopic	Ø Drainage Device 2 Monitoring Device 3 Infusion Device Y Other Device	Z No Qualifier
K Lung, Right L Lung, Left	X External	Ø Drainage Device 2 Monitoring Device 3 Infusion Device	Z No Qualifier
Q Pleura	Ø Open 3 Percutaneous 4 Percutaneous Endoscopic 7 Via Natural or Artificial Opening 8 Via Natural or Artificial Opening Endoscopic	Ø Drainage Device 2 Monitoring Device Y Other Device	Z No Qualifier
Q Pleura	X External	Ø Drainage Device 2 Monitoring Device	Z No Qualifier

DRG Non-OR ØBWØ[78][23D]Z *(proposed)*
DRG Non-OR ØBWK[78][Ø23D]Z *(proposed)*
DRG Non-OR ØBWL[78][Ø23]Z *(proposed)*

Non-OR ØBWØX[Ø237CDJK]Z
Non-OR ØBW1X[Ø27CDFJK]Z
Non-OR ØBW[KL]X[Ø23]Z
Non-OR ØBWQ[Ø3478][Ø2]Z

SECTION: Ø MEDICAL AND SURGICAL
BODY SYSTEM: B RESPIRATORY SYSTEM
OPERATION: W REVISION: *(continued)*

Correcting, to the extent possible, a portion of a malfunctioning device or the position of a displaced device

Body Part	Approach	Device	Qualifier
T Diaphragm	Ø Open 3 Percutaneous 4 Percutaneous Endoscopic 7 Via Natural or Artificial Opening 8 Via Natural or Artificial Opening Endoscopic	Ø Drainage Device 2 Monitoring Device 7 Autologous Tissue Substitute J Synthetic Substitute K Nonautologous Tissue Substitute M Diaphragmatic Pacemaker Lead Y Other Device	Z No Qualifier
T Diaphragm	X External	Ø Drainage Device 2 Monitoring Device 7 Autologous Tissue Substitute J Synthetic Substitute K Nonautologous Tissue Substitute M Diaphragmatic Pacemaker Lead	Z No Qualifier

Non-OR ØBWQX[Ø2]Z
Non-OR ØBWTX[Ø27JKM]Z

SECTION: Ø MEDICAL AND SURGICAL
BODY SYSTEM: B RESPIRATORY SYSTEM
OPERATION: Y TRANSPLANTATION: Putting in or on all or a portion of a living body part taken from another individual or animal to physically take the place and/or function of all or a portion of a similar body part

Body Part	Approach	Device	Qualifier
C Upper Lung Lobe, Right D Middle Lung Lobe, Right F Lower Lung Lobe, Right G Upper Lung Lobe, Left H Lung Lingula J Lower Lung Lobe, Left K Lung, Right L Lung, Left M Lungs, Bilateral	Ø Open	Z No Device	Ø Allogeneic 1 Syngeneic 2 Zooplastic

All Values

ØC. Mouth and Throat 227
ØCØ. Alteration 228
ØC2. Change 228
ØC5. Destruction 228
ØC7. Dilation 229
ØC9. Drainage 23Ø
ØCB. Excision 231
ØCC. Extirpation 232
ØCD. Extraction 232
ØCF. Fragmentation 233
ØCH. Insertion 233
ØCJ. Inspection 233
ØCL. Occlusion 234
ØCM. Reattachment 234
ØCN. Release 235
ØCP. Removal 236
ØCQ. Repair 237
ØCR. Replacement 238
ØCS. Reposition 238
ØCT. Resection 239
ØCU. Supplement 239
ØCV. Restriction 24Ø
ØCW. Revision 24Ø
ØCX. Transfer 241

SECTION: Ø MEDICAL AND SURGICAL
BODY SYSTEM: C MOUTH AND THROAT
OPERATION: Ø ALTERATION: Modifying the anatomic structure of a body part without affecting the function of the body part

Body Part	Approach	Device	Qualifier
Ø Upper Lip 1 Lower Lip	X External	7 Autologous Tissue Substitute J Synthetic Substitute K Nonautologous Tissue Substitute Z No Device	Z No Qualifier

SECTION: Ø MEDICAL AND SURGICAL
BODY SYSTEM: C MOUTH AND THROAT
OPERATION: 2 CHANGE: Taking out or off a device from a body part and putting back an identical or similar device in or on the same body part without cutting or puncturing the skin or a mucous membrane

Body Part	Approach	Device	Qualifier
A Salivary Gland S Larynx Y Mouth and Throat	X External	Ø Drainage Device Y Other Device	Z No Qualifier

Non-OR All Values

SECTION: Ø MEDICAL AND SURGICAL
BODY SYSTEM: C MOUTH AND THROAT
OPERATION: 5 DESTRUCTION: *(on multiple pages)*
Physical eradication of all or a portion of a body part by the use of direct energy, force, or a destructive agent

Body Part	Approach	Device	Qualifier
Ø Upper Lip 1 Lower Lip 2 Hard Palate 3 Soft Palate 4 Buccal Mucosa 5 Upper Gingiva 6 Lower Gingiva 7 Tongue N Uvula P Tonsils Q Adenoids	Ø Open 3 Percutaneous X External	Z No Device	Z No Qualifier

Non-OR ØC5[56][Ø3X]ZZ

SECTION: Ø MEDICAL AND SURGICAL
BODY SYSTEM: C MOUTH AND THROAT
OPERATION: 5 DESTRUCTION: *(continued)*

Physical eradication of all or a portion of a body part by the use of direct energy, force, or a destructive agent

Body Part	Approach	Device	Qualifier
8 Parotid Gland, Right 9 Parotid Gland, Left B Parotid Duct, Right C Parotid Duct, Left D Sublingual Gland, Right F Sublingual Gland, Left G Submaxillary Gland, Right H Submaxillary Gland, Left J Minor Salivary Gland	Ø Open 3 Percutaneous	Z No Device	Z No Qualifier
M Pharynx R Epiglottis S Larynx T Vocal Cord, Right V Vocal Cord, Left	Ø Open 3 Percutaneous 4 Percutaneous Endoscopic 7 Via Natural or Artificial Opening 8 Via Natural or Artificial Opening Endoscopic	Z No Device	Z No Qualifier
W Upper Tooth X Lower Tooth	Ø Open X External	Z No Device	Ø Single 1 Multiple 2 All

Non-OR ØC5[WX][ØX]Z[Ø12]

SECTION: Ø MEDICAL AND SURGICAL
BODY SYSTEM: C MOUTH AND THROAT
OPERATION: 7 DILATION: Expanding an orifice or the lumen of a tubular body part

Body Part	Approach	Device	Qualifier
B Parotid Duct, Right C Parotid Duct, Left	Ø Open 3 Percutaneous 7 Via Natural or Artificial Opening	D Intraluminal Device Z No Device	Z No Qualifier
M Pharynx	7 Via Natural or Artificial Opening 8 Via Natural or Artificial Opening Endoscopic	D Intraluminal Device Z No Device	Z No Qualifier
S Larynx	Ø Open 3 Percutaneous 4 Percutaneous Endoscopic 7 Via Natural or Artificial Opening 8 Via Natural or Artificial Opening Endoscopic	D Intraluminal Device Z No Device	Z No Qualifier

Non-OR ØC7[BC][Ø37][DZ]Z
Non-OR ØC7M[78][DZ]Z

SECTION: Ø MEDICAL AND SURGICAL

BODY SYSTEM: C MOUTH AND THROAT

OPERATION: 9 DRAINAGE: *(on multiple pages)*

Taking or letting out fluids and/or gases from a body part

Body Part	Approach	Device	Qualifier
Ø Upper Lip 1 Lower Lip 2 Hard Palate 3 Soft Palate 4 Buccal Mucosa 5 Upper Gingiva 6 Lower Gingiva 7 Tongue N Uvula P Tonsils Q Adenoids	Ø Open 3 Percutaneous X External	Ø Drainage Device	Z No Qualifier
Ø Upper Lip 1 Lower Lip 2 Hard Palate 3 Soft Palate 4 Buccal Mucosa 5 Upper Gingiva 6 Lower Gingiva 7 Tongue N Uvula P Tonsils Q Adenoids	Ø Open 3 Percutaneous X External	Z No Device	X Diagnostic Z No Qualifier
8 Parotid Gland, Right 9 Parotid Gland, Left B Parotid Duct, Right C Parotid Duct, Left D Sublingual Gland, Right F Sublingual Gland, Left G Submaxillary Gland, Right H Submaxillary Gland, Left J Minor Salivary Gland	Ø Open 3 Percutaneous	Ø Drainage Device	Z No Qualifier
8 Parotid Gland, Right 9 Parotid Gland, Left B Parotid Duct, Right C Parotid Duct, Left D Sublingual Gland, Right F Sublingual Gland, Left G Submaxillary Gland, Right H Submaxillary Gland, Left J Minor Salivary Gland	Ø Open 3 Percutaneous	Z No Device	X Diagnostic Z No Qualifier
M Pharynx R Epiglottis S Larynx T Vocal Cord, Right V Vocal Cord, Left	Ø Open 3 Percutaneous 4 Percutaneous Endoscopic 7 Via Natural or Artificial Opening 8 Via Natural or Artificial Opening Endoscopic	Ø Drainage Device	Z No Qualifier

Non-OR ØC9[Ø12347NPQ]3ØZ
Non-OR ØC9[Ø12347NPQ]3ZZ
Non-OR ØC9[56][Ø3X]ØZ
Non-OR ØC9[Ø1456][Ø3X]ZX
Non-OR ØC9[56][Ø3X]ZZ
Non-OR ØC97[3X]ZX
Non-OR ØC9[89BCDFGHJ][Ø3]ØZ
Non-OR ØC9[89BCDFGHJ]3ZX
Non-OR ØC9[89BCDFGHJ][Ø3]ZZ
Non-OR ØC9[MRSTV]3ØZ

SECTION: Ø MEDICAL AND SURGICAL
BODY SYSTEM: C MOUTH AND THROAT
OPERATION: 9 DRAINAGE: *(continued)*
Taking or letting out fluids and/or gases from a body part

Body Part	Approach	Device	Qualifier
M Pharynx R Epiglottis S Larynx T Vocal Cord, Right V Vocal Cord, Left	Ø Open 3 Percutaneous 4 Percutaneous Endoscopic 7 Via Natural or Artificial Opening 8 Via Natural or Artificial Opening Endoscopic	Z No Device	X Diagnostic Z No Qualifier
W Upper Tooth X Lower Tooth	Ø Open X External	Ø Drainage Device Z No Device	Ø Single 1 Multiple 2 All

Non-OR ØC9[MRSTV]3ZZ
Non-OR ØC9M[Ø3478]ZX
Non-OR ØC9[RSTV][3478]ZX
Non-OR ØC9[WX][ØX][ØZ][Ø12]

SECTION: Ø MEDICAL AND SURGICAL
BODY SYSTEM: C MOUTH AND THROAT
OPERATION: B EXCISION: Cutting out or off, without replacement, a portion of a body part

Body Part	Approach	Device	Qualifier
Ø Upper Lip 1 Lower Lip 2 Hard Palate 3 Soft Palate 4 Buccal Mucosa 5 Upper Gingiva 6 Lower Gingiva 7 Tongue N Uvula P Tonsils Q Adenoids	Ø Open 3 Percutaneous X External	Z No Device	X Diagnostic Z No Qualifier
8 Parotid Gland, Right 9 Parotid Gland, Left B Parotid Duct, Right C Parotid Duct, Left D Sublingual Gland, Right F Sublingual Gland, Left G Submaxillary Gland, Right H Submaxillary Gland, Left J Minor Salivary Gland	Ø Open 3 Percutaneous	Z No Device	X Diagnostic Z No Qualifier
M Pharynx R Epiglottis S Larynx T Vocal Cord, Right V Vocal Cord, Left	Ø Open 3 Percutaneous 4 Percutaneous Endoscopic 7 Via Natural or Artificial Opening 8 Via Natural or Artificial Opening Endoscopic	Z No Device	X Diagnostic Z No Qualifier
W Upper Tooth X Lower Tooth	Ø Open X External	Z No Device	Ø Single 1 Multiple 2 All

Non-OR ØCB[Ø1456][Ø3X]ZX
Non-OR ØCB[56][Ø3X]ZZ
Non-OR ØCB7[3X]ZX
Non-OR ØCB[89BCDFGHJ]3ZX
Non-OR ØCBM[Ø3478]ZX
Non-OR ØCB[RSTV][3478]ZX
Non-OR ØCB[WX][ØX]Z[Ø12]

Coding Clinic: 2Ø16, Q2, P2Ø – ØCBM8ZX
Coding Clinic: 2Ø16, Q3, P28 – ØCBM8ZZ

SECTION: Ø MEDICAL AND SURGICAL
BODY SYSTEM: C MOUTH AND THROAT
OPERATION: C EXTIRPATION: Taking or cutting out solid matter from a body part

Body Part	Approach	Device	Qualifier
Ø Upper Lip 1 Lower Lip 2 Hard Palate 3 Soft Palate 4 Buccal Mucosa 5 Upper Gingiva 6 Lower Gingiva 7 Tongue N Uvula P Tonsils Q Adenoids	Ø Open 3 Percutaneous X External	Z No Device	Z No Qualifier
8 Parotid Gland, Right 9 Parotid Gland, Left B Parotid Duct, Right C Parotid Duct, Left D Sublingual Gland, Right F Sublingual Gland, Left G Submaxillary Gland, Right H Submaxillary Gland, Left J Minor Salivary Gland	Ø Open 3 Percutaneous	Z No Device	Z No Qualifier
M Pharynx R Epiglottis S Larynx T Vocal Cord, Right V Vocal Cord, Left	Ø Open 3 Percutaneous 4 Percutaneous Endoscopic 7 Via Natural or Artificial Opening 8 Via Natural or Artificial Opening Endoscopic	Z No Device	Z No Qualifier
W Upper Tooth X Lower Tooth	Ø Open X External	Z No Device	Ø Single 1 Multiple 2 All

Non-OR ØCC[Ø12347NPQ]XZZ
Non-OR ØCC[56][Ø3X]ZZ
Non-OR ØCC[89BCDFGHJ][Ø3]ZZ
Non-OR ØCC[MS][78]ZZ
Non-OR ØCC[WX][ØX]Z[Ø12]

Coding Clinic: 2Ø16, Q2, P2Ø – ØCCH3ZZ

SECTION: Ø MEDICAL AND SURGICAL
BODY SYSTEM: C MOUTH AND THROAT
OPERATION: D EXTRACTION: Pulling or stripping out or off all or a portion of a body part by the use of force

Body Part	Approach	Device	Qualifier
T Vocal Cord, Right V Vocal Cord, Left	Ø Open 3 Percutaneous 4 Percutaneous Endoscopic 7 Via Natural or Artificial Opening 8 Via Natural or Artificial Opening Endoscopic	Z No Device	Z No Qualifier
W Upper Tooth X Lower Tooth	X External	Z No Device	Ø Single 1 Multiple 2 All

Non-OR ØCD[WX]XZ[Ø12]

SECTION: Ø MEDICAL AND SURGICAL
BODY SYSTEM: C MOUTH AND THROAT
OPERATION: F FRAGMENTATION: Breaking solid matter in a body part into pieces

Body Part	Approach	Device	Qualifier
B Parotid Duct, Right C Parotid Duct, Left	Ø Open 3 Percutaneous 7 Via Natural or Artificial Opening X External	Z No Device	Z No Qualifier

ØCF[BC]XZZ

Non-OR All Values

SECTION: Ø MEDICAL AND SURGICAL
BODY SYSTEM: C MOUTH AND THROAT
OPERATION: H INSERTION: Putting in a nonbiological appliance that monitors, assists, performs, or prevents a physiological function but does not physically take the place of a body part

Body Part	Approach	Device	Qualifier
7 Tongue	Ø Open 3 Percutaneous X External	1 Radioactive Element	Z No Qualifier
A Salivary Gland S Larynx	Ø Open 3 Percutaneous 7 Via Natural or Artificial Opening 8 Via Natural or Artificial Opening Endoscopic	1 Radioactive Element Y Other Device	Z No Qualifier
Y Mouth and Throat	Ø Open 3 Percutaneous	1 Radioactive Element Y Other Device	Z No Qualifier
Y Mouth and Throat	7 Via Natural or Artificial Opening 8 Via Natural or Artificial Opening Endoscopic	1 Radioactive Element B Intraluminal Device, Airway Y Other Device	Z No Qualifier

Non-OR ØCHY[78]BZ

SECTION: Ø MEDICAL AND SURGICAL
BODY SYSTEM: C MOUTH AND THROAT
OPERATION: J INSPECTION: Visually and/or manually exploring a body part

Body Part	Approach	Device	Qualifier
A Salivary Gland	Ø Open 3 Percutaneous X External	Z No Device	Z No Qualifier
S Larynx Y Mouth and Throat	Ø Open 3 Percutaneous 4 Percutaneous Endoscopic 7 Via Natural or Artificial Opening 8 Via Natural or Artificial Opening Endoscopic X External	Z No Device	Z No Qualifier

Non-OR All Values

SECTION: Ø MEDICAL AND SURGICAL
BODY SYSTEM: C MOUTH AND THROAT
OPERATION: L OCCLUSION: Completely closing an orifice or the lumen of a tubular body part

Body Part	Approach	Device	Qualifier
B Parotid Duct, Right C Parotid Duct, Left	Ø Open 3 Percutaneous 4 Percutaneous Endoscopic	C Extraluminal Device D Intraluminal Device Z No Device	Z No Qualifier
B Parotid Duct, Right C Parotid Duct, Left	7 Via Natural or Artificial Opening 8 Via Natural or Artificial Opening Endoscopic	D Intraluminal Device Z No Device	Z No Qualifier

SECTION: Ø MEDICAL AND SURGICAL
BODY SYSTEM: C MOUTH AND THROAT
OPERATION: M REATTACHMENT: Putting back in or on all or a portion of a separated body part to its normal location or other suitable location

Body Part	Approach	Device	Qualifier
Ø Upper Lip 1 Lower Lip 3 Soft Palate 7 Tongue N Uvula	Ø Open	Z No Device	Z No Qualifier
W Upper Tooth X Lower Tooth	Ø Open X External	Z No Device	Ø Single 1 Multiple 2 All

Non-OR ØCM[WX][ØX]Z[Ø12]

SECTION: Ø MEDICAL AND SURGICAL
BODY SYSTEM: C MOUTH AND THROAT
OPERATION: N RELEASE: Freeing a body part from an abnormal physical constraint by cutting or by the use of force

Body Part	Approach	Device	Qualifier
Ø Upper Lip 1 Lower Lip 2 Hard Palate 3 Soft Palate 4 Buccal Mucosa 5 Upper Gingiva 6 Lower Gingiva 7 Tongue N Uvula P Tonsils Q Adenoids	Ø Open 3 Percutaneous X External	Z No Device	Z No Qualifier
8 Parotid Gland, Right 9 Parotid Gland, Left B Parotid Duct, Right C Parotid Duct, Left D Sublingual Gland, Right F Sublingual Gland, Left G Submaxillary Gland, Right H Submaxillary Gland, Left J Minor Salivary Gland	Ø Open 3 Percutaneous	Z No Device	Z No Qualifier
M Pharynx R Epiglottis S Larynx T Vocal Cord, Right V Vocal Cord, Left	Ø Open 3 Percutaneous 4 Percutaneous Endoscopic 7 Via Natural or Artificial Opening 8 Via Natural or Artificial Opening Endoscopic	Z No Device	Z No Qualifier
W Upper Tooth X Lower Tooth	Ø Open X External	Z No Device	Ø Single 1 Multiple 2 All

Non-OR ØCN[Ø1567][Ø3X]ZZ
Non-OR ØCN[WX][ØX]Z[Ø12]

SECTION: Ø MEDICAL AND SURGICAL
BODY SYSTEM: C MOUTH AND THROAT
OPERATION: P REMOVAL: Taking out or off a device from a body part

Body Part	Approach	Device	Qualifier
A Salivary Gland	Ø Open 3 Percutaneous	Ø Drainage Device C Extraluminal Device Y Other Device	Z No Qualifier
A Salivary Gland	7 Via Natural or Artificial Opening 8 Via Natural or Artificial Opening Endoscopic	Y Other Device	Z No Qualifier
S Larynx	Ø Open 3 Percutaneous 7 Via Natural or Artificial Opening 8 Via Natural or Artificial Opening Endoscopic	Ø Drainage Device 7 Autologous Tissue Substitute D Intraluminal Device J Synthetic Substitute K Nonautologous Tissue Substitute Y Other Device	Z No Qualifier
S Larynx	X External	Ø Drainage Device 7 Autologous Tissue Substitute D Intraluminal Device J Synthetic Substitute K Nonautologous Tissue Substitute	Z No Qualifier
Y Mouth and Throat	Ø Open 3 Percutaneous 7 Via Natural or Artificial Opening 8 Via Natural or Artificial Opening Endoscopic	Ø Drainage Device 1 Radioactive Element 7 Autologous Tissue Substitute D Intraluminal Device J Synthetic Substitute K Nonautologous Tissue Substitute Y Other Device	Z No Qualifier
Y Mouth and Throat	X External	Ø Drainage Device 1 Radioactive Element 7 Autologous Tissue Substitute D Intraluminal Device J Synthetic Substitute K Nonautologous Tissue Substitute	Z No Qualifier

Non-OR ØCPA[Ø3][ØC]Z
Non-OR ØCPS[78][ØD]Z
Non-OR ØCPSX[Ø7DJK]Z
Non-OR ØCPY[78][ØD]Z
Non-OR ØCPYX[Ø17DJK]Z

SECTION: Ø MEDICAL AND SURGICAL
BODY SYSTEM: C MOUTH AND THROAT
OPERATION: Q REPAIR: Restoring, to the extent possible, a body part to its normal anatomic structure and function

Body Part	Approach	Device	Qualifier
Ø Upper Lip 1 Lower Lip 2 Hard Palate 3 Soft Palate 4 Buccal Mucosa 5 Upper Gingiva 6 Lower Gingiva 7 Tongue N Uvula P Tonsils Q Adenoids	Ø Open 3 Percutaneous X External	Z No Device	Z No Qualifier
8 Parotid Gland, Right 9 Parotid Gland, Left B Parotid Duct, Right C Parotid Duct, Left D Sublingual Gland, Right F Sublingual Gland, Left G Submaxillary Gland, Right H Submaxillary Gland, Left J Minor Salivary Gland	Ø Open 3 Percutaneous	Z No Device	Z No Qualifier
M Pharynx R Epiglottis S Larynx T Vocal Cord, Right V Vocal Cord, Left	Ø Open 3 Percutaneous 4 Percutaneous Endoscopic 7 Via Natural or Artificial Opening 8 Via Natural or Artificial Opening Endoscopic	Z No Device	Z No Qualifier
W Upper Tooth X Lower Tooth	Ø Open X External	Z No Device	Ø Single 1 Multiple 2 All

Non-OR ØCQ[Ø1]XZZ
Non-OR ØCQ[56][Ø3X]ZZ
Non-OR ØCQ[WX][ØX]Z[Ø12]

Coding Clinic: 2Ø17, Q1, P21 – ØCQ5ØZZ

SECTION: Ø MEDICAL AND SURGICAL
BODY SYSTEM: C MOUTH AND THROAT
OPERATION: R REPLACEMENT: Putting in or on biological or synthetic material that physically takes the place and/or function of all or a portion of a body part

Body Part	Approach	Device	Qualifier
Ø Upper Lip 1 Lower Lip 2 Hard Palate 3 Soft Palate 4 Buccal Mucosa 5 Upper Gingiva 6 Lower Gingiva 7 Tongue N Uvula	Ø Open 3 Percutaneous X External	7 Autologous Tissue Substitute J Synthetic Substitute K Nonautologous Tissue Substitute	Z No Qualifier
B Parotid Duct, Right C Parotid Duct, Left	Ø Open 3 Percutaneous	7 Autologous Tissue Substitute J Synthetic Substitute K Nonautologous Tissue Substitute	Z No Qualifier
M Pharynx R Epiglottis S Larynx T Vocal Cord, Right V Vocal Cord, Left	Ø Open 7 Via Natural or Artificial Opening 8 Via Natural or Artificial Opening Endoscopic	7 Autologous Tissue Substitute J Synthetic Substitute K Nonautologous Tissue Substitute	Z No Qualifier
W Upper Tooth X Lower Tooth	Ø Open X External	7 Autologous Tissue Substitute J Synthetic Substitute K Nonautologous Tissue Substitute	Ø Single 1 Multiple 2 All

Non-OR ØCR[WX][ØX][7JK][Ø12]

SECTION: Ø MEDICAL AND SURGICAL
BODY SYSTEM: C MOUTH AND THROAT
OPERATION: S REPOSITION: Moving to its normal location, or other suitable location, all or a portion of a body part

Body Part	Approach	Device	Qualifier
Ø Upper Lip 1 Lower Lip 2 Hard Palate 3 Soft Palate 7 Tongue N Uvula	Ø Open X External	Z No Device	Z No Qualifier
B Parotid Duct, Right C Parotid Duct, Left	Ø Open 3 Percutaneous	Z No Device	Z No Qualifier
R Epiglottis S Larynx T Vocal Cord, Right V Vocal Cord, Left	Ø Open 7 Via Natural or Artificial Opening 8 Via Natural or Artificial Opening Endoscopic	Z No Device	Z No Qualifier
W Upper Tooth X Lower Tooth	Ø Open X External	5 External Fixation Device Z No Device	Ø Single 1 Multiple 2 All

Non-OR 0CS[WX][0X][5Z][012]

Coding Clinic: 2016, Q3, P29 – 0CSR8ZZ

Coding Clinic: 2Ø22, Q2, P24 – ØCS[23]ØZZ

Coding Clinic: 2Ø23, Q4, P53 – ØCSSØZZ

SECTION: Ø MEDICAL AND SURGICAL
BODY SYSTEM: C MOUTH AND THROAT
OPERATION: T RESECTION: Cutting out or off, without replacement, all of a body part

Body Part	Approach	Device	Qualifier
Ø Upper Lip 1 Lower Lip 2 Hard Palate 3 Soft Palate 7 Tongue N Uvula P Tonsils Q Adenoids	Ø Open X External	Z No Device	Z No Qualifier
8 Parotid Gland, Right 9 Parotid Gland, Left B Parotid Duct, Right C Parotid Duct, Left D Sublingual Gland, Right F Sublingual Gland, Left G Submaxillary Gland, Right H Submaxillary Gland, Left J Minor Salivary Gland	Ø Open	Z No Device	Z No Qualifier
M Pharynx R Epiglottis S Larynx T Vocal Cord, Right V Vocal Cord, Left	Ø Open 4 Percutaneous Endoscopic 7 Via Natural or Artificial Opening 8 Via Natural or Artificial Opening Endoscopic	Z No Device	Z No Qualifier
W Upper Tooth X Lower Tooth	Ø Open	Z No Device	Ø Single 1 Multiple 2 All

Non-OR ØCT[WX]ØZ[Ø12]

Coding Clinic: 2Ø16, Q2, P13 – ØCT9ØZZ

SECTION: Ø MEDICAL AND SURGICAL
BODY SYSTEM: C MOUTH AND THROAT
OPERATION: U SUPPLEMENT: Putting in or on biological or synthetic material that physically reinforces and/or augments the function of a portion of a body part

Body Part	Approach	Device	Qualifier
Ø Upper Lip 1 Lower Lip 2 Hard Palate 3 Soft Palate 4 Buccal Mucosa 5 Upper Gingiva 6 Lower Gingiva 7 Tongue N Uvula	Ø Open 3 Percutaneous X External	7 Autologous Tissue Substitute J Synthetic Substitute K Nonautologous Tissue Substitute	Z No Qualifier
M Pharynx R Epiglottis S Larynx T Vocal Cord, Right V Vocal Cord, Left	Ø Open 7 Via Natural or Artificial Opening 8 Via Natural or Artificial Opening Endoscopic	7 Autologous Tissue Substitute J Synthetic Substitute K Nonautologous Tissue Substitute	Z No Qualifier

Non-OR ØCU2[Ø3]JZ

SECTION: Ø MEDICAL AND SURGICAL
BODY SYSTEM: C MOUTH AND THROAT
OPERATION: V RESTRICTION: Partially closing an orifice or the lumen of a tubular body part

Body Part	Approach	Device	Qualifier
B Parotid Duct, Right C Parotid Duct, Left	Ø Open 3 Percutaneous	C Extraluminal Device D Intraluminal Device Z No Device	Z No Qualifier
B Parotid Duct, Right C Parotid Duct, Left	7 Via Natural or Artificial Opening 8 Via Natural or Artificial Opening Endoscopic	D Intraluminal Device Z No Device	Z No Qualifier

SECTION: Ø MEDICAL AND SURGICAL
BODY SYSTEM: C MOUTH AND THROAT
OPERATION: W REVISION: *(on multiple pages)*
Correcting, to the extent possible, a portion of a malfunctioning device or the position of a displaced device

Body Part	Approach	Device	Qualifier
A Salivary Gland	Ø Open 3 Percutaneous	Ø Drainage Device C Extraluminal Device Y Other Device	Z No Qualifier
A Salivary Gland	7 Via Natural or Artificial Opening 8 Via Natural or Artificial Opening Endoscopic	Y Other Device	Z No Qualifier
A Salivary Gland	X External	Ø Drainage Device C Extraluminal Device	Z No Qualifier
S Larynx	Ø Open 3 Percutaneous 7 Via Natural or Artificial Opening 8 Via Natural or Artificial Opening Endoscopic	Ø Drainage Device 7 Autologous Tissue Substitute D Intraluminal Device J Synthetic Substitute K Nonautologous Tissue Substitute Y Other Device	Z No Qualifier
S Larynx	X External	Ø Drainage Device 7 Autologous Tissue Substitute D Intraluminal Device J Synthetic Substitute K Nonautologous Tissue Substitute	Z No Qualifier

Non-OR ØCWA[Ø3X][ØC]Z
Non-OR ØCWSX[Ø7DHJ]Z

SECTION: Ø MEDICAL AND SURGICAL
BODY SYSTEM: C MOUTH AND THROAT
OPERATION: W REVISION: *(continued)*
Correcting, to the extent possible, a portion of a malfunctioning device or the position of a displaced device

Body Part	Approach	Device	Qualifier
Y Mouth and Throat	Ø Open 3 Percutaneous 7 Via Natural or Artificial Opening 8 Via Natural or Artificial Opening Endoscopic	Ø Drainage Device 1 Radioactive Element 7 Autologous Tissue Substitute D Intraluminal Device J Synthetic Substitute K Nonautologous Tissue Substitute Y Other Device	Z No Qualifier
Y Mouth and Throat	X External	Ø Drainage Device 1 Radioactive Element 7 Autologous Tissue Substitute D Intraluminal Device J Synthetic Substitute K Nonautologous Tissue Substitute	Z No Qualifier

Non-OR ØCWYØ7Z
Non-OR ØCWYX[Ø17DJK]Z

SECTION: Ø MEDICAL AND SURGICAL
BODY SYSTEM: C MOUTH AND THROAT
OPERATION: X TRANSFER: Moving, without taking out, all or a portion of a body part to another location to take over the function of all or a portion of a body part

Body Part	Approach	Device	Qualifier
Ø Upper Lip 1 Lower Lip 3 Soft Palate 4 Buccal Mucosa 5 Upper Gingiva 6 Lower Gingiva 7 Tongue	Ø Open X External	Z No Device	Z No Qualifier

ØD. Gastrointestinal System 242
ØD1. Bypass 243
ØD2. Change 244
ØD5. Destruction 245
ØD7. Dilation 246
ØD8. Division 247
ØD9. Drainage 247
ØDB. Excision 249
ØDC. Extirpation 251
ØDD. Extraction 252
ØDF. Fragmentation 252
ØDH. Insertion 253
ØDJ. Inspection 254
ØDL. Occlusion 255
ØDM. Reattachment 256
ØDN. Release 257
ØDP. Removal 258
ØDQ. Repair 26Ø
ØDR. Replacement 261
ØDS. Reposition 261
ØDT. Resection 262
ØDU. Supplement 263
ØDV. Restriction 264
ØDW. Revision 265
ØDX. Transfer 267
ØDY. Transplantation 267

SECTION: Ø MEDICAL AND SURGICAL
BODY SYSTEM: D GASTROINTESTINAL SYSTEM
OPERATION: 1 BYPASS: *(on multiple pages)*
Altering the route of passage of the contents of a tubular body part

Body Part	Approach	Device	Qualifier
1 Esophagus, Upper 2 Esophagus, Middle 3 Esophagus, Lower 5 Esophagus	Ø Open 4 Percutaneous Endoscopic 8 Via Natural or Artificial Opening Endoscopic	7 Autologous Tissue Substitute J Synthetic Substitute K Nonautologous Tissue Substitute Z No Device	4 Cutaneous 6 Stomach 9 Duodenum A Jejunum B Ileum
1 Esophagus, Upper 2 Esophagus, Middle 3 Esophagus, Lower 5 Esophagus	3 Percutaneous	J Synthetic Substitute	4 Cutaneous
6 Stomach 9 Duodenum	Ø Open 4 Percutaneous Endoscopic 8 Via Natural or Artificial Opening Endoscopic	7 Autologous Tissue Substitute J Synthetic Substitute K Nonautologous Tissue Substitute Z No Device	4 Cutaneous 9 Duodenum A Jejunum B Ileum L Transverse Colon
6 Stomach 9 Duodenum	3 Percutaneous	J Synthetic Substitute	4 Cutaneous
8 Small Intestine	Ø Open 4 Percutaneous Endoscopic 8 Via Natural or Artificial Opening Endoscopic	7 Autologous Tissue Substitute J Synthetic Substitute K Nonautologous Tissue Substitute Z No Device	4 Cutaneous 8 Small Intestine H Cecum K Ascending Colon L Transverse Colon M Descending Colon N Sigmoid Colon P Rectum Q Anus
A Jejunum	Ø Open 4 Percutaneous Endoscopic 8 Via Natural or Artificial Opening Endoscopic	7 Autologous Tissue Substitute J Synthetic Substitute K Nonautologous Tissue Substitute Z No Device	4 Cutaneous A Jejunum B Ileum H Cecum K Ascending Colon L Transverse Colon M Descending Colon N Sigmoid Colon P Rectum Q Anus
A Jejunum	3 Percutaneous	J Synthetic Substitute	4 Cutaneous
B Ileum	Ø Open 4 Percutaneous Endoscopic 8 Via Natural or Artificial Opening Endoscopic	7 Autologous Tissue Substitute J Synthetic Substitute K Nonautologous Tissue Substitute Z No Device	4 Cutaneous B Ileum H Cecum K Ascending Colon L Transverse Colon M Descending Colon N Sigmoid Colon P Rectum Q Anus
B Ileum	3 Percutaneous	J Synthetic Substitute	4 Cutaneous
E Large Intestine	Ø Open 4 Percutaneous Endoscopic 8 Via Natural or Artificial Opening Endoscopic	7 Autologous Tissue Substitute J Synthetic Substitute K Nonautologous Tissue Substitute Z No Device	4 Cutaneous E Large Intestine P Rectum

Non-OR ØD16[Ø48][7JKZ]4
Non-OR ØD163J4

ØD16[Ø48][7JKZ][9ABL] when reported with Principal Diagnosis E66.Ø1 and Secondary Diagnosis K68.11, K95.Ø1, K95.81, T81.4ØXA, T8141XA, T8142XA, T8143XA, T8144XA, or T8149XA

Coding Clinic: 2Ø16, Q2, P31 – ØD194ZB
Coding Clinic: 2Ø17, Q2, P18 – ØD16ØZA

SECTION: Ø MEDICAL AND SURGICAL
BODY SYSTEM: D GASTROINTESTINAL SYSTEM
OPERATION: 1 BYPASS: *(continued)*
Altering the route of passage of the contents of a tubular body part

Body Part	Approach	Device	Qualifier
H Cecum	Ø Open 4 Percutaneous Endoscopic 8 Via Natural or Artificial Opening Endoscopic	7 Autologous Tissue Substitute J Synthetic Substitute K Nonautologous Tissue Substitute Z No Device	4 Cutaneous H Cecum K Ascending Colon L Transverse Colon M Descending Colon N Sigmoid Colon P Rectum
H Cecum	3 Percutaneous	J Synthetic Substitute	4 Cutaneous
K Ascending Colon	Ø Open 4 Percutaneous Endoscopic 8 Via Natural or Artificial Opening Endoscopic	7 Autologous Tissue Substitute J Synthetic Substitute K Nonautologous Tissue Substitute Z No Device	4 Cutaneous K Ascending Colon L Transverse Colon M Descending Colon N Sigmoid Colon P Rectum
K Ascending Colon	3 Percutaneous	J Synthetic Substitute	4 Cutaneous
L Transverse Colon	Ø Open 4 Percutaneous Endoscopic 8 Via Natural or Artificial Opening Endoscopic	7 Autologous Tissue Substitute J Synthetic Substitute K Nonautologous Tissue Substitute Z No Device	4 Cutaneous L Transverse Colon M Descending Colon N Sigmoid Colon P Rectum
L Transverse Colon	3 Percutaneous	J Synthetic Substitute	4 Cutaneous
M Descending Colon	Ø Open 4 Percutaneous Endoscopic 8 Via Natural or Artificial Opening Endoscopic	7 Autologous Tissue Substitute J Synthetic Substitute K Nonautologous Tissue Substitute Z No Device	4 Cutaneous M Descending Colon N Sigmoid Colon P Rectum
M Descending Colon	3 Percutaneous	J Synthetic Substitute	4 Cutaneous
N Sigmoid Colon	Ø Open 4 Percutaneous Endoscopic 8 Via Natural or Artificial Opening Endoscopic	7 Autologous Tissue Substitute J Synthetic Substitute K Nonautologous Tissue Substitute Z No Device	4 Cutaneous N Sigmoid Colon P Rectum
N Sigmoid Colon	3 Percutaneous	J Synthetic Substitute	4 Cutaneous

SECTION: Ø MEDICAL AND SURGICAL
BODY SYSTEM: D GASTROINTESTINAL SYSTEM
OPERATION: 2 CHANGE: Taking out or off a device from a body part and putting back an identical or similar device in or on the same body part without cutting or puncturing the skin or a mucous membrane

Body Part	Approach	Device	Qualifier
Ø Upper Intestinal Tract D Lower Intestinal Tract	X External	Ø Drainage Device U Feeding Device Y Other Device	Z No Qualifier
U Omentum V Mesentery W Peritoneum	X External	Ø Drainage Device Y Other Device	Z No Qualifier

Non-OR All Values

Coding Clinic: 2Ø19, Q1, P26 – ØD2DXUZ
Coding Clinic: 2Ø22, Q1, P45 – ØD2ØXYZ

SECTION: Ø MEDICAL AND SURGICAL
BODY SYSTEM: D GASTROINTESTINAL SYSTEM
OPERATION: 5 DESTRUCTION: *(on multiple pages)*

Physical eradication of all or a portion of a body part by the direct use of energy, force, or a destructive agent

Body Part	Approach	Device	Qualifier
1 Esophagus, Upper 2 Esophagus, Middle 3 Esophagus, Lower 4 Esophagogastric Junction 5 Esophagus 6 Stomach 7 Stomach, Pylorus 8 Small Intestine 9 Duodenum A Jejunum B Ileum C Ileocecal Valve E Large Intestine F Large Intestine, Right G Large Intestine, Left H Cecum J Appendix K Ascending Colon L Transverse Colon M Descending Colon N Sigmoid Colon P Rectum Q Anus	Ø Open 3 Percutaneous 4 Percutaneous Endoscopic	Z No Device	3 Laser Interstitial Thermal Therapy Z No Qualifier
1 Esophagus, Upper 2 Esophagus, Middle 3 Esophagus, Lower 4 Esophagogastric Junction 5 Esophagus 6 Stomach 7 Stomach, Pylorus 8 Small Intestine 9 Duodenum A Jejunum B Ileum C Ileocecal Valve E Large Intestine F Large Intestine, Right G Large Intestine, Left H Cecum J Appendix K Ascending Colon L Transverse Colon M Descending Colon N Sigmoid Colon P Rectum Q Anus	7 Via Natural or Artificial Opening 8 Via Natural or Artificial Opening Endoscopic	Z No Device	Z No Qualifier

Non-OR ØD5[12345679EFGHKLMN][48]ZZ
Non-OR ØD5P[Ø3478]ZZ
Non-OR ØD5Q[48]ZZ
Non-OR ØD5R4ZZ
Non-OR ØD5[123456789ABCEFGHJKLMNP][Ø34]Z3

Coding Clinic: 2017, Q1, P35 – 0D5W0ZZ

SECTION: Ø MEDICAL AND SURGICAL
BODY SYSTEM: D GASTROINTESTINAL SYSTEM
OPERATION: 5 DESTRUCTION: *(continued)*
Physical eradication of all or a portion of a body part by the direct use of energy, force, or a destructive agent

Body Part	Approach	Device	Qualifier
Q Anus	Ø Open 3 Percutaneous 4 Percutaneous Endoscopic	Z No Device	3 Laser Interstitial Thermal Therapy Z No Qualifier
Q Anus	7 Via Natural or Artificial Opening 8 Via Natural or Artificial Opening Endoscopic X External	Z No Device	Z No Qualifier
R Anal Sphincter U Omentum V Mesentery W Peritoneum	Ø Open 3 Percutaneous 4 Percutaneous Endoscopic	Z No Device	Z No Qualifier

SECTION: Ø MEDICAL AND SURGICAL
BODY SYSTEM: D GASTROINTESTINAL SYSTEM
OPERATION: 7 DILATION: Expanding an orifice or the lumen of a tubular body part

Body Part	Approach	Device	Qualifier
1 Esophagus, Upper 2 Esophagus, Middle 3 Esophagus, Lower 4 Esophagogastric Junction 5 Esophagus 6 Stomach 7 Stomach, Pylorus 8 Small Intestine 9 Duodenum A Jejunum B Ileum C Ileocecal Valve E Large Intestine F Large Intestine, Right G Large Intestine, Left H Cecum K Ascending Colon L Transverse Colon M Descending Colon N Sigmoid Colon P Rectum Q Anus	Ø Open 3 Percutaneous 4 Percutaneous Endoscopic 7 Via Natural or Artificial Opening 8 Via Natural or Artificial Opening Endoscopic	D Intraluminal Device Z No Device	Z No Qualifier

Non-OR ØD7[12345689ABCEFGHKLMNPQ][78][DZ]Z
Non-OR ØD77[478]DZ
Non-OR ØD778ZZ
Non-OR ØD7[89ABCEFGHKLMN][Ø34]DZ

SECTION: Ø MEDICAL AND SURGICAL
BODY SYSTEM: D GASTROINTESTINAL SYSTEM
OPERATION: 8 DIVISION: Cutting into a body part, without draining fluids and/or gases from the body part, in order to separate or transect a body part

Body Part	Approach	Device	Qualifier
4 Esophagogastric Junction 7 Stomach, Pylorus	Ø Open 3 Percutaneous 4 Percutaneous Endoscopic 7 Via Natural or Artificial Opening 8 Via Natural or Artificial Opening Endoscopic	Z No Device	Z No Qualifier
R Anal Sphincter	Ø Open 3 Percutaneous	Z No Device	Z No Qualifier

Coding Clinic: 2Ø17, Q3, P23-24 – ØD8[47]4ZZ
Coding Clinic: 2Ø19, Q2, P16 – ØD874ZZ

SECTION: Ø MEDICAL AND SURGICAL
BODY SYSTEM: D GASTROINTESTINAL SYSTEM
OPERATION: 9 DRAINAGE: *(on multiple pages)*
Taking or letting out fluids and/or gases from a body part

Body Part	Approach	Device	Qualifier
1 Esophagus, Upper 2 Esophagus, Middle 3 Esophagus, Lower 4 Esophagogastric Junction 5 Esophagus 6 Stomach 7 Stomach, Pylorus 8 Small Intestine 9 Duodenum A Jejunum B Ileum C Ileocecal Valve E Large Intestine F Large Intestine, Right G Large Intestine, Left H Cecum J Appendix K Ascending Colon L Transverse Colon M Descending Colon N Sigmoid Colon P Rectum	Ø Open 3 Percutaneous 4 Percutaneous Endoscopic 7 Via Natural or Artificial Opening 8 Via Natural or Artificial Opening Endoscopic	Ø Drainage Device	Z No Qualifier

DRG Non-OR ØD9[8ABC]3ØZ
DRG Non-OR ØD9[ABC]3ZZ
Non-OR ØD9[12345679EFGHJKLMNP]3ØZ
Non-OR ØD9[6789ABEFGHKLMNP][78]ØZ
Non-OR ØD9[123456789ABCEFGHKLMNP][3478]ZX
Non-OR ØD9[12345679EFGHJKLMNP]3ZZ

Coding Clinic: 2Ø15, Q2, P29 – ØD967ØZ
Coding Clinic: 2Ø24, Q1, P29 – ØD9Q7ØZ

SECTION: Ø MEDICAL AND SURGICAL

BODY SYSTEM: D GASTROINTESTINAL SYSTEM

OPERATION: 9 DRAINAGE: *(continued)*

Taking or letting out fluids and/or gases from a body part

Body Part	Approach	Device	Qualifier
1 Esophagus, Upper 2 Esophagus, Middle 3 Esophagus, Lower 4 Esophagogastric Junction 5 Esophagus 6 Stomach 7 Stomach, Pylorus 8 Small Intestine 9 Duodenum A Jejunum B Ileum C Ileocecal Valve E Large Intestine F Large Intestine, Right G Large Intestine, Left H Cecum J Appendix K Ascending Colon L Transverse Colon M Descending Colon N Sigmoid Colon P Rectum	Ø Open 3 Percutaneous 4 Percutaneous Endoscopic 7 Via Natural or Artificial Opening 8 Via Natural or Artificial Opening Endoscopic	Z No Device	X Diagnostic Z No Qualifier
Q Anus	Ø Open 3 Percutaneous 4 Percutaneous Endoscopic 7 Via Natural or Artificial Opening 8 Via Natural or Artificial Opening Endoscopic X External	Ø Drainage Device	Z No Qualifier
Q Anus	Ø Open 3 Percutaneous 4 Percutaneous Endoscopic 7 Via Natural or Artificial Opening 8 Via Natural or Artificial Opening Endoscopic X External	Z No Device	X Diagnostic Z No Qualifier
R Anal Sphincter U Omentum V Mesentery W Peritoneum	Ø Open 3 Percutaneous 4 Percutaneous Endoscopic	Ø Drainage Device	Z No Qualifier
R Anal Sphincter U Omentum V Mesentery W Peritoneum	Ø Open 3 Percutaneous 4 Percutaneous Endoscopic	Z No Device	X Diagnostic Z No Qualifier

DRG Non-OR ØD9[UVW]3ZX *(proposed)*
Non-OR ØD9Q3ØZ
Non-OR ØD9Q[Ø3478X]ZX
Non-OR ØD9Q3ZZ
Non-OR ØD9R3ØZ
Non-OR ØD9R3ZZ
Non-OR ØD9[UVW][34]ØZ
Non-OR ØD9R[Ø34]ZX
Non-OR ØD9[UVW][34]ZZ

SECTION: Ø MEDICAL AND SURGICAL
BODY SYSTEM: D GASTROINTESTINAL SYSTEM
OPERATION: B EXCISION: *(on multiple pages)*
Cutting out or off, without replacement, a portion of a body part

Body Part	Approach	Device	Qualifier
1 Esophagus, Upper 2 Esophagus, Middle 3 Esophagus, Lower 4 Esophagogastric Junction 5 Esophagus 7 Stomach, Pylorus 8 Small Intestine 9 Duodenum A Jejunum B Ileum C Ileocecal Valve E Large Intestine ~~F Large Intestine, Right~~ H Cecum ~~J Appendix~~ K Ascending Colon P Rectum	Ø Open 3 Percutaneous 4 Percutaneous Endoscopic 7 Via Natural or Artificial Opening 8 Via Natural or Artificial Opening Endoscopic	Z No Device	X Diagnostic Z No Qualifier
6 Stomach	Ø Open 3 Percutaneous 4 Percutaneous Endoscopic 7 Via Natural or Artificial Opening 8 Via Natural or Artificial Opening Endoscopic	Z No Device	3 Vertical X Diagnostic Z No Qualifier
F Large Intestine, Right J Appendix	Ø Open 3 Percutaneous 7 Via Natural or Artificial Opening 8 Via Natural or Artificial Opening Endoscopic	Z No Device	X Diagnostic Z No Qualifier
F Large Intestine, Right J Appendix	4 Percutaneous Endoscopic	Z No Device	G Hand-Assisted X Diagnostic Z No Qualifier
G Large Intestine, Left L Transverse Colon M Descending Colon N Sigmoid Colon	Ø Open 3 Percutaneous 7 Via Natural or Artificial Opening 8 Via Natural or Artificial Opening Endoscopic	Z No Device	X Diagnostic Z No Qualifier

Non-OR ØDB[12345789ABCEFHKP][3478]ZX
Non-OR ØDB[123579][48]ZZ
Non-OR ØDB[4EHKP]8ZZ
Non-OR ØDB6[3478]ZX
Non-OR ØDB6[48]ZZ
Non-OR ~~ØDB[GLMN][3478]ZX~~
Non-OR ~~ØDB[GLMN]8ZZ~~

Coding Clinic: 2016, Q1, P22 – 0DBP7ZZ
Coding Clinic: 2016, Q1, P24 – ØDB28ZX
Coding Clinic: 2016, Q2, P31 – ØDB64Z3
Coding Clinic: 2016, Q3, P5-7 – ØDBBØZZ
Coding Clinic: 2017, Q1, P16 – ØDBK8ZZ
Coding Clinic: 2017, Q2, P17 – ØDB6ØZZ
Coding Clinic: 2019, Q1, P5 – ØDB6[A]ØZZ
Coding Clinic: 2019, Q1, P6 – ØDB9ØZZ
Coding Clinic: 2019, Q1, P7 – ØDB6ØZZ
Coding Clinic: 2019, Q1, P27 – ØDBN[P]ØZZ
Coding Clinic: 2019, Q2, P16 – ØDBA4ZZ
Coding Clinic: 2021, Q2, P12 – ØDB8ØZZ
Coding Clinic: 2021, Q3, P29 – ØDBB4ZZ
Coding Clinic: 2023, Q1, P32 – ØDB18ZZ

SECTION: Ø MEDICAL AND SURGICAL
BODY SYSTEM: D GASTROINTESTINAL SYSTEM
OPERATION: B EXCISION: *(continued)* Cutting out or off, without replacement, a portion of a body part

Body Part	Approach	Device	Qualifier
G Large Intestine, Left L Transverse Colon M Descending Colon N Sigmoid Colon	4 Percutaneous Endoscopic	Z No Device	G Hand-Assisted X Diagnostic Z No Qualifier
~~G Large Intestine, Left~~ ~~L Transverse Colon~~ ~~M Descending Colon~~ ~~N Sigmoid Colon~~	~~Ø Open~~ ~~3 Percutaneous~~ ~~4 Percutaneous Endoscopic~~ ~~7 Via Natural or Artificial Opening~~ ~~8 Via Natural or Artificial Opening Endoscopic~~	~~Z No Device~~	~~X Diagnostic~~ ~~Z No Qualifier~~
G Large Intestine, Left L Transverse Colon M Descending Colon N Sigmoid Colon	F Via Natural or Artificial Opening With Percutaneous Endoscopic Assistance	Z No Device	Z No Qualifier
Q Anus	Ø Open 3 Percutaneous 4 Percutaneous Endoscopic 7 Via Natural or Artificial Opening 8 Via Natural or Artificial Opening Endoscopic X External	Z No Device	X Diagnostic Z No Qualifier
R Anal Sphincter U Omentum V Mesentery W Peritoneum	Ø Open 3 Percutaneous 4 Percutaneous Endoscopic	Z No Device	X Diagnostic Z No Qualifier

Non-OR ØDBQ[Ø3478X]ZX
Non-OR ØDBR[Ø34]ZX
Non-OR ØDB[UVW][34]ZX

Coding Clinic: 2Ø23, Q2, P24– ØDBQØZZ

SECTION: Ø MEDICAL AND SURGICAL
BODY SYSTEM: D GASTROINTESTINAL SYSTEM
OPERATION: C EXTIRPATION: Taking or cutting out solid matter from a body part

Body Part	Approach	Device	Qualifier
1 Esophagus, Upper 2 Esophagus, Middle 3 Esophagus, Lower 4 Esophagogastric Junction 5 Esophagus 6 Stomach 7 Stomach, Pylorus 8 Small Intestine 9 Duodenum A Jejunum B Ileum C Ileocecal Valve E Large Intestine F Large Intestine, Right G Large Intestine, Left H Cecum J Appendix K Ascending Colon L Transverse Colon M Descending Colon N Sigmoid Colon P Rectum	Ø Open 3 Percutaneous 4 Percutaneous Endoscopic 7 Via Natural or Artificial Opening 8 Via Natural or Artificial Opening Endoscopic	Z No Device	Z No Qualifier
Q Anus	Ø Open 3 Percutaneous 4 Percutaneous Endoscopic 7 Via Natural or Artificial Opening 8 Via Natural or Artificial Opening Endoscopic X External	Z No Device	Z No Qualifier
R Anal Sphincter U Omentum V Mesentery W Peritoneum	Ø Open 3 Percutaneous 4 Percutaneous Endoscopic	Z No Device	Z No Qualifier

Non-OR ØDC[123456789ABCEFGHKLMNP][78]ZZ
Non-OR ØDCQ[78X]ZZ

SECTION: Ø MEDICAL AND SURGICAL
BODY SYSTEM: D GASTROINTESTINAL SYSTEM
OPERATION: D EXTRACTION: Pulling or stripping out or off all or a portion of a body part by the use of force

Body Part	Approach	Device	Qualifier
1 Esophagus, Upper 2 Esophagus, Middle 3 Esophagus, Lower 4 Esophagogastric Junction 5 Esophagus 6 Stomach 7 Stomach, Pylorus 8 Small Intestine 9 Duodenum A Jejunum B Ileum C Ileocecal Valve E Large Intestine F Large Intestine, Right G Large Intestine, Left H Cecum J Appendix K Ascending Colon L Transverse Colon M Descending Colon N Sigmoid Colon P Rectum	3 Percutaneous 4 Percutaneous Endoscopic 8 Via Natural or Artificial Opening Endoscopic	Z No Device	X Diagnostic
Q Anus	3 Percutaneous 4 Percutaneous Endoscopic 8 Via Natural or Artificial Opening Endoscopic X External	Z No Device	X Diagnostic

Coding Clinic: 2Ø17, Q4, P42 – ØDD68ZX
Coding Clinic: 2Ø21, Q1, P21 – ØDDP8ZX

SECTION: Ø MEDICAL AND SURGICAL
BODY SYSTEM: D GASTROINTESTINAL SYSTEM
OPERATION: F FRAGMENTATION: Breaking solid matter in a body part into pieces

Body Part	Approach	Device	Qualifier
5 Esophagus 6 Stomach 8 Small Intestine 9 Duodenum A Jejunum B Ileum E Large Intestine F Large Intestine, Right G Large Intestine, Left H Cecum J Appendix K Ascending Colon L Transverse Colon M Descending Colon N Sigmoid Colon P Rectum Q Anus	Ø Open 3 Percutaneous 4 Percutaneous Endoscopic 7 Via Natural or Artificial Opening 8 Via Natural or Artificial Opening Endoscopic X External	Z No Device	Z No Qualifier

ØDF[5689ABEFGHJKLMNPQ]XZZ

Non-OR ØDF[5689ABEFGHJKLMNPQ]XZZ

SECTION: Ø MEDICAL AND SURGICAL
BODY SYSTEM: D GASTROINTESTINAL SYSTEM
OPERATION: H INSERTION: *(on multiple pages)*

Putting in a nonbiological appliance that monitors, assists, performs, or prevents a physiological function but does not physically take the place of a body part

Body Part	Approach	Device	Qualifier
Ø Upper Intestinal Tract D Lower Intestinal Tract	Ø Open 3 Percutaneous 4 Percutaneous Endoscopic 7 Via Natural or Artificial Opening 8 Via Natural or Artificial Opening Endoscopic	Y Other Device	Z No Qualifier
1 Esophagus, Upper 2 Esophagus, Middle 3 Esophagus, Lower	7 Via Natural or Artificial Opening	J Magnetic Lengthening Device	Z No Qualifier
5 Esophagus	Ø Open 3 Percutaneous 4 Percutaneous Endoscopic	1 Radioactive Element 2 Monitoring Device 3 Infusion Device D Intraluminal Device U Feeding Device Y Other Device	Z No Qualifier
5 Esophagus	7 Via Natural or Artificial Opening 8 Via Natural or Artificial Opening Endoscopic	1 Radioactive Element 2 Monitoring Device 3 Infusion Device B Airway D Intraluminal Device U Feeding Device Y Other Device	Z No Qualifier
6 Stomach ⊞	Ø Open 3 Percutaneous 4 Percutaneous Endoscopic	1 Radioactive Element 2 Monitoring Device 3 Infusion Device D Intraluminal Device M Stimulator Lead U Feeding Device Y Other Device	Z No Qualifier
6 Stomach	7 Via Natural or Artificial Opening 8 Via Natural or Artificial Opening Endoscopic	1 Radioactive Element 2 Monitoring Device 3 Infusion Device D Intraluminal Device U Feeding Device Y Other Device	Z No Qualifier
8 Small Intestine 9 Duodenum A Jejunum B Ileum	Ø Open 3 Percutaneous 4 Percutaneous Endoscopic 7 Via Natural or Artificial Opening 8 Via Natural or Artificial Opening Endoscopic	1 Radioactive Element 2 Monitoring Device 3 Infusion Device D Intraluminal Device U Feeding Device	Z No Qualifier
E Large Intestine P Rectum	Ø Open 3 Percutaneous 4 Percutaneous Endoscopic 7 Via Natural or Artificial Opening 8 Via Natural or Artificial Opening Endoscopic	1 Radioactive Element D Intraluminal Device	Z No Qualifier

⊞ ØDH6[Ø34][1M]Z
Non-OR ØDH5[Ø34][DU]Z
Non-OR ØDH5[78][23BDU]Z
Non-OR ØDH6[34]UZ
Non-OR ØDH6[78][23U]Z

Non-OR ØDH[89AB][Ø3478][DU]Z
Non-OR ØDH[89AB][78][23]Z
Non-OR ØDHE[Ø3478]DZ
Non-OR ØDHP[Ø3478]DZ

Coding Clinic: 2Ø16, Q26, P5 – ØDH67UZ
Coding Clinic: 2Ø19, Q2, P18 – ØDHØ8YZ
Coding Clinic: 2Ø22, Q1, P44 – ØDHØ8YZ
Coding Clinic: 2Ø23, Q3, P7 – ØDH5ØYZ

SECTION: Ø MEDICAL AND SURGICAL
BODY SYSTEM: D GASTROINTESTINAL SYSTEM
OPERATION: H INSERTION: *(continued)*

Putting in a nonbiological appliance that monitors, assists, performs, or prevents a physiological function but does not physically take the place of a body part

Body Part	Approach	Device	Qualifier
P Rectum	Ø Open 3 Percutaneous 4 Percutaneous Endoscopic 7 Via Natural or Artificial Opening 8 Via Natural or Artificial Opening Endoscopic	1 Radioactive Element D Intraluminal Device	Z No Qualifier
Q Anus	Ø Open 3 Percutaneous 4 Percutaneous Endoscopic	D Intraluminal Device L Artificial Sphincter	Z No Qualifier
Q Anus	7 Via Natural or Artificial Opening 8 Via Natural or Artificial Opening Endoscopic	D Intraluminal Device	Z No Qualifier
R Anal Sphincter	Ø Open 3 Percutaneous 4 Percutaneous Endoscopic	M Stimulator Lead	Z No Qualifier

SECTION: Ø MEDICAL AND SURGICAL
BODY SYSTEM: D GASTROINTESTINAL SYSTEM
OPERATION: J INSPECTION: Visually and/or manually exploring a body part

Body Part	Approach	Device	Qualifier
Ø Upper Intestinal Tract 6 Stomach D Lower Intestinal Tract	Ø Open 3 Percutaneous 4 Percutaneous Endoscopic 7 Via Natural or Artificial Opening 8 Via Natural or Artificial Opening Endoscopic X External	Z No Device	Z No Qualifier
U Omentum V Mesentery W Peritoneum	Ø Open 3 Percutaneous 4 Percutaneous Endoscopic X External	Z No Device	Z No Qualifier

DRG Non-OR ØDJ[UVW]3ZZ
Non-OR ØDJ[Ø6D][378X]ZZ
Non-OR ØDJ[UVW]XZZ

Coding Clinic: 2015, Q3, P25 – ØDJØ8ZZ
Coding Clinic: 2016, Q2, P21 – ØDJØ7ZZ
Coding Clinic: 2017, Q2, P15 – ØDJD8ZZ
Coding Clinic: 2019, Q1, P26 – ØDJDØZZ

SECTION: Ø MEDICAL AND SURGICAL
BODY SYSTEM: D GASTROINTESTINAL SYSTEM
OPERATION: L OCCLUSION: Completely closing an orifice or the lumen of a tubular body part

Body Part	Approach	Device	Qualifier
1 Esophagus, Upper 2 Esophagus, Middle 3 Esophagus, Lower 4 Esophagogastric Junction 5 Esophagus 6 Stomach 7 Stomach, Pylorus 8 Small Intestine 9 Duodenum A Jejunum B Ileum C Ileocecal Valve E Large Intestine F Large Intestine, Right G Large Intestine, Left H Cecum K Ascending Colon L Transverse Colon M Descending Colon N Sigmoid Colon P Rectum	Ø Open 3 Percutaneous 4 Percutaneous Endoscopic	C Extraluminal Device D Intraluminal Device Z No Device	Z No Qualifier
1 Esophagus, Upper 2 Esophagus, Middle 3 Esophagus, Lower 4 Esophagogastric Junction 5 Esophagus 6 Stomach 7 Stomach, Pylorus 8 Small Intestine 9 Duodenum A Jejunum B Ileum C Ileocecal Valve E Large Intestine F Large Intestine, Right G Large Intestine, Left H Cecum K Ascending Colon L Transverse Colon M Descending Colon N Sigmoid Colon P Rectum	7 Via Natural or Artificial Opening 8 Via Natural or Artificial Opening Endoscopic	D Intraluminal Device Z No Device	Z No Qualifier
Q Anus	Ø Open 3 Percutaneous 4 Percutaneous Endoscopic X External	C Extraluminal Device D Intraluminal Device Z No Device	Z No Qualifier
Q Anus	7 Via Natural or Artificial Opening 8 Via Natural or Artificial Opening Endoscopic	D Intraluminal Device Z No Device	Z No Qualifier

Non-OR ØDL[12345][Ø34][CDZ]Z
Non-OR ØDL[12345][78][DZ]Z

SECTION: Ø MEDICAL AND SURGICAL
BODY SYSTEM: D GASTROINTESTINAL SYSTEM
OPERATION: M REATTACHMENT: Putting back in or on all or a portion of a separated body part to its normal location or other suitable location

Body Part	Approach	Device	Qualifier
5 Esophagus 6 Stomach 8 Small Intestine 9 Duodenum A Jejunum B Ileum E Large Intestine F Large Intestine, Right G Large Intestine, Left H Cecum K Ascending Colon L Transverse Colon M Descending Colon N Sigmoid Colon P Rectum	Ø Open 4 Percutaneous Endoscopic	Z No Device	Z No Qualifier

SECTION: Ø MEDICAL AND SURGICAL
BODY SYSTEM: D GASTROINTESTINAL SYSTEM
OPERATION: N RELEASE: Freeing a body part from an abnormal physical constraint by cutting or by the use of force

Body Part	Approach	Device	Qualifier
1 Esophagus, Upper 2 Esophagus, Middle 3 Esophagus, Lower 4 Esophagogastric Junction 5 Esophagus 6 Stomach 7 Stomach, Pylorus 8 Small Intestine 9 Duodenum A Jejunum B Ileum C Ileocecal Valve E Large Intestine F Large Intestine, Right G Large Intestine, Left H Cecum J Appendix K Ascending Colon L Transverse Colon M Descending Colon N Sigmoid Colon P Rectum	Ø Open 3 Percutaneous 4 Percutaneous Endoscopic 7 Via Natural or Artificial Opening 8 Via Natural or Artificial Opening Endoscopic	Z No Device	Z No Qualifier
Q Anus	Ø Open 3 Percutaneous 4 Percutaneous Endoscopic 7 Via Natural or Artificial Opening 8 Via Natural or Artificial Opening Endoscopic X External	Z No Device	Z No Qualifier
R Anal Sphincter U Omentum V Mesentery W Peritoneum	Ø Open 3 Percutaneous 4 Percutaneous Endoscopic	Z No Device	Z No Qualifier

Non-OR ØDN[89ABEFGHKLMN][78]ZZ

Coding Clinic: 2Ø15, Q3, P15-16 – ØDN5ØZZ
Coding Clinic: 2Ø17, Q1, P35 – ØDNWØZZ
Coding Clinic: 2Ø17, Q4, P5Ø – ØDN8ØZZ

SECTION: Ø MEDICAL AND SURGICAL

BODY SYSTEM: D GASTROINTESTINAL SYSTEM

OPERATION: P REMOVAL: *(on multiple pages)*

Taking out or off a device from a body part

Body Part	Approach	Device	Qualifier
Ø Upper Intestinal Tract D Lower Intestinal Tract	Ø Open 3 Percutaneous 4 Percutaneous Endoscopic 7 Via Natural or Artificial Opening 8 Via Natural or Artificial Opening Endoscopic	Ø Drainage Device 2 Monitoring Device 3 Infusion Device 7 Autologous Tissue Substitute C Extraluminal Device D Intraluminal Device J Synthetic Substitute K Nonautologous Tissue Substitute U Feeding Device Y Other Device	Z No Qualifier
Ø Upper Intestinal Tract D Lower Intestinal Tract	X External	Ø Drainage Device 2 Monitoring Device 3 Infusion Device D Intraluminal Device U Feeding Device	Z No Qualifier
5 Esophagus	Ø Open 3 Percutaneous 4 Percutaneous Endoscopic	1 Radioactive Element 2 Monitoring Device 3 Infusion Device U Feeding Device Y Other Device	Z No Qualifier
5 Esophagus	7 Via Natural or Artificial Opening 8 Via Natural or Artificial Opening Endoscopic	1 Radioactive Element D Intraluminal Device Y Other Device	Z No Qualifier
5 Esophagus	X External	1 Radioactive Element 2 Monitoring Device 3 Infusion Device D Intraluminal Device U Feeding Device	Z No Qualifier
6 Stomach	Ø Open 3 Percutaneous 4 Percutaneous Endoscopic	Ø Drainage Device 2 Monitoring Device 3 Infusion Device 7 Autologous Tissue Substitute C Extraluminal Device D Intraluminal Device J Synthetic Substitute K Nonautologous Tissue Substitute M Stimulator Lead U Feeding Device Y Other Device	Z No Qualifier

Non-OR ØDP[ØD][78][Ø23D]Z
Non-OR ØDP[ØD]X[Ø23DU]Z
Non-OR ØDP5[78][1D]Z
Non-OR ØDP5X[123DU]Z

SECTION: Ø MEDICAL AND SURGICAL
BODY SYSTEM: D GASTROINTESTINAL SYSTEM
OPERATION: P REMOVAL: *(continued)*
Taking out or off a device from a body part

Body Part	Approach	Device	Qualifier
6 Stomach	7 Via Natural or Artificial Opening 8 Via Natural or Artificial Opening Endoscopic	Ø Drainage Device 2 Monitoring Device 3 Infusion Device 7 Autologous Tissue Substitute C Extraluminal Device D Intraluminal Device J Synthetic Substitute K Nonautologous Tissue Substitute U Feeding Device Y Other Device	Z No Qualifier
6 Stomach	X External	Ø Drainage Device 2 Monitoring Device 3 Infusion Device D Intraluminal Device U Feeding Device	Z No Qualifier
P Rectum	Ø Open 3 Percutaneous 4 Percutaneous Endoscopic 7 Via Natural or Artificial Opening 8 Via Natural or Artificial Opening Endoscopic X External	1 Radioactive Element	Z No Qualifier
Q Anus	Ø Open 3 Percutaneous 4 Percutaneous Endoscopic 7 Via Natural or Artificial Opening 8 Via Natural or Artificial Opening Endoscopic	L Artificial Sphincter	Z No Qualifier
R Anal Sphincter	Ø Open 3 Percutaneous 4 Percutaneous Endoscopic	M Stimulator Lead	Z No Qualifier
U Omentum V Mesentery W Peritoneum	Ø Open 3 Percutaneous 4 Percutaneous Endoscopic	Ø Drainage Device 1 Radioactive Element 7 Autologous Tissue Substitute J Synthetic Substitute K Nonautologous Tissue Substitute	Z No Qualifier

Non-OR ØDP6[78][Ø23D]Z
Non-OR ØDP6X[Ø23DU]Z
Non-OR ØDPP[78X]1Z

Coding Clinic: 2Ø19, Q2, P19 – ØDP68YZ

SECTION: Ø MEDICAL AND SURGICAL
BODY SYSTEM: D GASTROINTESTINAL SYSTEM
OPERATION: Q REPAIR: Restoring, to the extent possible, a body part to its normal anatomic structure and function

Body Part	Approach	Device	Qualifier
1 Esophagus, Upper 2 Esophagus, Middle 3 Esophagus, Lower 4 Esophagogastric Junction 5 Esophagus 6 Stomach 7 Stomach, Pylorus 8 Small Intestine ⊞ 9 Duodenum ⊞ A Jejunum ⊞ B Ileum ⊞ C Ileocecal Valve E Large Intestine ⊞ F Large Intestine, Right ⊞ G Large Intestine, Left ⊞ H Cecum ⊞ J Appendix K Ascending Colon ⊞ L Transverse Colon ⊞ M Descending Colon ⊞ N Sigmoid Colon ⊞ P Rectum	Ø Open 3 Percutaneous 4 Percutaneous Endoscopic 7 Via Natural or Artificial Opening 8 Via Natural or Artificial Opening Endoscopic	Z No Device	Z No Qualifier
Q Anus	Ø Open 3 Percutaneous 4 Percutaneous Endoscopic 7 Via Natural or Artificial Opening 8 Via Natural or Artificial Opening Endoscopic X External	Z No Device	Z No Qualifier
R Anal Sphincter U Omentum V Mesentery W Peritoneum	Ø Open 3 Percutaneous 4 Percutaneous Endoscopic	Z No Device	Z No Qualifier

⊞ ØDQ[89ABEFGHKLMN]ØZZ
⊞ ØDQW[Ø34]ZZ

Coding Clinic: 2Ø16, Q1, P7-8 – ØDQRØZZ, ØDQPØZZ
Coding Clinic: 2Ø18, Q1, P11 – ØDQV4ZZ
Coding Clinic: 2Ø19, Q2, P16 – ØDQ64ZZ
Coding Clinic: 2Ø24, Q1, P29 – ØDQ6ØZZ

SECTION: Ø MEDICAL AND SURGICAL
BODY SYSTEM: D GASTROINTESTINAL SYSTEM
OPERATION: R REPLACEMENT: Putting in or on biological or synthetic material that physically takes the place and/or function of all or a portion of a body part

Body Part	Approach	Device	Qualifier
5 Esophagus	Ø Open 4 Percutaneous Endoscopic 7 Via Natural or Artificial Opening 8 Via Natural or Artificial Opening Endoscopic	7 Autologous Tissue Substitute J Synthetic Substitute K Nonautologous Tissue Substitute	Z No Qualifier
R Anal Sphincter U Omentum V Mesentery W Peritoneum	Ø Open 4 Percutaneous Endoscopic	7 Autologous Tissue Substitute J Synthetic Substitute K Nonautologous Tissue Substitute	Z No Qualifier

SECTION: Ø MEDICAL AND SURGICAL
BODY SYSTEM: D GASTROINTESTINAL SYSTEM
OPERATION: S REPOSITION: Moving to its normal location, or other suitable location, all or a portion of a body part

Body Part	Approach	Device	Qualifier
5 Esophagus 6 Stomach 9 Duodenum A Jejunum B Ileum H Cecum K Ascending Colon L Transverse Colon M Descending Colon N Sigmoid Colon P Rectum Q Anus	Ø Open 4 Percutaneous Endoscopic 7 Via Natural or Artificial Opening 8 Via Natural or Artificial Opening Endoscopic X External	Z No Device	Z No Qualifier
8 Small Intestine E Large Intestine	Ø Open 4 Percutaneous Endoscopic 7 Via Natural or Artificial Opening 8 Via Natural or Artificial Opening Endoscopic	Z No Device	Z No Qualifier

Non-OR ØDS[69ABHKLMNP]XZZ

Coding Clinic: 2016, Q3, P5 – ØDSM4ZZ
Coding Clinic: 2017, Q3, P1Ø – ØDS[BK]7ZZ
Coding Clinic: 2019, Q1, P31; 2017, Q3, P18 – ØDSPØZZ
Coding Clinic: 2017, Q4, P5Ø – ØDS[8E]ØZZ

SECTION: Ø MEDICAL AND SURGICAL
BODY SYSTEM: D GASTROINTESTINAL SYSTEM
OPERATION: T RESECTION: Cutting out or off, without replacement, all of a body part

Body Part	Approach	Device	Qualifier
1 Esophagus, Upper 2 Esophagus, Middle 3 Esophagus, Lower 4 Esophagogastric Junction 5 Esophagus 6 Stomach 7 Stomach, Pylorus 8 Small Intestine 9 Duodenum ⊞ A Jejunum B Ileum C Ileocecal Valve E Large Intestine ~~F Large Intestine, Right~~ H Cecum ~~J Appendix~~ K Ascending Colon P Rectum Q Anus	Ø Open 4 Percutaneous Endoscopic 7 Via Natural or Artificial Opening 8 Via Natural or Artificial Opening Endoscopic	Z No Device	Z No Qualifier
~~G Large Intestine, Left~~ ~~L Transverse Colon~~ ~~M Descending Colon~~ ~~N Sigmoid Colon~~	~~Ø Open~~ ~~4 Percutaneous Endoscopic~~ ~~7 Via Natural or Artificial Opening~~ ~~8 Via Natural or Artificial Opening Endoscopic~~ ~~F Via Natural or Artificial Opening With Percutaneous Endoscopic Assistance~~	~~Z No Device~~	~~Z No Qualifier~~
F Large Intestine, Right J Appendix	Ø Open 7 Via Natural or Artificial Opening 8 Via Natural or Artificial Opening Endoscopic	Z No Device	Z No Qualifier
F Large Intestine, Right J Appendix	4 Percutaneous Endoscopic	Z No Device	G Hand-Assisted Z No Qualifier
G Large Intestine, Left L Transverse Colon M Descending Colon N Sigmoid Colon	Ø Open 7 Via Natural or Artificial Opening 8 Via Natural or Artificial Opening Endoscopic	Z No Device	Z No Qualifier
G Large Intestine, Left L Transverse Colon M Descending Colon N Sigmoid Colon	4 Percutaneous Endoscopic	Z No Device	G Hand-Assisted Z No Qualifier
R Anal Sphincter U Omentum	Ø Open 4 Percutaneous Endoscopic	Z No Device	Z No Qualifier

⊞ ØDT9ØZZ

Coding Clinic: 2Ø17, Q4, P5Ø – ØDTJØZZ
Coding Clinic: 2Ø19, Q1, P5, 7 – ØDT9ØZZ
Coding Clinic: 2Ø19, Q1, P15 – ØDT3ØZZ

SECTION: Ø MEDICAL AND SURGICAL
BODY SYSTEM: D GASTROINTESTINAL SYSTEM
OPERATION: U SUPPLEMENT: Putting in or on biological or synthetic material that physically reinforces and/or augments the function of a portion of a body part

Body Part	Approach	Device	Qualifier
1 Esophagus, Upper 2 Esophagus, Middle 3 Esophagus, Lower 4 Esophagogastric Junction 5 Esophagus 6 Stomach 7 Stomach, Pylorus 8 Small Intestine 9 Duodenum A Jejunum B Ileum C Ileocecal Valve E Large Intestine F Large Intestine, Right G Large Intestine, Left H Cecum K Ascending Colon L Transverse Colon M Descending Colon N Sigmoid Colon P Rectum	Ø Open 4 Percutaneous Endoscopic 7 Via Natural or Artificial Opening 8 Via Natural or Artificial Opening Endoscopic	7 Autologous Tissue Substitute J Synthetic Substitute K Nonautologous Tissue Substitute	Z No Qualifier
Q Anus	Ø Open 4 Percutaneous Endoscopic 7 Via Natural or Artificial Opening 8 Via Natural or Artificial Opening Endoscopic X External	7 Autologous Tissue Substitute J Synthetic Substitute K Nonautologous Tissue Substitute	Z No Qualifier
R Anal Sphincter U Omentum V Mesentery W Peritoneum	Ø Open 4 Percutaneous Endoscopic	7 Autologous Tissue Substitute J Synthetic Substitute K Nonautologous Tissue Substitute	Z No Qualifier

Coding Clinic: 2Ø19, Q1, P31 – ØDUPØJZ
Coding Clinic: 2Ø21, Q2, P21 – ØDUEØ7Z

SECTION: Ø MEDICAL AND SURGICAL
BODY SYSTEM: D GASTROINTESTINAL SYSTEM
OPERATION: V RESTRICTION: Partially closing an orifice or the lumen of a tubular body part

Body Part	Approach	Device	Qualifier
1 Esophagus, Upper 2 Esophagus, Middle 3 Esophagus, Lower 4 Esophagogastric Junction 5 Esophagus 6 Stomach 7 Stomach, Pylorus 8 Small Intestine 9 Duodenum A Jejunum B Ileum C Ileocecal Valve E Large Intestine F Large Intestine, Right G Large Intestine, Left H Cecum K Ascending Colon L Transverse Colon M Descending Colon N Sigmoid Colon P Rectum	Ø Open 3 Percutaneous 4 Percutaneous Endoscopic	C Extraluminal Device D Intraluminal Device Z No Device	Z No Qualifier
1 Esophagus, Upper 2 Esophagus, Middle 3 Esophagus, Lower 4 Esophagogastric Junction 5 Esophagus 6 Stomach 7 Stomach, Pylorus 8 Small Intestine 9 Duodenum A Jejunum B Ileum C Ileocecal Valve E Large Intestine F Large Intestine, Right G Large Intestine, Left H Cecum K Ascending Colon L Colon M Descending Colon N Sigmoid Colon P Rectum	7 Via Natural or Artificial Opening 8 Via Natural or Artificial Opening Endoscopic	D Intraluminal Device Z No Device	Z No Qualifier
Q Anus	Ø Open 3 Percutaneous 4 Percutaneous Endoscopic X External	C Extraluminal Device D Intraluminal Device Z No Device	Z No Qualifier
Q Anus	7 Via Natural or Artificial Opening 8 Via Natural or Artificial Opening Endoscopic	D Intraluminal Device Z No Device	Z No Qualifier

ØDV6[78]DZ

Non-OR ØDV6[78]DZ

ØDV64CZ when reported with Principal Diagnosis E66.Ø1 and Secondary Diagnosis K68.11, K95.Ø1, K95.81, or T81.4XXA

Coding Clinic: 2Ø16, Q2, P23 – ØDV4ØZZ **Coding Clinic: 2Ø17, Q3, P23 – ØDV44ZZ**

New/Revised Text in Green ~~deleted~~ Deleted ♀ Females Only ♂ Males Only Coding Clinic
Non-covered Limited Coverage Combination (See Appendix E) DRG Non-OR Non-OR Hospital-Acquired Condition

SECTION: Ø MEDICAL AND SURGICAL
BODY SYSTEM: D GASTROINTESTINAL SYSTEM
OPERATION: W REVISION: *(on multiple pages)*

Correcting, to the extent possible, a portion of a malfunctioning device or the position of a displaced device

Body Part	Approach	Device	Qualifier
Ø Upper Intestinal Tract D Lower Intestinal Tract	Ø Open 3 Percutaneous 4 Percutaneous Endoscopic 7 Via Natural or Artificial Opening 8 Via Natural or Artificial Opening Endoscopic	Ø Drainage Device 2 Monitoring Device 3 Infusion Device 7 Autologous Tissue Substitute C Extraluminal Device D Intraluminal Device J Synthetic Substitute K Nonautologous Tissue Substitute U Feeding Device Y Other Device	Z No Qualifier
Ø Upper Intestinal Tract D Lower Intestinal Tract	X External	Ø Drainage Device 2 Monitoring Device 3 Infusion Device 7 Autologous Tissue Substitute C Extraluminal Device D Intraluminal Device J Synthetic Substitute K Nonautologous Tissue Substitute U Feeding Device	Z No Qualifier
5 Esophagus	Ø Open 3 Percutaneous 4 Percutaneous Endoscopic	Y Other Device	Z No Qualifier
5 Esophagus	7 Via Natural or Artificial Opening 8 Via Natural or Artificial Opening Endoscopic	D Intraluminal Device Y Other Device	Z No Qualifier
5 Esophagus	X External	D Intraluminal Device	Z No Qualifier
6 Stomach	Ø Open 3 Percutaneous 4 Percutaneous Endoscopic	Ø Drainage Device 2 Monitoring Device 3 Infusion Device 7 Autologous Tissue Substitute C Extraluminal Device D Intraluminal Device J Synthetic Substitute K Nonautologous Tissue Substitute M Stimulator Lead U Feeding Device Y Other Device	Z No Qualifier
6 Stomach	7 Via Natural or Artificial Opening 8 Via Natural or Artificial Opening Endoscopic	Ø Drainage Device 2 Monitoring Device 3 Infusion Device 7 Autologous Tissue Substitute C Extraluminal Device D Intraluminal Device J Synthetic Substitute K Nonautologous Tissue Substitute U Feeding Device Y Other Device	Z No Qualifier

Non-OR ØDW[ØD]X[Ø237CDJKU]Z
Non-OR ØDW5XDZ
Non-OR ØDW6X[Ø237CDJKU]Z
Non-OR ØDW[UVW][Ø34]ØZ

Coding Clinic: 2018, Q1, P2Ø – ØDW63CZ

SECTION: Ø MEDICAL AND SURGICAL
BODY SYSTEM: D GASTROINTESTINAL SYSTEM
OPERATION: W REVISION: *(continued)*

Correcting, to the extent possible, a portion of a malfunctioning device or the position of a displaced device

Body Part	Approach	Device	Qualifier
6 Stomach	X External	Ø Drainage Device 2 Monitoring Device 3 Infusion Device 7 Autologous Tissue Substitute C Extraluminal Device D Intraluminal Device J Synthetic Substitute K Nonautologous Tissue Substitute U Feeding Device	Z No Qualifier
8 Small Intestine E Large Intestine	Ø Open 4 Percutaneous Endoscopic 7 Via Natural or Artificial Opening 8 Via Natural or Artificial Opening Endoscopic	7 Autologous Tissue Substitute J Synthetic Substitute K Nonautologous Tissue Substitute	Z No Qualifier
Q Anus	Ø Open 3 Percutaneous 4 Percutaneous Endoscopic 7 Via Natural or Artificial Opening 8 Via Natural or Artificial Opening Endoscopic	L Artificial Sphincter	Z No Qualifier
R Anal Sphincter	Ø Open 3 Percutaneous 4 Percutaneous Endoscopic	M Stimulator Lead	Z No Qualifier
U Omentum V Mesentery W Peritoneum	Ø Open 3 Percutaneous 4 Percutaneous Endoscopic	Ø Drainage Device 7 Autologous Tissue Substitute J Synthetic Substitute K Nonautologous Tissue Substitute	Z No Qualifier

Coding Clinic: 2Ø21, Q1, P2Ø – ØDW8Ø7Z

SECTION: Ø MEDICAL AND SURGICAL
BODY SYSTEM: D GASTROINTESTINAL SYSTEM
OPERATION: X TRANSFER: Moving, without taking out, all or a portion of a body part to another location to take over the function of all or a portion of a body part

Body Part	Approach	Device	Qualifier
6 Stomach	Ø Open 4 Percutaneous Endoscopic	Z No Device	5 Esophagus
8 Small Intestine	Ø Open 4 Percutaneous Endoscopic	Z No Device	5 Esophagus B Bladder C Ureter, Right D Ureter, Left F Ureters, Bilateral
E Large Intestine	Ø Open 4 Percutaneous Endoscopic	Z No Device	5 Esophagus 7 Vagina B Bladder
U Omentum	Ø Open 4 Percutaneous Endoscopic	Z No Device	V Thoracic Region W Abdominal Region X Pelvic Region Y Inguinal Region

Coding Clinic: 2017, Q2, P18; 2016, Q2, P24 – ØDX6ØZ5
Coding Clinic: 2019, Q1, P15 – ØDXEØZ5
Coding Clinic: 2019, Q4, P3Ø – ØDXEØZ7A
Coding Clinic: 2022, Q4, P57 – ØDX8ØZB

SECTION: Ø MEDICAL AND SURGICAL
BODY SYSTEM: D GASTROINTESTINAL SYSTEM
OPERATION: Y TRANSPLANTATION: Putting in or on all or a portion of a living body part taken from another individual or animal to physically take the place and/or function of all or a portion of a similar body part

Body Part	Approach	Device	Qualifier
5 Esophagus 6 Stomach 8 Small Intestine E Large Intestine	Ø Open	Z No Device	0 Allogeneic 1 Syngeneic 2 Zooplastic

ØDY[8E]ØZ[Ø12]
Non-OR ØDY5ØZ[Ø12]

ØF

ØF. Hepatobiliary System and Pancreas 268
ØF1. Bypass 269
ØF2. Change 269
ØF5. Destruction 27Ø
ØF7. Dilation 271
ØF8. Division 271
ØF9. Drainage 272
ØFB. Excision 273
ØFC. Extirpation 273
ØFD. Extraction 274
ØFF. Fragmentation 275
ØFH. Insertion 275
ØFJ. Inspection 276
ØFL. Occlusion 276
ØFM. Reattachment 277
ØFN. Release 277
ØFP. Removal 278
ØFQ. Repair 279
ØFR. Replacement 279
ØFS. Reposition 28Ø
ØFT. Resection 28Ø
ØFU. Supplement 281
ØFV. Restriction 281
ØFW. Revision 282
ØFY. Transplantation 283

SECTION: Ø MEDICAL AND SURGICAL
BODY SYSTEM: F HEPATOBILIARY SYSTEM AND PANCREAS
OPERATION: 1 BYPASS: Altering the route of passage of the contents of a tubular body part

Body Part	Approach	Device	Qualifier
4 Gallbladder 5 Hepatic Duct, Right 6 Hepatic Duct, Left 7 Hepatic Duct, Common 8 Cystic Duct 9 Common Bile Duct	Ø Open 4 Percutaneous Endoscopic	D Intraluminal Device Z No Device	3 Duodenum 4 Stomach 5 Hepatic Duct, Right 6 Hepatic Duct, Left 7 Hepatic Duct, Caudate 8 Cystic Duct 9 Common Bile Duct B Small Intestine
D Pancreatic Duct F Pancreatic Duct, Accessory G Pancreas	Ø Open 4 Percutaneous Endoscopic	D Intraluminal Device Z No Device	3 Duodenum B Small Intestine C Large Intestine
D Pancreatic Duct	Ø Open 4 Percutaneous Endoscopic	D Intraluminal Device Z No Device	3 Duodenum 4 Stomach B Small Intestine C Large Intestine
D Pancreatic Duct	Ø Open 4 Percutaneous Endoscopic	D Intraluminal Device Z No Device	3 Duodenum 4 Stomach B Small Intestine C Large Intestine
D Pancreatic Duct, Accessory G Pancreas	Ø Open 4 Percutaneous Endoscopic	D Intraluminal Device Z No Device	3 Duodenum B Small Intestine C Large Intestine

SECTION: Ø MEDICAL AND SURGICAL
BODY SYSTEM: F HEPATOBILIARY SYSTEM AND PANCREAS
OPERATION: 2 CHANGE: Taking out or off a device from a body part and putting back an identical or similar device in or on the same body part without cutting or puncturing the skin or a mucous membrane

Body Part	Approach	Device	Qualifier
Ø Liver 4 Gallbladder B Hepatobiliary Duct D Pancreatic Duct G Pancreas	X External	Ø Drainage Device Y Other Device	Z No Qualifier

Non-OR All Values

SECTION: Ø MEDICAL AND SURGICAL
BODY SYSTEM: F HEPATOBILIARY SYSTEM AND PANCREAS
OPERATION: 5 DESTRUCTION: Physical eradication of all or a portion of a body part by the direct use of energy, force, or a destructive agent

Body Part	Approach	Device	Qualifier
Ø Liver 1 Liver, Right Lobe 2 Liver, Left Lobe	Ø Open 3 Percutaneous 4 Percutaneous Endoscopic	Z No Device	3 Laser Interstitial Thermal Therapy F Irreversible Electroporation Z No Qualifier
4 Gallbladder	Ø Open 3 Percutaneous 4 Percutaneous Endoscopic	Z No Device	3 Laser Interstitial Thermal Therapy Z No Qualifier
4 Gallbladder	8 Via Natural or Artificial Opening Endoscopic	Z No Device	Z No Qualifier
5 Hepatic Duct, Right 6 Hepatic Duct, Left 7 Hepatic Duct, Common 8 Cystic Duct 9 Common Bile Duct C Ampulla of Vater D Pancreatic Duct F Pancreatic Duct, Accessory	Ø Open 3 Percutaneous 4 Percutaneous Endoscopic	Z No Device	3 Laser Interstitial Thermal Therapy Z No Qualifier
5 Hepatic Duct, Right 6 Hepatic Duct, Left 7 Hepatic Duct, Common 8 Cystic Duct 9 Common Bile Duct C Ampulla of Vater D Pancreatic Duct F Pancreatic Duct, Accessory	7 Via Natural or Artificial Opening 8 Via Natural or Artificial Opening Endoscopic	Z No Device	Z No Qualifier
G Pancreas	Ø Open 3 Percutaneous 4 Percutaneous Endoscopic	Z No Device	3 Laser Interstitial Thermal Therapy F Irreversible Electroporation Z No Qualifier
G Pancreas	8 Via Natural or Artificial Opening Endoscopic	Z No Device	Z No Qualifier

Non-OR ØF5G4ZZ
Non-OR ØF5[5689CDF][48]ZZ
Non-OR ØF5[56789CDFG]4Z3
Non-OR ØF5[Ø12345679CDFG][Ø34]Z3

Coding Clinic: 2Ø18, Q4, P4Ø – ØF5G4ZF

SECTION: Ø MEDICAL AND SURGICAL
BODY SYSTEM: F HEPATOBILIARY SYSTEM AND PANCREAS
OPERATION: 7 DILATION: Expanding an orifice or the lumen of a tubular body part

Body Part	Approach	Device	Qualifier
5 Hepatic Duct, Right 6 Hepatic Duct, Left 7 Hepatic Duct, Common 8 Cystic Duct 9 Common Bile Duct C Ampulla of Vater D Pancreatic Duct F Pancreatic Duct, Accessory	Ø Open 3 Percutaneous 4 Percutaneous Endoscopic 7 Via Natural or Artificial Opening 8 Via Natural or Artificial Opening Endoscopic	D Intraluminal Device Z No Device	Z No Qualifier

Non-OR ØF7[5689][34][DZ]Z
Non-OR ØF7[5689D][78]DZ
Non-OR ØF7[CF]8DZ
Non-OR ØF7[DF]4[DZ]Z
Non-OR ØF7[5689CDF]8ZZ

Coding Clinic: 2016, Q1, P25 – ØF798DZ, ØF7D8DZ
Coding Clinic: 2016, Q3, P28 – ØF7D8DZ

SECTION: Ø MEDICAL AND SURGICAL
BODY SYSTEM: F HEPATOBILIARY SYSTEM AND PANCREAS
OPERATION: 8 DIVISION: Cutting into a body part, without draining fluids and/or gases from the body part, in order to separate or transect a body part

Body Part	Approach	Device	Qualifier
Ø Liver 1 Liver, Right Lobe 2 Liver, Left Lobe G Pancreas	Ø Open 3 Percutaneous 4 Percutaneous Endoscopic	Z No Device	Z No Qualifier

Coding Clinic: 2021, Q4, P49 – ØF824ZZ

SECTION: Ø MEDICAL AND SURGICAL
BODY SYSTEM: F HEPATOBILIARY SYSTEM AND PANCREAS
OPERATION: 9 DRAINAGE: Taking or letting out fluids and/or gases from a body part

Body Part	Approach	Device	Qualifier
Ø Liver 1 Liver, Right Lobe 2 Liver, Left Lobe	Ø Open 3 Percutaneous 4 Percutaneous Endoscopic	Ø Drainage Device	Z No Qualifier
Ø Liver 1 Liver, Right Lobe 2 Liver, Left Lobe	Ø Open 3 Percutaneous 4 Percutaneous Endoscopic	Z No Device	X Diagnostic Z No Qualifier
4 Gallbladder G Pancreas	Ø Open 3 Percutaneous 4 Percutaneous Endoscopic 8 Via Natural or Artificial Opening Endoscopic	Ø Drainage Device	Z No Qualifier
4 Gallbladder G Pancreas	Ø Open 3 Percutaneous 4 Percutaneous Endoscopic 8 Via Natural or Artificial Opening Endoscopic	Z No Device	X Diagnostic Z No Qualifier
5 Hepatic Duct, Right 6 Hepatic Duct, Left 7 Hepatic Duct, Common 8 Cystic Duct 9 Common Bile Duct C Ampulla of Vater D Pancreatic Duct F Pancreatic Duct, Accessory	Ø Open 3 Percutaneous 4 Percutaneous Endoscopic 7 Via Natural or Artificial Opening 8 Via Natural or Artificial Opening Endoscopic	Ø Drainage Device	Z No Qualifier
5 Hepatic Duct, Right 6 Hepatic Duct, Left 7 Hepatic Duct, Common 8 Cystic Duct 9 Common Bile Duct C Ampulla of Vater D Pancreatic Duct F Pancreatic Duct, Accessory	Ø Open 3 Percutaneous 4 Percutaneous Endoscopic 7 Via Natural or Artificial Opening 8 Via Natural or Artificial Opening Endoscopic	Z No Device	X Diagnostic Z No Qualifier

Non-OR ØF9[Ø12][34]ØZ
Non-OR ØF9[4G]3ØZ
Non-OR ØF944ØZ
Non-OR ØF9G3ZZ
Non-OR ØF9[Ø124][34]Z[XZ]
Non-OR ØF9G[34]ZX
Non-OR ØF9[5689CDF]3ØZ
Non-OR ØF9[9DF]8ØZ
Non-OR ØF9C[48]ØZ
Non-OR ØF9[568][3478]ZX
Non-OR ØF99[3478]Z[XZ]
Non-OR ØF9[CDF][347]ZX
Non-OR ØF9[568CDF]3ZZ
Non-OR ØF994ZZ
Non-OR ØF9C8Z[XZ]
Non-OR ØF9[DF]8ZX

Coding Clinic: 2015, Q1, P32 – ØF963ØZ

SECTION: Ø MEDICAL AND SURGICAL
BODY SYSTEM: F HEPATOBILIARY SYSTEM AND PANCREAS
OPERATION: B EXCISION: Cutting out or off, without replacement, a portion of a body part

Body Part	Approach	Device	Qualifier
Ø Liver 1 Liver, Right Lobe 2 Liver, Left Lobe	Ø Open 3 Percutaneous ~~4 Percutaneous Endoscopic~~	Z No Device	X Diagnostic Z No Qualifier
Ø Liver 1 Liver, Right Lobe 2 Liver, Left Lobe	4 Percutaneous Endoscopic	Z No Device	G Hand-Assisted X Diagnostic Z No Qualifier
4 Gallbladder	Ø Open 3 Percutaneous 4 Percutaneous Endoscopic 8 Via Natural or Artificial Opening Endoscopic	Z No Device	X Diagnostic Z No Qualifier
4 Gallbladder ~~G Pancreas~~	Ø Open 3 Percutaneous 4 Percutaneous Endoscopic 8 Via Natural or Artificial Opening Endoscopic	Z No Device	X Diagnostic Z No Qualifier
5 Hepatic Duct, Right 6 Hepatic Duct, Left 7 Hepatic Duct, Common 8 Cystic Duct 9 Common Bile Duct C Ampulla of Vater D Pancreatic Duct F Pancreatic Duct, Accessory	Ø Open 3 Percutaneous 4 Percutaneous Endoscopic 7 Via Natural or Artificial Opening 8 Via Natural or Artificial Opening Endoscopic	Z No Device	X Diagnostic Z No Qualifier
G Pancreas	Ø Open 3 Percutaneous 8 Via Natural or Artificial Opening Endoscopic	Z No Device	X Diagnostic Z No Qualifier
G Pancreas	4 Percutaneous Endoscopic	Z No Device	G Hand-Assisted X Diagnostic Z No Qualifier

Non-OR ØFB[Ø12]3ZX
Non-OR ØFB[4G][34]ZX
Non-OR ØFB[5689CDF][3478]ZX
Non-OR ØFB[5689CDF][48]ZZ

Coding Clinic: 2016, Q1, P23, P25 – ØFB98ZX
Coding Clinic: 2016, Q1, P25 – ØFBD8ZX
Coding Clinic: 2016, Q3, P41 – ØFBØØZX
Coding Clinic: 2019, Q1, P5-8 – ØFBG[9]ØZZ

SECTION: Ø MEDICAL AND SURGICAL
BODY SYSTEM: F HEPATOBILIARY SYSTEM AND PANCREAS
OPERATION: C EXTIRPATION: Taking or cutting out solid matter from a body part

Body Part	Approach	Device	Qualifier
Ø Liver 1 Liver, Right Lobe 2 Liver, Left Lobe	Ø Open 3 Percutaneous 4 Percutaneous Endoscopic	Z No Device	Z No Qualifier
4 Gallbladder G Pancreas	Ø Open 3 Percutaneous 4 Percutaneous Endoscopic 8 Via Natural or Artificial Opening Endoscopic	Z No Device	Z No Qualifier

SECTION: Ø MEDICAL AND SURGICAL
BODY SYSTEM: F HEPATOBILIARY SYSTEM AND PANCREAS
OPERATION: C EXTIRPATION: *(continued)*
Taking or cutting out solid matter from a body part

Body Part	Approach	Device	Qualifier
5 Hepatic Duct, Right 6 Hepatic Duct, Left 7 Hepatic Duct, Common 8 Cystic Duct 9 Common Bile Duct C Ampulla of Vater D Pancreatic Duct F Pancreatic Duct, Accessory	Ø Open 3 Percutaneous 4 Percutaneous Endoscopic 7 Via Natural or Artificial Opening 8 Via Natural or Artificial Opening Endoscopic	Z No Device	Z No Qualifier

Non-OR ØFC[5689][3478]ZZ
Non-OR ØFCC[48]ZZ
Non-OR ØFC[DF][348]ZZ

Coding Clinic: 2023, Q2, P23 – ØFCG8ZZ

SECTION: Ø MEDICAL AND SURGICAL
BODY SYSTEM: F HEPATOBILIARY SYSTEM AND PANCREAS
OPERATION: D EXTRACTION: Pulling or stripping out or off all or a portion of a body part by the use of force

Body Part	Approach	Device	Qualifier
Ø Liver 1 Liver, Right Lobe 2 Liver, Left Lobe	3 Percutaneous 4 Percutaneous Endoscopic	Z No Device	X Diagnostic
4 Gallbladder 5 Hepatic Duct, Right 6 Hepatic Duct, Left 7 Hepatic Duct, Common 8 Cystic Duct 9 Common Bile Duct C Ampulla of Vater D Pancreatic Duct F Pancreatic Duct, Accessory G Pancreas	3 Percutaneous 4 Percutaneous Endoscopic 8 Via Natural or Artificial Opening Endoscopic	Z No Device	X Diagnostic

SECTION: Ø MEDICAL AND SURGICAL
BODY SYSTEM: F HEPATOBILIARY SYSTEM AND PANCREAS
OPERATION: F FRAGMENTATION: Breaking solid matter in a body part into pieces

Body Part	Approach	Device	Qualifier
4 Gallbladder (NC) 5 Hepatic Duct, Right (NC) 6 Hepatic Duct, Left (NC) 7 Hepatic Duct, Common 8 Cystic Duct (NC) 9 Common Bile Duct (NC) C Ampulla of Vater (NC) D Pancreatic Duct (NC) F Pancreatic Duct, Acessory (NC)	Ø Open 3 Percutaneous 4 Percutaneous Endoscopic 7 Via Natural or Artificial Opening 8 Via Natural or Artificial Opening Endoscopic X External	Z No Device	Z No Qualifier

(NC) ØFF[45689CDF]XZZ

Non-OR ØFF[45689C][8X]ZZ

Non-OR ØFF[DF]XZZ

SECTION: Ø MEDICAL AND SURGICAL
BODY SYSTEM: F HEPATOBILIARY SYSTEM AND PANCREAS
OPERATION: H INSERTION: Putting in a nonbiological appliance that monitors, assists, performs, or prevents a physiological function but does not physically take the place of a body part

Body Part	Approach	Device	Qualifier
Ø Liver 4 Gallbladder G Pancreas	Ø Open 3 Percutaneous 4 Percutaneous Endoscopic	1 Radioactive Element 2 Monitoring Device 3 Infusion Device Y Other Device	Z No Qualifier
1 Liver, Right Lobe 2 Liver, Left Lobe	Ø Open 3 Percutaneous 4 Percutaneous Endoscopic	2 Monitoring Device 3 Infusion Device	Z No Qualifier
B Hepatobiliary Duct D Pancreatic Duct	Ø Open 3 Percutaneous 4 Percutaneous Endoscopic 7 Via Natural or Artificial Opening 8 Via Natural or Artificial Opening Endoscopic	1 Radioactive Element 2 Monitoring Device 3 Infusion Device D Intraluminal Device Y Other Device	Z No Qualifier

Non-OR ØFH[Ø4G][Ø34]3Z

Non-OR ØFH[12][Ø34]3Z

Non-OR ØFH[BD][78][23]Z

Non-OR ØFH[BD][Ø3478]3Z

Non-OR ØFH[BD]4DZ

Non-OR ØFH[BD]8DZ

Coding Clinic: 2Ø22, Q2, P26 – ØFHØ31Z

SECTION: Ø **MEDICAL AND SURGICAL**
BODY SYSTEM: F **HEPATOBILIARY SYSTEM AND PANCREAS**
OPERATION: J **INSPECTION:** Visually and/or manually exploring a body part

Body Part	Approach	Device	Qualifier
Ø Liver	Ø Open 3 Percutaneous 4 Percutaneous Endoscopic X External	Z No Device	Z No Qualifier
4 Gallbladder G Pancreas	Ø Open 3 Percutaneous 4 Percutaneous Endoscopic 8 Via Natural or Artificial Opening Endoscopic X External	Z No Device	Z No Qualifier
B Hepatobiliary Duct D Pancreatic Duct	Ø Open 3 Percutaneous 4 Percutaneous Endoscopic 7 Via Natural or Artificial Opening 8 Via Natural or Artificial Opening Endoscopic	Z No Device	Z No Qualifier

DRG Non-OR ØFJØ3ZZ
DRG Non-OR ØFJG3ZZ
DRG Non-OR ØFJD[378]ZZ
Non-OR ØFJØXZZ
Non-OR ØFJ[4G]XZZ
Non-OR ØFJ43ZZ
Non-OR ØFJB[378]ZZ

SECTION: Ø **MEDICAL AND SURGICAL**
BODY SYSTEM: F **HEPATOBILIARY SYSTEM AND PANCREAS**
OPERATION: L **OCCLUSION:** Completely closing an orifice or the lumen of a tubular body part

Body Part	Approach	Device	Qualifier
5 Hepatic Duct, Right 6 Hepatic Duct, Left 7 Hepatic Duct, Common 8 Cystic Duct 9 Common Bile Duct C Ampulla of Vater D Pancreatic Duct F Pancreatic Duct, Accessory	Ø Open 3 Percutaneous 4 Percutaneous Endoscopic	C Extraluminal Device D Intraluminal Device Z No Device	Z No Qualifier
5 Hepatic Duct, Right 6 Hepatic Duct, Left 7 Hepatic Duct, Common 8 Cystic Duct 9 Common Bile Duct C Ampulla of Vater D Pancreatic Duct F Pancreatic Duct, Accessory	7 Via Natural or Artificial Opening 8 Via Natural or Artificial Opening Endoscopic	D Intraluminal Device Z No Device	Z No Qualifier

Non-OR ØFL[5689][34][CDZ]Z
Non-OR ØFL[5689][78][DZ]Z

SECTION: Ø MEDICAL AND SURGICAL
BODY SYSTEM: F HEPATOBILIARY SYSTEM AND PANCREAS
OPERATION: M REATTACHMENT: Putting back in or on all or a portion of a separated body part to its normal location or other suitable location

Body Part	Approach	Device	Qualifier
Ø Liver 1 Liver, Right Lobe 2 Liver, Left Lobe 4 Gallbladder 5 Hepatic Duct, Right 6 Hepatic Duct, Left 7 Hepatic Duct, Common 8 Cystic Duct 9 Common Bile Duct C Ampulla of Vater D Pancreatic Duct F Pancreatic Duct, Accessory G Pancreas	Ø Open 4 Percutaneous Endoscopic	Z No Device	Z No Qualifier

Non-OR ØFM[45689]4ZZ

SECTION: Ø MEDICAL AND SURGICAL
BODY SYSTEM: F HEPATOBILIARY SYSTEM AND PANCREAS
OPERATION: N RELEASE: Freeing a body part from an abnormal physical constraint by cutting or by the use of force

Body Part	Approach	Device	Qualifier
Ø Liver 1 Liver, Right Lobe 2 Liver, Left Lobe	Ø Open 3 Percutaneous 4 Percutaneous Endoscopic	Z No Device	Z No Qualifier
4 Gallbladder G Pancreas	Ø Open 3 Percutaneous 4 Percutaneous Endoscopic 8 Via Natural or Artificial Opening Endoscopic	Z No Device	Z No Qualifier
5 Hepatic Duct, Right 6 Hepatic Duct, Left 7 Hepatic Duct, Common 8 Cystic Duct 9 Common Bile Duct C Ampulla of Vater D Pancreatic Duct F Pancreatic Duct, Accessory	Ø Open 3 Percutaneous 4 Percutaneous Endoscopic 7 Via Natural or Artificial Opening 8 Via Natural or Artificial Opening Endoscopic	Z No Device	Z No Qualifier

SECTION: Ø MEDICAL AND SURGICAL
BODY SYSTEM: F HEPATOBILIARY SYSTEM AND PANCREAS
OPERATION: P REMOVAL: Taking out or off a device from a body part

Body Part	Approach	Device	Qualifier
Ø Liver	Ø Open 3 Percutaneous 4 Percutaneous Endoscopic	Ø Drainage Device 2 Monitoring Device 3 Infusion Device Y Other Device	Z No Qualifier
Ø Liver	X External	Ø Drainage Device 2 Monitoring Device 3 Infusion Device	Z No Qualifier
4 Gallbladder G Pancreas	Ø Open 3 Percutaneous 4 Percutaneous Endoscopic	Ø Drainage Device 2 Monitoring Device 3 Infusion Device D Intraluminal Device Y Other Device	Z No Qualifier
4 Gallbladder G Pancreas	8 Via Natural or Artificial Opening Endoscopic	Ø Drainage Device	Z No Qualifier
4 Gallbladder G Pancreas	X External	Ø Drainage Device 2 Monitoring Device 3 Infusion Device D Intraluminal Device	Z No Qualifier
B Hepatobiliary Duct D Pancreatic Duct	Ø Open 3 Percutaneous 4 Percutaneous Endoscopic 7 Via Natural or Artificial Opening 8 Via Natural or Artificial Opening Endoscopic	Ø Drainage Device 1 Radioactive Element 2 Monitoring Device 3 Infusion Device 7 Autologous Tissue Substitute C Extraluminal Device D Intraluminal Device J Synthetic Substitute K Nonautologous Tissue Substitute Y Other Device	Z No Qualifier
B Hepatobiliary Duct D Pancreatic Duct	X External	Ø Drainage Device 1 Radioactive Element 2 Monitoring Device 3 Infusion Device D Intraluminal Device	Z No Qualifier

Non-OR ØFPØX[Ø23]Z
Non-OR ØFP4X[Ø23D]Z
Non-OR ØFPGX[Ø23]Z
Non-OR ØFP[BD][78][Ø23D]Z
Non-OR ØFP[BD]X[Ø123D]Z

SECTION: Ø MEDICAL AND SURGICAL
BODY SYSTEM: F HEPATOBILIARY SYSTEM AND PANCREAS
OPERATION: Q REPAIR: Restoring, to the extent possible, a body part to its normal anatomic structure and function

Body Part	Approach	Device	Qualifier
Ø Liver 1 Liver, Right Lobe 2 Liver, Left Lobe	Ø Open 3 Percutaneous 4 Percutaneous Endoscopic	Z No Device	Z No Qualifier
4 Gallbladder G Pancreas	Ø Open 3 Percutaneous 4 Percutaneous Endoscopic 8 Via Natural or Artificial Opening Endoscopic	Z No Device	Z No Qualifier
5 Hepatic Duct, Right 6 Hepatic Duct, Left 7 Hepatic Duct, Common 8 Cystic Duct 9 Common Bile Duct C Ampulla of Vater D Pancreatic Duct F Pancreatic Duct, Accessory	Ø Open 3 Percutaneous 4 Percutaneous Endoscopic 7 Via Natural or Artificial Opening 8 Via Natural or Artificial Opening Endoscopic	Z No Device	Z No Qualifier

Coding Clinic: 2Ø16, Q3, P27 – ØFQ9ØZZ

SECTION: Ø MEDICAL AND SURGICAL
BODY SYSTEM: F HEPATOBILIARY SYSTEM AND PANCREAS
OPERATION: R REPLACEMENT: Putting in or on biological or synthetic material that physically takes the place and/or function of all or a portion of a body part

Body Part	Approach	Device	Qualifier
5 Hepatic Duct, Right 6 Hepatic Duct, Left 7 Hepatic Duct, Common 8 Cystic Duct 9 Common Bile Duct C Ampulla of Vater D Pancreatic Duct F Pancreatic Duct, Accessory	Ø Open 4 Percutaneous Endoscopic 8 Via Natural or Artificial Opening Endoscopic	7 Autologous Tissue Substitute J Synthetic Substitute K Nonautologous Tissue Substitute	Z No Qualifier

SECTION: Ø MEDICAL AND SURGICAL
BODY SYSTEM: F HEPATOBILIARY SYSTEM AND PANCREAS
OPERATION: S REPOSITION: Moving to its normal location, or other suitable location, all or a portion of a body part

Body Part	Approach	Device	Qualifier
Ø Liver 4 Gallbladder 5 Hepatic Duct, Right 6 Hepatic Duct, Left 7 Hepatic Duct, Common 8 Cystic Duct 9 Common Bile Duct C Ampulla of Vater D Pancreatic Duct F Pancreatic Duct, Accessory G Pancreas	Ø Open 4 Percutaneous Endoscopic	Z No Device	Z No Qualifier

SECTION: Ø MEDICAL AND SURGICAL
BODY SYSTEM: F HEPATOBILIARY SYSTEM AND PANCREAS
OPERATION: T RESECTION: Cutting out or off, without replacement, all of a body part

Body Part	Approach	Device	Qualifier
Ø Liver 1 Liver, Right Lobe 2 Liver, Left Lobe 4 Gallbladder G Pancreas ⊞	Ø Open ~~4 Percutaneous Endoscopic~~	Z No Device	Z No Qualifier
Ø Liver 1 Liver, Right Lobe 2 Liver, Left Lobe 4 Gallbladder G Pancreas	4 Percutaneous Endoscopic	Z No Device	G Hand-Assisted Z No Qualifier
5 Hepatic Duct, Right 6 Hepatic Duct, Left 7 Hepatic Duct, Common 8 Cystic Duct 9 Common Bile Duct C Ampulla of Vater D Pancreatic Duct F Pancreatic Duct, Accessory	Ø Open 4 Percutaneous Endoscopic 7 Via Natural or Artificial Opening 8 Via Natural or Artificial Opening Endoscopic	Z No Device	Z No Qualifier

⊞ ØFTGØZZ

Non-OR ØFT[DF][48]ZZ

Coding Clinic: 2012, Q4, P1ØØ – ØFTØØZZ
Coding Clinic: 2019, Q1, P5 – ØFT4ØZZ
Coding Clinic: 2021, Q4, P49 – ØFT44ZZ

SECTION: Ø MEDICAL AND SURGICAL
BODY SYSTEM: F HEPATOBILIARY SYSTEM AND PANCREAS
OPERATION: U SUPPLEMENT: Putting in or on biological or synthetic material that physically reinforces and/or augments the function of a portion of a body part

Body Part	Approach	Device	Qualifier
5 Hepatic Duct, Right 6 Hepatic Duct, Left 7 Hepatic Duct, Common 8 Cystic Duct 9 Common Bile Duct C Ampulla of Vater D Pancreatic Duct F Pancreatic Duct, Accessory	Ø Open 3 Percutaneous 4 Percutaneous Endoscopic 8 Via Natural or Artificial Opening Endoscopic	7 Autologous Tissue Substitute J Synthetic Substitute K Nonautologous Tissue Substitute	Z No Qualifier

SECTION: Ø MEDICAL AND SURGICAL
BODY SYSTEM: F HEPATOBILIARY SYSTEM AND PANCREAS
OPERATION: V RESTRICTION: Partially closing an orifice or the lumen of a tubular body part

Body Part	Approach	Device	Qualifier
5 Hepatic Duct, Right 6 Hepatic Duct, Left 7 Hepatic Duct, Common 8 Cystic Duct 9 Common Bile Duct C Ampulla of Vater D Pancreatic Duct F Pancreatic Duct, Accessory	Ø Open 3 Percutaneous 4 Percutaneous Endoscopic	C Extraluminal Device D Intraluminal Device Z No Device	Z No Qualifier
5 Hepatic Duct, Right 6 Hepatic Duct, Left 7 Hepatic Duct, Common 8 Cystic Duct 9 Common Bile Duct C Ampulla of Vater D Pancreatic Duct F Pancreatic Duct, Accessory	7 Via Natural or Artificial Opening 8 Via Natural or Artificial Opening Endoscopic	D Intraluminal Device Z No Device	Z No Qualifier

Non-OR ØFV[5689][34][CDZ]Z
Non-OR ØFV[5689][78][DZ]Z

SECTION: Ø MEDICAL AND SURGICAL
BODY SYSTEM: F HEPATOBILIARY SYSTEM AND PANCREAS
OPERATION: W REVISION: Correcting, to the extent possible, a portion of a malfunctioning device or the position of a displaced device

Body Part	Approach	Device	Qualifier
Ø Liver	Ø Open 3 Percutaneous 4 Percutaneous Endoscopic	Ø Drainage Device 2 Monitoring Device 3 Infusion Device Y Other Device	Z No Qualifier
Ø Liver	X External	Ø Drainage Device 2 Monitoring Device 3 Infusion Device	Z No Qualifier
4 Gallbladder G Pancreas	Ø Open 3 Percutaneous 4 Percutaneous Endoscopic	Ø Drainage Device 2 Monitoring Device 3 Infusion Device D Intraluminal Device Y Other Device	Z No Qualifier
4 Gallbladder G Pancreas	8 Via Natural or Artificial Opening Endoscopic	Ø Drainage Device	Z No Qualifier
4 Gallbladder G Pancreas	X External	Ø Drainage Device 2 Monitoring Device 3 Infusion Device D Intraluminal Device	Z No Qualifier
B Hepatobiliary Duct D Pancreatic Duct	Ø Open 3 Percutaneous 4 Percutaneous Endoscopic 7 Via Natural or Artificial Opening 8 Via Natural or Artificial Opening Endoscopic	Ø Drainage Device 2 Monitoring Device 3 Infusion Device 7 Autologous Tissue Substitute C Extraluminal Device D Intraluminal Device J Synthetic Substitute K Nonautologous Tissue Substitute Y Other Device	Z No Qualifier
B Hepatobiliary Duct D Pancreatic Duct	X External	Ø Drainage Device 2 Monitoring Device 3 Infusion Device 7 Autologous Tissue Substitute C Extraluminal Device D Intraluminal Device J Synthetic Substitute K Nonautologous Tissue Substitute	Z No Qualifier

Non-OR ØFWØX[Ø23]Z
Non-OR ØFW[4G]X[Ø23D]Z
Non-OR ØFW[BD]X[Ø237CDJK]Z

SECTION: Ø MEDICAL AND SURGICAL
BODY SYSTEM: F HEPATOBILIARY SYSTEM AND PANCREAS
OPERATION: Y TRANSPLANTATION: Putting in or on all or a portion of a living body part taken from another individual or animal to physically take the place and/or function of all or a portion of a similar body part

Body Part	Approach	Device	Qualifier
Ø Liver G Pancreas	Ø Open	Z No Device	Ø Allogeneic 1 Syngeneic 2 Zooplastic

ØFYGØZ2

ØFYGØZØ, ØFYGØZ1 alone [without kidney transplant codes (ØTYØØZ[Ø1], ØTY1ØZ[Ø12])], except when ØFYGØZØ or ØFYGØZ1 is combined with at least one principal or secondary diagnosis code from the following list:

E1Ø.1Ø	E1Ø.321	E1Ø.359	E1Ø.44	E1Ø.62Ø	E1Ø.649
E1Ø.11	E1Ø.329	E1Ø.36	E1Ø.49	E1Ø.621	E1Ø.65
E1Ø.21	E1Ø.331	E1Ø.39	E1Ø.51	E1Ø.622	E1Ø.69
E1Ø.22	E1Ø.339	E1Ø.4Ø	E1Ø.52	E1Ø.628	E1Ø.8
E1Ø.29	E1Ø.341	E1Ø.41	E1Ø.59	E1Ø.63Ø	E1Ø.9
E1Ø.311	E1Ø.349	E1Ø.42	E1Ø.61Ø	E1Ø.638	E89.1
E1Ø.319	E1Ø.351	E1Ø.43	E1Ø.618	E1Ø.641	

ØFYØØZ[Ø12]
ØFYGØZ[Ø1]
ØFYGØZ[Ø12]

Coding Clinic: 2Ø12, Q4, P1ØØ – ØFYØØZØ

ØG. Endocrine System 284
ØG2. Change 285
ØG5. Destruction 285
ØG8. Division 285
ØG9. Drainage 286
ØGB. Excision 287
ØGC. Extirpation 287
ØGH. Insertion 288
ØGJ. Inspection 288
ØGM. Reattachment 288
ØGN. Release 289
ØGP. Removal 289
ØGQ. Repair 29Ø
ØGS. Reposition 29Ø
ØGT. Resection 291
ØGW. Revision 291

New/Revised Text in Green ~~deleted~~ Deleted ♀ Females Only ♂ Males Only **Coding Clinic**
Non-covered Limited Coverage Combination (See Appendix E) DRG Non-OR Non-OR Hospital-Acquired Condition

SECTION: Ø MEDICAL AND SURGICAL
BODY SYSTEM: G ENDOCRINE SYSTEM
OPERATION: 2 CHANGE: Taking out or off a device from a body part and putting back an identical or similar device in or on the same body part without cutting or puncturing the skin or a mucous membrane

Body Part	Approach	Device	Qualifier
Ø Pituitary Gland 1 Pineal Body 5 Adrenal Gland K Thyroid Gland R Parathyroid Gland S Endocrine Gland	X External	Ø Drainage Device Y Other Device	Z No Qualifier

Non-OR All Values

SECTION: Ø MEDICAL AND SURGICAL
BODY SYSTEM: G ENDOCRINE SYSTEM
OPERATION: 5 DESTRUCTION: Physical eradication of all or a portion of a body part by the direct use of energy, force, or a destructive agent

Body Part	Approach	Device	Qualifier
Ø Pituitary Gland 1 Pineal Body 2 Adrenal Gland, Left 3 Adrenal Gland, Right 4 Adrenal Glands, Bilateral 6 Carotid Body, Left 7 Carotid Body, Right 8 Carotid Bodies, Bilateral 9 Para-aortic Body B Coccygeal Glomus C Glomus Jugulare D Aortic Body F Paraganglion Extremity G Thyroid Gland Lobe, Left H Thyroid Gland Lobe, Right K Thyroid Gland L Superior Parathyroid Gland, Right M Superior Parathyroid Gland, Left N Inferior Parathyroid Gland, Right P Inferior Parathyroid Gland, Left Q Parathyroid Glands, Multiple R Parathyroid Gland	Ø Open 3 Percutaneous 4 Percutaneous Endoscopic	Z No Device	3 Laser Interstitial Thermal Therapy Z No Qualifier

Non-OR All Values

SECTION: Ø MEDICAL AND SURGICAL
BODY SYSTEM: G ENDOCRINE SYSTEM
OPERATION: 8 DIVISION: Cutting into a body part, without draining fluids and/or gases from the body part, in order to separate or transect a body part

Body Part	Approach	Device	Qualifier
Ø Pituitary Gland J Thyroid Gland Isthmus	Ø Open 3 Percutaneous 4 Percutaneous Endoscopic	Z No Device	Z No Qualifier

SECTION: Ø MEDICAL AND SURGICAL
BODY SYSTEM: G ENDOCRINE SYSTEM
OPERATION: 9 DRAINAGE: Taking or letting out fluids and/or gases from a body part

Body Part	Approach	Device	Qualifier
Ø Pituitary Gland 1 Pineal Body 2 Adrenal Gland, Left 3 Adrenal Gland, Right 4 Adrenal Glands, Bilateral 6 Carotid Body, Left 7 Carotid Body, Right 8 Carotid Bodies, Bilateral 9 Para-aortic Body B Coccygeal Glomus C Glomus Jugulare D Aortic Body F Paraganglion Extremity G Thyroid Gland Lobe, Left H Thyroid Gland Lobe, Right K Thyroid Gland L Superior Parathyroid Gland, Right M Superior Parathyroid Gland, Left N Inferior Parathyroid Gland, Right P Inferior Parathyroid Gland, Left Q Parathyroid Glands, Multiple R Parathyroid Gland	Ø Open 3 Percutaneous 4 Percutaneous Endoscopic	Ø Drainage Device	Z No Qualifier
Ø Pituitary Gland 1 Pineal Body 2 Adrenal Gland, Left 3 Adrenal Gland, Right 4 Adrenal Glands, Bilateral 6 Carotid Body, Left 7 Carotid Body, Right 8 Carotid Bodies, Bilateral 9 Para-aortic Body B Coccygeal Glomus C Glomus Jugulare D Aortic Body F Paraganglion Extremity G Thyroid Gland Lobe, Left H Thyroid Gland Lobe, Right K Thyroid Gland L Superior Parathyroid Gland, Right M Superior Parathyroid Gland, Left N Inferior Parathyroid Gland, Right P Inferior Parathyroid Gland, Left Q Parathyroid Glands, Multiple R Parathyroid Gland	Ø Open 3 Percutaneous 4 Percutaneous Endoscopic	Z No Device	X Diagnostic Z No Qualifier

Non-OR ØG9[Ø12346789BCDF]3ØZ
Non-OR ØG9[GHKLMNPQR][34]ØZ
Non-OR ØG9[234GHK][34]ZX
Non-OR ØG9[Ø12346789BCDF]3ZZ
Non-OR ØG9[GHKLMNPQR][34]ZZ

SECTION: Ø MEDICAL AND SURGICAL
BODY SYSTEM: G ENDOCRINE SYSTEM
OPERATION: B EXCISION: Cutting out or off, without replacement, a portion of a body part

Body Part	Approach	Device	Qualifier
Ø Pituitary Gland 1 Pineal Body 2 Adrenal Gland, Left 3 Adrenal Gland, Right 4 Adrenal Glands, Bilateral 6 Carotid Body, Left 7 Carotid Body, Right 8 Carotid Bodies, Bilateral 9 Para-aortic Body B Coccygeal Glomus C Glomus Jugulare D Aortic Body F Paraganglion Extremity G Thyroid Gland Lobe, Left H Thyroid Gland Lobe, Right J Thyroid Gland Isthmus L Superior Parathyroid Gland, Right M Superior Parathyroid Gland, Left N Inferior Parathyroid Gland, Right P Inferior Parathyroid Gland, Left Q Parathyroid Glands, Multiple R Parathyroid Gland	Ø Open 3 Percutaneous 4 Percutaneous Endoscopic	Z No Device	X Diagnostic Z No Qualifier

Non-OR ØGB[234GH][34]ZX

Coding Clinic: 2017, Q2, P2Ø – ØGB[GH]ØZZ
Coding Clinic: 2021, Q2, P7– ØGB9ØZZ

SECTION: Ø MEDICAL AND SURGICAL
BODY SYSTEM: G ENDOCRINE SYSTEM
OPERATION: C EXTIRPATION: Taking or cutting out solid matter from a body part

Body Part	Approach	Device	Qualifier
Ø Pituitary Gland 1 Pineal Body 2 Adrenal Gland, Left 3 Adrenal Gland, Right 4 Adrenal Glands, Bilateral 6 Carotid Body, Left 7 Carotid Body, Right 8 Carotid Bodies, Bilateral 9 Para-aortic Body B Coccygeal Glomus C Glomus Jugulare D Aortic Body F Paraganglion Extremity G Thyroid Gland Lobe, Left H Thyroid Gland Lobe, Right K Thyroid Gland L Superior Parathyroid Gland, Right M Superior Parathyroid Gland, Left N Inferior Parathyroid Gland, Right P Inferior Parathyroid Gland, Left Q Parathyroid Glands, Multiple R Parathyroid Gland	Ø Open 3 Percutaneous 4 Percutaneous Endoscopic	Z No Device	Z No Qualifier

SECTION: Ø MEDICAL AND SURGICAL
BODY SYSTEM: G ENDOCRINE SYSTEM
OPERATION: H INSERTION: Putting in a nonbiological appliance that monitors, assists, performs, or prevents a physiological function but does not physically take the place of a body part

Body Part	Approach	Device	Qualifier
S Endocrine Gland	Ø Open 3 Percutaneous 4 Percutaneous Endoscopic	1 Radioactive Element 2 Monitoring Device 3 Infusion Device Y Other Device	Z No Qualifier

SECTION: Ø MEDICAL AND SURGICAL
BODY SYSTEM: G ENDOCRINE SYSTEM
OPERATION: J INSPECTION: Visually and/or manually exploring a body part

Body Part	Approach	Device	Qualifier
Ø Pituitary Gland 1 Pineal Body 5 Adrenal Gland K Thyroid Gland R Parathyroid Gland S Endocrine Gland	Ø Open 3 Percutaneous 4 Percutaneous Endoscopic	Z No Device	Z No Qualifier

Non-OR ØGJ[Ø15KRS]3ZZ

SECTION: Ø MEDICAL AND SURGICAL
BODY SYSTEM: G ENDOCRINE SYSTEM
OPERATION: M REATTACHMENT: Putting back in or on all or a portion of a separated body part to its normal location or other suitable location

Body Part	Approach	Device	Qualifier
2 Adrenal Gland, Left 3 Adrenal Gland, Right G Thyroid Gland Lobe, Left H Thyroid Gland Lobe, Right L Superior Parathyroid Gland, Right M Superior Parathyroid Gland, Left N Inferior Parathyroid Gland, Right P Inferior Parathyroid Gland, Left Q Parathyroid Glands, Multiple R Parathyroid Gland	Ø Open 4 Percutaneous Endoscopic	Z No Device	Z No Qualifier

SECTION: Ø MEDICAL AND SURGICAL
BODY SYSTEM: G ENDOCRINE SYSTEM
OPERATION: N RELEASE: Freeing a body part from an abnormal physical constraint by cutting or by the use of force

Body Part	Approach	Device	Qualifier
Ø Pituitary Gland 1 Pineal Body 2 Adrenal Gland, Left 3 Adrenal Gland, Right 4 Adrenal Glands, Bilateral 6 Carotid Body, Left 7 Carotid Body, Right 8 Carotid Bodies, Bilateral 9 Para-aortic Body B Coccygeal Glomus C Glomus Jugulare D Aortic Body F Paraganglion Extremity G Thyroid Gland Lobe, Left H Thyroid Gland Lobe, Right K Thyroid Gland L Superior Parathyroid Gland, Right M Superior Parathyroid Gland, Left N Inferior Parathyroid Gland, Right P Inferior Parathyroid Gland, Left Q Parathyroid Glands, Multiple R Parathyroid Gland	Ø Open 3 Percutaneous 4 Percutaneous Endoscopic	Z No Device	Z No Qualifier

SECTION: Ø MEDICAL AND SURGICAL
BODY SYSTEM: G ENDOCRINE SYSTEM
OPERATION: P REMOVAL: Taking out or off a device from a body part

Body Part	Approach	Device	Qualifier
Ø Pituitary Gland 1 Pineal Body 5 Adrenal Gland K Thyroid Gland R Parathyroid Gland	Ø Open 3 Percutaneous 4 Percutaneous Endoscopic X External	Ø Drainage Device	Z No Qualifier
S Endocrine Gland	Ø Open 3 Percutaneous 4 Percutaneous Endoscopic	Ø Drainage Device 2 Monitoring Device 3 Infusion Device Y Other Device	Z No Qualifier
S Endocrine Gland	X External	Ø Drainage Device 2 Monitoring Device 3 Infusion Device	Z No Qualifier

Non-OR ØGP[Ø15KR]XØZ
Non-OR ØGPSX[Ø23]Z

SECTION: Ø MEDICAL AND SURGICAL
BODY SYSTEM: G ENDOCRINE SYSTEM
OPERATION: Q REPAIR: Restoring, to the extent possible, a body part to its normal anatomic structure and function

Body Part	Approach	Device	Qualifier
Ø Pituitary Gland 1 Pineal Body 2 Adrenal Gland, Left 3 Adrenal Gland, Right 4 Adrenal Glands, Bilateral 6 Carotid Body, Left 7 Carotid Body, Right 8 Carotid Bodies, Bilateral 9 Para-aortic Body B Coccygeal Glomus C Glomus Jugulare D Aortic Body F Paraganglion Extremity G Thyroid Gland Lobe, Left H Thyroid Gland Lobe, Right J Thyroid Gland Isthmus K Thyroid Gland L Superior Parathyroid Gland, Right M Superior Parathyroid Gland, Left N Inferior Parathyroid Gland, Right P Inferior Parathyroid Gland, Left Q Parathyroid Glands, Multiple R Parathyroid Gland	Ø Open 3 Percutaneous 4 Percutaneous Endoscopic	Z No Device	Z No Qualifier

SECTION: Ø MEDICAL AND SURGICAL
BODY SYSTEM: G ENDOCRINE SYSTEM
OPERATION: S REPOSITION: Moving to its normal location, or other suitable location, all or a portion of a body part

Body Part	Approach	Device	Qualifier
2 Adrenal Gland, Left 3 Adrenal Gland, Right G Thyroid Gland Lobe, Left H Thyroid Gland Lobe, Right L Superior Parathyroid Gland, Right M Superior Parathyroid Gland, Left N Inferior Parathyroid Gland, Right P Inferior Parathyroid Gland, Left Q Parathyroid Glands, Multiple R Parathyroid Gland	Ø Open 4 Percutaneous Endoscopic	Z No Device	Z No Qualifier

SECTION: Ø MEDICAL AND SURGICAL
BODY SYSTEM: G ENDOCRINE SYSTEM
OPERATION: T RESECTION: Cutting out or off, without replacement, all of a body part

Body Part	Approach	Device	Qualifier
Ø Pituitary Gland 1 Pineal Body 2 Adrenal Gland, Left 3 Adrenal Gland, Right 4 Adrenal Glands, Bilateral 6 Carotid Body, Left 7 Carotid Body, Right 8 Carotid Bodies, Bilateral 9 Para-aortic Body B Coccygeal Glomus C Glomus Jugulare D Aortic Body F Paraganglion Extremity G Thyroid Gland Lobe, Left H Thyroid Gland Lobe, Right J Thyroid Gland Isthmus K Thyroid Gland L Superior Parathyroid Gland, Right M Superior Parathyroid Gland, Left N Inferior Parathyroid Gland, Right P Inferior Parathyroid Gland, Left Q Parathyroid Glands, Multiple R Parathyroid Gland	Ø Open 4 Percutaneous Endoscopic	Z No Device	Z No Qualifier

SECTION: Ø MEDICAL AND SURGICAL
BODY SYSTEM: G ENDOCRINE SYSTEM
OPERATION: W REVISION: Correcting, to the extent possible, a portion of a malfunctioning device or the position of a displaced device

Body Part	Approach	Device	Qualifier
Ø Pituitary Gland 1 Pineal Body 5 Adrenal Gland K Thyroid Gland R Parathyroid Gland	Ø Open 3 Percutaneous 4 Percutaneous Endoscopic X External	Ø Drainage Device	Z No Qualifier
S Endocrine Gland	Ø Open 3 Percutaneous 4 Percutaneous Endoscopic	Ø Drainage Device 2 Monitoring Device 3 Infusion Device Y Other Device	Z No Qualifier
S Endocrine Gland	X External	Ø Drainage Device 2 Monitoring Device 3 Infusion Device	Z No Qualifier

Non-OR ØGW[Ø15KR]XØZ
Non-OR ØGWSX[Ø23]Z

ØH. Skin and Breast 292
ØHØ. Alteration 293
ØH2. Change 293
ØH5. Destruction 294
ØH8. Division 295
ØH9. Drainage 296
ØHB. Excision 297
ØHC. Extirpation 298
ØHD. Extraction 299
ØHH. Insertion 300
ØHJ. Inspection 300
ØHM. Reattachment 301
ØHN. Release 302
ØHP. Removal 303
ØHQ. Repair 304
ØHR. Replacement 305
ØHS. Reposition 307
ØHT. Resection 307
ØHU. Supplement 307
ØHW. Revision 308
ØHX. Transfer 309

New/Revised Text in Green ~~deleted~~ Deleted ♀ Females Only ♂ Males Only Coding Clinic
Non-covered Limited Coverage Combination (See Appendix E) DRG Non-OR Non-OR Hospital-Acquired Condition

SECTION: Ø MEDICAL AND SURGICAL
BODY SYSTEM: H SKIN AND BREAST
OPERATION: Ø ALTERATION: Modifying the anatomic structure of a body part without affecting the function of the body part

Body Part	Approach	Device	Qualifier
T Breast, Right U Breast, Left V Breast, Bilateral	Ø Open 3 Percutaneous X External	7 Autologous Tissue Substitute J Synthetic Substitute K Nonautologous Tissue Substitute Z No Device	Z No Qualifier

Coding Clinic: 2Ø22, Q1, P15 – ØHØTØZZ

SECTION: Ø MEDICAL AND SURGICAL
BODY SYSTEM: H SKIN AND BREAST
OPERATION: 2 CHANGE: Taking out or off a device from a body part and putting back an identical or similar device in or on the same body part without cutting or puncturing the skin or a mucous membrane

Body Part	Approach	Device	Qualifier
P Skin T Breast, Right U Breast, Left	X External	Ø Drainage Device Y Other Device	Z No Qualifier

Non-OR All Values

SECTION: Ø MEDICAL AND SURGICAL
BODY SYSTEM: H SKIN AND BREAST
OPERATION: 5 DESTRUCTION: Physical eradication of all or a portion of a body part by the direct use of energy, force, or a destructive agent

Body Part	Approach	Device	Qualifier
Ø Skin, Scalp 1 Skin, Face 2 Skin, Right Ear 3 Skin, Left Ear 4 Skin, Neck 5 Skin, Chest 6 Skin, Back 7 Skin, Abdomen 8 Skin, Buttock 9 Skin, Perineum A Skin, Inguinal B Skin, Right Upper Arm C Skin, Left Upper Arm D Skin, Right Lower Arm E Skin, Left Lower Arm F Skin, Right Hand G Skin, Left Hand H Skin, Right Upper Leg J Skin, Left Upper Leg K Skin, Right Lower Leg L Skin, Left Lower Leg M Skin, Right Foot N Skin, Left Foot	X External	Z No Device	D Multiple Z No Qualifier
Q Finger Nail R Toe Nail	X External	Z No Device	Z No Qualifier
T Breast, Right U Breast, Left V Breast, Bilateral	Ø Open 3 Percutaneous	Z No Device	3 Laser Interstitial Thermal Therapy Z No Qualifier
T Breast, Right U Breast, Left V Breast, Bilateral	7 Via Natural or Artificial Opening 8 Via Natural or Artificial Opening Endoscopic	Z No Device	Z No Qualifier
W Nipple, Right X Nipple, Left	Ø Open 3 Percutaneous 7 Via Natural or Artificial Opening 8 Via Natural or Artificial Opening Endoscopic X External	Z No Device	Z No Qualifier

DRG Non-OR ØH5[Ø1456789ABCDEFGHJKLMN]XZ[DZ]
DRG Non-OR ØH5[QR]XZZ
Non-OR ØH5[23]XZ[DZ]
Non-OR ØH5[TUV][Ø3]Z[3Z]

SECTION: Ø MEDICAL AND SURGICAL
BODY SYSTEM: H SKIN AND BREAST
OPERATION: 8 DIVISION: Cutting into a body part, without draining fluids and/or gases from the body part, in order to separate or transect a body part

Body Part	Approach	Device	Qualifier
Ø Skin, Scalp 1 Skin, Face 2 Skin, Right Ear 3 Skin, Left Ear 4 Skin, Neck 5 Skin, Chest 6 Skin, Back 7 Skin, Abdomen 8 Skin, Buttock 9 Skin, Perineum A Skin, Inguinal B Skin, Right Upper Arm C Skin, Left Upper Arm D Skin, Right Lower Arm E Skin, Left Lower Arm F Skin, Right Hand G Skin, Left Hand H Skin, Right Upper Leg J Skin, Left Upper Leg K Skin, Right Lower Leg L Skin, Left Lower Leg M Skin, Right Foot N Skin, Left Foot	X External	Z No Device	Z No Qualifier

DRG Non-OR ØH8[Ø1456789ABCDEFGHJKLMN]XZZ
Non-OR ØH8[23]XZZ

SECTION: Ø MEDICAL AND SURGICAL
BODY SYSTEM: H SKIN AND BREAST
OPERATION: 9 DRAINAGE: *(on multiple pages)*
Taking or letting out fluids and/or gases from a body part

Body Part	Approach	Device	Qualifier
Ø Skin, Scalp 1 Skin, Face 2 Skin, Right Ear 3 Skin, Left Ear 4 Skin, Neck 5 Skin, Chest 6 Skin, Back 7 Skin, Abdomen 8 Skin, Buttock 9 Skin, Perineum A Skin, Inguinal B Skin, Right Upper Arm C Skin, Left Upper Arm D Skin, Right Lower Arm E Skin, Left Lower Arm F Skin, Right Hand G Skin, Left Hand H Skin, Right Upper Leg J Skin, Left Upper Leg K Skin, Right Lower Leg L Skin, Left Lower Leg M Skin, Right Foot N Skin, Left Foot Q Finger Nail R Toe Nail	X External	Ø Drainage Device	Z No Qualifier
Ø Skin, Scalp 1 Skin, Face 2 Skin, Right Ear 3 Skin, Left Ear 4 Skin, Neck 5 Skin, Chest 6 Skin, Back 7 Skin, Abdomen 8 Skin, Buttock 9 Skin, Perineum A Skin, Inguinal B Skin, Right Upper Arm C Skin, Left Upper Arm D Skin, Right Lower Arm E Skin, Left Lower Arm F Skin, Right Hand G Skin, Left Hand H Skin, Right Upper Leg J Skin, Left Upper Leg K Skin, Right Lower Leg L Skin, Left Lower Leg M Skin, Right Foot N Skin, Left Foot Q Finger Nail R Toe Nail	X External	Z No Device	X Diagnostic Z No Qualifier

Non-OR ØH9[Ø12345678ABCDEFGHJKLMNQR]XØZ
Non-OR ØH9[Ø123456789ABCDEFGHJKLMNQR]XZX
Non-OR ØH9[Ø12345678ABCDEFGHJKLMNQR]XZZ

New/Revised Text in Green ~~deleted~~ Deleted ♀ Females Only ♂ Males Only Coding Clinic
Non-covered Limited Coverage ⊞ Combination (See Appendix E) DRG Non-OR Non-OR Hospital-Acquired Condition

SECTION: Ø MEDICAL AND SURGICAL
BODY SYSTEM: H SKIN AND BREAST
OPERATION: 9 DRAINAGE: *(continued)*
Taking or letting out fluids and/or gases from a body part

Body Part	Approach	Device	Qualifier
T Breast, Right U Breast, Left V Breast, Bilateral	Ø Open 3 Percutaneous 7 Via Natural or Artificial Opening 8 Via Natural or Artificial Opening Endoscopic X External	Ø Drainage Device	Z No Qualifier
T Breast, Right U Breast, Left V Breast, Bilateral	Ø Open 3 Percutaneous 7 Via Natural or Artificial Opening 8 Via Natural or Artificial Opening Endoscopic X External	Z No Device	X Diagnostic Z No Qualifier
W Nipple, Right X Nipple, Left	Ø Open 3 Percutaneous 7 Via Natural or Artificial Opening 8 Via Natural or Artificial Opening Endoscopic X External	Ø Drainage Device	Z No Qualifier
W Nipple, Right X Nipple, Left	Ø Open 3 Percutaneous 7 Via Natural or Artificial Opening 8 Via Natural or Artificial Opening Endoscopic X External	Z No Device	X Diagnostic Z No Qualifier

Non-OR ØH9[TUVWX][Ø378X]ØZ Non-OR ØH9[TUVWX][378X]ZX Non-OR ØH9[TUVWX][Ø378X]ZZ

SECTION: Ø MEDICAL AND SURGICAL
BODY SYSTEM: H SKIN AND BREAST
OPERATION: B EXCISION: *(on multiple pages)*
Cutting out or off, without replacement, a portion of a body part

Body Part	Approach	Device	Qualifier
Ø Skin, Scalp 1 Skin, Face 2 Skin, Right Ear 3 Skin, Left Ear 4 Skin, Neck 5 Skin, Chest 6 Skin, Back 7 Skin, Abdomen 8 Skin, Buttock 9 Skin, Perineum A Skin, Inguinal B Skin, Right Upper Arm C Skin, Left Upper Arm D Skin, Right Lower Arm E Skin, Left Lower Arm F Skin, Right Hand G Skin, Left Hand H Skin, Right Upper Leg J Skin, Left Upper Leg K Skin, Right Lower Leg L Skin, Left Lower Leg M Skin, Right Foot N Skin, Left Foot Q Finger Nail R Toe Nail	X External	Z No Device	X Diagnostic Z No Qualifier

DRG Non-OR ØHB9XZZ
DRG Non-OR ØHB[Ø145678ABCDEFGHJKLMN]XZZ
Non-OR ØHB[Ø12456789ABCDEFGHJKLMNQR]XZX
Non-OR ØHB[23QR]XZZ
Coding Clinic: 2Ø16, Q3, P29 – ØHBJXZZ
Coding Clinic: 2Ø2Ø, Q1, P31 – ØHBHXZZ

SECTION: Ø MEDICAL AND SURGICAL
BODY SYSTEM: H SKIN AND BREAST
OPERATION: B EXCISION: *(continued)*
Cutting out or off, without replacement, a portion of a body part

Body Part	Approach	Device	Qualifier
T Breast, Right U Breast, Left V Breast, Bilateral Y Supernumerary Breast	Ø Open 3 Percutaneous 7 Via Natural or Artificial Opening 8 Via Natural or Artificial Opening Endoscopic X External	Z No Device	X Diagnostic Z No Qualifier
W Nipple, Right X Nipple, Left	Ø Open 3 Percutaneous 7 Via Natural or Artificial Opening 8 Via Natural or Artificial Opening Endoscopic X External	Z No Device	X Diagnostic Z No Qualifier

Non-OR ØHB[TUVWXY][378X]ZX

Coding Clinic: 2015, Q3, P3 – ØHB8XZZ
Coding Clinic: 2018, Q1, P15 – ØHBTØZZ
Coding Clinic: 2022, Q1, P14 – ØHBUØZZ

SECTION: Ø MEDICAL AND SURGICAL
BODY SYSTEM: H SKIN AND BREAST
OPERATION: C EXTIRPATION: *(on multiple pages)*
Taking or cutting out solid matter from a body part

Body Part	Approach	Device	Qualifier
Ø Skin, Scalp 1 Skin, Face 2 Skin, Right Ear 3 Skin, Left Ear 4 Skin, Neck 5 Skin, Chest 6 Skin, Back 7 Skin, Abdomen 8 Skin, Buttock 9 Skin, Perineum A Skin, Inguinal B Skin, Right Upper Arm C Skin, Left Upper Arm D Skin, Right Lower Arm E Skin, Left Lower Arm F Skin, Right Hand G Skin, Left Hand H Skin, Right Upper Leg J Skin, Left Upper Leg K Skin, Right Lower Leg L Skin, Left Lower Leg M Skin, Right Foot N Skin, Left Foot Q Finger Nail R Toe Nail	X External	Z No Device	Z No Qualifier
T Breast, Right U Breast, Left V Breast, Bilateral	Ø Open 3 Percutaneous 7 Via Natural or Artificial Opening 8 Via Natural or Artificial Opening Endoscopic X External	Z No Device	Z No Qualifier

Non-OR All Values

SECTION: Ø MEDICAL AND SURGICAL
BODY SYSTEM: H SKIN AND BREAST
OPERATION: C EXTIRPATION: *(continued)*
Taking or cutting out solid matter from a body part

Body Part	Approach	Device	Qualifier
W Nipple, Right X Nipple, Left	Ø Open 3 Percutaneous 7 Via Natural or Artificial Opening 8 Via Natural or Artificial Opening Endoscopic X External	Z No Device	Z No Qualifier

SECTION: Ø MEDICAL AND SURGICAL
BODY SYSTEM: H SKIN AND BREAST
OPERATION: D EXTRACTION: Pulling or stripping out or off all or a portion of a body part by the use of force

Body Part	Approach	Device	Qualifier
Ø Skin, Scalp 1 Skin, Face 2 Skin, Right Ear 3 Skin, Left Ear 4 Skin, Neck 5 Skin, Chest 6 Skin, Back 7 Skin, Abdomen 8 Skin, Buttock 9 Skin, Perineum A Skin, Inguinal B Skin, Right Upper Arm C Skin, Left Upper Arm D Skin, Right Lower Arm E Skin, Left Lower Arm F Skin, Right Hand G Skin, Left Hand H Skin, Right Upper Leg J Skin, Left Upper Leg K Skin, Right Lower Leg L Skin, Left Lower Leg M Skin, Right Foot N Skin, Left Foot Q Finger Nail R Toe Nail S Hair	X External	Z No Device	Z No Qualifier
T Breast, Right U Breast, Left V Breast, Bilateral Y Supernumerary Breast	Ø Open	Z No Device	Z No Qualifier

Non-OR All Values

Coding Clinic: 2015, Q3, P5-6 – ØHD[6H]XZZ

SECTION: Ø MEDICAL AND SURGICAL
BODY SYSTEM: H SKIN AND BREAST
OPERATION: H INSERTION: Putting in a nonbiological appliance that monitors, assists, performs, or prevents a physiological function but does not physically take the place of a body part

Body Part	Approach	Device	Qualifier
P Skin	X External	Y Other Device	Z No Qualifier
T Breast, Right U Breast, Left	Ø Open 3 Percutaneous 7 Via Natural or Artificial Opening 8 Via Natural or Artificial Opening Endoscopic	1 Radioactive Element N Tissue Expander Y Other Device	Z No Qualifier
T Breast, Right U Breast, Left	X External	1 Radioactive Element	Z No Qualifier
V Breast, Bilateral	Ø Open 3 Percutaneous 7 Via Natural or Artificial Opening 8 Via Natural or Artificial Opening Endoscopic	1 Radioactive Element N Tissue Expander	Z No Qualifier
W Nipple, Right X Nipple, Left	Ø Open 3 Percutaneous 7 Via Natural or Artificial Opening 8 Via Natural or Artificial Opening Endoscopic	1 Radioactive Element N Tissue Expander	Z No Qualifier
W Nipple, Right X Nipple, Left	X External	1 Radioactive Element	Z No Qualifier

Coding Clinic: 2Ø17, Q4, P67 – ØHHTØNZ

SECTION: Ø MEDICAL AND SURGICAL
BODY SYSTEM: H SKIN AND BREAST
OPERATION: J INSPECTION: Visually and/or manually exploring a body part

Body Part	Approach	Device	Qualifier
P Skin Q Finger Nail R Toe Nail	X External	Z No Device	Z No Qualifier
T Breast, Right U Breast, Left	Ø Open 3 Percutaneous 7 Via Natural or Artificial Opening 8 Via Natural or Artificial Opening Endoscopic	Z No Device	Z No Qualifier

Non-OR All Values

SECTION: Ø MEDICAL AND SURGICAL
BODY SYSTEM: H SKIN AND BREAST
OPERATION: M REATTACHMENT: Putting back in or on all or a portion of a separated body part to its normal location or other suitable location

Body Part	Approach	Device	Qualifier
Ø Skin, Scalp 1 Skin, Face 2 Skin, Right Ear 3 Skin, Left Ear 4 Skin, Neck 5 Skin, Chest 6 Skin, Back 7 Skin, Abdomen 8 Skin, Buttock 9 Skin, Perineum A Skin, Inguinal B Skin, Right Upper Arm C Skin, Left Upper Arm D Skin, Right Lower Arm E Skin, Left Lower Arm F Skin, Right Hand G Skin, Left Hand H Skin, Right Upper Leg J Skin, Left Upper Leg K Skin, Right Lower Leg L Skin, Left Lower Leg M Skin, Right Foot N Skin, Left Foot T Breast, Right U Breast, Left V Breast, Bilateral W Nipple, Right X Nipple, Left	X External	Z No Device	Z No Qualifier

Non-OR ØHMØXZZ

SECTION: Ø MEDICAL AND SURGICAL
BODY SYSTEM: H SKIN AND BREAST
OPERATION: N RELEASE: Freeing a body part from an abnormal physical constraint by cutting or by the use of force

Body Part	Approach	Device	Qualifier
Ø Skin, Scalp 1 Skin, Face 2 Skin, Right Ear 3 Skin, Left Ear 4 Skin, Neck 5 Skin, Chest 6 Skin, Back 7 Skin, Abdomen 8 Skin, Buttock 9 Skin, Perineum A Skin, Inguinal B Skin, Right Upper Arm C Skin, Left Upper Arm D Skin, Right Lower Arm E Skin, Left Lower Arm F Skin, Right Hand G Skin, Left Hand H Skin, Right Upper Leg J Skin, Left Upper Leg K Skin, Right Lower Leg L Skin, Left Lower Leg M Skin, Right Foot N Skin, Left Foot Q Finger Nail R Toe Nail	X External	Z No Device	Z No Qualifier
T Breast, Right U Breast, Left V Breast, Bilateral	Ø Open 3 Percutaneous 7 Via Natural or Artificial Opening 8 Via Natural or Artificial Opening Endoscopic X External	Z No Device	Z No Qualifier
W Nipple, Right X Nipple, Left	Ø Open 3 Percutaneous 7 Via Natural or Artificial Opening 8 Via Natural or Artificial Opening Endoscopic X External	Z No Device	Z No Qualifier

SECTION: Ø MEDICAL AND SURGICAL
BODY SYSTEM: H SKIN AND BREAST
OPERATION: P REMOVAL: Taking out or off a device from a body part

Body Part	Approach	Device	Qualifier
P Skin	X External	Ø Drainage Device 7 Autologous Tissue Substitute J Synthetic Substitute K Nonautologous Tissue Substitute Y Other Device	Z No Qualifier
Q Finger Nail R Toe Nail	X External	Ø Drainage Device 7 Autologous Tissue Substitute J Synthetic Substitute K Nonautologous Tissue Substitute	Z No Qualifier
S Hair	X External	7 Autologous Tissue Substitute J Synthetic Substitute K Nonautologous Tissue Substitute	Z No Qualifier
T Breast, Right U Breast, Left	Ø Open 3 Percutaneous 7 Via Natural or Artificial Opening 8 Via Natural or Artificial Opening Endoscopic	Ø Drainage Device 1 Radioactive Element 7 Autologous Tissue Substitute J Synthetic Substitute K Nonautologous Tissue Substitute N Tissue Expander Y Other Device	Z No Qualifier

Non-OR ØPHPX[Ø7JK]Z
Non-OR ØHP[QR]X[Ø7JK]Z
Non-OR ØHPSX[7JK]Z
Non-OR ØHP[TU][Ø3][Ø17K]Z
Non-OR ØHP[TU][78][Ø17JKN]Z

Coding Clinic: 2016, Q2, P27 – ØHP[TU]Ø7Z
Coding Clinic: 2022, Q3, P21 – ØHP[TU]ØNZ

Ø: M/S H: SKIN AND BREAST P: REMOVAL

SECTION: Ø MEDICAL AND SURGICAL
BODY SYSTEM: H SKIN AND BREAST
OPERATION: Q REPAIR: Restoring, to the extent possible, a body part to its normal anatomic structure and function

Body Part	Approach	Device	Qualifier
Ø Skin, Scalp 1 Skin, Face 2 Skin, Right Ear 3 Skin, Left Ear 4 Skin, Neck 5 Skin, Chest 6 Skin, Back 7 Skin, Abdomen 8 Skin, Buttock 9 Skin, Perineum A Skin, Inguinal B Skin, Right Upper Arm C Skin, Left Upper Arm D Skin, Right Lower Arm E Skin, Left Lower Arm F Skin, Right Hand G Skin, Left Hand H Skin, Right Upper Leg J Skin, Left Upper Leg K Skin, Right Lower Leg L Skin, Left Lower Leg M Skin, Right Foot N Skin, Left Foot Q Finger Nail R Toe Nail	X External	Z No Device	Z No Qualifier
T Breast, Right U Breast, Left V Breast, Bilateral Y Supernumerary Breast	Ø Open 3 Percutaneous 7 Via Natural or Artificial Opening 8 Via Natural or Artificial Opening Endoscopic X External	Z No Device	Z No Qualifier
W Nipple, Right X Nipple, Left	Ø Open 3 Percutaneous 7 Via Natural or Artificial Opening 8 Via Natural or Artificial Opening Endoscopic X External	Z No Device	Z No Qualifier

DRG Non-OR ØHQ9XZZ
Non-OR ØHQ[Ø12345678ABCDEFGHJKLMN]XZZ
Non-OR ØHQ[TUVY]XZZ

Coding Clinic: 2Ø16, Q1, P7 – ØHQ9XZZ

SECTION: Ø MEDICAL AND SURGICAL
BODY SYSTEM: H SKIN AND BREAST
OPERATION: R REPLACEMENT: *(on multiple pages)*

Putting in or on biological or synthetic material that physically takes the place and/or function of all or a portion of a body part

Body Part	Approach	Device	Qualifier
Ø Skin, Scalp 1 Skin, Face 2 Skin, Right Ear 3 Skin, Left Ear 4 Skin, Neck 5 Skin, Chest 6 Skin, Back 7 Skin, Abdomen 8 Skin, Buttock 9 Skin, Perineum A Skin, Inguinal B Skin, Right Upper Arm C Skin, Left Upper Arm D Skin, Right Lower Arm E Skin, Left Lower Arm F Skin, Right Hand G Skin, Left Hand H Skin, Right Upper Leg J Skin, Left Upper Leg K Skin, Right Lower Leg L Skin, Left Lower Leg M Skin, Right Foot N Skin, Left Foot	X External	7 Autologous Tissue Substitute	2 Cell Suspension Technique 3 Full Thickness 4 Partial Thickness
Ø Skin, Scalp 1 Skin, Face 2 Skin, Right Ear 3 Skin, Left Ear 4 Skin, Neck 5 Skin, Chest 6 Skin, Back 7 Skin, Abdomen 8 Skin, Buttock 9 Skin, Perineum A Skin, Inguinal B Skin, Right Upper Arm C Skin, Left Upper Arm D Skin, Right Lower Arm E Skin, Left Lower Arm F Skin, Right Hand G Skin, Left Hand H Skin, Right Upper Leg J Skin, Left Upper Leg K Skin, Right Lower Leg L Skin, Left Lower Leg M Skin, Right Foot N Skin, Left Foot	X External	J Synthetic Substitute	3 Full Thickness 4 Partial Thickness Z No Qualifier

Non-OR ØHRSX7Z

Coding Clinic: 2Ø17, Q1, P36 – ØHRMXK3

SECTION: Ø MEDICAL AND SURGICAL
BODY SYSTEM: H SKIN AND BREAST
OPERATION: R REPLACEMENT: *(continued)*

Putting in or on biological or synthetic material that physically takes the place and/or function of all or a portion of a body part

Body Part	Approach	Device	Qualifier
Ø Skin, Scalp 1 Skin, Face 2 Skin, Right Ear 3 Skin, Left Ear 4 Skin, Neck 5 Skin, Chest 6 Skin, Back 7 Skin, Abdomen 8 Skin, Buttock 9 Skin, Perineum A Skin, Inguinal B Skin, Right Upper Arm C Skin, Left Upper Arm D Skin, Right Lower Arm E Skin, Left Lower Arm F Skin, Right Hand G Skin, Left Hand H Skin, Right Upper Leg J Skin, Left Upper Leg K Skin, Right Lower Leg L Skin, Left Lower Leg M Skin, Right Foot N Skin, Left Foot	X External	K Nonautologous Tissue Substitute	3 Full Thickness 4 Partial Thickness
Q Finger Nail R Toe Nail S Hair	X External	7 Autologous Tissue Substitute J Synthetic Substitute K Nonautologous Tissue Substitute	Z No Qualifier
T Breast, Right U Breast, Left V Breast, Bilateral	Ø Open	7 Autologous Tissue Substitute	5 Latissimus Dorsi Myocutaneous Flap 6 Transverse Rectus Abdominis Myocutaneous Flap 7 Deep Inferior Epigastric Artery Perforator Flap 8 Superficial Inferior Epigastric Artery Flap 9 Gluteal Artery Perforator Flap B Lumbar Artery Perforator Flap Z No Qualifier
T Breast, Right U Breast, Left V Breast, Bilateral	Ø Open	J Synthetic Substitute K Nonautologous Tissue Substitute	Z No Qualifier
T Breast, Right ⊞ U Breast, Left ⊞ V Breast, Bilateral ⊞	3 Percutaneous	7 Autologous Tissue Substitute J Synthetic Substitute K Nonautologous Tissue Substitute	Z No Qualifier
W Nipple, Right X Nipple, Left	Ø Open 3 Percutaneous X External	7 Autologous Tissue Substitute J Synthetic Substitute K Nonautologous Tissue Substitute	Z No Qualifier

⊞ ØHR[TUV]37Z

Coding Clinic: 2020, Q1, P27 – ØHRU07Z

Coding Clinic: 2022, Q1, P15 – ØHRX07Z

New/Revised Text in Green ~~deleted~~ Deleted ♀ Females Only ♂ Males Only Coding Clinic
Non-covered Limited Coverage ⊞ Combination (See Appendix E) DRG Non-OR Non-OR Hospital-Acquired Condition

SECTION: Ø MEDICAL AND SURGICAL
BODY SYSTEM: H SKIN AND BREAST
OPERATION: S REPOSITION: Moving to its normal location, or other suitable location, all or a portion of a body part

Body Part	Approach	Device	Qualifier
S Hair W Nipple, Right X Nipple, Left	X External	Z No Device	Z No Qualifier
T Breast, Right U Breast, Left V Breast, Bilateral	Ø Open	Z No Device	Z No Qualifier

Non-OR ØHSSXZZ

SECTION: Ø MEDICAL AND SURGICAL
BODY SYSTEM: H SKIN AND BREAST
OPERATION: T RESECTION: Cutting out or off, without replacement, all of a body part

Body Part	Approach	Device	Qualifier
Q Finger Nail R Toe Nail W Nipple, Right X Nipple, Left	X External	Z No Device	Z No Qualifier
T Breast, Right ⊞ U Breast, Left ⊞ V Breast, Bilateral ⊞ Y Supernumerary Breast	Ø Open	Z No Device	Z No Qualifier

⊞ ØHT[TUV]ØZZ
Non-OR ØHT[QR]XZZ

Coding Clinic: 2021, Q2, P16 – ØHTVØZZ

SECTION: Ø MEDICAL AND SURGICAL
BODY SYSTEM: H SKIN AND BREAST
OPERATION: U SUPPLEMENT: Putting in or on biological or synthetic material that physically reinforces and/or augments the function of a portion of a body part

Body Part	Approach	Device	Qualifier
T Breast, Right U Breast, Left V Breast, Bilateral	Ø Open 3 Percutaneous 7 Via Natural of Artificial Opening 8 Via Natural or Artificial Opening Endoscopic	7 Autologous Tissue Substitute J Synthetic Substitute K Nonautologous Tissue Substitute	Z No Qualifier
W Nipple, Right X Nipple, Left	Ø Open 3 Percutaneous 7 Via Natural or Artificial Opening 8 Via Natural or Artificial Opening Endoscopic X External	7 Autologous Tissue Substitute J Synthetic Substitute K Nonautologous Tissue Substitute	Z No Qualifier

SECTION: Ø MEDICAL AND SURGICAL
BODY SYSTEM: H SKIN AND BREAST
OPERATION: W REVISION: Correcting, to the extent possible, a portion of a malfunctioning device or the position of a displaced device

Body Part	Approach	Device	Qualifier
P Skin	X External	Ø Drainage Device 7 Autologous Tissue Substitute J Synthetic Substitute K Nonautologous Tissue Substitute Y Other Device	Z No Qualifier
Q Finger Nail R Toe Nail	X External	Ø Drainage Device 7 Autologous Tissue Substitute J Synthetic Substitute K Nonautologous Tissue Substitute	Z No Qualifier
S Hair	X External	7 Autologous Tissue Substitute J Synthetic Substitute K Nonautologous Tissue Substitute	Z No Qualifier
T Breast, Right U Breast, Left	Ø Open 3 Percutaneous 7 Via Natural or Artificial Opening 8 Via Natural or Artificial Opening Endoscopic	Ø Drainage Device 7 Autologous Tissue Substitute J Synthetic Substitute K Nonautologous Tissue Substitute N Tissue Expander Y Other Device	Z No Qualifier

Non-OR ØHWPX[Ø7JK]Z
Non-OR ØHW[QR]X[Ø7JK]Z
Non-OR ØHWSX[7JK]Z
Non-OR ØHW[TU][Ø3][Ø7KN]Z
Non-OR ØHW[TU][78][Ø7JKN]Z

SECTION: Ø MEDICAL AND SURGICAL
BODY SYSTEM: H SKIN AND BREAST
OPERATION: X TRANSFER: Moving, without taking out, all or a portion of a body part to another location to take over the function of all or a portion of a body part

Body Part	Approach	Device	Qualifier
Ø Skin, Scalp 1 Skin, Face 2 Skin, Right Ear 3 Skin, Left Ear 4 Skin, Neck 5 Skin, Chest 6 Skin, Back 7 Skin, Abdomen 8 Skin, Buttock 9 Skin, Perineum A Skin, Inguinal B Skin, Right Upper Arm C Skin, Left Upper Arm D Skin, Right Lower Arm E Skin, Left Lower Arm F Skin, Right Hand G Skin, Left Hand H Skin, Right Upper Leg J Skin, Left Upper Leg K Skin, Right Lower Leg L Skin, Left Lower Leg M Skin, Right Foot N Skin, Left Foot	X External	Z No Device	Z No Qualifier

Coding Clinic: 2Ø23, Q2, P24,31; 2Ø22, Q3, P14 – ØHX9XZZ

ØJ. Subcutaneous Tissue and Fascia 31Ø
ØJØ. Alteration 311
ØJ2. Change 311
ØJ5. Destruction 312
ØJ8. Division 313
ØJ9. Drainage 314
ØJB. Excision 316
ØJC. Extirpation 317
ØJD. Extraction 318
ØJH. Insertion 319
ØJJ. Inspection 321
ØJN. Release 321
ØJP. Removal 322
ØJQ. Repair 323
ØJR. Replacement 324
ØJU. Supplement 325
ØJW. Revision 326
ØJX. Transfer 328

SECTION: Ø MEDICAL AND SURGICAL
BODY SYSTEM: J SUBCUTANEOUS TISSUE AND FASCIA
OPERATION: Ø ALTERATION: Modifying the anatomic structure of a body part without affecting the function of the body part

Body Part	Approach	Device	Qualifier
1 Subcutaneous Tissue and Fascia, Face 4 Subcutaneous Tissue and Fascia, Right Neck 5 Subcutaneous Tissue and Fascia, Left Neck 6 Subcutaneous Tissue and Fascia, Chest 7 Subcutaneous Tissue and Fascia, Back 8 Subcutaneous Tissue and Fascia, Abdomen 9 Subcutaneous Tissue and Fascia, Buttock D Subcutaneous Tissue and Fascia, Right Upper Arm F Subcutaneous Tissue and Fascia, Left Upper Arm G Subcutaneous Tissue and Fascia, Right Lower Arm H Subcutaneous Tissue and Fascia, Left Lower Arm L Subcutaneous Tissue and Fascia, Right Upper Leg M Subcutaneous Tissue and Fascia, Left Upper Leg N Subcutaneous Tissue and Fascia, Right Lower Leg P Subcutaneous Tissue and Fascia, Left Lower Leg	Ø Open 3 Percutaneous	Z No Device	Z No Qualifier

SECTION: Ø MEDICAL AND SURGICAL
BODY SYSTEM: J SUBCUTANEOUS TISSUE AND FASCIA
OPERATION: 2 CHANGE: Taking out or off a device from a body part and putting back an identical or similar device in or on the same body part without cutting or puncturing the skin or a mucous membrane

Body Part	Approach	Device	Qualifier
S Subcutaneous Tissue and Fascia, Head and Neck T Subcutaneous Tissue and Fascia, Trunk V Subcutaneous Tissue and Fascia, Upper Extremity W Subcutaneous Tissue and Fascia, Lower Extremity	X External	Ø Drainage Device Y Other Device	Z No Qualifier

Non-OR All Values

Coding Clinic: 2017, Q2, P25 – ØJ2TXYZ

SECTION: Ø MEDICAL AND SURGICAL
BODY SYSTEM: J SUBCUTANEOUS TISSUE AND FASCIA
OPERATION: 5 DESTRUCTION: Physical eradication of all or a portion of a body part by the direct use of energy, force, or a destructive agent

Body Part	Approach	Device	Qualifier
Ø Subcutaneous Tissue and Fascia, Scalp 1 Subcutaneous Tissue and Fascia, Face 4 Subcutaneous Tissue and Fascia, Right Neck 5 Subcutaneous Tissue and Fascia, Left Neck 6 Subcutaneous Tissue and Fascia, Chest 7 Subcutaneous Tissue and Fascia, Back 8 Subcutaneous Tissue and Fascia, Abdomen 9 Subcutaneous Tissue and Fascia, Buttock B Subcutaneous Tissue and Fascia, Perineum C Subcutaneous Tissue and Fascia, Pelvic Region D Subcutaneous Tissue and Fascia, Right Upper Arm F Subcutaneous Tissue and Fascia, Left Upper Arm G Subcutaneous Tissue and Fascia, Right Lower Arm H Subcutaneous Tissue and Fascia, Left Lower Arm J Subcutaneous Tissue and Fascia, Right Hand K Subcutaneous Tissue and Fascia, Left Hand L Subcutaneous Tissue and Fascia, Right Upper Leg M Subcutaneous Tissue and Fascia, Left Upper Leg N Subcutaneous Tissue and Fascia, Right Lower Leg P Subcutaneous Tissue and Fascia, Left Lower Leg Q Subcutaneous Tissue and Fascia, Right Foot R Subcutaneous Tissue and Fascia, Left Foot	Ø Open 3 Percutaneous	Z No Device	Z No Qualifier

DRG Non-OR All Values

SECTION: Ø MEDICAL AND SURGICAL
BODY SYSTEM: J SUBCUTANEOUS TISSUE AND FASCIA
OPERATION: 8 DIVISION: Cutting into a body part, without draining fluids and/or gases from the body part, in order to separate or transect a body part

Body Part	Approach	Device	Qualifier
Ø Subcutaneous Tissue and Fascia, Scalp 1 Subcutaneous Tissue and Fascia, Face 4 Subcutaneous Tissue and Fascia, Right Neck 5 Subcutaneous Tissue and Fascia, Left Neck 6 Subcutaneous Tissue and Fascia, Chest 7 Subcutaneous Tissue and Fascia, Back 8 Subcutaneous Tissue and Fascia, Abdomen 9 Subcutaneous Tissue and Fascia, Buttock B Subcutaneous Tissue and Fascia, Perineum C Subcutaneous Tissue and Fascia, Pelvic Region D Subcutaneous Tissue and Fascia, Right Upper Arm F Subcutaneous Tissue and Fascia, Left Upper Arm G Subcutaneous Tissue and Fascia, Right Lower Arm H Subcutaneous Tissue and Fascia, Left Lower Arm J Subcutaneous Tissue and Fascia, Right Hand K Subcutaneous Tissue and Fascia, Left Hand L Subcutaneous Tissue and Fascia, Right Upper Leg M Subcutaneous Tissue and Fascia, Left Upper Leg N Subcutaneous Tissue and Fascia, Right Lower Leg P Subcutaneous Tissue and Fascia, Left Lower Leg Q Subcutaneous Tissue and Fascia, Right Foot R Subcutaneous Tissue and Fascia, Left Foot S Subcutaneous Tissue and Fascia, Head and Neck T Subcutaneous Tissue and Fascia, Trunk V Subcutaneous Tissue and Fascia, Upper Extremity W Subcutaneous Tissue and Fascia, Lower Extremity	Ø Open 3 Percutaneous	Z No Device	Z No Qualifier

SECTION: Ø MEDICAL AND SURGICAL
BODY SYSTEM: J SUBCUTANEOUS TISSUE AND FASCIA
OPERATION: 9 DRAINAGE: *(on multiple pages)*
Taking or letting out fluids and/or gases from a body part

Body Part	Approach	Device	Qualifier
Ø Subcutaneous Tissue and Fascia, Scalp 1 Subcutaneous Tissue and Fascia, Face 4 Subcutaneous Tissue and Fascia, Right Neck 5 Subcutaneous Tissue and Fascia, Left Neck 6 Subcutaneous Tissue and Fascia, Chest 7 Subcutaneous Tissue and Fascia, Back 8 Subcutaneous Tissue and Fascia, Abdomen 9 Subcutaneous Tissue and Fascia, Buttock B Subcutaneous Tissue and Fascia, Perineum C Subcutaneous Tissue and Fascia, Pelvic Region D Subcutaneous Tissue and Fascia, Right Upper Arm F Subcutaneous Tissue and Fascia, Left Upper Arm G Subcutaneous Tissue and Fascia, Right Lower Arm H Subcutaneous Tissue and Fascia, Left Lower Arm J Subcutaneous Tissue and Fascia, Right Hand K Subcutaneous Tissue and Fascia, Left Hand L Subcutaneous Tissue and Fascia, Right Upper Leg M Subcutaneous Tissue and Fascia, Left Upper Leg N Subcutaneous Tissue and Fascia, Right Lower Leg P Subcutaneous Tissue and Fascia, Left Lower Leg Q Subcutaneous Tissue and Fascia, Right Foot R Subcutaneous Tissue and Fascia, Left Foot	Ø Open 3 Percutaneous	Ø Drainage Device	Z No Qualifier

DRG Non-OR ØJ9[1]ØØZ
Non-OR ØJ9[1JK]3ØZ
Non-OR ØJ9[Ø456789BCDFGHJKLMNPQR][Ø3]ØZ

SECTION: Ø MEDICAL AND SURGICAL
BODY SYSTEM: J SUBCUTANEOUS TISSUE AND FASCIA
OPERATION: 9 DRAINAGE: *(continued)*
Taking or letting out fluids and/or gases from a body part

Body Part	Approach	Device	Qualifier
Ø Subcutaneous Tissue and Fascia, Scalp 1 Subcutaneous Tissue and Fascia, Face 4 Subcutaneous Tissue and Fascia, Right Neck 5 Subcutaneous Tissue and Fascia, Left Neck 6 Subcutaneous Tissue and Fascia, Chest 7 Subcutaneous Tissue and Fascia, Back 8 Subcutaneous Tissue and Fascia, Abdomen 9 Subcutaneous Tissue and Fascia, Buttock B Subcutaneous Tissue and Fascia, Perineum C Subcutaneous Tissue and Fascia, Pelvic Region D Subcutaneous Tissue and Fascia, Right Upper Arm F Subcutaneous Tissue and Fascia, Left Upper Arm G Subcutaneous Tissue and Fascia, Right Lower Arm H Subcutaneous Tissue and Fascia, Left Lower Arm J Subcutaneous Tissue and Fascia, Right Hand K Subcutaneous Tissue and Fascia, Left Hand L Subcutaneous Tissue and Fascia, Right Upper Leg M Subcutaneous Tissue and Fascia, Left Upper Leg N Subcutaneous Tissue and Fascia, Right Lower Leg P Subcutaneous Tissue and Fascia, Left Lower Leg Q Subcutaneous Tissue and Fascia, Right Foot R Subcutaneous Tissue and Fascia, Left Foot	Ø Open 3 Percutaneous	Z No Device	X Diagnostic Z No Qualifier

DRG Non-OR ØJ9[Ø1456789BCDFGHLMNPQR]ØZZ
Non-OR ØJ9[Ø1456789BCDFGHJKLMNPQR][Ø3]ZX
Non-OR ØJ9[Ø1456789BCDFGHJKLMNPQR]3ZZ

Coding Clinic: 2Ø15, Q3, P24 – ØJ9[6CDFLM]ØZZ

SECTION: Ø MEDICAL AND SURGICAL
BODY SYSTEM: J SUBCUTANEOUS TISSUE AND FASCIA
OPERATION: B EXCISION: Cutting out or off, without replacement, a portion of a body part

Body Part	Approach	Device	Qualifier
Ø Subcutaneous Tissue and Fascia, Scalp 1 Subcutaneous Tissue and Fascia, Face 4 Subcutaneous Tissue and Fascia, Right Neck 5 Subcutaneous Tissue and Fascia, Left Neck 6 Subcutaneous Tissue and Fascia, Chest 7 Subcutaneous Tissue and Fascia, Back 8 Subcutaneous Tissue and Fascia, Abdomen 9 Subcutaneous Tissue and Fascia, Buttock B Subcutaneous Tissue and Fascia, Perineum C Subcutaneous Tissue and Fascia, Pelvic Region D Subcutaneous Tissue and Fascia, Right Upper Arm F Subcutaneous Tissue and Fascia, Left Upper Arm G Subcutaneous Tissue and Fascia, Right Lower Arm H Subcutaneous Tissue and Fascia, Left Lower Arm J Subcutaneous Tissue and Fascia, Right Hand K Subcutaneous Tissue and Fascia, Left Hand L Subcutaneous Tissue and Fascia, Right Upper Leg M Subcutaneous Tissue and Fascia, Left Upper Leg N Subcutaneous Tissue and Fascia, Right Lower Leg P Subcutaneous Tissue and Fascia, Left Lower Leg Q Subcutaneous Tissue and Fascia, Right Foot R Subcutaneous Tissue and Fascia, Left Foot	Ø Open 3 Percutaneous	Z No Device	X Diagnostic Z No Qualifier

DRG Non-OR ØJB[Ø456789BCDFGHLMNPQR]3ZZ
Non-OR ØJB[Ø1456789BCDFGHJKLMNPQR][Ø3]ZX

Coding Clinic: 2015, Q1, P3Ø – ØJBBØZZ
Coding Clinic: 2015, Q2, P13 – ØJBHØZZ
Coding Clinic: 2015, Q3, P7 – ØJB9ØZZ
Coding Clinic: 2023, Q2, P3Ø; 2018, Q1, P7 – ØJB7ØZZ
Coding Clinic: 2019, Q3, P25 – ØJB93ZZ
Coding Clinic: 202Ø, Q1, P31 – ØJB8ØZZ
Coding Clinic: 2022, Q3, P13 – ØJBLØZZ

SECTION: Ø MEDICAL AND SURGICAL
BODY SYSTEM: J SUBCUTANEOUS TISSUE AND FASCIA
OPERATION: C EXTIRPATION: Taking or cutting out solid matter from a body part

Body Part	Approach	Device	Qualifier
Ø Subcutaneous Tissue and Fascia, Scalp 1 Subcutaneous Tissue and Fascia, Face 4 Subcutaneous Tissue and Fascia, Right Neck 5 Subcutaneous Tissue and Fascia, Left Neck 6 Subcutaneous Tissue and Fascia, Chest 7 Subcutaneous Tissue and Fascia, Back 8 Subcutaneous Tissue and Fascia, Abdomen 9 Subcutaneous Tissue and Fascia, Buttock B Subcutaneous Tissue and Fascia, Perineum C Subcutaneous Tissue and Fascia, Pelvic Region D Subcutaneous Tissue and Fascia, Right Upper Arm F Subcutaneous Tissue and Fascia, Left Upper Arm G Subcutaneous Tissue and Fascia, Right Lower Arm H Subcutaneous Tissue and Fascia, Left Lower Arm J Subcutaneous Tissue and Fascia, Right Hand K Subcutaneous Tissue and Fascia, Left Hand L Subcutaneous Tissue and Fascia, Right Upper Leg M Subcutaneous Tissue and Fascia, Left Upper Leg N Subcutaneous Tissue and Fascia, Right Lower Leg P Subcutaneous Tissue and Fascia, Left Lower Leg Q Subcutaneous Tissue and Fascia, Right Foot R Subcutaneous Tissue and Fascia, Left Foot	Ø Open 3 Percutaneous	Z No Device	Z No Qualifier

Non-OR All Values

Coding Clinic: 2Ø17, Q3, P22 – ØJC8ØZZ

SECTION: Ø MEDICAL AND SURGICAL
BODY SYSTEM: J SUBCUTANEOUS TISSUE AND FASCIA
OPERATION: D EXTRACTION: Pulling or stripping out or off all or a portion of a body part by the use of force

Body Part	Approach	Device	Qualifier
Ø Subcutaneous Tissue and Fascia, Scalp 1 Subcutaneous Tissue and Fascia, Face 4 Subcutaneous Tissue and Fascia, Right Neck 5 Subcutaneous Tissue and Fascia, Left Neck 6 Subcutaneous Tissue and Fascia, Chest ⊞ 7 Subcutaneous Tissue and Fascia, Back ⊞ 8 Subcutaneous Tissue and Fascia, Abdomen ⊞ 9 Subcutaneous Tissue and Fascia, Buttock ⊞ B Subcutaneous Tissue and Fascia, Perineum C Subcutaneous Tissue and Fascia, Pelvic Region D Subcutaneous Tissue and Fascia, Right Upper Arm F Subcutaneous Tissue and Fascia, Left Upper Arm G Subcutaneous Tissue and Fascia, Right Lower Arm H Subcutaneous Tissue and Fascia, Left Lower Arm J Subcutaneous Tissue and Fascia, Right Hand K Subcutaneous Tissue and Fascia, Left Hand L Subcutaneous Tissue and Fascia, Right Upper Leg ⊞ M Subcutaneous Tissue and Fascia, Left Upper Leg ⊞ N Subcutaneous Tissue and Fascia, Right Lower Leg P Subcutaneous Tissue and Fascia, Left Lower Leg Q Subcutaneous Tissue and Fascia, Right Foot R Subcutaneous Tissue and Fascia, Left Foot	Ø Open 3 Percutaneous	Z No Device	Z No Qualifier

⊞ ØJD[6789LM]3ZZ
DRG Non-OR ØJD[Ø1456789BCDFGHJKLMNPQR][Ø3]ZZ

Coding Clinic: 2Ø15, Q1, P23 – ØJDCØZZ
Coding Clinic: 2Ø16, Q1, P4Ø – ØJDLØZZ
Coding Clinic: 2Ø16, Q3, P21-22 – ØJD[7NR]ØZZ
Coding Clinic: 2Ø23, Q1, P36 – ØJDRØZZ

SECTION: Ø MEDICAL AND SURGICAL
BODY SYSTEM: J SUBCUTANEOUS TISSUE AND FASCIA
OPERATION: H INSERTION: *(on multiple pages)*

Putting in a nonbiological appliance that monitors, assists, performs, or prevents a physiological function but does not physically take the place of a body part

Body Part	Approach	Device	Qualifier
Ø Subcutaneous Tissue and Fascia, Scalp 1 Subcutaneous Tissue and Fascia, Face 4 Subcutaneous Tissue and Fascia, Right Neck 5 Subcutaneous Tissue and Fascia, Left Neck 9 Subcutaneous Tissue and Fascia, Buttock B Subcutaneous Tissue and Fascia, Perineum C Subcutaneous Tissue and Fascia, Pelvic Region J Subcutaneous Tissue and Fascia, Right Hand K Subcutaneous Tissue and Fascia, Left Hand Q Subcutaneous Tissue and Fascia, Right Foot R Subcutaneous Tissue and Fascia, Left Foot	Ø Open 3 Percutaneous	N Tissue Expander	Z No Qualifer
6 Subcutaneous Tissue and Fascia, Chest	Ø Open 3 Percutaneous	Ø Monitoring Device, Hemodynamic 2 Monitoring Device 4 Pacemaker, Single Chamber 5 Pacemaker, Single Chamber Rate Responsive 6 Pacemaker, Dual Chamber 7 Cardiac Resynchronization Pacemaker Pulse Generator 8 Defibrillator Generator 9 Cardiac Resynchronization Defibrillator Pulse Generator A Contractility Modulation Device B Stimulator Generator, Single Array C Stimulator Generator, Single Array Rechargeable D Stimulator Generator, Multiple Array E Stimulator Generator, Multiple Array Rechargeable F Subcutaneous Defibrillator Lead H Contraceptive Device M Stimulator Generator N Tissue Expander P Cardiac Rhythm Related Device V Infusion Device, Pump W Vascular Access Device, Totally Implantable X Vascular Access Device, Tunneled Y Other Device	Z No Qualifier
7 Subcutaneous Tissue and Fascia, Back	Ø Open 3 Percutaneous	B Stimulator Generator, Single Array C Stimulator Generator, Single Array Rechargeable D Stimulator Generator, Multiple Array E Stimulator Generator, Multiple Array Rechargeable M Stimulator Generator N Tissue Expander V Infusion Device, Pump Y Other Device	Z No Qualifier

ØJH[7][Ø3]MZ
ØJH[6][Ø3][Ø456789ABCDEF]Z
ØJH7[3][BCDE]Z
DRG Non-OR ØJH[6][Ø3][4567HPWX]Z
ØJH[6][Ø3][456789P]Z when reported with Secondary Diagnosis K68.11, T81.4XXA, or T82.7XXA, except ØJH63XZ
ØJH63XZ when reported with Secondary Diagnosis J95.811

Coding Clinic: 2Ø15, Q2, P33 – ØJH6ØXZ
Coding Clinic: 2Ø15, Q4, P15 – ØJH63VZ
Coding Clinic: 2Ø17, Q2, P25; 2Ø16, Q2, P16; 2Ø15, Q4, P31-32 – ØJH63XZ
Coding Clinic: 2Ø16, Q4, P99 – ØJH6ØMZ
Coding Clinic: 2Ø17, Q4, P64 – ØJH6ØWZ
Coding Clinic: 2Ø2Ø, Q2, P16 – ØJHS33Z
Coding Clinic: 2Ø2Ø, Q2, P17 – ØØHTØ3Z
Coding Clinic: 2Ø24, Q2, P3Ø – ØHJ637Z

SECTION: Ø MEDICAL AND SURGICAL
BODY SYSTEM: J SUBCUTANEOUS TISSUE AND FASCIA
OPERATION: H INSERTION: *(continued)*

Putting in a nonbiological appliance that monitors, assists, performs, or prevents a physiological function but does not physically take the place of a body part

Body Part	Approach	Device	Qualifier
8 Subcutaneous Tissue and Fascia, Abdomen ⊞	Ø Open 3 Percutaneous	Ø Monitoring Device, Hemodynamic 2 Monitoring Device 4 Pacemaker, Single Chamber 5 Pacemaker, Single Chamber Rate Responsive 6 Pacemaker, Dual Chamber 7 Cardiac Resynchronization Pacemaker Pulse Generator 8 Defibrillator Generator 9 Cardiac Resynchronization Defibrillator Pulse Generator A Contractility Modulation Device B Stimulator Generator, Single Array C Stimulator Generator, Single Array Rechargeable D Stimulator Generator, Multiple Array E Stimulator Generator, Multiple Array Rechargeable H Contraceptive Device M Stimulator Generator N Tissue Expander P Cardiac Rhythm Related Device V Infusion Device, Pump W Vascular Access Device, Totally Implantable X Vascular Access Device, Tunneled Y Other Device	Z No Qualifier
D Subcutaneous Tissue and Fascia, Right Upper Arm F Subcutaneous Tissue and Fascia, Left Upper Arm G Subcutaneous Tissue and Fascia, Right Lower Arm H Subcutaneous Tissue and Fascia, Left Lower Arm L Subcutaneous Tissue and Fascia, Right Upper Leg M Subcutaneous Tissue and Fascia, Left Upper Leg N Subcutaneous Tissue and Fascia, Right Lower Leg P Subcutaneous Tissue and Fascia, Left Lower Leg	Ø Open 3 Percutaneous	H Contraceptive Device N Tissue Expander V Infusion Device, Pump W Vascular Access Device, Totally Implantable X Vascular Access Device, Tunneled	Z No Qualifier
S Subcutaneous Tissue and Fascia, Head and Neck V Subcutaneous Tissue and Fascia, Upper Extremity W Subcutaneous Tissue and Fascia, Lower Extremity	Ø Open 3 Percutaneous	1 Radioactive Element 3 Infusion Device Y Other Device	Z No Qualifier
T Subcutaneous Tissue and Fascia, Trunk	Ø Open 3 Percutaneous	1 Radioactive Element 3 Infusion Device V Infusion Device, Pump Y Other Device	Z No Qualifier

ØJH[8][Ø3]MZ
⊞ ØJH8[Ø3][Ø456789ABCDEP]Z
DRG Non-OR ØJH[DFGHLM][Ø3][WX]Z
DRG Non-OR ØJHNØ[WX]Z
DRG Non-OR ØJHN3[HWX]Z
DRG Non-OR ØJHP[Ø3][HWX]Z
DRG Non-OR ØJH[SVW][Ø3]3Z
DRG Non-OR ØJHT[Ø3]3Z
DRG Non-OR ØJH8[Ø3][2456789ABCDEHPWX]Z

Non-OR ØJH[DFGHLM][Ø3]HZ
Non-OR ØJHNØHZ
Non-OR ØJH[SVW][Ø3]3Z
Non-OR ØJHT[Ø3]3Z

ØJH8[Ø3][89]Z

Coding Clinic: 2012, Q4, P1Ø5 – ØJH6Ø8Z & ØJH6ØPZ
Coding Clinic: 2016, Q2, P14 – ØJH8ØWZ
Coding Clinic: 2018, Q4, P43 – ØJHTØYZ

SECTION: Ø MEDICAL AND SURGICAL
BODY SYSTEM: J SUBCUTANEOUS TISSUE AND FASCIA
OPERATION: J INSPECTION: Visually and/or manually exploring a body part

Body Part	Approach	Device	Qualifier
S Subcutaneous Tissue and Fascia, Head and Neck T Subcutaneous Tissue and Fascia, Trunk V Subcutaneous Tissue and Fascia, Upper Extremity W Subcutaneous Tissue and Fascia, Lower Extremity	Ø Open 3 Percutaneous X External	Z No Device	Z No Qualifier

Non-OR All Values

SECTION: Ø MEDICAL AND SURGICAL
BODY SYSTEM: J SUBCUTANEOUS TISSUE AND FASCIA
OPERATION: N RELEASE: Freeing a body part from an abnormal physical constraint by cutting or by the use of force

Body Part	Approach	Device	Qualifier
Ø Subcutaneous Tissue and Fascia, Scalp 1 Subcutaneous Tissue and Fascia, Face 4 Subcutaneous Tissue and Fascia, Right Neck 5 Subcutaneous Tissue and Fascia, Left Neck 6 Subcutaneous Tissue and Fascia, Chest 7 Subcutaneous Tissue and Fascia, Back 8 Subcutaneous Tissue and Fascia, Abdomen 9 Subcutaneous Tissue and Fascia, Buttock B Subcutaneous Tissue and Fascia, Perineum C Subcutaneous Tissue and Fascia, Pelvic Region D Subcutaneous Tissue and Fascia, Right Upper Arm F Subcutaneous Tissue and Fascia, Left Upper Arm G Subcutaneous Tissue and Fascia, Right Lower Arm H Subcutaneous Tissue and Fascia, Left Lower Arm J Subcutaneous Tissue and Fascia, Right Hand K Subcutaneous Tissue and Fascia, Left Hand L Subcutaneous Tissue and Fascia, Right Upper Leg M Subcutaneous Tissue and Fascia, Left Upper Leg N Subcutaneous Tissue and Fascia, Right Lower Leg P Subcutaneous Tissue and Fascia, Left Lower Leg Q Subcutaneous Tissue and Fascia, Right Foot R Subcutaneous Tissue and Fascia, Left Foot	Ø Open 3 Percutaneous X External	Z No Device	Z No Qualifier

Non-OR ØJN[1456789BCDFGHJKLMNPQR]XZZ

Coding Clinic: 2017, Q3, P12 – ØJN[LMNPQR]ØZZ

SECTION: Ø MEDICAL AND SURGICAL
BODY SYSTEM: J SUBCUTANEOUS TISSUE AND FASCIA
OPERATION: P REMOVAL: Taking out or off a device from a body part

Body Part	Approach	Device	Qualifier
S Subcutaneous Tissue and Fascia, Head and Neck	Ø Open 3 Percutaneous	Ø Drainage Device 1 Radioactive Element 3 Infusion Device 7 Autologous Tissue Substitute J Synthetic Substitute K Nonautologous Tissue Substitute N Tissue Expander Y Other Device	Z No Qualifier
S Subcutaneous Tissue and Fascia, Head and Neck	X External	Ø Drainage Device 1 Radioactive Element 3 Infusion Device	Z No Qualifier
T Subcutaneous Tissue and Fascia, Trunk	Ø Open 3 Percutaneous	Ø Drainage Device 1 Radioactive Element 2 Monitoring Device 3 Infusion Device 7 Autologous Tissue Substitute F Subcutaneous Defibrillator H Contraceptive Device J Synthetic Substitute K Nonautologous Tissue Substitute M Stimulator Generator N Tissue Expander P Cardiac Rhythm Related Device V Infusion Device, Pump W Vascular Access Device, Totally Implantable X Vascular Access Device, Tunneled Y Other Device	Z No Qualifier
T Subcutaneous Tissue and Fascia, Trunk	X External	Ø Drainage Device 1 Radioactive Element 2 Monitoring Device 3 Infusion Device H Contraceptive Device V Infusion Device, Pump X Vascular Access Device, Tunneled	Z No Qualifier
V Subcutaneous Tissue and Fascia, Upper Extremity W Subcutaneous Tissue and Fascia, Lower Extremity	Ø Open 3 Percutaneous	Ø Drainage Device 1 Radioactive Element 3 Infusion Device 7 Autologous Tissue Substitute H Contraceptive Device J Synthetic Substitute K Nonautologous Tissue Substitute N Tissue Expander V Infusion Device, Pump W Vascular Access Device, Totally Implantable X Vascular Access Device, Tunneled Y Other Device	Z No Qualifier
V Subcutaneous Tissue and Fascia, Upper Extremity W Subcutaneous Tissue and Fascia, Lower Extremity	X External	Ø Drainage Device 1 Radioactive Element 3 Infusion Device H Contraceptive Device V Infusion Pump X Vascular Access Device, Tunneled	Z No Qualifier

Non-OR ØJPS[Ø3][Ø137JKN]Z
Non-OR ØJPSX[Ø13]Z
Non-OR ØJPT[Ø3][Ø1237HJKMNVWX]Z
Non-OR ØJPTX[Ø123HVX]Z

Non-OR ØJP[VW][Ø3][Ø137HJKNVWX]Z
Non-OR ØJP[VW]X[Ø13HVX]Z
ØJPT[Ø3][FP]Z when reported with Secondary Diagnosis K68.11, T81.4XXA, T82.6XXA, or T82.7XXA

Coding Clinic: 2012, Q4, P1Ø5 – ØJPTØPZ
Coding Clinic: 2016, Q2, P15; 2015, Q4, P32 – ØJPTØXZ
Coding Clinic: 2018, Q4, P86 – ØJPT3JZ

SECTION: Ø MEDICAL AND SURGICAL
BODY SYSTEM: J SUBCUTANEOUS TISSUE AND FASCIA
OPERATION: Q REPAIR: Restoring, to the extent possible, a body part to its normal anatomic structure and function

Body Part	Approach	Device	Qualifier
Ø Subcutaneous Tissue and Fascia, Scalp 1 Subcutaneous Tissue and Fascia, Face 4 Subcutaneous Tissue and Fascia, Right Neck 5 Subcutaneous Tissue and Fascia, Left Neck 6 Subcutaneous Tissue and Fascia, Chest 7 Subcutaneous Tissue and Fascia, Back 8 Subcutaneous Tissue and Fascia, Abdomen 9 Subcutaneous Tissue and Fascia, Buttock B Subcutaneous Tissue and Fascia, Perineum C Subcutaneous Tissue and Fascia, Pelvic Region D Subcutaneous Tissue and Fascia, Right Upper Arm F Subcutaneous Tissue and Fascia, Left Upper Arm G Subcutaneous Tissue and Fascia, Right Lower Arm H Subcutaneous Tissue and Fascia, Left Lower Arm J Subcutaneous Tissue and Fascia, Right Hand K Subcutaneous Tissue and Fascia, Left Hand L Subcutaneous Tissue and Fascia, Right Upper Leg M Subcutaneous Tissue and Fascia, Left Upper Leg N Subcutaneous Tissue and Fascia, Right Lower Leg P Subcutaneous Tissue and Fascia, Left Lower Leg Q Subcutaneous Tissue and Fascia, Right Foot R Subcutaneous Tissue and Fascia, Left Foot	Ø Open 3 Percutaneous	Z No Device	Z No Qualifier

DRG Non-OR ØJQ[Ø1456789BCDFGHJKLMNPQR][Ø3]ZZ
Non-OR ØJQ[Ø1456789BCDFGHJKLMNPQR]3ZZ

Coding Clinic: 2017, Q3, P19 – ØJQCØZZ
Coding Clinic: 2022, Q3, P25 – ØJQ8ØZZ

SECTION: Ø MEDICAL AND SURGICAL
BODY SYSTEM: J SUBCUTANEOUS TISSUE AND FASCIA
OPERATION: R REPLACEMENT: Putting in or on biological or synthetic material that physically takes the place and/or function of all or a portion of a body part

Body Part	Approach	Device	Qualifier
Ø Subcutaneous Tissue and Fascia, Scalp 1 Subcutaneous Tissue and Fascia, Face 4 Subcutaneous Tissue and Fascia, Right Neck 5 Subcutaneous Tissue and Fascia, Left Neck 6 Subcutaneous Tissue and Fascia, Chest 7 Subcutaneous Tissue and Fascia, Back 8 Subcutaneous Tissue and Fascia, Abdomen 9 Subcutaneous Tissue and Fascia, Buttock B Subcutaneous Tissue and Fascia, Perineum C Subcutaneous Tissue and Fascia, Pelvic Region D Subcutaneous Tissue and Fascia, Right Upper Arm F Subcutaneous Tissue and Fascia, Left Upper Arm G Subcutaneous Tissue and Fascia, Right Lower Arm H Subcutaneous Tissue and Fascia, Left Lower Arm J Subcutaneous Tissue and Fascia, Right Hand K Subcutaneous Tissue and Fascia, Left Hand L Subcutaneous Tissue and Fascia, Right Upper Leg M Subcutaneous Tissue and Fascia, Left Upper Leg N Subcutaneous Tissue and Fascia, Right Lower Leg P Subcutaneous Tissue and Fascia, Left Lower Leg Q Subcutaneous Tissue and Fascia, Right Foot R Subcutaneous Tissue and Fascia, Left Foot	Ø Open 3 Percutaneous	7 Autologous Tissue Substitute J Synthetic Substitute K Nonautologous Tissue Substitute	Z No Qualifier

Coding Clinic: 2015, Q2, P13 – ØJR1Ø7Z

SECTION: Ø MEDICAL AND SURGICAL
BODY SYSTEM: J SUBCUTANEOUS TISSUE AND FASCIA
OPERATION: U SUPPLEMENT: Putting in or on biological or synthetic material that physically reinforces and/or augments the function of a portion of a body part

Body Part	Approach	Device	Qualifier
Ø Subcutaneous Tissue and Fascia, Scalp 1 Subcutaneous Tissue and Fascia, Face 4 Subcutaneous Tissue and Fascia, Right Neck 5 Subcutaneous Tissue and Fascia, Left Neck 6 Subcutaneous Tissue and Fascia, Chest 7 Subcutaneous Tissue and Fascia, Back 8 Subcutaneous Tissue and Fascia, Abdomen 9 Subcutaneous Tissue and Fascia, Buttock B Subcutaneous Tissue and Fascia, Perineum C Subcutaneous Tissue and Fascia, Pelvic Region D Subcutaneous Tissue and Fascia, Right Upper Arm F Subcutaneous Tissue and Fascia, Left Upper Arm G Subcutaneous Tissue and Fascia, Right Lower Arm H Subcutaneous Tissue and Fascia, Left Lower Arm J Subcutaneous Tissue and Fascia, Right Hand K Subcutaneous Tissue and Fascia, Left Hand L Subcutaneous Tissue and Fascia, Right Upper Leg M Subcutaneous Tissue and Fascia, Left Upper Leg N Subcutaneous Tissue and Fascia, Right Lower Leg P Subcutaneous Tissue and Fascia, Left Lower Leg Q Subcutaneous Tissue and Fascia, Right Foot R Subcutaneous Tissue and Fascia, Left Foot	Ø Open 3 Percutaneous	7 Autologous Tissue Substitute J Synthetic Substitute K Nonautologous Tissue Substitute	Z No Qualifier

Coding Clinic: 2018, Q1, P7 – ØJU7Ø7Z
Coding Clinic: 2018, Q2, P2Ø – ØJUHØKZ

SECTION: Ø MEDICAL AND SURGICAL
BODY SYSTEM: J SUBCUTANEOUS TISSUE AND FASCIA
OPERATION: W REVISION: *(on multiple pages)*

Correcting, to the extent possible, a portion of a malfunctioning device or the position of a displaced device

Body Part	Approach	Device	Qualifier
S Subcutaneous Tissue and Fascia, Head and Neck	Ø Open 3 Percutaneous	Ø Drainage Device 3 Infusion Device 7 Autologous Tissue Substitute J Synthetic Substitute K Nonautologous Tissue Substitute N Tissue Expander Y Other Device	Z No Qualifier
S Subcutaneous Tissue and Fascia, Head and Neck	X External	Ø Drainage Device 3 Infusion Device 7 Autologous Tissue Substitute J Synthetic Substitute K Nonautologous Tissue Substitute N Tissue Expander	Z No Qualifier
T Subcutaneous Tissue and Fascia, Trunk	Ø Open 3 Percutaneous	Ø Drainage Device 2 Monitoring Device 3 Infusion Device 7 Autologous Tissue Substitute F Subcutaneous Defibrillator H Contraceptive Device J Synthetic Substitute K Nonautologous Tissue Substitute M Stimulator Generator N Tissue Expander P Cardiac Rhythm Related Device V Infusion Device, Pump W Vascular Access Device, Totally Implantable X Vascular Access Device, Tunneled Y Other Device	Z No Qualifier
T Subcutaneous Tissue and Fascia, Trunk	X External	Ø Drainage Device 2 Monitoring Device 3 Infusion Device 7 Autologous Tissue Substitute F Subcutaneous Defibrillator H Contraceptive Device J Synthetic Substitute K Nonautologous Tissue Substitute M Stimulator Generator N Tissue Expander P Cardiac Rhythm Related Device V Infusion Device, Pump W Vascular Access Device, Totally Implantable X Vascular Access Device, Tunneled	Z No Qualifier

DRG Non-OR ØJWS[Ø3][Ø37JKNY]Z
DRG Non-OR ØJWT[Ø3X][Ø37HJKMNVWX]Z
Non-OR ØJWSX[Ø37JKN]Z
Non-OR ØJWTX[Ø237HJKNPVWX]Z
ØJWT[Ø3]PZ when reported with Secondary Diagnosis K68.11, T81.4XXA, T82.6XXA, or T82.7XXA

Coding Clinic: 2Ø12, Q4, P1Ø6 – ØJWTØPZ
Coding Clinic: 2Ø15, Q2, P1Ø – ØJWSØJZ
Coding Clinic: 2Ø15, Q4, P33 – ØJWT33Z
Coding Clinic: 2Ø18, Q1, P9 – ØJWTØJZ
Coding Clinic: 2Ø22, Q3, P25 – ØJWTØ3Z

SECTION: Ø MEDICAL AND SURGICAL
BODY SYSTEM: J SUBCUTANEOUS TISSUE AND FASCIA
OPERATION: W REVISION: *(continued)*

Correcting, to the extent possible, a portion of a malfunctioning device or the position of a displaced device

Body Part	Approach	Device	Qualifier
V Subcutaneous Tissue and Fascia, Upper Extremity W Subcutaneous Tissue and Fascia, Lower Extremity	Ø Open 3 Percutaneous	Ø Drainage Device 3 Infusion Device 7 Autologous Tissue Substitute H Contraceptive Device J Synthetic Substitute K Nonautologous Tissue Substitute N Tissue Expander V Infusion Device, Pump W Vascular Access Device, Totally Implantable X Vascular Access Device, Tunneled Y Other Device	Z No Qualifier
V Subcutaneous Tissue and Fascia, Upper Extremity W Subcutaneous Tissue and Fascia, Lower Extremity	X External	Ø Drainage Device 3 Infusion Device 7 Autologous Tissue Substitute H Contraceptive Device J Synthetic Substitute K Nonautologous Tissue Substitute N Tissue Expander V Infusion Device, Pump W Vascular Access Device, Totally Implantable X Vascular Access Device, Tunneled	Z No Qualifier

DRG Non-OR ØJW[VW][Ø3][Ø37HJKNVWXY]Z
Non-OR ØJW[VW]X[Ø37HJKNVWX]Z

SECTION: Ø MEDICAL AND SURGICAL
BODY SYSTEM: J SUBCUTANEOUS TISSUE AND FASCIA
OPERATION: X TRANSFER: Moving, without taking out, all or a portion of a body part to another location to take over the function of all or a portion of a body part

Body Part	Approach	Device	Qualifier
Ø Subcutaneous Tissue and Fascia, Scalp 1 Subcutaneous Tissue and Fascia, Face 4 Subcutaneous Tissue and Fascia, Right Neck 5 Subcutaneous Tissue and Fascia, Left Neck 6 Subcutaneous Tissue and Fascia, Chest 7 Subcutaneous Tissue and Fascia, Back 8 Subcutaneous Tissue and Fascia, Abdomen 9 Subcutaneous Tissue and Fascia, Buttock B Subcutaneous Tissue and Fascia, Perineum C Subcutaneous Tissue and Fascia, Pelvic Region D Subcutaneous Tissue and Fascia, Right Upper Arm F Subcutaneous Tissue and Fascia, Left Upper Arm G Subcutaneous Tissue and Fascia, Right Lower Arm H Subcutaneous Tissue and Fascia, Left Lower Arm J Subcutaneous Tissue and Fascia, Right Hand K Subcutaneous Tissue and Fascia, Left Hand L Subcutaneous Tissue and Fascia, Right Upper Leg M Subcutaneous Tissue and Fascia, Left Upper Leg N Subcutaneous Tissue and Fascia, Right Lower Leg P Subcutaneous Tissue and Fascia, Left Lower Leg Q Subcutaneous Tissue and Fascia, Right Foot R Subcutaneous Tissue and Fascia, Left Foot	Ø Open 3 Percutaneous	Z No Device	B Skin and Subcutaneous Tissue C Skin, Subcutaneous Tissue and Fascia Z No Qualifier

Coding Clinic: 2018, Q1, P1Ø – ØJXØØZC
Coding Clinic: 2021, Q2, P17 – ØJX6ØZB
Coding Clinic: 2021, Q3, P2Ø – ØJXFØZZ
Coding Clinic: 2022, Q3, P12 – ØJXLØZZ

ØK. Muscles 329
ØK2. Change 33Ø
ØK5. Destruction 33Ø
ØK8. Division 331
ØK9. Drainage 332
ØKB. Excision 334
ØKC. Extirpation 335
ØKD. Extraction 336
ØKH. Insertion 336
ØKJ. Inspection 337
ØKM. Reattachment 337
ØKN. Release 338
ØKP. Removal 338
ØKQ. Repair 339
ØKR. Replacement 34Ø
ØKS. Reposition 341
ØKT. Resection 342
ØKU. Supplement 343
ØKW. Revision 343
ØKX. Transfer 344

SECTION: Ø MEDICAL AND SURGICAL
BODY SYSTEM: K MUSCLES
OPERATION: 2 CHANGE: Taking out or off a device from a body part and putting back an identical or similar device in or on the same body part without cutting or puncturing the skin or a mucous membrane

Body Part	Approach	Device	Qualifier
X Upper Muscle Y Lower Muscle	X External	Ø Drainage Device Y Other Device	Z No Qualifier

Non-OR All Values

SECTION: Ø MEDICAL AND SURGICAL
BODY SYSTEM: K MUSCLES
OPERATION: 5 DESTRUCTION: Physical eradication of all or a portion of a body part by the direct use of energy, force, or a destructive agent

Body Part	Approach	Device	Qualifier
Ø Head Muscle 1 Facial Muscle 2 Neck Muscle, Right 3 Neck Muscle, Left 4 Tongue, Palate, Pharynx Muscle 5 Shoulder Muscle, Right 6 Shoulder Muscle, Left 7 Upper Arm Muscle, Right 8 Upper Arm Muscle, Left 9 Lower Arm and Wrist Muscle, Right B Lower Arm and Wrist Muscle, Left C Hand Muscle, Right D Hand Muscle, Left F Trunk Muscle, Right G Trunk Muscle, Left H Thorax Muscle, Right J Thorax Muscle, Left K Abdomen Muscle, Right L Abdomen Muscle, Left M Perineum Muscle N Hip Muscle, Right P Hip Muscle, Left Q Upper Leg Muscle, Right R Upper Leg Muscle, Left S Lower Leg Muscle, Right T Lower Leg Muscle, Left V Foot Muscle, Right W Foot Muscle, Left	Ø Open 3 Percutaneous 4 Percutaneous Endoscopic	Z No Device	Z No Qualifier

SECTION: Ø MEDICAL AND SURGICAL
BODY SYSTEM: K MUSCLES
OPERATION: 8 DIVISION: Cutting into a body part, without draining fluids and/or gases from the body part, in order to separate or transect a body part

Body Part	Approach	Device	Qualifier
Ø Head Muscle 1 Facial Muscle 2 Neck Muscle, Right 3 Neck Muscle, Left 5 Shoulder Muscle, Right 6 Shoulder Muscle, Left 7 Upper Arm Muscle, Right 8 Upper Arm Muscle, Left 9 Lower Arm and Wrist Muscle, Right B Lower Arm and Wrist Muscle, Left C Hand Muscle, Right D Hand Muscle, Left F Trunk Muscle, Right G Trunk Muscle, Left H Thorax Muscle, Right J Thorax Muscle, Left K Abdomen Muscle, Right L Abdomen Muscle, Left M Perineum Muscle N Hip Muscle, Right P Hip Muscle, Left Q Upper Leg Muscle, Right R Upper Leg Muscle, Left S Lower Leg Muscle, Right T Lower Leg Muscle, Left V Foot Muscle, Right W Foot Muscle, Left	Ø Open 3 Percutaneous 4 Percutaneous Endoscopic	Z No Device	Z No Qualifier
4 Tongue, Palate, Pharynx Muscle	Ø Open 3 Percutaneous 4 Percutaneous Endoscopic 7 Via Natural or Artificial Opening 8 Via Natural or Artificial Opening Endoscopic	Z No Device	Z No Qualifier

Coding Clinic: 2020, Q2, P25 – ØK844ZZ

SECTION: Ø MEDICAL AND SURGICAL
BODY SYSTEM: K MUSCLES
OPERATION: 9 DRAINAGE: *(on multiple pages)*
Taking or letting out fluids and/or gases from a body part

Body Part	Approach	Device	Qualifier
Ø Head Muscle 1 Facial Muscle 2 Neck Muscle, Right 3 Neck Muscle, Left 4 Tongue, Palate, Pharynx Muscle 5 Shoulder Muscle, Right 6 Shoulder Muscle, Left 7 Upper Arm Muscle, Right 8 Upper Arm Muscle, Left 9 Lower Arm and Wrist Muscle, Right B Lower Arm and Wrist Muscle, Left C Hand Muscle, Right D Hand Muscle, Left F Trunk Muscle, Right G Trunk Muscle, Left H Thorax Muscle, Right J Thorax Muscle, Left K Abdomen Muscle, Right L Abdomen Muscle, Left M Perineum Muscle N Hip Muscle, Right P Hip Muscle, Left Q Upper Leg Muscle, Right R Upper Leg Muscle, Left S Lower Leg Muscle, Right T Lower Leg Muscle, Left V Foot Muscle, Right W Foot Muscle, Left	Ø Open 3 Percutaneous 4 Percutaneous Endoscopic	Ø Drainage Device	Z No Qualifier

Non-OR ØK9[Ø123456789BCDFGHJKLMNPQRSTVW]3ØZ

SECTION: Ø MEDICAL AND SURGICAL
BODY SYSTEM: K MUSCLES
OPERATION: 9 DRAINAGE: *(continued)*
Taking or letting out fluids and/or gases from a body part

Body Part	Approach	Device	Qualifier
Ø Head Muscle 1 Facial Muscle 2 Neck Muscle, Right 3 Neck Muscle, Left 4 Tongue, Palate, Pharynx Muscle 5 Shoulder Muscle, Right 6 Shoulder Muscle, Left 7 Upper Arm Muscle, Right 8 Upper Arm Muscle, Left 9 Lower Arm and Wrist Muscle, Right B Lower Arm and Wrist Muscle, Left C Hand Muscle, Right D Hand Muscle, Left F Trunk Muscle, Right G Trunk Muscle, Left H Thorax Muscle, Right J Thorax Muscle, Left K Abdomen Muscle, Right L Abdomen Muscle, Left M Perineum Muscle N Hip Muscle, Right P Hip Muscle, Left Q Upper Leg Muscle, Right R Upper Leg Muscle, Left S Lower Leg Muscle, Right T Lower Leg Muscle, Left V Foot Muscle, Right W Foot Muscle, Left	Ø Open 3 Percutaneous 4 Percutaneous Endoscopic	Z No Device	X Diagnostic Z No Qualifier

Non-OR ØK9[Ø123456789BFGHJKLMNPQRSTVW]3ZZ
Non-OR ØK9[CD][34]ZZ

Ø: M/S K: MUSCLES 9: DRAINAGE

SECTION: Ø MEDICAL AND SURGICAL
BODY SYSTEM: K MUSCLES
OPERATION: B EXCISION: Cutting out or off, without replacement, a portion of a body part

Body Part	Approach	Device	Qualifier
Ø Head Muscle 1 Facial Muscle 2 Neck Muscle, Right 3 Neck Muscle, Left 4 Tongue, Palate, Pharynx Muscle 5 Shoulder Muscle, Right 6 Shoulder Muscle, Left 7 Upper Arm Muscle, Right 8 Upper Arm Muscle, Left 9 Lower Arm and Wrist Muscle, Right B Lower Arm and Wrist Muscle, Left C Hand Muscle, Right D Hand Muscle, Left F Trunk Muscle, Right G Trunk Muscle, Left H Thorax Muscle, Right J Thorax Muscle, Left K Abdomen Muscle, Right L Abdomen Muscle, Left M Perineum Muscle N Hip Muscle, Right P Hip Muscle, Left Q Upper Leg Muscle, Right R Upper Leg Muscle, Left S Lower Leg Muscle, Right T Lower Leg Muscle, Left V Foot Muscle, Right W Foot Muscle, Left	Ø Open 3 Percutaneous 4 Percutaneous Endoscopic	Z No Device	X Diagnostic Z No Qualifier

Non-OR ØKB[NP]3Z[XZ]

Coding Clinic: 2Ø16, Q3, P2Ø – ØKB[NP]ØZZ
Coding Clinic: 2Ø19, Q4, P44 – ØKBPØZZ
Coding Clinic: 2Ø2Ø, Q1, P28 – ØKBRØZZ
Coding Clinic: 2Ø23, Q1, P33 – ØKB44ZZ

SECTION: Ø MEDICAL AND SURGICAL
BODY SYSTEM: K MUSCLES
OPERATION: C EXTIRPATION: Taking or cutting out solid matter from a body part

Body Part	Approach	Device	Qualifier
Ø Head Muscle 1 Facial Muscle 2 Neck Muscle, Right 3 Neck Muscle, Left 4 Tongue, Palate, Pharynx Muscle 5 Shoulder Muscle, Right 6 Shoulder Muscle, Left 7 Upper Arm Muscle, Right 8 Upper Arm Muscle, Left 9 Lower Arm and Wrist Muscle, Right B Lower Arm and Wrist Muscle, Left C Hand Muscle, Right D Hand Muscle, Left F Trunk Muscle, Right G Trunk Muscle, Left H Thorax Muscle, Right J Thorax Muscle, Left K Abdomen Muscle, Right L Abdomen Muscle, Left M Perineum Muscle N Hip Muscle, Right P Hip Muscle, Left Q Upper Leg Muscle, Right R Upper Leg Muscle, Left S Lower Leg Muscle, Right T Lower Leg Muscle, Left V Foot Muscle, Right W Foot Muscle, Left	Ø Open 3 Percutaneous 4 Percutaneous Endoscopic	Z No Device	Z No Qualifier

SECTION: Ø MEDICAL AND SURGICAL
BODY SYSTEM: K MUSCLES
OPERATION: D EXTRACTION: Pulling or stripping out or off all or a portion of a body part by the use of force

Body Part	Approach	Device	Qualifier
Ø Head Muscle 1 Facial Muscle 2 Neck Muscle, Right 3 Neck Muscle, Left 4 Tongue, Palate, Pharynx Muscle 5 Shoulder Muscle, Right 6 Shoulder Muscle, Left 7 Upper Arm Muscle, Right 8 Upper Arm Muscle, Left 9 Lower Arm and Wrist Muscle, Right B Lower Arm and Wrist Muscle, Left C Hand Muscle, Right D Hand Muscle, Left F Trunk Muscle, Right G Trunk Muscle, Left H Thorax Muscle, Right J Thorax Muscle, Left K Abdomen Muscle, Right L Abdomen Muscle, Left M Perineum Muscle N Hip Muscle, Right P Hip Muscle, Left Q Upper Leg Muscle, Right R Upper Leg Muscle, Left S Lower Leg Muscle, Right T Lower Leg Muscle, Left V Foot Muscle, Right W Foot Muscle, Left	Ø Open	Z No Device	Z No Qualifier

Coding Clinic: 2Ø17, Q4, P42 – ØKDSØZZ

SECTION: Ø MEDICAL AND SURGICAL
BODY SYSTEM: K MUSCLES
OPERATION: H INSERTION: Putting in a nonbiological appliance that monitors, assists, performs, or prevents a physiological function but does not physically take the place of a body part

Body Part	Approach	Device	Qualifier
X Upper Muscle Y Lower Muscle	Ø Open 3 Percutaneous 4 Percutaneous Endoscopic	M Stimulator Lead Y Other Device	Z No Qualifier

SECTION: Ø MEDICAL AND SURGICAL
BODY SYSTEM: K MUSCLES
OPERATION: J INSPECTION: Visually and/or manually exploring a body part

Body Part	Approach	Device	Qualifier
X Upper Muscle Y Lower Muscle	Ø Open 3 Percutaneous 4 Percutaneous Endoscopic X External	Z No Device	Z No Qualifier

Non-OR ØKJ[XY][3X]ZZ

SECTION: Ø MEDICAL AND SURGICAL
BODY SYSTEM: K MUSCLES
OPERATION: M REATTACHMENT: Putting back in or on all or a portion of a separated body part to its normal location or other suitable location

Body Part	Approach	Device	Qualifier
Ø Head Muscle 1 Facial Muscle 2 Neck Muscle, Right 3 Neck Muscle, Left 4 Tongue, Palate, Pharynx Muscle 5 Shoulder Muscle, Right 6 Shoulder Muscle, Left 7 Upper Arm Muscle, Right 8 Upper Arm Muscle, Left 9 Lower Arm and Wrist Muscle, Right B Lower Arm and Wrist Muscle, Left C Hand Muscle, Right D Hand Muscle, Left F Trunk Muscle, Right G Trunk Muscle, Left H Thorax Muscle, Right J Thorax Muscle, Left K Abdomen Muscle, Right L Abdomen Muscle, Left M Perineum Muscle N Hip Muscle, Right P Hip Muscle, Left Q Upper Leg Muscle, Right R Upper Leg Muscle, Left S Lower Leg Muscle, Right T Lower Leg Muscle, Left V Foot Muscle, Right W Foot Muscle, Left	Ø Open 4 Percutaneous Endoscopic	Z No Device	Z No Qualifier

SECTION: Ø MEDICAL AND SURGICAL
BODY SYSTEM: K MUSCLES
OPERATION: N **RELEASE:** Freeing a body part from an abnormal physical constraint by cutting or by the use of force

Body Part	Approach	Device	Qualifier
Ø Head Muscle 1 Facial Muscle 2 Neck Muscle, Right 3 Neck Muscle, Left 4 Tongue, Palate, Pharynx Muscle 5 Shoulder Muscle, Right 6 Shoulder Muscle, Left 7 Upper Arm Muscle, Right 8 Upper Arm Muscle, Left 9 Lower Arm and Wrist Muscle, Right B Lower Arm and Wrist Muscle, Left C Hand Muscle, Right D Hand Muscle, Left F Trunk Muscle, Right G Trunk Muscle, Left H Thorax Muscle, Right J Thorax Muscle, Left K Abdomen Muscle, Right L Abdomen Muscle, Left M Perineum Muscle N Hip Muscle, Right P Hip Muscle, Left Q Upper Leg Muscle, Right R Upper Leg Muscle, Lefta S Lower Leg Muscle, Right T Lower Leg Muscle, Left V Foot Muscle, Right W Foot Muscle, Left	Ø Open 3 Percutaneous 4 Percutaneous Endoscopic X External	Z No Device	Z No Qualifier

Non-OR ØKN[Ø123456789BCDFGHJKLMNPQRSTVW]XZZ

Coding Clinic: 2015, Q2, P22 – ØKN84ZZ
Coding Clinic: 2017, Q2, P13 – ØKNVØZZ
Coding Clinic: 2017, Q2, P14 – ØKNTØZZ

SECTION: Ø MEDICAL AND SURGICAL
BODY SYSTEM: K MUSCLES
OPERATION: P **REMOVAL:** Taking out or off a device from a body part

Body Part	Approach	Device	Qualifier
X Upper Muscle Y Lower Muscle	Ø Open 3 Percutaneous 4 Percutaneous Endoscopic	Ø Drainage Device 7 Autologous Tissue Substitute J Synthetic Substitute K Nonautologous Tissue Substitute M Stimulator Lead Y Other Device	Z No Qualifier
X Upper Muscle Y Lower Muscle	X External	Ø Drainage Device M Stimulator Lead	Z No Qualifier

Non-OR ØKP[XY]X[ØM]Z

SECTION: Ø MEDICAL AND SURGICAL
BODY SYSTEM: K MUSCLES
OPERATION: Q REPAIR: Restoring, to the extent possible, a body part to its normal anatomic structure and function

Body Part	Approach	Device	Qualifier
Ø Head Muscle 1 Facial Muscle 2 Neck Muscle, Right 3 Neck Muscle, Left 4 Tongue, Palate, Pharynx Muscle 5 Shoulder Muscle, Right 6 Shoulder Muscle, Left 7 Upper Arm Muscle, Right 8 Upper Arm Muscle, Left 9 Lower Arm and Wrist Muscle, Right B Lower Arm and Wrist Muscle, Left C Hand Muscle, Right D Hand Muscle, Left F Trunk Muscle, Right G Trunk Muscle, Left H Thorax Muscle, Right J Thorax Muscle, Left K Abdomen Muscle, Right L Abdomen Muscle, Left M Perineum Muscle N Hip Muscle, Right P Hip Muscle, Left Q Upper Leg Muscle, Right R Upper Leg Muscle, Left S Lower Leg Muscle, Right T Lower Leg Muscle, Left V Foot Muscle, Right W Foot Muscle, Left	Ø Open 3 Percutaneous 4 Percutaneous Endoscopic	Z No Device	Z No Qualifier

Coding Clinic: 2Ø22, Q3, P14; 2Ø16, Q2, P35, Q1, P7 – ØKQMØZZ

SECTION: Ø MEDICAL AND SURGICAL

BODY SYSTEM: K MUSCLES

OPERATION: R REPLACEMENT: Putting in or on biological or synthetic material that physically takes the place and/or function of all or a portion of a body part

Body Part	Approach	Device	Qualifier
Ø Head Muscle 1 Facial Muscle 2 Neck Muscle, Right 3 Neck Muscle, Left 4 Tongue, Palate, Pharynx Muscle 5 Shoulder Muscle, Right 6 Shoulder Muscle, Left 7 Upper Arm Muscle, Right 8 Upper Arm Muscle, Left 9 Lower Arm and Wrist Muscle, Right B Lower Arm and Wrist Muscle, Left C Hand Muscle, Right D Hand Muscle, Left F Trunk Muscle, Right G Trunk Muscle, Left H Thorax Muscle, Right J Thorax Muscle, Left K Abdomen Muscle, Right L Abdomen Muscle, Left M Perineum Muscle N Hip Muscle, Right P Hip Muscle, Left Q Upper Leg Muscle, Right R Upper Leg Muscle, Left S Lower Leg Muscle, Right T Lower Leg Muscle, Left V Foot Muscle, Right W Foot Muscle, Left	Ø Open 4 Percutaneous Endoscopic	7 Autologous Tissue Substitute J Synthetic Substitute K Nonautologous Tissue Substitute	Z No Qualifier

ØKS

SECTION: Ø MEDICAL AND SURGICAL
BODY SYSTEM: K MUSCLES
OPERATION: S REPOSITION: Moving to its normal location, or other suitable location, all or a portion of a body part

Body Part	Approach	Device	Qualifier
Ø Head Muscle 1 Facial Muscle 2 Neck Muscle, Right 3 Neck Muscle, Left 4 Tongue, Palate, Pharynx Muscle 5 Shoulder Muscle, Right 6 Shoulder Muscle, Left 7 Upper Arm Muscle, Right 8 Upper Arm Muscle, Left 9 Lower Arm and Wrist Muscle, Right B Lower Arm and Wrist Muscle, Left C Hand Muscle, Right D Hand Muscle, Left F Trunk Muscle, Right G Trunk Muscle, Left H Thorax Muscle, Right J Thorax Muscle, Left K Abdomen Muscle, Right L Abdomen Muscle, Left M Perineum Muscle N Hip Muscle, Right P Hip Muscle, Left Q Upper Leg Muscle, Right R Upper Leg Muscle, Left S Lower Leg Muscle, Right T Lower Leg Muscle, Left V Foot Muscle, Right W Foot Muscle, Left	Ø Open 4 Percutaneous Endoscopic	Z No Device	Z No Qualifier

Coding Clinic: 2Ø22, Q3, P12 – ØKSQØZZ

SECTION: Ø MEDICAL AND SURGICAL
BODY SYSTEM: K MUSCLES
OPERATION: T RESECTION: Cutting out or off, without replacement, all of a body part

Body Part	Approach	Device	Qualifier
Ø Head Muscle 1 Facial Muscle 2 Neck Muscle, Right 3 Neck Muscle, Left 4 Tongue, Palate, Pharynx Muscle 5 Shoulder Muscle, Right 6 Shoulder Muscle, Left 7 Upper Arm Muscle, Right 8 Upper Arm Muscle, Left 9 Lower Arm and Wrist Muscle, Right B Lower Arm and Wrist Muscle, Left C Hand Muscle, Right D Hand Muscle, Left F Trunk Muscle, Right G Trunk Muscle, Left H Thorax Muscle, Right ⊞ J Thorax Muscle, Left ⊞ K Abdomen Muscle, Right L Abdomen Muscle, Left M Perineum Muscle N Hip Muscle, Right P Hip Muscle, Left Q Upper Leg Muscle, Right R Upper Leg Muscle, Left S Lower Leg Muscle, Right T Lower Leg Muscle, Left V Foot Muscle, Right W Foot Muscle, Left	Ø Open 4 Percutaneous Endoscopic	Z No Device	Z No Qualifier

⊞ ØKT[HJ]ØZZ

Coding Clinic: 2Ø15, Q1, P38 – ØKTMØZZ
Coding Clinic: 2Ø16, Q2, P13 – ØKT3ØZZ

Ø: M/S K: MUSCLES T: RESECTION

New/Revised Text in Green ~~deleted~~ Deleted ♀ Females Only ♂ Males Only Coding Clinic
Non-covered Limited Coverage ⊞ Combination (See Appendix E) DRG Non-OR Non-OR Hospital-Acquired Condition

SECTION: Ø MEDICAL AND SURGICAL
BODY SYSTEM: K MUSCLES
OPERATION: U SUPPLEMENT: Putting in or on biological or synthetic material that physically reinforces and/or augments the function of a portion of a body part

Body Part	Approach	Device	Qualifier
Ø Head Muscle 1 Facial Muscle 2 Neck Muscle, Right 3 Neck Muscle, Left 4 Tongue, Palate, Pharynx Muscle 5 Shoulder Muscle, Right 6 Shoulder Muscle, Left 7 Upper Arm Muscle, Right 8 Upper Arm Muscle, Left 9 Lower Arm and Wrist Muscle, Right B Lower Arm and Wrist Muscle, Left C Hand Muscle, Right D Hand Muscle, Left F Trunk Muscle, Right G Trunk Muscle, Left H Thorax Muscle, Right J Thorax Muscle, Left K Abdomen Muscle, Right L Abdomen Muscle, Left M Perineum Muscle N Hip Muscle, Right P Hip Muscle, Left Q Upper Leg Muscle, Right R Upper Leg Muscle, Left S Lower Leg Muscle, Right T Lower Leg Muscle, Left V Foot Muscle, Right W Foot Muscle, Left	Ø Open 4 Percutaneous Endoscopic	7 Autologous Tissue Substitute J Synthetic Substitute K Nonautologous Tissue Substitute	Z No Qualifier

SECTION: Ø MEDICAL AND SURGICAL
BODY SYSTEM: K MUSCLES
OPERATION: W REVISION: Correcting, to the extent possible, a portion of a malfunctioning device or the position of a displaced device

Body Part	Approach	Device	Qualifier
X Upper Muscle Y Lower Muscle	Ø Open 3 Percutaneous 4 Percutaneous Endoscopic	Ø Drainage Device 7 Autologous Tissue Substitute J Synthetic Substitute K Nonautologous Tissue Substitute M Stimulator Lead Y Other device	Z No Qualifier
X Upper Muscle Y Lower Muscle	X External	Ø Drainage Device 7 Autologous Tissue Substitute J Synthetic Substitute K Nonautologous Tissue Substitute M Stimulator Lead	Z No Qualifier

Non-OR ØKW[XY]X[Ø7JKM]Z

SECTION: Ø MEDICAL AND SURGICAL
BODY SYSTEM: K MUSCLES
OPERATION: X TRANSFER: Moving, without taking out, all or a portion of a body part to another location to take over the function of all or a portion of a body part

Body Part	Approach	Device	Qualifier
Ø Head Muscle 1 Facial Muscle 2 Neck Muscle, Right 3 Neck Muscle, Left 4 Tongue, Palate, Pharynx Muscle 5 Shoulder Muscle, Right 6 Shoulder Muscle, Left 7 Upper Arm Muscle, Right 8 Upper Arm Muscle, Left 9 Lower Arm and Wrist Muscle, Right B Lower Arm and Wrist Muscle, Left C Hand Muscle, Right D Hand Muscle, Left H Thorax Muscle, Right J Thorax Muscle, Left M Perineum Muscle N Hip Muscle, Right P Hip Muscle, Left Q Upper Leg Muscle, Right R Upper Leg Muscle, Left S Lower Leg Muscle, Right T Lower Leg Muscle, Left V Foot Muscle, Right W Foot Muscle, Left	Ø Open 4 Percutaneous Endoscopic	Z No Device	Ø Skin 1 Subcutaneous Tissue 2 Skin and Subcutaneous Tissue Z No Qualifier
F Trunk Muscle, Right G Trunk Muscle, Left	Ø Open 4 Percutaneous Endoscopic	Z No Device	Ø Skin 1 Subcutaneous Tissue 2 Skin and Subcutaneous Tissue 5 Latissimus Dorsi Myocutaneous Flap 7 Deep Inferior Epigastric Artery Perforator Flap 8 Superficial Inferior Epigastric Artery Flap 9 Gluteal Artery Perforator Flap Z No Qualifier
K Abdomen Muscle, Right L Abdomen Muscle, Left	Ø Open 4 Percutaneous Endoscopic	Z No Device	Ø Skin 1 Subcutaneous Tissue 2 Skin and Subcutaneous Tissue 6 Transverse Rectus Abdominis Myocutaneous Flap Z No Qualifier

Coding Clinic: 2Ø15, Q2, P26 – ØKX4ØZ2
Coding Clinic: 2Ø15, Q3, P33 – ØKX1ØZ2
Coding Clinic: 2Ø16, Q3, P3Ø-31 – ØKX[QR]ØZZ
Coding Clinic: 2Ø17, Q4, P67 – ØKXFØZ5

ØL. Tendons 345
ØL2. Change 346
ØL5. Destruction 346
ØL8. Division 347
ØL9. Drainage 348
ØLB. Excision 349
ØLC. Extirpation 35Ø
ØLD. Extraction 351
ØLH. Insertion 351
ØLJ. Inspection 352
ØLM. Reattachment 352
ØLN. Release 353
ØLP. Removal 353
ØLQ. Repair 354
ØLR. Replacement 355
ØLS. Reposition 356
ØLT. Resection 357
ØLU. Supplement 358
ØLW. Revision 358
ØLX. Transfer 359

SECTION: Ø MEDICAL AND SURGICAL
BODY SYSTEM: L TENDONS
OPERATION: 2 CHANGE: Taking out or off a device from a body part and putting back an identical or similar device in or on the same body part without cutting or puncturing the skin or a mucous membrane

Body Part	Approach	Device	Qualifier
X Upper Tendon Y Lower Tendon	X External	Ø Drainage Device Y Other Device	Z No Qualifier

Non-OR All Values

SECTION: Ø MEDICAL AND SURGICAL
BODY SYSTEM: L TENDONS
OPERATION: 5 DESTRUCTION: Physical eradication of all or a portion of a body part by the direct use of energy, force, or a destructive agent

Body Part	Approach	Device	Qualifier
Ø Head and Neck Tendon 1 Shoulder Tendon, Right 2 Shoulder Tendon, Left 3 Upper Arm Tendon, Right 4 Upper Arm Tendon, Left 5 Lower Arm and Wrist Tendon, Right 6 Lower Arm and Wrist Tendon, Left 7 Hand Tendon, Right 8 Hand Tendon, Left 9 Trunk Tendon, Right B Trunk Tendon, Left C Thorax Tendon, Right D Thorax Tendon, Left F Abdomen Tendon, Right G Abdomen Tendon, Left H Perineum Tendon J Hip Tendon, Right K Hip Tendon, Left L Upper Leg Tendon, Right M Upper Leg Tendon, Left N Lower Leg Tendon, Right P Lower Leg Tendon, Left Q Knee Tendon, Right R Knee Tendon, Left S Ankle Tendon, Right T Ankle Tendon, Left V Foot Tendon, Right W Foot Tendon, Left	Ø Open 3 Percutaneous 4 Percutaneous Endoscopic	Z No Device	Z No Qualifier

SECTION: Ø MEDICAL AND SURGICAL
BODY SYSTEM: L TENDONS
OPERATION: 8 DIVISION: Cutting into a body part, without draining fluids and/or gases from the body part, in order to separate or transect a body part

Body Part	Approach	Device	Qualifier
Ø Head and Neck Tendon 1 Shoulder Tendon, Right 2 Shoulder Tendon, Left 3 Upper Arm Tendon, Right 4 Upper Arm Tendon, Left 5 Lower Arm and Wrist Tendon, Right 6 Lower Arm and Wrist Tendon, Left 7 Hand Tendon, Right 8 Hand Tendon, Left 9 Trunk Tendon, Right B Trunk Tendon, Left C Thorax Tendon, Right D Thorax Tendon, Left F Abdomen Tendon, Right G Abdomen Tendon, Left H Perineum Tendon J Hip Tendon, Right K Hip Tendon, Left L Upper Leg Tendon, Right M Upper Leg Tendon, Left N Lower Leg Tendon, Right P Lower Leg Tendon, Left Q Knee Tendon, Right R Knee Tendon, Left S Ankle Tendon, Right T Ankle Tendon, Left V Foot Tendon, Right W Foot Tendon, Left	Ø Open 3 Percutaneous 4 Percutaneous Endoscopic	Z No Device	Z No Qualifier

Coding Clinic: 2Ø16, Q3, P31 – ØL8JØZZ

SECTION: Ø MEDICAL AND SURGICAL
BODY SYSTEM: L TENDONS
OPERATION: 9 DRAINAGE: Taking or letting out fluids and/or gases from a body part

Body Part	Approach	Device	Qualifier
Ø Head and Neck Tendon 1 Shoulder Tendon, Right 2 Shoulder Tendon, Left 3 Upper Arm Tendon, Right 4 Upper Arm Tendon, Left 5 Lower Arm and Wrist Tendon, Right 6 Lower Arm and Wrist Tendon, Left 7 Hand Tendon, Right 8 Hand Tendon, Left 9 Trunk Tendon, Right B Trunk Tendon, Left C Thorax Tendon, Right D Thorax Tendon, Left F Abdomen Tendon, Right G Abdomen Tendon, Left H Perineum Tendon J Hip Tendon, Right K Hip Tendon, Left L Upper Leg Tendon, Right M Upper Leg Tendon, Left N Lower Leg Tendon, Right P Lower Leg Tendon, Left Q Knee Tendon, Right R Knee Tendon, Left S Ankle Tendon, Right T Ankle Tendon, Left V Foot Tendon, Right W Foot Tendon, Left	Ø Open 3 Percutaneous 4 Percutaneous Endoscopic	Ø Drainage Device	Z No Qualifier
Ø Head and Neck Tendon 1 Shoulder Tendon, Right 2 Shoulder Tendon, Left 3 Upper Arm Tendon, Right 4 Upper Arm Tendon, Left 5 Lower Arm and Wrist Tendon, Right 6 Lower Arm and Wrist Tendon, Left 7 Hand Tendon, Right 8 Hand Tendon, Left 9 Trunk Tendon, Right B Trunk Tendon, Left C Thorax Tendon, Right D Thorax Tendon, Left F Abdomen Tendon, Right G Abdomen Tendon, Left H Perineum Tendon J Hip Tendon, Right K Hip Tendon, Left L Upper Leg Tendon, Right M Upper Leg Tendon, Left N Lower Leg Tendon, Right P Lower Leg Tendon, Left Q Knee Tendon, Right R Knee Tendon, Left S Ankle Tendon, Right T Ankle Tendon, Left V Foot Tendon, Right W Foot Tendon, Left	Ø Open 3 Percutaneous 4 Percutaneous Endoscopic	Z No Device	X Diagnostic Z No Qualifier

Non-OR ØL9[Ø123456789BCDFGHJKLMNPQRSTVW]3ØZ
Non-OR ØL9[Ø1234569BCDFGHJKLMNPQRSTVW]3ZZ
Non-OR ØL9[78][34]ZZ

New/Revised Text in Green ~~deleted~~ Deleted ♀ Females Only ♂ Males Only Coding Clinic
Non-covered Limited Coverage Combination (See Appendix E) DRG Non-OR Non-OR Hospital-Acquired Condition

SECTION: Ø MEDICAL AND SURGICAL
BODY SYSTEM: L TENDONS
OPERATION: B EXCISION: Cutting out or off, without replacement, a portion of a body part

Body Part	Approach	Device	Qualifier
Ø Head and Neck Tendon 1 Shoulder Tendon, Right 2 Shoulder Tendon, Left 3 Upper Arm Tendon, Right 4 Upper Arm Tendon, Left 5 Lower Arm and Wrist Tendon, Right 6 Lower Arm and Wrist Tendon, Left 7 Hand Tendon, Right 8 Hand Tendon, Left 9 Trunk Tendon, Right B Trunk Tendon, Left C Thorax Tendon, Right D Thorax Tendon, Left F Abdomen Tendon, Right G Abdomen Tendon, Left H Perineum Tendon J Hip Tendon, Right K Hip Tendon, Left L Upper Leg Tendon, Right M Upper Leg Tendon, Left N Lower Leg Tendon, Right P Lower Leg Tendon, Left Q Knee Tendon, Right R Knee Tendon, Left S Ankle Tendon, Right T Ankle Tendon, Left V Foot Tendon, Right W Foot Tendon, Left	Ø Open 3 Percutaneous 4 Percutaneous Endoscopic	Z No Device	X Diagnostic Z No Qualifier

Coding Clinic: 2Ø15, Q3, P27 – ØLB6ØZZ
Coding Clinic: 2Ø17, Q2, P22 – ØLBLØZZ

Ø: M/S L: TENDONS B: EXCISION

SECTION: Ø MEDICAL AND SURGICAL
BODY SYSTEM: L TENDONS
OPERATION: C EXTIRPATION: Taking or cutting out solid matter from a body part

Body Part	Approach	Device	Qualifier
Ø Head and Neck Tendon 1 Shoulder Tendon, Right 2 Shoulder Tendon, Left 3 Upper Arm Tendon, Right 4 Upper Arm Tendon, Left 5 Lower Arm and Wrist Tendon, Right 6 Lower Arm and Wrist Tendon, Left 7 Hand Tendon, Right 8 Hand Tendon, Left 9 Trunk Tendon, Right B Trunk Tendon, Left C Thorax Tendon, Right D Thorax Tendon, Left F Abdomen Tendon, Right G Abdomen Tendon, Left H Perineum Tendon J Hip Tendon, Right K Hip Tendon, Left L Upper Leg Tendon, Right M Upper Leg Tendon, Left N Lower Leg Tendon, Right P Lower Leg Tendon, Left Q Knee Tendon, Right R Knee Tendon, Left S Ankle Tendon, Right T Ankle Tendon, Left V Foot Tendon, Right W Foot Tendon, Left	Ø Open 3 Percutaneous 4 Percutaneous Endoscopic	Z No Device	Z No Qualifier

SECTION: Ø MEDICAL AND SURGICAL
BODY SYSTEM: L TENDONS
OPERATION: D EXTRACTION: Pulling or stripping out or off all or a portion of a body part by the use of force

Body Part	Approach	Device	Qualifier
Ø Head and Neck Tendon 1 Shoulder Tendon, Right 2 Shoulder Tendon, Left 3 Upper Arm Tendon, Right 4 Upper Arm Tendon, Left 5 Lower Arm and Wrist Tendon, Right 6 Lower Arm and Wrist Tendon, Left 7 Hand Tendon, Right 8 Hand Tendon, Left 9 Trunk Tendon, Right B Trunk Tendon, Left C Thorax Tendon, Right D Thorax Tendon, Left F Abdomen Tendon, Right G Abdomen Tendon, Left H Perineum Tendon J Hip Tendon, Right K Hip Tendon, Left L Upper Leg Tendon, Right M Upper Leg Tendon, Left N Lower Leg Tendon, Right P Lower Leg Tendon, Left Q Knee Tendon, Right R Knee Tendon, Left S Ankle Tendon, Right T Ankle Tendon, Left V Foot Tendon, Right W Foot Tendon, Left	Ø Open	Z No Device	Z No Qualifier

SECTION: Ø MEDICAL AND SURGICAL
BODY SYSTEM: L TENDONS
OPERATION: H INSERTION: Putting in a nonbiological appliance that monitors, assists, performs, or prevents a physiological function but does not physically take the place of a body part

Body Part	Approach	Device	Qualifier
X Upper Tendon Y Lower Tendon	Ø Open 3 Percutaneous 4 Percutaneous Endoscopic	Y Other Device	Z No Qualifier

SECTION: Ø MEDICAL AND SURGICAL
BODY SYSTEM: L TENDONS
OPERATION: J INSPECTION: Visually and/or manually exploring a body part

Body Part	Approach	Device	Qualifier
X Upper Tendon Y Lower Tendon	Ø Open 3 Percutaneous 4 Percutaneous Endoscopic X External	Z No Device	Z No Qualifier

Non-OR ØLJ[XY][3X]ZZ

SECTION: Ø MEDICAL AND SURGICAL
BODY SYSTEM: L TENDONS
OPERATION: M REATTACHMENT: Putting back in or on all or a portion of a separated body part to its normal location or other suitable location

Body Part	Approach	Device	Qualifier
Ø Head and Neck Tendon 1 Shoulder Tendon, Right 2 Shoulder Tendon, Left 3 Upper Arm Tendon, Right 4 Upper Arm Tendon, Left 5 Lower Arm and Wrist Tendon, Right 6 Lower Arm and Wrist Tendon, Left 7 Hand Tendon, Right 8 Hand Tendon, Left 9 Trunk Tendon, Right B Trunk Tendon, Left C Thorax Tendon, Right D Thorax Tendon, Left F Abdomen Tendon, Right G Abdomen Tendon, Left H Perineum Tendon J Hip Tendon, Right K Hip Tendon, Left L Upper Leg Tendon, Right M Upper Leg Tendon, Left N Lower Leg Tendon, Right P Lower Leg Tendon, Left Q Knee Tendon, Right R Knee Tendon, Left S Ankle Tendon, Right T Ankle Tendon, Left V Foot Tendon, Right W Foot Tendon, Left	Ø Open 4 Percutaneous Endoscopic	Z No Device	Z No Qualifier

SECTION: Ø MEDICAL AND SURGICAL
BODY SYSTEM: L TENDONS
OPERATION: N RELEASE: Freeing a body part from an abnormal physical constraint by cutting or by the use of force

Body Part	Approach	Device	Qualifier
Ø Head and Neck Tendon 1 Shoulder Tendon, Right 2 Shoulder Tendon, Left 3 Upper Arm Tendon, Right 4 Upper Arm Tendon, Left 5 Lower Arm and Wrist Tendon, Right 6 Lower Arm and Wrist Tendon, Left 7 Hand Tendon, Right 8 Hand Tendon, Left 9 Trunk Tendon, Right B Trunk Tendon, Left C Thorax Tendon, Right D Thorax Tendon, Left F Abdomen Tendon, Right G Abdomen Tendon, Left H Perineum Tendon J Hip Tendon, Right K Hip Tendon, Left L Upper Leg Tendon, Right M Upper Leg Tendon, Left N Lower Leg Tendon, Right P Lower Leg Tendon, Left Q Knee Tendon, Right R Knee Tendon, Left S Ankle Tendon, Right T Ankle Tendon, Left V Foot Tendon, Right W Foot Tendon, Left	Ø Open 3 Percutaneous 4 Percutaneous Endoscopic X External	Z No Device	Z No Qualifier

Non-OR ØLN[Ø123456789BCDFGHJKLMNPQRSTVW]XZZ

SECTION: Ø MEDICAL AND SURGICAL
BODY SYSTEM: L TENDONS
OPERATION: P REMOVAL: Taking out or off a device from a body part

Body Part	Approach	Device	Qualifier
X Upper Tendon Y Lower Tendon	Ø Open 3 Percutaneous 4 Percutaneous Endoscopic	Ø Drainage Device 7 Autologous Tissue Substitute J Synthetic Substitute K Nonautologous Tissue Substitute Y Other Device	Z No Qualifier
X Upper Tendon Y Lower Tendon	X External	Ø Drainage Device	Z No Qualifier

Non-OR ØLP[XY]3ØZ
Non-OR ØLP[XY]XØZ

SECTION: Ø MEDICAL AND SURGICAL
BODY SYSTEM: L TENDONS
OPERATION: Q REPAIR: Restoring, to the extent possible, a body part to its normal anatomic structure and function

Body Part	Approach	Device	Qualifier
Ø Head and Neck Tendon 1 Shoulder Tendon, Right 2 Shoulder Tendon, Left 3 Upper Arm Tendon, Right 4 Upper Arm Tendon, Left 5 Lower Arm and Wrist Tendon, Right 6 Lower Arm and Wrist Tendon, Left 7 Hand Tendon, Right 8 Hand Tendon, Left 9 Trunk Tendon, Right B Trunk Tendon, Left C Thorax Tendon, Right D Thorax Tendon, Left F Abdomen Tendon, Right G Abdomen Tendon, Left H Perineum Tendon J Hip Tendon, Right K Hip Tendon, Left L Upper Leg Tendon, Right M Upper Leg Tendon, Left N Lower Leg Tendon, Right P Lower Leg Tendon, Left Q Knee Tendon, Right R Knee Tendon, Left S Ankle Tendon, Right T Ankle Tendon, Left V Foot Tendon, Right W Foot Tendon, Left	Ø Open 3 Percutaneous 4 Percutaneous Endoscopic	Z No Device	Z No Qualifier

Coding Clinic: 2Ø13, Q3, P21 – ØLQ14ZZ
Coding Clinic: 2Ø16, Q3, P33 – ØLQ14ZZ

SECTION: Ø MEDICAL AND SURGICAL
BODY SYSTEM: L TENDONS
OPERATION: R REPLACEMENT: Putting in or on biological or synthetic material that physically takes the place and/or function of all or a portion of a body part

Body Part	Approach	Device	Qualifier
Ø Head and Neck Tendon 1 Shoulder Tendon, Right 2 Shoulder Tendon, Left 3 Upper Arm Tendon, Right 4 Upper Arm Tendon, Left 5 Lower Arm and Wrist Tendon, Right 6 Lower Arm and Wrist Tendon, Left 7 Hand Tendon, Right 8 Hand Tendon, Left 9 Trunk Tendon, Right B Trunk Tendon, Left C Thorax Tendon, Right D Thorax Tendon, Left F Abdomen Tendon, Right G Abdomen Tendon, Left H Perineum Tendon J Hip Tendon, Right K Hip Tendon, Left L Upper Leg Tendon, Right M Upper Leg Tendon, Left N Lower Leg Tendon, Right P Lower Leg Tendon, Left Q Knee Tendon, Right R Knee Tendon, Left S Ankle Tendon, Right T Ankle Tendon, Left V Foot Tendon, Right W Foot Tendon, Left	Ø Open 4 Percutaneous Endoscopic	7 Autologous Tissue Substitute J Synthetic Substitute K Nonautologous Tissue Substitute	Z No Qualifier

SECTION: Ø MEDICAL AND SURGICAL
BODY SYSTEM: L TENDONS
OPERATION: S REPOSITION: Moving to its normal location, or other suitable location, all or a portion of a body part

Body Part	Approach	Device	Qualifier
Ø Head and Neck Tendon 1 Shoulder Tendon, Right 2 Shoulder Tendon, Left 3 Upper Arm Tendon, Right 4 Upper Arm Tendon, Left 5 Lower Arm and Wrist Tendon, Right 6 Lower Arm and Wrist Tendon, Left 7 Hand Tendon, Right 8 Hand Tendon, Left 9 Trunk Tendon, Right B Trunk Tendon, Left C Thorax Tendon, Right D Thorax Tendon, Left F Abdomen Tendon, Right G Abdomen Tendon, Left H Perineum Tendon J Hip Tendon, Right K Hip Tendon, Left L Upper Leg Tendon, Right M Upper Leg Tendon, Left N Lower Leg Tendon, Right P Lower Leg Tendon, Left Q Knee Tendon, Right R Knee Tendon, Left S Ankle Tendon, Right T Ankle Tendon, Left V Foot Tendon, Right W Foot Tendon, Left	Ø Open 4 Percutaneous Endoscopic	Z No Device	Z No Qualifier

Coding Clinic: 2Ø15, Q3, P15 – ØLS4ØZZ
Coding Clinic: 2Ø16, Q3, P33 – ØLS3ØZZ

SECTION: Ø MEDICAL AND SURGICAL
BODY SYSTEM: L TENDONS
OPERATION: T RESECTION: Cutting out or off, without replacement, all of a body part

Body Part	Approach	Device	Qualifier
Ø Head and Neck Tendon 1 Shoulder Tendon, Right 2 Shoulder Tendon, Left 3 Upper Arm Tendon, Right 4 Upper Arm Tendon, Left 5 Lower Arm and Wrist Tendon, Right 6 Lower Arm and Wrist Tendon, Left 7 Hand Tendon, Right 8 Hand Tendon, Left 9 Trunk Tendon, Right B Trunk Tendon, Left C Thorax Tendon, Right D Thorax Tendon, Left F Abdomen Tendon, Right G Abdomen Tendon, Left H Perineum Tendon J Hip Tendon, Right K Hip Tendon, Left L Upper Leg Tendon, Right M Upper Leg Tendon, Left N Lower Leg Tendon, Right P Lower Leg Tendon, Left Q Knee Tendon, Right R Knee Tendon, Left S Ankle Tendon, Right T Ankle Tendon, Left V Foot Tendon, Right W Foot Tendon, Left	Ø Open 4 Percutaneous Endoscopic	Z No Device	Z No Qualifier

SECTION: Ø **MEDICAL AND SURGICAL**
BODY SYSTEM: L **TENDONS**
OPERATION: U **SUPPLEMENT:** Putting in or on biological or synthetic material that physically reinforces and/or augments the function of a portion of a body part

Body Part	Approach	Device	Qualifier
Ø Head and Neck Tendon 1 Shoulder Tendon, Right 2 Shoulder Tendon, Left 3 Upper Arm Tendon, Right 4 Upper Arm Tendon, Left 5 Lower Arm and Wrist Tendon, Right 6 Lower Arm and Wrist Tendon, Left 7 Hand Tendon, Right 8 Hand Tendon, Left 9 Trunk Tendon, Right B Trunk Tendon, Left C Thorax Tendon, Right D Thorax Tendon, Left F Abdomen Tendon, Right G Abdomen Tendon, Left H Perineum Tendon J Hip Tendon, Right K Hip Tendon, Left L Upper Leg Tendon, Right M Upper Leg Tendon, Left N Lower Leg Tendon, Right P Lower Leg Tendon, Left Q Knee Tendon, Right R Knee Tendon, Left S Ankle Tendon, Right T Ankle Tendon, Left V Foot Tendon, Right W Foot Tendon, Left	Ø Open 4 Percutaneous Endoscopic	7 Autologous Tissue Substitute J Synthetic Substitute K Nonautologous Tissue Substitute	Z No Qualifier

Coding Clinic: 2Ø15, Q2, P11 – ØLU[QM]ØKZ

SECTION: Ø **MEDICAL AND SURGICAL**
BODY SYSTEM: L **TENDONS**
OPERATION: W **REVISION:** Correcting, to the extent possible, a portion of a malfunctioning device or the position of a displaced device

Body Part	Approach	Device	Qualifier
X Upper Tendon Y Lower Tendon	Ø Open 3 Percutaneous 4 Percutaneous Endoscopic	Ø Drainage Device 7 Autologous Tissue Substitute J Synthetic Substitute K Nonautologous Tissue Substitute Y Other Device	Z No Qualifier
X Upper Tendon Y Lower Tendon	X External	Ø Drainage Device 7 Autologous Tissue Substitute J Synthetic Substitute K Nonautologous Tissue Substitute	Z No Qualifier

Non-OR ØLW[XY]X[Ø7JK]Z

SECTION: Ø MEDICAL AND SURGICAL
BODY SYSTEM: L TENDONS
OPERATION: X TRANSFER: Moving, without taking out, all or a portion of a body part to another location to take over the function of all or a portion of a body part

Body Part	Approach	Device	Qualifier
Ø Head and Neck Tendon 1 Shoulder Tendon, Right 2 Shoulder Tendon, Left 3 Upper Arm Tendon, Right 4 Upper Arm Tendon, Left 5 Lower Arm and Wrist Tendon, Right 6 Lower Arm and Wrist Tendon, Left 7 Hand Tendon, Right 8 Hand Tendon, Left 9 Trunk Tendon, Right B Trunk Tendon, Left C Thorax Tendon, Right D Thorax Tendon, Left F Abdomen Tendon, Right G Abdomen Tendon, Left H Perineum Tendon J Hip Tendon, Right K Hip Tendon, Left L Upper Leg Tendon, Right M Upper Leg Tendon, Left N Lower Leg Tendon, Right P Lower Leg Tendon, Left Q Knee Tendon, Right R Knee Tendon, Left S Ankle Tendon, Right T Ankle Tendon, Left V Foot Tendon, Right W Foot Tendon, Left	Ø Open 4 Percutaneous Endoscopic	Z No Device	Z No Qualifier

ØM. Bursae and Ligaments 36Ø
ØM2. Change 361
ØM5. Destruction 361
ØM8. Division 362
ØM9. Drainage 363
ØMB. Excision 364
ØMC. Extirpation 365
ØMD. Extraction 366
ØMH. Insertion 366
ØMJ. Inspection 367
ØMM. Reattachment 367
ØMN. Release 368
ØMP. Removal 368
ØMQ. Repair 369
ØMR. Replacement 37Ø
ØMS. Reposition 371
ØMT. Resection 372
ØMU. Supplement 373
ØMW. Revision 373
ØMX. Transfer 374

SECTION: Ø MEDICAL AND SURGICAL
BODY SYSTEM: M BURSAE AND LIGAMENTS
OPERATION: 2 CHANGE: Taking out or off a device from a body part and putting back an identical or similar device in or on the same body part without cutting or puncturing the skin or a mucous membrane

Body Part	Approach	Device	Qualifier
X Upper Bursa and Ligament Y Lower Bursa and Ligament	X External	Ø Drainage Device Y Other Device	Z No Qualifier

Non-OR All Values

SECTION: Ø MEDICAL AND SURGICAL
BODY SYSTEM: M BURSAE AND LIGAMENTS
OPERATION: 5 DESTRUCTION: Physical eradication of all or a portion of a body part by the direct use of energy, force, or a destructive agent

Body Part	Approach	Device	Qualifier
Ø Head and Neck Bursa and Ligament 1 Shoulder Bursa and Ligament, Right 2 Shoulder Bursa and Ligament, Left 3 Elbow Bursa and Ligament, Right 4 Elbow Bursa and Ligament, Left 5 Wrist Bursa and Ligament, Right 6 Wrist Bursa and Ligament, Left 7 Hand Bursa and Ligament, Right 8 Hand Bursa and Ligament, Left 9 Upper Extremity Bursa and Ligament, Right B Upper Extremity Bursa and Ligament, Left C Upper Spine Bursa and Ligament D Lower Spine Bursa and Ligament F Sternum Bursa and Ligament G Rib(s) Bursa and Ligament H Abdomen Bursa and Ligament, Right J Abdomen Bursa and Ligament, Left K Perineum Bursa and Ligament L Hip Bursa and Ligament, Right M Hip Bursa and Ligament, Left N Knee Bursa and Ligament, Right P Knee Bursa and Ligament, Left Q Ankle Bursa and Ligament, Right R Ankle Bursa and Ligament, Left S Foot Bursa and Ligament, Right T Foot Bursa and Ligament, Left V Lower Extremity Bursa and Ligament, Right W Lower Extremity Bursa and Ligament, Left	Ø Open 3 Percutaneous 4 Percutaneous Endoscopic	Z No Device	Z No Qualifier

SECTION: Ø MEDICAL AND SURGICAL
BODY SYSTEM: M BURSAE AND LIGAMENTS
OPERATION: 8 DIVISION: Cutting into a body part, without draining fluids and/or gases from the body part, in order to separate or transect a body part

Body Part	Approach	Device	Qualifier
Ø Head and Neck Bursa and Ligament 1 Shoulder Bursa and Ligament, Right 2 Shoulder Bursa and Ligament, Left 3 Elbow Bursa and Ligament, Right 4 Elbow Bursa and Ligament, Left 5 Wrist Bursa and Ligament, Right 6 Wrist Bursa and Ligament, Left 7 Hand Bursa and Ligament, Right 8 Hand Bursa and Ligament, Left 9 Upper Extremity Bursa and Ligament, Right B Upper Extremity Bursa and Ligament, Left C Upper Spine Bursa and Ligament D Lower Spine Bursa and Ligament F Sternum Bursa and Ligament G Rib(s) Bursa and Ligament H Abdomen Bursa and Ligament, Right J Abdomen Bursa and Ligament, Left K Perineum Bursa and Ligament L Hip Bursa and Ligament, Right M Hip Bursa and Ligament, Left N Knee Bursa and Ligament, Right P Knee Bursa and Ligament, Left Q Ankle Bursa and Ligament, Right R Ankle Bursa and Ligament, Left S Foot Bursa and Ligament, Right T Foot Bursa and Ligament, Left V Lower Extremity Bursa and Ligament, Right W Lower Extremity Bursa and Ligament, Left	Ø Open 3 Percutaneous 4 Percutaneous Endoscopic	Z No Device	Z No Qualifier

SECTION: Ø MEDICAL AND SURGICAL
BODY SYSTEM: M BURSAE AND LIGAMENTS
OPERATION: 9 DRAINAGE: Taking or letting out fluids and/or gases from a body part

Body Part	Approach	Device	Qualifier
Ø Head and Neck Bursa and Ligament 1 Shoulder Bursa and Ligament, Right 2 Shoulder Bursa and Ligament, Left 3 Elbow Bursa and Ligament, Right 4 Elbow Bursa and Ligament, Left 5 Wrist Bursa and Ligament, Right 6 Wrist Bursa and Ligament, Left 7 Hand Bursa and Ligament, Right 8 Hand Bursa and Ligament, Left 9 Upper Extremity Bursa and Ligament, Right B Upper Extremity Bursa and Ligament, Left C Upper Spine Bursa and Ligament D Lower Spine Bursa and Ligament F Sternum Bursa and Ligament G Rib(s) Bursa and Ligament H Abdomen Bursa and Ligament, Right J Abdomen Bursa and Ligament, Left K Perineum Bursa and Ligament L Hip Bursa and Ligament, Right M Hip Bursa and Ligament, Left N Knee Bursa and Ligament, Right P Knee Bursa and Ligament, Left Q Ankle Bursa and Ligament, Right R Ankle Bursa and Ligament, Left S Foot Bursa and Ligament, Right T Foot Bursa and Ligament, Left V Lower Extremity Bursa and Ligament, Right W Lower Extremity Bursa and Ligament, Left	Ø Open 3 Percutaneous 4 Percutaneous Endoscopic	Ø Drainage Device	Z No Qualifier
Ø Head and Neck Bursa and Ligament 1 Shoulder Bursa and Ligament, Right 2 Shoulder Bursa and Ligament, Left 3 Elbow Bursa and Ligament, Right 4 Elbow Bursa and Ligament, Left 5 Wrist Bursa and Ligament, Right 6 Wrist Bursa and Ligament, Left 7 Hand Bursa and Ligament, Right 8 Hand Bursa and Ligament, Left 9 Upper Extremity Bursa and Ligament, Right B Upper Extremity Bursa and Ligament, Left C Upper Spine Bursa and Ligament D Lower Spine Bursa and Ligament F Sternum Bursa and Ligament G Rib(s) Bursa and Ligament H Abdomen Bursa and Ligament, Right J Abdomen Bursa and Ligament, Left K Perineum Bursa and Ligament L Hip Bursa and Ligament, Right M Hip Bursa and Ligament, Left N Knee Bursa and Ligament, Right P Knee Bursa and Ligament, Left Q Ankle Bursa and Ligament, Right R Ankle Bursa and Ligament, Left S Foot Bursa and Ligament, Right T Foot Bursa and Ligament, Left V Lower Extremity Bursa and Ligament, Right W Lower Extremity Bursa and Ligament, Left	Ø Open 3 Percutaneous 4 Percutaneous Endoscopic	Z No Device	X Diagnostic Z No Qualifier

Non-OR ØM9[1234789BCDFGHJKLMVW][34]ØZ
Non-OR ØM9[Ø56NPQRST]3ØZ
Non-OR ØM9[Ø12345678CDFGLMNPQRST][Ø34]ZX
Non-OR ØM9[Ø56789BCDFGHJKNPQRSTVW][34]ZZ
Non-OR ØM9[1234LM]3ZZ

SECTION: Ø MEDICAL AND SURGICAL
BODY SYSTEM: M BURSAE AND LIGAMENTS
OPERATION: B EXCISION: Cutting out or off, without replacement, a portion of a body part

Body Part	Approach	Device	Qualifier
Ø Head and Neck Bursa and Ligament 1 Shoulder Bursa and Ligament, Right 2 Shoulder Bursa and Ligament, Left 3 Elbow Bursa and Ligament, Right 4 Elbow Bursa and Ligament, Left 5 Wrist Bursa and Ligament, Right 6 Wrist Bursa and Ligament, Left 7 Hand Bursa and Ligament, Right 8 Hand Bursa and Ligament, Left 9 Upper Extremity Bursa and Ligament, Right B Upper Extremity Bursa and Ligament, Left C Upper Spine Bursa and Ligament D Lower Spine Bursa and Ligament F Sternum Bursa and Ligament G Rib(s) Bursa and Ligament H Abdomen Bursa and Ligament, Right J Abdomen Bursa and Ligament, Left K Perineum Bursa and Ligament L Hip Bursa and Ligament, Right M Hip Bursa and Ligament, Left N Knee Bursa and Ligament, Right P Knee Bursa and Ligament, Left Q Ankle Bursa and Ligament, Right R Ankle Bursa and Ligament, Left S Foot Bursa and Ligament, Right T Foot Bursa and Ligament, Left V Lower Extremity Bursa and Ligament, Right W Lower Extremity Bursa and Ligament, Left	Ø Open 3 Percutaneous 4 Percutaneous Endoscopic	Z No Device	X Diagnostic Z No Qualifier

Non-OR ØMB[Ø12345678BCDFGLMNPQRST][Ø34]ZX
Non-OR ØMB94ZX

SECTION: Ø MEDICAL AND SURGICAL
BODY SYSTEM: M BURSAE AND LIGAMENTS
OPERATION: C EXTIRPATION: Taking or cutting out solid matter from a body part

Body Part	Approach	Device	Qualifier
Ø Head and Neck Bursa and Ligament 1 Shoulder Bursa and Ligament, Right 2 Shoulder Bursa and Ligament, Left 3 Elbow Bursa and Ligament, Right 4 Elbow Bursa and Ligament, Left 5 Wrist Bursa and Ligament, Right 6 Wrist Bursa and Ligament, Left 7 Hand Bursa and Ligament, Right 8 Hand Bursa and Ligament, Left 9 Upper Extremity Bursa and Ligament, Right B Upper Extremity Bursa and Ligament, Left C Upper Spine Bursa and Ligament D Lower Spine Bursa and Ligament F Sternum Bursa and Ligament G Rib(s) Bursa and Ligament H Abdomen Bursa and Ligament, Right J Abdomen Bursa and Ligament, Left K Perineum Bursa and Ligament L Hip Bursa and Ligament, Right M Hip Bursa and Ligament, Left N Knee Bursa and Ligament, Right P Knee Bursa and Ligament, Left Q Ankle Bursa and Ligament, Right R Ankle Bursa and Ligament, Left S Foot Bursa and Ligament, Right T Foot Bursa and Ligament, Left V Lower Extremity Bursa and Ligament, Right W Lower Extremity Bursa and Ligament, Left	Ø Open 3 Percutaneous 4 Percutaneous Endoscopic	Z No Device	Z No Qualifier

SECTION: Ø MEDICAL AND SURGICAL
BODY SYSTEM: M BURSAE AND LIGAMENTS
OPERATION: D EXTRACTION: Pulling or stripping out or off all or a portion of a body part by the use of force

Body Part	Approach	Device	Qualifier
Ø Head and Neck Bursa and Ligament 1 Shoulder Bursa and Ligament, Right 2 Shoulder Bursa and Ligament, Left 3 Elbow Bursa and Ligament, Right 4 Elbow Bursa and Ligament, Left 5 Wrist Bursa and Ligament, Right 6 Wrist Bursa and Ligament, Left 7 Hand Bursa and Ligament, Right 8 Hand Bursa and Ligament, Left 9 Upper Extremity Bursa and Ligament, Right B Upper Extremity Bursa and Ligament, Left C Upper Spine Bursa and Ligament D Lower Spine Bursa and Ligament F Sternum Bursa and Ligament G Rib(s) Bursa and Ligament H Abdomen Bursa and Ligament, Right J Abdomen Bursa and Ligament, Left K Perineum Bursa and Ligament L Hip Bursa and Ligament, Right M Hip Bursa and Ligament, Left N Knee Bursa and Ligament, Right P Knee Bursa and Ligament, Left Q Ankle Bursa and Ligament, Right R Ankle Bursa and Ligament, Left S Foot Bursa and Ligament, Right T Foot Bursa and Ligament, Left V Lower Extremity Bursa and Ligament, Right W Lower Extremity Bursa and Ligament, Left	Ø Open 3 Percutaneous 4 Percutaneous Endoscopic	Z No Device	Z No Qualifier

SECTION: Ø MEDICAL AND SURGICAL
BODY SYSTEM: M BURSAE AND LIGAMENTS
OPERATION: H INSERTION: Putting in a nonbiological appliance that monitors, assists, performs, or prevents a physiological function but does not physically take the place of a body part

Body Part	Approach	Device	Qualifier
X Upper Bursa and Ligament Y Lower Bursa and Ligament	Ø Open 3 Percutaneous 4 Percutaneous Endoscopic	Y Other Device	Z No Qualifier

SECTION: Ø MEDICAL AND SURGICAL
BODY SYSTEM: M BURSAE AND LIGAMENTS
OPERATION: J INSPECTION: Visually and/or manually exploring a body part

Body Part	Approach	Device	Qualifier
X Upper Bursa and Ligament Y Lower Bursa and Ligament	Ø Open 3 Percutaneous 4 Percutaneous Endoscopic X External	Z No Device	Z No Qualifier

Non-OR ØMJ[XY][3X]ZZ

SECTION: Ø MEDICAL AND SURGICAL
BODY SYSTEM: M BURSAE AND LIGAMENTS
OPERATION: M REATTACHMENT: Putting back in or on all or a portion of a separated body part to its normal location or other suitable location

Body Part	Approach	Device	Qualifier
Ø Head and Neck Bursa and Ligament 1 Shoulder Bursa and Ligament, Right 2 Shoulder Bursa and Ligament, Left 3 Elbow Bursa and Ligament, Right 4 Elbow Bursa and Ligament, Left 5 Wrist Bursa and Ligament, Right 6 Wrist Bursa and Ligament, Left 7 Hand Bursa and Ligament, Right 8 Hand Bursa and Ligament, Left 9 Upper Extremity Bursa and Ligament, Right B Upper Extremity Bursa and Ligament, Left C Upper Spine Bursa and Ligament D Lower Spine Bursa and Ligament F Sternum Bursa and Ligament G Rib(s) Bursa and Ligament H Abdomen Bursa and Ligament, Right J Abdomen Bursa and Ligament, Left K Perineum Bursa and Ligament L Hip Bursa and Ligament, Right M Hip Bursa and Ligament, Left N Knee Bursa and Ligament, Right P Knee Bursa and Ligament, Left Q Ankle Bursa and Ligament, Right R Ankle Bursa and Ligament, Left S Foot Bursa and Ligament, Right T Foot Bursa and Ligament, Left V Lower Extremity Bursa and Ligament, Right W Lower Extremity Bursa and Ligament, Left	Ø Open 4 Percutaneous Endoscopic	Z No Device	Z No Qualifier

Coding Clinic: 2Ø13, Q3, P22 – ØMM14ZZ

SECTION: Ø MEDICAL AND SURGICAL
BODY SYSTEM: M BURSAE AND LIGAMENTS
OPERATION: N RELEASE: Freeing a body part from an abnormal physical constraint by cutting or by the use of force

Body Part	Approach	Device	Qualifier
Ø Head and Neck Bursa and Ligament 1 Shoulder Bursa and Ligament, Right 2 Shoulder Bursa and Ligament, Left 3 Elbow Bursa and Ligament, Right 4 Elbow Bursa and Ligament, Left 5 Wrist Bursa and Ligament, Right 6 Wrist Bursa and Ligament, Left 7 Hand Bursa and Ligament, Right 8 Hand Bursa and Ligament, Left 9 Upper Extremity Bursa and Ligament, Right B Upper Extremity Bursa and Ligament, Left C Upper Spine Bursa and Ligament D Lower Spine Bursa and Ligament F Sternum Bursa and Ligament G Rib(s) Bursa and Ligament H Abdomen Bursa and Ligament, Right J Abdomen Bursa and Ligament, Left K Perineum Bursa and Ligament L Hip Bursa and Ligament, Right M Hip Bursa and Ligament, Left N Knee Bursa and Ligament, Right P Knee Bursa and Ligament, Left Q Ankle Bursa and Ligament, Right R Ankle Bursa and Ligament, Left S Foot Bursa and Ligament, Right T Foot Bursa and Ligament, Left V Lower Extremity Bursa and Ligament, Right W Lower Extremity Bursa and Ligament, Left	Ø Open 3 Percutaneous 4 Percutaneous Endoscopic X External	Z No Device	Z No Qualifier

Non-OR ØMN[Ø123456789BCDFGHJKLMNPQRSTVW]XZZ

SECTION: Ø MEDICAL AND SURGICAL
BODY SYSTEM: M BURSAE AND LIGAMENTS
OPERATION: P REMOVAL: Taking out or off a device from a body part

Body Part	Approach	Device	Qualifier
X Upper Bursa and Ligament Y Lower Bursa and Ligament	Ø Open 3 Percutaneous 4 Percutaneous Endoscopic	Ø Drainage Device 7 Autologous Tissue Substitute J Synthetic Substitute K Nonautologous Tissue Substitute Y Other Device	Z No Qualifier
X Upper Bursa and Ligament Y Lower Bursa and Ligament	X External	Ø Drainage Device	Z No Qualifier

Non-OR ØMP[XY]3ØZ
Non-OR ØMP[XY]XØZ

SECTION: Ø MEDICAL AND SURGICAL
BODY SYSTEM: M BURSAE AND LIGAMENTS
OPERATION: Q REPAIR: Restoring, to the extent possible, a body part to its normal anatomic structure and function

Body Part	Approach	Device	Qualifier
Ø Head and Neck Bursa and Ligament 1 Shoulder Bursa and Ligament, Right 2 Shoulder Bursa and Ligament, Left 3 Elbow Bursa and Ligament, Right 4 Elbow Bursa and Ligament, Left 5 Wrist Bursa and Ligament, Right 6 Wrist Bursa and Ligament, Left 7 Hand Bursa and Ligament, Right 8 Hand Bursa and Ligament, Left 9 Upper Extremity Bursa and Ligament, Right B Upper Extremity Bursa and Ligament, Left C Upper Spine Bursa and Ligament D Lower Spine Bursa and Ligament F Sternum Bursa and Ligament G Rib(s) Bursa and Ligament H Abdomen Bursa and Ligament, Right J Abdomen Bursa and Ligament, Left K Perineum Bursa and Ligament L Hip Bursa and Ligament, Right M Hip Bursa and Ligament, Left N Knee Bursa and Ligament, Right P Knee Bursa and Ligament, Left Q Ankle Bursa and Ligament, Right R Ankle Bursa and Ligament, Left S Foot Bursa and Ligament, Right T Foot Bursa and Ligament, Left V Lower Extremity Bursa and Ligament, Right W Lower Extremity Bursa and Ligament, Left	Ø Open 3 Percutaneous 4 Percutaneous Endoscopic	Z No Device	Z No Qualifier

SECTION: Ø MEDICAL AND SURGICAL
BODY SYSTEM: M BURSAE AND LIGAMENTS
OPERATION: R REPLACEMENT: Putting in or on biological or synthetic material that physically takes the place and/or function of all or a portion of a body part

Body Part	Approach	Device	Qualifier
Ø Head and Neck Bursa and Ligament 1 Shoulder Bursa and Ligament, Right 2 Shoulder Bursa and Ligament, Left 3 Elbow Bursa and Ligament, Right 4 Elbow Bursa and Ligament, Left 5 Wrist Bursa and Ligament, Right 6 Wrist Bursa and Ligament, Left 7 Hand Bursa and Ligament, Right 8 Hand Bursa and Ligament, Left 9 Upper Extremity Bursa and Ligament, Right B Upper Extremity Bursa and Ligament, Left C Upper Spine Bursa and Ligament D Lower Spine Bursa and Ligament F Sternum Bursa and Ligament G Rib(s) Bursa and Ligament H Abdomen Bursa and Ligament, Right J Abdomen Bursa and Ligament, Left K Perineum Bursa and Ligament L Hip Bursa and Ligament, Right M Hip Bursa and Ligament, Left N Knee Bursa and Ligament, Right P Knee Bursa and Ligament, Left Q Ankle Bursa and Ligament, Right R Ankle Bursa and Ligament, Left S Foot Bursa and Ligament, Right T Foot Bursa and Ligament, Left V Lower Extremity Bursa and Ligament, Right W Lower Extremity Bursa and Ligament, Left	Ø Open 4 Percutaneous Endoscopic	7 Autologous Tissue Substitute J Synthetic Substitute K Nonautologous Tissue Substitute	Z No Qualifier

SECTION: Ø MEDICAL AND SURGICAL
BODY SYSTEM: M BURSAE AND LIGAMENTS
OPERATION: S REPOSITION: Moving to its normal location, or other suitable location, all or a portion of a body part

Body Part	Approach	Device	Qualifier
Ø Head and Neck Bursa and Ligament 1 Shoulder Bursa and Ligament, Right 2 Shoulder Bursa and Ligament, Left 3 Elbow Bursa and Ligament, Right 4 Elbow Bursa and Ligament, Left 5 Wrist Bursa and Ligament, Right 6 Wrist Bursa and Ligament, Left 7 Hand Bursa and Ligament, Right 8 Hand Bursa and Ligament, Left 9 Upper Extremity Bursa and Ligament, Right B Upper Extremity Bursa and Ligament, Left C Upper Spine Bursa and Ligament D Lower Spine Bursa and Ligament F Sternum Bursa and Ligament G Rib(s) Bursa and Ligament H Abdomen Bursa and Ligament, Right J Abdomen Bursa and Ligament, Left K Perineum Bursa and Ligament L Hip Bursa and Ligament, Right M Hip Bursa and Ligament, Left N Knee Bursa and Ligament, Right P Knee Bursa and Ligament, Left Q Ankle Bursa and Ligament, Right R Ankle Bursa and Ligament, Left S Foot Bursa and Ligament, Right T Foot Bursa and Ligament, Left V Lower Extremity Bursa and Ligament, Right W Lower Extremity Bursa and Ligament, Left	Ø Open 4 Percutaneous Endoscopic	Z No Device	Z No Qualifier

SECTION: Ø MEDICAL AND SURGICAL
BODY SYSTEM: M BURSAE AND LIGAMENTS
OPERATION: T RESECTION: Cutting out or off, without replacement, all of a body part

Body Part	Approach	Device	Qualifier
Ø Head and Neck Bursa and Ligament 1 Shoulder Bursa and Ligament, Right 2 Shoulder Bursa and Ligament, Left 3 Elbow Bursa and Ligament, Right 4 Elbow Bursa and Ligament, Left 5 Wrist Bursa and Ligament, Right 6 Wrist Bursa and Ligament, Left 7 Hand Bursa and Ligament, Right 8 Hand Bursa and Ligament, Left 9 Upper Extremity Bursa and Ligament, Right B Upper Extremity Bursa and Ligament, Left C Upper Spine Bursa and Ligament D Lower Spine Bursa and Ligament F Sternum Bursa and Ligament G Rib(s) Bursa and Ligament H Abdomen Bursa and Ligament, Right J Abdomen Bursa and Ligament, Left K Perineum Bursa and Ligament L Hip Bursa and Ligament, Right M Hip Bursa and Ligament, Left N Knee Bursa and Ligament, Right P Knee Bursa and Ligament, Left Q Ankle Bursa and Ligament, Right R Ankle Bursa and Ligament, Left S Foot Bursa and Ligament, Right T Foot Bursa and Ligament, Left V Lower Extremity Bursa and Ligament, Right W Lower Extremity Bursa and Ligament, Left	Ø Open 4 Percutaneous Endoscopic	Z No Device	Z No Qualifier

SECTION: Ø MEDICAL AND SURGICAL
BODY SYSTEM: M BURSAE AND LIGAMENTS
OPERATION: U SUPPLEMENT: Putting in or on biological or synthetic material that physically reinforces and/or augments the function of a portion of a body part

Body Part	Approach	Device	Qualifier
Ø Head and Neck Bursa and Ligament 1 Shoulder Bursa and Ligament, Right 2 Shoulder Bursa and Ligament, Left 3 Elbow Bursa and Ligament, Right 4 Elbow Bursa and Ligament, Left 5 Wrist Bursa and Ligament, Right 6 Wrist Bursa and Ligament, Left 7 Hand Bursa and Ligament, Right 8 Hand Bursa and Ligament, Left 9 Upper Extremity Bursa and Ligament, Right B Upper Extremity Bursa and Ligament, Left C Upper Spine Bursa and Ligament D Lower Spine Bursa and Ligament F Sternum Bursa and Ligament G Rib(s) Bursa and Ligament H Abdomen Bursa and Ligament, Right J Abdomen Bursa and Ligament, Left K Perineum Bursa and Ligament L Hip Bursa and Ligament, Right M Hip Bursa and Ligament, Left N Knee Bursa and Ligament, Right P Knee Bursa and Ligament, Left Q Ankle Bursa and Ligament, Right R Ankle Bursa and Ligament, Left S Foot Bursa and Ligament, Right T Foot Bursa and Ligament, Left V Lower Extremity Bursa and Ligament, Right W Lower Extremity Bursa and Ligament, Left	Ø Open 4 Percutaneous Endoscopic	7 Autologous Tissue Substitute J Synthetic Substitute K Nonautologous Tissue Substitute	Z No Qualifier

Coding Clinic: 2017, Q2, P22 – ØMUN47Z

SECTION: Ø MEDICAL AND SURGICAL
BODY SYSTEM: M BURSAE AND LIGAMENTS
OPERATION: W REVISION: Correcting, to the extent possible, a portion of a malfunctioning device or the position of a displaced device

Body Part	Approach	Device	Qualifier
X Upper Bursa and Ligament Y Lower Bursa and Ligament	Ø Open 3 Percutaneous 4 Percutaneous Endoscopic	Ø Drainage Device 7 Autologous Tissue Substitute J Synthetic Substitute K Nonautologous Tissue Substitute Y Other Device	Z No Qualifier
X Upper Bursa and Ligament Y Lower Bursa and Ligament	X External	Ø Drainage Device 7 Autologous Tissue Substitute J Synthetic Substitute K Nonautologous Tissue Substitute	Z No Qualifier

Non-OR ØMW[XY]X[Ø7JK]Z

SECTION: Ø MEDICAL AND SURGICAL
BODY SYSTEM: M BURSAE AND LIGAMENTS
OPERATION: X TRANSFER: Moving, without taking out, all or a portion of a body part to another location to take over the function of all or a portion of a body part

Body Part	Approach	Device	Qualifier
Ø Head and Neck Bursa and Ligament 1 Shoulder Bursa and Ligament, Right 2 Shoulder Bursa and Ligament, Left 3 Elbow Bursa and Ligament, Right 4 Elbow Bursa and Ligament, Left 5 Wrist Bursa and Ligament, Right 6 Wrist Bursa and Ligament, Left 7 Hand Bursa and Ligament, Right 8 Hand Bursa and Ligament, Left 9 Upper Extremity Bursa and Ligament, Right B Upper Extremity Bursa and Ligament, Left C Upper Spine Bursa and Ligament D Lower Spine Bursa and Ligament F Sternum Bursa and Ligament G Rib(s) Bursa and Ligament H Abdomen Bursa and Ligament, Right J Abdomen Bursa and Ligament, Left K Perineum Bursa and Ligament L Hip Bursa and Ligament, Right M Hip Bursa and Ligament, Left N Knee Bursa and Ligament, Right P Knee Bursa and Ligament, Left Q Ankle Bursa and Ligament, Right R Ankle Bursa and Ligament, Left S Foot Bursa and Ligament, Right T Foot Bursa and Ligament, Left V Lower Extremity Bursa and Ligament, Right W Lower Extremity Bursa and Ligament, Left	Ø Open 4 Percutaneous Endoscopic	Z No Device	Z No Qualifier

ØN. Head and Facial Bones 375
ØN2. Change 376
ØN5. Destruction 376
ØN8. Division 377
ØN9. Drainage 378
ØNB. Excision 379
ØNC. Extirpation 38Ø
ØND. Extraction 38Ø
ØNH. Insertion 381
ØNJ. Inspection 382
ØNN. Release 382
ØNP. Removal 383
ØNQ. Repair 384
ØNR. Replacement 385
ØNS. Reposition 385
ØNT. Resection 387
ØNU. Supplement 388
ØNW. Revision 389

SECTION: Ø MEDICAL AND SURGICAL
BODY SYSTEM: N HEAD AND FACIAL BONES
OPERATION: 2 CHANGE: Taking out or off a device from a body part and putting back an identical or similar device in or on the same body part without cutting or puncturing the skin or a mucous membrane

Body Part	Approach	Device	Qualifier
Ø Skull B Nasal Bone W Facial Bone	X External	Ø Drainage Device Y Other Device	Z No Qualifier

Non-OR All Values

SECTION: Ø MEDICAL AND SURGICAL
BODY SYSTEM: N HEAD AND FACIAL BONES
OPERATION: 5 DESTRUCTION: Physical eradication of all or a portion of a body part by the direct use of energy, force, or a destructive agent

Body Part	Approach	Device	Qualifier
Ø Skull 1 Frontal Bone 3 Parietal Bone, Right 4 Parietal Bone, Left 5 Temporal Bone, Right 6 Temporal Bone, Left 7 Occipital Bone B Nasal Bone C Sphenoid Bone F Ethmoid Bone, Right G Ethmoid Bone, Left H Lacrimal Bone, Right J Lacrimal Bone, Left K Palatine Bone, Right L Palatine Bone, Left M Zygomatic Bone, Right N Zygomatic Bone, Left P Orbit, Right Q Orbit, Left R Maxilla T Mandible, Right V Mandible, Left X Hyoid Bone	Ø Open 3 Percutaneous 4 Percutaneous Endoscopic	Z No Device	Z No Qualifier

SECTION: Ø MEDICAL AND SURGICAL
BODY SYSTEM: N HEAD AND FACIAL BONES
OPERATION: 8 DIVISION: Cutting into a body part, without draining fluids and/or gases from the body part, in order to separate or transect a body part

Body Part	Approach	Device	Qualifier
Ø Skull 1 Frontal Bone 3 Parietal Bone, Right 4 Parietal Bone, Left 5 Temporal Bone, Right 6 Temporal Bone, Left 7 Occipital Bonet B Nasal Bone C Sphenoid Bone F Ethmoid Bone, Right G Ethmoid Bone, Left H Lacrimal Bone, Right J Lacrimal Bone, Left K Palatine Bone, Right L Palatine Bone, Left M Zygomatic Bone, Right N Zygomatic Bone, Left P Orbit, Right Q Orbit, Left R Maxilla T Mandible, Right V Mandible, Left X Hyoid Bone	Ø Open 3 Percutaneous 4 Percutaneous Endoscopic	Z No Device	Z No Qualifier

Non-OR ØN8B[Ø34]ZZ

SECTION: Ø MEDICAL AND SURGICAL
BODY SYSTEM: N HEAD AND FACIAL BONES
OPERATION: 9 DRAINAGE: Taking or letting out fluids and/or gases from a body part

Body Part	Approach	Device	Qualifier
Ø Skull 1 Frontal Bone 3 Parietal Bone, Right 4 Parietal Bone, Left 5 Temporal Bone, Right 6 Temporal Bone, Left 7 Occipital Bone B Nasal Bone C Sphenoid Bone F Ethmoid Bone, Right G Ethmoid Bone, Left H Lacrimal Bone, Right J Lacrimal Bone, Left K Palatine Bone, Right L Palatine Bone, Left M Zygomatic Bone, Right N Zygomatic Bone, Left P Orbit, Right Q Orbit, Left R Maxilla T Mandible, Right V Mandible, Left X Hyoid Bone	Ø Open 3 Percutaneous 4 Percutaneous Endoscopic	Ø Drainage Device	Z No Qualifier
Ø Skull 1 Frontal Bone 3 Parietal Bone, Right 4 Parietal Bone, Left 5 Temporal Bone, Right 6 Temporal Bone, Left 7 Occipital Bone B Nasal Bone C Sphenoid Bone F Ethmoid Bone, Right G Ethmoid Bone, Left H Lacrimal Bone, Right J Lacrimal Bone, Left K Palatine Bone, Right L Palatine Bone, Left M Zygomatic Bone, Right N Zygomatic Bone, Left P Orbit, Right Q Orbit, Left R Maxilla T Mandible, Right V Mandible, Left X Hyoid Bone	Ø Open 3 Percutaneous 4 Percutaneous Endoscopic	Z No Device	X Diagnostic Z No Qualifier

Non-OR ØN9[Ø134567CFGHJKLMNPQX]3ØZ
Non-OR ØN9[BRTV][Ø34]ØZ
Non-OR ØN9[Ø134567CFGHJKLMNPQX]3ZZ
Non-OR ØN9B[Ø34]ZX
Non-OR ØN9[BRTV][Ø34]ZZ

SECTION: Ø MEDICAL AND SURGICAL
BODY SYSTEM: N HEAD AND FACIAL BONES
OPERATION: B EXCISION: Cutting out or off, without replacement, a portion of a body part

Body Part	Approach	Device	Qualifier
Ø Skull 1 Frontal Bone 3 Parietal Bone, Right 4 Parietal Bone, Left 5 Temporal Bone, Right 6 Temporal Bone, Left 7 Occipital Bone B Nasal Bone C Sphenoid Bone F Ethmoid Bone, Right G Ethmoid Bone, Left H Lacrimal Bone, Right J Lacrimal Bone, Left K Palatine Bone, Right L Palatine Bone, Left M Zygomatic Bone, Right N Zygomatic Bone, Left P Orbit, Right Q Orbit, Left R Maxilla T Mandible, Right V Mandible, Left X Hyoid Bone	Ø Open 3 Percutaneous 4 Percutaneous Endoscopic	Z No Device	X Diagnostic Z No Qualifier

Non-OR ØNB[BRTV][Ø34]ZX

Coding Clinic: 2Ø15, Q2, P13 – ØNBQØZZ
Coding Clinic: 2Ø17, Q1, P2Ø – ØNBBØZZ
Coding Clinic: 2Ø22, Q2, P18; 2Ø21, Q1, P21 – ØNBRØZZ
Coding Clinic: 2Ø21, Q3, P2Ø – ØNBXØZZ
Coding Clinic: 2Ø24, Q2, P18 – ØNBC4ZZ

SECTION: Ø MEDICAL AND SURGICAL
BODY SYSTEM: N HEAD AND FACIAL BONES
OPERATION: C EXTIRPATION: Taking or cutting out solid matter from a body part

Body Part	Approach	Device	Qualifier
1 Frontal Bone 3 Parietal Bone, Right 4 Parietal Bone, Left 5 Temporal Bone, Right 6 Temporal Bone, Left 7 Occipital Bone B Nasal Bone C Sphenoid Bone F Ethmoid Bone, Right G Ethmoid Bone, Left H Lacrimal Bone, Right J Lacrimal Bone, Left K Palatine Bone, Right L Palatine Bone, Left M Zygomatic Bone, Right N Zygomatic Bone, Left P Orbit, Right Q Orbit, Left R Maxilla T Mandible, Right V Mandible, Left X Hyoid Bone	Ø Open 3 Percutaneous 4 Percutaneous Endoscopic	Z No Device	Z No Qualifier

Non-OR ØNC[BRTV][Ø34]ZZ

SECTION: Ø MEDICAL AND SURGICAL
BODY SYSTEM: N HEAD AND FACIAL BONES
OPERATION: D EXTRACTION: Pulling or stripping out or off all or a portion of a body part by the use of force

Body Part	Approach	Device	Qualifier
Ø Skull 1 Frontal Bone 3 Parietal Bone, Right 4 Parietal Bone, Left 5 Temporal Bone, Right 6 Temporal Bone, Left 7 Occipital Bone B Nasal Bone C Sphenoid Bone F Ethmoid Bone, Right G Ethmoid Bone, Left H Lacrimal Bone, Right J Lacrimal Bone, Left K Palatine Bone, Right L Palatine Bone, Left M Zygomatic Bone, Right N Zygomatic Bone, Left P Orbit, Right Q Orbit, Left R Maxilla T Mandible, Right V Mandible, Left X Hyoid Bone	Ø Open	Z No Device	Z No Qualifier

SECTION: Ø MEDICAL AND SURGICAL
BODY SYSTEM: N HEAD AND FACIAL BONES
OPERATION: H INSERTION: Putting in a nonbiological appliance that monitors, assists, performs, or prevents a physiological function but does not physically take the place of a body part

Body Part	Approach	Device	Qualifier
Ø Skull ⊞	Ø Open	3 Infusion Device 4 Internal Fixation Device 5 External Fixation Device M Bone Growth Stimulator N Neurostimulator Generator	Z No Qualifier
Ø Skull	3 Percutaneous 4 Percutaneous Endoscopic	3 Infusion Device 4 Internal Fixation Device 5 External Fixation Device M Bone Growth Stimulator	Z No Qualifier
1 Frontal Bone 3 Parietal Bone, Right 4 Parietal Bone, Left 7 Occipital Bone C Sphenoid Bone F Ethmoid Bone, Right G Ethmoid Bone, Left H Lacrimal Bone, Right J Lacrimal Bone, Left K Palatine Bone, Right L Palatine Bone, Left M Zygomatic Bone, Right N Zygomatic Bone, Left P Orbit, Right Q Orbit, Left X Hyoid Bone	Ø Open 3 Percutaneous 4 Percutaneous Endoscopic	4 Internal Fixation Device	Z No Qualifier
5 Temporal Bone, Right 6 Temporal Bone, Left	Ø Open 3 Percutaneous 4 Percutaneous Endoscopic	4 Internal Fixation Device S Hearing Device	Z No Qualifier
B Nasal Bone	Ø Open 3 Percutaneous 4 Percutaneous Endoscopic	4 Internal Fixation Device M Bone Growth Stimulator	Z No Qualifier
R Maxilla T Mandible, Right V Mandible, Left	Ø Open 3 Percutaneous 4 Percutaneous Endoscopic	4 Internal Fixation Device 5 External Fixation Device	Z No Qualifier
W Facial Bone	Ø Open 3 Percutaneous 4 Percutaneous Endoscopic	M Bone Growth Stimulator	Z No Qualifier

⊞ ØNHØØNZ
Non-OR ØNHØØ5Z
Non-OR ØNHØ[34]5Z
Non-OR ØNHB[Ø34][4M]Z

Coding Clinic: 2Ø15, Q3, P14 – ØNHØØ4Z

SECTION: Ø MEDICAL AND SURGICAL
BODY SYSTEM: N HEAD AND FACIAL BONES
OPERATION: J INSPECTION: Visually and/or manually exploring a body part

Body Part	Approach	Device	Qualifier
Ø Skull B Nasal Bone W Facial Bone	Ø Open 3 Percutaneous 4 Percutaneous Endoscopic X External	Z No Device	Z No Qualifier

Non-OR ØNJ[ØBW][3X]ZZ

SECTION: Ø MEDICAL AND SURGICAL
BODY SYSTEM: N HEAD AND FACIAL BONES
OPERATION: N RELEASE: Freeing a body part from an abnormal physical constraint by cutting or by the use of force

Body Part	Approach	Device	Qualifier
1 Frontal Bone 3 Parietal Bone, Right 4 Parietal Bone, Left 5 Temporal Bone, Right 6 Temporal Bone, Left 7 Occipital Bone B Nasal Bone C Sphenoid Bone F Ethmoid Bone, Right G Ethmoid Bone, Left H Lacrimal Bone, Right J Lacrimal Bone, Left K Palatine Bone, Right L Palatine Bone, Left M Zygomatic Bone, Right N Zygomatic Bone, Left P Orbit, Right Q Orbit, Left R Maxilla T Mandible, Right V Mandible, Left X Hyoid Bone	Ø Open 3 Percutaneous 4 Percutaneous Endoscopic	Z No Device	Z No Qualifier

Non-OR ØNNB[Ø34]ZZ

SECTION: Ø MEDICAL AND SURGICAL
BODY SYSTEM: N HEAD AND FACIAL BONES
OPERATION: P REMOVAL: Taking out or off a device from a body part

Body Part	Approach	Device	Qualifier
Ø Skull	Ø Open	Ø Drainage Device 3 Infusion Device 4 Internal Fixation Device 5 External Fixation Device 7 Autologous Tissue Substitute J Synthetic Substitute K Nonautologous Tissue Substitute M Bone Growth Stimulator N Neurostimulator Generator S Hearing Device	Z No Qualifier
Ø Skull	3 Percutaneous 4 Percutaneous Endoscopic	Ø Drainage Device 3 Infusion Device 4 Internal Fixation Device 5 External Fixation Device 7 Autologous Tissue Substitute J Synthetic Substitute K Nonautologous Tissue Substitute M Bone Growth Stimulator S Hearing Device	Z No Qualifier
Ø Skull	X External	Ø Drainage Device 3 Infusion Device 4 Internal Fixation Device 5 External Fixation Device M Bone Growth Stimulator S Hearing Device	Z No Qualifier
B Nasal Bone W Facial Bone	Ø Open 3 Percutaneous 4 Percutaneous Endoscopic	Ø Drainage Device 4 Internal Fixation Device 5 External Fixation Device 7 Autologous Tissue Substitute J Synthetic Substitute K Nonautologous Tissue Substitute M Bone Growth Stimulator	Z No Qualifier
B Nasal Bone W Facial Bone	X External	Ø Drainage Device 4 Internal Fixation Device 5 External Fixation Device M Bone Growth Stimulator	Z No Qualifier

Non-OR ØNPØ[34]5Z
Non-OR ØNPØX[Ø5]Z
Non-OR ØNPB[Ø34][Ø47JKM]Z
Non-OR ØNPBX[Ø4M]Z
Non-OR ØNPWX[ØM]Z
Non-OR ØNPØ[Ø34]3Z

Coding Clinic: 2Ø15, Q3, P14 – ØNPØØ4Z
Coding Clinic: 2Ø23, Q1, P32 – ØNPØØ7Z

SECTION: Ø MEDICAL AND SURGICAL
BODY SYSTEM: N HEAD AND FACIAL BONES
OPERATION: Q REPAIR: Restoring, to the extent possible, a body part to its normal anatomic structure and function

Body Part	Approach	Device	Qualifier
Ø Skull 1 Frontal Bone 3 Parietal Bone, Right 4 Parietal Bone, Left 5 Temporal Bone, Right 6 Temporal Bone, Left 7 Occipital Bone B Nasal Bone C Sphenoid Bone F Ethmoid Bone, Right G Ethmoid Bone, Left H Lacrimal Bone, Right J Lacrimal Bone, Left K Palatine Bone, Right L Palatine Bone, Left M Zygomatic Bone, Right N Zygomatic Bone, Left P Orbit, Right Q Orbit, Left R Maxilla T Mandible, Right V Mandible, Left X Hyoid Bone	Ø Open 3 Percutaneous 4 Percutaneous Endoscopic X External	Z No Device	Z No Qualifier

DRG Non-OR ØNQ[Ø12345678BCDFGHJKLMNPQRSTVX]XZZ

Coding Clinic: 2Ø16, Q3, P29 – ØNQSØZZ

SECTION: Ø MEDICAL AND SURGICAL
BODY SYSTEM: N HEAD AND FACIAL BONES
OPERATION: R REPLACEMENT: Putting in or on biological or synthetic material that physically takes the place and/or function of all or a portion of a body part

Body Part	Approach	Device	Qualifier
Ø Skull 1 Frontal Bone 3 Parietal Bone, Right 4 Parietal Bone, Left 5 Temporal Bone, Right 6 Temporal Bone, Left 7 Occipital Bone B Nasal Bone C Sphenoid Bone F Ethmoid Bone, Right G Ethmoid Bone, Left H Lacrimal Bone, Right J Lacrimal Bone, Left K Palatine Bone, Right L Palatine Bone, Left M Zygomatic Bone, Right N Zygomatic Bone, Left P Orbit, Right Q Orbit, Left R Maxilla T Mandible, Right V Mandible, Left X Hyoid Bone	Ø Open 3 Percutaneous 4 Percutaneous Endoscopic	7 Autologous Tissue Substitute J Synthetic Substitute K Nonautologous Tissue Substitute	Z No Qualifier

Coding Clinic: 2Ø17, Q1, P24 – ØNRVØ[7J]Z
Coding Clinic: 2Ø17, Q3, P17 – ØNR8ØJZ
Coding Clinic: 2Ø21, Q1, P22 - ØNRRØJZ
Coding Clinic: 2Ø21, Q3, P3Ø – ØNR5ØJZ

SECTION: Ø MEDICAL AND SURGICAL
BODY SYSTEM: N HEAD AND FACIAL BONES
OPERATION: S REPOSITION: *(on multiple pages)*
Moving to its normal location, or other suitable location, all or a portion of a body part

Body Part	Approach	Device	Qualifier
Ø Skull R Maxilla T Mandible, Right V Mandible, Left	Ø Open 3 Percutaneous 4 Percutaneous Endoscopic	4 Internal Fixation Device 5 External Fixation Device Z No Device	Z No Qualifier
Ø Skull R Maxilla T Mandible, Right V Mandible, Left	X External	Z No Device	Z No Qualifier

Non-OR ØNS[RTV][34][45Z]Z
Non-OR ØNS[RTV]XZZ

Coding Clinic: 2Ø16, Q2, P3Ø; 2Ø15, Q3, P18 – ØNSØØZZ
Coding Clinic: 2Ø17, Q1, P21 – ØNS[RS]ØZZ
Coding Clinic: 2Ø17, Q3, P22 – ØNSØØ4Z

SECTION: Ø MEDICAL AND SURGICAL
BODY SYSTEM: N HEAD AND FACIAL BONES
OPERATION: S REPOSITION: *(continued)*
Moving to its normal location, or other suitable location, all or a portion of a body part

Body Part	Approach	Device	Qualifier
1 Frontal Bone 3 Parietal Bone, Right 4 Parietal Bone, Left 5 Temporal Bone, Right 6 Temporal Bone, Left 7 Occipital Bone B Nasal Bone C Sphenoid Bone F Ethmoid Bone, Right G Ethmoid Bone, Left H Lacrimal Bone, Right J Lacrimal Bone, Left K Palatine Bone, Right L Palatine Bone, Left M Zygomatic Bone, Right N Zygomatic Bone, Left P Orbit, Right Q Orbit, Left X Hyoid Bone	Ø Open 3 Percutaneous 4 Percutaneous Endoscopic	4 Internal Fixation Device Z No Device	Z No Qualifier
1 Frontal Bone 3 Parietal Bone, Right 4 Parietal Bone, Left 5 Temporal Bone, Right 6 Temporal Bone, Left 7 Occipital Bone B Nasal Bone C Sphenoid Bone F Ethmoid Bone, Right G Ethmoid Bone, Left H Lacrimal Bone, Right J Lacrimal Bone, Left K Palatine Bone, Right L Palatine Bone, Left M Zygomatic Bone, Right N Zygomatic Bone, Left P Orbit, Right Q Orbit, Left X Hyoid Bone	X External	Z No Device	Z No Qualifier

Non-OR ØNS[BCFGHJKLMNPQX][34][4Z]Z
Non-OR ØNS[BCFGHJKLMNPQX]XZZ

Coding Clinic: 2013, Q3, P25 – ØNSØØ5Z, ØNS1Ø4Z
Coding Clinic: 2015, Q3, P28 – ØNS5Ø4Z

SECTION: Ø MEDICAL AND SURGICAL
BODY SYSTEM: N HEAD AND FACIAL BONES
OPERATION: T RESECTION: Cutting out or off, without replacement, all of a body part

Body Part	Approach	Device	Qualifier
1 Frontal Bone 3 Parietal Bone, Right 4 Parietal Bone, Left 5 Temporal Bone, Right 6 Temporal Bone, Left 7 Occipital Bone B Nasal Bone C Sphenoid Bone F Ethmoid Bone, Right G Ethmoid Bone, Left H Lacrimal Bone, Right J Lacrimal Bone, Left K Palatine Bone, Right L Palatine Bone, Left M Zygomatic Bone, Right N Zygomatic Bone, Left P Orbit, Right Q Orbit, Left R Maxilla T Mandible, Right V Mandible, Left X Hyoid Bone	Ø Open	Z No Device	Z No Qualifier

SECTION: Ø MEDICAL AND SURGICAL
BODY SYSTEM: N HEAD AND FACIAL BONES
OPERATION: U SUPPLEMENT: Putting in or on biological or synthetic material that physically reinforces and/or augments the function of a portion of a body part

Body Part	Approach	Device	Qualifier
Ø Skull 1 Frontal Bone 3 Parietal Bone, Right 4 Parietal Bone, Left 5 Temporal Bone, Right 6 Temporal Bone, Left 7 Occipital Bone B Nasal Bone C Sphenoid Bone F Ethmoid Bone, Right G Ethmoid Bone, Left H Lacrimal Bone, Right J Lacrimal Bone, Left K Palatine Bone, Right L Palatine Bone, Left M Zygomatic Bone, Right N Zygomatic Bone, Left P Orbit, Right Q Orbit, Left R Maxilla T Mandible, Right V Mandible, Left X Hyoid Bone	Ø Open 3 Percutaneous 4 Percutaneous Endoscopic	7 Autologous Tissue Substitute J Synthetic Substitute K Nonautologous Tissue Substitute	Z No Qualifier

Coding Clinic: 2Ø13, Q3, P25 – ØNUØØJZ
Coding Clinic: 2Ø16, Q3, P29 – ØNURØ7Z
Coding Clinic: 2Ø21, Q1, P22 – ØDUP47Z
Coding Clinic: 2Ø21, Q3, P3Ø – ØNU5ØKZ
Coding Clinic: 2Ø23, Q2, P2Ø – ØNU5ØJZ

SECTION: Ø MEDICAL AND SURGICAL
BODY SYSTEM: N HEAD AND FACIAL BONES
OPERATION: W REVISION: Correcting, to the extent possible, a portion of a malfunctioning device or the position of a displaced device

Body Part	Approach	Device	Qualifier
Ø Skull	Ø Open	Ø Drainage Device 3 Infusion Device 4 Internal Fixation Device 5 External Fixation Device 7 Autologous Tissue Substitute J Synthetic Substitute K Nonautologous Tissue Substitute M Bone Growth Stimulator N Neurostimulator Generator S Hearing Device	Z No Qualifier
Ø Skull	3 Percutaneous 4 Percutaneous Endoscopic X External	Ø Drainage Device 3 Infusion Device 4 Internal Fixation Device 5 External Fixation Device 7 Autologous Tissue Substitute J Synthetic Substitute K Nonautologous Tissue Substitute M Bone Growth Stimulator S Hearing Device	Z No Qualifier
B Nasal Bone W Facial Bone	Ø Open 3 Percutaneous 4 Percutaneous Endoscopic X External	Ø Drainage Device 4 Internal Fixation Device 5 External Fixation Device 7 Autologous Tissue Substitute J Synthetic Substitute K Nonautologous Tissue Substitute M Bone Growth Stimulator	Z No Qualifier

Non-OR ØNWØX[Ø457JKMS]Z
Non-OR ØNWB[Ø34X][Ø47JKM]Z
Non-OR ØNWWX[Ø47JKM]Z

ØP. Upper Bones 390
ØP2. Change 391
ØP5. Destruction 391
ØP8. Division 392
ØP9. Drainage 393
ØPB. Excision 394
ØPC. Extirpation 395
ØPD. Extraction 396
ØPH. Insertion 397
ØPJ. Inspection 398
ØPN. Release 398
ØPP. Removal 399
ØPQ. Repair 401
ØPR. Replacement 402
ØPS. Reposition 402
ØPT. Resection 404
ØPU. Supplement 405
ØPW. Revision 406

SECTION: Ø MEDICAL AND SURGICAL
BODY SYSTEM: P UPPER BONES
OPERATION: 2 CHANGE: Taking out or off a device from a body part and putting back an identical or similar device in or on the same body part without cutting or puncturing the skin or a mucous membrane

Body Part	Approach	Device	Qualifier
Y Upper Bone	X External	Ø Drainage Device Y Other Device	Z No Qualifier

Non-OR All Values

SECTION: Ø MEDICAL AND SURGICAL
BODY SYSTEM: P UPPER BONES
OPERATION: 5 DESTRUCTION: Physical eradication of all or a portion of a body part by the direct use of energy, force, or a destructive agent

Body Part	Approach	Device	Qualifier
Ø Sternum 1 Rib, 1 to 2 2 Rib, 3 or More 5 Scapula, Right 6 Scapula, Left 7 Glenoid Cavity, Right 8 Glenoid Cavity, Left 9 Clavicle, Right B Clavicle, Left C Humeral Head, Right D Humeral Head, Left F Humeral Shaft, Right G Humeral Shaft, Left H Radius, Right J Radius, Left K Ulna, Right L Ulna, Left M Carpal, Right N Carpal, Left P Metacarpal, Right Q Metacarpal, Left R Thumb Phalanx, Right S Thumb Phalanx, Left T Finger Phalanx, Right V Finger Phalanx, Left	Ø Open 3 Percutaneous 4 Percutaneous Endoscopic	Z No Device	Z No Qualifier
3 Cervical Vertebra 4 Thoracic Vertebra	Ø Open 3 Percutaneous 4 Percutaneous Endoscopic	Z No Device	3 Laser Interstitial Thermal Z No Qualifier

SECTION: Ø MEDICAL AND SURGICAL
BODY SYSTEM: P UPPER BONES
OPERATION: 8 DIVISION: Cutting into a body part, without draining fluids and/or gases from the body part, in order to separate or transect a body part

Body Part	Approach	Device	Qualifier
Ø Sternum 1 Rib, 1 to 2 2 Rib, 3 or More 3 Cervical Vertebra 4 Thoracic Vertebra 5 Scapula, Right 6 Scapula, Left 7 Glenoid Cavity, Right 8 Glenoid Cavity, Left 9 Clavicle, Right B Clavicle, Left C Humeral Head, Right D Humeral Head, Left F Humeral Shaft, Right G Humeral Shaft, Left H Radius, Right J Radius, Left K Ulna, Right L Ulna, Left M Carpal, Right N Carpal, Left P Metacarpal, Right Q Metacarpal, Left R Thumb Phalanx, Right S Thumb Phalanx, Left T Finger Phalanx, Right V Finger Phalanx, Left	Ø Open 3 Percutaneous 4 Percutaneous Endoscopic	Z No Device	Z No Qualifier

SECTION: Ø MEDICAL AND SURGICAL
BODY SYSTEM: P UPPER BONES
OPERATION: 9 DRAINAGE: Taking or letting out fluids and/or gases from a body part

Body Part	Approach	Device	Qualifier
Ø Sternum 1 Rib, 1 to 2 2 Rib, 3 or More 3 Cervical Vertebra 4 Thoracic Vertebra 5 Scapula, Right 6 Scapula, Left 7 Glenoid Cavity, Right 8 Glenoid Cavity, Left 9 Clavicle, Right B Clavicle, Left C Humeral Head, Right D Humeral Head, Left F Humeral Shaft, Right G Humeral Shaft, Left H Radius, Right J Radius, Left K Ulna, Right L Ulna, Left M Carpal, Right N Carpal, Left P Metacarpal, Right Q Metacarpal, Left R Thumb Phalanx, Right S Thumb Phalanx, Left T Finger Phalanx, Right V Finger Phalanx, Left	Ø Open 3 Percutaneous 4 Percutaneous Endoscopic	Ø Drainage Device	Z No Qualifier
Ø Sternum 1 Rib, 1 to 2 2 Rib, 3 or More 3 Cervical Vertebra 4 Thoracic Vertebra 5 Scapula, Right 6 Scapula, Left 7 Glenoid Cavity, Right 8 Glenoid Cavity, Left 9 Clavicle, Right B Clavicle, Left C Humeral Head, Right D Humeral Head, Left F Humeral Shaft, Right G Humeral Shaft, Left H Radius, Right J Radius, Left K Ulna, Right L Ulna, Left M Carpal, Right N Carpal, Left P Metacarpal, Right Q Metacarpal, Left R Thumb Phalanx, Right S Thumb Phalanx, Left T Finger Phalanx, Right V Finger Phalanx, Left	Ø Open 3 Percutaneous 4 Percutaneous Endoscopic	Z No Device	X Diagnostic Z No Qualifier

Non-OR ØP9[Ø123456789BCDFGHJKLMNPQRSTV]3ØZ
Non-OR ØP9[Ø123456789BCDFGHJKLMNPQRSTV]3ZZ

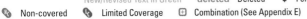

SECTION: Ø MEDICAL AND SURGICAL
BODY SYSTEM: P UPPER BONES
OPERATION: B EXCISION: Cutting out or off, without replacement, a portion of a body part

Body Part	Approach	Device	Qualifier
Ø Sternum 1 Rib, 1 to 2 2 Rib, 3 or More 3 Cervical Vertebra 4 Thoracic Vertebra 5 Scapula, Right 6 Scapula, Left 7 Glenoid Cavity, Right 8 Glenoid Cavity, Left 9 Clavicle, Right B Clavicle, Left C Humeral Head, Right D Humeral Head, Left F Humeral Shaft, Right G Humeral Shaft, Left H Radius, Right J Radius, Left K Ulna, Right L Ulna, Left M Carpal, Right N Carpal, Left P Metacarpal, Right Q Metacarpal, Left R Thumb Phalanx, Right S Thumb Phalanx, Left T Finger Phalanx, Right V Finger Phalanx, Left	Ø Open 3 Percutaneous 4 Percutaneous Endoscopic	Z No Device	X Diagnostic Z No Qualifier

Coding Clinic: 2Ø12, Q4, P1Ø1 – ØPB1ØZZ
Coding Clinic: 2Ø13, Q3, P22 – ØPB54ZZ

SECTION: Ø MEDICAL AND SURGICAL
BODY SYSTEM: P UPPER BONES
OPERATION: C EXTIRPATION: Taking or cutting out solid matter from a body part

Body Part	Approach	Device	Qualifier
Ø Sternum 1 Rib, 1 to 2 2 Rib, 3 or More 3 Cervical Vertebra 4 Thoracic Vertebra 5 Scapula, Right 6 Scapula, Left 7 Glenoid Cavity, Right 8 Glenoid Cavity, Left 9 Clavicle, Right B Clavicle, Left C Humeral Head, Right D Humeral Head, Left F Humeral Shaft, Right G Humeral Shaft, Left H Radius, Right J Radius, Left K Ulna, Right L Ulna, Left M Carpal, Right N Carpal, Left P Metacarpal, Right Q Metacarpal, Left R Thumb Phalanx, Right S Thumb Phalanx, Left T Finger Phalanx, Right V Finger Phalanx, Left	Ø Open 3 Percutaneous 4 Percutaneous Endoscopic	Z No Device	Z No Qualifier

Coding Clinic: 2019, Q3, P19 – ØPCØØZZ
Coding Clinic: 2021, Q3, P16 – ØPC[CD]3ZZ

SECTION: Ø MEDICAL AND SURGICAL
BODY SYSTEM: P UPPER BONES
OPERATION: D EXTRACTION: Pulling or stripping out or off all or a portion of a body part by the use of force

Body Part	Approach	Device	Qualifier
Ø Sternum 1 Rib, 1 to 2 2 Rib, 3 or More 3 Cervical Vertebra 4 Thoracic Vertebra 5 Scapula, Right 6 Scapula, Left 7 Glenoid Cavity, Right 8 Glenoid Cavity, Left 9 Clavicle, Right B Clavicle, Left C Humeral Head, Right D Humeral Head, Left F Humeral Shaft, Right G Humeral Shaft, Left H Radius, Right J Radius, Left K Ulna, Right L Ulna, Left M Carpal, Right N Carpal, Left P Metacarpal, Right Q Metacarpal, Left R Thumb Phalanx, Right S Thumb Phalanx, Left T Finger Phalanx, Right V Finger Phalanx, Left	Ø Open	Z No Device	Z No Qualifier

SECTION: Ø MEDICAL AND SURGICAL
BODY SYSTEM: P UPPER BONES
OPERATION: H INSERTION: Putting in a nonbiological appliance that monitors, assists, performs, or prevents a physiological function but does not physically take the place of a body part

Body Part	Approach	Device	Qualifier
Ø Sternum	Ø Open 3 Percutaneous 4 Percutaneous Endoscopic	Ø Internal Fixation Device, Rigid Plate 4 Internal Fixation Device	Z No Qualifier
1 Rib, 1 to 2 2 Rib, 3 or More 3 Cervical Vertebra 4 Thoracic Vertebra 5 Scapula, Right 6 Scapula, Left 7 Glenoid Cavity, Right 8 Glenoid Cavity, Left 9 Clavicle, Right B Clavicle, Left	Ø Open 3 Percutaneous 4 Percutaneous Endoscopic	4 Internal Fixation Device	Z No Qualifier
C Humeral Head, Right D Humeral Head, Left H Radius, Right J Radius, Left K Ulna, Right L Ulna, Left	Ø Open 3 Percutaneous 4 Percutaneous Endoscopic	4 Internal Fixation Device 5 External Fixation Device 6 Internal Fixation Device, Intramedullary 8 External Fixation Device, Limb Lengthening B External Fixation Device, Monoplanar C External Fixation Device, Ring D External Fixation Device, Hybrid	Z No Qualifier
F Humeral Shaft, Right G Humeral Shaft, Left	Ø Open 3 Percutaneous 4 Percutaneous Endoscopic	4 Internal Fixation Device 5 External Fixation Device 6 Internal Fixation Device, Intramedullary 7 Internal Fixation Device, Intramedullary Limb Lengthening 8 External Fixation Device, Limb Lengthening B External Fixation Device, Monoplanar C External Fixation Device, Ring D External Fixation Device, Hybrid	Z No Qualifier
M Carpal, Right N Carpal, Left P Metacarpal, Right Q Metacarpal, Left R Thumb Phalanx, Right S Thumb Phalanx, Left T Finger Phalanx, Right V Finger Phalanx, Left	Ø Open 3 Percutaneous 4 Percutaneous Endoscopic	4 Internal Fixation Device 5 External Fixation Device	Z No Qualifier
Y Upper Bone	Ø Open 3 Percutaneous 4 Percutaneous Endoscopic	M Bone Growth Stimulator	Z No Qualifier
Y Upper Bone	Ø Open 3 Percutaneous 4 Percutaneous Endoscopic X External	Z No Device	Z No Qualifier

Non-OR ØPH[CDFGHJKL][Ø34]8Z

Coding Clinic: 2018, Q4, P12 – ØPH5Ø4Z
Coding Clinic: 2020, Q1, P3Ø – ØPHØØØZ

SECTION: Ø MEDICAL AND SURGICAL
BODY SYSTEM: P UPPER BONES
OPERATION: J INSPECTION: Visually and/or manually exploring a body part

Body Part	Approach	Device	Qualifier
Y Upper Bone	Ø Open 3 Percutaneous 4 Percutaneous Endoscopic X External	Z No Device	Z No Qualifier

Non-OR ØPJY[3X]ZZ

SECTION: Ø MEDICAL AND SURGICAL
BODY SYSTEM: P UPPER BONES
OPERATION: N RELEASE: Freeing a body part from an abnormal physical constraint by cutting or by the use of force

Body Part	Approach	Device	Qualifier
Ø Sternum 1 Rib, 1 to 2 2 Rib, 3 or More 3 Cervical Vertebra 4 Thoracic Vertebra 5 Scapula, Right 6 Scapula, Left 7 Glenoid Cavity, Right 8 Glenoid Cavity, Left 9 Clavicle, Right B Clavicle, Left C Humeral Head, Right D Humeral Head, Left F Humeral Shaft, Right G Humeral Shaft, Left H Radius, Right J Radius, Left K Ulna, Right L Ulna, Left M Carpal, Right N Carpal, Left P Metacarpal, Right Q Metacarpal, Left R Thumb Phalanx, Right S Thumb Phalanx, Left T Finger Phalanx, Right V Finger Phalanx, Left	Ø Open 3 Percutaneous 4 Percutaneous Endoscopic	Z No Device	Z No Qualifier

SECTION: Ø MEDICAL AND SURGICAL
BODY SYSTEM: P UPPER BONES
OPERATION: P REMOVAL: *(on multiple pages)*

Taking out or off a device from a body part

Body Part	Approach	Device	Qualifier
Ø Sternum 1 Rib, 1 to 2 2 Rib, 3 or More 3 Cervical Vertebra 4 Thoracic Vertebra 5 Scapula, Right 6 Scapula, Left 7 Glenoid Cavity, Right 8 Glenoid Cavity, Left 9 Clavicle, Right B Clavicle, Left	Ø Open 3 Percutaneous 4 Percutaneous Endoscopic	4 Internal Fixation Device 7 Autologous Tissue Substitute J Synthetic Substitute K Nonautologous Tissue Substitute	Z No Qualifier
Ø Sternum 1 Rib, 1 to 2 2 Rib, 3 or More 3 Cervical Vertebra 4 Thoracic Vertebra 5 Scapula, Right 6 Scapula, Left 7 Glenoid Cavity, Right 8 Glenoid Cavity, Left 9 Clavicle, Right B Clavicle, Left	X External	4 Internal Fixation Device	Z No Qualifier
C Humeral Head, Right D Humeral Head, Left F Humeral Shaft, Right G Humeral Shaft, Left H Radius, Right J Radius, Left K Ulna, Right L Ulna, Left M Carpal, Right N Carpal, Left P Metacarpal, Right Q Metacarpal, Left R Thumb Phalanx, Right S Thumb Phalanx, Left T Finger Phalanx, Right V Finger Phalanx, Left	Ø Open 3 Percutaneous 4 Percutaneous Endoscopic	4 Internal Fixation Device 5 External Fixation Device 7 Autologous Tissue Substitute J Synthetic Substitute K Nonautologous Tissue Substitute	Z No Qualifier

Non-OR ØPP[Ø123456789B]X4Z

SECTION: Ø MEDICAL AND SURGICAL
BODY SYSTEM: P UPPER BONES
OPERATION: P REMOVAL: *(continued)*

Taking out or off a device from a body part

Body Part	Approach	Device	Qualifier
C Humeral Head, Right D Humeral Head, Left F Humeral Shaft, Right G Humeral Shaft, Left H Radius, Right J Radius, Left K Ulna, Right L Ulna, Left M Carpal, Right N Carpal, Left P Metacarpal, Right Q Metacarpal, Left R Thumb Phalanx, Right S Thumb Phalanx, Left T Finger Phalanx, Right V Finger Phalanx, Left	X External	4 Internal Fixation Device 5 External Fixation Device	Z No Qualifier
Y Upper Bone	Ø Open 3 Percutaneous 4 Percutaneous Endoscopic X External	Ø Drainage Device M Bone Growth Stimulator	Z No Qualifier

Non-OR ØPP[CDFGHJKLMNPQRSTV]X[45]Z
Non-OR ØPPY3ØZ
Non-OR ØPPYX[ØM]Z

SECTION: Ø MEDICAL AND SURGICAL
BODY SYSTEM: P UPPER BONES
OPERATION: Q REPAIR: Restoring, to the extent possible, a body part to its normal anatomic structure and function

Body Part	Approach	Device	Qualifier
Ø Sternum 1 Rib, 1 to 2 2 Rib, 3 or More 3 Cervical Vertebra 4 Thoracic Vertebra 5 Scapula, Right 6 Scapula, Left 7 Glenoid Cavity, Right 8 Glenoid Cavity, Left 9 Clavicle, Right B Clavicle, Left C Humeral Head, Right D Humeral Head, Left F Humeral Shaft, Right G Humeral Shaft, Left H Radius, Right J Radius, Left K Ulna, Right L Ulna, Left M Carpal, Right N Carpal, Left P Metacarpal, Right Q Metacarpal, Left R Thumb Phalanx, Right S Thumb Phalanx, Left T Finger Phalanx, Right V Finger Phalanx, Left	Ø Open 3 Percutaneous 4 Percutaneous Endoscopic X External	Z No Device	Z No Qualifier

DRG Non-OR ØPQ[Ø123456789BCDFGHJKLMNPQRSTV]XZZ

SECTION: Ø MEDICAL AND SURGICAL
BODY SYSTEM: P UPPER BONES
OPERATION: R REPLACEMENT: Putting in or on biological or synthetic material that physically takes the place and/or function of all or a portion of a body part

Body Part	Approach	Device	Qualifier
Ø Sternum 1 Rib, 1 to 2 2 Rib, 3 or More 3 Cervical Vertebra 4 Thoracic Vertebra 5 Scapula, Right 6 Scapula, Left 7 Glenoid Cavity, Right 8 Glenoid Cavity, Left 9 Clavicle, Right B Clavicle, Left C Humeral Head, Right D Humeral Head, Left F Humeral Shaft, Right G Humeral Shaft, Left H Radius, Right J Radius, Left K Ulna, Right L Ulna, Left M Carpal, Right N Carpal, Left P Metacarpal, Right Q Metacarpal, Left R Thumb Phalanx, Right S Thumb Phalanx, Left T Finger Phalanx, Right V Finger Phalanx, Left	Ø Open 3 Percutaneous 4 Percutaneous Endoscopic	7 Autologous Tissue Substitute J Synthetic Substitute K Nonautologous Tissue Substitute	Z No Qualifier

Coding Clinic: 2018, Q4, P92 – ØPRHØJZ

SECTION: Ø MEDICAL AND SURGICAL
BODY SYSTEM: P UPPER BONES
OPERATION: S REPOSITION: *(on multiple pages)* Moving to its normal location, or other suitable location, all or a portion of a body part

Body Part	Approach	Device	Qualifier
Ø Sternum	Ø Open 3 Percutaneous 4 Percutaneous Endoscopic	Ø Internal Fixation Device, Rigid Plate 4 Internal Fixation Device Z No Device	Z No Qualifier
Ø Sternum	X External	Z No Device	Z No Qualifier
1 Rib, 1 to 2 2 Rib, 3 or More 3 Cervical Vertebra ⊞ 5 Scapula, Right 6 Scapula, Left 7 Glenoid Cavity, Right 8 Glenoid Cavity, Left 9 Clavicle, Right B Clavicle, Left	Ø Open 3 Percutaneous 4 Percutaneous Endoscopic	4 Internal Fixation Device Z No Device	Z No Qualifier

⊞ ØPS3[34]ZZ
Non-OR ØPSØ[34]ZZ
Non-OR ØPSØXZZ

Non-OR ØPS[1256789B][34]ZZ

Coding Clinic: 2015, Q4, P34 – ØPSØØZZ
Coding Clinic: 2016, Q1, P21 – ØPS4XZZ
Coding Clinic: 2017, Q4, P53 – ØPS2Ø4Z
Coding Clinic: 2020, Q1, P33 – ØPS4Ø4Z

SECTION: Ø MEDICAL AND SURGICAL
BODY SYSTEM: P UPPER BONES
OPERATION: S REPOSITION: *(on multiple pages)*

Moving to its normal location, or other suitable location, all or a portion of a body part

Body Part	Approach	Device	Qualifier
1 Rib, 1 to 2 2 Rib, 3 or More 3 Cervical Vertebra 5 Scapula, Right 6 Scapula, Left 7 Glenoid Cavity, Right 8 Glenoid Cavity, Left 9 Clavicle, Right B Clavicle, Left	X External	Z No Device	Z No Qualifier
4 Thoracic Vertebra	Ø Open 4 Percutaneous Endoscopic	3 Spinal Stabilization Device, Vertebral Body Tether 4 Internal Fixation Device Z No Device	Z No Qualifier
4 Thoracic Vertebra	3 Percutaneous	4 Internal Fixation Device Z No Device	Z No Qualifier
4 Thoracic Vertebra	X External	Z No Device	Z No Qualifier
C Humeral Head, Right D Humeral Head, Left F Humeral Shaft, Right G Humeral Shaft, Left H Radius, Right J Radius, Left K Ulna, Right L Ulna, Left	Ø Open 3 Percutaneous 4 Percutaneous Endoscopic	4 Internal Fixation Device 5 External Fixation Device 6 Internal Fixation Device, Intramedullary B External Fixation Device, Monoplanar C External Fixation Device, Ring D External Fixation Device, Hybrid Z No Device	Z No Qualifier
C Humeral Head, Right D Humeral Head, Left F Humeral Shaft, Right G Humeral Shaft, Left H Radius, Right J Radius, Left K Ulna, Right L Ulna, Left	X External	Z No Device	Z No Qualifier
M Carpal, Right N Carpal, Left P Metacarpal, Right Q Metacarpal, Left R Thumb Phalanx, Right S Thumb Phalanx, Left T Finger Phalanx, Right V Finger Phalanx, Left	Ø Open 3 Percutaneous 4 Percutaneous Endoscopic	4 Internal Fixation Device 5 External Fixation Device Z No Device	Z No Qualifier

SECTION: Ø MEDICAL AND SURGICAL
BODY SYSTEM: P UPPER BONES
OPERATION: S REPOSITION: *(continued)*
Moving to its normal location, or other suitable location, all or a portion of a body part

Body Part	Approach	Device	Qualifier
M Carpal, Right N Carpal, Left P Metacarpal, Right Q Metacarpal, Left R Thumb Phalanx, Right S Thumb Phalanx, Left T Finger Phalanx, Right V Finger Phalanx, Left	X External	Z No Device	Z No Qualifier

Non-OR ØPS[1256789B]XZZ
Non-OR ØPS[CDFGHJKL][34]ZZ
Non-OR ØPS[CDFGHJKL]XZZ
Non-OR ØPS[MNPQRSTV][34]ZZ
Non-OR ØPS[MNPQRSTV]XZZ

Coding Clinic: 2Ø15, Q2, P35 – ØPS3XZZ

SECTION: Ø MEDICAL AND SURGICAL
BODY SYSTEM: P UPPER BONES
OPERATION: T RESECTION: Cutting out or off, without replacement, all of a body part

Body Part	Approach	Device	Qualifier
Ø Sternum 1 Rib, 1 to 2 2 Rib, 3 or More 5 Scapula, Right 6 Scapula, Left 7 Glenoid Cavity, Right 8 Glenoid Cavity, Left 9 Clavicle, Right B Clavicle, Left C Humeral Head, Right D Humeral Head, Left F Humeral Shaft, Right G Humeral Shaft, Left H Radius, Right J Radius, Left K Ulna, Right L Ulna, Left M Carpal, Right N Carpal, Left P Metacarpal, Right Q Metacarpal, Left R Thumb Phalanx, Right S Thumb Phalanx, Left T Finger Phalanx, Right V Finger Phalanx, Left	Ø Open	Z No Device	Z No Qualifier

Coding Clinic: 2Ø15, Q3, P27 – ØPTNØZZ

SECTION: Ø MEDICAL AND SURGICAL
BODY SYSTEM: P UPPER BONES
OPERATION: U SUPPLEMENT: Putting in or on biological or synthetic material that physically reinforces and/or augments the function of a portion of a body part

Body Part	Approach	Device	Qualifier
Ø Sternum 1 Rib, 1 to 2 2 Rib, 3 or More 3 Cervical Vertebra ⊞ 4 Thoracic Vertebra ⊞ 5 Scapula, Right 6 Scapula, Left 7 Glenoid Cavity, Right 8 Glenoid Cavity, Left 9 Clavicle, Right B Clavicle, Left C Humeral Head, Right D Humeral Head, Left F Humeral Shaft, Right G Humeral Shaft, Left H Radius, Right J Radius, Left K Ulna, Right L Ulna, Left M Carpal, Right N Carpal, Left P Metacarpal, Right Q Metacarpal, Left R Thumb Phalanx, Right S Thumb Phalanx, Left T Finger Phalanx, Right V Finger Phalanx, Left	Ø Open 3 Percutaneous 4 Percutaneous Endoscopic	7 Autologous Tissue Substitute J Synthetic Substitute K Nonautologous Tissue Substitute	Z No Qualifier

⊞ ØPU[34]3JZ

Coding Clinic: 2Ø15, Q2, P2Ø – ØPU3ØKZ
Coding Clinic: 2Ø18, Q4, P12 – ØPU5Ø7Z, ØPU5ØKZ
Coding Clinic: 2Ø21, Q3, P16 – ØPU[CD]3JZ
Coding Clinic: 2Ø23, Q2, P25 – ØPUC47Z

Ø: M/S P: UPPER BONES U: SUPPLEMENT

SECTION: Ø MEDICAL AND SURGICAL
BODY SYSTEM: P UPPER BONES
OPERATION: W REVISION: Correcting, to the extent possible, a portion of a malfunctioning device or the position of a displaced device

Body Part	Approach	Device	Qualifier
Ø Sternum 1 Rib, 1 to 2 2 Rib, 3 or More 3 Cervical Vertebra 4 Thoracic Vertebra 5 Scapula, Right 6 Scapula, Left 7 Glenoid Cavity, Right 8 Glenoid Cavity, Left 9 Clavicle, Right B Clavicle, Left	Ø Open 3 Percutaneous 4 Percutaneous Endoscopic X External	4 Internal Fixation Device 7 Autologous Tissue Substitute J Synthetic Substitute K Nonautologous Tissue Substitute	Z No Qualifier
C Humeral Head, Right D Humeral Head, Left F Humeral Shaft, Right G Humeral Shaft, Left H Radius, Right J Radius, Left K Ulna, Right L Ulna, Left M Carpal, Right N Carpal, Left P Metacarpal, Right Q Metacarpal, Left R Thumb Phalanx, Right S Thumb Phalanx, Left T Finger Phalanx, Right V Finger Phalanx, Left	Ø Open 3 Percutaneous 4 Percutaneous Endoscopic X External	4 Internal Fixation Device 5 External Fixation Device 7 Autologous Tissue Substitute J Synthetic Substitute K Nonautologous Tissue Substitute	Z No Qualifier
Y Upper Bone	Ø Open 3 Percutaneous 4 Percutaneous Endoscopic X External	Ø Drainage Device M Bone Growth Stimulator	Z No Qualifier

Non-OR ØPW[Ø123456789B]X[47JK]Z
Non-OR ØPW[CDFGHJKLMNPQRSTV]X[457JK]Z
Non-OR ØPWYX[ØM]Z

ØQ. Lower Bones 407
ØQ2. Change 408
ØQ5. Destruction 408
ØQ8. Division 409
ØQ9. Drainage 41Ø
ØQB. Excision 411
ØQC. Extirpation 412
ØQD. Extraction 412
ØQH. Insertion 413
ØQJ. Inspection 414
ØQN. Release 414
ØQP. Removal 415
ØQQ. Repair 417
ØQR. Replacement 418
ØQS. Reposition 419
ØQT. Resection 42Ø
ØQU. Supplement 421
ØQW. Revision 422

SECTION: Ø MEDICAL AND SURGICAL
BODY SYSTEM: Q LOWER BONES
OPERATION: 2 CHANGE: Taking out or off a device from a body part and putting back an identical or similar device in or on the same body part without cutting or puncturing the skin or a mucous membrane

Body Part	Approach	Device	Qualifier
Y Lower Bone	X External	Ø Drainage Device Y Other Device	Z No Qualifier

Non-OR All Values

SECTION: Ø MEDICAL AND SURGICAL
BODY SYSTEM: Q LOWER BONES
OPERATION: 5 DESTRUCTION: Physical eradication of all or a portion of a body part by the direct use of energy, force, or a destructive agent

Body Part	Approach	Device	Qualifier
Ø Lumbar Vertebra 1 Sacrum	Ø Open 3 Percutaneous 4 Percutaneous Endoscopic	Z No Device	3 Laser Interstitial Thermal Therapy Z No Qualifier
2 Pelvic Bone, Right 3 Pelvic Bone, Left 4 Acetabulum, Right 5 Acetabulum, Left 6 Upper Femur, Right 7 Upper Femur, Left 8 Femoral Shaft, Right 9 Femoral Shaft, Left B Lower Femur, Right C Lower Femur, Left D Patella, Right F Patella, Left G Tibia, Right H Tibia, Left J Fibula, Right K Fibula, Left L Tarsal, Right M Tarsal, Left N Metatarsal, Right P Metatarsal, Left Q Toe Phalanx, Right R Toe Phalanx, Left S Coccyx	Ø Open 3 Percutaneous 4 Percutaneous Endoscopic	Z No Device	Z No Qualifier

SECTION: Ø MEDICAL AND SURGICAL
BODY SYSTEM: Q LOWER BONES
OPERATION: 8 DIVISION: Cutting into a body part, without draining fluids and/or gases from the body part, in order to separate or transect a body part

Body Part	Approach	Device	Qualifier
Ø Lumbar Vertebra 1 Sacrum 2 Pelvic Bone, Right 3 Pelvic Bone, Left 4 Acetabulum, Right 5 Acetabulum, Left 6 Upper Femur, Right 7 Upper Femur, Left 8 Femoral Shaft, Right 9 Femoral Shaft, Left B Lower Femur, Right C Lower Femur, Left D Patella, Right F Patella, Left G Tibia, Right H Tibia, Left J Fibula, Right K Fibula, Left L Tarsal, Right M Tarsal, Left N Metatarsal, Right P Metatarsal, Left Q Toe Phalanx, Right R Toe Phalanx, Left S Coccyx	Ø Open 3 Percutaneous 4 Percutaneous Endoscopic	Z No Device	Z No Qualifier

Coding Clinic: 2Ø16, Q2, P32 – ØQ83ØZZ

SECTION: Ø MEDICAL AND SURGICAL
BODY SYSTEM: Q LOWER BONES
OPERATION: 9 DRAINAGE: Taking or letting out fluids and/or gases from a body part

Body Part	Approach	Device	Qualifier
Ø Lumbar Vertebra 1 Sacrum 2 Pelvic Bone, Right 3 Pelvic Bone, Left 4 Acetabulum, Right 5 Acetabulum, Left 6 Upper Femur, Right 7 Upper Femur, Left 8 Femoral Shaft, Right 9 Femoral Shaft, Left B Lower Femur, Right C Lower Femur, Left D Patella, Right F Patella, Left G Tibia, Right H Tibia, Left J Fibula, Right K Fibula, Left L Tarsal, Right M Tarsal, Left N Metatarsal, Right P Metatarsal, Left Q Toe Phalanx, Right R Toe Phalanx, Left S Coccyx	Ø Open 3 Percutaneous 4 Percutaneous Endoscopic	Ø Drainage Device	Z No Qualifier
Ø Lumbar Vertebra 1 Sacrum 2 Pelvic Bone, Right 3 Pelvic Bone, Left 4 Acetabulum, Right 5 Acetabulum, Left 6 Upper Femur, Right 7 Upper Femur, Left 8 Femoral Shaft, Right 9 Femoral Shaft, Left B Lower Femur, Right C Lower Femur, Left D Patella, Right F Patella, Left G Tibia, Right H Tibia, Left J Fibula, Right K Fibula, Left L Tarsal, Right M Tarsal, Left N Metatarsal, Right P Metatarsal, Left Q Toe Phalanx, Right R Toe Phalanx, Left S Coccyx	Ø Open 3 Percutaneous 4 Percutaneous Endoscopic	Z No Device	X Diagnostic Z No Qualifier

Non-OR ØQ9[Ø123456789BCDFGHJKLMNPQRS]3ØZ
Non-OR ØQ9[Ø123456789BCDFGHJKLMNPQRS]3ZZ

Coding Clinic: 2022, Q1, P32 – ØQ9[23]3ZX

SECTION: Ø MEDICAL AND SURGICAL
BODY SYSTEM: Q LOWER BONES
OPERATION: B EXCISION: Cutting out or off, without replacement, a portion of a body part

Body Part	Approach	Device	Qualifier
Ø Lumbar Vertebra 1 Sacrum 2 Pelvic Bone, Right 3 Pelvic Bone, Left 4 Acetabulum, Right 5 Acetabulum, Left 6 Upper Femur, Right 7 Upper Femur, Left 8 Femoral Shaft, Right 9 Femoral Shaft, Left B Lower Femur, Right C Lower Femur, Left D Patella, Right F Patella, Left G Tibia, Right H Tibia, Left J Fibula, Right K Fibula, Left L Tarsal, Right M Tarsal, Left Q Toe Phalanx, Right R Toe Phalanx, Left S Coccyx	Ø Open 3 Percutaneous 4 Percutaneous Endoscopic	Z No Device	X Diagnostic Z No Qualifier
N Metatarsal, Right P Metatarsal, Left	Ø Open 3 Percutaneous 4 Percutaneous Endoscopic	Z No Device	2 Sesamoid Bone(s) 1st Toe X Diagnostic Z No Qualifier

Coding Clinic: 2Ø13, Q2, P4Ø – ØQBKØZZ
Coding Clinic: 2Ø15, Q3, P4 – ØQBSØZZ
Coding Clinic: 2Ø17, Q1, P24 – ØQBJØZZ
Coding Clinic: 2Ø19, Q2, P2Ø – ØQB3ØZZ
Coding Clinic: 2Ø2Ø, Q2, P26 – ØQB1ØZZ
Coding Clinic: 2Ø21, Q2, P18 – ØQBNØZZ

SECTION: Ø MEDICAL AND SURGICAL
BODY SYSTEM: Q LOWER BONES
OPERATION: C EXTIRPATION: Taking or cutting out solid matter from a body part

Body Part	Approach	Device	Qualifier
Ø Lumbar Vertebra 1 Sacrum 2 Pelvic Bone, Right 3 Pelvic Bone, Left 4 Acetabulum, Right 5 Acetabulum, Left 6 Upper Femur, Right 7 Upper Femur, Left 8 Femoral Shaft, Right 9 Femoral Shaft, Left B Lower Femur, Right C Lower Femur, Left D Patella, Right F Patella, Left G Tibia, Right H Tibia, Left J Fibula, Right K Fibula, Left L Tarsal, Right M Tarsal, Left N Metatarsal, Right P Metatarsal, Left Q Toe Phalanx, Right R Toe Phalanx, Left S Coccyx	Ø Open 3 Percutaneous 4 Percutaneous Endoscopic	Z No Device	Z No Qualifier

SECTION: Ø MEDICAL AND SURGICAL
BODY SYSTEM: Q LOWER BONES
OPERATION: D EXTRACTION: Pulling or stripping out or off all or a portion of a body part by the use of force

Body Part	Approach	Device	Qualifier
Ø Lumbar Vertebra 1 Sacrum 2 Pelvic Bone, Right 3 Pelvic Bone, Left 4 Acetabulum, Right 5 Acetabulum, Left 6 Upper Femur, Right 7 Upper Femur, Left 8 Femoral Shaft, Right 9 Femoral Shaft, Left B Lower Femur, Right C Lower Femur, Left D Patella, Right F Patella, Left G Tibia, Right H Tibia, Left J Fibula, Right K Fibula, Left L Tarsal, Right M Tarsal, Left N Metatarsal, Right P Metatarsal, Left Q Toe Phalanx, Right R Toe Phalanx, Left S Coccyx	Ø Open	Z No Device	Z No Qualifier

SECTION: Ø MEDICAL AND SURGICAL
BODY SYSTEM: Q LOWER BONES
OPERATION: H INSERTION: Putting in a nonbiological appliance that monitors, assists, performs, or prevents a physiological function but does not physically take the place of a body part

Body Part	Approach	Device	Qualifier
Ø Lumbar Vertebra 1 Sacrum 2 Pelvic Bone, Right 3 Pelvic Bone, Left 4 Acetabulum, Right 5 Acetabulum, Left D Patella, Right F Patella, Left L Tarsal, Right M Tarsal, Left N Metatarsal, Right P Metatarsal, Left Q Toe Phalanx, Right R Toe Phalanx, Left S Coccyx	Ø Open 3 Percutaneous 4 Percutaneous Endoscopic	4 Internal Fixation Device 5 External Fixation Device	Z No Qualifier
6 Upper Femur, Right 7 Upper Femur, Left B Lower Femur, Right C Lower Femur, Left J Fibula, Right K Fibula, Left	Ø Open 3 Percutaneous 4 Percutaneous Endoscopic	4 Internal Fixation Device 5 External Fixation Device 6 Internal Fixation Device, Intramedullary 8 External Fixation Device, Limb Lengthening B External Fixation Device, Monoplanar C External Fixation Device, Ring D External Fixation Device, Hybrid	Z No Qualifier
8 Femoral Shaft, Right 9 Femoral Shaft, Left G Tibia, Right H Tibia, Leftt	Ø Open 3 Percutaneous 4 Percutaneous Endoscopic	4 Internal Fixation Device 5 External Fixation Device 6 Internal Fixation Device, Intramedullary 7 Internal Fixation Device, Intramedullary Limb Lengthening 8 External Fixation Device, Limb Lengthening B External Fixation Device, Monoplanar C External Fixation Device, Ring D External Fixation Device, Hybrid	Z No Qualifier
Y Lower Bone	Ø Open 3 Percutaneous 4 Percutaneous Endoscopic	M Bone Growth Stimulator	Z No Qualifier

Non-OR ØQH[6789BCGHJK][Ø34]8Z

Coding Clinic: 2Ø16, Q3, P35 – ØQH[GJ]Ø4Z
Coding Clinic: 2Ø17, Q1, P22 – ØQH[23]Ø4Z
Coding Clinic: 2Ø22, Q2, P21 – ØQH[HK]38Z

SECTION: Ø MEDICAL AND SURGICAL
BODY SYSTEM: Q LOWER BONES
OPERATION: J INSPECTION: Visually and/or manually exploring a body part

Body Part	Approach	Device	Qualifier
Y Lower Bone	Ø Open 3 Percutaneous 4 Percutaneous Endoscopic X External	Z No Device	Z No Qualifier

Non-OR ØQJY[3X]ZZ

SECTION: Ø MEDICAL AND SURGICAL
BODY SYSTEM: Q LOWER BONES
OPERATION: N RELEASE: Freeing a body part from an abnormal physical constraint by cutting or by the use of force

Body Part	Approach	Device	Qualifier
Ø Lumbar Vertebra 1 Sacrum 2 Pelvic Bone, Right 3 Pelvic Bone, Left 4 Acetabulum, Right 5 Acetabulum, Left 6 Upper Femur, Right 7 Upper Femur, Left 8 Femoral Shaft, Right 9 Femoral Shaft, Left B Lower Femur, Right C Lower Femur, Left D Patella, Right F Patella, Left G Tibia, Right H Tibia, Left J Fibula, Right K Fibula, Left L Tarsal, Right M Tarsal, Left N Metatarsal, Right P Metatarsal, Left Q Toe Phalanx, Right R Toe Phalanx, Left S Coccyx	Ø Open 3 Percutaneous 4 Percutaneous Endoscopic	Z No Device	Z No Qualifier

SECTION: Ø MEDICAL AND SURGICAL
BODY SYSTEM: Q LOWER BONES
OPERATION: P REMOVAL: *(on multiple pages)*
Taking out or off a device from a body part

Body Part	Approach	Device	Qualifier
Ø Lumbar Vertebra 1 Sacrum 4 Acetabulum, Right 5 Acetabulum, Left S Coccyx	Ø Open 3 Percutaneous 4 Percutaneous Endoscopic	4 Internal Fixation Device 7 Autologous Tissue Substitute J Synthetic Substitute K Nonautologous Tissue Substitute	Z No Qualifier
Ø Lumbar Vertebra 1 Sacrum 4 Acetabulum, Right 5 Acetabulum, Left S Coccyx	X External	4 Internal Fixation Device	Z No Qualifier
Ø Lumbar Vertebra 1 Sacrum 2 Pelvic Bone, Right 3 Pelvic Bone, Left 4 Acetabulum, Right 5 Acetabulum, Left 6 Upper Femur, Right 7 Upper Femur, Left 8 Femoral Shaft, Right 9 Femoral Shaft, Left B Lower Femur, Right C Lower Femur, Left D Patella, Right F Patella, Left G Tibia, Right H Tibia, Left J Fibula, Right K Fibula, Left L Tarsal, Right M Tarsal, Left N Metatarsal, Right P Metatarsal, Left Q Toe Phalanx, Right R Toe Phalanx, Left S Coccyx	Ø Open 3 Percutaneous 4 Percutaneous Endoscopic	4 Internal Fixation Device 5 External Fixation Device 7 Autologous Tissue Substitute J Synthetic Substitute K Nonautologous Tissue Substitute	Z No Qualifier

Non-OR ØQP[Ø145S]X4Z

Coding Clinic: 2Ø15, Q2, P6 – ØQPGØ4Z
Coding Clinic: 2Ø17, Q4, P75 – ØQPØØ4Z
Coding Clinic: 2Ø23, Q1, P34 – ØQP1Ø4Z

SECTION: Ø MEDICAL AND SURGICAL
BODY SYSTEM: Q LOWER BONES
OPERATION: P REMOVAL: *(continued)*
Taking out or off a device from a body part

Body Part	Approach	Device	Qualifier
Ø Lumbar Vertebra 1 Sacrum 2 Pelvic Bone, Right 3 Pelvic Bone, Left 4 Acetabulum, Right 5 Acetabulum, Left 6 Upper Femur, Right 7 Upper Femur, Left 8 Femoral Shaft, Right 9 Femoral Shaft, Left B Lower Femur, Right C Lower Femur, Left D Patella, Right F Patella, Left G Tibia, Right H Tibia, Left J Fibula, Right K Fibula, Left L Tarsal, Right M Tarsal, Left N Metatarsal, Right P Metatarsal, Left Q Toe Phalanx, Right R Toe Phalanx, Left S Coccyx	X External	4 Internal Fixation Device 5 External Fixation Device	Z No Qualifier
Y Lower Bone	Ø Open 3 Percutaneous 4 Percutaneous Endoscopic X External	Ø Drainage Device M Bone Growth Stimulator	Z No Qualifier

Non-OR ØQP[Ø123456789BCDFGHJKLMNPQRS]X[45]Z
Non-OR ØQPY3ØZ
Non-OR ØQPYX[ØM]Z

SECTION: Ø MEDICAL AND SURGICAL
BODY SYSTEM: Q LOWER BONES
OPERATION: Q REPAIR: Restoring, to the extent possible, a body part to its normal anatomic structure and function

Body Part	Approach	Device	Qualifier
Ø Lumbar Vertebra 1 Sacrum 2 Pelvic Bone, Right 3 Pelvic Bone, Left 4 Acetabulum, Right 5 Acetabulum, Left 6 Upper Femur, Right 7 Upper Femur, Left 8 Femoral Shaft, Right 9 Femoral Shaft, Left B Lower Femur, Right C Lower Femur, Left D Patella, Right F Patella, Left G Tibia, Right H Tibia, Left J Fibula, Right K Fibula, Left L Tarsal, Right M Tarsal, Left N Metatarsal, Right P Metatarsal, Left Q Toe Phalanx, Right R Toe Phalanx, Left S Coccyx	Ø Open 3 Percutaneous 4 Percutaneous Endoscopic X External	Z No Device	Z No Qualifier

DRG Non-OR ØQQ[Ø123456789BCDFGHJKLMNPQRS]XZZ

Coding Clinic: 2Ø18, Q1, P15 – ØQQ[23]ØZZ

SECTION: Ø MEDICAL AND SURGICAL
BODY SYSTEM: Q LOWER BONES
OPERATION: R REPLACEMENT: Putting in or on biological or synthetic material that physically takes the place and/or function of all or a portion of a body part

Body Part	Approach	Device	Qualifier
Ø Lumbar Vertebra 1 Sacrum 2 Pelvic Bone, Right 3 Pelvic Bone, Left 4 Acetabulum, Right 5 Acetabulum, Left 6 Upper Femur, Right 7 Upper Femur, Left 8 Femoral Shaft, Right 9 Femoral Shaft, Left B Lower Femur, Right C Lower Femur, Left D Patella, Right F Patella, Left G Tibia, Right H Tibia, Left J Fibula, Right K Fibula, Left L Tarsal, Right M Tarsal, Left N Metatarsal, Right P Metatarsal, Left Q Toe Phalanx, Right R Toe Phalanx, Left S Coccyx	Ø Open 3 Percutaneous 4 Percutaneous Endoscopic	7 Autologous Tissue Substitute J Synthetic Substitute K Nonautologous Tissue Substitute	Z No Qualifier

SECTION: Ø MEDICAL AND SURGICAL
BODY SYSTEM: Q LOWER BONES
OPERATION: S REPOSITION: *(on multiple pages)*

Moving to its normal location, or other suitable location, all or a portion of a body part

Body Part	Approach	Device	Qualifier
Ø Lumbar Vertebra	Ø Open 4 Percutaneous Endoscopic	3 Spinal Stabilization Device, Vertebral Body Tether 4 Internal Fixation Device Z No Device	Z No Qualifier
Ø Lumbar Vertebra	3 Percutaneous	4 Internal Fixation Device Z No Device	Z No Qualifier
Ø Lumbar Vertebra	X External	Z No Device	Z No Qualifier
1 Sacrum ⊞ 4 Acetabulum, Right 5 Acetabulum, Left S Coccyx ⊞	Ø Open 3 Percutaneous 4 Percutaneous Endoscopic	4 Internal Fixation Device Z No Device	Z No Qualifier
1 Sacrum 4 Acetabulum, Right 5 Acetabulum, Left S Coccyx	X External	Z No Device	Z No Qualifier
2 Pelvic Bone, Right 3 Pelvic Bone, Left D Patella, Right F Patella, Left L Tarsal, Right M Tarsal, Left Q Toe Phalanx, Right R Toe Phalanx, Left	Ø Open 3 Percutaneous 4 Percutaneous Endoscopic	4 Internal Fixation Device 5 External Fixation Device Z No Device	Z No Qualifier
2 Pelvic Bone, Right 3 Pelvic Bone, Left D Patella, Right F Patella, Left L Tarsal, Right M Tarsal, Left Q Toe Phalanx, Right R Toe Phalanx, Left	X External	Z No Device	Z No Qualifier
6 Upper Femur, Right 7 Upper Femur, Left 8 Femoral Shaft, Right 9 Femoral Shaft, Left B Lower Femur, Right C Lower Femur, Left G Tibia, Right H Tibia, Left J Fibula, Right K Fibula, Left	Ø Open 3 Percutaneous 4 Percutaneous Endoscopic	4 Internal Fixation Device 5 External Fixation Device 6 Internal Fixation Device, Intramedullary B External Fixation Device, Monoplanar C External Fixation Device, Ring D External Fixation Device, Hybrid Z No Device	Z No Qualifier

⊞ ØQS[Ø1S]3ZZ
Non-OR ØQS[45][34]ZZ
Non-OR ØQS[45]XZZ
Non-OR ØQS[23DFLMQR][34]ZZ
Non-OR ØQS[23DFLMQR]XZZ
Non-OR ØQS[6789BCGHJK][34]ZZ

Coding Clinic: 2Ø16, Q3, P35 – ØQS[FH]Ø4Z
Coding Clinic: 2Ø16, Q3, P35 – ØQSKØZZ
Coding Clinic: 2Ø18, Q1, P13 – ØQS[LM]Ø4Z
Coding Clinic: 2Ø19, Q3, P26 – ØQS9Ø4Z
Coding Clinic: 2Ø2Ø, Q1, P34 – ØQSØØ4Z
Coding Clinic: 2Ø22, Q2, P21 – ØQS[HK]3CZ

SECTION: Ø MEDICAL AND SURGICAL
BODY SYSTEM: Q LOWER BONES
OPERATION: S REPOSITION: *(continued)*
Moving to its normal location, or other suitable location, all or a portion of a body part

Body Part	Approach	Device	Qualifier
6 Upper Femur, Right 7 Upper Femur, Left 8 Femoral Shaft, Right 9 Femoral Shaft, Left B Lower Femur, Right C Lower Femur, Left G Tibia, Right H Tibia, Left J Fibula, Right K Fibula, Left	X External	Z No Device	Z No Qualifier
N Metatarsal, Right P Metatarsal, Left	Ø Open 3 Percutaneous 4 Percutaneous Endoscopic	4 Internal Fixation Device 5 External Fixation Device Z No Device	2 Sesamoid Bone(s) 1st Toe Z No Qualifier
N Metatarsal, Right P Metatarsal, Left	X External	Z No Device	2 Sesamoid Bone(s) 1st Toe Z No Qualifier

Non-OR ØQS[6789BCGHJK]XZZ Non-OR ØQS[NP][34]ZZ Non-OR ØQS[NP]XZZ

SECTION: Ø MEDICAL AND SURGICAL
BODY SYSTEM: Q LOWER BONES
OPERATION: T RESECTION: Cutting out or off, without replacement, all of a body part

Body Part	Approach	Device	Qualifier
2 Pelvic Bone, Right 3 Pelvic Bone, Left 4 Acetabulum, Right 5 Acetabulum, Left 6 Upper Femur, Right 7 Upper Femur, Left 8 Femoral Shaft, Right 9 Femoral Shaft, Left B Lower Femur, Right C Lower Femur, Left D Patella, Right F Patella, Left G Tibia, Right H Tibia, Left J Fibula, Right K Fibula, Left L Tarsal, Right M Tarsal, Left N Metatarsal, Right P Metatarsal, Left Q Toe Phalanx, Right R Toe Phalanx, Left S Coccyx	Ø Open	Z No Device	Z No Qualifier

Coding Clinic: 2Ø15, Q3, P26 – ØQT7ØZZ
Coding Clinic: 2Ø16, Q3, P3Ø – ØQT[67]ØZZ

SECTION: Ø MEDICAL AND SURGICAL
BODY SYSTEM: Q LOWER BONES
OPERATION: U SUPPLEMENT: Putting in or on biological or synthetic material that physically reinforces and/or augments the function of a portion of a body part

Body Part	Approach	Device	Qualifier
Ø Lumbar Vertebra ⊞ 1 Sacrum ⊞ 2 Pelvic Bone, Right 3 Pelvic Bone, Left 4 Acetabulum, Right 5 Acetabulum, Left 6 Upper Femur, Right 7 Upper Femur, Left 8 Femoral Shaft, Right 9 Femoral Shaft, Left B Lower Femur, Right C Lower Femur, Left D Patella, Right F Patella, Left G Tibia, Right H Tibia, Left J Fibula, Right K Fibula, Left L Tarsal, Right M Tarsal, Left N Metatarsal, Right P Metatarsal, Left Q Toe Phalanx, Right R Toe Phalanx, Left S Coccyx ⊞	Ø Open 3 Percutaneous 4 Percutaneous Endoscopic	7 Autologous Tissue Substitute J Synthetic Substitute K Nonautologous Tissue Substitute	Z No Qualifier

⊞ ØQU[Ø1S]3JZ

Coding Clinic: 2013, Q2, P36 – ØQU2ØJZ
Coding Clinic: 2015, Q3, P19 – ØQU5ØJZ
Coding Clinic: 2019, Q2, P35 – ØQUØ3JZ
Coding Clinic: 2019, Q3, P26 – ØQU9ØKZ
Coding Clinic: 2023, Q3, P23 – ØQUFØJZ

SECTION: Ø MEDICAL AND SURGICAL
BODY SYSTEM: Q LOWER BONES
OPERATION: W REVISION: Correcting, to the extent possible, a portion of a malfunctioning device or the position of a displaced device

Body Part	Approach	Device	Qualifier
Ø Lumbar Vertebra 1 Sacrum 4 Acetabulum, Right 5 Acetabulum, Left S Coccyx	Ø Open 3 Percutaneous 4 Percutaneous Endoscopic X External	4 Internal Fixation Device 7 Autologous Tissue Substitute J Synthetic Substitute K Nonautologous Tissue Substitute	Z No Qualifier
2 Pelvic Bone, Right 3 Pelvic Bone, Left 6 Upper Femur, Right 7 Upper Femur, Left 8 Femoral Shaft, Right 9 Femoral Shaft, Left B Lower Femur, Right C Lower Femur, Left D Patella, Right F Patella, Left G Tibia, Right H Tibia, Left J Fibula, Right K Fibula, Left L Tarsal, Right M Tarsal, Left N Metatarsal, Right P Metatarsal, Left Q Toe Phalanx, Right R Toe Phalanx, Left	Ø Open 3 Percutaneous 4 Percutaneous Endoscopic X External	4 Internal Fixation Device 5 External Fixation Device 7 Autologous Tissue Substitute J Synthetic Substitute K Nonautologous Tissue Substitute	Z No Qualifier
Y Lower Bone	Ø Open 3 Percutaneous 4 Percutaneous Endoscopic X External	Ø Drainage Device M Bone Growth Stimulator	Z No Qualifier

Non-OR ØQW[Ø145S]X[47JK]Z
Non-OR ØQW[236789BCDFGHJKLMNPQR]X[457JK]Z
Non-OR ØQWYX[ØM]Z

Coding Clinic: 2Ø17, Q4, P75 – ØQWØ34Z

New/Revised Text in Green ~~deleted~~ Deleted ♀ Females Only ♂ Males Only **Coding Clinic**
Non-covered 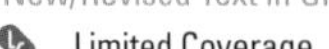 Limited Coverage ⊞ Combination (See Appendix E) DRG Non-OR Non-OR Hospital-Acquired Condition

ØR. Upper Joints 423
ØR2. Change 424
ØR5. Destruction 424
ØR9. Drainage 425
ØRB. Excision 427
ØRC. Extirpation 428
ØRG. Fusion 429
ØRH. Insertion 430
ØRJ. Inspection 431
ØRN. Release 432
ØRP. Removal 432
ØRQ. Repair 434
ØRR. Replacement 435
ØRS. Reposition 436
ØRT. Resection 437
ØRU. Supplement 438
ØRW. Revision 439

SECTION: Ø MEDICAL AND SURGICAL
BODY SYSTEM: R UPPER JOINTS
OPERATION: 2 **CHANGE:** Taking out or off a device from a body part and putting back an identical or similar device in or on the same body part without cutting or puncturing the skin or a mucous membrane

Body Part	Approach	Device	Qualifier
Y Upper Joint	X External	Ø Drainage Device Y Other Device	Z No Qualifier

Non-OR All Values

SECTION: Ø MEDICAL AND SURGICAL
BODY SYSTEM: R UPPER JOINTS
OPERATION: 5 **DESTRUCTION:** Physical eradication of all or a portion of a body part by the direct use of energy, force, or destructive agent

Body Part	Approach	Device	Qualifier
Ø Occipital-cervical Joint 1 Cervical Vertebral Joint 3 Cervical Vertebral Disc 4 Cervicothoracic Vertebral Joint 5 Cervicothoracic Vertebral Disc 6 Thoracic Vertebral Joint 9 Thoracic Vertebral Disc A Thoracolumbar Vertebral Joint B Thoracolumbar Vertebral Disc C Temporomandibular Joint, Right D Temporomandibular Joint, Left E Sternoclavicular Joint, Right F Sternoclavicular Joint, Left G Acromioclavicular Joint, Right H Acromioclavicular Joint, Left J Shoulder Joint, Right K Shoulder Joint, Left L Elbow Joint, Right M Elbow Joint, Left N Wrist Joint, Right P Wrist Joint, Left Q Carpal Joint, Right R Carpal Joint, Left S Carpometacarpal Joint, Right T Carpometacarpal Joint, Left U Metacarpophalangeal Joint, Right V Metacarpophalangeal Joint, Left W Finger Phalangeal Joint, Right X Finger Phalangeal Joint, Left	Ø Open 3 Percutaneous 4 Percutaneous Endoscopic	Z No Device	Z No Qualifier

Non-OR ØR5[359B][34]ZZ

SECTION: Ø MEDICAL AND SURGICAL
BODY SYSTEM: R UPPER JOINTS
OPERATION: 9 DRAINAGE: *(on multiple pages)*
Taking or letting out fluids and/or gases from a body part

Body Part	Approach	Device	Qualifier
Ø Occipital-cervical Joint 1 Cervical Vertebral Joint 3 Cervical Vertebral Disc 4 Cervicothoracic Vertebral Joint 5 Cervicothoracic Vertebral Disc 6 Thoracic Vertebral Joint 9 Thoracic Vertebral Disc A Thoracolumbar Vertebral Joint B Thoracolumbar Vertebral Disc C Temporomandibular Joint, Right D Temporomandibular Joint, Left E Sternoclavicular Joint, Right F Sternoclavicular Joint, Left G Acromioclavicular Joint, Right H Acromioclavicular Joint, Left J Shoulder Joint, Right K Shoulder Joint, Left L Elbow Joint, Right M Elbow Joint, Left N Wrist Joint, Right P Wrist Joint, Left Q Carpal Joint, Right R Carpal Joint, Left S Carpometacarpal Joint, Right T Carpometacarpal Joint, Left U Metacarpophalangeal Joint, Right V Metacarpophalangeal Joint, Left W Finger Phalangeal Joint, Right X Finger Phalangeal Joint, Left	Ø Open 3 Percutaneous 4 Percutaneous Endoscopic	Ø Drainage Device	Z No Qualifier

Non-OR ØR9[CD]3ØZ
Non-OR ØR9[Ø134569ABEFGHJKLMNPQRSTUVWX][34]ØZ

SECTION: Ø MEDICAL AND SURGICAL
BODY SYSTEM: R UPPER JOINTS
OPERATION: 9 DRAINAGE: *(continued)*
Taking or letting out fluids and/or gases from a body part

Body Part	Approach	Device	Qualifier
Ø Occipital-cervical Joint 1 Cervical Vertebral Joint 3 Cervical Vertebral Disc 4 Cervicothoracic Vertebral Joint 5 Cervicothoracic Vertebral Disc 6 Thoracic Vertebral Joint 9 Thoracic Vertebral Disc A Thoracolumbar Vertebral Joint B Thoracolumbar Vertebral Disc C Temporomandibular Joint, Right D Temporomandibular Joint, Left E Sternoclavicular Joint, Right F Sternoclavicular Joint, Left G Acromioclavicular Joint, Right H Acromioclavicular Joint, Left J Shoulder Joint, Right K Shoulder Joint, Left L Elbow Joint, Right M Elbow Joint, Left N Wrist Joint, Right P Wrist Joint, Left Q Carpal Joint, Right R Carpal Joint, Left S Carpometacarpal Joint, Right T Carpometacarpal Joint, Left U Metacarpophalangeal Joint, Right V Metacarpophalangeal Joint, Left W Finger Phalangeal Joint, Right X Finger Phalangeal Joint, Left	Ø Open 3 Percutaneous 4 Percutaneous Endoscopic	Z No Device	X Diagnostic Z No Qualifier

DRG Non-OR ØR9[CD]3ZZ
Non-OR ØR9[Ø134569ABEFGHJKLMNPQRSTUVWX][Ø34]ZX
Non-OR ØR9[Ø134569ABEFGHJKLMNPQRSTUVWX][34]ZZ

SECTION: Ø MEDICAL AND SURGICAL
BODY SYSTEM: R UPPER JOINTS
OPERATION: B EXCISION: Cutting out or off, without replacement, a portion of a body part

Body Part	Approach	Device	Qualifier
Ø Occipital-cervical Joint 1 Cervical Vertebral Joint 3 Cervical Vertebral Disc 4 Cervicothoracic Vertebral Joint 5 Cervicothoracic Vertebral Disc 6 Thoracic Vertebral Joint 9 Thoracic Vertebral Disc A Thoracolumbar Vertebral Joint B Thoracolumbar Vertebral Disc C Temporomandibular Joint, Right D Temporomandibular Joint, Left E Sternoclavicular Joint, Right F Sternoclavicular Joint, Left G Acromioclavicular Joint, Right H Acromioclavicular Joint, Left J Shoulder Joint, Right K Shoulder Joint, Left L Elbow Joint, Right M Elbow Joint, Left N Wrist Joint, Right P Wrist Joint, Left Q Carpal Joint, Right R Carpal Joint, Left S Carpometacarpal Joint, Right T Carpometacarpal Joint, Left U Metacarpophalangeal Joint, Right V Metacarpophalangeal Joint, Left W Finger Phalangeal Joint, Right X Finger Phalangeal Joint, Left	Ø Open 3 Percutaneous 4 Percutaneous Endoscopic	Z No Device	X Diagnostic Z No Qualifier

Non-OR ØRB[Ø134569ABEFGHJKLMNPQRSTUVWX][Ø34]ZX

SECTION: Ø MEDICAL AND SURGICAL
BODY SYSTEM: R UPPER JOINTS
OPERATION: C EXTIRPATION: Taking or cutting out solid matter from a body part

Body Part	Approach	Device	Qualifier
Ø Occipital-cervical Joint 1 Cervical Vertebral Joint 3 Cervical Vertebral Disc 4 Cervicothoracic Vertebral Joint 5 Cervicothoracic Vertebral Disc 6 Thoracic Vertebral Joint 9 Thoracic Vertebral Disc A Thoracolumbar Vertebral Joint B Thoracolumbar Vertebral Disc C Temporomandibular Joint, Right D Temporomandibular Joint, Left E Sternoclavicular Joint, Right F Sternoclavicular Joint, Left G Acromioclavicular Joint, Right H Acromioclavicular Joint, Left J Shoulder Joint, Right K Shoulder Joint, Left L Elbow Joint, Right M Elbow Joint, Left N Wrist Joint, Right P Wrist Joint, Left Q Carpal Joint, Right R Carpal Joint, Left S Carpometacarpal Joint, Right T Carpometacarpal Joint, Left U Metacarpophalangeal Joint, Right V Metacarpophalangeal Joint, Left W Finger Phalangeal Joint, Right X Finger Phalangeal Joint, Left	Ø Open 3 Percutaneous 4 Percutaneous Endoscopic	Z No Device	Z No Qualifier

SECTION: Ø MEDICAL AND SURGICAL
BODY SYSTEM: R UPPER JOINTS
OPERATION: G FUSION: Joining together portions of an articular body part, rendering the articular body part immobile

Body Part	Approach	Device	Qualifier
Ø Occipital-cervical Joint 1 Cervical Vertebral Joint 2 Cervical Vertebral Joints, 2 or more 4 Cervicothoracic Vertebral Joint 6 Thoracic Vertebral Joint 7 Thoracic Vertebral Joint, 2 to 7 8 Thoracic Vertebral Joint, 8 or more A Thoracolumbar Vertebral Joint	Ø Open 3 Percutaneous 4 Percutaneous Endoscopic	7 Autologous Tissue Substitute J Synthetic Substitute K Nonautologous Tissue Substitute	Ø Anterior Approach, Anterior Column 1 Posterior Approach, Posterior Column J Posterior Approach, Anterior Column
Ø Occipital-cervical Joint 1 Cervical Vertebral Joint 2 Cervical Vertebral Joints, 2 or more 4 Cervicothoracic Vertebral Joint 6 Thoracic Vertebral Joint 7 Thoracic Vertebral Joints, 2 to 7 8 Thoracic Vertebral Joints, 8 or more A Thoracolumbar Vertebral Joint	Ø Open 3 Percutaneous 4 Percutaneous Endoscopic	A Interbody Fusion Device	Ø Anterior Approach, Anterior Column J Posterior Approach, Anterior Column
C Temporomandibular Joint, Right D Temporomandibular Joint, Left E Sternoclavicular Joint, Right F Sternoclavicular Joint, Left G Acromioclavicular Joint, Right H Acromioclavicular Joint, Left J Shoulder Joint, Right K Shoulder Joint, Left	Ø Open 3 Percutaneous 4 Percutaneous Endoscopic	4 Internal Fixation Device 7 Autologous Tissue Substitute J Synthetic Substitute K Nonautologous Tissue Substitute	Z No Qualifier
L Elbow Joint, Right M Elbow Joint, Left N Wrist Joint, Right P Wrist Joint, Left Q Carpal Joint, Right R Carpal Joint, Left S Carpometacarpal Joint, Right T Carpometacarpal Joint, Left U Metacarpophalangeal Joint, Right V Metacarpophalangeal Joint, Left W Finger Phalangeal Joint, Right X Finger Phalangeal Joint, Left	Ø Open 3 Percutaneous 4 Percutaneous Endoscopic	3 Internal Fixation Device, Sustained Compression 4 Internal Fixation Device 5 External Fixation Device 7 Autologous Tissue Substitute J Synthetic Substitute K Nonautologous Tissue Substitute	Z No Qualifier

ØRG7[Ø34][7JKZ][Ø1J]
ØRG7[Ø34]A[ØJ]
ØRG[Ø124678A][Ø34][7JK][Ø1J] when reported with Secondary Diagnosis K68.11, T81.4XXA, or T84.6ØXA-T84.7XXA
ØRG[Ø124678A][Ø34]A[ØJ] when reported with Secondary Diagnosis K68.11, T81.4XXA, or T84.6ØXA-T84.7XXA
ØRG[EFGHJK][Ø34][47JK]Z when reported with Secondary Diagnosis K68.11, T81.4XXA, or T84.6ØXA-T84.7XXA
ØRG[LM][Ø34][3457JK]Z when reported with Secondary Diagnosis K68.11, T81.4XXA, or T84.6ØXA-T84.7XXA

Coding Clinic: 2Ø13, Q1, P29 – ØRG4ØAØ
Coding Clinic: 2Ø13, Q1, P22 – ØRG7Ø71, ØRGAØ71
Coding Clinic: 2Ø17, Q4, P62 – ØRGWØ4Z
Coding Clinic: 2Ø19, Q2, P19 – ØDG2371
Coding Clinic: 2Ø19, Q3, P28 – ØRG2ØAØ

SECTION: Ø MEDICAL AND SURGICAL
BODY SYSTEM: R UPPER JOINTS
OPERATION: H INSERTION: Putting in a nonbiological appliance that monitors, assists, performs, or prevents a physiological function but does not physically take the place of a body part

Body Part	Approach	Device	Qualifier
Ø Occipital-cervical Joint 1 Cervical Vertebral Joint 4 Cervicothoracic Vertebral Joint 6 Thoracic Vertebral Joint A Thoracolumbar Vertebral Joint	Ø Open 3 Percutaneous 4 Percutaneous Endoscopic	3 Infusion Device 4 Internal Fixation Device 8 Spacer B Spinal Stabilization Device, Interspinous Process C Spinal Stabilization Device, Pedicle-Based D Spinal Stabilization Device, Facet Replacement	Z No Qualifier
3 Cervical Vertebral Disc 5 Cervicothoracic Vertebral Disc 9 Thoracic Vertebral Disc B Thoracolumbar Vertebral Disc	Ø Open 3 Percutaneous 4 Percutaneous Endoscopic	3 Infusion Device	Z No Qualifier
C Temporomandibular Joint, Right D Temporomandibular Joint, Left E Sternoclavicular Joint, Right F Sternoclavicular Joint, Left G Acromioclavicular Joint, Right H Acromioclavicular Joint, Left J Shoulder Joint, Right K Shoulder Joint, Left	Ø Open 3 Percutaneous 4 Percutaneous Endoscopic	3 Infusion Device 4 Internal Fixation Device 8 Spacer	Z No Qualifier
L Elbow Joint, Right M Elbow Joint, Left N Wrist Joint, Right P Wrist Joint, Left Q Carpal Joint, Right R Carpal Joint, Left S Carpometacarpal Joint, Right T Carpometacarpal Joint, Left U Metacarpophalangeal Joint, Right V Metacarpophalangeal Joint, Left W Finger Phalangeal Joint, Right X Finger Phalangeal Joint, Left	Ø Open 3 Percutaneous 4 Percutaneous Endoscopic	3 Infusion Device 4 Internal Fixation Device 5 External Fixation Device 8 Spacer	Z No Qualifier

DRG Non-OR ØRH[Ø146A][34]3Z
DRG Non-OR ØRH[359B][34]3Z
DRG Non-OR ØRH[EFGHJK][34]3Z
DRG Non-OR ØRH[LMNPQRSTUVWX][34]3Z
Non-OR ØRH[Ø146A][Ø34][38]Z
Non-OR ØRH[359B][Ø34]3Z
Non-OR ØRH[CD]33Z
Non-OR ØRH[CD][Ø34]8Z
Non-OR ØRH[EFGHJK][Ø34][38]Z
Non-OR ØRH[LMNPQRSTUVWX][Ø34][38]Z

Coding Clinic: 2Ø16, Q3, P33 – ØRHJØ4ZZ
Coding Clinic: 2Ø17, Q2, P24 – ØRH1Ø4Z

SECTION: Ø MEDICAL AND SURGICAL
BODY SYSTEM: R UPPER JOINTS
OPERATION: J INSPECTION: Visually and/or manually exploring a body part

Body Part	Approach	Device	Qualifier
Ø Occipital-cervical Joint 1 Cervical Vertebral Joint 3 Cervical Vertebral Disc 4 Cervicothoracic Vertebral Joint 5 Cervicothoracic Vertebral Disc 6 Thoracic Vertebral Joint 9 Thoracic Vertebral Disc A Thoracolumbar Vertebral Joint B Thoracolumbar Vertebral Disc C Temporomandibular Joint, Right D Temporomandibular Joint, Left E Sternoclavicular Joint, Right F Sternoclavicular Joint, Left G Acromioclavicular Joint, Right H Acromioclavicular Joint, Left J Shoulder Joint, Right K Shoulder Joint, Left L Elbow Joint, Right M Elbow Joint, Left N Wrist Joint, Right P Wrist Joint, Left Q Carpal Joint, Right R Carpal Joint, Left S Carpometacarpal Joint, Right T Carpometacarpal Joint, Left U Metacarpophalangeal Joint, Right V Metacarpophalangeal Joint, Left W Finger Phalangeal Joint, Right X Finger Phalangeal Joint, Left	Ø Open 3 Percutaneous 4 Percutaneous Endoscopic X External	Z No Device	Z No Qualifier

Non-OR ØRJ[Ø134569ABCDEFGHJKLMNPQRSTUVWX][3X]ZZ

SECTION: Ø MEDICAL AND SURGICAL
BODY SYSTEM: R UPPER JOINTS
OPERATION: N RELEASE: Freeing a body part from an abnormal physical constraint by cutting or by the use of force

Body Part	Approach	Device	Qualifier
Ø Occipital-cervical Joint 1 Cervical Vertebral Joint 3 Cervical Vertebral Disc 4 Cervicothoracic Vertebral Joint 5 Cervicothoracic Vertebral Disc 6 Thoracic Vertebral Joint 9 Thoracic Vertebral Disc A Thoracolumbar Vertebral Joint B Thoracolumbar Vertebral Disc C Temporomandibular Joint, Right D Temporomandibular Joint, Left E Sternoclavicular Joint, Right F Sternoclavicular Joint, Left G Acromioclavicular Joint, Right H Acromioclavicular Joint, Left J Shoulder Joint, Right K Shoulder Joint, Left L Elbow Joint, Right M Elbow Joint, Left N Wrist Joint, Right P Wrist Joint, Left Q Carpal Joint, Right R Carpal Joint, Left S Carpometacarpal Joint, Right T Carpometacarpal Joint, Left U Metacarpophalangeal Joint, Right V Metacarpophalangeal Joint, Left W Finger Phalangeal Joint, Right X Finger Phalangeal Joint, Left	Ø Open 3 Percutaneous 4 Percutaneous Endoscopic X External	Z No Device	Z No Qualifier

Non-OR ØRN[Ø134569ABCDEFGHJKLMNPQRSTUVWX]XZZ

Coding Clinic: 2015, Q2, P23 – ØRNK4ZZ
Coding Clinic: 2016, Q3, P33 – ØRNJ4ZZ

SECTION: Ø MEDICAL AND SURGICAL
BODY SYSTEM: R UPPER JOINTS
OPERATION: P REMOVAL: *(on multiple pages)* Taking out or off a device from a body part

Body Part	Approach	Device	Qualifier
Ø Occipital-cervical Joint 1 Cervical Vertebral Joint 4 Cervicothoracic Vertebral Joint 6 Thoracic Vertebral Joint A Thoracolumbar Vertebral Joint	Ø Open 3 Percutaneous 4 Percutaneous Endoscopic	Ø Drainage Device 3 Infusion Device 4 Internal Fixation Device 7 Autologous Tissue Substitute 8 Spacer A Interbody Fusion Device J Synthetic Substitute K Nonautologous Tissue Substitute	Z No Qualifier
Ø Occipital-cervical Joint 1 Cervical Vertebral Joint 4 Cervicothoracic Vertebral Joint 6 Thoracic Vertebral Joint A Thoracolumbar Vertebral Joint	X External	Ø Drainage Device 3 Infusion Device 4 Internal Fixation Device	Z No Qualifier

DRG Non-OR ØRQ[Ø134569ABEFGHJKLMNPQRSTUVWX]XZZ
Non-OR ØRP[Ø146A][Ø34]8Z
Non-OR ØRP[Ø146A]3[Ø3]Z

SECTION: Ø MEDICAL AND SURGICAL
BODY SYSTEM: R UPPER JOINTS
OPERATION: P REMOVAL: *(continued)*
Taking out or off a device from a body part

Body Part	Approach	Device	Qualifier
3 Cervical Vertebral Disc 5 Cervicothoracic Vertebral Disc 9 Thoracic Vertebral Disc B Thoracolumbar Vertebral Disc	Ø Open 3 Percutaneous 4 Percutaneous Endoscopic	Ø Drainage Device 3 Infusion Device 7 Autologous Tissue Substitute J Synthetic Substitute K Nonautologous Tissue Substitute	Z No Qualifier
3 Cervical Vertebral Disc 5 Cervicothoracic Vertebral Disc 9 Thoracic Vertebral Disc B Thoracolumbar Vertebral Disc	X External	Ø Drainage Device 3 Infusion Device	Z No Qualifier
C Temporomandibular Joint, Right D Temporomandibular Joint, Left E Sternoclavicular Joint, Right F Sternoclavicular Joint, Left G Acromioclavicular Joint, Right H Acromioclavicular Joint, Left	Ø Open 3 Percutaneous 4 Percutaneous Endoscopic	Ø Drainage Device 3 Infusion Device 4 Internal Fixation Device 7 Autologous Tissue Substitute 8 Spacer J Synthetic Substitute K Nonautologous Tissue Substitute	Z No Qualifier
C Temporomandibular Joint, Right D Temporomandibular Joint, Left E Sternoclavicular Joint, Right F Sternoclavicular Joint, Left G Acromioclavicular Joint, Right H Acromioclavicular Joint, Left	X External	Ø Drainage Device 3 Infusion Device 4 Internal Fixation Device	Z No Qualifier
J Shoulder Joint, Right K Shoulder Joint, Left	Ø Open 3 Percutaneous 4 Percutaneous Endoscopic	Ø Drainage Device 3 Infusion Device 4 Internal Fixation Device 7 Autologous Tissue Substitute 8 Spacer K Nonautologous Tissue Substitute	Z No Qualifier
J Shoulder Joint, Right K Shoulder Joint, Left	Ø Open 3 Percutaneous 4 Percutaneous Endoscopic	J Synthetic Substitute	6 Humeral Surface 7 Glenoid Surface Z No Qualifier
J Shoulder Joint, Right K Shoulder Joint, Left	X External	Ø Drainage Device 3 Infusion Device 4 Internal Fixation Device	Z No Qualifier
L Elbow Joint, Right M Elbow Joint, Left N Wrist Joint, Right P Wrist Joint, Left Q Carpal Joint, Right R Carpal Joint, Left S Carpometacarpal Joint, Right T Carpometacarpal Joint, Left U Metacarpophalangeal Joint, Right V Metacarpophalangeal Joint, Left W Finger Phalangeal Joint, Right X Finger Phalangeal Joint, Left	Ø Open 3 Percutaneous 4 Percutaneous Endoscopic	Ø Drainage Device 3 Infusion Device 4 Internal Fixation Device 5 External Fixation Device 7 Autologous Tissue Substitute 8 Spacer J Synthetic Substitute K Nonautologous Tissue Substitute	Z No Qualifier

Non-OR ØRP[Ø146A]X[Ø34]Z
Non-OR ØRP[359B]3[Ø3]Z
Non-OR ØRP[359B]X[Ø3]Z
Non-OR ØRP[CDEFGHJK][Ø34]8Z
Non-OR ØRP[CDEFGHJK]3[Ø3]Z
Non-OR ØRP[CD]X[Ø3]Z
Non-OR ØRP[EFGHJK]X[Ø34]Z
Non-OR ØRP[LMNPQRSTUVWX]3[Ø3]Z
Non-OR ØRP[LMNPQRSTUVWX][Ø34]8Z

SECTION: Ø MEDICAL AND SURGICAL
BODY SYSTEM: R UPPER JOINTS
OPERATION: P REMOVAL: *(continued)*
Taking out or off a device from a body part

Body Part	Approach	Device	Qualifier
L Elbow Joint, Right M Elbow Joint, Left N Wrist Joint, Right P Wrist Joint, Left Q Carpal Joint, Right R Carpal Joint, Left S Carpometacarpal Joint, Right T Carpometacarpal Joint, Left U Metacarpophalangeal Joint, Right V Metacarpophalangeal Joint, Left W Finger Phalangeal Joint, Right X Finger Phalangeal Joint, Left	X External	Ø Drainage Device 3 Infusion Device 4 Internal Fixation Device 5 External Fixation Device	Z No Qualifier

Non-OR ØRP[LMNPQRSTUVWX]X[Ø345]Z

SECTION: Ø MEDICAL AND SURGICAL
BODY SYSTEM: R UPPER JOINTS
OPERATION: Q REPAIR: Restoring, to the extent possible, a body part to its normal anatomic structure and function

Body Part	Approach	Device	Qualifier
Ø Occipital-cervical Joint 1 Cervical Vertebral Joint 3 Cervical Vertebral Disc 4 Cervicothoracic Vertebral Joint 5 Cervicothoracic Vertebral Disc 6 Thoracic Vertebral Joint 9 Thoracic Vertebral Disc A Thoracolumbar Vertebral Joint B Thoracolumbar Vertebral Disc C Temporomandibular Joint, Right D Temporomandibular Joint, Left E Sternoclavicular Joint, Right F Sternoclavicular Joint, Left G Acromioclavicular Joint, Right H Acromioclavicular Joint, Left J Shoulder Joint, Right K Shoulder Joint, Left L Elbow Joint, Right M Elbow Joint, Left N Wrist Joint, Right P Wrist Joint, Left Q Carpal Joint, Right R Carpal Joint, Left S Carpometacarpal Joint, Right T Carpometacarpal Joint, Left U Metacarpophalangeal Joint, Right V Metacarpophalangeal Joint, Left W Finger Phalangeal Joint, Right X Finger Phalangeal Joint, Left	Ø Open 3 Percutaneous 4 Percutaneous Endoscopic X External	Z No Device	Z No Qualifier

DRG Non-OR ØRQ[EFGHJKLM]XZZ
Non-OR ØRQ[CD]XZZ

ØRQ[EFGHJKLM][Ø34X]ZZ when reported with Secondary Diagnosis K68.11, T81.4ØXA-T81.49XA, or T82.7XXA

Coding Clinic: 2016, Q1, P3Ø – ØRQJ4ZZ

SECTION: Ø MEDICAL AND SURGICAL
BODY SYSTEM: R UPPER JOINTS
OPERATION: R REPLACEMENT: Putting in or on biological or synthetic material that physically takes the place and/or function of all or a portion of a body part

Body Part	Approach	Device	Qualifier
Ø Occipital-cervical Joint 1 Cervical Vertebral Joint 3 Cervical Vertebral Disc 4 Cervicothoracic Vertebral Joint 5 Cervicothoracic Vertebral Disc 6 Thoracic Vertebral Joint 9 Thoracic Vertebral Disc A Thoracolumbar Vertebral Joint B Thoracolumbar Vertebral Disc C Temporomandibular Joint, Right D Temporomandibular Joint, Left E Sternoclavicular Joint, Right F Sternoclavicular Joint, Left G Acromioclavicular Joint, Right H Acromioclavicular Joint, Left L Elbow Joint, Right M Elbow Joint, Left N Wrist Joint, Right P Wrist Joint, Left Q Carpal Joint, Right R Carpal Joint, Left S Carpometacarpal Joint, Right T Carpometacarpal Joint, Left U Metacarpophalangeal Joint, Right V Metacarpophalangeal Joint, Left W Finger Phalangeal Joint, Right X Finger Phalangeal Joint, Left	Ø Open	7 Autologous Tissue Substitute J Synthetic Substitute K Nonautologous Tissue Substitute	Z No Qualifier
J Shoulder Joint, Right K Shoulder Joint, Left	Ø Open	Ø Synthetic Substitute, Reverse Ball and Socket 7 Autologous Tissue Substitute K Nonautologous Tissue Substitute	Z No Qualifier
J Shoulder Joint, Right K Shoulder Joint, Left	Ø Open	J Synthetic Substitute	6 Humeral Surface 7 Glenoid Surface Z No Qualifier

Coding Clinic: 2Ø15, Q1, P27 – ØRRJØØZ
Coding Clinic: 2Ø15, Q3, P15 – ØRRKØJ6

SECTION: Ø MEDICAL AND SURGICAL

BODY SYSTEM: R UPPER JOINTS

OPERATION: S REPOSITION: Moving to its normal location, or other suitable location, all or a portion of a body part

Body Part	Approach	Device	Qualifier
Ø Occipital-cervical Joint 1 Cervical Vertebral Joint 4 Cervicothoracic Vertebral Joint 6 Thoracic Vertebral Joint A Thoracolumbar Vertebral Joint C Temporomandibular Joint, Right D Temporomandibular Joint, Left E Sternoclavicular Joint, Right F Sternoclavicular Joint, Left G Acromioclavicular Joint, Right H Acromioclavicular Joint, Left J Shoulder Joint, Right K Shoulder Joint, Left	Ø Open 3 Percutaneous 4 Percutaneous Endoscopic X External	4 Internal Fixation Device Z No Device	Z No Qualifier
L Elbow Joint, Right M Elbow Joint, Left N Wrist Joint, Right P Wrist Joint, Left Q Carpal Joint, Right R Carpal Joint, Left S Carpometacarpal Joint, Right T Carpometacarpal Joint, Left U Metacarpophalangeal Joint, Right V Metacarpophalangeal Joint, Left W Finger Phalangeal Joint, Right X Finger Phalangeal Joint, Left	Ø Open 3 Percutaneous 4 Percutaneous Endoscopic X External	4 Internal Fixation Device 5 External Fixation Device Z No Device	Z No Qualifier

Non-OR ØRS[Ø146ACDEFGHJK][34X][4Z]Z
Non-OR ØRS[LMNPQRSTUVWX][34X][45Z]Z

Coding Clinic: 2Ø15, Q2, P35; 2Ø13, Q2, P39 – ØRS1XZZ
Coding Clinic: 2Ø19, Q3, P27 – ØRSHØ4Z

New/Revised Text in Green ~~deleted~~ Deleted ♀ Females Only ♂ Males Only Coding Clinic
Non-covered Limited Coverage Combination (See Appendix E) DRG Non-OR Non-OR Hospital-Acquired Condition

SECTION: Ø MEDICAL AND SURGICAL
BODY SYSTEM: R UPPER JOINTS
OPERATION: T RESECTION: Cutting out or off, without replacement, all of a body part

Body Part	Approach	Device	Qualifier
3 Cervical Vertebral Disc 4 Cervicothoracic Vertebral Joint 5 Cervicothoracic Vertebral Disc 9 Thoracic Vertebral Disc B Thoracolumbar Vertebral Disc C Temporomandibular Joint, Right D Temporomandibular Joint, Left E Sternoclavicular Joint, Right F Sternoclavicular Joint, Left G Acromioclavicular Joint, Right H Acromioclavicular Joint, Left J Shoulder Joint, Right K Shoulder Joint, Left L Elbow Joint, Right M Elbow Joint, Left N Wrist Joint, Right P Wrist Joint, Left Q Carpal Joint, Right R Carpal Joint, Left S Carpometacarpal Joint, Right T Carpometacarpal Joint, Left U Metacarpophalangeal Joint, Right V Metacarpophalangeal Joint, Left W Finger Phalangeal Joint, Right X Finger Phalangeal Joint, Left	Ø Open	Z No Device	Z No Qualifier

SECTION: Ø MEDICAL AND SURGICAL
BODY SYSTEM: R UPPER JOINTS
OPERATION: U SUPPLEMENT: Putting in or on biological or synthetic material that physically reinforces and/or augments the function of a portion of a body part

Body Part	Approach	Device	Qualifier
Ø Occipital-cervical Joint 1 Cervical Vertebral Joint 3 Cervical Vertebral Disc 4 Cervicothoracic Vertebral Joint 5 Cervicothoracic Vertebral Disc 6 Thoracic Vertebral Joint 9 Thoracic Vertebral Disc A Thoracolumbar Vertebral Joint B Thoracolumbar Vertebral Disc C Temporomandibular Joint, Right D Temporomandibular Joint, Left E Sternoclavicular Joint, Right F Sternoclavicular Joint, Left G Acromioclavicular Joint, Right H Acromioclavicular Joint, Left J Shoulder Joint, Right K Shoulder Joint, Left L Elbow Joint, Right M Elbow Joint, Left N Wrist Joint, Right P Wrist Joint, Left Q Carpal Joint, Right R Carpal Joint, Left S Carpometacarpal Joint, Right T Carpometacarpal Joint, Left U Metacarpophalangeal Joint, Right V Metacarpophalangeal Joint, Left W Finger Phalangeal Joint, Right X Finger Phalangeal Joint, Left	Ø Open 3 Percutaneous 4 Percutaneous Endoscopic	7 Autologous Tissue Substitute J Synthetic Substitute K Nonautologous Tissue Substitute	Z No Qualifier

ØRU[EFGHJKLM][Ø34][7JK]Z when reported with Secondary Diagnosis K68.11, T81.4XXA, or T84.6ØXA-T84.7XXA

Coding Clinic: 2Ø15, Q3, P27 – ØRUTØ7Z
Coding Clinic: 2Ø19, Q3, P27 – ØRUHØKZ

SECTION: Ø MEDICAL AND SURGICAL
BODY SYSTEM: R UPPER JOINTS
OPERATION: W REVISION: Correcting, to the extent possible, a portion of a malfunctioning device or the position of a displaced device

Body Part	Approach	Device	Qualifier
Ø Occipital-cervical Joint 1 Cervical Vertebral Joint 4 Cervicothoracic Vertebral Joint 6 Thoracic Vertebral Joint A Thoracolumbar Vertebral Joint	Ø Open 3 Percutaneous 4 Percutaneous Endoscopic X External	Ø Drainage Device 3 Infusion Device 4 Internal Fixation Device 7 Autologous Tissue Substitute 8 Spacer A Interbody Fusion Device J Synthetic Substitute K Nonautologous Tissue Substitute	Z No Qualifier
3 Cervical Vertebral Disc 5 Cervicothoracic Vertebral Disc 9 Thoracic Vertebral Disc B Thoracolumbar Vertebral Disc	Ø Open 3 Percutaneous 4 Percutaneous Endoscopic X External	Ø Drainage Device 3 Infusion Device 7 Autologous Tissue Substitute J Synthetic Substitute K Nonautologous Tissue Substitute	Z No Qualifier
C Temporomandibular Joint, Right D Temporomandibular Joint, Left E Sternoclavicular Joint, Right F Sternoclavicular Joint, Left G Acromioclavicular Joint, Right H Acromioclavicular Joint, Left	Ø Open 3 Percutaneous 4 Percutaneous Endoscopic X External	Ø Drainage Device 3 Infusion Device 4 Internal Fixation Device 7 Autologous Tissue Substitute 8 Spacer J Synthetic Substitute K Nonautologous Tissue Substitute	Z No Qualifier
J Shoulder Joint, Right K Shoulder Joint, Left	Ø Open 3 Percutaneous 4 Percutaneous Endoscopic X External	Ø Drainage Device 3 Infusion Device 4 Internal Fixation Device 7 Autologous Tissue Substitute 8 Spacer K Nonautologous Tissue Substitute	Z No Qualifier
J Shoulder Joint, Right K Shoulder Joint, Left	Ø Open 3 Percutaneous 4 Percutaneous Endoscopic	J Synthetic Substitute	6 Humeral Surface 7 Glenoid Surface Z No Qualifier
L Elbow Joint, Right M Elbow Joint, Left N Wrist Joint, Right P Wrist Joint, Left Q Carpal Joint, Right R Carpal Joint, Left S Carpometacarpal Joint, Right T Carpometacarpal Joint, Left U Metacarpophalangeal Joint, Right V Metacarpophalangeal Joint, Left W Finger Phalangeal Joint, Right X Finger Phalangeal Joint, Left	Ø Open 3 Percutaneous 4 Percutaneous Endoscopic X External	Ø Drainage Device 3 Infusion Device 4 Internal Fixation Device 5 External Fixation Device 7 Autologous Tissue Substitute 8 Spacer J Synthetic Substitute K Nonautologous Tissue Substitute	Z No Qualifier

Non-OR ØRW[Ø146A]X[Ø3478AJK]Z
Non-OR ØRW[359B]X[Ø37JK]Z
Non-OR ØRW[CDEFGHJK]X[Ø3478JK]Z
Non-OR ØRW[LMNPQRSTUVWX]X[Ø34578JK]Z

ØS. Lower Joints 440
ØS2. Change 441
ØS5. Destruction 441
ØS9. Drainage 442
ØSB. Excision 443
ØSC. Extirpation 443
ØSG. Fusion 444
ØSH. Insertion 445
ØSJ. Inspection 446
ØSN. Release 446
ØSP. Removal 447
ØSQ. Repair 450
ØSR. Replacement 451
ØSS. Reposition 453
ØST. Resection 453
ØSU. Supplement 454
ØSW. Revision 455

SECTION: Ø MEDICAL AND SURGICAL
BODY SYSTEM: S LOWER JOINTS
OPERATION: 2 CHANGE: Taking out or off a device from a body part and putting back an identical or similar device in or on the same body part without cutting or puncturing the skin or a mucous membrane

Body Part	Approach	Device	Qualifier
Y Lower Joint	X External	Ø Drainage Device Y Other Device	Z No Qualifier

Non-OR All Values

SECTION: Ø MEDICAL AND SURGICAL
BODY SYSTEM: S LOWER JOINTS
OPERATION: 5 DESTRUCTION: Physical eradication of all or a portion of a body part by the direct use of energy, force, or destructive agent

Body Part	Approach	Device	Qualifier
Ø Lumbar Vertebral Joint 2 Lumbar Vertebral Disc 3 Lumbosacral Joint 4 Lumbosacral Disc 5 Sacrococcygeal Joint 6 Coccygeal Joint 7 Sacroiliac Joint, Right 8 Sacroiliac Joint, Left 9 Hip Joint, Right B Hip Joint, Left C Knee Joint, Right D Knee Joint, Left F Ankle Joint, Right G Ankle Joint, Left H Tarsal Joint, Right J Tarsal Joint, Left K Tarsometatarsal Joint, Right L Tarsometatarsal Joint, Left M Metatarsal-Phalangeal Joint, Right N Metatarsal-Phalangeal Joint, Left P Toe Phalangeal Joint, Right Q Toe Phalangeal Joint, Left	Ø Open 3 Percutaneous 4 Percutaneous Endoscopic	Z No Device	Z No Qualifier

SECTION: Ø MEDICAL AND SURGICAL
BODY SYSTEM: S LOWER JOINTS
OPERATION: 9 DRAINAGE: Taking or letting out fluids and/or gases from a body part

Body Part	Approach	Device	Qualifier
Ø Lumbar Vertebral Joint 2 Lumbar Vertebral Disc 3 Lumbosacral Joint 4 Lumbosacral Disc 5 Sacrococcygeal Joint 6 Coccygeal Joint 7 Sacroiliac Joint, Right 8 Sacroiliac Joint, Left 9 Hip Joint, Right B Hip Joint, Left C Knee Joint, Right D Knee Joint, Left F Ankle Joint, Right G Ankle Joint, Left H Tarsal Joint, Right J Tarsal Joint, Left K Tarsometatarsal Joint, Right L Tarsometatarsal Joint, Left M Metatarsal-Phalangeal Joint, Right N Metatarsal-Phalangeal Joint, Left P Toe Phalangeal Joint, Right Q Toe Phalangeal Joint, Left	Ø Open 3 Percutaneous 4 Percutaneous Endoscopic	Ø Drainage Device	Z No Qualifier
Ø Lumbar Vertebral Joint 2 Lumbar Vertebral Disc 3 Lumbosacral Joint 4 Lumbosacral Disc 5 Sacrococcygeal Joint 6 Coccygeal Joint 7 Sacroiliac Joint, Right 8 Sacroiliac Joint, Left 9 Hip Joint, Right B Hip Joint, Left C Knee Joint, Right D Knee Joint, Left F Ankle Joint, Right G Ankle Joint, Left H Tarsal Joint, Right J Tarsal Joint, Left K Tarsometatarsal Joint, Right L Tarsometatarsal Joint, Left M Metatarsal-Phalangeal Joint, Right N Metatarsal-Phalangeal Joint, Left P Toe Phalangeal Joint, Right Q Toe Phalangeal Joint, Left	Ø Open 3 Percutaneous 4 Percutaneous Endoscopic	Z No Device	X Diagnostic Z No Qualifier

Non-OR ØS9[Ø23456789BCDFGHJKLMNPQ][34]ØZ
Non-OR ØS9[Ø23456789BCDFGHJKLMNPQ][Ø34]ZX
Non-OR ØS9[Ø23456789BCDFGHJKLMNPQ][34]ZZ

Coding Clinic: 2Ø18, Q2, P17 – ØS9D4ZZ

SECTION: Ø MEDICAL AND SURGICAL
BODY SYSTEM: S LOWER JOINTS
OPERATION: B EXCISION: Cutting out or off, without replacement, a portion of a body part

Body Part	Approach	Device	Qualifier
Ø Lumbar Vertebral Joint 2 Lumbar Vertebral Disc 3 Lumbosacral Joint 4 Lumbosacral Disc 5 Sacrococcygeal Joint 6 Coccygeal Joint 7 Sacroiliac Joint, Right 8 Sacroiliac Joint, Left 9 Hip Joint, Right B Hip Joint, Left C Knee Joint, Right D Knee Joint, Left F Ankle Joint, Right G Ankle Joint, Left H Tarsal Joint, Right J Tarsal Joint, Left K Tarsometatarsal Joint, Right L Tarsometatarsal Joint, Left M Metatarsal-Phalangeal Joint, Right N Metatarsal-Phalangeal Joint, Left P Toe Phalangeal Joint, Right Q Toe Phalangeal Joint, Left	Ø Open 3 Percutaneous 4 Percutaneous Endoscopic	Z No Device	X Diagnostic Z No Qualifier

Non-OR ØSB[Ø23456789BCDFGHJKLMNPQ][Ø34]ZX

Coding Clinic: 2Ø15, Q1, P34 – ØSBD4ZZ
Coding Clinic: 2Ø17, Q4, P76; 2Ø16, Q2, P16 – ØSB2ØZZ
Coding Clinic: 2Ø17, Q4, P76 – ØSB4ØZZ

SECTION: Ø MEDICAL AND SURGICAL
BODY SYSTEM: S LOWER JOINTS
OPERATION: C EXTIRPATION: Taking or cutting out solid matter from a body part

Body Part	Approach	Device	Qualifier
Ø Lumbar Vertebral Joint 2 Lumbar Vertebral Disc 3 Lumbosacral Joint 4 Lumbosacral Disc 5 Sacrococcygeal Joint 6 Coccygeal Joint 7 Sacroiliac Joint, Right 8 Sacroiliac Joint, Left 9 Hip Joint, Right B Hip Joint, Left C Knee Joint, Right D Knee Joint, Left F Ankle Joint, Right G Ankle Joint, Left H Tarsal Joint, Right J Tarsal Joint, Left K Tarsometatarsal Joint, Right L Tarsometatarsal Joint, Left M Metatarsal-Phalangeal Joint, Right N Metatarsal-Phalangeal Joint, Left P Toe Phalangeal Joint, Right Q Toe Phalangeal Joint, Left	Ø Open 3 Percutaneous 4 Percutaneous Endoscopic	Z No Device	Z No Qualifier

SECTION: Ø MEDICAL AND SURGICAL
BODY SYSTEM: S LOWER JOINTS
OPERATION: G FUSION: Joining together portions of an articular body part, rendering the articular body part immobile

Body Part	Approach	Device	Qualifier
Ø Lumbar Vertebral Joint 1 Lumbar Vertebral Joints, 2 or more 3 Lumbosacral Joint	Ø Open 3 Percutaneous 4 Percutaneous Endoscopic	7 Autologous Tissue Substitute J Synthetic Substitute K Nonautologous Tissue Substitute	Ø Anterior Approach, Anterior Column 1 Posterior Approach, Posterior Column J Posterior Approach, Anterior Column
Ø Lumbar Vertebral Joint 1 Lumbar Vertebral Joints, 2 or more 3 Lumbosacral Joint	Ø Open 3 Percutaneous 4 Percutaneous Endoscopic	A Interbody Fusion Device	Ø Anterior Approach, Anterior Column J Posterior Approach, Anterior Column
5 Sacrococcygeal Joint 6 Coccygeal Joint 7 Sacroiliac Joint, Right 8 Sacroiliac Joint, Left	Ø Open 3 Percutaneous 4 Percutaneous Endoscopic	4 Internal Fixation Device 7 Autologous Tissue Substitute J Synthetic Substitute K Nonautologous Tissue Substitute	Z No Qualifier
9 Hip Joint, Right B Hip Joint, Left C Knee Joint, Right D Knee Joint, Left F Ankle Joint, Right G Ankle Joint, Left H Tarsal Joint, Right J Tarsal Joint, Left K Tarsometatarsal Joint, Right L Tarsometatarsal Joint, Left M Metatarsal-Phalangeal Joint, Right N Metatarsal-Phalangeal Joint, Left P Toe Phalangeal Joint, Right Q Toe Phalangeal Joint, Left	Ø Open 3 Percutaneous 4 Percutaneous Endoscopic	3 Internal Fixation Device, Sustained Compression 4 Internal Fixation Device 5 External Fixation Device 7 Autologous Tissue Substitute J Synthetic Substitute K Nonautologous Tissue Substitute	Z No Qualifier

ØSG1[Ø34][7JKZ][Ø1J]
ØSG1[Ø34]A[ØJ]
ØSG[Ø13][Ø34][7JK][Ø1J] when reported with Secondary Diagnosis K68.11, T814XA-T8149XA, or T84.6ØXA-T84.7XXA
ØSG[Ø13][Ø34]A[ØJ] when reported with Secondary Diagnosis K68.11, T814XA-T8149XA, or T84.6ØXA-T84.7XXA
ØSG[78][Ø34][47JK]Z when reported with Secondary Diagnosis K68.11, T814XA-T8149XA, or T84.6ØXA-T84.7XXA

Coding Clinic: 2Ø13, Q3, P26, Q1, P23 – ØSGØØ71
Coding Clinic: 2Ø13, Q3, P26 – ØSGØØAJ
Coding Clinic: 2Ø13, Q2, P4Ø – ØSGGØ4Z, ØSGGØ7Z
Coding Clinic: 2Ø21, Q3, P24 – ØSGJØ[47]Z, ØSGLØ[47]Z
Coding Clinic: 2Ø21, Q3, P25 – ØSGØØK1
Coding Clinic: 2Ø22, Q2, P23 – ØSG834Z
Coding Clinic: 2Ø22, Q3, P22 – ØSGØØAJ
Coding Clinic: 2Ø23, Q2, P26 – ØSG1ØK1

SECTION: Ø MEDICAL AND SURGICAL
BODY SYSTEM: S LOWER JOINTS
OPERATION: H INSERTION: Putting in a nonbiological appliance that monitors, assists, performs, or prevents a physiological function but does not physically take the place of a body part

Body Part	Approach	Device	Qualifier
Ø Lumbar Vertebral Joint 3 Lumbosacral Joint	Ø Open 3 Percutaneous 4 Percutaneous Endoscopic	3 Infusion Device 4 Internal Fixation Device 8 Spacer B Spinal Stabilization Device, Interspinous Process C Spinal Stabilization Device, Pedicle-Based D Spinal Stabilization Device, Facet Replacement	Z No Qualifier
2 Lumbar Vertebral Disc 4 Lumbosacral Disc	Ø Open 3 Percutaneous 4 Percutaneous Endoscopic	3 Infusion Device 8 Spacer	Z No Qualifier
5 Sacrococcygeal Joint 6 Coccygeal Joint 7 Sacroiliac Joint, Right 8 Sacroiliac Joint, Left	Ø Open 3 Percutaneous 4 Percutaneous Endoscopic	3 Infusion Device 4 Internal Fixation Device 8 Spacer	Z No Qualifier
9 Hip Joint, Right B Hip Joint, Left C Knee Joint, Right D Knee Joint, Left F Ankle Joint, Right G Ankle Joint, Left H Tarsal Joint, Right J Tarsal Joint, Left K Tarsometatarsal Joint, Right L Tarsometatarsal Joint, Left M Metatarsal-Phalangeal Joint, Right N Metatarsal-Phalangeal Joint, Left P Toe Phalangeal Joint, Right Q Toe Phalangeal Joint, Left	Ø Open 3 Percutaneous 4 Percutaneous Endoscopic	3 Infusion Device 4 Internal Fixation Device 5 External Fixation Device 8 Spacer	Z No Qualifier

DRG Non-OR ØSH[Ø3][34]3Z
DRG Non-OR ØSH[24][34]3Z
DRG Non-OR ØSH[5678][34]3Z
DRG Non-OR ØSH[9BCDFGHJKLMNPQ][34]3Z
Non-OR ØSH[Ø3]Ø3Z
Non-OR ØSH[Ø3][Ø34]8Z
Non-OR ØSH[24]Ø3Z
Non-OR ØSH[24][Ø34]8Z
Non-OR ØSH[5678]Ø3Z
Non-OR ØSH[5678][Ø34]8Z
Non-OR ØSH[9BCDFGHJKLMNPQ]Ø3Z
Non-OR ØSH[9BCDFGHJKLMNPQ][Ø34]8Z

Coding Clinic: 2Ø21, Q1, P19 - ØSH4Ø8Z
Coding Clinic: 2Ø21, Q3, P25 – ØSHØØBZ

SECTION: Ø MEDICAL AND SURGICAL
BODY SYSTEM: S LOWER JOINTS
OPERATION: J INSPECTION: Visually and/or manually exploring a body part

Body Part	Approach	Device	Qualifier
Ø Lumbar Vertebral Joint 2 Lumbar Vertebral Disc 3 Lumbosacral Joint 4 Lumbosacral Disc 5 Sacrococcygeal Joint 6 Coccygeal Joint 7 Sacroiliac Joint, Right 8 Sacroiliac Joint, Left 9 Hip Joint, Right B Hip Joint, Left C Knee Joint, Right D Knee Joint, Left F Ankle Joint, Right G Ankle Joint, Left H Tarsal Joint, Right J Tarsal Joint, Left K Tarsometatarsal Joint, Right L Tarsometatarsal Joint, Left M Metatarsal-Phalangeal Joint, Right N Metatarsal-Phalangeal Joint, Left P Toe Phalangeal Joint, Right Q Toe Phalangeal Joint, Left	Ø Open 3 Percutaneous 4 Percutaneous Endoscopic X External	Z No Device	Z No Qualifier

Non-OR ØSJ[Ø23456789BCDFGHJKLMNPQ][3X]ZZ

Coding Clinic: 2Ø17, Q1, P5Ø – ØSJG3ZZ

SECTION: Ø MEDICAL AND SURGICAL
BODY SYSTEM: S LOWER JOINTS
OPERATION: N RELEASE: Freeing a body part from an abnormal physical constraint by cutting or by the use of force

Body Part	Approach	Device	Qualifier
Ø Lumbar Vertebral Joint 2 Lumbar Vertebral Disc 3 Lumbosacral Joint 4 Lumbosacral Disc 5 Sacrococcygeal Joint 6 Coccygeal Joint 7 Sacroiliac Joint, Right 8 Sacroiliac Joint, Left 9 Hip Joint, Right B Hip Joint, Left C Knee Joint, Right D Knee Joint, Left F Ankle Joint, Right G Ankle Joint, Left H Tarsal Joint, Right J Tarsal Joint, Left K Tarsometatarsal Joint, Right L Tarsometatarsal Joint, Left M Metatarsal-Phalangeal Joint, Right N Metatarsal-Phalangeal Joint, Left P Toe Phalangeal Joint, Right Q Toe Phalangeal Joint, Left	Ø Open 3 Percutaneous 4 Percutaneous Endoscopic X External	Z No Device	Z No Qualifier

Non-OR ØSN[Ø23456789BCDFGHJKLMNPQ]XZZ

Coding Clinic: 2Ø2Ø, Q2, P27 – ØSNC4ZZ

SECTION: Ø MEDICAL AND SURGICAL
BODY SYSTEM: S LOWER JOINTS
OPERATION: P REMOVAL: *(on multiple pages)*
Taking out or off a device from a body part

Body Part	Approach	Device	Qualifier
Ø Lumbar Vertebral Joint 3 Lumbosacral Joint	Ø Open 3 Percutaneous 4 Percutaneous Endoscopic	Ø Drainage Device 3 Infusion Device 4 Internal Fixation Device 7 Autologous Tissue Substitute 8 Spacer A Interbody Fusion Device J Synthetic Substitute K Nonautologous Tissue Substitute	Z No Qualifier
Ø Lumbar Vertebral Joint 3 Lumbosacral Joint	X External	Ø Drainage Device 3 Infusion Device 4 Internal Fixation Device	Z No Qualifier
2 Lumbar Vertebral Disc 4 Lumbosacral Disc	Ø Open 3 Percutaneous 4 Percutaneous Endoscopic	Ø Drainage Device 3 Infusion Device 7 Autologous Tissue Substitute J Synthetic Substitute K Nonautologous Tissue Substitute	Z No Qualifier
2 Lumbar Vertebral Disc 4 Lumbosacral Disc	X External	Ø Drainage Device 3 Infusion Device	Z No Qualifier
5 Sacrococcygeal Joint 6 Coccygeal Joint 7 Sacroiliac Joint, Right 8 Sacroiliac Joint, Left	Ø Open 3 Percutaneous 4 Percutaneous Endoscopic	Ø Drainage Device 3 Infusion Device 4 Internal Fixation Device 7 Autologous Tissue Substitute 8 Spacer J Synthetic Substitute K Nonautologous Tissue Substitute	Z No Qualifier
5 Sacrococcygeal Joint 6 Coccygeal Joint 7 Sacroiliac Joint, Right 8 Sacroiliac Joint, Left	X External	Ø Drainage Device 3 Infusion Device 4 Internal Fixation Device	Z No Qualifier
9 Hip Joint, Right ⊞ B Hip Joint, Left ⊞	Ø Open	Ø Drainage Device 3 Infusion Device 4 Internal Fixation Device 5 External Fixation Device 7 Autologous Tissue Substitute 8 Spacer 9 Liner B Resurfacing Device E Articulating Spacer J Synthetic Substitute K Nonautologous Tissue Substitute	Z No Qualifier
9 Hip Joint, Right ⊞ B Hip Joint, Left ⊞	3 Percutaneous 4 Percutaneous Endoscopic	Ø Drainage Device 3 Infusion Device 4 Internal Fixation Device 5 External Fixation Device 7 Autologous Tissue Substitute 8 Spacer J Synthetic Substitute K Nonautologous Tissue Substitute	Z No Qualifier

⊞ ØSP[9B]Ø[89BJ]Z
⊞ ØSP[9B]4[8J]Z
DRG Non-OR ØSP[9B]Ø8Z
DRG Non-OR ØSP[9B]48Z
Non-OR ØSP[Ø3][Ø34]8Z
Non-OR ØSP[Ø3]3[Ø3]Z
Non-OR ØSP[Ø3]X[Ø34]Z
Non-OR ØSP[24]3[Ø3]Z
Non-OR ØSP[24]X[Ø3]Z
Non-OR ØSP[5678][Ø34]8Z
Non-OR ØSP[5678]3[Ø3]Z
Non-OR ØSP[5678]X[Ø34]Z
Non-OR ØSP[9B]3[Ø38]Z

Coding Clinic: 2Ø15, Q2, P2Ø – ØSP9Ø9Z
Coding Clinic: 2Ø16, Q4, P112 – ØSP9Ø9Z

SECTION: Ø MEDICAL AND SURGICAL
BODY SYSTEM: S LOWER JOINTS
OPERATION: P REMOVAL: *(continued)*
Taking out or off a device from a body part

Body Part	Approach	Device	Qualifier
9 Hip Joint, Right B Hip Joint, Left	X External	Ø Drainage Device 3 Infusion Device 4 Internal Fixation Device 5 External Fixation Device	Z No Qualifier
A Hip Joint, Acetabular Surface, Right ⊞ E Hip Joint, Acetabular Surface, Left ⊞ R Hip Joint, Femoral Surface, Right ⊞ S Hip Joint, Femoral Surface, Left ⊞ T Knee Joint, Femoral Surface, Right ⊞ U Knee Joint, Femoral Surface, Left ⊞ V Knee Joint, Tibial Surface, Right ⊞ W Knee Joint, Tibial Surface, Left ⊞	Ø Open 3 Percutaneous 4 Percutaneous Endoscopic	J Synthetic Substitute	Z No Qualifier
C Knee Joint, Right ⊞ D Knee Joint, Left ⊞	Ø Open	Ø Drainage Device 3 Infusion Device 4 Internal Fixation Device 5 External Fixation Device 7 Autologous Tissue Substitute 8 Spacer 9 Liner E Articulating Spacer K Nonautologous Tissue Substitute L Synthetic Substitute, Unicondylar Medial M Synthetic Substitute, Unicondylar Lateral N Synthetic Substitute, Patellofemoral	Z No Qualifier
C Knee Joint, Right ⊞ D Knee Joint, Left ⊞	Ø Open	J Synthetic Substitute	C Patellar Surface Z No Qualifier
C Knee Joint, Right ⊞ D Knee Joint, Left ⊞	3 Percutaneous 4 Percutaneous Endoscopic	Ø Drainage Device 3 Infusion Device 4 Internal Fixation Device 5 External Fixation Device 7 Autologous Tissue Substitute 8 Spacer K Nonautologous Tissue Substitute L Synthetic Substitute, Unicondylar Medial M Synthetic Substitute, Unicondylar Lateral N Synthetic Substitute, Patellofemoral	Z No Qualifier
C Knee Joint, Right ⊞ D Knee Joint, Left ⊞	3 Percutaneous 4 Percutaneous Endoscopic	J Synthetic Substitute	C Patellar Surface Z No Qualifier
C Knee Joint, Right D Knee Joint, Left	X External	Ø Drainage Device 3 Infusion Device 4 Internal Fixation Device 5 External Fixation Device	Z No Qualifier

⊞ ØSP[AERSTUVW][Ø4]JZ
⊞ ØSP[CD]Ø[89]Z
⊞ ØSP[CD]ØJ[CZ]
⊞ ØSP[CD][34]8Z
⊞ ØSP[CD]4J[CZ]

DRG Non-OR ØSP[CD]Ø8Z
DRG Non-OR ØSP[CD][34]8Z
Non-OR ØSP[9B]X[Ø345]Z
Non-OR ØSP[CD]3[Ø3]Z
Non-OR ØSP[CD]X[Ø345]Z

Coding Clinic: 2Ø15, Q2, P18 – ØSPCØJZ
Coding Clinic: 2Ø15, Q2, P2Ø – ØSP9ØJZ
Coding Clinic: 2Ø16, Q4, P112 – ØSPRØJZ
Coding Clinic: 2Ø18, Q2, P16 – ØSPWØJZ
Coding Clinic: 2Ø21, Q3, P26– ØSPDØJZ
Coding Clinic: 2Ø23, Q3, P23 – ØSPDØ9Z

SECTION: Ø MEDICAL AND SURGICAL
BODY SYSTEM: S LOWER JOINTS
OPERATION: P REMOVAL: *(continued)*
Taking out or off a device from a body part

Body Part	Approach	Device	Qualifier
F Ankle Joint, Right G Ankle Joint, Left H Tarsal Joint, Right J Tarsal Joint, Left K Tarsometatarsal Joint, Right L Tarsometatarsal Joint, Left M Metatarsal-Phalangeal Joint, Right N Metatarsal-Phalangeal Joint, Left P Toe Phalangeal Joint, Right Q Toe Phalangeal Joint, Left	Ø Open 3 Percutaneous 4 Percutaneous Endoscopic	Ø Drainage Device 3 Infusion Device 4 Internal Fixation Device 5 External Fixation Device 7 Autologous Tissue Substitute 8 Spacer J Synthetic Substitute K Nonautologous Tissue Substitute	Z No Qualifier
F Ankle Joint, Right G Ankle Joint, Left H Tarsal Joint, Right J Tarsal Joint, Left K Tarsometatarsal Joint, Right L Tarsometatarsal Joint, Left M Metatarsal-Phalangeal Joint, Right N Metatarsal-Phalangeal Joint, Left P Toe Phalangeal Joint, Right Q Toe Phalangeal Joint, Left	X External	Ø Drainage Device 3 Infusion Device 4 Internal Fixation Device 5 External Fixation Device	Z No Qualifier

Non-OR ØSP[FGHJKLMNPQ]3[Ø3]Z
Non-OR ØSP[FGHJKLMNPQ][Ø34]8Z
Non-OR ØSP[FGHJKLMNPQ]X[Ø345]Z

Coding Clinic: 2Ø13, Q2, P4Ø – ØSPGØ4Z
Coding Clinic: 2Ø16, Q4, P111 – ØSP
Coding Clinic: 2Ø21, Q1, P18; 2Ø17, Q4, P1Ø8 – ØSPFØJZ

Ø: M/S S: LOWER JOINTS P: REMOVAL

SECTION: Ø MEDICAL AND SURGICAL
BODY SYSTEM: S LOWER JOINTS
OPERATION: Q REPAIR: Restoring, to the extent possible, a body part to its normal anatomic structure and function

Body Part	Approach	Device	Qualifier
Ø Lumbar Vertebral Joint 2 Lumbar Vertebral Disc 3 Lumbosacral Joint 4 Lumbosacral Disc 5 Sacrococcygeal Joint 6 Coccygeal Joint 7 Sacroiliac Joint, Right 8 Sacroiliac Joint, Left 9 Hip Joint, Right B Hip Joint, Left C Knee Joint, Right D Knee Joint, Left F Ankle Joint, Right G Ankle Joint, Left H Tarsal Joint, Right J Tarsal Joint, Left K Tarsometatarsal Joint, Right L Tarsometatarsal Joint, Left M Metatarsal-Phalangeal Joint, Right N Metatarsal-Phalangeal Joint, Left P Toe Phalangeal Joint, Right Q Toe Phalangeal Joint, Left	Ø Open 3 Percutaneous 4 Percutaneous Endoscopic X External	Z No Device	Z No Qualifier

DRG Non-OR ØSQ[Ø23456789BCDFGHJKLMNPQ]XZZ

SECTION: Ø MEDICAL AND SURGICAL
BODY SYSTEM: S LOWER JOINTS
OPERATION: R REPLACEMENT: *(on multiple pages)*

Putting in or on biological or synthetic material that physically takes the place and/or function of all or a portion of a body part

Body Part	Approach	Device	Qualifier
Ø Lumbar Vertebral Joint 2 Lumbar Vertebral Disc 3 Lumbosacral Joint 4 Lumbosacral Disc 5 Sacrococcygeal Joint 6 Coccygeal Joint 7 Sacroiliac Joint, Right 8 Sacroiliac Joint, Left H Tarsal Joint, Right J Tarsal Joint, Left K Tarsometatarsal Joint, Right L Tarsometatarsal Joint, Left M Metatarsal-Phalangeal Joint, Right N Metatarsal-Phalangeal Joint, Left P Toe Phalangeal Joint, Right Q Toe Phalangeal Joint, Left	Ø Open	7 Autologous Tissue Substitute J Synthetic Substitute K Nonautologous Tissue Substitute	Z No Qualifier
9 Hip Joint, Right B Hip Joint, Left	Ø Open	1 Synthetic Substitute, Metal 2 Synthetic Substitute, Metal on Polyethylene 3 Synthetic Substitute, Ceramic 4 Synthetic Substitute, Ceramic on Polyethylene 6 Synthetic Substitute, Oxidized Zirconium on Polyethylene J Synthetic Substitute	9 Cemented A Uncemented Z No Qualifier
9 Hip Joint, Right B Hip Joint, Left	Ø Open	7 Autologous Tissue Substitute E Articulating Spacer K Nonautologous Tissue Substitute	Z No Qualifier
A Hip Joint, Acetabular Surface, Right E Hip Joint, Acetabular Surface, Left	Ø Open	Ø Synthetic Substitute, Polyethylene 1 Synthetic Substitute, Metal 3 Synthetic Substitute, Ceramic J Synthetic Substitute	9 Cemented A Uncemented Z No Qualifier
A Hip Joint, Acetabular Surface, Right E Hip Joint, Acetabular Surface, Left	Ø Open	7 Autologous Tissue Substitute K Nonautologous Tissue Substitute	Z No Qualifier

ØSR[24]Ø[7JK]Z when the beneficiary is over age 6Ø
ØSR[24]ØJZ when beneficiary is over age 6Ø
ØSR[9B]Ø[1234J][9AZ]
ØSR[AE]Ø[Ø13J][9AZ]
ØSR[9B]Ø[1234J][9AZ] when reported with Secondary Diagnosis from I26.Ø2-I26.Ø9, I26.92-I26.99, or I82.4Ø1-I82.4Z9
ØSR[9B]Ø[7K]Z when reported with Secondary Diagnosis from I26.Ø2-I26.Ø9, I26.92-I26.99, or I82.4Ø1-I82.4Z9
ØSR[AE]Ø[Ø13J][9AZ] when reported with Secondary Diagnosis from I26.Ø2-I26.Ø9, I26.92-I26.99, or I82.4Ø1-I82.4Z9
ØSR[AE]Ø[7K]Z when reported with Secondary Diagnosis from I26.Ø2-I26.Ø9, I26.92-I26.99, or I82.4Ø1-I82.4Z9

Coding Clinic: 2Ø16, Q4, P1Ø9 – ØSR
Coding Clinic: 2Ø17, Q4, P39 – ØSRBØ6Z
Coding Clinic: 2Ø22, Q1, P39 – ØSRBØ2A

SECTION: Ø MEDICAL AND SURGICAL
BODY SYSTEM: S LOWER JOINTS
OPERATION: R REPLACEMENT: *(continued)*

Putting in or on biological or synthetic material that physically takes the place and/or function of all or a portion of a body part

Body Part	Approach	Device	Qualifier
C Knee Joint, Right D Knee Joint, Left	Ø Open	6 Synthetic Substitute, Oxidized Zirconium on Polyethylene J Synthetic Substitute L Synthetic Substitute, Unicondylar Medial M Synthetic Substitute, Unicondylar Lateral N Synthetic Substitute, Patellofemoral	9 Cemented A Uncemented Z No Qualifier
C Knee Joint, Right D Knee Joint, Left	Ø Open	7 Autologous Tissue Substitute E Articulating Spacer K Nonautologous Tissue Substitute	Z No Qualifier
F Ankle Joint, Right G Ankle Joint, Left T Knee Joint, Femoral Surface, Right U Knee Joint, Femoral Surface, Left V Knee Joint, Tibial Surface, Right W Knee Joint, Tibial Surface, Left	Ø Open	7 Autologous Tissue Substitute K Nonautologous Tissue Substitute	Z No Qualifier
F Ankle Joint, Right G Ankle Joint, Left T Knee Joint, Femoral Surface, Right U Knee Joint, Femoral Surface, Left V Knee Joint, Tibial Surface, Right W Knee Joint, Tibial Surface, Left	Ø Open	J Synthetic Substitute	9 Cemented A Uncemented Z No Qualifier
R Hip Joint, Femoral Surface, Right S Hip Joint, Femoral Surface, Left	Ø Open	1 Synthetic Substitute, Metal 3 Synthetic Substitute, Ceramic J Synthetic Substitute	9 Cemented A Uncemented Z No Qualifier
R Hip Joint, Femoral Surface, Right S Hip Joint, Femoral Surface, Left	Ø Open	7 Autologous Tissue Substitute K Nonautologous Tissue Substitute	Z No Qualifier

ØSR[CDTUVW]ØJ[9AZ]
ØSR[CD]ØL[9AZ]
ØSR[RS]Ø[13J][9AZ]
ØSR[CD]Ø[7K]Z when reported with Secondary Diagnosis from I26.Ø2-I26.Ø9, I26.92-I26.99, or I82.4Ø1-I82.4Z9
ØSR[CD]ØL[9AZ] when reported with Secondary Diagnosis from I26.Ø2-I26.Ø9, I26.92-I26.99, or I82.4Ø1-I82.4Z9
ØSR[TUVW]Ø[7K]Z when reported with Secondary Diagnosis from I26.Ø2-I26.Ø9, I26.92-I26.99, or I82.4Ø1-I82.4Z9
ØSR[CD]ØJ[9AZ] when reported with Secondary Diagnosis from I26.Ø2-I26.Ø9, I26.92-I26.99, or I82.4Ø1-I82.4Z9
ØSR[TUVW]ØJ[9AZ] when reported with Secondary Diagnosis from I26.Ø2-I26.Ø9, I26.92-I26.99, or I82.4Ø1-I82.4Z9
ØSR[RS]Ø[13J][9AZ] when reported with Secondary Diagnosis from I26.Ø2-I26.Ø9, I26.92-I26.99, or I82.4Ø1-I82.4Z9
ØSR[RS]Ø[7K]Z when reported with Secondary Diagnosis from I26.Ø2-I26.Ø9, I26.92-I26.99, or I82.4Ø1-I82.4Z9

Coding Clinic: 2015, Q2, P18 – ØSRCØJ9
Coding Clinic: 2015, Q2, P2Ø – ØSRRØ3A
Coding Clinic: 2015, Q3, P19 – ØSRBØJ9
Coding Clinic: 2016, Q4, P11Ø – ØSRDØ[JL]Z
Coding Clinic: 2016, Q4, P111 – ØSRRØJ9
Coding Clinic: 2017, Q4, P1Ø8 – ØSRFØJA
Coding Clinic: 2018, Q2, P16 – ØSRWØJZ
Coding Clinic: 2021, Q3, P26 – ØSRDØJ9

SECTION: Ø MEDICAL AND SURGICAL
BODY SYSTEM: S LOWER JOINTS
OPERATION: S REPOSITION: Moving to its normal location, or other suitable location, all or a portion of a body part

Body Part	Approach	Device	Qualifier
Ø Lumbar Vertebral Joint 3 Lumbosacral Joint 5 Sacrococcygeal Joint 6 Coccygeal Joint 7 Sacroiliac Joint, Right 8 Sacroiliac Joint, Left	Ø Open 3 Percutaneous 4 Percutaneous Endoscopic X External	4 Internal Fixation Device Z No Device	Z No Qualifier
9 Hip Joint, Right B Hip Joint, Left C Knee Joint, Right D Knee Joint, Left F Ankle Joint, Right G Ankle Joint, Left H Tarsal Joint, Right J Tarsal Joint, Left K Tarsometatarsal Joint, Right L Tarsometatarsal Joint, Left M Metatarsal-Phalangeal Joint, Right N Metatarsal-Phalangeal Joint, Left P Toe Phalangeal Joint, Right Q Toe Phalangeal Joint, Left	Ø Open 3 Percutaneous 4 Percutaneous Endoscopic X External	4 Internal Fixation Device 5 External Fixation Device Z No Device	Z No Qualifier

Non-OR ØSS[Ø35678][34X][4Z]Z
Non-OR ØSS[9BCDFGHJKLMNPQ][34X][45Z]Z

Coding Clinic: 2Ø16, Q2, P32 – ØSSBØ4Z
Coding Clinic: 2Ø22, Q2, P22 – ØSSG35Z
Coding Clinic: 2Ø22, Q3, P27 – ØSS[GJ]35Z

SECTION: Ø MEDICAL AND SURGICAL
BODY SYSTEM: S LOWER JOINTS
OPERATION: T RESECTION: Cutting out or off, without replacement, all of a body part

Body Part	Approach	Device	Qualifier
2 Lumbar Vertebral Disc 4 Lumbosacral Disc 5 Sacrococcygeal Joint 6 Coccygeal Joint 7 Sacroiliac Joint, Right 8 Sacroiliac Joint, Left 9 Hip Joint, Right B Hip Joint, Left C Knee Joint, Right D Knee Joint, Left F Ankle Joint, Right G Ankle Joint, Left H Tarsal Joint, Right J Tarsal Joint, Left K Tarsometatarsal Joint, Right L Tarsometatarsal Joint, Left M Metatarsal-Phalangeal Joint, Right N Metatarsal-Phalangeal Joint, Left P Toe Phalangeal Joint, Right Q Toe Phalangeal Joint, Left	Ø Open	Z No Device	Z No Qualifier

Coding Clinic: 2Ø16, Q1, P2Ø – ØSTMØZZ

SECTION: Ø MEDICAL AND SURGICAL
BODY SYSTEM: S LOWER JOINTS
OPERATION: U SUPPLEMENT: Putting in or on biological or synthetic material that physically reinforces and/or augments the function of a portion of a body part

Body Part	Approach	Device	Qualifier
Ø Lumbar Vertebral Joint 2 Lumbar Vertebral Disc 3 Lumbosacral Joint 4 Lumbosacral Disc 5 Sacrococcygeal Joint 6 Coccygeal Joint 7 Sacroiliac Joint, Right 8 Sacroiliac Joint, Left F Ankle Joint, Right G Ankle Joint, Left H Tarsal Joint, Right J Tarsal Joint, Left K Tarsometatarsal Joint, Right L Tarsometatarsal Joint, Left M Metatarsal-Phalangeal Joint, Right N Metatarsal-Phalangeal Joint, Left P Toe Phalangeal Joint, Right Q Toe Phalangeal Joint, Left	Ø Open 3 Percutaneous 4 Percutaneous Endoscopic	7 Autologous Tissue Substitute J Synthetic Substitute K Nonautologous Tissue Substitute	Z No Qualifier
9 Hip Joint, Right ⊞ ⊗ B Hip Joint, Left ⊞ ⊗	Ø Open	7 Autologous Tissue Substitute 9 Liner B Resurfacing Device J Synthetic Substitute K Nonautologous Tissue Substitute	Z No Qualifier
9 Hip Joint, Right B Hip Joint, Left	3 Percutaneous 4 Percutaneous Endoscopic	7 Autologous Tissue Substitute J Synthetic Substitute K Nonautologous Tissue Substitute	Z No Qualifier
A Hip Joint, Acetabular Surface, Right ⊞ ⊗ E Hip Joint, Acetabular Surface, Left ⊞ ⊗ R Hip Joint, Femoral Surface, Right ⊞ ⊗ S Hip Joint, Femoral Surface, Left ⊞ ⊗	Ø Open	9 Liner B Resurfacing Device	Z No Qualifier
C Knee Joint, Right D Knee Joint, Left	Ø Open	7 Autologous Tissue Substitute J Synthetic Substitute K Nonautologous Tissue Substitute	Z No Qualifier
C Knee Joint, Right D Knee Joint, Left	Ø Open	9 Liner	C Patellar Surface Z No Qualifier
C Knee Joint, Right D Knee Joint, Left	3 Percutaneous 4 Percutaneous Endoscopic	7 Autologous Tissue Substitute J Synthetic Substitute K Nonautologous Tissue Substitute	Z No Qualifier
T Knee Joint, Femoral Surface, Right U Knee Joint, Femoral Surface, Left V Knee Joint, Tibial Surface, Right ⊞ W Knee Joint, Tibial Surface, Left ⊞	Ø Open	9 Liner	Z No Qualifier

⊞ ØSU[9B]Ø9Z
⊞ ØSU[AERS]Ø9Z
⊞ ØSU[VW]Ø9Z
⊗ ØSU[9B]ØBZ when reported with Secondary Diagnosis from I26.Ø2-I26.Ø9, I26.92-I26.99, or I82.4Ø1-I82.4Z9
⊗ ØSU[AERS]ØBZ when reported with Secondary Diagnosis from I26.Ø2-I26.Ø9, I26.92-I26.99, or I82.4Ø1-I82.4Z9

Coding Clinic: 2Ø15, Q2, P2Ø – ØSUAØ9Z
Coding Clinic: 2Ø16, Q4, P112 – ØSUAØ9Z
Coding Clinic: 2Ø21, Q1, P18 – ØSUFØJZ
Coding Clinic: 2Ø22, Q1, P47 – ØSUCØ7Z
Coding Clinic: 2Ø23, Q3, P23 – ØSUWØ9Z

Ø: M/S S: LOWER JOINTS U: SUPPLEMENT

SECTION: Ø MEDICAL AND SURGICAL
BODY SYSTEM: S LOWER JOINTS
OPERATION: W REVISION: *(on multiple pages)*
Correcting, to the extent possible, a portion of a malfunctioning device or the position of a displaced device

Body Part	Approach	Device	Qualifier
Ø Lumbar Vertebral Joint 3 Lumbosacral Joint	Ø Open 3 Percutaneous 4 Percutaneous Endoscopic X External	Ø Drainage Device 3 Infusion Device 4 Internal Fixation Device 7 Autologous Tissue Substitute 8 Spacer A Interbody Fusion Device J Synthetic Substitute K Nonautologous Tissue Substitute	Z No Qualifier
2 Lumbar Vertebral Disc 4 Lumbosacral Disc	Ø Open 3 Percutaneous 4 Percutaneous Endoscopic X External	Ø Drainage Device 3 Infusion Device 7 Autologous Tissue Substitute J Synthetic Substitute K Nonautologous Tissue Substitute	Z No Qualifier
5 Sacrococcygeal Joint 6 Coccygeal Joint 7 Sacroiliac Joint, Right 8 Sacroiliac Joint, Left	Ø Open 3 Percutaneous 4 Percutaneous Endoscopic X External	Ø Drainage Device 3 Infusion Device 4 Internal Fixation Device 7 Autologous Tissue Substitute 8 Spacer J Synthetic Substitute K Nonautologous Tissue Substitute	Z No Qualifier
9 Hip Joint, Right B Hip Joint, Left	Ø Open	Ø Drainage Device 3 Infusion Device 4 Internal Fixation Device 5 External Fixation Device 7 Autologous Tissue Substitute 8 Spacer 9 Liner B Resurfacing Device J Synthetic Substitute K Nonautologous Tissue Substitute	Z No Qualifier
9 Hip Joint, Right B Hip Joint, Left	3 Percutaneous 4 Percutaneous Endoscopic X External	Ø Drainage Device 3 Infusion Device 4 Internal Fixation Device 5 External Fixation Device 7 Autologous Tissue Substitute 8 Spacer J Synthetic Substitute K Nonautologous Tissue Substitute	Z No Qualifier

Non-OR ØSW[Ø3]X[Ø3478AJK]Z
Non-OR ØSW[24]X[Ø37JK]Z
Non-OR ØSW[5678]X[Ø3478JK]Z
Non-OR ØSW[9B]X[Ø34578JK]Z

Coding Clinic: 2Ø16, Q4, P111 – ØSW

SECTION: Ø MEDICAL AND SURGICAL
BODY SYSTEM: S LOWER JOINTS
OPERATION: W REVISION: *(continued)*

Correcting, to the extent possible, a portion of a malfunctioning device or the position of a displaced device

Body Part	Approach	Device	Qualifier
A Hip Joint, Acetabular Surface, Right E Hip Joint, Acetabular Surface, Left R Hip Joint, Femoral Surface, Right S Hip Joint, Femoral Surface, Left T Knee Joint, Femoral Surface, Right U Knee Joint, Femoral Surface, Left V Knee Joint, Tibial Surface, Right W Knee Joint, Tibial Surface, Left	Ø Open 3 Percutaneous 4 Percutaneous Endoscopic X External	J Synthetic Substitute	Z No Qualifier
C Knee Joint, Right D Knee Joint, Left	Ø Open	Ø Drainage Device 3 Infusion Device 4 Internal Fixation Device 5 External Fixation Device 7 Autologous Tissue Substitute 8 Spacer 9 Liner K Nonautologous Tissue Substitute	Z No Qualifier
C Knee Joint, Right D Knee Joint, Left	Ø Open	J Synthetic Substitute	C Patellar Surface Z No Qualifier
C Knee Joint, Right D Knee Joint, Left	3 Percutaneous 4 Percutaneous Endoscopic X External	Ø Drainage Device 3 Infusion Device 4 Internal Fixation Device 5 External Fixation Device 7 Autologous Tissue Substitute 8 Spacer K Nonautologous Tissue Substitute	Z No Qualifier
C Knee Joint, Right D Knee Joint, Left	3 Percutaneous 4 Percutaneous Endoscopic X External	J Synthetic Substitute	C Patellar Surface Z No Qualifier
F Ankle Joint, Right G Ankle Joint, Left H Tarsal Joint, Right J Tarsal Joint, Left K Tarsometatarsal Joint, Right L Tarsometatarsal Joint, Left M Metatarsal-Phalangeal Joint, Right N Metatarsal-Phalangeal Joint, Left P Toe Phalangeal Joint, Right Q Toe Phalangeal Joint, Left	Ø Open 3 Percutaneous 4 Percutaneous Endoscopic X External	Ø Drainage Device 3 Infusion Device 4 Internal Fixation Device 5 External Fixation Device 7 Autologous Tissue Substitute 8 Spacer J Synthetic Substitute K Nonautologous Tissue Substitute	Z No Qualifier

Non-OR ØSW[AERSTUVW]XJZ
Non-OR ØSW[CD]X[Ø34578K]Z
Non-OR ØSW[CD]XJZ
Non-OR ØSW[FGHJKLMNPQ]X[Ø34578JK]Z

Coding Clinic: 2Ø16, Q4, P112 – ØSWWØJZ
Coding Clinic: 2Ø17, Q4, P1Ø7 – ØSWFØJZ

ØT. Urinary System 457
ØT1. Bypass 458
ØT2. Change 458
ØT5. Destruction 459
ØT7. Dilation 459
ØT8. Division 459
ØT9. Drainage 46Ø
ØTB. Excision 461
ØTC. Extirpation 461
ØTD. Extraction 461
ØTF. Fragmentation 462
ØTH. Insertion 462
ØTJ. Inspection 463
ØTL. Occlusion 463
ØTM. Reattachment 464
ØTN. Release 464
ØTP. Removal 465
ØTQ. Repair 466
ØTR. Replacement 467
ØTS. Reposition 467
ØTT. Resection 468
ØTU. Supplement 468
ØTV. Restriction 469
ØTW. Revision 47Ø
ØTY. Transplantation 472

SECTION: Ø MEDICAL AND SURGICAL
BODY SYSTEM: T URINARY SYSTEM
OPERATION: 1 **BYPASS:** Altering the route of passage of the contents of a tubular body part

Body Part	Approach	Device	Qualifier
3 Kidney Pelvis, Right 4 Kidney Pelvis, Left	Ø Open 4 Percutaneous Endoscopic	7 Autologous Tissue Substitute J Synthetic Substitute K Nonautologous Tissue Substitute Z No Device	3 Kidney Pelvis, Right 4 Kidney Pelvis, Left 6 Ureter, Right 7 Ureter, Left 8 Colon 9 Colocutaneous A Ileum B Bladder C Ileocutaneous D Cutaneous
3 Kidney Pelvis, Right 4 Kidney Pelvis, Left	3 Percutaneous	J Synthetic Substitute	D Cutaneous
6 Ureter, Right 7 Ureter, Left 8 Ureters, Bilateral	Ø Open 4 Percutaneous Endoscopic	7 Autologous Tissue Substitute J Synthetic Substitute K Nonautologous Tissue Substitute Z No Device	6 Ureter, Right 7 Ureter, Left 8 Colon 9 Colocutaneous A Ileum B Bladder C Ileocutaneous D Cutaneous
6 Ureter, Right 7 Ureter, Left 8 Ureters, Bilateral	3 Percutaneous	J Synthetic Substitute	D Cutaneous
B Bladder	Ø Open 4 Percutaneous Endoscopic	7 Autologous Tissue Substitute J Synthetic Substitute K Nonautologous Tissue Substitute Z No Device	9 Colocutaneous C Ileocutaneous D Cutaneous
B Bladder	3 Percutaneous	J Synthetic Substitute	D Cutaneous

Coding Clinic: 2Ø15, Q3, P35 – ØT17ØZB
Coding Clinic: 2Ø17, Q3, P21-22 – ØT1[8B]ØZ[9C]

SECTION: Ø MEDICAL AND SURGICAL
BODY SYSTEM: T URINARY SYSTEM
OPERATION: 2 **CHANGE:** Taking out or off a device from a body part and putting back an identical or similar device in or on the same body part without cutting or puncturing the skin or a mucous membrane

Body Part	Approach	Device	Qualifier
5 Kidney 9 Ureter B Bladder D Urethra	X External	Ø Drainage Device Y Other Device	Z No Qualifier

Non-OR All Values

SECTION: Ø MEDICAL AND SURGICAL
BODY SYSTEM: T URINARY SYSTEM
OPERATION: 5 DESTRUCTION: Physical eradication of all or a portion of a body part by the direct use of energy, force, or a destructive agent

Body Part	Approach	Device	Qualifier
Ø Kidney, Right 1 Kidney, Left 3 Kidney Pelvis, Right 4 Kidney Pelvis, Left 6 Ureter, Right 7 Ureter, Left B Bladder C Bladder Neck	Ø Open 3 Percutaneous 4 Percutaneous Endoscopic 7 Via Natural or Artificial Opening 8 Via Natural or Artificial Opening Endoscopic	Z No Device	Z No Qualifier
D Urethra	Ø Open 3 Percutaneous 4 Percutaneous Endoscopic 7 Via Natural or Artificial Opening 8 Via Natural or Artificial Opening Endoscopic X External	Z No Device	Z No Qualifier

Non-OR ØT5D[Ø3478X]ZZ

SECTION: Ø MEDICAL AND SURGICAL
BODY SYSTEM: T URINARY SYSTEM
OPERATION: 7 DILATION: Expanding an orifice or the lumen of a tubular body part

Body Part	Approach	Device	Qualifier
3 Kidney Pelvis, Right 4 Kidney Pelvis, Left 6 Ureter, Right 7 Ureter, Left 8 Ureters, Bilateral B Bladder C Bladder Neck D Urethra	Ø Open 3 Percutaneous 4 Percutaneous Endoscopic 7 Via Natural or Artificial Opening 8 Via Natural or Artificial Opening Endoscopic	D Intraluminal Device Z No Device	Z No Qualifier

Non-OR ØT7[67][Ø3478]DZ
Non-OR ØT7[8D][Ø34]DZ
Non-OR ØT7[8D][78][DZ]Z
Non-OR ØT7C[Ø3478][DZ]Z

Coding Clinic: 2Ø16, Q2, P28 – ØT767DZ

SECTION: Ø MEDICAL AND SURGICAL
BODY SYSTEM: T URINARY SYSTEM
OPERATION: 8 DIVISION: Cutting into a body part, without draining fluids and/or gases from the body part, in order to separate or transect a body part

Body Part	Approach	Device	Qualifier
2 Kidneys, Bilateral C Bladder Neck	Ø Open 3 Percutaneous 4 Percutaneous Endoscopic	Z No Device	Z No Qualifier

SECTION: Ø MEDICAL AND SURGICAL
BODY SYSTEM: T URINARY SYSTEM
OPERATION: 9 DRAINAGE: Taking or letting out fluids and/or gases from a body part

Body Part	Approach	Device	Qualifier
Ø Kidney, Right 1 Kidney, Left 3 Kidney Pelvis, Right 4 Kidney Pelvis, Left 6 Ureter, Right 7 Ureter, Left 8 Ureters, Bilateral B Bladder C Bladder Neck	Ø Open 3 Percutaneous 4 Percutaneous Endoscopic 7 Via Natural or Artificial Opening 8 Via Natural or Artificial Opening Endoscopic	Ø Drainage Device	Z No Qualifier
Ø Kidney, Right 1 Kidney, Left 3 Kidney Pelvis, Right 4 Kidney Pelvis, Left 6 Ureter, Right 7 Ureter, Left 8 Ureters, Bilateral B Bladder C Bladder Neck	Ø Open 3 Percutaneous 4 Percutaneous Endoscopic 7 Via Natural or Artificial Opening 8 Via Natural or Artificial Opening Endoscopic	Z No Device	X Diagnostic Z No Qualifier
D Urethra	Ø Open 3 Percutaneous 4 Percutaneous Endoscopic 7 Via Natural or Artificial Opening 8 Via Natural or Artificial Opening Endoscopic X External	Ø Drainage Device	Z No Qualifier
D Urethra	Ø Open 3 Percutaneous 4 Percutaneous Endoscopic 7 Via Natural or Artificial Opening 8 Via Natural or Artificial Opening Endoscopic X External	Z No Device	X Diagnostic Z No Qualifier

DRG Non-OR ØT9[34]3ØZ
Non-OR ØT9[678][Ø3478]ØZ
Non-OR ØT9[678]3ZZ
Non-OR ØT9[BC][3478]ØZ
Non-OR ØT9[Ø134678][3478]ZX
Non-OR ØT9[Ø134][34]ZZ
Non-OR ØT9[BC][3478]ZZ
Non-OR ØT9D[Ø3478X]ZX
Non-OR ØT9D3ØZ
Non-OR ØT9D3ZZ

Coding Clinic: 2Ø17, Q3, P2Ø – ØT968ØZ

SECTION: Ø MEDICAL AND SURGICAL
BODY SYSTEM: T URINARY SYSTEM
OPERATION: B EXCISION: Cutting out or off, without replacement, a portion of a body part

Body Part	Approach	Device	Qualifier
Ø Kidney, Right 1 Kidney, Left 3 Kidney Pelvis, Right 4 Kidney Pelvis, Left 6 Ureter, Right 7 Ureter, Left B Bladder C Bladder Neck	Ø Open 3 Percutaneous 4 Percutaneous Endoscopic 7 Via Natural or Artificial Opening 8 Via Natural or Artificial Opening Endoscopic	Z No Device	X Diagnostic Z No Qualifier
D Urethra	Ø Open 3 Percutaneous 4 Percutaneous Endoscopic 7 Via Natural or Artificial Opening 8 Via Natural or Artificial Opening Endoscopic X External	Z No Device	X Diagnostic Z No Qualifier

Non-OR ØTB[Ø13467][3478]ZX
Non-OR ØTBD[Ø3478X]ZX

Coding Clinic: 2Ø15, Q3, P34 – ØTBD8ZZ
Coding Clinic: 2Ø16, Q1, P19 – ØTBB8ZX

SECTION: Ø MEDICAL AND SURGICAL
BODY SYSTEM: T URINARY SYSTEM
OPERATION: C EXTIRPATION: Taking or cutting out solid matter from a body part

Body Part	Approach	Device	Qualifier
Ø Kidney, Right 1 Kidney, Left 3 Kidney Pelvis, Right 4 Kidney Pelvis, Left 6 Ureter, Right 7 Ureter, Left B Bladder C Bladder Neck	Ø Open 3 Percutaneous 4 Percutaneous Endoscopic 7 Via Natural or Artificial Opening 8 Via Natural or Artificial Opening Endoscopic	Z No Device	Z No Qualifier
D Urethra	Ø Open 3 Percutaneous 4 Percutaneous Endoscopic 7 Via Natural or Artificial Opening 8 Via Natural or Artificial Opening Endoscopic X External	Z No Device	Z No Qualifier

Non-OR ØTC[BC][78]ZZ
Non-OR ØTCD[78X]ZZ

Coding Clinic: 2Ø15, Q2, P8 – ØTC48ZZ
Coding Clinic: 2Ø15, Q2, P9 – ØTC18ZZ, ØTC78ZZ, ØTCB8ZZ, ØTC78DZ
Coding Clinic: 2Ø19, Q3, P4; 2Ø16, Q3, P24 – ØTCB8ZZ

SECTION: Ø MEDICAL AND SURGICAL
BODY SYSTEM: T URINARY SYSTEM
OPERATION: D EXTRACTION: Pulling or stripping out or off all or a portion of a body part by the use of force

Body Part	Approach	Device	Qualifier
Ø Kidney, Right 1 Kidney, Left	Ø Open 3 Percutaneous 4 Percutaneous Endoscopic	Z No Device	Z No Qualifier

SECTION: Ø MEDICAL AND SURGICAL
BODY SYSTEM: T URINARY SYSTEM
OPERATION: F FRAGMENTATION: Breaking solid matter in a body part into pieces

Body Part	Approach	Device	Qualifier
3 Kidney Pelvis, Right 4 Kidney Pelvis, Left 6 Ureter, Right 7 Ureter, Left B Bladder C Bladder Neck D Urethra	Ø Open 3 Percutaneous 4 Percutaneous Endoscopic 7 Via Natural or Artificial Opening 8 Via Natural or Artificial Opening Endoscopic X External	Z No Device	Z No Qualifier

ØTFDXZZ
Non-OR ØTF[34][Ø78]ZZ
Non-OR ØTF[67BC][Ø3478]ZZ
Non-OR ØTFD[Ø3478X]ZZ

SECTION: Ø MEDICAL AND SURGICAL
BODY SYSTEM: T URINARY SYSTEM
OPERATION: H INSERTION: Putting in a nonbiological appliance that monitors, assists, performs, or prevents a physiological function but does not physically take the place of a body part

Body Part	Approach	Device	Qualifier
5 Kidney	Ø Open 3 Percutaneous 4 Percutaneous Endoscopic 7 Via Natural or Artificial Opening 8 Via Natural or Artificial Opening Endoscopic	1 Radioactive Element 2 Monitoring Device 3 Infusion Device Y Other Device	Z No Qualifier
9 Ureter	Ø Open 3 Percutaneous 4 Percutaneous Endoscopic 7 Via Natural or Artificial Opening 8 Via Natural or Artificial Opening Endoscopic	1 Radioactive Element 2 Monitoring Device 3 Infusion Device M Stimulator Lead Y Other Device	Z No Qualifier
B Bladder	Ø Open 3 Percutaneous 4 Percutaneous Endoscopic 7 Via Natural or Artificial Opening 8 Via Natural or Artificial Opening Endoscopic	1 Radioactive Element 2 Monitoring Device 3 Infusion Device L Artificial Sphincter M Stimulator Lead Y Other Device	Z No Qualifier
C Bladder Neck	Ø Open 3 Percutaneous 4 Percutaneous Endoscopic 7 Via Natural or Artificial Opening 8 Via Natural or Artificial Opening Endoscopic	L Artificial Sphincter	Z No Qualifier
D Urethra	Ø Open 3 Percutaneous 4 Percutaneous Endoscopic 7 Via Natural or Artificial Opening 8 Via Natural or Artificial Opening Endoscopic	1 Radioactive Element 2 Monitoring Device 3 Infusion Device L Artificial Sphincter Y Other Device	Z No Qualifier
D Urethra	X External	2 Monitoring Device 3 Infusion Device L Artificial Sphincter	Z No Qualifier

ØTHB[Ø3478]MZ
Non-OR ØTH5[Ø3478]3Z
Non-OR ØTH5[78]2Z
Non-OR ØTH9[Ø3478]3Z
Non-OR ØTH9[78]2Z
Non-OR ØTHB[Ø3478]3Z
Non-OR ØTHB[78]2Z
Non-OR ØTHD[Ø3478]3Z
Non-OR ØTHD[78]2Z
Non-OR ØTHDX3Z

SECTION: Ø MEDICAL AND SURGICAL
BODY SYSTEM: T URINARY SYSTEM
OPERATION: J INSPECTION: Visually and/or manually exploring a body part

Body Part	Approach	Device	Qualifier
5 Kidney 9 Ureter B Bladder D Urethra	Ø Open 3 Percutaneous 4 Percutaneous Endoscopic 7 Via Natural or Artificial Opening 8 Via Natural or Artificial Opening Endoscopic X External	Z No Device	Z No Qualifier

DRG Non-OR ØTJ[5B][37]ZZ
Non-OR ØTJ9[37]ZZ
Non-OR ØTJ[59][48X]ZZ
Non-OR ØTJB[8X]ZZ
Non-OR ØTJD[3478X]ZZ

SECTION: Ø MEDICAL AND SURGICAL
BODY SYSTEM: T URINARY SYSTEM
OPERATION: L OCCLUSION: Completely closing an orifice or the lumen of a tubular body part

Body Part	Approach	Device	Qualifier
3 Kidney Pelvis, Right 4 Kidney Pelvis, Left 6 Ureter, Right 7 Ureter, Left B Bladder C Bladder Neck	Ø Open 3 Percutaneous 4 Percutaneous Endoscopic	C Extraluminal Device D Intraluminal Device Z No Device	Z No Qualifier
3 Kidney Pelvis, Right 4 Kidney Pelvis, Left 6 Ureter, Right 7 Ureter, Left B Bladder C Bladder Neck	7 Via Natural or Artificial Opening 8 Via Natural or Artificial Opening Endoscopic	D Intraluminal Device Z No Device	Z No Qualifier
D Urethra	Ø Open 3 Percutaneous 4 Percutaneous Endoscopic X External	C Extraluminal Device D Intraluminal Device Z No Device	Z No Qualifier
D Urethra	7 Via Natural or Artificial Opening 8 Via Natural or Artificial Opening Endoscopic	D Intraluminal Device Z No Device	Z No Qualifier

SECTION: Ø **MEDICAL AND SURGICAL**
BODY SYSTEM: T **URINARY SYSTEM**
OPERATION: M **REATTACHMENT:** Putting back in or on all or a portion of a separated body part to its normal location or other suitable location

Body Part	Approach	Device	Qualifier
Ø Kidney, Right 1 Kidney, Left 2 Kidneys, Bilateral 3 Kidney Pelvis, Right 4 Kidney Pelvis, Left 6 Ureter, Right 7 Ureter, Left 8 Ureters, Bilateral B Bladder C Bladder Neck D Urethra	Ø Open 4 Percutaneous Endoscopic	Z No Device	Z No Qualifier

SECTION: Ø **MEDICAL AND SURGICAL**
BODY SYSTEM: T **URINARY SYSTEM**
OPERATION: N **RELEASE:** Freeing a body part from an abnormal physical constraint by cutting or by the use of force

Body Part	Approach	Device	Qualifier
Ø Kidney, Right 1 Kidney, Left 3 Kidney Pelvis, Right 4 Kidney Pelvis, Left 6 Ureter, Right 7 Ureter, Left B Bladder C Bladder Neck	Ø Open 3 Percutaneous 4 Percutaneous Endoscopic 7 Via Natural or Artificial Opening 8 Via Natural or Artificial Opening Endoscopic	Z No Device	Z No Qualifier
D Urethra	Ø Open 3 Percutaneous 4 Percutaneous Endoscopic 7 Via Natural or Artificial Opening 8 Via Natural or Artificial Opening Endoscopic X External	Z No Device	Z No Qualifier

SECTION: Ø MEDICAL AND SURGICAL
BODY SYSTEM: T URINARY SYSTEM
OPERATION: P REMOVAL: *(on multiple pages)*
Taking out or off a device from a body part

Body Part	Approach	Device	Qualifier
5 Kidney	Ø Open 3 Percutaneous 4 Percutaneous Endoscopic 7 Via Natural or Artificial Opening 8 Via Natural or Artificial Opening Endoscopic	Ø Drainage Device 2 Monitoring Device 3 Infusion Device 7 Autologous Tissue Substitute C Extraluminal Device D Intraluminal Device J Synthetic Substitute K Nonautologous Tissue Substitute Y Other Device	Z No Qualifier
5 Kidney	X External	Ø Drainage Device 2 Monitoring Device 3 Infusion Device D Intraluminal Device	Z No Qualifier
9 Ureter	Ø Open 3 Percutaneous 4 Percutaneous Endoscopic 7 Via Natural or Artificial Opening 8 Via Natural or Artificial Opening Endoscopic	Ø Drainage Device 2 Monitoring Device 3 Infusion Device 7 Autologous Tissue Substitute C Extraluminal Device D Intraluminal Device J Synthetic Substitute K Nonautologous Tissue Substitute M Stimulator Lead Y Other Device	Z No Qualifier
9 Ureter	X External	Ø Drainage Device 2 Monitoring Device 3 Infusion Device D Intraluminal Device M Stimulator Lead	Z No Qualifier
B Bladder	Ø Open 3 Percutaneous 4 Percutaneous Endoscopic 7 Via Natural or Artificial Opening 8 Via Natural or Artificial Opening Endoscopic	Ø Drainage Device 2 Monitoring Device 3 Infusion Device 7 Autologous Tissue Substitute C Extraluminal Device D Intraluminal Device J Synthetic Substitute K Nonautologous Tissue Substitute L Artificial Sphincter M Stimulator Lead Y Other Device	Z No Qualifier
B Bladder	X External	Ø Drainage Device 2 Monitoring Device 3 Infusion Device D Intraluminal Device L Artificial Sphincter M Stimulator Lead	Z No Qualifier

ØTPB[Ø3478]MZ
Non-OR ØTP5[78][Ø23D]Z
Non-OR ØTP5X[Ø23D]Z
Non-OR ØTP9[78][Ø23D]Z
Non-OR ØTP9X[Ø23D]Z
Non-OR ØTPB[78][Ø23D]Z
Non-OR ØTPBX[Ø23DL]Z

Coding Clinic: 2016, Q2, P28 – Ø2P98DZ

New/Revised Text in Green ~~deleted~~ Deleted ♀ Females Only ♂ Males Only Coding Clinic
Non-covered Limited Coverage Combination (See Appendix E) DRG Non-OR Non-OR Hospital-Acquired Condition

SECTION: Ø MEDICAL AND SURGICAL
BODY SYSTEM: T URINARY SYSTEM
OPERATION: P REMOVAL: *(continued)*
Taking out or off a device from a body part

Body Part	Approach	Device	Qualifier
D Urethra	Ø Open 3 Percutaneous 4 Percutaneous Endoscopic 7 Via Natural or Artificial Opening 8 Via Natural or Artificial Opening Endoscopic	Ø Drainage Device 2 Monitoring Device 3 Infusion Device 7 Autologous Tissue Substitute C Extraluminal Device D Intraluminal Device J Synthetic Substitute K Nonautologous Tissue Substitute L Artificial Sphincter Y Other Device	Z No Qualifier
D Urethra	X External	Ø Drainage Device 2 Monitoring Device 3 Infusion Device D Intraluminal Device L Artificial Sphincter	Z No Qualifier

Non-OR ØTPD[78][Ø23D]Z
Non-OR ØTPDX[Ø23D]Z

SECTION: Ø MEDICAL AND SURGICAL
BODY SYSTEM: T URINARY SYSTEM
OPERATION: Q REPAIR: Restoring, to the extent possible, a body part to its normal anatomic structure and function

Body Part	Approach	Device	Qualifier
Ø Kidney, Right 1 Kidney, Left 3 Kidney Pelvis, Right 4 Kidney Pelvis, Left 6 Ureter, Right 7 Ureter, Left B Bladder ⊞ C Bladder Neck	Ø Open 3 Percutaneous 4 Percutaneous Endoscopic 7 Via Natural or Artificial Opening 8 Via Natural or Artificial Opening Endoscopic	Z No Device	Z No Qualifier
D Urethra	Ø Open 3 Percutaneous 4 Percutaneous Endoscopic 7 Via Natural or Artificial Opening 8 Via Natural or Artificial Opening Endoscopic X External	Z No Device	Z No Qualifier

Non-OR ØTQB[Ø34]ZZ

Coding Clinic: 2017, Q1, P38 – ØTQDØZZ

SECTION: Ø MEDICAL AND SURGICAL
BODY SYSTEM: T URINARY SYSTEM
OPERATION: R **REPLACEMENT:** Putting in or on biological or synthetic material that physically takes the place and/or function of all or a portion of a body part

Body Part	Approach	Device	Qualifier
3 Kidney Pelvis, Right 4 Kidney Pelvis, Left 6 Ureter, Right 7 Ureter, Left B Bladder C Bladder Neck	Ø Open 4 Percutaneous Endoscopic 7 Via Natural or Artificial Opening 8 Via Natural or Artificial Opening Endoscopic	7 Autologous Tissue Substitute J Synthetic Substitute K Nonautologous Tissue Substitute	Z No Qualifier
D Urethra	Ø Open 4 Percutaneous Endoscopic 7 Via Natural or Artificial Opening 8 Via Natural or Artificial Opening Endoscopic X External	7 Autologous Tissue Substitute J Synthetic Substitute K Nonautologous Tissue Substitute	Z No Qualifier

Coding Clinic: 2Ø17, Q3, P2Ø – ØTRBØ7Z

SECTION: Ø MEDICAL AND SURGICAL
BODY SYSTEM: T URINARY SYSTEM
OPERATION: S **REPOSITION:** Moving to its normal location, or other suitable location, all or a portion of a body part

Body Part	Approach	Device	Qualifier
Ø Kidney, Right 1 Kidney, Left 2 Kidneys, Bilateral 3 Kidney Pelvis, Right 4 Kidney Pelvis, Left 6 Ureter, Right 7 Ureter, Left 8 Ureters, Bilateral B Bladder C Bladder Neck D Urethra	Ø Open 4 Percutaneous Endoscopic	Z No Device	Z No Qualifier

Coding Clinic: 2Ø16, Q1, P15 – ØTSDØZZ
Coding Clinic: 2Ø19, Q1, P3Ø; 2Ø17, Q1, P37 – ØTS6ØZZ

SECTION: Ø MEDICAL AND SURGICAL
BODY SYSTEM: T URINARY SYSTEM
OPERATION: T RESECTION: Cutting out or off, without replacement, all of a body part

Body Part	Approach	Device	Qualifier
Ø Kidney, Right 1 Kidney, Left 2 Kidneys, Bilateral	Ø Open ~~4 Percutaneous Endoscopic~~	Z No Device	Z No Qualifier
Ø Kidney, Right 1 Kidney, Left 2 Kidneys, Bilateral	4 Percutaneous Endoscopic	Z No Device	G Hand-Assisted Z No Qualifier
3 Kidney Pelvis, Right 4 Kidney Pelvis, Left 6 Ureter, Right 7 Ureter, Left B Bladder ⊞ C Bladder Neck D Urethra ⊞	Ø Open 4 Percutaneous Endoscopic 7 Via Natural or Artificial Opening 8 Via Natural or Artificial Opening Endoscopic	Z No Device	Z No Qualifier

Non-OR ØTTD[Ø478]ZZ
⊞ ØTT[BD]ØZZ

SECTION: Ø MEDICAL AND SURGICAL
BODY SYSTEM: T URINARY SYSTEM
OPERATION: U SUPPLEMENT: Putting in or on biological or synthetic material that physically reinforces and/or augments the function of a portion of a body part

Body Part	Approach	Device	Qualifier
3 Kidney Pelvis, Right 4 Kidney Pelvis, Left 6 Ureter, Right 7 Ureter, Left B Bladder C Bladder Neck	Ø Open 4 Percutaneous Endoscopic 7 Via Natural or Artificial Opening 8 Via Natural or Artificial Opening Endoscopic	7 Autologous Tissue Substitute J Synthetic Substitute K Nonautologous Tissue Substitute	Z No Qualifier
D Urethra	Ø Open 4 Percutaneous Endoscopic 7 Via Natural or Artificial Opening 8 Via Natural or Artificial Opening Endoscopic X External	7 Autologous Tissue Substitute J Synthetic Substitute K Nonautologous Tissue Substitute	Z No Qualifier

Coding Clinic: 2Ø17, Q3, P21 – ØTUBØ7Z

SECTION: Ø MEDICAL AND SURGICAL
BODY SYSTEM: T URINARY SYSTEM
OPERATION: V RESTRICTION: Partially closing an orifice or the lumen of a tubular body part

Body Part	Approach	Device	Qualifier
3 Kidney Pelvis, Right 4 Kidney Pelvis, Left 6 Ureter, Right 7 Ureter, Left B Bladder C Bladder Neck	Ø Open 3 Percutaneous 4 Percutaneous Endoscopic	C Extraluminal Device D Intraluminal Device Z No Device	Z No Qualifier
3 Kidney Pelvis, Right 4 Kidney Pelvis, Left 6 Ureter, Right 7 Ureter, Left B Bladder C Bladder Neck	7 Via Natural or Artificial Opening 8 Via Natural or Artificial Opening Endoscopic	D Intraluminal Device Z No Device	Z No Qualifier
D Urethra	Ø Open 3 Percutaneous 4 Percutaneous Endoscopic	C Extraluminal Device D Intraluminal Device Z No Device	Z No Qualifier
D Urethra	7 Via Natural or Artificial Opening 8 Via Natural or Artificial Opening Endoscopic	D Intraluminal Device Z No Device	Z No Qualifier
D Urethra	X External	Z No Device	Z No Qualifier

Coding Clinic: 2Ø15, Q2, P12 – ØTV[67]8ZZ

SECTION: Ø MEDICAL AND SURGICAL
BODY SYSTEM: T URINARY SYSTEM
OPERATION: W REVISION: *(on multiple pages)*

Correcting, to the extent possible, a portion of a malfunctioning device or the position of a displaced device

Body Part	Approach	Device	Qualifier
5 Kidney	Ø Open 3 Percutaneous 4 Percutaneous Endoscopic 7 Via Natural or Artificial Opening 8 Via Natural or Artificial Opening Endoscopic	Ø Drainage Device 2 Monitoring Device 3 Infusion Device 7 Autologous Tissue Substitute C Extraluminal Device D Intraluminal Device J Synthetic Substitute K Nonautologous Tissue Substitute Y Other Device	Z No Qualifier
5 Kidney	X External	Ø Drainage Device 2 Monitoring Device 3 Infusion Device 7 Autologous Tissue Substitute C Extraluminal Device D Intraluminal Device J Synthetic Substitute K Nonautologous Tissue Substitute	Z No Qualifier
9 Ureter	Ø Open 3 Percutaneous 4 Percutaneous Endoscopic 7 Via Natural or Artificial Opening 8 Via Natural or Artificial Opening Endoscopic	Ø Drainage Device 2 Monitoring Device 3 Infusion Device 7 Autologous Tissue Substitute C Extraluminal Device D Intraluminal Device J Synthetic Substitute K Nonautologous Tissue Substitute M Stimulator Lead Y Other Device	Z No Qualifier
9 Ureter	X External	Ø Drainage Device 2 Monitoring Device 3 Infusion Device 7 Autologous Tissue Substitute C Extraluminal Device D Intraluminal Device J Synthetic Substitute K Nonautologous Tissue Substitute M Stimulator Lead	Z No Qualifier

Non-OR ØTW5X[Ø237CDJK]Z

SECTION: Ø MEDICAL AND SURGICAL
BODY SYSTEM: T URINARY SYSTEM
OPERATION: W REVISION: *(continued)*

Correcting, to the extent possible, a portion of a malfunctioning device or the position of a displaced device

Body Part	Approach	Device	Qualifier
B Bladder	Ø Open 3 Percutaneous 4 Percutaneous Endoscopic 7 Via Natural or Artificial Opening 8 Via Natural or Artificial Opening Endoscopic	Ø Drainage Device 2 Monitoring Device 3 Infusion Device 7 Autologous Tissue Substitute C Extraluminal Device D Intraluminal Device J Synthetic Substitute K Nonautologous Tissue Substitute L Artificial Sphincter M Stimulator Lead Y Other Device	Z No Qualifier
B Bladder	X External	Ø Drainage Device 2 Monitoring Device 3 Infusion Device 7 Autologous Tissue Substitute C Extraluminal Device D Intraluminal Device J Synthetic Substitute K Nonautologous Tissue Substitute L Artificial Sphincter M Stimulator Lead	Z No Qualifier
D Urethra	Ø Open 3 Percutaneous 4 Percutaneous Endoscopic 7 Via Natural or Artificial Opening 8 Via Natural or Artificial Opening Endoscopic	Ø Drainage Device 2 Monitoring Device 3 Infusion Device 7 Autologous Tissue Substitute C Extraluminal Device D Intraluminal Device J Synthetic Substitute K Nonautologous Tissue Substitute L Artificial Sphincter Y Other Device	Z No Qualifier
D Urethra	X External	Ø Drainage Device 2 Monitoring Device 3 Infusion Device 7 Autologous Tissue Substitute C Extraluminal Device D Intraluminal Device J Synthetic Substitute K Nonautologous Tissue Substitute L Artificial Sphincter	Z No Qualifier

Non-OR ØTW9X[Ø237CDJKM]Z
Non-OR ØTWBX[Ø237CDJKLM]Z
Non-OR ØTWDX[Ø237CDJKL]Z

SECTION: Ø MEDICAL AND SURGICAL
BODY SYSTEM: T URINARY SYSTEM
OPERATION: Y TRANSPLANTATION: Putting in or on all or a portion of a living body part taken from another individual or animal to physically take the place and/or function of all or a portion of a similar body part

Body Part	Approach	Device	Qualifier
Ø Kidney, Right 1 Kidney, Left	Ø Open	Z No Device	Ø Allogeneic 1 Syngeneic 2 Zooplastic

ØTY[Ø1]ØZ[Ø12]
ØTY[Ø1]ØZ[Ø12]

ØU. Female Reproductive System....473
ØU1. Bypass....474
ØU2. Change....474
ØU5. Destruction....475
ØU7. Dilation....476
ØU8. Division....476
ØU9. Drainage....477
ØUB. Excision....478
ØUC. Extirpation....479
ØUD. Extraction....480
ØUF. Fragmentation....480
ØUH. Insertion....481
ØUJ. Inspection....482
ØUL. Occlusion....482
ØUM. Reattachment....483
ØUN. Release....483
ØUP. Removal....484
ØUQ. Repair....485
ØUS. Reposition....486
ØUT. Resection....486
ØUU. Supplement....487
ØUV. Restriction....487
ØUW. Revision....488
ØUY. Transplantation....489

SECTION: Ø **MEDICAL AND SURGICAL**
BODY SYSTEM: U **FEMALE REPRODUCTIVE SYSTEM**
OPERATION: 1 **BYPASS:** Altering the route of passage of the contents of a tubular body part

Body Part	Approach	Device	Qualifier
5 Fallopian Tube, Right ♀ 6 Fallopian Tube, Left ♀	Ø Open 4 Percutaneous Endoscopic	7 Autologous Tissue Substitute J Synthetic Substitute K Nonautologous Tissue Substitute Z No Device	5 Fallopian Tube, Right 6 Fallopian Tube, Left 9 Uterus

SECTION: Ø **MEDICAL AND SURGICAL**
BODY SYSTEM: U **FEMALE REPRODUCTIVE SYSTEM**
OPERATION: 2 **CHANGE:** Taking out or off a device from a body part and putting back an identical or similar device in or on the same body part without cutting or puncturing the skin or a mucous membrane

Body Part	Approach	Device	Qualifier
3 Ovary ♀ 8 Fallopian Tube ♀ M Vulva ♀	X External	Ø Drainage Device Y Other Device	Z No Qualifier
D Uterus and Cervix ♀	X External	Ø Drainage Device H Contraceptive Device Y Other Device	Z No Qualifier
H Vagina and Cul-de-sac ♀	X External	Ø Drainage Device G Intraluminal Device, Pessary Y Other Device	Z No Qualifier

Non-OR All Values

SECTION: Ø MEDICAL AND SURGICAL
BODY SYSTEM: U FEMALE REPRODUCTIVE SYSTEM
OPERATION: 5 DESTRUCTION: Physical eradication of all or a portion of a body part by the direct use of energy, force, or a destructive agent

Body Part	Approach	Device	Qualifier
Ø Ovary, Right ♀ 1 Ovary, Left ♀ 2 Ovaries, Bilateral ♀ 4 Uterine Supporting Structure ♀	Ø Open 3 Percutaneous 4 Percutaneous Endoscopic 8 Via Natural or Artificial Opening Endoscopic	Z No Device	Z No Qualifier
5 Fallopian Tube, Right ♀ 6 Fallopian Tube, Left ♀ 7 Fallopian Tubes, Bilateral ♀ 9 Uterus ♀ B Endometrium ♀ C Cervix ♀ F Cul-de-sac ♀	Ø Open 3 Percutaneous 4 Percutaneous Endoscopic 7 Via Natural or Artificial Opening 8 Via Natural or Artificial Opening Endoscopic	Z No Device	Z No Qualifier
G Vagina ♀ K Hymen ♀	Ø Open 3 Percutaneous 4 Percutaneous Endoscopic 7 Via Natural or Artificial Opening 8 Via Natural or Artificial Opening Endoscopic X External	Z No Device	Z No Qualifier
J Clitoris ♀ L Vestibular Gland ♀ M Vulva ♀	Ø Open X External	Z No Device	Z No Qualifier

ØU57[Ø3478]ZZ when Z3Ø.2 is listed as the principal diagnosis

SECTION: Ø MEDICAL AND SURGICAL
BODY SYSTEM: U FEMALE REPRODUCTIVE SYSTEM
OPERATION: 7 DILATION: Expanding an orifice or the lumen of a tubular body part

Body Part	Approach	Device	Qualifier
5 Fallopian Tube, Right ♀ 6 Fallopian Tube, Left ♀ 7 Fallopian Tubes, Bilateral ♀ 9 Uterus ♀ C Cervix ♀ G Vagina ♀	Ø Open 3 Percutaneous 4 Percutaneous Endoscopic 7 Via Natural or Artificial Opening 8 Via Natural or Artificial Opening Endoscopic	D Intraluminal Device Z No Device	Z No Qualifier
K Hymen ♀	Ø Open 3 Percutaneous 4 Percutaneous Endoscopic 7 Via Natural or Artificial Opening 8 Via Natural or Artificial Opening Endoscopic X External	D Intraluminal Device Z No Device	Z No Qualifier

Non-OR ØU7C[Ø3478][DZ]Z
Non-OR ØU7G[78][DZ]Z

Coding Clinic: 2020, Q2, P30 – ØU7C7ZZ

SECTION: Ø MEDICAL AND SURGICAL
BODY SYSTEM: U FEMALE REPRODUCTIVE SYSTEM
OPERATION: 8 DIVISION: Cutting into a body part, without draining fluids and/or gases from the body part, in order to separate or transect a body part

Body Part	Approach	Device	Qualifier
Ø Ovary, Right ♀ 1 Ovary, Left ♀ 2 Ovaries, Bilateral ♀ 4 Uterine Supporting Structure ♀	Ø Open 3 Percutaneous 4 Percutaneous Endoscopic	Z No Device	Z No Qualifier
K Hymen ♀	7 Via Natural or Artificial Opening 8 Via Natural or Artificial Opening Endoscopic X External	Z No Device	Z No Qualifier

Non-OR ØU8K[78X]ZZ

SECTION: Ø MEDICAL AND SURGICAL
BODY SYSTEM: U FEMALE REPRODUCTIVE SYSTEM
OPERATION: 9 DRAINAGE: *(on multiple pages)*
Taking or letting out fluids and/or gases from a body part

Body Part	Approach	Device	Qualifier
Ø Ovary, Right ♀ 1 Ovary, Left ♀ 2 Ovaries, Bilateral ♀	Ø Open 3 Percutaneous 4 Percutaneous Endoscopic 8 Via Natural or Artificial Opening Endoscopic	Ø Drainage Device	Z No Qualifier
Ø Ovary, Right ♀ 1 Ovary, Left ♀ 2 Ovaries, Bilateral ♀	Ø Open 3 Percutaneous 4 Percutaneous Endoscopic 8 Via Natural or Artificial Opening Endoscopic	Z No Device	X Diagnostic Z No Qualifier
Ø Ovary, Right ♀ 1 Ovary, Left ♀ 2 Ovaries, Bilateral ♀	X External	Z No Device	Z No Qualifier
4 Uterine Supporting Structure ♀	Ø Open 3 Percutaneous 4 Percutaneous Endoscopic 8 Via Natural or Artificial Opening Endoscopic	Ø Drainage Device	Z No Qualifier
4 Uterine Supporting Structure ♀	Ø Open 3 Percutaneous 4 Percutaneous Endoscopic 8 Via Natural or Artificial Opening Endoscopic	Z No Device	X Diagnostic Z No Qualifier
5 Fallopian Tube, Right ♀ 6 Fallopian Tube, Left ♀ 7 Fallopian Tubes, Bilateral ♀ 9 Uterus ♀ C Cervix ♀ F Cul-de-sac ♀	Ø Open 3 Percutaneous 4 Percutaneous Endoscopic 7 Via Natural or Artificial Opening 8 Via Natural or Artificial Opening Endoscopic	Ø Drainage Device	Z No Qualifier
5 Fallopian Tube, Right ♀ 6 Fallopian Tube, Left ♀ 7 Fallopian Tubes, Bilateral ♀ 9 Uterus ♀ C Cervix ♀ F Cul-de-sac ♀	Ø Open 3 Percutaneous 4 Percutaneous Endoscopic 7 Via Natural or Artificial Opening 8 Via Natural or Artificial Opening Endoscopic	Z No Device	X Diagnostic Z No Qualifier
G Vagina ♀ K Hymen ♀	Ø Open 3 Percutaneous 4 Percutaneous Endoscopic 7 Via Natural or Artificial Opening 8 Via Natural or Artificial Opening Endoscopic X External	Ø Drainage Device	Z No Qualifier

Non-OR ØU9[Ø12]3ØZ
Non-OR ØU9[Ø12]3ZZ
Non-OR ØU943ØZ
Non-OR ØU943ZZ
Non-OR ØU9[5679C]3ØZ
Non-OR ØU9F[34]ØZ
Non-OR ØU9[567][3478]ZZ
Non-OR ØU9F[34]ZZ
Non-OR ØU9K[Ø3478X]ØZ
Non-OR ØU9K[Ø3478X]ZZ
Non-OR ØU9[9C]3ZZ
Non-OR ØU9G3ØZ
Non-OR ØU9G3ZZ

SECTION: Ø MEDICAL AND SURGICAL
BODY SYSTEM: U FEMALE REPRODUCTIVE SYSTEM
OPERATION: 9 DRAINAGE: *(continued)*
Taking or letting out fluids and/or gases from a body part

Body Part	Approach	Device	Qualifier
G Vagina ♀ K Hymen ♀	Ø Open 3 Percutaneous 4 Percutaneous Endoscopic 7 Via Natural or Artificial Opening 8 Via Natural or Artificial Opening Endoscopic X External	Z No Device	X Diagnostic Z No Qualifier
J Clitoris ♀ L Vestibular Gland ♀ M Vulva ♀	Ø Open X External	Ø Drainage Device	Z No Qualifier
J Clitoris ♀ L Vestibular Gland ♀ M Vulva ♀	Ø Open X External	Z No Device	X Diagnostic Z No Qualifier

Non-OR ØU9L[ØX]ØZ
Non-OR ØU9L[ØX]ZZ

SECTION: Ø MEDICAL AND SURGICAL
BODY SYSTEM: U FEMALE REPRODUCTIVE SYSTEM
OPERATION: B EXCISION: Cutting out or off, without replacement, a portion of a body part

Body Part	Approach	Device	Qualifier
Ø Ovary, Right ♀ 1 Ovary, Left ♀ 2 Ovaries, Bilateral ♀ 4 Uterine Supporting Structure ♀ 5 Fallopian Tube, Right ♀ 6 Fallopian Tube, Left ♀ 7 Fallopian Tubes, Bilateral ♀ 9 Uterus ♀ C Cervix ♀ F Cul-de-sac ♀	Ø Open 3 Percutaneous 4 Percutaneous Endoscopic 7 Via Natural or Artificial Opening 8 Via Natural or Artificial Opening Endoscopic	Z No Device	X Diagnostic Z No Qualifier
G Vagina ♀ K Hymen ♀	Ø Open 3 Percutaneous 4 Percutaneous Endoscopic 7 Via Natural or Artificial Opening 8 Via Natural or Artificial Opening Endoscopic X External	Z No Device	X Diagnostic Z No Qualifier
J Clitoris ♀ L Vestibular Gland ♀ M Vulva ♀	Ø Open X External	Z No Device	X Diagnostic Z No Qualifier

Coding Clinic: 2Ø15, Q3, P31 – ØUB7ØZZ
Coding Clinic: 2Ø15, Q3, P32 – ØUB64ZZ

SECTION: Ø MEDICAL AND SURGICAL
BODY SYSTEM: U FEMALE REPRODUCTIVE SYSTEM
OPERATION: C EXTIRPATION: Taking or cutting out solid matter from a body part

Body Part	Approach	Device	Qualifier
Ø Ovary, Right ♀ 1 Ovary, Left ♀ 2 Ovaries, Bilateral ♀ 4 Uterine Supporting Structure ♀	Ø Open 3 Percutaneous 4 Percutaneous Endoscopic 8 Via Natural or Artificial Opening Endoscopic	Z No Device	Z No Qualifier
5 Fallopian Tube, Right ♀ 6 Fallopian Tube, Left ♀ 7 Fallopian Tubes, Bilateral ♀ 9 Uterus ♀ B Endometrium ♀ C Cervix ♀ F Cul-de-sac ♀	Ø Open 3 Percutaneous 4 Percutaneous Endoscopic 7 Via Natural or Artificial Opening 8 Via Natural or Artificial Opening Endoscopic	Z No Device	Z No Qualifier
G Vagina ♀ K Hymen ♀	Ø Open 3 Percutaneous 4 Percutaneous Endoscopic 7 Via Natural or Artificial Opening 8 Via Natural or Artificial Opening Endoscopic X External	Z No Device	Z No Qualifier
J Clitoris ♀ L Vestibular Gland ♀ M Vulva ♀	Ø Open X External	Z No Device	Z No Qualifier

Non-OR ØUC9[78]ZZ
Non-OR ØUCG[78X]ZZ
Non-OR ØUCK[Ø3478X]ZZ
Non-OR ØUCMXZZ

Coding Clinic: 2Ø13, Q2, P38 – ØUC97ZZ
Coding Clinic: 2Ø15, Q3, P3Ø-31 – ØUCC[78]ZZ

SECTION: Ø MEDICAL AND SURGICAL
BODY SYSTEM: U FEMALE REPRODUCTIVE SYSTEM
OPERATION: D EXTRACTION: Pulling or stripping out or off all or a portion of a body part by the use of force

Body Part	Approach	Device	Qualifier
B Endometrium ♀	7 Via Natural or Artificial Opening 8 Via Natural or Artificial Opening Endoscopic	Z No Device	X Diagnostic Z No Qualifier
N Ova ♀	Ø Open 3 Percutaneous 4 Percutaneous Endoscopic	Z No Device	Z No Qualifier

SECTION: Ø MEDICAL AND SURGICAL
BODY SYSTEM: U FEMALE REPRODUCTIVE SYSTEM
OPERATION: F FRAGMENTATION: Breaking solid matter in a body part into pieces

Body Part	Approach	Device	Qualifier
5 Fallopian Tube, Right ♀ 6 Fallopian Tube, Left ♀ 7 Fallopian Tubes, Bilateral ♀ 9 Uterus ♀	Ø Open 3 Percutaneous 4 Percutaneous Endoscopic 7 Via Natural or Artificial Opening 8 Via Natural or Artificial Opening Endoscopic X External	Z No Device	Z No Qualifier

ØUF[5679]XZZ

Non-OR ØUF[5679]XZZ

SECTION: Ø MEDICAL AND SURGICAL

BODY SYSTEM: U FEMALE REPRODUCTIVE SYSTEM

OPERATION: H INSERTION: Putting in a nonbiological appliance that monitors, assists, performs, or prevents a physiological function but does not physically take the place of a body part

Body Part	Approach	Device	Qualifier
3 Ovary ♀	Ø Open 3 Percutaneous 4 Percutaneous Endoscopic	1 Radioactive Element 3 Infusion Device Y Other Device	Z No Qualifier
3 Ovary ♀	7 Via Natural or Artificial Opening 8 Via Natural or Artificial Opening Endoscopic	1 Radioactive Element Y Other Device	Z No Qualifier
8 Fallopian Tube ♀ D Uterus and Cervix ♀ H Vagina and Cul-de-sac ♀	Ø Open 3 Percutaneous 4 Percutaneous Endoscopic 7 Via Natural or Artificial Opening 8 Via Natural or Artificial Opening Endoscopic	3 Infusion Device Y Other Device	Z No Qualifier
9 Uterus ♀	Ø Open 7 Via Natural or Artificial Opening 8 Via Natural or Artificial Opening Endoscopic	1 Radioactive Element H Contraceptive Device	Z No Qualifier
C Cervix ♀	Ø Open 3 Percutaneous 4 Percutaneous Endoscopic	1 Radioactive Element	Z No Qualifier
C Cervix ♀	7 Via Natural or Artificial Opening 8 Via Natural or Artificial Opening Endoscopic	1 Radioactive Element H Contraceptive Device	Z No Qualifier
F Cul-de-sac ♀	7 Via Natural or Artificial Opening 8 Via Natural or Artificial Opening Endoscopic	G Intraluminal Device, Pessary	Z No Qualifier
G Vagina ♀	Ø Open 3 Percutaneous 4 Percutaneous Endoscopic X External	1 Radioactive Element	Z No Qualifier
G Vagina ♀	7 Via Natural or Artificial Opening 8 Via Natural or Artificial Opening Endoscopic	1 Radioactive Element G Intraluminal Device, Pessary	Z No Qualifier

Non-OR ØUH3[Ø34]3Z
Non-OR ØUH[8D][Ø3478]3Z
Non-OR ØUHH[78]3Z
Non-OR ØUH9[78]HZ
Non-OR ØUHC[78]HZ
Non-OR ØUHF[78]GZ
Non-OR ØUHG[78]GZ

Coding Clinic: 2013, Q2, P34 – ØUH97HZ

SECTION: Ø MEDICAL AND SURGICAL
BODY SYSTEM: U FEMALE REPRODUCTIVE SYSTEM
OPERATION: J INSPECTION: Visually and/or manually exploring a body part

Body Part	Approach	Device	Qualifier
3 Ovary ♀	Ø Open 3 Percutaneous 4 Percutaneous Endoscopic 8 Via Natural or Artificial Opening Endoscopic X External	Z No Device	Z No Qualifier
8 Fallopian Tube ♀ D Uterus and Cervix ♀ H Vagina and Cul-de-sac ♀	Ø Open 3 Percutaneous 4 Percutaneous Endoscopic 7 Via Natural or Artificial Opening 8 Via Natural or Artificial Opening Endoscopic X External	Z No Device	Z No Qualifier
M Vulva ♀	Ø Open X External	Z No Device	Z No Qualifier

Non-OR ØUJ8[378]ZZ
Non-OR ØUJD3ZZ
Non-OR ØUJ3[3X]ZZ
Non-OR ØUJ8XZZ
Non-OR ØUJD[78X]ZZ
Non-OR ØUJH[378X]ZZ
Non-OR ØUJMXZZ

Coding Clinic: 2Ø15, Q1, P34 – ØUJD4ZZ

SECTION: Ø MEDICAL AND SURGICAL
BODY SYSTEM: U FEMALE REPRODUCTIVE SYSTEM
OPERATION: L OCCLUSION: Completely closing an orifice or the lumen of a tubular body part

Body Part	Approach	Device	Qualifier
5 Fallopian Tube, Right ♀ 6 Fallopian Tube, Left ♀ 7 Fallopian Tubes, Bilateral ♀	Ø Open 3 Percutaneous 4 Percutaneous Endoscopic	C Extraluminal Device D Intraluminal Device Z No Device	Z No Qualifier
5 Fallopian Tube, Right ♀ 6 Fallopian Tube, Left ♀ 7 Fallopian Tubes, Bilateral ♀	7 Via Natural or Artificial Opening 8 Via Natural or Artificial Opening Endoscopic	D Intraluminal Device Z No Device	Z No Qualifier
F Cul-de-sac ♀ G Vagina ♀	7 Via Natural or Artificial Opening 8 Via Natural or Artificial Opening Endoscopic	D Intraluminal Device Z No Device	Z No Qualifier

ØUL7[Ø34][CDZ]Z when Z3Ø.2 is listed as the principal diagnosis
ØUL7[78][DZ]Z when Z3Ø.2 is listed as the principal diagnosis

SECTION: Ø MEDICAL AND SURGICAL
BODY SYSTEM: U FEMALE REPRODUCTIVE SYSTEM
OPERATION: M REATTACHMENT: Putting back in or on all or a portion of a separated body part to its normal location or other suitable location

Body Part	Approach	Device	Qualifier
Ø Ovary, Right ♀ 1 Ovary, Left ♀ 2 Ovaries, Bilateral ♀ 4 Uterine Supporting Structure ♀ 5 Fallopian Tube, Right ♀ 6 Fallopian Tube, Left ♀ 7 Fallopian Tubes, Bilateral ♀ 9 Uterus ♀ C Cervix ♀ F Cul-de-sac ♀ G Vagina ♀	Ø Open 4 Percutaneous Endoscopic	Z No Device	Z No Qualifier
J Clitoris ♀ M Vulva ♀	X External	Z No Device	Z No Qualifier
K Hymen ♀	Ø Open 4 Percutaneous Endoscopic X External	Z No Device	Z No Qualifier

SECTION: Ø MEDICAL AND SURGICAL
BODY SYSTEM: U FEMALE REPRODUCTIVE SYSTEM
OPERATION: N RELEASE: Freeing a body part from an abnormal physical constraint by cutting or by the use of force

Body Part	Approach	Device	Qualifier
Ø Ovary, Right ♀ 1 Ovary, Left ♀ 2 Ovaries, Bilateral ♀ 4 Uterine Supporting Structure ♀	Ø Open 3 Percutaneous 4 Percutaneous Endoscopic 8 Via Natural or Artificial Opening Endoscopic	Z No Device	Z No Qualifier
5 Fallopian Tube, Right ♀ 6 Fallopian Tube, Left ♀ 7 Fallopian Tubes, Bilateral ♀ 9 Uterus ♀ C Cervix ♀ F Cul-de-sac ♀	Ø Open 3 Percutaneous 4 Percutaneous Endoscopic 7 Via Natural or Artificial Opening 8 Via Natural or Artificial Opening Endoscopic	Z No Device	Z No Qualifier
G Vagina ♀ K Hymen ♀	Ø Open 3 Percutaneous 4 Percutaneous Endoscopic 7 Via Natural or Artificial Opening 8 Via Natural or Artificial Opening Endoscopic X External	Z No Device	Z No Qualifier
J Clitoris ♀ L Vestibular Gland ♀ M Vulva ♀	Ø Open X External	Z No Device	Z No Qualifier

SECTION: Ø MEDICAL AND SURGICAL
BODY SYSTEM: U FEMALE REPRODUCTIVE SYSTEM
OPERATION: P REMOVAL: *(on multiple pages)*
Taking out or off a device from a body part

Body Part	Approach	Device	Qualifier
3 Ovary ♀	Ø Open 3 Percutaneous 4 Percutaneous Endoscopic	Ø Drainage Device 3 Infusion Device Y Other Device	Z No Qualifier
3 Ovary ♀	7 Via Natural or Artificial Opening 8 Via Natural or Artificial Opening Endoscopic	Y Other Device	Z No Qualifier
3 Ovary ♀	X External	Ø Drainage Device 3 Infusion Device	Z No Qualifier
8 Fallopian Tube ♀	Ø Open 3 Percutaneous 4 Percutaneous Endoscopic 7 Via Natural or Artificial Opening 8 Via Natural or Artificial Opening Endoscopic	Ø Drainage Device 3 Infusion Device 7 Autologous Tissue Substitute C Extraluminal Device D Intraluminal Device J Synthetic Substitute K Nonautologous Tissue Substitute Y Other Device	Z No Qualifier
8 Fallopian Tube ♀	X External	Ø Drainage Device 3 Infusion Device D Intraluminal Device	Z No Qualifier
D Uterus and Cervix ♀	Ø Open 3 Percutaneous 4 Percutaneous Endoscopic 7 Via Natural or Artificial Opening 8 Via Natural or Artificial Opening Endoscopic	Ø Drainage Device 1 Radioactive Element 3 Infusion Device 7 Autologous Tissue Substitute C Extraluminal Device D Intraluminal Device H Contraceptive Device J Synthetic Substitute K Nonautologous Tissue Substitute Y Other Device	Z No Qualifier
D Uterus and Cervix ♀	X External	Ø Drainage Device 3 Infusion Device D Intraluminal Device H Contraceptive Device	Z No Qualifier
H Vagina and Cul-de-sac ♀	Ø Open 3 Percutaneous 4 Percutaneous Endoscopic 7 Via Natural or Artificial Opening 8 Via Natural or Artificial Opening Endoscopic	Ø Drainage Device 1 Radioactive Element 3 Infusion Device 7 Autologous Tissue Substitute D Intraluminal Device J Synthetic Substitute K Nonautologous Tissue Substitute Y Other Device	Z No Qualifier

Non-OR ØUP3X[Ø3]Z
Non-OR ØUP8[78][Ø3D]Z
Non-OR ØUP8X[Ø3D]Z
Non-OR ØUPD[34]CZ
Non-OR ØUPD[78][Ø3CDH]Z
Non-OR ØUPDX[Ø3DH]Z
Non-OR ØUPH[78][Ø3D]Z

Coding Clinic: 2022, Q3, P14 – ØUPH77Z

SECTION: Ø MEDICAL AND SURGICAL
BODY SYSTEM: U FEMALE REPRODUCTIVE SYSTEM
OPERATION: P REMOVAL: *(continued)*
Taking out or off a device from a body part

Body Part	Approach	Device	Qualifier
H Vagina and Cul-de-sac ♀	X External	Ø Drainage Device 1 Radioactive Element 3 Infusion Device D Intraluminal Device	Z No Qualifier
M Vulva ♀	Ø Open	Ø Drainage Device 7 Autologous Tissue Substitute J Synthetic Substitute K Nonautologous Tissue Substitute	Z No Qualifier
M Vulva ♀	X External	Ø Drainage Device	Z No Qualifier

Non-OR ØUPHX[Ø13D]Z
Non-OR ØUPMXØZ

SECTION: Ø MEDICAL AND SURGICAL
BODY SYSTEM: U FEMALE REPRODUCTIVE SYSTEM
OPERATION: Q REPAIR: Restoring, to the extent possible, a body part to its normal anatomic structure and function

Body Part	Approach	Device	Qualifier
Ø Ovary, Right ♀ 1 Ovary, Left ♀ 2 Ovaries, Bilateral ♀ 4 Uterine Supporting Structure ♀	Ø Open 3 Percutaneous 4 Percutaneous Endoscopic 8 Via Natural or Artificial Opening Endoscopic	Z No Device	Z No Qualifier
5 Fallopian Tube, Right ♀ 6 Fallopian Tube, Left ♀ 7 Fallopian Tubes, Bilateral ♀ 9 Uterus ♀ C Cervix ♀ F Cul-de-sac ♀	Ø Open 3 Percutaneous 4 Percutaneous Endoscopic 7 Via Natural or Artificial Opening 8 Via Natural or Artificial Opening Endoscopic	Z No Device	Z No Qualifier
G Vagina ♀ K Hymen ♀	Ø Open 3 Percutaneous 4 Percutaneous Endoscopic 7 Via Natural or Artificial Opening 8 Via Natural or Artificial Opening Endoscopic X External	Z No Device	Z No Qualifier
J Clitoris ♀ L Vestibular Gland ♀ M Vulva ♀	Ø Open X External	Z No Device	Z No Qualifier

SECTION: Ø MEDICAL AND SURGICAL
BODY SYSTEM: U FEMALE REPRODUCTIVE SYSTEM
OPERATION: S **REPOSITION:** Moving to its normal location, or other suitable location, all or a portion of a body part

Body Part	Approach	Device	Qualifier
Ø Ovary, Right ♀ 1 Ovary, Left ♀ 2 Ovaries, Bilateral ♀ 4 Uterine Supporting Structure ♀ 5 Fallopian Tube, Right ♀ 6 Fallopian Tube, Left ♀ 7 Fallopian Tubes, Bilateral ♀ C Cervix ♀ F Cul-de-sac ♀	Ø Open 4 Percutaneous Endoscopic 8 Via Natural or Artificial Opening Endoscopic	Z No Device	Z No Qualifier
9 Uterus ♀ G Vagina ♀	Ø Open 4 Percutaneous Endoscopic 7 Via Natural or Artificial Opening 8 Via Natural or Artificial Opening Endoscopic X External	Z No Device	Z No Qualifier

Non-OR ØUS9XZZ

Coding Clinic: 2Ø16, Q1, P9 – ØUS9XZZ
Coding Clinic: 2Ø17, Q4, P68 – ØUT9[Ø7]Z[LZ]
Coding Clinic: 2Ø22, Q1, P21 – ØUT[79]ØZZ

SECTION: Ø MEDICAL AND SURGICAL
BODY SYSTEM: U FEMALE REPRODUCTIVE SYSTEM
OPERATION: T **RESECTION:** Cutting out or off, without replacement, all of a body part

Body Part	Approach	Device	Qualifier
Ø Ovary, Right ♀ 1 Ovary, Left ♀ 2 Ovaries, Bilateral ♀ ⊞ 5 Fallopian Tube, Right ♀ 6 Fallopian Tube, Left ♀ 7 Fallopian Tubes, Bilateral ♀	Ø Open 4 Percutaneous Endoscopic 7 Via Natural or Artificial Opening 8 Via Natural or Artificial Opening Endoscopic F Via Natural or Artificial Opening With Percutaneous Endoscopic Assistance	Z No Device	Z No Qualifier
4 Uterine Supporting Structure ♀ ⊞ C Cervix ♀ ⊞ F Cul-de-sac ♀ G Vagina ♀ ⊞	Ø Open 4 Percutaneous Endoscopic 7 Via Natural or Artificial Opening 8 Via Natural or Artificial Opening Endoscopic	Z No Device	Z No Qualifier
9 Uterus ♀ ⊞	Ø Open 4 Percutaneous Endoscopic 7 Via Natural or Artificial Opening 8 Via Natural or Artificial Opening Endoscopic F Via Natural or Artificial Opening With Percutaneous Endoscopic Assistance	Z No Device	L Supracervical Z No Qualifier
J Clitoris ♀ L Vestibular Gland ♀ M Vulva ♀ ⊞	Ø Open X External	Z No Device	Z No Qualifier
K Hymen ♀	Ø Open 4 Percutaneous Endoscopic 7 Via Natural or Artificial Opening 8 Via Natural or Artificial Opening Endoscopic X External	Z No Device	Z No Qualifier

⊞ ØUT9[Ø478F]ZZ
⊞ ØUT[24CG][Ø478]ZZ
⊞ ØUTM[ØX]ZZ

Coding Clinic: 2Ø13, Q1, P24 – ØUTØØZZ
Coding Clinic: 2Ø15, Q1, P33-34; 2Ø13, Q3, P28 – ØUT9ØZZ, ØUTCØZZ
Coding Clinic: 2Ø15, Q1, P34 – ØUT2ØZZ, ØUT7ØZZ

SECTION: Ø MEDICAL AND SURGICAL
BODY SYSTEM: U FEMALE REPRODUCTIVE SYSTEM
OPERATION: U SUPPLEMENT: Putting in or on biological or synthetic material that physically reinforces and/or augments the function of a portion of a body part

Body Part	Approach	Device	Qualifier
4 Uterine Supporting Structure ♀	Ø Open 4 Percutaneous Endoscopic	7 Autologous Tissue Substitute J Synthetic Substitute K Nonautologous Tissue Substitute	Z No Qualifier
5 Fallopian Tube Right ♀ 6 Fallopian Tube, Left ♀ 7 Fallopian Tubes, Bilateral ♀ F Cul-de-sac ♀	Ø Open 4 Percutaneous Endoscopic 7 Via Natural or Artificial Opening 8 Via Natural or Artificial Opening Endoscopic	7 Autologous Tissue Substitute J Synthetic Substitute K Nonautologous Tissue Substitute	Z No Qualifier
G Vagina ♀ K Hymen ♀	Ø Open 4 Percutaneous Endoscopic 7 Via Natural or Artificial Opening 8 Via Natural or Artificial Opening Endoscopic X External	7 Autologous Tissue Substitute J Synthetic Substitute K Nonautologous Tissue Substitute	Z No Qualifier
J Clitoris ♀ M Vulva ♀	Ø Open X External	7 Autologous Tissue Substitute J Synthetic Substitute K Nonautologous Tissue Substitute	Z No Qualifier

SECTION: Ø MEDICAL AND SURGICAL
BODY SYSTEM: U FEMALE REPRODUCTIVE SYSTEM
OPERATION: V RESTRICTION: Partially closing an orifice or the lumen of a tubular body part

Body Part	Approach	Device	Qualifier
C Cervix ♀	Ø Open 3 Percutaneous 4 Percutaneous Endoscopic	C Extraluminal Device D Intraluminal Device Z No Device	Z No Qualifier
C Cervix ♀	7 Via Natural or Artificial Opening 8 Via Natural or Artificial Opening Endoscopic	D Intraluminal Device Z No Device	Z No Qualifier

Coding Clinic: 2Ø15, Q3, P3Ø – ØUVC7ZZ

SECTION: Ø MEDICAL AND SURGICAL
BODY SYSTEM: U FEMALE REPRODUCTIVE SYSTEM
OPERATION: W REVISION: *(on multiple pages)*

Correcting, to the extent possible, a portion of a malfunctioning device or the position of a displaced device

Body Part	Approach	Device	Qualifier
3 Ovary ♀	Ø Open 3 Percutaneous 4 Percutaneous Endoscopic	Ø Drainage Device 3 Infusion Device Y Other Device	Z No Qualifier
3 Ovary ♀	7 Via Natural or Artificial Opening 8 Via Natural or Artificial Opening Endoscopic	Y Other Device	Z No Qualifier
3 Ovary ♀	X External	Ø Drainage Device 3 Infusion Device	Z No Qualifier
8 Fallopian Tube ♀	Ø Open 3 Percutaneous 4 Percutaneous Endoscopic 7 Via Natural or Artificial Opening 8 Via Natural or Artificial Opening Endoscopic	Ø Drainage Device 3 Infusion Device 7 Autologous Tissue Substitute C Extraluminal Device D Intraluminal Device J Synthetic Substitute K Nonautologous Tissue Substitute Y Other Device	Z No Qualifier
8 Fallopian Tube ♀	X External	Ø Drainage Device 3 Infusion Device 7 Autologous Tissue Substitute C Extraluminal Device D Intraluminal Device J Synthetic Substitute K Nonautologous Tissue Substitute	Z No Qualifier
D Uterus and Cervix ♀	Ø Open 3 Percutaneous 4 Percutaneous Endoscopic 7 Via Natural or Artificial Opening 8 Via Natural or Artificial Opening Endoscopic	Ø Drainage Device 1 Radioactive Element 3 Infusion Device 7 Autologous Tissue Substitute C Extraluminal Device D Intraluminal Device H Contraceptive Device J Synthetic Substitute K Nonautologous Tissue Substitute Y Other Device	Z No Qualifier
D Uterus and Cervix ♀	X External	Ø Drainage Device 3 Infusion Device 7 Autologous Tissue Substitute C Extraluminal Device D Intraluminal Device H Contraceptive Device J Synthetic Substitute K Nonautologous Tissue Substitute	Z No Qualifier
H Vagina and Cul-de-sac ♀	Ø Open 3 Percutaneous 4 Percutaneous Endoscopic 7 Via Natural or Artificial Opening 8 Via Natural or Artificial Opening Endoscopic	Ø Drainage Device 1 Radioactive Element 3 Infusion Device 7 Autologous Tissue Substitute D Intraluminal Device J Synthetic Substitute K Nonautologous Tissue Substitute Y Other Device	Z No Qualifier

Non-OR ØUW3X[Ø3]Z Non-OR ØUW8X[Ø37CDJK]Z Non-OR ØUWDX[Ø37CDHJK]Z

SECTION: Ø MEDICAL AND SURGICAL
BODY SYSTEM: U FEMALE REPRODUCTIVE SYSTEM
OPERATION: W REVISION: *(continued)*
Correcting, to the extent possible, a portion of a malfunctioning device or the position of a displaced device

Body Part	Approach	Device	Qualifier
H Vagina and Cul-de-sac ♀	X External	Ø Drainage Device 3 Infusion Device 7 Autologous Tissue Substitute D Intraluminal Device J Synthetic Substitute K Nonautologous Tissue Substitute	Z No Qualifier
M Vulva ♀	Ø Open X External	Ø Drainage Device 7 Autologous Tissue Substitute J Synthetic Substitute K Nonautologous Tissue Substitute	Z No Qualifier

Non-OR ØUWHX[Ø37DJK]Z
Non-OR ØUWMX[Ø7JK]Z

SECTION: Ø MEDICAL AND SURGICAL
BODY SYSTEM: U FEMALE REPRODUCTIVE SYSTEM
OPERATION: Y TRANSPLANTATION: Putting in or on all or a portion of a living body part taken from another individual or animal to physically take the place and/or function of all or a portion of a similar body part

Body Part	Approach	Device	Qualifier
Ø Ovary, Right ♀ 1 Ovary, Left ♀ 9 Uterus ♀	Ø Open	Z No Device	Ø Allogeneic 1 Syngeneic 2 Zooplastic

ØV. Male Reproductive System 49Ø
ØV1. Bypass 491
ØV2. Change 491
ØV5. Destruction 492
ØV7. Dilation 492
ØV9. Drainage 493
ØVB. Excision 494
ØVC. Extirpation 495
ØVH. Insertion 496
ØVJ. Inspection 496
ØVL. Occlusion 497
ØVM. Reattachment 497
ØVN. Release 498
ØVP. Removal 499
ØVQ. Repair 5ØØ
ØVR. Replacement 5ØØ
ØVS. Reposition 5Ø1
ØVT. Resection 5Ø1
ØVU. Supplement 5Ø2
ØVW. Revision 5Ø3
ØVX. Transfer 5Ø4
ØVY. Transplantation 5Ø4

SECTION: Ø MEDICAL AND SURGICAL
BODY SYSTEM: V MALE REPRODUCTIVE SYSTEM
OPERATION: 1 BYPASS: Altering the route of passage of the contents of a tubular body part

Body Part	Approach	Device	Qualifier
N Vas Deferens, Right ♂ P Vas Deferens, Left ♂ Q Vas Deferens, Bilateral ♂	Ø Open 4 Percutaneous Endoscopic	7 Autologous Tissue Substitute J Synthetic Substitute K Nonautologous Tissue Substitute Z No Device	J Epididymis, Right K Epididymis, Left N Vas Deferens, Right P Vas Deferens, Left

SECTION: Ø MEDICAL AND SURGICAL
BODY SYSTEM: V MALE REPRODUCTIVE SYSTEM
OPERATION: 2 CHANGE: Taking out or off a device from a body part and putting back an identical or similar device in or on the same body part without cutting or puncturing the skin or a mucous membrane

Body Part	Approach	Device	Qualifier
4 Prostate and Seminal Vesicles ♂ 8 Scrotum and Tunica Vaginalis ♂ D Testis ♂ M Epididymis and Spermatic Cord ♂ R Vas Deferens ♂ S Penis ♂	X External	Ø Drainage Device Y Other Device	Z No Qualifier

Non-OR All Values

SECTION: Ø MEDICAL AND SURGICAL
BODY SYSTEM: V MALE REPRODUCTIVE SYSTEM
OPERATION: 5 DESTRUCTION: Physical eradication of all or a portion of a body part by the direct use of energy, force, or a destructive agent

Body Part	Approach	Device	Qualifier
Ø Prostate ♂	Ø Open 3 Percutaneous 4 Percutaneous Endoscopic	Z No Device	3 Laser Interstitial Thermal Therapy Z No Qualifier
Ø Prostate ♂	7 Via Natural or Artificial Opening 8 Via Natural or Artificial Opening Endoscopic	Z No Device	Z No Qualifier
1 Seminal Vesicle, Right ♂ 2 Seminal Vesicle, Left ♂ 3 Seminal Vesicles, Bilateral ♂ 6 Tunica Vaginalis, Right ♂ 7 Tunica Vaginalis, Left ♂ 9 Testis, Right ♂ B Testis, Left ♂ C Testes, Bilateral ♂	Ø Open 3 Percutaneous 4 Percutaneous Endoscopic	Z No Device	Z No Qualifier
5 Scrotum ♂ S Penis ♂ T Prepuce ♂	Ø Open 3 Percutaneous 4 Percutaneous Endoscopic X External	Z No Device	Z No Qualifier
F Spermatic Cord, Right ♂ G Spermatic Cord, Left ♂ H Spermatic Cords, Bilateral ♂ J Epididymis, Right ♂ K Epididymis, Left ♂ L Epididymis, Bilateral ♂ N Vas Deferens, Right ♂ NC P Vas Deferens, Left ♂ NC Q Vas Deferens, Bilateral ♂ NC	Ø Open 3 Percutaneous 4 Percutaneous Endoscopic 8 Via Natural or Artificial Opening Endoscopic	Z No Device	Z No Qualifier

NC ØV5[NPQ][Ø34]ZZ when Z3Ø.2 is listed as the principal diagnosis
Non-OR ØV5[NPQ][Ø34]ZZ
Non-OR ØV55[Ø34X]ZZ
Non-OR ØV5Ø[Ø34]3Z

SECTION: Ø MEDICAL AND SURGICAL
BODY SYSTEM: V MALE REPRODUCTIVE SYSTEM
OPERATION: 7 DILATION: Expanding an orifice or the lumen of a tubular body part

Body Part	Approach	Device	Qualifier
N Vas Deferens, Right ♂ P Vas Deferens, Left ♂ Q Vas Deferens, Bilateral ♂	Ø Open 3 Percutaneous 4 Percutaneous Endoscopic	D Intraluminal Device Z No Device	Z No Qualifier

SECTION: Ø MEDICAL AND SURGICAL
BODY SYSTEM: V MALE REPRODUCTIVE SYSTEM
OPERATION: 9 DRAINAGE: *(on multiple pages)*
Taking or letting out fluids and/or gases from a body part

Body Part	Approach	Device	Qualifier
Ø Prostate ♂	Ø Open 3 Percutaneous 4 Percutaneous Endoscopic 7 Via Natural or Artificial Opening 8 Via Natural or Artificial Opening Endoscopic	Ø Drainage Device	Z No Qualifier
Ø Prostate ♂	Ø Open 3 Percutaneous 4 Percutaneous Endoscopic 7 Via Natural or Artificial Opening 8 Via Natural or Artificial Opening Endoscopic	Z No Device	X Diagnostic Z No Qualifier
1 Seminal Vesicle, Right ♂ 2 Seminal Vesicle, Left ♂ 3 Seminal Vesicles, Bilateral ♂ 6 Tunica Vaginalis, Right ♂ 7 Tunica Vaginalis, Left ♂ 9 Testis, Right ♂ B Testis, Left ♂ C Testes, Bilateral ♂ F Spermatic Cord, Right ♂ G Spermatic Cord, Left ♂ H Spermatic Cords, Bilateral ♂ J Epididymis, Right ♂ K Epididymis, Left ♂ L Epididymis, Bilateral ♂ N Vas Deferens, Right ♂ P Vas Deferens, Left ♂ Q Vas Deferens, Bilateral ♂	Ø Open 3 Percutaneous 4 Percutaneous Endoscopic	Ø Drainage Device	Z No Qualifier
1 Seminal Vesicle, Right ♂ 2 Seminal Vesicle, Left ♂ 3 Seminal Vesicles, Bilateral ♂ 6 Tunica Vaginalis, Right ♂ 7 Tunica Vaginalis, Left ♂ 9 Testis, Right ♂ B Testis, Left ♂ C Testes, Bilateral ♂ F Spermatic Cord, Right ♂ G Spermatic Cord, Left ♂ H Spermatic Cords, Bilateral ♂ J Epididymis, Right ♂ K Epididymis, Left ♂ L Epididymis, Bilateral ♂ N Vas Deferens, Right ♂ P Vas Deferens, Left ♂ Q Vas Deferens, Bilateral ♂	Ø Open 3 Percutaneous 4 Percutaneous Endoscopic	Z No Device	X Diagnostic Z No Qualifier

SECTION: Ø MEDICAL AND SURGICAL
BODY SYSTEM: V MALE REPRODUCTIVE SYSTEM
OPERATION: 9 DRAINAGE: *(continued)*

Taking or letting out fluids and/or gases from a body part

Body Part	Approach	Device	Qualifier
5 Scrotum ♂ S Penis ♂ T Prepuce ♂	Ø Open 3 Percutaneous 4 Percutaneous Endoscopic X External	Ø Drainage Device	Z No Qualifier
5 Scrotum ♂ S Penis ♂ T Prepuce ♂	Ø Open 3 Percutaneous 4 Percutaneous Endoscopic X External	Z No Device	X Diagnostic Z No Qualifier

Non-OR ØV9[ST]3ØZ
Non-OR ØV9[ST]3ZZ
Non-OR ØV95[Ø34X]Z[XZ]

SECTION: Ø MEDICAL AND SURGICAL
BODY SYSTEM: V MALE REPRODUCTIVE SYSTEM
OPERATION: B EXCISION: *(on multiple pages)*

Cutting out or off, without replacement, a portion of a body part

Body Part	Approach	Device	Qualifier
Ø Prostate ♂	Ø Open 3 Percutaneous 4 Percutaneous Endoscopic 7 Via Natural or Artificial Opening 8 Via Natural or Artificial Opening Endoscopic	Z No Device	X Diagnostic Z No Qualifier
1 Seminal Vesicle, Right ♂ 2 Seminal Vesicle, Left ♂ 3 Seminal Vesicles, Bilateral ♂ 6 Tunica Vaginalis, Right ♂ 7 Tunica Vaginalis, Left ♂ 9 Testis, Right ♂ B Testis, Left ♂ C Testes, Bilateral ♂	Ø Open 3 Percutaneous 4 Percutaneous Endoscopic	Z No Device	X Diagnostic Z No Qualifier
5 Scrotum ♂ S Penis ♂ T Prepuce ♂	Ø Open 3 Percutaneous 4 Percutaneous Endoscopic X External	Z No Device	X Diagnostic Z No Qualifier

ØVB[NPQ][Ø34]ZZ when Z3Ø.2 is listed as the principal diagnosis
Non-OR ØVBØ[3478]ZX
Non-OR ØVB[1239BC][34]ZX
Non-OR ØVB[67F][Ø34]ZX
Non-OR ØVB5[Ø34X]Z[XZ]

Coding Clinic: 2016, Q1, P23 – ØVBQ4ZZ

SECTION: Ø MEDICAL AND SURGICAL
BODY SYSTEM: V MALE REPRODUCTIVE SYSTEM
OPERATION: B EXCISION: *(continued)*
Cutting out or off, without replacement, a portion of a body part

Body Part	Approach	Device	Qualifier
F Spermatic Cord, Right ♂ G Spermatic Cord, Left ♂ H Spermatic Cords, Bilateral ♂ J Epididymis, Right ♂ K Epididymis, Left ♂ L Epididymis, Bilateral ♂ N Vas Deferens, Right ♂ P Vas Deferens, Left ♂ Q Vas Deferens, Bilateral ♂	Ø Open 3 Percutaneous 4 Percutaneous Endoscopic 8 Via Natural or Artificial Opening Endoscopic	Z No Device	X Diagnostic Z No Qualifier

Non-OR ØVB[GHJKL][Ø34]ZX
Non-OR ØVB[NPQ][Ø34]Z[XZ]

SECTION: Ø MEDICAL AND SURGICAL
BODY SYSTEM: V MALE REPRODUCTIVE SYSTEM
OPERATION: C EXTIRPATION: Taking or cutting out solid matter from a body part

Body Part	Approach	Device	Qualifier
Ø Prostate ♂	Ø Open 3 Percutaneous 4 Percutaneous Endoscopic 7 Via Natural or Artificial Opening 8 Via Natural or Artificial Opening Endoscopic	Z No Device	Z No Qualifier
1 Seminal Vesicle, Right ♂ 2 Seminal Vesicle, Left ♂ 3 Seminal Vesicles, Bilateral ♂ 6 Tunica Vaginalis, Right ♂ 7 Tunica Vaginalis, Left ♂ 9 Testis, Right ♂ B Testis, Left ♂ C Testes, Bilateral ♂ F Spermatic Cord, Right ♂ G Spermatic Cord, Left ♂ H Spermatic Cords, Bilateral ♂ J Epididymis, Right ♂ K Epididymis, Left ♂ L Epididymis, Bilateral ♂ N Vas Deferens, Right ♂ P Vas Deferens, Left ♂ Q Vas Deferens, Bilateral ♂	Ø Open 3 Percutaneous 4 Percutaneous Endoscopic	Z No Device	Z No Qualifier
5 Scrotum ♂ S Penis ♂ T Prepuce ♂	Ø Open 3 Percutaneous 4 Percutaneous Endoscopic X External	Z No Device	Z No Qualifier

Non-OR ØVC[67NPQ][Ø34]ZZ
Non-OR ØVC5[Ø34X]ZZ
Non-OR ØVCSXZZ

SECTION: Ø MEDICAL AND SURGICAL
BODY SYSTEM: V MALE REPRODUCTIVE SYSTEM
OPERATION: H INSERTION: Putting in a nonbiological appliance that monitors, assists, performs, or prevents a physiological function but does not physically take the place of a body part

Body Part	Approach	Device	Qualifier
Ø Prostate ♂	Ø Open 3 Percutaneous 4 Percutaneous Endoscopic 7 Via Natural or Artificial Opening 8 Via Natural or Artificial Opening Endoscopic	1 Radioactive Element	Z No Qualifier
4 Prostate and Seminal Vesicles ♂ 8 Scrotum and Tunica Vaginalis ♂ M Epididymis and Spermatic Cord ♂ R Vas Deferens ♂	Ø Open 3 Percutaneous 4 Percutaneous Endoscopic 7 Via Natural or Artificial Opening 8 Via Natural or Artificial Opening Endoscopic	3 Infusion Device Y Other Device	Z No Qualifier
D Testis	Ø Open 3 Percutaneous 4 Percutaneous Endoscopic 7 Via Natural or Artificial Opening 8 Via Natural or Artificial Opening Endoscopic	1 Radioactive Element 3 Infusion Device Y Other Device	Z No Qualifier
S Penis ♂	Ø Open 3 Percutaneous 4 Percutaneous Endoscopic	3 Infusion Device Y Other Device	Z No Qualifier
S Penis ♂	7 Via Natural or Artificial Opening 8 Via Natural or Artificial Opening Endoscopic	Y Other Device	Z No Qualifier
S Penis ♂	X External	3 Infusion Device	Z No Qualifier

DRG Non-OR ØVH[48DMR][Ø3478]3Z
DRG Non-OR ØVHS[Ø34]3Z
DRG Non-OR ØVHSX3Z

SECTION: Ø MEDICAL AND SURGICAL
BODY SYSTEM: V MALE REPRODUCTIVE SYSTEM
OPERATION: J INSPECTION: Visually and/or manually exploring a body part

Body Part	Approach	Device	Qualifier
4 Prostate and Seminal Vesicles ♂ 8 Scrotum and Tunica Vaginalis ♂ D Testis ♂ M Epididymis and Spermatic Cord ♂ R Vas Deferens ♂ S Penis ♂	Ø Open 3 Percutaneous 4 Percutaneous Endoscopic X External	Z No Device	Z No Qualifier

Non-OR ØVJ[4DMR][3X]ZZ
Non-OR ØVJ[8S][Ø34X]ZZ

SECTION: Ø MEDICAL AND SURGICAL
BODY SYSTEM: V MALE REPRODUCTIVE SYSTEM
OPERATION: L OCCLUSION: Completely closing an orifice or the lumen of a tubular body part

Body Part	Approach	Device	Qualifier
F Spermatic Cord, Right ♂ G Spermatic Cord, Left ♂ H Spermatic Cords, Bilateral ♂ N Vas Deferens, Right ♂ P Vas Deferens, Left ♂ Q Vas Deferens, Bilateral ♂	Ø Open 3 Percutaneous 4 Percutaneous Endoscopic 8 Via Natural or Artificial Opening Endoscopic	C Extraluminal Device D Intraluminal Device Z No Device	Z No Qualifier

ØVL[FGH][Ø34][CDZ]Z when Z3Ø.2 is listed as the principal diagnosis
ØVL[NPQ][Ø34][CZ]Z when Z3Ø.2 is listed as the principal diagnosis
Non-OR ØVL[FGH][Ø34][CDZ]Z
Non-OR ØVL[NPQ][Ø34][CZ]Z

SECTION: Ø MEDICAL AND SURGICAL
BODY SYSTEM: V MALE REPRODUCTIVE SYSTEM
OPERATION: M REATTACHMENT: Putting back in or on all or a portion of a separated body part to its normal location or other suitable location

Body Part	Approach	Device	Qualifier
5 Scrotum ♂ S Penis ♂	X External	Z No Device	Z No Qualifier
6 Tunica Vaginalis, Right ♂ 7 Tunica Vaginalis, Left ♂ 9 Testis, Right ♂ B Testis, Left ♂ C Testes, Bilateral ♂ F Spermatic Cord, Right ♂ G Spermatic Cord, Left ♂ H Spermatic Cords, Bilateral ♂	Ø Open 4 Percutaneous Endoscopic	Z No Device	Z No Qualifier

SECTION: Ø MEDICAL AND SURGICAL
BODY SYSTEM: V MALE REPRODUCTIVE SYSTEM
OPERATION: N RELEASE: Freeing a body part from an abnormal physical restraint by cutting or by the use of force

Body Part	Approach	Device	Qualifier
Ø Prostate ♂	Ø Open 3 Percutaneous 4 Percutaneous Endoscopic 7 Via Natural or Artificial Opening 8 Via Natural or Artificial Opening Endoscopic	Z No Device	Z No Qualifier
1 Seminal Vesicle, Right ♂ 2 Seminal Vesicle, Left ♂ 3 Seminal Vesicles, Bilateral ♂ 6 Tunica Vaginalis, Right ♂ 7 Tunica Vaginalis, Left ♂ 9 Testis, Right ♂ B Testis, Left ♂ C Testes, Bilateral ♂	Ø Open 3 Percutaneous 4 Percutaneous Endoscopic	Z No Device	Z No Qualifier
5 Scrotum ♂ S Penis ♂ T Prepuce ♂	Ø Open 3 Percutaneous 4 Percutaneous Endoscopic X External	Z No Device	Z No Qualifier
F Spermatic Cord, Right ♂ G Spermatic Cord, Left ♂ H Spermatic Cords, Bilateral ♂ J Epididymis, Right ♂ K Epididymis, Left ♂ L Epididymis, Bilateral ♂ N Vas Deferens, Right ♂ P Vas Deferens, Left ♂ Q Vas Deferens, Bilateral ♂	Ø Open 3 Percutaneous 4 Percutaneous Endoscopic 8 Via Natural or Artificial Opening Endoscopic	Z No Device	Z No Qualifier

Non-OR ØVN[9BC][Ø34]ZZ
Non-OR ØVNT[Ø34X]ZZ

SECTION: Ø MEDICAL AND SURGICAL
BODY SYSTEM: V MALE REPRODUCTIVE SYSTEM
OPERATION: P REMOVAL: Taking out or off a device from a body part

Body Part	Approach	Device	Qualifier
4 Prostate and Seminal Vesicles ♂	Ø Open 3 Percutaneous 4 Percutaneous Endoscopic 7 Via Natural or Artificial Opening 8 Via Natural or Artificial Opening Endoscopic	Ø Drainage Device 1 Radioactive Element 3 Infusion Device 7 Autologous Tissue Substitute J Synthetic Substitute K Nonautologous Tissue Substitute Y Other Device	Z No Qualifier
4 Prostate and Seminal Vesicles ♂	X External	Ø Drainage Device 1 Radioactive Element 3 Infusion Device	Z No Qualifier
8 Scrotum and Tunica Vaginalis ♂ D Testis ♂ S Penis ♂	Ø Open 3 Percutaneous 4 Percutaneous Endoscopic 7 Via Natural or Artificial Opening 8 Via Natural or Artificial Opening Endoscopic	Ø Drainage Device 3 Infusion Device 7 Autologous Tissue Substitute J Synthetic Substitute K Nonautologous Tissue Substitute Y Other Device	Z No Qualifier
8 Scrotum and Tunica Vaginalis ♂ D Testis ♂ S Penis ♂	X External	Ø Drainage Device 3 Infusion Device	Z No Qualifier
M Epididymis and Spermatic Cord ♂	Ø Open 3 Percutaneous 4 Percutaneous Endoscopic 7 Via Natural or Artificial Opening 8 Via Natural or Artificial Opening Endoscopic	Ø Drainage Device 3 Infusion Device 7 Autologous Tissue Substitute C Extraluminal Device J Synthetic Substitute K Nonautologous Tissue Substitute Y Other Device	Z No Qualifier
M Epididymis and Spermatic Cord ♂	X External	Ø Drainage Device 3 Infusion Device	Z No Qualifier
R Vas Deferens ♂	Ø Open 3 Percutaneous 4 Percutaneous Endoscopic 7 Via Natural or Artificial Opening 8 Via Natural or Artificial Opening Endoscopic	Ø Drainage Device 3 Infusion Device 7 Autologous Tissue Substitute C Extraluminal Device D Intraluminal Device J Synthetic Substitute K Nonautologous Tissue Substitute Y Other Device	Z No Qualifier
R Vas Deferens ♂	X External	Ø Drainage Device 3 Infusion Device D Intraluminal Device	Z No Qualifier

Non-OR ØVP4[78][Ø3]Z
Non-OR ØVP4X[Ø13]Z
Non-OR ØVP8[Ø3478][Ø37JK]Z
Non-OR ØVPD[78][Ø3]Z
Non-OR ØVPS[78][Ø3]Z
Non-OR ØVP[8DS]X[Ø3]Z
Non-OR ØVPM[78][Ø3]Z
Non-OR ØVPMX[Ø3]Z
Non-OR ØVPR[Ø3478][Ø37CDJK]Z
Non-OR ØVPR[78]DZ
Non-OR ØVPRX[Ø3D]Z

Coding Clinic: 2016, Q2, P28 – ØVPSØJZ

SECTION: Ø MEDICAL AND SURGICAL
BODY SYSTEM: V MALE REPRODUCTIVE SYSTEM
OPERATION: Q REPAIR: Restoring, to the extent possible, a body part to its normal anatomic structure and function

Body Part	Approach	Device	Qualifier
Ø Prostate ♂	Ø Open 3 Percutaneous 4 Percutaneous Endoscopic 7 Via Natural or Artificial Opening 8 Via Natural or Artificial Opening Endoscopic	Z No Device	Z No Qualifier
1 Seminal Vesicle, Right ♂ 2 Seminal Vesicle, Left ♂ 3 Seminal Vesicles, Bilateral ♂ 6 Tunica Vaginalis, Right ♂ 7 Tunica Vaginalis, Left ♂ 9 Testis, Right ♂ B Testis, Left ♂ C Testes, Bilateral ♂	Ø Open 3 Percutaneous 4 Percutaneous Endoscopic	Z No Device	Z No Qualifier
5 Scrotum ♂ S Penis ♂ T Prepuce ♂	Ø Open 3 Percutaneous 4 Percutaneous Endoscopic X External	Z No Device	Z No Qualifier
F Spermatic Cord, Right ♂ G Spermatic Cord, Left ♂ H Spermatic Cords, Bilateral ♂ J Epididymis, Right ♂ K Epididymis, Left ♂ L Epididymis, Bilateral ♂ N Vas Deferens, Right ♂ P Vas Deferens, Left ♂ Q Vas Deferens, Bilateral ♂	Ø Open 3 Percutaneous 4 Percutaneous Endoscopic 8 Via Natural or Artificial Opening Endoscopic	Z No Device	Z No Qualifier

Non-OR ØVQ[67][Ø34]ZZ
Non-OR ØVQ5[Ø34X]ZZ

SECTION: Ø MEDICAL AND SURGICAL
BODY SYSTEM: V MALE REPRODUCTIVE SYSTEM
OPERATION: R REPLACEMENT: Putting in or on biological or synthetic material that physically takes the place and/or function of all or a portion of a body part

Body Part	Approach	Device	Qualifier
9 Testis, Right ♂ B Testis, Left ♂ C Testis, Bilateral ♂	Ø Open	J Synthetic Substitute	Z No Qualifier

SECTION: Ø MEDICAL AND SURGICAL
BODY SYSTEM: V MALE REPRODUCTIVE SYSTEM
OPERATION: S REPOSITION: Moving to its normal location or other suitable location all or a portion of a body part

Body Part	Approach	Device	Qualifier
9 Testis, Right ♂ B Testis, Left ♂ C Testes, Bilateral ♂ F Spermatic Cord, Right ♂ G Spermatic Cord, Left ♂ H Spermatic Cords, Bilateral ♂	Ø Open 3 Percutaneous 4 Percutaneous Endoscopic 8 Via Natural or Artificial Opening Endoscopic	Z No Device	Z No Qualifier

SECTION: Ø MEDICAL AND SURGICAL
BODY SYSTEM: V MALE REPRODUCTIVE SYSTEM
OPERATION: T RESECTION: Cutting out or off, without replacement, all of a body part

Body Part	Approach	Device	Qualifier
Ø Prostate ♂ ⊞	Ø Open 4 Percutaneous Endoscopic 7 Via Natural or Artificial Opening 8 Via Natural or Artificial Opening Endoscopic	Z No Device	Z No Qualifier
1 Seminal Vesicle, Right ♂ 2 Seminal Vesicle, Left ♂ 3 Seminal Vesicles, Bilateral ♂ ⊞ 6 Tunica Vaginalis, Right ♂ 7 Tunica Vaginalis, Left ♂ 9 Testis, Right ♂ B Testis, Left ♂ C Testes, Bilateral ♂ F Spermatic Cord, Right ♂ G Spermatic Cord, Left ♂ H Spermatic Cords, Bilateral ♂ J Epididymis, Right ♂ K Epididymis, Left ♂ L Epididymis, Bilateral ♂ N Vas Deferens, Right ♂ Non-covered P Vas Deferens, Left ♂ Non-covered Q Vas Deferens, Bilateral ♂ Non-covered	Ø Open 4 Percutaneous Endoscopic	Z No Device	Z No Qualifier
5 Scrotum ♂ S Penis ♂ T Prepuce ♂	Ø Open 4 Percutaneous Endoscopic X External	Z No Device	Z No Qualifier

Non-covered ØVT[NPQ][Ø4]ZZ when Z3Ø.2 is listed as the principal diagnosis
⊞ ØVTØ[Ø478]ZZ
⊞ ØVT3[Ø4]ZZ
Non-OR ØVT[NPQ][Ø4]ZZ
Non-OR ØVT[5T][Ø4X]ZZ

SECTION: Ø MEDICAL AND SURGICAL
BODY SYSTEM: V MALE REPRODUCTIVE SYSTEM
OPERATION: U SUPPLEMENT: Putting in or on biological or synthetic material that physically reinforces and/or augments the function of a portion of a body part

Body Part	Approach	Device	Qualifier
1 Seminal Vesicle, Right ♂ 2 Seminal Vesicle, Left ♂ 3 Seminal Vesicles, Bilateral ♂ 6 Tunica Vaginalis, Right ♂ 7 Tunica Vaginalis, Left ♂ F Spermatic Cord, Right ♂ G Spermatic Cord, Left ♂ H Spermatic Cords, Bilateral ♂ J Epididymis, Right ♂ K Epididymis, Left ♂ L Epididymis, Bilateral ♂ N Vas Deferens, Right ♂ P Vas Deferens, Left ♂ Q Vas Deferens, Bilateral ♂	Ø Open 4 Percutaneous Endoscopic 8 Via Natural or Artificial Opening Endoscopic	7 Autologous Tissue Substitute J Synthetic Substitute K Nonautologous Tissue Substitute	Z No Qualifier
5 Scrotum ♂ S Penis ♂ T Prepuce ♂	Ø Open 4 Percutaneous Endoscopic X External	7 Autologous Tissue Substitute J Synthetic Substitute K Nonautologous Tissue Substitute	Z No Qualifier
9 Testis, Right ♂ B Testis, Left ♂ C Testis, Bilateral ♂	Ø Open	7 Autologous Tissue Substitute J Synthetic Substitute K Nonautologous Tissue Substitute	Z No Qualifier

Non-OR ØVUSX[7JK]Z

Coding Clinic: 2016, Q2, P29; 2015, Q3, P25 – ØVUSØJZ

SECTION: Ø MEDICAL AND SURGICAL
BODY SYSTEM: V MALE REPRODUCTIVE SYSTEM
OPERATION: W REVISION: Correcting, to the extent possible, a portion of a malfunctioning device or the position of a displaced device

Body Part	Approach	Device	Qualifier
4 Prostate and Seminal Vesicles ♂ 8 Scrotum and Tunica Vaginalis ♂ D Testis @ ♂ S Penis @ ♂	Ø Open 3 Percutaneous 4 Percutaneous Endoscopic 7 Via Natural or Artificial Opening 8 Via Natural or Artificial Opening Endoscopic	Ø Drainage Device 3 Infusion Device 7 Autologous Tissue Substitute J Synthetic Substitute K Nonautologous Tissue Substitute Y Other Device	Z No Qualifier
4 Prostate and Seminal Vesicles ♂ 8 Scrotum and Tunica Vaginalis ♂ D Testis ♂ S Penis ♂	X External	Ø Drainage Device 3 Infusion Device 7 Autologous Tissue Substitute J Synthetic Substitute K Nonautologous Tissue Substitute	Z No Qualifier
M Epididymis and Spermatic Cord ♂	Ø Open 3 Percutaneous 4 Percutaneous Endoscopic 7 Via Natural or Artificial Opening 8 Via Natural or Artificial Opening Endoscopic	Ø Drainage Device 3 Infusion Device 7 Autologous Tissue Substitute C Extraluminal Device J Synthetic Substitute K Nonautologous Tissue Substitute Y Other Device	Z No Qualifier
M Epididymis and Spermatic Cord ♂	X External	Ø Drainage Device 3 Infusion Device 7 Autologous Tissue Substitute C Extraluminal Device J Synthetic Substitute K Nonautologous Tissue Substitute	Z No Qualifier
R Vas Deferens ♂	Ø Open 3 Percutaneous 4 Percutaneous Endoscopic 7 Via Natural or Artificial Opening 8 Via Natural or Artificial Opening Endoscopic	Ø Drainage Device 3 Infusion Device 7 Autologous Tissue Substitute C Extraluminal Device D Intraluminal Device J Synthetic Substitute K Nonautologous Tissue Substitute Y Other Device	Z No Qualifier
R Vas Deferens ♂	X External	Ø Drainage Device 3 Infusion Device 7 Autologous Tissue Substitute C Extraluminal Device D Intraluminal Device J Synthetic Substitute K Nonautologous Tissue Substitute	Z No Qualifier

Non-OR ØVW[4DS]X[Ø37JK]Z
Non-OR ØVW8[Ø3478][Ø37JK]Z
Non-OR ØVW8X[Ø37]Z
Non-OR ØVWMX[Ø37CJK]Z
Non-OR ØVWR[Ø3478][Ø37CDJK]Z
Non-OR ØVWRX[Ø37CDJK]Z

Ø: M/S V: MALE REPRODUCTIVE SYSTEM W: REVISION

SECTION: Ø MEDICAL AND SURGICAL
BODY SYSTEM: V MALE REPRODUCTIVE SYSTEM
OPERATION: X TRANSFER: Moving, without taking out, all or a portion of a body part to another location to take over the function of all or a portion of a body part

Body Part	Approach	Device	Qualifier
T Prepuce ♂	Ø Open X External	Z No Device	D Urethra S Penis

SECTION: Ø MEDICAL AND SURGICAL
BODY SYSTEM: V MALE REPRODUCTIVE SYSTEM
OPERATION: Y TRANSPLANTATION: Putting in or on all or a portion of a living body part taken from another individual or animal to physically take the place and/or function of all or a portion of a similar body part

Body Part	Approach	Device	Qualifier
5 Scrotum S Penis	Ø Open	Z No Device	Ø Allogeneic 1 Syngeneic 2 Zooplastic

Coding Clinic: 2020, Q1, P31 – ØVYSØ7Z

ØW. Anatomical Regions, General 5Ø5
ØWØ. Alteration 5Ø6
ØW1. Bypass 5Ø6
ØW2. Change 5Ø7
ØW3. Control 5Ø7
ØW4. Creation 5Ø8
ØW8. Division 5Ø8
ØW9. Drainage 5Ø9
ØWB. Excision 51Ø
ØWC. Extirpation 51Ø
ØWF. Fragmentation 511
ØWH. Insertion 512
ØWJ. Inspection 513
ØWM. Reattachment 513
ØWP. Removal 514
ØWQ. Repair 515
ØWU. Supplement 515
ØWW. Revision 516
ØWY. Transplantation 516

SECTION: Ø MEDICAL AND SURGICAL
BODY SYSTEM: W ANATOMICAL REGIONS, GENERAL
OPERATION: Ø **ALTERATION:** Modifying the anatomic structure of a body part without affecting the function of the body part

Body Part	Approach	Device	Qualifier
Ø Head 2 Face 4 Upper Jaw 5 Lower Jaw 6 Neck 8 Chest Wall F Abdominal Wall K Upper Back L Lower Back M Perineum, Male ♂ N Perineum, Female ♀	Ø Open 3 Percutaneous 4 Percutaneous Endoscopic	7 Autologous Tissue Substitute J Synthetic Substitute K Nonautologous Tissue Substitute Z No Device	Z No Qualifier

Coding Clinic: 2Ø15, Q1, P31 – ØWØ2ØZZ

SECTION: Ø MEDICAL AND SURGICAL
BODY SYSTEM: W ANATOMICAL REGIONS, GENERAL
OPERATION: 1 **BYPASS:** Altering the route of passage of the contents of a tubular body part

Body Part	Approach	Device	Qualifier
1 Cranial Cavity	Ø Open	J Synthetic Substitute	9 Pleural Cavity, Right B Pleural Cavity, Left G Peritoneal Cavity J Pelvic Cavity
9 Pleural Cavity, Right B Pleural Cavity, Left J Pelvic Cavity	Ø Open 3 Percutaneous 4 Percutaneous Endoscopic	J Synthetic Substitute	4 Cutaneous 9 Pleural Cavity, Right B Pleural Cavity, Left G Peritoneal Cavity J Pelvic Cavity W Upper Vein Y Lower Vein
G Peritoneal Cavity	Ø Open 3 Percutaneous 4 Percutaneous Endoscopic	J Synthetic Substitute	4 Cutaneous 6 Bladder 9 Pleural Cavity, Right B Pleural Cavity, Left G Peritoneal Cavity J Pelvic Cavity W Upper Vein Y Lower Vein
9 Pleural Cavity, Right B Pleural Cavity, Left G Peritoneal Cavity J Pelvic Cavity	3 Percutaneous	J Synthetic Substitute	4 Cutaneous

Non-OR ØW1[9B][Ø4]J[4GY]
Non-OR ØW1G[Ø4]J[9BGJ]
Non-OR ØW1J[Ø4]J[4Y]
Non-OR ØW1[9BGJ]3J4

Coding Clinic: 2Ø18, Q4, P42 – ØW1G3JW

SECTION: Ø MEDICAL AND SURGICAL
BODY SYSTEM: W ANATOMICAL REGIONS, GENERAL
OPERATION: 2 CHANGE: Taking out or off a device from a body part and putting back an identical or similar device in or on the same body part without cutting or puncturing the skin or a mucous membrane

Body Part	Approach	Device	Qualifier
Ø Head 1 Cranial Cavity 2 Face 4 Upper Jaw 5 Lower Jaw 6 Neck 8 Chest Wall 9 Pleural Cavity, Right B Pleural Cavity, Left C Mediastinum D Pericardial Cavity F Abdominal Wall G Peritoneal Cavity H Retroperitoneum J Pelvic Cavity K Upper Back L Lower Back M Perineum, Male ♂ N Perineum, Female ♀	X External	Ø Drainage Device Y Other Device	Z No Qualifier

Non-OR All Values

SECTION: Ø MEDICAL AND SURGICAL
BODY SYSTEM: W ANATOMICAL REGIONS, GENERAL
OPERATION: 3 CONTROL: *(on multiple pages)* Stopping, or attempting to stop, postprocedure or other acute bleeding

Body Part	Approach	Device	Qualifier
Ø Head 1 Cranial Cavity 2 Face 3 Oral Cavity and Throat 4 Upper Jaw 5 Lower Jaw 6 Neck 8 Chest Wall 9 Pleural Cavity, Right B Pleural Cavity, Left C Mediastinum D Pericardial Cavity F Abdominal Wall G Peritoneal Cavity H Retroperitoneum J Pelvic Cavity K Upper Back L Lower Back M Perineum, Male ♂ N Perineum, Female ♀	Ø Open 3 Percutaneous 4 Percutaneous Endoscopic	Z No Device	Z No Qualifier

SECTION: Ø MEDICAL AND SURGICAL
BODY SYSTEM: W ANATOMICAL REGIONS, GENERAL
OPERATION: 3 CONTROL: *(continued)*
Stopping, or attempting to stop, postprocedure or other acute bleeding

Body Part	Approach	Device	Qualifier
3 Oral Cavity and Throat	Ø Open 3 Percutaneous 4 Percutaneous Endoscopic 7 Via Natural or Artificial Opening 8 Via Natural or Artificial Opening Endoscopic X External	Z No Device	Z No Qualifier
P Gastrointestinal Tract Q Respiratory Tract R Genitourinary Tract	Ø Open 3 Percutaneous 4 Percutaneous Endoscopic 7 Via Natural or Artificial Opening 8 Via Natural or Artificial Opening Endoscopic	Z No Device	Z No Qualifier

Non-OR ØW3P8ZZ

Coding Clinic: 2018, Q1, P19-20 – ØW3[PQ]8ZZ
Coding Clinic: 2023, Q3, P7; 2023, Q2, P27 – ØW3P8ZZ
Coding Clinic: 2023, Q3, P6 – ØW3R7ZZ

SECTION: Ø MEDICAL AND SURGICAL
BODY SYSTEM: W ANATOMICAL REGIONS, GENERAL
OPERATION: 4 CREATION: Putting in or on biological or synthetic material to form a new body part that to the extent possible replicates the anatomic structure or function of an absent body part

Body Part	Approach	Device	Qualifier
M Perineum, Male ♂	Ø Open	7 Autologous Tissue Substitute J Synthetic Substitute K Nonautologous Tissue Substitute	Ø Vagina
N Perineum, Female ♀	Ø Open	7 Autologous Tissue Substitute J Synthetic Substitute K Nonautologous Tissue Substitute	1 Penis

Coding Clinic: 2016, Q4, P1Ø1 – ØW4

SECTION: Ø MEDICAL AND SURGICAL
BODY SYSTEM: W ANATOMICAL REGIONS, GENERAL
OPERATION: 8 DIVISION: Cutting into a body part, without draining fluids and/or gases from the body part, in order to separate or transect a body part

Body Part	Approach	Device	Qualifier
N Perineum, Female ♀	X External	Z No Device	Z No Qualifier

Non-OR ØW8NXZZ

SECTION: Ø MEDICAL AND SURGICAL
BODY SYSTEM: W ANATOMICAL REGIONS, GENERAL
OPERATION: 9 DRAINAGE: Taking or letting out fluids and/or gases from a body part

Body Part	Approach	Device	Qualifier
Ø Head 1 Cranial Cavity 2 Face 3 Oral Cavity and Throat 4 Upper Jaw 5 Lower Jaw 8 Chest Wall 9 Pleural Cavity, Right B Pleural Cavity, Left C Mediastinum D Pericardial Cavity F Abdominal Wall G Peritoneal Cavity H Retroperitoneum K Upper Back L Lower Back M Perineum, Male ♂ N Perineum, Female ♀	Ø Open 3 Percutaneous 4 Percutaneous Endoscopic	Ø Drainage Device	Z No Qualifier
Ø Head 1 Cranial Cavity 2 Face 3 Oral Cavity and Throat 4 Upper Jaw 5 Lower Jaw 8 Chest Wall 9 Pleural Cavity, Right B Pleural Cavity, Left C Mediastinum D Pericardial Cavity F Abdominal Wall G Peritoneal Cavity H Retroperitoneum K Upper Back L Lower Back M Perineum, Male ♂ N Perineum, Female ♀	Ø Open 3 Percutaneous 4 Percutaneous Endoscopic	Z No Device	X Diagnostic Z No Qualifier
6 Neck J Pelvic Cavity	Ø Open 3 Percutaneous 4 Percutaneous Endoscopic 7 Via Natural or Artificial Opening 8 Via Natural or Artificial Opening Endoscopic	Ø Drainage Device	Z No Qualifier
6 Neck J Pelvic Cavity	Ø Open 3 Percutaneous 4 Percutaneous Endoscopic 7 Via Natural or Artificial Opening 8 Via Natural or Artificial Opening Endoscopic	Z No Device	X Diagnostic Z No Qualifier

DRG Non-OR ØW9H3ØZ
DRG Non-OR ØW9H3ZZ
Non-OR ØW9[Ø8KLM][Ø34]ØZ
Non-OR ØW9[9B][Ø3]ØZ
Non-OR ØW9[1DFG][34]ØZ
Non-OR ØW9J3ØZ
Non-OR ØW9[Ø234568KLMN][Ø34]ZX
Non-OR ØW9G3ZX
Non-OR ØW9[9B][Ø3]ZZ
Non-OR ØW9[Ø8KLM][Ø34]ZZ
Non-OR ØW9[9B][Ø3]ZZ
Non-OR ØW9[1CD][34]ZX
Non-OR ØW9[1DFG][34]ZZ
Non-OR ØW9J3ZZ

Coding Clinic: 2017, Q2, P17 – 0W930ZZ
Coding Clinic: 2Ø17, Q3, P13 – ØW9G3ZZ
Coding Clinic: 2Ø21, Q3, P18,22 – ØW96ØZZ
Coding Clinic: 2Ø21, Q3, P27 – ØW9DØZZ
Coding Clinic: 2Ø22, Q4, P57 – ØW968ZZ

SECTION: Ø MEDICAL AND SURGICAL
BODY SYSTEM: W ANATOMICAL REGIONS, GENERAL
OPERATION: B EXCISION: Cutting out or off, without replacement, a portion of a body part

Body Part	Approach	Device	Qualifier
Ø Head 2 Face 3 Oral Cavity and Throat 4 Upper Jaw 5 Lower Jaw 8 Chest Wall K Upper Back L Lower Back M Perineum, Male ♂ N Perineum, Female ♀	Ø Open 3 Percutaneous 4 Percutaneous Endoscopic X External	Z No Device	X Diagnostic Z No Qualifier
6 Neck F Abdominal Wall	Ø Open 3 Percutaneous 4 Percutaneous Endoscopic	Z No Device	X Diagnostic Z No Qualifier
6 Neck F Abdominal Wall	X External	Z No Device	2 Stoma X Diagnostic Z No Qualifier
C Mediastinum H Retroperitoneum	Ø Open 3 Percutaneous 4 Percutaneous Endoscopic	Z No Device	X Diagnostic Z No Qualifier

Non-OR ØWB[Ø2458KLM][Ø34X]ZX
Non-OR ØWB6[Ø34]ZX
Non-OR ØWB6XZX
Non-OR ØWB[CH][34]ZX

Coding Clinic: 2Ø16, Q1, P22 – ØWBF4ZZ
Coding Clinic: 2Ø19, Q1, P27 – ØWBHØZZ
Coding Clinic: 2Ø21, Q3, P21 – ØWB6ØZZ

SECTION: Ø MEDICAL AND SURGICAL
BODY SYSTEM: W ANATOMICAL REGIONS, GENERAL
OPERATION: C EXTIRPATION: Taking or cutting out solid matter from a body part

Body Part	Approach	Device	Qualifier
1 Cranial Cavity 3 Oral Cavity and Throat 9 Pleural Cavity, Right B Pleural Cavity, Left C Mediastinum D Pericardial Cavity G Peritoneal Cavity H Retroperitoneum J Pelvic Cavity	Ø Open 3 Percutaneous 4 Percutaneous Endoscopic X External	Z No Device	Z No Qualifier
4 Upper Jaw 5 Lower Jaw	Ø Open 3 Percutaneous 4 Percutaneous Endoscopic	Z No Device	Z No Qualifier
P Gastrointestinal Tract Q Respiratory Tract R Genitourinary Tract	Ø Open 3 Percutaneous 4 Percutaneous Endoscopic 7 Via Natural or Artificial Opening 8 Via Natural or Artificial Opening Endoscopic X External	Z No Device	Z No Qualifier

Non-OR ØWC[13]XZZ
Non-OR ØWC[9B][Ø34X]ZZ
Non-OR ØWC[CDGJ]XZZ
Non-OR ØWCP[78X]ZZ
Non-OR ØWCQ[Ø34X]ZZ
Non-OR ØWCR[78X]ZZ

Coding Clinic: 2Ø17, Q2, P16 – ØWC3ØZZ
Coding Clinic: 2Ø22, Q1, P43 – ØWC[HJ]ØZZ

SECTION: Ø MEDICAL AND SURGICAL
BODY SYSTEM: W ANATOMICAL REGIONS, GENERAL
OPERATION: F FRAGMENTATION: Breaking solid matter in a body part into pieces

Body Part	Approach	Device	Qualifier
1 Cranial Cavity 3 Oral Cavity and Throat 9 Pleural Cavity, Right B Pleural Cavity, Left C Mediastinum D Pericardial Cavity G Peritoneal Cavity J Pelvic Cavity	Ø Open 3 Percutaneous 4 Percutaneous Endoscopic X External	Z No Device	Z No Qualifier
P Gastrointestinal Tract Q Respiratory Tract R Genitourinary Tract	Ø Open 3 Percutaneous 4 Percutaneous Endoscopic 7 Via Natural or Artificial Opening 8 Via Natural or Artificial Opening Endoscopic X External	Z No Device	Z No Qualifier

ØWF[139BCGJ]XZZ
ØWF[PQ]XZZ
Non-OR ØWF[139BCG]XZZ
Non-OR ØWFJ[Ø34X]ZZ
Non-OR ØWFP[Ø3478X]ZZ
Non-OR ØWFQXZZ
Non-OR ØWFR[Ø3478]ZZ

SECTION: Ø MEDICAL AND SURGICAL
BODY SYSTEM: W ANATOMICAL REGIONS, GENERAL
OPERATION: H INSERTION: Putting in a nonbiological appliance that monitors, assists, performs, or prevents a physiological function but does not physically take the place of a body part

Body Part	Approach	Device	Qualifier
Ø Head 1 Cranial Cavity 2 Face 3 Oral Cavity and Throat 4 Upper Jaw 5 Lower Jaw 6 Neck 8 Chest Wall 9 Pleural Cavity, Right B Pleural Cavity, Left D Pericardial Cavity F Abdominal Wall G Peritoneal Cavity H Retroperitoneum J Pelvic Cavity K Upper Back L Lower Back M Perineum, Male ♂ N Perineum, Female ♀	Ø Open 3 Percutaneous 4 Percutaneous Endoscopic	1 Radioactive Element 3 Infusion Device Y Other Device	Z No Qualifier
C Mediastinum	Ø Open 3 Percutaneous 4 Percutaneous Endoscopic	1 Radioactive Element 3 Infusion Device G Defibrillator Lead Y Other Device	Z No Qualifier
P Gastrointestinal Tract Q Respiratory Tract R Genitourinary Tract	Ø Open 3 Percutaneous 4 Percutaneous Endoscopic 7 Via Natural or Artificial Opening 8 Via Natural or Artificial Opening Endoscopic	1 Radioactive Element 3 Infusion Device Y Other Device	Z No Qualifier

DRG Non-OR ØWH[Ø2456KLM][Ø34][3Y]Z
Non-OR ØWH1[Ø34]3Z
Non-OR ØWH[89B][Ø34][3Y]Z
Non-OR ØWHPØYZ
Non-OR ØWHP[3478][3Y]Z
Non-OR ØWHQ[Ø78][3Y]Z
Non-OR ØWHR[Ø3478][3Y]Z

Coding Clinic: 2Ø16, Q2, P14 – ØWHG33Z
Coding Clinic: 2Ø17, Q4, P1Ø4 – ØUHD7YZ
Coding Clinic: 2Ø19, Q4, P44 – ØWHJØ1Z
Coding Clinic: 2Ø21, Q2, P14 – ØWHGØ3Z

SECTION: Ø MEDICAL AND SURGICAL
BODY SYSTEM: W ANATOMICAL REGIONS, GENERAL
OPERATION: J INSPECTION: Visually and/or manually exploring a body part

Body Part	Approach	Device	Qualifier
Ø Head 2 Face 3 Oral Cavity and Throat 4 Upper Jaw 5 Lower Jaw 6 Neck 8 Chest Wall F Abdominal Wall K Upper Back L Lower Back M Perineum, Male ♂ N Perineum, Female ♀	Ø Open 3 Percutaneous 4 Percutaneous Endoscopic X External	Z No Device	Z No Qualifier
1 Cranial Cavity 9 Pleural Cavity, Right B Pleural Cavity, Left C Mediastinum D Pericardial Cavity G Peritoneal Cavity H Retroperitoneum J Pelvic Cavity	Ø Open 3 Percutaneous 4 Percutaneous Endoscopic	Z No Device	Z No Qualifier
P Gastrointestinal Tract Q Respiratory Tract R Genitourinary Tract	Ø Open 3 Percutaneous 4 Percutaneous Endoscopic 7 Via Natural or Artificial Opening 8 Via Natural or Artificial Opening Endoscopic	Z No Device	Z No Qualifier

DRG Non-OR ØWJ[Ø245KLM]ØZZ
DRG Non-OR ØWJF3ZZ
DRG Non-OR ØWJM[Ø4]ZZ
DRG Non-OR ØWJ[1GHJ]3ZZ
DRG Non-OR ØWJ[PR][378]ZZ
Non-OR ØWJ[Ø245KL][34X]ZZ
Non-OR ØWJ[68]3ZZ
Non-OR ØWJ3[Ø34X]ZZ
Non-OR ØWJ[68FN]XZZ
Non-OR OWJM[3X]ZZ
Non-OR ØWJ[9BC]3ZZ
Non-OR ØWJD[Ø3]ZZ
Non-OR ØWJQ[378]ZZ
Coding Clinic: 2Ø13, Q2, P37 – ØWJG4ZZ
Coding Clinic: 2Ø21, Q2, P2Ø; 2Ø19, Q1, P5, 25 – ØWJG4ZZ

SECTION: Ø MEDICAL AND SURGICAL
BODY SYSTEM: W ANATOMICAL REGIONS, GENERAL
OPERATION: M REATTACHMENT: Putting back in or on all or a portion of a separated body part to its normal location or other suitable location

Body Part	Approach	Device	Qualifier
2 Face 4 Upper Jaw 5 Lower Jaw 6 Neck 8 Chest Wall F Abdominal Wall K Upper Back L Lower Back M Perineum, Male ♂ N Perineum, Female ♀	Ø Open	Z No Device	Z No Qualifier

SECTION: Ø MEDICAL AND SURGICAL
BODY SYSTEM: W ANATOMICAL REGIONS, GENERAL
OPERATION: P REMOVAL: Taking out or off a device from a body part

Body Part	Approach	Device	Qualifier
Ø Head 2 Face 4 Upper Jaw 5 Lower Jaw 6 Neck 8 Chest Wall F Abdominal Wall K Upper Back L Lower Back M Perineum, Male ♂ N Perineum, Female ♀	Ø Open 3 Percutaneous 4 Percutaneous Endoscopic X External	Ø Drainage Device 1 Radioactive Element 3 Infusion Device 7 Autologous Tissue Substitute J Synthetic Substitute K Nonautologous Tissue Substitute Y Other Device	Z No Qualifier
1 Cranial Cavity 9 Pleural Cavity, Right B Pleural Cavity, Left G Peritoneal Cavity J Pelvic Cavity	Ø Open 3 Percutaneous 4 Percutaneous Endoscopic	Ø Drainage Device 1 Radioactive Element 3 Infusion Device J Synthetic Substitute Y Other Device	Z No Qualifier
1 Cranial Cavity 9 Pleural Cavity, Right B Pleural Cavity, Left G Peritoneal Cavity J Pelvic Cavity	X External	Ø Drainage Device 1 Radioactive Element 3 Infusion Device	Z No Qualifier
C Mediastinum	Ø Open 3 Percutaneous 4 Percutaneous Endoscopic X External	Ø Drainage Device 1 Radioactive Element 3 Infusion Device 7 Autologous Tissue Substitute G Defibrillator Lead J Synthetic Substitute K Nonautologous Tissue Substitute Y Other Device	Z No Qualifier
D Pericardial Cavity H Retroperitoneum	Ø Open 3 Percutaneous 4 Percutaneous Endoscopic	Ø Drainage Device 1 Radioactive Element 3 Infusion Device Y Other Device	Z No Qualifier
D Pericardial Cavity H Retroperitoneum	X External	Ø Drainage Device 1 Radioactive Element 3 Infusion Device	Z No Qualifier
P Gastrointestinal Tract Q Respiratory Tract R Genitourinary Tract	Ø Open 3 Percutaneous 4 Percutaneous Endoscopic 7 Via Natural or Artificial Opening 8 Via Natural or Artificial Opening Endoscopic X External	1 Radioactive Element 3 Infusion Device Y Other Device	Z No Qualifier

Non-OR OWP[Ø24568KL][Ø34X][Ø137JKY]Z
Non-OR OWPM[Ø34][Ø13JY]Z
Non-OR OWPMX[Ø13Y]Z
Non-OR OWP[CFN]X[Ø137JKY]Z
Non-OR OWP1[Ø34]3Z
Non-OR OWP[9BJ][Ø34][Ø13JY]Z
Non-OR OWP[19BGJ]X[Ø13]Z
Non-OR OWP[DH]X[Ø13]Z
Non-OR OWPP[3478X][13Y]Z
Non-OR ØWPQ73Z
Non-OR OWPQ8[3Y]Z
Non-OR OWPQ[ØX][13Y]Z
Non-OR OWPR[Ø3478X][13Y]Z

New/Revised Text in Green ~~deleted~~ Deleted ♀ Females Only ♂ Males Only Coding Clinic
Non-covered Limited Coverage Combination (See Appendix E) DRG Non-OR Non-OR Hospital-Acquired Condition

SECTION: Ø MEDICAL AND SURGICAL
BODY SYSTEM: W ANATOMICAL REGIONS, GENERAL
OPERATION: Q REPAIR: Restoring, to the extent possible, a body part to its normal anatomic structure and function

Body Part	Approach	Device	Qualifier
Ø Head 2 Face 3 Oral Cavity and Throat 4 Upper Jaw 5 Lower Jaw 8 Chest Wall K Upper Back L Lower Back M Perineum, Male ♂ N Perineum, Female ♀	Ø Open 3 Percutaneous 4 Percutaneous Endoscopic X External	Z No Device	Z No Qualifier
6 Neck F Abdominal Wall	Ø Open 3 Percutaneous 4 Percutaneous Endoscopic	Z No Device	Z No Qualifier
6 Neck F Abdominal Wall ⊞	X External	Z No Device	2 Stoma Z No Qualifier
C Mediastinum	Ø Open 3 Percutaneous 4 Percutaneous Endoscopic	Z No Device	Z No Qualifier

⊞ ØWQFXZ[2Z]
Non-OR ØWQNXZZ

Coding Clinic: 2Ø16, Q3, P6 – ØWQFØZZ
Coding Clinic: 2Ø17, Q3, P9 – ØWQFØZZ

SECTION: Ø MEDICAL AND SURGICAL
BODY SYSTEM: W ANATOMICAL REGIONS, GENERAL
OPERATION: U SUPPLEMENT: Putting in or on biological or synthetic material that physically reinforces and/or augments the function of a portion of a body part

Body Part	Approach	Device	Qualifier
Ø Head 2 Face 4 Upper Jaw 5 Lower Jaw 6 Neck 8 Chest Wall C Mediastinum F Abdominal Wall K Upper Back L Lower Back M Perineum, Male ♂ N Perineum, Female ♀	Ø Open 4 Percutaneous Endoscopic	7 Autologous Tissue Substitute J Synthetic Substitute K Nonautologous Tissue Substitute	Z No Qualifier

Coding Clinic: 2Ø12, Q4, P1Ø1 – ØWU8ØJZ
Coding Clinic: 2Ø16, Q3, P41 – ØWUFØ7Z
Coding Clinic: 2Ø17, Q3, P8 – ØWUFØJZ

SECTION: Ø MEDICAL AND SURGICAL
BODY SYSTEM: W ANATOMICAL REGIONS, GENERAL
OPERATION: W REVISION: Correcting, to the extent possible, a portion of a malfunctioning device or the position of a displaced device

Body Part	Approach	Device	Qualifier
Ø Head 2 Face 4 Upper Jaw 5 Lower Jaw 6 Neck 8 Chest Wall F Abdominal Wall K Upper Back L Lower Back M Perineum, Male ♂ N Perineum, Female ♀	Ø Open 3 Percutaneous 4 Percutaneous Endoscopic X External	Ø Drainage Device 1 Radioactive Element 3 Infusion Device 7 Autologous Tissue Substitute J Synthetic Substitute K Nonautologous Tissue Substitute Y Other Device	Z No Qualifier
1 Cranial Cavity 9 Pleural Cavity, Right B Pleural Cavity, Left G Peritoneal Cavity J Pelvic Cavity	Ø Open 3 Percutaneous 4 Percutaneous Endoscopic X External	Ø Drainage Device 1 Radioactive Element 3 Infusion Device J Synthetic Substitute Y Other Device	Z No Qualifier
C Mediastinum	Ø Open 3 Percutaneous 4 Percutaneous Endoscopic X External	Ø Drainage Device 1 Radioactive Element 3 Infusion Device 7 Autologous Tissue Substitute G Defibrillator Lead J Synthetic Substitute K Nonautologous Tissue Substitute Y Other Device	Z No Qualifier
D Pericardial Cavity H Retroperitoneum	Ø Open 3 Percutaneous 4 Percutaneous Endoscopic X External	Ø Drainage Device 1 Radioactive Element 3 Infusion Device Y Other Device	Z No Qualifier
P Gastrointestinal Tract Q Respiratory Tract R Genitourinary Tract	Ø Open 3 Percutaneous 4 Percutaneous Endoscopic 7 Via Natural or Artificial Opening 8 Via Natural or Artificial Opening Endoscopic X External	1 Radioactive Element 3 Infusion Device Y Other Device	Z No Qualifier

DRG Non-OR ØWW[Ø2456KL][Ø34][Ø137JKY]Z
DRG Non-OR ØWWM[Ø34][Ø13JY]Z
Non-OR OWW[Ø2456CFKLMN]X[Ø137JKY]Z
Non-OR OWW8[Ø34X][Ø137JKY]Z
Non-OR OWW[1GJ]X[Ø13JY]Z
Non-OR OWW[9B][Ø34X][Ø13JY]Z
Non-OR OWW[DH]X[Ø13Y]Z
Non-OR OWWP[3478X][13Y]Z
Non-OR OWWQ[ØX][13Y]Z
Non-OR OWWR[Ø3478X][13Y]Z

Coding Clinic: 2015, Q2, P1Ø – ØWWG4JZ
Coding Clinic: 2016, Q4, P112 – ØWY

SECTION: Ø MEDICAL AND SURGICAL
BODY SYSTEM: W ANATOMICAL REGIONS, GENERAL
OPERATION: Y TRANSPLANTATION: Putting in or on all or a portion of a living body part taken from another individual or animal to physically take the place and/or function of all or a portion of a similar body part

Body Part	Approach	Device	Qualifier
2 Face	Ø Open	Z No Device	Ø Allogeneic 1 Syngeneic

ØX. Anatomical Regions, Upper Extremities 517
ØXØ. Alteration 518
ØX2. Change 518
ØX3. Control 518
ØX6. Detachment 519
ØX9. Drainage 52Ø
ØXB. Excision 521
ØXH. Insertion 521
ØXJ. Inspection 522
ØXM. Reattachment 522
ØXP. Removal 523
ØXQ. Repair 523
ØXR. Replacement 524
ØXU. Supplement 524
ØXW. Revision 525
ØXX. Transfer 525
ØXY. Transplantation 525

SECTION: Ø MEDICAL AND SURGICAL
BODY SYSTEM: X ANATOMICAL REGIONS, UPPER EXTREMITIES
OPERATION: Ø ALTERATION: Modifying the anatomic structure of a body part without affecting the function of the body part

Body Part	Approach	Device	Qualifier
2 Shoulder Region, Right 3 Shoulder Region, Left 4 Axilla, Right 5 Axilla, Left 6 Upper Extremity, Right 7 Upper Extremity, Left 8 Upper Arm, Right 9 Upper Arm, Left B Elbow Region, Right C Elbow Region, Left D Lower Arm, Right F Lower Arm, Left G Wrist Region, Right H Wrist Region, Left	Ø Open 3 Percutaneous 4 Percutaneous Endoscopic	7 Autologous Tissue Substitute J Synthetic Substitute K Nonautologous Tissue Substitute Z No Device	Z No Qualifier

SECTION: Ø MEDICAL AND SURGICAL
BODY SYSTEM: X ANATOMICAL REGIONS, UPPER EXTREMITIES
OPERATION: 2 CHANGE: Taking out or off a device from a body part and putting back an identical or similar device in or on the same body part without cutting or puncturing the skin or a mucous membrane

Body Part	Approach	Device	Qualifier
6 Upper Extremity, Right 7 Upper Extremity, Left	X External	Ø Drainage Device Y Other Device	Z No Qualifier

Non-OR All Values

SECTION: Ø MEDICAL AND SURGICAL
BODY SYSTEM: X ANATOMICAL REGIONS, UPPER EXTREMITIES
OPERATION: 3 CONTROL: Stopping, or attempting to stop, postprocedure or other acute bleeding

Body Part	Approach	Device	Qualifier
2 Shoulder Region, Right 3 Shoulder Region, Left 4 Axilla, Right 5 Axilla, Left 6 Upper Extremity, Right 7 Upper Extremity, Left 8 Upper Arm, Right 9 Upper Arm, Left B Elbow Region, Right C Elbow Region, Left D Lower Arm, Right F Lower Arm, Left G Wrist Region, Right H Wrist Region, Left J Hand, Right K Hand, Left	Ø Open 3 Percutaneous 4 Percutaneous Endoscopic	Z No Device	Z No Qualifier

Coding Clinic: 2Ø15, Q1, P35 – ØX37ØZZ
Coding Clinic: 2Ø16, Q4, P99 – ØX3

SECTION: Ø MEDICAL AND SURGICAL
BODY SYSTEM: X ANATOMICAL REGIONS, UPPER EXTREMITIES
OPERATION: 6 DETACHMENT: Cutting off all or a portion of the upper or lower extremities

Body Part	Approach	Device	Qualifier
Ø Forequarter, Right 1 Forequarter, Left 2 Shoulder Region, Right 3 Shoulder Region, Left B Elbow Region, Right C Elbow Region, Left	Ø Open	Z No Device	Z No Qualifier
8 Upper Arm, Right 9 Upper Arm, Left D Lower Arm, Right F Lower Arm, Left	Ø Open	Z No Device	1 High 2 Mid 3 Low
J Hand, Right K Hand, Left	Ø Open	Z No Device	Ø Complete 4 Complete 1st Ray 5 Complete 2nd Ray 6 Complete 3rd Ray 7 Complete 4th Ray 8 Complete 5th Ray 9 Partial 1st Ray B Partial 2nd Ray C Partial 3rd Ray D Partial 4th Ray F Partial 5th Ray
L Thumb, Right M Thumb, Left	Ø Open	Z No Device	Ø Complete 1 High 3 Low
~~L Thumb, Right~~ ~~M Thumb, Left~~ N Index Finger, Right P Index Finger, Left Q Middle Finger, Right R Middle Finger, Left S Ring Finger, Right T Ring Finger, Left V Little Finger, Right W Little Finger, Left	Ø Open	Z No Device	Ø Complete 1 High 2 Mid 3 Low

Coding Clinic: 2016, Q3, P34 – ØX6[MTW]ØZ1
Coding Clinic: 2017, Q1, P52 – ØX6[MTW]ØZ3
Coding Clinic: 2017, Q2, P19 – ØX6VØZØ

SECTION: Ø MEDICAL AND SURGICAL
BODY SYSTEM: X ANATOMICAL REGIONS, UPPER EXTREMITIES
OPERATION: 9 DRAINAGE: Taking or letting out fluids and/or gases from a body part

Body Part	Approach	Device	Qualifier
2 Shoulder Region, Right 3 Shoulder Region, Left 4 Axilla, Right 5 Axilla, Left 6 Upper Extremity, Right 7 Upper Extremity, Left 8 Upper Arm, Right 9 Upper Arm, Left B Elbow Region, Right C Elbow Region, Left D Lower Arm, Right F Lower Arm, Left G Wrist Region, Right H Wrist Region, Left J Hand, Right K Hand, Left	Ø Open 3 Percutaneous 4 Percutaneous Endoscopic	Ø Drainage Device	Z No Qualifier
2 Shoulder Region, Right 3 Shoulder Region, Left 4 Axilla, Right 5 Axilla, Left 6 Upper Extremity, Right 7 Upper Extremity, Left 8 Upper Arm, Right 9 Upper Arm, Left B Elbow Region, Right C Elbow Region, Left D Lower Arm, Right F Lower Arm, Left G Wrist Region, Right H Wrist Region, Left J Hand, Right K Hand, Left	Ø Open 3 Percutaneous 4 Percutaneous Endoscopic	Z No Device	X Diagnostic Z No Qualifier

Non-OR All Values

SECTION: Ø MEDICAL AND SURGICAL
BODY SYSTEM: X ANATOMICAL REGIONS, UPPER EXTREMITIES
OPERATION: B EXCISION: Cutting out or off, without replacement, a portion of a body part

Body Part	Approach	Device	Qualifier
2 Shoulder Region, Right 3 Shoulder Region, Left 4 Axilla, Right 5 Axilla, Left 6 Upper Extremity, Right 7 Upper Extremity, Left 8 Upper Arm, Right 9 Upper Arm, Left B Elbow Region, Right C Elbow Region, Left D Lower Arm, Right F Lower Arm, Left G Wrist Region, Right H Wrist Region, Left J Hand, Right K Hand, Left	Ø Open 3 Percutaneous 4 Percutaneous Endoscopic	Z No Device	X Diagnostic Z No Qualifier

Non-OR ØXB[23456789BCDFGHJK][Ø34]ZX

SECTION: Ø MEDICAL AND SURGICAL
BODY SYSTEM: X ANATOMICAL REGIONS, UPPER EXTREMITIES
OPERATION: H INSERTION: Putting in a nonbiological appliance that monitors, assists, performs, or prevents a physiological function but does not physically take the place of a body part

Body Part	Approach	Device	Qualifier
2 Shoulder Region, Right 3 Shoulder Region, Left 4 Axilla, Right 5 Axilla, Left 6 Upper Extremity, Right 7 Upper Extremity, Left 8 Upper Arm, Right 9 Upper Arm, Left B Elbow Region, Right C Elbow Region, Left D Lower Arm, Right F Lower Arm, Left G Wrist Region, Right H Wrist Region, Left J Hand, Right K Hand, Left	Ø Open 3 Percutaneous 4 Percutaneous Endoscopic	1 Radioactive Element 3 Infusion Device Y Other Device	Z No Qualifier

DRG Non-OR ØXH[23456789BCDFGHJK][Ø34][3Y]Z

Coding Clinic: 2017, Q2, P21 – ØXH9ØYZ

SECTION: Ø MEDICAL AND SURGICAL
BODY SYSTEM: X ANATOMICAL REGIONS, UPPER EXTREMITIES
OPERATION: J INSPECTION: Visually and/or manually exploring a body part

Body Part	Approach	Device	Qualifier
2 Shoulder Region, Right 3 Shoulder Region, Left 4 Axilla, Right 5 Axilla, Left 6 Upper Extremity, Right 7 Upper Extremity, Left 8 Upper Arm, Right 9 Upper Arm, Left B Elbow Region, Right C Elbow Region, Left D Lower Arm, Right F Lower Arm, Left G Wrist Region, Right H Wrist Region, Left J Hand, Right K Hand, Left	Ø Open 3 Percutaneous 4 Percutaneous Endoscopic X External	Z No Device	Z No Qualifier

DRG Non-OR ØXJ[23456789BCDFGHJK]ØZZ
Non-OR ØXJ[23456789BCDFGH][34X]ZZ
Non-OR ØXJ[JK]3ZZ
Non-OR ØXJ[JK]XZZ

SECTION: Ø MEDICAL AND SURGICAL
BODY SYSTEM: X ANATOMICAL REGIONS, UPPER EXTREMITIES
OPERATION: M REATTACHMENT: Putting back in or on all or a portion of a separated body part to its normal location or other suitable location

Body Part	Approach	Device	Qualifier
Ø Forequarter, Right 1 Forequarter, Left 2 Shoulder Region, Right 3 Shoulder Region, Left 4 Axilla, Right 5 Axilla, Left 6 Upper Extremity, Right 7 Upper Extremity, Left 8 Upper Arm, Right 9 Upper Arm, Left B Elbow Region, Right C Elbow Region, Left D Lower Arm, Right F Lower Arm, Left G Wrist Region, Right H Wrist Region, Left J Hand, Right K Hand, Left L Thumb, Right M Thumb, Left N Index Finger, Right P Index Finger, Left Q Middle Finger, Right R Middle Finger, Left S Ring Finger, Right T Ring Finger, Left V Little Finger, Right W Little Finger, Left	Ø Open	Z No Device	Z No Qualifier

SECTION: Ø MEDICAL AND SURGICAL
BODY SYSTEM: X ANATOMICAL REGIONS, UPPER EXTREMITIES
OPERATION: P REMOVAL: Taking out or off a device from a body part

Body Part	Approach	Device	Qualifier
6 Upper Extremity, Right 7 Upper Extremity, Left	Ø Open 3 Percutaneous 4 Percutaneous Endoscopic X External	Ø Drainage Device 1 Radioactive Element 3 Infusion Device 7 Autologous Tissue Substitute J Synthetic Substitute K Nonautologous Tissue Substitute Y Other Device	Z No Qualifier

Non-OR All Values

Coding Clinic: 2017, Q2, P21 – ØXP7ØYZ

SECTION: Ø MEDICAL AND SURGICAL
BODY SYSTEM: X ANATOMICAL REGIONS, UPPER EXTREMITIES
OPERATION: Q REPAIR: Restoring, to the extent possible, a body part to its normal anatomic structure and function

Body Part	Approach	Device	Qualifier
2 Shoulder Region, Right 3 Shoulder Region, Left 4 Axilla, Right 5 Axilla, Left 6 Upper Extremity, Right 7 Upper Extremity, Left 8 Upper Arm, Right 9 Upper Arm, Left B Elbow Region, Right C Elbow Region, Left D Lower Arm, Right F Lower Arm, Left G Wrist Region, Right H Wrist Region, Left J Hand, Right K Hand, Left L Thumb, Right M Thumb, Left N Index Finger, Right P Index Finger, Left Q Middle Finger, Right R Middle Finger, Left S Ring Finger, Right T Ring Finger, Left V Little Finger, Right W Little Finger, Left	Ø Open 3 Percutaneous 4 Percutaneous Endoscopic X External	Z No Device	Z No Qualifier

SECTION: Ø **MEDICAL AND SURGICAL**
BODY SYSTEM: X **ANATOMICAL REGIONS, UPPER EXTREMITIES**
OPERATION: R **REPLACEMENT:** Putting in or on biological or synthetic material that physically takes the place and/or function of all or a portion of a body part

Body Part	Approach	Device	Qualifier
L Thumb, Right M Thumb, Left	Ø Open 4 Percutaneous Endoscopic	7 Autologous Tissue Substitute	N Toe, Right P Toe, Left

SECTION: Ø **MEDICAL AND SURGICAL**
BODY SYSTEM: X **ANATOMICAL REGIONS, UPPER EXTREMITIES**
OPERATION: U **SUPPLEMENT:** Putting in or on biological or synthetic material that physically reinforces and/or augments the function of a portion of a body part

Body Part	Approach	Device	Qualifier
2 Shoulder Region, Right 3 Shoulder Region, Left 4 Axilla, Right 5 Axilla, Left 6 Upper Extremity, Right 7 Upper Extremity, Left 8 Upper Arm, Right 9 Upper Arm, Left B Elbow Region, Right C Elbow Region, Left D Lower Arm, Right F Lower Arm, Left G Wrist Region, Right H Wrist Region, Left J Hand, Right K Hand, Left L Thumb, Right M Thumb, Left N Index Finger, Right P Index Finger, Left Q Middle Finger, Right R Middle Finger, Left S Ring Finger, Right T Ring Finger, Left V Little Finger, Right W Little Finger, Left	Ø Open 4 Percutaneous Endoscopic	7 Autologous Tissue Substitute J Synthetic Substitute K Nonautologous Tissue Substitute	Z No Qualifier

SECTION: Ø MEDICAL AND SURGICAL
BODY SYSTEM: X ANATOMICAL REGIONS, UPPER EXTREMITIES
OPERATION: W REVISION: Correcting, to the extent possible, a portion of a malfunctioning device or the position of displaced device

Body Part	Approach	Device	Qualifier
6 Upper Extremity, Right 7 Upper Extremity, Left	Ø Open 3 Percutaneous 4 Percutaneous Endoscopic X External	Ø Drainage Device 3 Infusion Device 7 Autologous Tissue Substitute J Synthetic Substitute K Nonautologous Tissue Substitute Y Other Device	Z No Qualifier

DRG Non-OR ØXW[67][Ø34][Ø37JKY]Z
Non-OR ØXW[67]X[Ø37JKY]Z

SECTION: Ø MEDICAL AND SURGICAL
BODY SYSTEM: X ANATOMICAL REGIONS, UPPER EXTREMITIES
OPERATION: X TRANSFER: Moving, without taking out, all or a portion of a body part to another location to take over the function of all or a portion of a body part

Body Part	Approach	Device	Qualifier
N Index Finger, Right	Ø Open	Z No Device	L Thumb, Right
P Index Finger, Left	Ø Open	Z No Device	M Thumb, Left

SECTION: Ø MEDICAL AND SURGICAL
BODY SYSTEM: X ANATOMICAL REGIONS, UPPER EXTREMITIES
OPERATION: Y TRANSPLANTATION: Putting in or on all or a portion of a living body part taken from another individual or animal to physically take the place and/or function of all or a portion of a similar body part

Body Part	Approach	Device	Qualifier
J Hand, Right K Hand, Left	Ø Open	Z No Device	Ø Allogeneic 1 Syngeneic

Coding Clinic: 2Ø16, Q4, P112 – ØXY

ØY. Anatomical Regions, Lower Extremities 526
ØYØ. Alteration 527
ØY2. Change 527
ØY3. Control 527
ØY6. Detachment 528
ØY9. Drainage 529
ØYB. Excision 53Ø
ØYH. Insertion 53Ø
ØYJ. Inspection 531
ØYM. Reattachment 532
ØYP. Removal 532
ØYQ. Repair 533
ØYU. Supplement 534
ØYW. Revision 534

SECTION: Ø MEDICAL AND SURGICAL
BODY SYSTEM: Y ANATOMICAL REGIONS, LOWER EXTREMITIES
OPERATION: Ø ALTERATION: Modifying the anatomic structure of a body part without affecting the function of the body part

Body Part	Approach	Device	Qualifier
Ø Buttock, Right 1 Buttock, Left 9 Lower Extremity, Right B Lower Extremity, Left C Upper Leg, Right D Upper Leg, Left F Knee Region, Right G Knee Region, Left H Lower Leg, Right J Lower Leg, Left K Ankle Region, Right L Ankle Region, Left	Ø Open 3 Percutaneous 4 Percutaneous Endoscopic	7 Autologous Tissue Substitute J Synthetic Substitute K Nonautologous Tissue Substitute Z No Device	Z No Qualifier

SECTION: Ø MEDICAL AND SURGICAL
BODY SYSTEM: Y ANATOMICAL REGIONS, LOWER EXTREMITIES
OPERATION: 2 CHANGE: Taking out or off a device from a body part and putting back an identical or similar device in or on the same body part without cutting or puncturing the skin or a mucous membrane

Body Part	Approach	Device	Qualifier
9 Lower Extremity, Right B Lower Extremity, Left	X External	Ø Drainage Device Y Other Device	Z No Qualifier

Non-OR All Values

SECTION: Ø MEDICAL AND SURGICAL
BODY SYSTEM: Y ANATOMICAL REGIONS, LOWER EXTREMITIES
OPERATION: 3 CONTROL: Stopping, or attempting to stop, postprocedure or other acute bleeding

Body Part	Approach	Device	Qualifier
Ø Buttock, Right 1 Buttock, Left 5 Inguinal Region, Right 6 Inguinal Region, Left 7 Femoral Region, Right 8 Femoral Region, Left 9 Lower Extremity, Right B Lower Extremity, Left C Upper Leg, Right D Upper Leg, Left F Knee Region, Right G Knee Region, Left H Lower Leg, Right J Lower Leg, Left K Ankle Region, Right L Ankle Region, Left M Foot, Right N Foot, Left	Ø Open 3 Percutaneous 4 Percutaneous Endoscopic	Z No Device	Z No Qualifier

Coding Clinic: 2Ø16, Q4, P99 – ØY3

SECTION: Ø MEDICAL AND SURGICAL
BODY SYSTEM: Y ANATOMICAL REGIONS, LOWER EXTREMITIES
OPERATION: 6 DETACHMENT: Cutting off all or a portion of the upper or lower extremities

Body Part	Approach	Device	Qualifier
2 Hindquarter, Right 3 Hindquarter, Left 4 Hindquarter, Bilateral 7 Femoral Region, Right 8 Femoral Region, Left F Knee Region, Right G Knee Region, Left	Ø Open	Z No Device	Z No Qualifier
C Upper Leg, Right D Upper Leg, Left H Lower Leg, Right J Lower Leg, Left	Ø Open	Z No Device	1 High 2 Mid 3 Low
M Foot, Right N Foot, Left	Ø Open	Z No Device	Ø Complete 4 Complete 1st Ray 5 Complete 2nd Ray 6 Complete 3rd Ray 7 Complete 4th Ray 8 Complete 5th Ray 9 Partial 1st Ray B Partial 2nd Ray C Partial 3rd Ray D Partial 4th Ray F Partial 5th Ray
P 1st Toe, Right Q 1st Toe, Left	Ø Open	Z No Device	Ø Complete 1 High 3 Low
~~P 1st Toe, Right~~ ~~Q 1st Toe, Left~~ R 2nd Toe, Right S 2nd Toe, Left T 3rd Toe, Right U 3rd Toe, Left V 4th Toe, Right W 4th Toe, Left X 5th Toe, Right Y 5th Toe, Left	Ø Open	Z No Device	Ø Complete 1 High 2 Mid 3 Low

Coding Clinic: 2Ø15, Q1, P28 – ØY6NØZØ
Coding Clinic: 2Ø15, Q2, P29 – ØY6[PQ]ØZ3
Coding Clinic: 2Ø17, Q1, P23 – ØY6NØZØ

SECTION: Ø MEDICAL AND SURGICAL
BODY SYSTEM: Y ANATOMICAL REGIONS, LOWER EXTREMITIES
OPERATION: 9 DRAINAGE: Taking or letting out fluids and/or gases from a body part

Body Part	Approach	Device	Qualifier
Ø Buttock, Right 1 Buttock, Left 5 Inguinal Region, Right 6 Inguinal Region, Left 7 Femoral Region, Right 8 Femoral Region, Left 9 Lower Extremity, Right B Lower Extremity, Left C Upper Leg, Right D Upper Leg, Left F Knee Region, Right G Knee Region, Left H Lower Leg, Right J Lower Leg, Left K Ankle Region, Right L Ankle Region, Left M Foot, Right N Foot, Left	Ø Open 3 Percutaneous 4 Percutaneous Endoscopic	Ø Drainage Device	Z No Qualifier
Ø Buttock, Right 1 Buttock, Left 5 Inguinal Region, Right 6 Inguinal Region, Left 7 Femoral Region, Right 8 Femoral Region, Left 9 Lower Extremity, Right B Lower Extremity, Left C Upper Leg, Right D Upper Leg, Left F Knee Region, Right G Knee Region, Left H Lower Leg, Right J Lower Leg, Left K Ankle Region, Right L Ankle Region, Left M Foot, Right N Foot, Left	Ø Open 3 Percutaneous 4 Percutaneous Endoscopic	Z No Device	X Diagnostic Z No Qualifier

DRG Non-OR ØY9[56]3ØZ
DRG Non-OR ØY9[56]3ZZ
Non-OR ØY9[Ø1789BCDFGHJKLMN][Ø34]ØZ
Non-OR ØY9[Ø1789BCDFGHJKLMN][Ø34]Z[XZ]

Coding Clinic: 2015, Q1, P22-23 – ØY98ØZZ

SECTION: Ø **MEDICAL AND SURGICAL**
BODY SYSTEM: Y **ANATOMICAL REGIONS, LOWER EXTREMITIES**
OPERATION: B **EXCISION:** Cutting out or off, without replacement, a portion of a body part

Body Part	Approach	Device	Qualifier
Ø Buttock, Right 1 Buttock, Left 5 Inguinal Region, Right 6 Inguinal Region, Left 7 Femoral Region, Right 8 Femoral Region, Left 9 Lower Extremity, Right B Lower Extremity, Left C Upper Leg, Right D Upper Leg, Left F Knee Region, Right G Knee Region, Left H Lower Leg, Right J Lower Leg, Left K Ankle Region, Right L Ankle Region, Left M Foot, Right N Foot, Left	Ø Open 3 Percutaneous 4 Percutaneous Endoscopic	Z No Device	X Diagnostic Z No Qualifier

Non-OR ØYB[Ø19BCDFGHJKLMN][Ø34]ZX

SECTION: Ø **MEDICAL AND SURGICAL**
BODY SYSTEM: Y **ANATOMICAL REGIONS, LOWER EXTREMITIES**
OPERATION: H **INSERTION:** Putting in a nonbiological appliance that monitors, assists, performs, or prevents a physiological function but does not physically take the place of a body part

Body Part	Approach	Device	Qualifier
Ø Buttock, Right 1 Buttock, Left 5 Inguinal Region, Right 6 Inguinal Region, Left 7 Femoral Region, Right 8 Femoral Region, Left 9 Lower Extremity, Right B Lower Extremity, Left C Upper Leg, Right D Upper Leg, Left F Knee Region, Right G Knee Region, Left H Lower Leg, Right J Lower Leg, Left K Ankle Region, Right L Ankle Region, Left M Foot, Right N Foot, Left	Ø Open 3 Percutaneous 4 Percutaneous Endoscopic	1 Radioactive Element 3 Infusion Device Y Other Device	Z No Qualifier

DRG Non-OR ØYH[Ø156789BCDFGHJKLMN][Ø34][3Y]Z

Coding Clinic: 2Ø23, Q1, P28-29 – ØYH[CD]ØYZ

SECTION: Ø MEDICAL AND SURGICAL
BODY SYSTEM: Y ANATOMICAL REGIONS, LOWER EXTREMITIES
OPERATION: J INSPECTION: Visually and/or manually exploring a body part

Body Part	Approach	Device	Qualifier
Ø Buttock, Right 1 Buttock, Left 5 Inguinal Region, Right 6 Inguinal Region, Left 7 Femoral Region, Right 8 Femoral Region, Left 9 Lower Extremity, Right A Inguinal Region, Bilateral B Lower Extremity, Left C Upper Leg, Right D Upper Leg, Left E Femoral Region, Bilateral F Knee Region, Right G Knee Region, Left H Lower Leg, Right J Lower Leg, Left K Ankle Region, Right L Ankle Region, Left M Foot, Right N Foot, Left	Ø Open 3 Percutaneous 4 Percutaneous Endoscopic X External	Z No Device	Z No Qualifier

DRG Non-OR ØYJ[Ø19BCDFGHJKLMN]ØZZ
DRG Non-OR ØYJ[567A]3ZZ
DRG Non-OR ØYJ[8E][Ø3]ZZ
Non-OR ØYJ[Ø19BCDFGHJKLMN][34X]ZZ
Non-OR ØYJ[5678AE]XZZ

SECTION: Ø **MEDICAL AND SURGICAL**
BODY SYSTEM: Y **ANATOMICAL REGIONS, LOWER EXTREMITIES**
OPERATION: M **REATTACHMENT:** Putting back in or on all or a portion of a separated body part to its normal location or other suitable location

Body Part	Approach	Device	Qualifier
Ø Buttock, Right 1 Buttock, Left 2 Hindquarter, Right 3 Hindquarter, Left 4 Hindquarter, Bilateral 5 Inguinal Region, Right 6 Inguinal Region, Left 7 Femoral Region, Right 8 Femoral Region, Left 9 Lower Extremity, Right B Lower Extremity, Left C Upper Leg, Right D Upper Leg, Left F Knee Region, Right G Knee Region, Left H Lower Leg, Right J Lower Leg, Left K Ankle Region, Right L Ankle Region, Left M Foot, Right N Foot, Left P 1st Toe, Right Q 1st Toe, Left R 2nd Toe, Right S 2nd Toe, Left T 3rd Toe, Right U 3rd Toe, Left V 4th Toe, Right W 4th Toe, Left X 5th Toe, Right Y 5th Toe, Left	Ø Open	Z No Device	Z No Qualifier

SECTION: Ø **MEDICAL AND SURGICAL**
BODY SYSTEM: Y **ANATOMICAL REGIONS, LOWER EXTREMITIES**
OPERATION: P **REMOVAL:** Taking out or off a device from a body part

Body Part	Approach	Device	Qualifier
9 Lower Extremity, Right B Lower Extremity, Left	Ø Open 3 Percutaneous 4 Percutaneous Endoscopic X External	Ø Drainage Device 1 Radioactive Element 3 Infusion Device 7 Autologous Tissue Substitute J Synthetic Substitute K Nonautologous Tissue Substitute Y Other Device	Z No Qualifier

Non-OR All Values

SECTION: Ø MEDICAL AND SURGICAL
BODY SYSTEM: Y ANATOMICAL REGIONS, LOWER EXTREMITIES
OPERATION: Q REPAIR: Restoring, to the extent possible, a body part to its normal anatomic structure and function

Body Part	Approach	Device	Qualifier
Ø Buttock, Right 1 Buttock, Left 5 Inguinal Region, Right 6 Inguinal Region, Left 7 Femoral Region, Right 8 Femoral Region, Left 9 Lower Extremity, Right A Inguinal Region, Bilateral B Lower Extremity, Left C Upper Leg, Right D Upper Leg, Left E Femoral Region, Bilateral F Knee Region, Right G Knee Region, Left H Lower Leg, Right J Lower Leg, Left K Ankle Region, Right L Ankle Region, Left M Foot, Right N Foot, Left P 1st Toe, Right Q 1st Toe, Left R 2nd Toe, Right S 2nd Toe, Left T 3rd Toe, Right U 3rd Toe, Left V 4th Toe, Right W 4th Toe, Left X 5th Toe, Right Y 5th Toe, Left	Ø Open 3 Percutaneous 4 Percutaneous Endoscopic X External	Z No Device	Z No Qualifier

Non-OR ØYQ[5678AE]XZZ

SECTION: Ø MEDICAL AND SURGICAL
BODY SYSTEM: Y ANATOMICAL REGIONS, LOWER EXTREMITIES
OPERATION: U SUPPLEMENT: Putting in or on biological or synthetic material that physically reinforces and/or augments the function of a portion of a body part

Body Part	Approach	Device	Qualifier
Ø Buttock, Right 1 Buttock, Left 5 Inguinal Region, Right 6 Inguinal Region, Left 7 Femoral Region, Right 8 Femoral Region, Left 9 Lower Extremity, Right A Inguinal Region, Bilateral B Lower Extremity, Left C Upper Leg, Right D Upper Leg, Left E Femoral Region, Bilateral F Knee Region, Right G Knee Region, Left H Lower Leg, Right J Lower Leg, Left K Ankle Region, Right L Ankle Region, Left M Foot, Right N Foot, Left P 1st Toe, Right Q 1st Toe, Left R 2nd Toe, Right S 2nd Toe, Left T 3rd Toe, Right U 3rd Toe, Left V 4th Toe, Right W 4th Toe, Left X 5th Toe, Right Y 5th Toe, Left	Ø Open 4 Percutaneous Endoscopic	7 Autologous Tissue Substitute J Synthetic Substitute K Nonautologous Tissue Substitute	Z No Qualifier

SECTION: Ø MEDICAL AND SURGICAL
BODY SYSTEM: Y ANATOMICAL REGIONS, LOWER EXTREMITIES
OPERATION: W REVISION: Correcting, to the extent possible, a portion of a malfunctioning device or the position of a displaced device

Body Part	Approach	Device	Qualifier
9 Lower Extremity, Right B Lower Extremity, Left	Ø Open 3 Percutaneous 4 Percutaneous Endoscopic X External	Ø Drainage Device 3 Infusion Device 7 Autologous Tissue Substitute J Synthetic Substitute K Nonautologous Tissue Substitute Y Other Device	Z No Qualifier

DRG Non-OR ØYW[9B][Ø34][Ø37JKY]Z
Non-OR ØYW[9B]X[Ø37JKY]Z

1 **Obstetrics** 535
1Ø2. Pregnancy, Change 536
1Ø9. Pregnancy, Drainage 536
1ØA. Pregnancy, Abortion 536
1ØD. Pregnancy, Extraction 537
1ØE. Pregnancy, Delivery 537
1ØH. Pregnancy, Insertion 537
1ØJ. Pregnancy, Inspection 538
1ØP. Pregnancy, Removal 538
1ØQ. Pregnancy, Repair 538
1ØS. Pregnancy, Reposition 539
1ØT. Pregnancy, Resection 539
1ØY. Pregnancy, Transplantation 539

ICD-10-PCS Coding Guidelines

Obstetric Section Guidelines (section 1)

C. Obstetrics Section

Products of conception

C1

Procedures performed on the products of conception are coded to the Obstetrics section. Procedures performed on the pregnant female other than the products of conception are coded to the appropriate root operation in the Medical and Surgical section.

Example: Amniocentesis is coded to the products of conception body part in the Obstetrics section. Repair of obstetric urethral laceration is coded to the urethra body part in the Medical and Surgical section.

Procedures following delivery or abortion

C2

Procedures performed following a delivery or abortion for curettage of the endometrium or evacuation of retained products of conception are all coded in the Obstetrics section, to the root operation Extraction and the body part Products of Conception, Retained. Diagnostic or therapeutic dilation and curettage performed during times other than the postpartum or post-abortion period are all coded in the Medical and Surgical section, to the root operation Extraction and the body part Endometrium.

SECTION: 1 OBSTETRICS
BODY SYSTEM: Ø PREGNANCY
OPERATION: 2 CHANGE: Taking out or off a device from a body part and putting back an identical or similar device in or on the same body part without cutting or puncturing the skin or a mucous membrane

Body Part	Approach	Device	Qualifier
Ø Products of Conception ♀	7 Via Natural or Artificial Opening	3 Monitoring Electrode Y Other Device	Z No Qualifier

Non-OR All Values

SECTION: 1 OBSTETRICS
BODY SYSTEM: Ø PREGNANCY
OPERATION: 9 DRAINAGE: Taking or letting out fluids and/or gases from a body part

Body Part	Approach	Device	Qualifier
Ø Products of Conception ♀	Ø Open 3 Percutaneous 4 Percutaneous Endoscopic 7 Via Natural or Artificial Opening 8 Via Natural or Artificial Opening Endoscopic	Z No Device	9 Fetal Blood A Fetal Cerebrospinal Fluid B Fetal Fluid, Other C Amniotic Fluid, Therapeutic D Fluid, Other U Amniotic Fluid, Diagnostic

Non-OR All Values

SECTION: 1 OBSTETRICS
BODY SYSTEM: Ø PREGNANCY
OPERATION: A ABORTION: Artificially terminating a pregnancy

Body Part	Approach	Device	Qualifier
Ø Products of Conception ♀	Ø Open 3 Percutaneous 4 Percutaneous Endoscopic 8 Via Natural or Artificial Opening Endoscopic	Z No Device	Z No Qualifier
Ø Products of Conception ♀	7 Via Natural or Artificial Opening	Z No Device	6 Vacuum W Laminaria X Abortifacient Z No Qualifier

DRG Non-OR 1ØAØ7Z6
Non-OR 1ØAØ7Z[WX]
Coding Clinic: 2022, Q1, P42 – 1ØAØ7ZZ

SECTION: 1 OBSTETRICS
BODY SYSTEM: Ø PREGNANCY
OPERATION: D EXTRACTION: Pulling or stripping out or off all or a portion of a body part by the use of force

Body Part	Approach	Device	Qualifier
Ø Products of Conception ♀	Ø Open	Z No Device	Ø High 1 Low 2 Extraperitoneal
Ø Products of Conception ♀	7 Via Natural or Artificial Opening	Z No Device	3 Low Forceps 4 Mid Forceps 5 High Forceps 6 Vacuum 7 Internal Version 8 Other
1 Products of Conception, Retained ♀	7 Via Natural or Artificial Opening 8 Via Natural or Artificial Opening Endoscopic	Z No Device	9 Manual Z No Qualifier
2 Products of Conception, Ectopic ♀	Ø Open 4 Percutaneous Endoscopic 7 Via Natural or Artificial Opening 8 Via Natural or Artificial Opening Endoscopic	Z No Device	Z No Qualifier

DRG Non-OR 1ØDØ7Z[345678]

Coding Clinic: 2016, Q1, P1Ø – 1ØDØ7Z3

Coding Clinic: 2018, Q4, P51; 2018, Q2, P18 – 1ØDØØZØ

Coding Clinic: 2022, Q1, P19 – 1ØD17ZZ

SECTION: 1 OBSTETRICS
BODY SYSTEM: Ø PREGNANCY
OPERATION: E DELIVERY: Assisting the passage of the products of conception from the genital canal

Body Part	Approach	Device	Qualifier
Ø Products of Conception ♀	X External	Z No Device	Z No Qualifier

DRG Non-OR 1ØEØXZZ

Coding Clinic: 2016, Q2, P34-35 – 1ØEØXZZ

Coding Clinic: 2017, Q3, P5 – 1ØEØXZZ

SECTION: 1 OBSTETRICS
BODY SYSTEM: Ø PREGNANCY
OPERATION: H INSERTION: Putting in a nonbiological appliance that monitors, assists, performs, or prevents a physiological function but does not physically take the place of a body part

Body Part	Approach	Device	Qualifier
Ø Products of Conception ♀	Ø Open 7 Via Natural or Artificial Opening	3 Monitoring Electrode Y Other Device	Z No Qualifier

Non-OR 1ØHØ7[3Y]Z

Coding Clinic: 2013, Q2, P36 – 1ØHØ7YZ

SECTION: 1 OBSTETRICS
BODY SYSTEM: Ø PREGNANCY
OPERATION: J INSPECTION: Visually and/or manually exploring a body part

Body Part	Approach	Device	Qualifier
Ø Products of Conception ♀ 1 Products of Conception, Retained ♀ 2 Products of Conception, Ectopic ♀	Ø Open 3 Percutaneous 4 Percutaneous Endoscopic 7 Via Natural or Artificial Opening 8 Via Natural or Artificial Opening Endoscopic X External	Z No Device	Z No Qualifier

Non-OR All Values

SECTION: 1 OBSTETRICS
BODY SYSTEM: Ø PREGNANCY
OPERATION: P REMOVAL: Taking out or off a device from a body part, region or orifice

Body Part	Approach	Device	Qualifier
Ø Products of Conception ♀	Ø Open 7 Via Natural or Artificial Opening	3 Monitoring Electrode Y Other Device	Z No Qualifier

Non-OR 1ØP7[3Y]Z

SECTION: 1 OBSTETRICS
BODY SYSTEM: Ø PREGNANCY
OPERATION: Q REPAIR: Restoring, to the extent possible, a body part to its normal anatomic structure and function

Body Part	Approach	Device	Qualifier
Ø Products of Conception ♀	Ø Open 3 Percutaneous 4 Percutaneous Endoscopic 7 Via Natural or Artificial Opening 8 Via Natural or Artificial Opening Endoscopic	Y Other Device Z No Device	E Nervous System F Cardiovascular System G Lymphatics and Hemic H Eye J Ear, Nose, and Sinus K Respiratory System L Mouth and Throat M Gastrointestinal System N Hepatobiliary and Pancreas P Endocrine System Q Skin R Musculoskeletal System S Urinary System T Female Reproductive System V Male Reproductive System Y Other Body System

Non-OR 1ØQØ[Ø3478][YZ][EFGHJKLMNPQRSTVY]

Coding Clinic: 2021, Q2, P22 – 1ØQØØZK

SECTION: 1 OBSTETRICS
BODY SYSTEM: Ø PREGNANCY
OPERATION: S REPOSITION: Moving to its normal location or other suitable location all or a portion of a body part

Body Part	Approach	Device	Qualifier
Ø Products of Conception ♀	7 Via Natural or Artificial Opening X External	Z No Device	Z No Qualifier
2 Products of Conception, Ectopic ♀	Ø Open 3 Percutaneous 4 Percutaneous Endoscopic 7 Via Natural or Artificial Opening 8 Via Natural or Artificial Opening Endoscopic	Z No Device	Z No Qualifier

DRG Non-OR 1ØSØ7ZZ
Non-OR 1ØSØXZZ

SECTION: 1 OBSTETRICS
BODY SYSTEM: Ø PREGNANCY
OPERATION: T RESECTION: Cutting out or off, without replacement, all of a body part

Body Part	Approach	Device	Qualifier
2 Products of Conception, Ectopic ♀	Ø Open 3 Percutaneous 4 Percutaneous Endoscopic 7 Via Natural or Artificial Opening 8 Via Natural or Artificial Opening Endoscopic	Z No Device	Z No Qualifier

Coding Clinic: 2015, Q3, P32 – 1ØT24ZZ

SECTION: 1 OBSTETRICS
BODY SYSTEM: Ø PREGNANCY
OPERATION: Y TRANSPLANTATION: Putting in or on all or a portion of a living body part taken from another individual or animal to physically take the place and/or function of all or a portion of a similar body part

Body Part	Approach	Device	Qualifier
Ø Products of Conception ♀	3 Percutaneous 4 Percutaneous Endoscopic 7 Via Natural or Artificial Opening	Z No Device	E Nervous System F Cardiovascular System G Lymphatics and Hemic H Eye J Ear, Nose, and Sinus K Respiratory System L Mouth and Throat M Gastrointestinal System N Hepatobiliary and Pancreas P Endocrine System Q Skin R Musculoskeletal System S Urinary System T Female Reproductive System V Male Reproductive System Y Other Body System

Non-OR 1ØYØ[347]Z[EFGHJKLMNPQRSTVY]

2 Placement ... **54Ø**
2W. Anatomical Regions ... 541
2WØ. Change ... 541
2W1. Compression ... 542
2W2. Dressing ... 543
2W3. Immobilization ... 544
2W4. Packing ... 545
2W5. Removal ... 546
2W6. Traction ... 547
2Y. Anatomical Orifices ... 548
2YØ. Change ... 548
2Y4. Packing ... 548
2Y5. Removal ... 548

2WØ

SECTION: 2 PLACEMENT

BODY SYSTEM: W ANATOMICAL REGIONS

OPERATION: Ø CHANGE: Taking out or off a device from a body part and putting back an identical or similar device in or on the same body part without cutting or puncturing the skin or a mucous membrane

Body Region	Approach	Device	Qualifier
Ø Head 2 Neck 3 Abdominal Wall 4 Chest Wall 5 Back 6 Inguinal Region, Right 7 Inguinal Region, Left 8 Upper Extremity, Right 9 Upper Extremity, Left A Upper Arm, Right B Upper Arm, Left C Lower Arm, Right D Lower Arm, Left E Hand, Right F Hand, Left G Thumb, Right H Thumb, Left J Finger, Right K Finger, Left L Lower Extremity, Right M Lower Extremity, Left N Upper Leg, Right P Upper Leg, Left Q Lower Leg, Right R Lower Leg, Left S Foot, Right T Foot, Left U Toe, Right V Toe, Left	X External	Ø Traction Apparatus 1 Splint 2 Cast 3 Brace 4 Bandage 5 Packing Material 6 Pressure Dressing 7 Intermittent Pressure Device Y Other Device	Z No Qualifier
1 Face	X External	Ø Traction Apparatus 1 Splint 2 Cast 3 Brace 4 Bandage 5 Packing Material 6 Pressure Dressing 7 Intermittent Pressure Device 9 Wire Y Other Device	Z No Qualifier

SECTION: 2 PLACEMENT
BODY SYSTEM: W ANATOMICAL REGIONS
OPERATION: 1 COMPRESSION: Putting pressure on a body region

Body Region	Approach	Device	Qualifier
Ø Head 1 Face 2 Neck 3 Abdominal Wall 4 Chest Wall 5 Back 6 Inguinal Region, Right 7 Inguinal Region, Left 8 Upper Extremity, Right 9 Upper Extremity, Left A Upper Arm, Right B Upper Arm, Left C Lower Arm, Right D Lower Arm, Left E Hand, Right F Hand, Left G Thumb, Right H Thumb, Left J Finger, Right K Finger, Left L Lower Extremity, Right M Lower Extremity, Left N Upper Leg, Right P Upper Leg, Left Q Lower Leg, Right R Lower Leg, Left S Foot, Right T Foot, Left U Toe, Right V Toe, Left	X External	6 Pressure Dressing 7 Intermittent Pressure Device	Z No Qualifier

SECTION: 2 PLACEMENT
BODY SYSTEM: W ANATOMICAL REGIONS
OPERATION: 2 DRESSING: Putting material on a body region for protection

Body Region	Approach	Device	Qualifier
Ø Head 1 Face 2 Neck 3 Abdominal Wall 4 Chest Wall 5 Back 6 Inguinal Region, Right 7 Inguinal Region, Left 8 Upper Extremity, Right 9 Upper Extremity, Left A Upper Arm, Right B Upper Arm, Left C Lower Arm, Right D Lower Arm, Left E Hand, Right F Hand, Left G Thumb, Right H Thumb, Left J Finger, Right K Finger, Left L Lower Extremity, Right M Lower Extremity, Left N Upper Leg, Right P Upper Leg, Left Q Lower Leg, Right R Lower Leg, Left S Foot, Right T Foot, Left U Toe, Right V Toe, Left	X External	4 Bandage	Z No Qualifier

SECTION: 2 PLACEMENT
BODY SYSTEM: W ANATOMICAL REGIONS
OPERATION: 3 IMMOBILIZATION: Limiting or preventing motion of a body region

Body Region	Approach	Device	Qualifier
Ø Head 2 Neck 3 Abdominal Wall 4 Chest Wall 5 Back 6 Inguinal Region, Right 7 Inguinal Region, Left 8 Upper Extremity, Right 9 Upper Extremity, Left A Upper Arm, Right B Upper Arm, Left C Lower Arm, Right D Lower Arm, Left E Hand, Right F Hand, Left G Thumb, Right H Thumb, Left J Finger, Right K Finger, Left L Lower Extremity, Right M Lower Extremity, Left N Upper Leg, Right P Upper Leg, Left Q Lower Leg, Right R Lower Leg, Left S Foot, Right T Foot, Left U Toe, Right V Toe, Left	X External	1 Splint 2 Cast 3 Brace Y Other Device	Z No Qualifier
1 Face	X External	1 Splint 2 Cast 3 Brace 9 Wire Y Other Device	Z No Qualifier

SECTION: 2 PLACEMENT
BODY SYSTEM: W ANATOMICAL REGIONS
OPERATION: 4 PACKING: Putting material in a body region or orifice

Body Region	Approach	Device	Qualifier
Ø Head 1 Face 2 Neck 3 Abdominal Wall 4 Chest Wall 5 Back 6 Inguinal Region, Right 7 Inguinal Region, Left 8 Upper Extremity, Right 9 Upper Extremity, Left A Upper Arm, Right B Upper Arm, Left C Lower Arm, Right D Lower Arm, Left E Hand, Right F Hand, Left G Thumb, Right H Thumb, Left J Finger, Right K Finger, Left L Lower Extremity, Right M Lower Extremity, Left N Upper Leg, Right P Upper Leg, Left Q Lower Leg, Right R Lower Leg, Left S Foot, Right T Foot, Left U Toe, Right V Toe, Left	X External	5 Packing Material	Z No Qualifier

SECTION: 2 PLACEMENT

BODY SYSTEM: W ANATOMICAL REGIONS

OPERATION: 5 REMOVAL: Taking out or off a device from a body part

Body Region	Approach	Device	Qualifier
Ø Head 2 Neck 3 Abdominal Wall 4 Chest Wall 5 Back 6 Inguinal Region, Right 7 Inguinal Region, Left 8 Upper Extremity, Right 9 Upper Extremity, Left A Upper Arm, Right B Upper Arm, Left C Lower Arm, Right D Lower Arm, Left E Hand, Right F Hand, Left G Thumb, Right H Thumb, Left J Finger, Right K Finger, Left L Lower Extremity, Right M Lower Extremity, Left N Upper Leg, Right P Upper Leg, Left Q Lower Leg, Right R Lower Leg, Left S Foot, Right T Foot, Left U Toe, Right V Toe, Left	X External	Ø Traction Apparatus 1 Splint 2 Cast 3 Brace 4 Bandage 5 Packing Material 6 Pressure Dressing 7 Intermittent Pressure Device Y Other Device	Z No Qualifier
1 Face	X External	Ø Traction Apparatus 1 Splint 2 Cast 3 Brace 4 Bandage 5 Packing Material 6 Pressure Dressing 7 Intermittent Pressure Device 9 Wire Y Other Device	Z No Qualifier

2: PLACEMENT W: ANATOMICAL REGIONS 5: REMOVAL

New/Revised Text in Green ~~deleted~~ Deleted ♀ Females Only ♂ Males Only Coding Clinic
Non-covered Limited Coverage Combination (See Appendix E) DRG Non-OR Non-OR Hospital-Acquired Condition

SECTION: 2 PLACEMENT
BODY SYSTEM: W ANATOMICAL REGIONS
OPERATION: 6 TRACTION: Exerting a pulling force on a body region in a distal direction

Body Region	Approach	Device	Qualifier
Ø Head 1 Face 2 Neck 3 Abdominal Wall 4 Chest Wall 5 Back 6 Inguinal Region, Right 7 Inguinal Region, Left 8 Upper Extremity, Right 9 Upper Extremity, Left A Upper Arm, Right B Upper Arm, Left C Lower Arm, Right D Lower Arm, Left E Hand, Right F Hand, Left G Thumb, Right H Thumb, Left J Finger, Right K Finger, Left L Lower Extremity, Right M Lower Extremity, Left N Upper Leg, Right P Upper Leg, Left Q Lower Leg, Right R Lower Leg, Left S Foot, Right T Foot, Left U Toe, Right V Toe, Left	X External	Ø Traction Apparatus Z No Device	Z No Qualifier

Coding Clinic: 2Ø15, Q2, P35; 2Ø13, Q2, P39 – 2W6ØXØZ
Coding Clinic: 2Ø15, Q2, P35 – 2W62XØZ

SECTION: 2 PLACEMENT
BODY SYSTEM: Y ANATOMICAL ORIFICES
OPERATION: Ø CHANGE: Taking out or off a device from a body part and putting back an identical or similar device in or on the same body part without cutting or puncturing the skin or a mucous membrane

Body Region	Approach	Device	Qualifier
Ø Mouth and Pharynx 1 Nasal 2 Ear 3 Anorectal 4 Female Genital Tract ♀ 5 Urethra	X External	5 Packing Material	Z No Qualifier

SECTION: 2 PLACEMENT
BODY SYSTEM: Y ANATOMICAL ORIFICES
OPERATION: 4 PACKING: Putting material in a body region or orifice

Body Region	Approach	Device	Qualifier
Ø Mouth and Pharynx 1 Nasal 2 Ear 3 Anorectal 4 Female Genital Tract ♀ 5 Urethra	X External	5 Packing Material	Z No Qualifier

Coding Clinic: 2Ø18, Q4, P38; 2Ø17, Q4, P1Ø6 – 2Y41X5Z

SECTION: 2 PLACEMENT
BODY SYSTEM: Y ANATOMICAL ORIFICES
OPERATION: 5 REMOVAL: Taking out or off a device from a body part

Body Region	Approach	Device	Qualifier
Ø Mouth and Pharynx 1 Nasal 2 Ear 3 Anorectal 4 Female Genital Tract ♀ 5 Urethra	X External	5 Packing Material	Z No Qualifier

3 Administration **549**
30. Circulatory 550
302. Transfusion 550
3C. Indwelling Device 552
3C1. Irrigation 552
3E. Physiological Systems and Anatomical Regions 552
3E0. Introduction 552
3E1. Irrigation 566

SECTION: 3 ADMINISTRATION
BODY SYSTEM: Ø CIRCULATORY
OPERATION: 2 TRANSFUSION: *(on multiple pages)*
Putting in blood or blood products

Body System / Region	Approach	Substance	Qualifier
3 Peripheral Vein 4 Central Vein	3 Percutaneous	A Stem Cells, Embryonic	Z No Qualifier
3 Peripheral Vein 4 Central Vein	3 Percutaneous	C Hematopoietic Stem/ Progenitor Cells, Genetically Modified	Ø Autologous
3 Peripheral Vein 4 Central Vein	3 Percutaneous	D Pathogen Reduced Cryoprecipitated Fibrinogen Complex	1 Nonautologous
3 Peripheral Vein 4 Central Vein	3 Percutaneous	G Bone Marrow X Stem Cells, Cord Blood Y Stem Cells, Hematopoietic	Ø Autologous 2 Allogeneic, Related 3 Allogeneic, Unrelated 4 Allogeneic, Unspecified
3 Peripheral Vein 4 Central Vein	3 Percutaneous	H Whole Blood J Serum Albumin K Frozen Plasma L Fresh Plasma M Plasma Cryoprecipitate N Red Blood Cells P Frozen Red Cells Q White Cells R Platelets S Globulin T Fibrinogen V Antihemophilic Factors W Factor IX	Ø Autologous 1 Nonautologous
3 Peripheral Vein 4 Central Vein	3 Percutaneous	U Stem Cells, T-cell Depleted Hematopoietic	2 Allogeneic, Related 3 Allogeneic, Unrelated 4 Allogeneic, Unspecified

302[34][3]AZ is identified as non-covered when a code from the diagnosis list below is present as a principal or secondary diagnosis

C91ØØ	C924Ø	C93ØØ
C92ØØ	C925Ø	C94ØØ
C921Ø	C926Ø	C95ØØ
C9211	C92AØ	

Non-OR 3Ø2[34][Ø3][HJKLMNPQRSTUVWX][Ø1234]

New/Revised Text in Green ~~deleted~~ Deleted ♀ Females Only ♂ Males Only Coding Clinic
Non-covered Limited Coverage Combination (See Appendix E) DRG Non-OR Non-OR Hospital-Acquired Condition

3: ADMINISTRATION Ø: CIRCULATORY 2: TRANSFUSION

SECTION: 3 ADMINISTRATION
BODY SYSTEM: Ø CIRCULATORY
OPERATION: 2 TRANSFUSION: *(continued)*
Putting in blood or blood products

Body System / Region	Approach	Substance	Qualifier
7 Products of Conception, Circulatory ♀	3 Percutaneous 7 Via Natural or Artificial Opening	H Whole Blood J Serum Albumin K Frozen Plasma L Fresh Plasma M Plasma Cryoprecipitate N Red Blood Cells P Frozen Red Cells Q White Cells R Platelets S Globulin T Fibrinogen V Antihemophilic Factors W Factor IX	1 Nonautologous
8 Vein	3 Percutaneous	B 4-Factor Prothrombin Complex Concentrate	1 Nonautologous
A Bone Marrow	3 Percutaneous	H Whole Blood J Serum Albumin K Frozen Plasma L Fresh Plasma N Red Blood Cells P Frozen Red Cells R Platelets	Ø Autologous 1 Nonautologous

Non-OR 3Ø27[37][HJKLMNPQRSTVW]1
Non-OR 3Ø28[Ø3]B1

Coding Clinic: 2Ø23, Q1, P11 – 3Ø2A3H1

SECTION: 3 ADMINISTRATION
BODY SYSTEM: C INDWELLING DEVICE
OPERATION: 1 IRRIGATION: Putting in or on a cleansing substance

Body System / Region	Approach	Substance	Qualifier
Z None	X External	8 Irrigating Substance	Z No Qualifier

SECTION: 3 ADMINISTRATION
BODY SYSTEM: E PHYSIOLOGICAL SYSTEMS AND ANATOMICAL REGIONS
OPERATION: Ø INTRODUCTION: *(on multiple pages)*

Putting in or on a therapeutic, diagnostic, nutritional, physiological, or prophylactic substance except blood or blood products

Body System / Region	Approach	Substance	Qualifier
Ø Skin and Mucous Membranes	X External	Ø Antineoplastic	5 Other Antineoplastic M Monoclonal Antibody
Ø Skin and Mucous Membranes	X External	2 Anti-infective	8 Oxazolidinones 9 Other Anti-infective
Ø Skin and Mucous Membranes	X External	3 Anti-inflammatory 4 Serum, Toxoid and Vaccine B Anesthetic Agent K Other Diagnostic Substance M Pigment N Analgesics, Hypnotics, Sedatives T Destructive Agent	Z No Qualifier
Ø Skin and Mucous Membranes	X External	G Other Therapeutic Substance	C Other Substance
1 Subcutaneous Tissue	Ø Open	2 Anti-infective	A Anti-Infective Envelope
1 Subcutaneous Tissue	3 Percutaneous	Ø Antineoplastic	5 Other Antineoplastic M Monoclonal Antibody
1 Subcutaneous Tissue	3 Percutaneous	2 Anti-infective	8 Oxazolidinones 9 Other Anti-infective A Anti-Infective Envelope
1 Subcutaneous Tissue	3 Percutaneous	3 Anti-inflammatory 6 Nutritional Substance 7 Electrolytic and Water Balance Substance B Anesthetic Agent H Radioactive Substance K Other Diagnostic Substance N Analgesics, Hypnotics, Sedatives T Destructive Agent	Z No Qualifier
1 Subcutaneous Tissue	3 Percutaneous	4 Serum, Toxoid and Vaccine	Ø Influenza Vaccine Z No Qualifier
1 Subcutaneous Tissue	3 Percutaneous	G Other Therapeutic Substance	C Other Substance
1 Subcutaneous Tissue	3 Percutaneous	V Hormone	G Insulin J Other Hormone
2 Muscle	3 Percutaneous	Ø Antineoplastic	5 Other Antineoplastic M Monoclonal Antibody

SECTION: 3 ADMINISTRATION
BODY SYSTEM: E PHYSIOLOGICAL SYSTEMS AND ANATOMICAL REGIONS
OPERATION: Ø INTRODUCTION: *(continued)*

Putting in or on a therapeutic, diagnostic, nutritional, physiological, or prophylactic substance except blood or blood products

Body System / Region	Approach	Substance	Qualifier
2 Muscle	3 Percutaneous	2 Anti-infective	8 Oxazolidinones 9 Other Anti-infective
2 Muscle	3 Percutaneous	3 Anti-inflammatory 6 Nutritional Substance 7 Electrolytic and Water Balance Substance B Anesthetic Agent H Radioactive Substance K Other Diagnostic Substance N Analgesics, Hypnotics, Sedatives T Destructive Agent	Z No Qualifier
2 Muscle	3 Percutaneous	4 Serum, Toxoid and Vaccine	Ø Influenza Vaccine Z No Qualifier
2 Muscle	3 Percutaneous	G Other Therapeutic Substance	C Other Substance
3 Peripheral Vein	Ø Open	Ø Antineoplastic	2 High-dose Interleukin-2 3 Low-dose Interleukin-2 5 Other Antineoplastic M Monoclonal Antibody P Clofarabine
3 Peripheral Vein	Ø Open	1 Thrombolytic	6 Recombinant Human-activated Protein C 7 Other Thrombolytic
3 Peripheral Vein	Ø Open	2 Anti-infective	8 Oxazolidinones 9 Other Anti-infective
3 Peripheral Vein	Ø Open	3 Anti-inflammatory 4 Serum, Toxoid and Vaccine 6 Nutritional Substance 7 Electrolytic and Water Balance Substance F Intracirculatory Anesthetic H Radioactive Substance K Other Diagnostic Substance N Analgesics, Hypnotics, Sedatives P Platelet Inhibitor R Antiarrhythmic T Destructive Agent X Vasopressor	Z No Qualifier
3 Peripheral Vein	Ø Open	G Other Therapeutic Substance	C Other Substance N Blood Brain Barrier Disruption
3 Peripheral Vein	Ø Open	U Pancreatic Islet Cells	Ø Autologous 1 Nonautologous
3 Peripheral Vein	Ø Open	V Hormone	G Insulin H Human B-type Natriuretic Peptide J Other Hormone
3 Peripheral Vein	Ø Open	W Immunotherapeutic	K Immunostimulator L Immunosuppressive

DRG Non-OR 3EØ3ØØ2
DRG Non-OR 3EØ3Ø17
DRG Non-OR 3EØ3ØU[Ø1]

SECTION: 3 ADMINISTRATION
BODY SYSTEM: E PHYSIOLOGICAL SYSTEMS AND ANATOMICAL REGIONS
OPERATION: Ø INTRODUCTION: *(continued)*

Putting in or on a therapeutic, diagnostic, nutritional, physiological, or prophylactic substance except blood or blood products

Body System / Region	Approach	Substance	Qualifier
3 Peripheral Vein	3 Percutaneous	Ø Antineoplastic	2 High-dose Interleukin-2 3 Low-dose Interleukin-2 5 Other Antineoplastic M Monoclonal Antibody P Clofarabine
3 Peripheral Vein	3 Percutaneous	1 Thrombolytic	6 Recombinant Human-activated Protein C 7 Other Thrombolytic
3 Peripheral Vein	3 Percutaneous	2 Anti-infective	8 Oxazolidinones 9 Other Anti-infective
3 Peripheral Vein	3 Percutaneous	3 Anti-inflammatory 4 Serum, Toxoid and Vaccine 6 Nutritional Substance 7 Electrolytic and Water Balance Substance F Intracirculatory Anesthetic H Radioactive Substance K Other Diagnostic Substance N Analgesics, Hypnotics, Sedatives P Platelet Inhibitor R Antiarrhythmic T Destructive Agent X Vasopressor	Z No Qualifier
3 Peripheral Vein	3 Percutaneous	G Other Therapeutic Substance	C Other Substance N Blood Brain Barrier Disruption Q Glucarpidase R Other Therapeutic Monoclonal Antibody
3 Peripheral Vein	3 Percutaneous	U Pancreatic Islet Cells	Ø Autologous 1 Nonautologous
3 Peripheral Vein	3 Percutaneous	V Hormone	G Insulin H Human B-type Natriuretic Peptide J Other Hormone
3 Peripheral Vein	3 Percutaneous	W Immunotherapeutic	K Immunostimulator L Immunosuppressive
4 Central Vein	Ø Open	Ø Antineoplastic	2 High-dose Interleukin-2 3 Low-dose Interleukin-2 5 Other Antineoplastic M Monoclonal Antibody P Clofarabine
4 Central Vein	Ø Open	1 Thrombolytic	6 Recombinant Human-activated Protein C 7 Other Thrombolytic
4 Central Vein	Ø Open	2 Anti-infective	8 Oxazolidinones 9 Other Anti-infective

DRG Non-OR 3EØ33Ø2
DRG Non-OR 3EØ3317
DRG Non-OR 3EØ33U[Ø1]
DRG Non-OR 3EØ4ØØ2
DRG Non-OR 3EØ417
DRG Non-OR 3EØ33TZ *(proposed)*

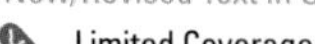
New/Revised Text in Green ~~deleted~~ Deleted ♀ Females Only ♂ Males Only Coding Clinic
Non-covered Limited Coverage Combination (See Appendix E) DRG Non-OR Non-OR Hospital-Acquired Condition

SECTION: 3 ADMINISTRATION
BODY SYSTEM: E PHYSIOLOGICAL SYSTEMS AND ANATOMICAL REGIONS
OPERATION: Ø INTRODUCTION: *(continued)*

Putting in or on a therapeutic, diagnostic, nutritional, physiological, or prophylactic substance except blood or blood products

Body System / Region	Approach	Substance	Qualifier
4 Central Vein	Ø Open	3 Anti-inflammatory 4 Serum, Toxoid and Vaccine 6 Nutritional Substance 7 Electrolytic and Water Balance Substance F Intracirculatory Anesthetic H Radioactive Substance K Other Diagnostic Substance N Analgesics, Hypnotics, Sedatives P Platelet Inhibitor R Antiarrhythmic T Destructive Agent X Vasopressor	Z No Qualifier
4 Central Vein	Ø Open	G Other Therapeutic Substance	C Other Substance N Blood Brain Barrier Disruption
4 Central Vein	Ø Open	V Hormone	G Insulin H Human B-type Natriuretic Peptide J Other Hormone
4 Central Vein	Ø Open	W Immunotherapeutic	K Immunostimulator L Immunosuppressive
4 Central Vein	3 Percutaneous	Ø Antineoplastic	2 High-dose Interleukin-2 3 Low-dose Interleukin-2 5 Other Antineoplastic M Monoclonal Antibody P Clofarabine
4 Central Vein	3 Percutaneous	1 Thrombolytic	6 Recombinant Human-activated Protein C 7 Other Thrombolytic
4 Central Vein	3 Percutaneous	2 Anti-infective	8 Oxazolidinones 9 Other Anti-infective
4 Central Vein	3 Percutaneous	3 Anti-inflammatory 4 Serum, Toxoid and Vaccine 6 Nutritional Substance 7 Electrolytic and Water Balance Substance F Intracirculatory Anesthetic H Radioactive Substance K Other Diagnostic Substance N Analgesics, Hypnotics, Sedatives P Platelet Inhibitor R Antiarrhythmic T Destructive Agent X Vasopressor	Z No Qualifier
4 Central Vein	3 Percutaneous	G Other Therapeutic Substance	C Other Substance N Blood Brain Barrier Disruption Q Glucarpidase R Other Therapeutic Monoclonal Antibody
4 Central Vein	3 Percutaneous	V Hormone	G Insulin H Human B-type Natriuretic Peptide J Other Hormone

DRG Non-OR 3EØ43Ø2 DRG Non-OR 3EØ4317 DRG Non-OR 3EØ43TZ *(proposed)*

Coding Clinic: 2022, Q3, P26 – 3EØ43GC

SECTION: 3 ADMINISTRATION
BODY SYSTEM: E PHYSIOLOGICAL SYSTEMS AND ANATOMICAL REGIONS
OPERATION: Ø INTRODUCTION: *(continued)*

Putting in or on a therapeutic, diagnostic, nutritional, physiological, or prophylactic substance except blood or blood products

Body System / Region	Approach	Substance	Qualifier
4 Central Vein	3 Percutaneous	W Immunotherapeutic	K Immunostimulator L Immunosuppressive
5 Peripheral Artery 6 Central Artery	Ø Open 3 Percutaneous	Ø Antineoplastic	2 High-dose Interleukin-2 3 Low-dose Interleukin-2 5 Other Antineoplastic M Monoclonal Antibody P Clofarabine
5 Peripheral Artery 6 Central Artery	Ø Open 3 Percutaneous	1 Thrombolytic	6 Recombinant Human-activated Protein C 7 Other Thrombolytic
5 Peripheral Artery 6 Central Artery	Ø Open 3 Percutaneous	2 Anti-infective	8 Oxazolidinones 9 Other Anti-infective
5 Peripheral Artery 6 Central Artery	Ø Open 3 Percutaneous	3 Anti-inflammatory 4 Serum, Toxoid and Vaccine 6 Nutritional Substance 7 Electrolytic and Water Balance Substance F Intracirculatory Anesthetic H Radioactive Substance K Other Diagnostic Substance N Analgesics, Hypnotics, Sedatives P Platelet Inhibitor R Antiarrhythmic T Destructive Agent X Vasopressor	Z No Qualifier
5 Peripheral Artery 6 Central Artery	Ø Open 3 Percutaneous	G Other Therapeutic Substance	C Other Substance N Blood Brain Barrier Disruption
5 Peripheral Artery 6 Central Artery	Ø Open 3 Percutaneous	V Hormone	G Insulin H Human B-type Natriuretic Peptide J Other Hormone
5 Peripheral Artery 6 Central Artery	Ø Open 3 Percutaneous	W Immunotherapeutic	K Immunostimulator L Immunosuppressive
7 Coronary Artery 8 Heart	Ø Open 3 Percutaneous	1 Thrombolytic	6 Recombinant Human-activated Protein C 7 Other Thrombolytic
7 Coronary Artery 8 Heart	Ø Open 3 Percutaneous	G Other Therapeutic Substance	C Other Substance
7 Coronary Artery 8 Heart	Ø Open 3 Percutaneous	K Other Diagnostic Substance P Platelet Inhibitor	Z No Qualifier
7 Coronary Artery 8 Heart	4 Percutaneous Endoscopic	G Other Therapeutic Substance	C Other Substance
9 Nose	3 Percutaneous 7 Via Natural or Artificial Opening X External	Ø Antineoplastic	5 Other Antineoplastic M Monoclonal Antibody
9 Nose	3 Percutaneous 7 Via Natural or Artificial Opening X External	2 Anti-infective	8 Oxazolidinones 9 Other Anti-infective

DRG Non-OR 3EØ[56][Ø3]Ø2
DRG Non-OR 3EØ[56][Ø3]17
DRG Non-OR 3EØ8[Ø3]17

SECTION: 3 ADMINISTRATION
BODY SYSTEM: E PHYSIOLOGICAL SYSTEMS AND ANATOMICAL REGIONS
OPERATION: Ø INTRODUCTION: *(continued)*

Putting in or on a therapeutic, diagnostic, nutritional, physiological, or prophylactic substance except blood or blood products

Body System / Region	Approach	Substance	Qualifier
9 Nose	3 Percutaneous 7 Via Natural or Artificial Opening X External	3 Anti-inflammatory 4 Serum, Toxoid and Vaccine B Anesthetic Agent H Radioactive Substance K Other Diagnostic Substance N Analgesics, Hypnotics, Sedatives T Destructive Agent	Z No Qualifier
9 Nose	3 Percutaneous 7 Via Natural or Artificial Opening X External	G Other Therapeutic Substance	C Other Substance
A Bone Marrow	3 Percutaneous	Ø Antineoplastic	5 Other Antineoplastic M Monoclonal Antibody
A Bone Marrow	3 Percutaneous	G Other Therapeutic Substance	C Other Substance
B Ear	3 Percutaneous 7 Via Natural or Artificial Opening X External	Ø Antineoplastic	4 Liquid Brachytherapy Radioisotope 5 Other Antineoplastic M Monoclonal Antibody
B Ear	3 Percutaneous 7 Via Natural or Artificial Opening X External	2 Anti-infective	8 Oxazolidinones 9 Other Anti-infective
B Ear	3 Percutaneous 7 Via Natural or Artificial Opening X External	3 Anti-inflammatory B Anesthetic Agent H Radioactive Substance K Other Diagnostic Substance N Analgesics, Hypnotics, Sedatives T Destructive Agent	Z No Qualifier
B Ear	3 Percutaneous 7 Via Natural or Artificial Opening X External	G Other Therapeutic Substance	C Other Substance
C Eye	3 Percutaneous 7 Via Natural or Artificial Opening X External	Ø Antineoplastic	4 Liquid Brachytherapy Radioisotope 5 Other Antineoplastic M Monoclonal Antibody
C Eye	3 Percutaneous 7 Via Natural or Artificial Opening X External	2 Anti-infective	8 Oxazolidinones 9 Other Anti-infective
C Eye	3 Percutaneous 7 Via Natural or Artificial Opening X External	3 Anti-inflammatory B Anesthetic Agent H Radioactive Substance K Other Diagnostic Substance M Pigment N Analgesics, Hypnotics, Sedatives T Destructive Agent	Z No Qualifier
C Eye	3 Percutaneous 7 Via Natural or Artificial Opening X External	G Other Therapeutic Substance	C Other Substance

DRG Non-OR 3EØB329 *(proposed)*
DRG Non-OR 3EØB33Z *(proposed)*
DRG Non-OR 3EØB3[GHKT]C *(proposed)*
DRG Non-OR 3EØB[7X]29 *(proposed)*
DRG Non-OR 3EØB[7X][3BHKT]Z *(proposed)*
DRG Non-OR 3EØB[7X]GC *(proposed)*
DRG Non-OR 3EØC[37X][3BHKMT]Z *(proposed)*
DRG Non-OR 3EØC[37X]GC *(proposed)*
DRG Non-OR 3EØC[37X]SF *(proposed)*
DRG Non-OR 3EØC[7X]29 *(proposed)*

SECTION: 3 ADMINISTRATION
BODY SYSTEM: E PHYSIOLOGICAL SYSTEMS AND ANATOMICAL REGIONS
OPERATION: Ø INTRODUCTION: *(continued)*

Putting in or on a therapeutic, diagnostic, nutritional, physiological, or prophylactic substance except blood or blood products

Body System / Region	Approach	Substance	Qualifier
C Eye	3 Percutaneous 7 Via Natural or Artificial Opening X External	S Gas	F Other Gas
D Mouth and Pharynx	3 Percutaneous 7 Via Natural or Artificial Opening X External	Ø Antineoplastic	4 Liquid Brachytherapy Radioisotope 5 Other Antineoplastic M Monoclonal Antibody
D Mouth and Pharynx	3 Percutaneous 7 Via Natural or Artificial Opening X External	2 Anti-infective	8 Oxazolidinones 9 Other Anti-infective
D Mouth and Pharynx	3 Percutaneous 7 Via Natural or Artificial Opening X External	3 Anti-inflammatory 4 Serum, Toxoid and Vaccine 6 Nutritional Substance 7 Electrolytic and Water Balance Substance B Anesthetic Agent H Radioactive Substance K Other Diagnostic Substance N Analgesics, Hypnotics, Sedatives R Antiarrhythmic T Destructive Agent	Z No Qualifier
D Mouth and Pharynx	3 Percutaneous 7 Via Natural or Artificial Opening X External	G Other Therapeutic Substance	C Other Substance
E Products of Conception ♀ G Upper GI H Lower GI K Genitourinary Tract N Male Reproductive ♂	3 Percutaneous 7 Via Natural or Artificial Opening 8 Via Natural or Artificial Opening Endoscopic	Ø Antineoplastic	4 Liquid Brachytherapy Radioisotope 5 Other Antineoplastic M Monoclonal Antibody
E Products of Conception ♀ G Upper GI H Lower GI K Genitourinary Tract N Male Reproductive ♂	3 Percutaneous 7 Via Natural or Artificial Opening 8 Via Natural or Artificial Opening Endoscopic	2 Anti-infective	8 Oxazolidinones 9 Other Anti-infective
E Products of Conception ♀ G Upper GI H Lower GI K Genitourinary Tract N Male Reproductive ♂	3 Percutaneous 7 Via Natural or Artificial Opening 8 Via Natural or Artificial Opening Endoscopic	3 Anti-inflammatory 6 Nutritional Substance 7 Electrolytic and Water Balance Substance B Anesthetic Agent H Radioactive Substance K Other Diagnostic Substance N Analgesics, Hypnotics, Sedatives T Destructive Agent	Z No Qualifier
E Products of Conception ♀ G Upper GI H Lower GI K Genitourinary Tract N Male Reproductive ♂	3 Percutaneous 7 Via Natural or Artificial Opening 8 Via Natural or Artificial Opening Endoscopic	G Other Therapeutic Substance	C Other Substance

Coding Clinic: 2023, Q2, P34 – 3EØE3KZ

SECTION: 3 ADMINISTRATION
BODY SYSTEM: E PHYSIOLOGICAL SYSTEMS AND ANATOMICAL REGIONS
OPERATION: Ø INTRODUCTION: *(continued)*

Putting in or on a therapeutic, diagnostic, nutritional, physiological, or prophylactic substance except blood or blood products

Body System / Region	Approach	Substance	Qualifier
E Products of Conception ♀ G Upper GI H Lower GI K Genitourinary Tract N Male Reproductive ♂	3 Percutaneous 7 Via Natural or Artificial Opening 8 Via Natural or Artificial Opening Endoscopic	S Gas	F Other Gas
E Products of Conception ♀ G Upper GI H Lower GI K Genitourinary Tract N Male Reproductive ♂	4 Percutaneous Endoscopic	G Other Therapeutic Substance	C Other Substance
F Respiratory Tract	3 Percutaneous 7 Via Natural or Artificial Opening 8 Via Natural or Artificial Opening Endoscopic	Ø Antineoplastic	4 Liquid Brachytherapy Radioisotope 5 Other Antineoplastic M Monoclonal Antibody
F Respiratory Tract	3 Percutaneous 7 Via Natural or Artificial Opening 8 Via Natural or Artificial Opening Endoscopic	2 Anti-infective	8 Oxazolidinones 9 Other Anti-infective
F Respiratory Tract	3 Percutaneous 7 Via Natural or Artificial Opening 8 Via Natural or Artificial Opening Endoscopic	3 Anti-inflammatory 6 Nutritional Substance 7 Electrolytic and Water Balance Substance B Anesthetic Agent H Radioactive Substance K Other Diagnostic Substance N Analgesics, Hypnotics, Sedatives T Destructive Agent	Z No Qualifier
F Respiratory Tract	3 Percutaneous 7 Via Natural or Artificial Opening 8 Via Natural or Artificial Opening Endoscopic	G Other Therapeutic Substance	C Other Substance
F Respiratory Tract	3 Percutaneous 7 Via Natural or Artificial Opening 8 Via Natural or Artificial Opening Endoscopic	S Gas	D Nitric Oxide F Other Gas
F Respiratory Tract	4 Percutaneous Endoscopic	G Other Therapeutic Substance	C Other Substance
J Biliary and Pancreatic Tract	3 Percutaneous 7 Via Natural or Artificial Opening 8 Via Natural or Artificial Opening Endoscopic	Ø Antineoplastic	4 Liquid Brachytherapy Radioisotope 5 Other Antineoplastic M Monoclonal Antibody
J Biliary and Pancreatic Tract	3 Percutaneous 7 Via Natural or Artificial Opening 8 Via Natural or Artificial Opening Endoscopic	2 Anti-infective	8 Oxazolidinones 9 Other Anti-infective
J Biliary and Pancreatic Tract	3 Percutaneous 7 Via Natural or Artificial Opening 8 Via Natural or Artificial Opening Endoscopic	3 Anti-inflammatory 6 Nutritional Substance 7 Electrolytic and Water Balance Substance B Anesthetic Agent H Radioactive Substance K Other Diagnostic Substance N Analgesics, Hypnotics, Sedatives T Destructive Agent	Z No Qualifier

New/Revised Text in Green ~~deleted~~ Deleted ♀ Females Only ♂ Males Only Coding Clinic
Non-covered Limited Coverage Combination (See Appendix E) DRG Non-OR Non-OR Hospital-Acquired Condition

SECTION: 3 ADMINISTRATION
BODY SYSTEM: E PHYSIOLOGICAL SYSTEMS AND ANATOMICAL REGIONS
OPERATION: Ø INTRODUCTION: *(continued)*

Putting in or on a therapeutic, diagnostic, nutritional, physiological, or prophylactic substance except blood or blood products

Body System / Region	Approach	Substance	Qualifier
J Biliary and Pancreatic Tract	3 Percutaneous 7 Via Natural or Artificial Opening 8 Via Natural or Artificial Opening Endoscopic	G Other Therapeutic Substance	C Other Substance
J Biliary and Pancreatic Tract	3 Percutaneous 7 Via Natural or Artificial Opening 8 Via Natural or Artificial Opening Endoscopic	S Gas	F Other Gas
J Biliary and Pancreatic Tract	3 Percutaneous 7 Via Natural or Artificial Opening 8 Via Natural or Artificial Opening Endoscopic	U Pancreatic Islet Cells	Ø Autologous 1 Nonautologous
J Biliary and Pancreatic Tract	4 Percutaneous Endoscopic	G Other Therapeutic Substance	C Other Substance
L Pleural Cavity ~~M Peritoneal Cavity~~	Ø Open	5 Adhesion Barrier	Z No Qualifier
L Pleural Cavity	3 Percutaneous	Ø Antineoplastic	4 Liquid Brachytherapy Radioisotope 5 Other Antineoplastic M Monoclonal Antibody
L Pleural Cavity	3 Percutaneous	1 Thrombolytic	7 Other Thrombolytic
L Pleural Cavity	3 Percutaneous	2 Anti-infective	8 Oxazolidinones 9 Other Anti-infective
L Pleural Cavity	3 Percutaneous	3 Anti-inflammatory 5 Adhesion Barrier 6 Nutritional Substance 7 Electrolytic and Water Balance Substance B Anesthetic Agent H Radioactive Substance K Other Diagnostic Substance N Analgesics, Hypnotics, Sedatives T Destructive Agent	Z No Qualifier
L Pleural Cavity	3 Percutaneous	G Other Therapeutic Substance	C Other Substance
L Pleural Cavity	3 Percutaneous	S Gas	F Other Gas
L Pleural Cavity	4 Percutaneous Endoscopic	5 Adhesion Barrier	Z No Qualifier
L Pleural Cavity	4 Percutaneous Endoscopic	G Other Therapeutic Substance	C Other Substance
L Pleural Cavity	7 Via Natural or Artificial Opening	Ø Antineoplastic	4 Liquid Brachytherapy Radioisotope 5 Other Antineoplastic M Monoclonal Antibody
L Pleural Cavity	7 Via Natural or Artificial Opening	S Gas	F Other Gas
M Peritoneal Cavity	Ø Open	5 Adhesion Barrier	Z No Qualifier
M Peritoneal Cavity	3 Percutaneous	Ø Antineoplastic	4 Liquid Brachytherapy Radioisotope 5 Other Antineoplastic M Monoclonal Antibody Y Hyperthermic

DRG Non-OR 3EØJ[378]U[Ø1]

Coding Clinic: 2019, Q4, P37 – 3EØM3ØY

SECTION: 3 ADMINISTRATION
BODY SYSTEM: E PHYSIOLOGICAL SYSTEMS AND ANATOMICAL REGIONS
OPERATION: Ø INTRODUCTION: *(continued)*

Putting in or on a therapeutic, diagnostic, nutritional, physiological, or prophylactic substance except blood or blood products

Body System / Region	Approach	Substance	Qualifier
M Peritoneal Cavity	3 Percutaneous	2 Anti-infective	8 Oxazolidinones 9 Other Anti-infective
M Peritoneal Cavity	3 Percutaneous	3 Anti-inflammatory 5 Adhesion Barrier 6 Nutritional Substance 7 Electrolytic and Water Balance Substance B Anesthetic Agent H Radioactive Substance K Other Diagnostic Substance N Analgesics, Hypnotics, Sedatives T Destructive Agent	Z No Qualifier
M Peritoneal Cavity	3 Percutaneous	G Other Therapeutic Substance	C Other Substance
M Peritoneal Cavity	3 Percutaneous	S Gas	F Other Gas
M Peritoneal Cavity	4 Percutaneous Endoscopic	5 Adhesion Barrier	Z No Qualifier
M Peritoneal Cavity	4 Percutaneous Endoscopic	G Other Therapeutic Substance	C Other Substance
M Peritoneal Cavity	7 Via Natural or Artificial Opening	Ø Antineoplastic	4 Liquid Brachytherapy Radioisotope 5 Other Antineoplastic M Monoclonal Antibody
M Peritoneal Cavity	7 Via Natural or Artificial Opening	S Gas	F Other Gas
P Female Reproductive ♀	Ø Open	5 Adhesion Barrier	Z No Qualifier
P Female Reproductive ♀	3 Percutaneous	Ø Antineoplastic	4 Liquid Brachytherapy Radioisotope 5 Other Antineoplastic M Monoclonal Antibody
P Female Reproductive ♀	3 Percutaneous	2 Anti-infective	8 Oxazolidinones 9 Other Anti-infective
P Female Reproductive ♀	3 Percutaneous	3 Anti-inflammatory 5 Adhesion Barrier 6 Nutritional Substance 7 Electrolytic and Water Balance Substance B Anesthetic Agent H Radioactive Substance K Other Diagnostic Substance L Sperm N Analgesics, Hypnotics, Sedatives T Destructive Agent V Hormone	Z No Qualifier
P Female Reproductive ♀	3 Percutaneous	G Other Therapeutic Substance	C Other Substance
P Female Reproductive ♀	3 Percutaneous	Q Fertilized Ovum	Ø Autologous 1 Nonautologous
P Female Reproductive ♀	3 Percutaneous	S Gas	F Other Gas
P Female Reproductive ♀	4 Percutaneous Endoscopic	5 Adhesion Barrier	Z No Qualifier
P Female Reproductive ♀	4 Percutaneous Endoscopic	G Other Therapeutic Substance	C Other Substance
P Female Reproductive ♀	7 Via Natural or Artificial Opening	Ø Antineoplastic	4 Liquid Brachytherapy Radioisotope 5 Other Antineoplastic M Monoclonal Antibody

Coding Clinic: 2Ø17, Q2, P15; 2Ø15, Q2, P31 – 3EØL3GC

SECTION: 3 ADMINISTRATION
BODY SYSTEM: E PHYSIOLOGICAL SYSTEMS AND ANATOMICAL REGIONS
OPERATION: Ø INTRODUCTION: *(continued)*
Putting in or on a therapeutic, diagnostic, nutritional, physiological, or prophylactic substance except blood or blood products

Body System / Region	Approach	Substance	Qualifier
P Female Reproductive ♀	7 Via Natural or Artificial Opening	2 Anti-infective	8 Oxazolidinones 9 Other Anti-infective
P Female Reproductive ♀	7 Via Natural or Artificial Opening	3 Anti-inflammatory 6 Nutritional Substance 7 Electrolytic and Water Balance Substance B Anesthetic Agent H Radioactive Substance K Other Diagnostic Substance L Sperm N Analgesics, Hypnotics, Sedatives T Destructive Agent V Hormone	Z No Qualifier
P Female Reproductive ♀	7 Via Natural or Artificial Opening	G Other Therapeutic Substance	C Other Substance
P Female Reproductive ♀	7 Via Natural or Artificial Opening	Q Fertilized Ovum	Ø Autologous 1 Nonautologous
P Female Reproductive ♀	7 Via Natural or Artificial Opening	S Gas	F Other Gas
P Female Reproductive ♀	8 Via Natural or Artificial Opening Endoscopic	Ø Antineoplastic	4 Liquid Brachytherapy Radioisotope 5 Other Antineoplastic M Monoclonal Antibody
P Female Reproductive ♀	8 Via Natural or Artificial Opening Endoscopic	2 Anti-infective	8 Oxazolidinones 9 Other Anti-infective
P Female Reproductive ♀	8 Via Natural or Artificial Opening Endoscopic	3 Anti-inflammatory 6 Nutritional Substance 7 Electrolytic and Water Balance Substance B Anesthetic Agent H Radioactive Substance K Other Diagnostic Substance N Analgesics, Hypnotics, Sedatives T Destructive Agent	Z No Qualifier
P Female Reproductive ♀	8 Via Natural or Artificial Opening Endoscopic	G Other Therapeutic Substance	C Other Substance
P Female Reproductive ♀	8 Via Natural or Artificial Opening Endoscopic	S Gas	F Other Gas
Q Cranial Cavity and Brain	Ø Open 3 Percutaneous	Ø Antineoplastic	4 Liquid Brachytherapy Radioisotope 5 Other Antineoplastic M Monoclonal Antibody
Q Cranial Cavity and Brain	Ø Open 3 Percutaneous	2 Anti-infective	8 Oxazolidinones 9 Other Anti-infective
Q Cranial Cavity and Brain	Ø Open 3 Percutaneous	3 Anti-inflammatory 6 Nutritional Substance 7 Electrolytic and Water Balance Substance A Stem Cells, Embryonic B Anesthetic Agent H Radioactive Substance K Other Diagnostic Substance N Analgesics, Hypnotics, Sedatives T Destructive Agent	Z No Qualifier

DRG Non-OR 3EØQ[Ø3]Ø5
DRG Non-OR 3EØP73Z *(proposed)*

Coding Clinic: 2016, Q4, P114 – 3EØQØØ5

SECTION: 3 ADMINISTRATION
BODY SYSTEM: E PHYSIOLOGICAL SYSTEMS AND ANATOMICAL REGIONS
OPERATION: Ø INTRODUCTION: *(continued)*

Putting in or on a therapeutic, diagnostic, nutritional, physiological, or prophylactic substance except blood or blood products

Body System / Region	Approach	Substance	Qualifier
Q Cranial Cavity and Brain	Ø Open 3 Percutaneous	E Stem Cells, Somatic	Ø Autologous 1 Nonautologous
Q Cranial Cavity and Brain	Ø Open 3 Percutaneous	G Other Therapeutic Substance	C Other Substance
Q Cranial Cavity and Brain	Ø Open 3 Percutaneous	S Gas	F Other Gas
Q Cranial Cavity and Brain	7 Via Natural or Artificial Opening	Ø Antineoplastic	4 Liquid Brachytherapy Radioisotope 5 Other Antineoplastic M Monoclonal Antibody
Q Cranial Cavity and Brain	7 Via Natural or Artificial Opening	S Gas	F Other Gas
R Spinal Canal	Ø Open	A Stem Cells, Embryonic	Z No Qualifier
R Spinal Canal	Ø Open	A Stem Cells, Somatic	Ø Autologous 1 Nonautologous
R Spinal Canal	3 Percutaneous	Ø Antineoplastic	2 High-dose Interleukin-2 3 Low-dose Interleukin-2 4 Liquid Brachytherapy Radioisotope 5 Other Antineoplastic M Monoclonal Antibody
R Spinal Canal	3 Percutaneous	2 Anti-infective	8 Oxazolidinones 9 Other Anti-infective
R Spinal Canal	3 Percutaneous	3 Anti-inflammatory 6 Nutritional Substance 7 Electrolytic and Water Balance Substance A Stem Cells, Embryonic B Anesthetic Agent H Radioactive Substance K Other Diagnostic Substance N Analgesics, Hypnotics, Sedatives T Destructive Agent	Z No Qualifier
R Spinal Canal	3 Percutaneous	E Stem Cells, Somatic	Ø Autologous 1 Nonautologous
R Spinal Canal	3 Percutaneous	G Other Therapeutic Substance	C Other Substance
R Spinal Canal	3 Percutaneous	S Gas	F Other Gas
R Spinal Canal	7 Via Natural or Artificial Opening	S Gas	F Other Gas
S Epidural Space	3 Percutaneous	Ø Antineoplastic	2 High-dose Interleukin-2 3 Low-dose Interleukin-2 4 Liquid Brachytherapy Radioisotope 5 Other Antineoplastic M Monoclonal Antibody
S Epidural Space	3 Percutaneous	2 Anti-infective	8 Oxazolidinones 9 Other Anti-infective

DRG Non-OR 3EØQ7Ø5
DRG Non-OR 3EØR3Ø2

SECTION: 3 ADMINISTRATION
BODY SYSTEM: E PHYSIOLOGICAL SYSTEMS AND ANATOMICAL REGIONS
OPERATION: Ø INTRODUCTION: *(continued)*

Putting in or on a therapeutic, diagnostic, nutritional, physiological, or prophylactic substance except blood or blood products

Body System / Region	Approach	Substance	Qualifier
S Epidural Space	3 Percutaneous	3 Anti-inflammatory 6 Nutritional Substance 7 Electrolytic and Water Balance Substance B Anesthetic Agent H Radioactive Substance K Other Diagnostic Substance N Analgesics, Hypnotics, Sedatives T Destructive Agent	Z No Qualifier
S Epidural Space	3 Percutaneous	G Other Therapeutic Substance	C Other Substance
S Epidural Space	3 Percutaneous	S Gas	F Other Gas
S Epidural Space	7 Via Natural or Artificial Opening	S Gas	F Other Gas
T Peripheral Nerves and Plexi X Cranial Nerves	3 Percutaneous	3 Anti-inflammatory B Anesthetic Agent T Destructive Agent	Z No Qualifier
T Peripheral Nerves and Plexi X Cranial Nerves	3 Percutaneous	G Other Therapeutic Substance	C Other Substance
U Joints	Ø Open	2 Anti-infective	8 Oxazolidinones 9 Other Anti-infective
U Joints	Ø Open	G Other Therapeutic Substance	B Recombinant Bone Morphogenetic Protein
U Joints	3 Percutaneous	Ø Antineoplastic	4 Liquid Brachytherapy Radioisotope 5 Other Antineoplastic M Monoclonal Antibody
U Joints	3 Percutaneous	2 Anti-infective	8 Oxazolidinones 9 Other Anti-infective
U Joints	3 Percutaneous	3 Anti-inflammatory 6 Nutritional Substance 7 Electrolytic and Water Balance Substance B Anesthetic Agent H Radioactive Substance K Other Diagnostic Substance N Analgesics, Hypnotics, Sedatives T Destructive Agent	Z No Qualifier
U Joints	3 Percutaneous	G Other Therapeutic Substance	B Recombinant Bone Morphogenetic Protein C Other Substance
U Joints	3 Percutaneous	S Gas	F Other Gas
U Joints	3 Percutaneous Endoscopic	G Other Therapeutic Substance	C Other Substance

DRG Non-OR 3EØS3Ø2

Coding Clinic: 2Ø18, Q1, P8 – 3EØUØGB

SECTION: 3 ADMINISTRATION
BODY SYSTEM: E PHYSIOLOGICAL SYSTEMS AND ANATOMICAL REGIONS
OPERATION: Ø INTRODUCTION: *(continued)*

Putting in or on a therapeutic, diagnostic, nutritional, physiological, or prophylactic substance except blood or blood products

Body System / Region	Approach	Substance	Qualifier
V Bones	Ø Open	G Other Therapeutic Substance	B Recombinant Bone Morphogenetic Protein C Other Substance
V Bones	3 Percutaneous	Ø Antineoplastic	5 Other Antineoplastic M Monoclonal Antibody
V Bones	3 Percutaneous	2 Anti-infective	8 Oxazolidinones 9 Other Anti-infective
V Bones	3 Percutaneous	3 Anti-inflammatory 6 Nutritional Substance 7 Electrolytic and Water Balance Substance B Anesthetic Agent H Radioactive Substance K Other Diagnostic Substance N Analgesics, Hypnotics, Sedatives T Destructive Agent	Z No Qualifier
V Bones	3 Percutaneous	G Other Therapeutic Substance	B Recombinant Bone Morphogenetic Protein C Other Substance
V Bones	4 Percutaneous Endoscopic	G Other Therapeutic Substance	C Other Substance
W Lymphatics	3 Percutaneous	Ø Antineoplastic	5 Other Antineoplastic M Monoclonal Antibody
W Lymphatics	3 Percutaneous	2 Anti-infective	8 Oxazolidinones 9 Other Anti-infective
W Lymphatics	3 Percutaneous	3 Anti-inflammatory 6 Nutritional Substance 7 Electrolytic and Water Balance Substance B Anesthetic Agent H Radioactive Substance K Other Diagnostic Substance N Analgesics, Hypnotics, Sedatives T Destructive Agent	Z No Qualifier
W Lymphatics	3 Percutaneous	G Other Therapeutic Substance	C Other Substance
Y Pericardial Cavity	3 Percutaneous	Ø Antineoplastic	4 Liquid Brachytherapy Radioisotope 5 Other Antineoplastic M Monoclonal Antibody
Y Pericardial Cavity	3 Percutaneous	2 Anti-infective	8 Oxazolidinones 9 Other Anti-infective
Y Pericardial Cavity	3 Percutaneous	3 Anti-inflammatory 6 Nutritional Substance 7 Electrolytic and Water Balance Substance B Anesthetic Agent H Radioactive Substance K Other Diagnostic Substance N Analgesics, Hypnotics, Sedatives T Destructive Agent	Z No Qualifier

Coding Clinic: 2Ø16, Q3, P3Ø – 3EØVØGB

SECTION: 3 ADMINISTRATION
BODY SYSTEM: E PHYSIOLOGICAL SYSTEMS AND ANATOMICAL REGIONS
OPERATION: Ø INTRODUCTION: *(continued)*

Putting in or on a therapeutic, diagnostic, nutritional, physiological, or prophylactic substance except blood or blood products

Body System / Region	Approach	Substance	Qualifier
Y Pericardial Cavity	3 Percutaneous	G Other Therapeutic Substance	C Other Substance
Y Pericardial Cavity	3 Percutaneous	S Gas	F Other Gas
Y Pericardial Cavity	3 Percutaneous Endoscopic	G Other Therapeutic Substance	C Other Substance
Y Pericardial Cavity	7 Via Natural or Artificial Opening	Ø Antineoplastic	4 Liquid Brachytherapy Radioisotope 5 Other Antineoplastic M Monoclonal Antibody
Y Pericardial Cavity	7 Via Natural or Artificial Opening	S Gas	F Other Gas

Coding Clinic: 2Ø13, Q1, P27 – 3EØG8TZ
Coding Clinic: 2Ø15, Q1, P31 – 3EØR3Ø5
Coding Clinic: 2Ø15, Q1, P38 – 3EØ53Ø5

SECTION: 3 ADMINISTRATION
BODY SYSTEM: E PHYSIOLOGICAL SYSTEMS AND ANATOMICAL REGIONS
OPERATION: 1 IRRIGATION: Putting in or on a cleansing substance

Body System / Region	Approach	Substance	Qualifier
Ø Skin and Mucous Membranes C Eye	3 Percutaneous X External	8 Irrigating Substance	X Diagnostic Z No Qualifier
9 Nose B Ear F Respiratory Tract G Upper GI H Lower GI J Biliary and Pancreatic Tract K Genitourinary Tract N Male Reproductive ♂ P Female Reproductive ♀	3 Percutaneous 7 Via Natural or Artificial Opening 8 Via Natural or Artificial Opening Endoscopic	8 Irrigating Substance	X Diagnostic Z No Qualifier
L Pleural Cavity Q Cranial Cavity and Brain R Spinal Canal S Epidural Space Y Pericardial Cavity	3 Percutaneous	8 Irrigating Substance	X Diagnostic Z No Qualifier
M Peritoneal Cavity	3 Percutaneous	8 Irrigating Substance	X Diagnostic Z No Qualifier
M Peritoneal Cavity	3 Percutaneous	9 Dialysate	Z No Qualifier
M Peritoneal Cavity	4 Percutaneous Endoscopic	8 Irrigating Substance	X Diagnostic Z No Qualifier
U Joints	3 Percutaneous 4 Percutaneous Endoscopic	8 Irrigating Substance	X Diagnostic Z No Qualifier

4 Measurement and Monitoring **567**
4A. Physiological Systems 568
4AØ. Measurement 568
4A1. Monitoring 57Ø
4B. Physiological Devices 572
4BØ. Measurement 572

SECTION: 4 MEASUREMENT AND MONITORING
BODY SYSTEM: A PHYSIOLOGICAL SYSTEMS
OPERATION: Ø MEASUREMENT: *(on multiple pages)*
Determining the level of a physiological or physical function at a point in time

Body System	Approach	Function / Device	Qualifier
Ø Central Nervous	Ø Open	2 Conductivity 4 Electrical Activity B Pressure	Z No Qualifier
Ø Central Nervous	3 Percutaneous 7 Via Natural or Artificial Opening 8 Via Natural or Artificial Opening Endoscopic	4 Electrical Activity	Z No Qualifier
Ø Central Nervous	3 Percutaneous 7 Via Natural or Artificial Opening 8 Via Natural or Artificial Opening Endoscopic	B Pressure K Temperature R Saturation	D Intracranial
Ø Central Nervous	X External	2 Conductivity 4 Electrical Activity	Z No Qualifier
1 Peripheral Nervous	Ø Open 3 Percutaneous 7 Via Natural or Artificial Opening 8 Via Natural or Artificial Opening Endoscopic X External	2 Conductivity	9 Sensory B Motor
1 Peripheral Nervous	Ø Open 3 Percutaneous 7 Via Natural or Artificial Opening 8 Via Natural or Artificial Opening Endoscopic X External	4 Electrical Activity	Z No Qualifier
2 Cardiac	Ø Open 3 Percutaneous 7 Via Natural or Artificial Opening 8 Via Natural or Artificial Opening Endoscopic	4 Electrical Activity 9 Output C Rate F Rhythm H Sound P Action Currents	Z No Qualifier
2 Cardiac	Ø Open 3 Percutaneous 7 Via Natural or Artificial Opening 8 Via Natural or Artificial Opening Endoscopic	N Sampling and Pressure	6 Right Heart 7 Left Heart 8 Bilateral
2 Cardiac	X External	4 Electrical Activity	A Guidance Z No Qualifier
2 Cardiac	X External	9 Output C Rate F Rhythm H Sound P Action Currents	Z No Qualifier
2 Cardiac	X External	M Total Activity	4 Stress
3 Arterial	Ø Open 3 Percutaneous	5 Flow J Pulse	1 Peripheral 3 Pulmonary C Coronary
3 Arterial	Ø Open 3 Percutaneous	B Pressure	1 Peripheral 3 Pulmonary C Coronary F Other Thoracic

DRG Non-OR 4AØ2[378]FZ
DRG Non-OR 4AØ2[Ø378]N[678]
Non-OR 4AØ2X4A

Coding Clinic: 2Ø15, Q3, P29 – 4AØ2X4Z
Coding Clinic: 2Ø16, Q3, P37 – 4AØ33BC
Coding Clinic: 2Ø18, Q1, P13 – 4AØ23N8
Coding Clinic: 2Ø19, Q3, P32 – 4AØ23N6
Coding Clinic: 2Ø22, Q1, P46 – 4AØ234Z

SECTION: 4 MEASUREMENT AND MONITORING
BODY SYSTEM: A PHYSIOLOGICAL SYSTEMS
OPERATION: Ø MEASUREMENT: *(continued)*
Determining the level of a physiological or physical function at a point in time

Body System	Approach	Function / Device	Qualifier
3 Arterial	Ø Open 3 Percutaneous	H Sound R Saturation	1 Peripheral
3 Arterial	X External	5 Flow	1 Peripheral D Intracranial
3 Arterial	X External	B Pressure H Sound J Pulse R Saturation	1 Peripheral
4 Venous	Ø Open 3 Percutaneous	5 Flow B Pressure J Pulse	Ø Central 1 Peripheral 2 Portal 3 Pulmonary
4 Venous	Ø Open 3 Percutaneous	R Saturation	1 Peripheral
4 Venous	4 Percutaneous Endoscopic	B Pressure	2 Portal
4 Venous	X External	5 Flow B Pressure J Pulse R Saturation	1 Peripheral
5 Circulatory	X External	L Volume	Z No Qualifier
6 Lymphatic	Ø Open 3 Percutaneous 7 Via Natural or Artificial Opening 8 Via Natural or Artificial Opening Endoscopic	5 Flow B Pressure	Z No Qualifier
7 Visual	X External	Ø Acuity 7 Mobility B Pressure	Z No Qualifier
8 Olfactory	X External	Ø Acuity	Z No Qualifier
9 Respiratory	7 Via Natural or Artificial Opening 8 Via Natural or Artificial Opening Endoscopic X External	1 Capacity 5 Flow C Rate D Resistance L Volume M Total Activity	Z No Qualifier
B Gastrointestinal	7 Via Natural or Artificial Opening 8 Via Natural or Artificial Opening Endoscopic	8 Motility B Pressure G Secretion	Z No Qualifier
C Biliary	3 Percutaneous 4 Percutaneous Endoscopic 7 Via Natural or Artificial Opening 8 Via Natural or Artificial Opening Endoscopic	5 Flow B Pressure	Z No Qualifier
D Urinary	7 Via Natural or Artificial Opening 8 Via Natural or Artificial Opening Endoscopic	3 Contractility 5 Flow B Pressure D Resistance L Volume	Z No Qualifier
F Musculoskeletal	3 Percutaneous	3 Contractility	Z No Qualifier
F Musculoskeletal	3 Percutaneous	B Pressure	E Compartment

SECTION: 4 MEASUREMENT AND MONITORING
BODY SYSTEM: A PHYSIOLOGICAL SYSTEMS
OPERATION: Ø MEASUREMENT: *(continued)*

Determining the level of a physiological or physical function at a point in time

Body System	Approach	Function / Device	Qualifier
F Musculoskeletal	X External	3 Contractility	Z No Qualifier
H Products of Conception, Cardiac ♀	7 Via Natural or Artificial Opening 8 Via Natural or Artificial Opening Endoscopic X External	4 Electrical Activity C Rate F Rhythm H Sound	Z No Qualifier
J Products of Conception, Nervous ♀	7 Via Natural or Artificial Opening 8 Via Natural or Artificial Opening Endoscopic X External	2 Conductivity 4 Electrical Activity B Pressure	Z No Qualifier
Z None	7 Via Natural or Artificial Opening	6 Metabolism K Temperature	Z No Qualifier
Z None	X External	6 Metabolism K Temperature Q Sleep	Z No Qualifier

SECTION: 4 MEASUREMENT AND MONITORING
BODY SYSTEM: A PHYSIOLOGICAL SYSTEMS
OPERATION: 1 MONITORING: *(on multiple pages)*

Determining the level of a physiological or physical function repetitively over a period of time

Body System	Approach	Function / Device	Qualifier
Ø Central Nervous	Ø Open	2 Conductivity B Pressure	Z No Qualifier
Ø Central Nervous	Ø Open	4 Electrical Activity	G Intraoperative Z No Qualifier
Ø Central Nervous	3 Percutaneous 7 Via Natural or Artificial Opening 8 Via Natural or Artificial Opening Endoscopic	4 Electrical Activity	G Intraoperative Z No Qualifier
Ø Central Nervous	3 Percutaneous 7 Via Natural or Artificial Opening 8 Via Natural or Artificial Opening Endoscopic	B Pressure K Temperature R Saturation	D Intracranial
Ø Central Nervous	X External	2 Conductivity	Z No Qualifier
Ø Central Nervous	X External	4 Electrical Activity	G Intraoperative Z No Qualifier
1 Peripheral Nervous	Ø Open 3 Percutaneous 7 Via Natural or Artificial Opening 8 Via Natural or Artificial Opening Endoscopic X External	2 Conductivity	9 Sensory B Motor
1 Peripheral Nervous	Ø Open 3 Percutaneous 7 Via Natural or Artificial Opening 8 Via Natural or Artificial Opening Endoscopic X External	4 Electrical Activity	G Intraoperative Z No Qualifier

Coding Clinic: 2Ø15, Q2, P14 – 4A11X4G
Coding Clinic: 2Ø16, Q2, P29 – 4A1Ø3BD

SECTION: 4 MEASUREMENT AND MONITORING
BODY SYSTEM: A PHYSIOLOGICAL SYSTEMS
OPERATION: 1 MONITORING: *(continued)*

Determining the level of a physiological or physical function repetitively over a period of time

Body System	Approach	Function / Device	Qualifier
2 Cardiac	Ø Open 3 Percutaneous 7 Via Natural or Artificial Opening 8 Via Natural or Artificial Opening Endoscopic	4 Electrical Activity 9 Output C Rate F Rhythm H Sound	Z No Qualifier
2 Cardiac	X External	4 Electrical Activity	5 Ambulatory Z No Qualifier
2 Cardiac	X External	9 Output C Rate F Rhythm H Sound	Z No Qualifier
2 Cardiac	X External	M Total Activity	4 Stress
2 Cardiac	X External	S Vascular Perfusion	H Indocyanine Green Dye
3 Arterial	Ø Open 3 Percutaneous	5 Flow B Pressure J Pulse	1 Peripheral 3 Pulmonary C Coronary
3 Arterial	Ø Open 3 Percutaneous	H Sound R Saturation	1 Peripheral
3 Arterial	X External	5 Flow B Pressure H Sound J Pulse R Saturation	1 Peripheral
4 Venous	Ø Open 3 Percutaneous	5 Flow B Pressure J Pulse	Ø Central 1 Peripheral 2 Portal 3 Pulmonary
4 Venous	Ø Open 3 Percutaneous	R Saturation	Ø Central 2 Portal 3 Pulmonary
4 Venous	X External	5 Flow B Pressure J Pulse	1 Peripheral
6 Lymphatic	Ø Open 3 Percutaneous 7 Via Natural or Artificial Opening 8 Via Natural or Artificial Opening Endoscopic	5 Flow	H Indocyanine Green Dye Z No Qualifier
6 Lymphatic	Ø Open 3 Percutaneous 7 Via Natural or Artificial Opening 8 Via Natural or Artificial Opening Endoscopic	B Pressure	Z No Qualifier

Coding Clinic: 2Ø15, Q3, P35 – 4A1239Z, 4A133B3
Coding Clinic: 2Ø16, Q2, P33 – 4A133[BJ]1

SECTION: 4 MEASUREMENT AND MONITORING
BODY SYSTEM: A PHYSIOLOGICAL SYSTEMS
OPERATION: 1 MONITORING: *(continued)*
Determining the level of a physiological or physical function repetitively over a period of time

Body System	Approach	Function / Device	Qualifier
9 Respiratory	7 Via Natural or Artificial Opening X External	1 Capacity 5 Flow C Rate D Resistance L Volume	Z No Qualifier
B Gastrointestinal	7 Via Natural or Artificial Opening 8 Via Natural or Artificial Opening Endoscopic	8 Motility B Pressure G Secretion	Z No Qualifier
B Gastrointestinal	X External	S Vascular Perfusion	H Indocyanine Green Dye
D Urinary	7 Via Natural or Artificial Opening 8 Via Natural or Artificial Opening Endoscopic	3 Contractility 5 Flow B Pressure D Resistance L Volume	Z No Qualifier
G Skin and Breast	X External	S Vascular Perfusion	H Indocyanine Green Dye
H Products of Conception, Cardiac ♀	7 Via Natural or Artificial Opening 8 Via Natural or Artificial Opening Endoscopic X External	4 Electrical Activity C Rate F Rhythm H Sound	Z No Qualifier
J Products of Conception, Nervous ♀	7 Via Natural or Artificial Opening 8 Via Natural or Artificial Opening Endoscopic X External	2 Conductivity 4 Electrical Activity B Pressure	Z No Qualifier
Z None	7 Via Natural or Artificial Opening	K Temperature	Z No Qualifier
Z None	X External	K Temperature Q Sleep	Z No Qualifier

Coding Clinic: 2Ø15, Q1, P26 – 4A11X4G

SECTION: 4 MEASUREMENT AND MONITORING
BODY SYSTEM: B PHYSIOLOGICAL DEVICES
OPERATION: Ø MEASUREMENT: Determining the level of a physiological or physical function at a point in time

Body System	Approach	Function / Device	Qualifier
Ø Central Nervous	X External	V Stimulator	Z No Qualifier
Ø Central Nervous	X External	W Cerebrospinal Fluid Shunt	Ø Wireless Sensor
1 Peripheral Nervous F Musculoskeletal	X External	V Stimulator	Z No Qualifier
2 Cardiac	X External	S Pacemaker T Defibrillator	Z No Qualifier
9 Respiratory	X External	S Pacemaker	Z No Qualifier

5 Extracorporeal or Systemic Assistance and Performance 573
5A. Physiological Systems 574
5AØ. Assistance 574
5A1. Performance 575
5A2. Restoration 575

SECTION: 5 EXTRACORPOREAL OR SYSTEMIC ASSISTANCE AND PERFORMANCE

BODY SYSTEM: A PHYSIOLOGICAL SYSTEMS

OPERATION: Ø ASSISTANCE: Taking over a portion of a physiological function by extracorporeal means

Body System	Duration	Function	Qualifier
2 Cardiac	1 Intermittent	1 Output	Ø Balloon Pump 5 Pulsatile Compression 6 Pump D Impeller Pump
2 Cardiac	2 Continuous	1 Output	Ø Balloon Pump 5 Pulsatile Compression 6 Other Pump D Impeller Pump
2 Cardiac	2 Continuous	2 Oxygenation	C Supersaturated
5 Circulatory	1 Intermittent 2 Continuous	2 Oxygenation	1 Hyperbaric
5 Circulatory	A Intraoperative	Ø Filtration	L Peripheral Veno-venous
9 Respiratory	2 Continuous	Ø Filtration	Z No Qualifier
9 Respiratory	3 Less than 24 Consecutive Hours 4 24-96 Consecutive Hours 5 Greater than 96 Consecutive Hours	5 Ventilation	7 Continuous Positive Airway Pressure 8 Intermittent Positive Airway Pressure 9 Continuous Negative Airway Pressure A High Nasal Flow/Velocity Cannula B Intermittent Negative Airway Pressure Z No Qualifier
9 Respiratory	B Less than 8 Consecutive Hours C 8-24 Consecutive Hours D Greater than 24 Consecutive Hours	5 Ventilation	K Intubated Prone Positioning

Coding Clinic: 2022, Q3, P24; 2021, Q2, P12; 2013, Q3, P19 – 5A02210
Coding Clinic: 2017, Q1, P10-11, 29; 2016, Q4, P137 – 5AØ
Coding Clinic: 2017, Q1, P11-12; 2016, Q4, P139 – 5A0221D
Coding Clinic: 2017, Q4, P44-45 – 5A0221D
Coding Clinic: 2018, Q2, P4-5 – 5A02210
Coding Clinic: 2020, Q1, P11 – 5A09357
Coding Clinic: 2024, Q1, P30 – 5A02216

SECTION: 5 EXTRACORPOREAL OR SYSTEMIC ASSISTANCE AND PERFORMANCE
BODY SYSTEM: A PHYSIOLOGICAL SYSTEMS
OPERATION: 1 PERFORMANCE: Completely taking over a physiological function by extracorporeal means

Body System	Duration	Function	Qualifier
2 Cardiac	Ø Single	1 Output	2 Manual
2 Cardiac	1 Intermittent	3 Pacing	Z No Qualifier
2 Cardiac	2 Continuous	1 Output	J Automated Z No Qualifier
2 Cardiac	2 Continuous	3 Pacing	Z No Qualifier
5 Circulatory	2 Continuous A Intraoperative	2 Oxygenation	F Membrane, Central G Membrane, Peripheral Veno-arterial H Membrane, Peripheral Veno-venous
9 Respiratory	Ø Single	5 Ventilation	4 Nonmechanical
9 Respiratory	3 Less than 24 Consecutive Hours 4 24-96 Consecutive Hours 5 Greater than 96 Consecutive Hours	5 Ventilation	Z No Qualifier
C Biliary	Ø Single 6 Multiple	Ø Filtration	Z No Qualifier
D Urinary	7 Intermittent, Less than 6 Hours Per Day 8 Prolonged Intermittent, 6-18 Hours Per Day 9 Continuous, Greater than 18 Hours Per Day	Ø Filtration	Z No Qualifier

DRG Non-OR 5A19[345]5Z
DRG Non-OR 5A1522[GH]
DRG Non-OR 5A1D[789]ØZ
NOTE: **5A1955Z** should only be coded on claims when the respiratory ventilation is provided for greater than 4 consecutive days during the length of stay.

Coding Clinic: 2013, Q3, P19 – 5A1223Z
Coding Clinic: 2015, Q4, P23-25; 2013, Q3, P19 – 5A1221Z
Coding Clinic: 2016, Q1, P28 – 5A1221Z
Coding Clinic: 2016, Q1, P29 – 5A1CØØZ, 5A1D6ØZ
Coding Clinic: 2017, Q1, P2Ø – 5A1221Z
Coding Clinic: 2017, Q3, P7 – 5A1221Z
Coding Clinic: 2017, Q4, P72-73 – 51AD[789]ØZ
Coding Clinic: 2018, Q1, P14 – 5A1935Z
Coding Clinic: 2018, Q4, P53-54 – 5A1522H
Coding Clinic: 2018, Q4, P54 – 5A1522G
Coding Clinic: 2019, Q2, P36 – 5A1522F
Coding Clinic: 2019, Q4, P4Ø – 5A15A2G
Coding Clinic: 2022, Q2, P25 – 51A1223Z

SECTION: 5 EXTRACORPOREAL OR SYSTEMIC ASSISTANCE AND PERFORMANCE
BODY SYSTEM: A PHYSIOLOGICAL SYSTEMS
OPERATION: 2 RESTORATION: Returning, or attempting to return, a physiological function to its original state by extracorporeal means

Body System	Duration	Function	Qualifier
2 Cardiac	Ø Single	4 Rhythm	Z No Qualifier

Coding Clinic: 2022, Q1, P46 – 5A22Ø4Z

6 Extracorporeal or Systemic Therapies **576**
6A. Physiological Systems 577
6AØ. Atmospheric Control 577
6A1. Decompression 577
6A2. Electromagnetic Therapy 577
6A3. Hyperthermia 577
6A4. Hypothermia 577
6A5. Pheresis 578
6A6. Phototherapy 578
6A7. Ultrasound Therapy 578
6A8. Ultraviolet Light Therapy 578
6A9. Shock Wave Therapy 579
6AB. Perfusion 579

SECTION: 6 EXTRACORPOREAL OR SYSTEMIC THERAPIES
BODY SYSTEM: A PHYSIOLOGICAL SYSTEMS
OPERATION: Ø ATMOSPHERIC CONTROL: Extracorporeal control of atmospheric pressure and composition

Body System	Duration	Qualifier	Qualifier
Z None	Ø Single 1 Multiple	Z No Qualifier	Z No Qualifier

SECTION: 6 EXTRACORPOREAL OR SYSTEMIC THERAPIES
BODY SYSTEM: A PHYSIOLOGICAL SYSTEMS
OPERATION: 1 DECOMPRESSION: Extracorporeal elimination of undissolved gas from body fluids

Body System	Duration	Qualifier	Qualifier
5 Circulatory	Ø Single 1 Multiple	Z No Qualifier	Z No Qualifier

SECTION: 6 EXTRACORPOREAL OR SYSTEMIC THERAPIES
BODY SYSTEM: A PHYSIOLOGICAL SYSTEMS
OPERATION: 2 ELECTROMAGNETIC THERAPY: Extracorporeal treatment by electromagnetic rays

Body System	Duration	Qualifier	Qualifier
1 Urinary 2 Central Nervous	Ø Single 1 Multiple	Z No Qualifier	Z No Qualifier

SECTION: 6 EXTRACORPOREAL OR SYSTEMIC THERAPIES
BODY SYSTEM: A PHYSIOLOGICAL SYSTEMS
OPERATION: 3 HYPERTHERMIA: Extracorporeal raising of body temperature

Body System	Duration	Qualifier	Qualifier
Z None	Ø Single 1 Multiple	Z No Qualifier	Z No Qualifier

SECTION: 6 EXTRACORPOREAL OR SYSTEMIC THERAPIES
BODY SYSTEM: A PHYSIOLOGICAL SYSTEMS
OPERATION: 4 HYPOTHERMIA: Extracorporeal lowering of body temperature

Body System	Duration	Qualifier	Qualifier
Z None	Ø Single 1 Multiple	Z No Qualifier	Z No Qualifier

Coding Clinic: 2Ø19, Q2, P18 – 6A4ZØZZ

SECTION: 6 EXTRACORPOREAL OR SYSTEMIC THERAPIES
BODY SYSTEM: A PHYSIOLOGICAL SYSTEMS
OPERATION: 5 PHERESIS: Extracorporeal separation of blood products

Body System	Duration	Qualifier	Qualifier
5 Circulatory	Ø Single 1 Multiple	Z No Qualifier	Ø Erythrocytes 1 Leukocytes 2 Platelets 3 Plasma T Stem Cells, Cord Blood V Stem Cells, Hematopoietic

Coding Clinic: 2022, Q1, P48 – 6A55ØZT

SECTION: 6 EXTRACORPOREAL OR SYSTEMIC THERAPIES
BODY SYSTEM: A PHYSIOLOGICAL SYSTEMS
OPERATION: 6 PHOTOTHERAPY: Extracorporeal treatment by light rays

Body System	Duration	Qualifier	Qualifier
Ø Skin 5 Circulatory	Ø Single 1 Multiple	Z No Qualifier	Z No Qualifier

SECTION: 6 EXTRACORPOREAL OR SYSTEMIC THERAPIES
BODY SYSTEM: A PHYSIOLOGICAL SYSTEMS
OPERATION: 7 ULTRASOUND THERAPY: Extracorporeal treatment by ultrasound

Body System	Duration	Qualifier	Qualifier
5 Circulatory	Ø Single 1 Multiple	Z No Qualifier	4 Head and Neck Vessels 5 Heart 6 Peripheral Vessels 7 Other Vessels Z No Qualifier

SECTION: 6 EXTRACORPOREAL OR SYSTEMIC THERAPIES
BODY SYSTEM: A PHYSIOLOGICAL SYSTEMS
OPERATION: 8 ULTRAVIOLET LIGHT THERAPY: Extracorporeal treatment by ultraviolet light

Body System	Duration	Qualifier	Qualifier
Ø Skin	Ø Single 1 Multiple	Z No Qualifier	Z No Qualifier

SECTION: 6 EXTRACORPOREAL OR SYSTEMIC THERAPIES
BODY SYSTEM: A PHYSIOLOGICAL SYSTEMS
OPERATION: 9 SHOCK WAVE THERAPY: Extracorporeal treatment by shock waves

Body System	Duration	Qualifier	Qualifier
3 Musculoskeletal	Ø Single 1 Multiple	Z No Qualifier	Z No Qualifier

SECTION: 6 EXTRACORPOREAL OR SYSTEMIC THERAPIES
BODY SYSTEM: A PHYSIOLOGICAL SYSTEMS
OPERATION: B PERFUSION: Extracorporeal treatment by diffusion of therapeutic fluid

Body System	Duration	Qualifier	Qualifier
5 Circulatory B Respiratory System F Hepatobiliary System and Pancreas T Urinary System	Ø Single	B Donor Organ	Z No Qualifier

7 Osteopathic **58Ø**
7W. Anatomical Regions 581
7WØ. Treatment 581

SECTION: 7 OSTEOPATHIC
BODY SYSTEM: W ANATOMICAL REGIONS
OPERATION: Ø TREATMENT: Manual treatment to eliminate or alleviate somatic dysfunction and related disorders

Body Region	Approach	Method	Qualifier
Ø Head 1 Cervical 2 Thoracic 3 Lumbar 4 Sacrum 5 Pelvis 6 Lower Extremities 7 Upper Extremities 8 Rib Cage 9 Abdomen	X External	Ø Articulatory-Raising 1 Fascial Release 2 General Mobilization 3 High Velocity-Low Amplitude 4 Indirect 5 Low Velocity-High Amplitude 6 Lymphatic Pump 7 Muscle Energy-Isometric 8 Muscle Energy-Isotonic 9 Other Method	Z None

8 **Other Procedures** **582**
8C. Indwelling Device 583
8CØ. Other Procedures 583
8E. Physiological Systems and Anatomical Regions 583
8EØ. Other Procedures 583

New/Revised Text in Green ~~deleted~~ Deleted ♀ Females Only ♂ Males Only Coding Clinic
Non-covered Limited Coverage Combination (See Appendix E) DRG Non-OR Non-OR Hospital-Acquired Condition

SECTION: 8 OTHER PROCEDURES
BODY SYSTEM: C INDWELLING DEVICE
OPERATION: Ø OTHER PROCEDURES: Methodologies which attempt to remediate or cure a disorder or disease

Body Region	Approach	Method	Qualifier
1 Nervous System	X External	6 Collection	J Cerebrospinal Fluid L Other Fluid
2 Circulatory System	X External	6 Collection	K Blood L Other Fluid

SECTION: 8 OTHER PROCEDURES
BODY SYSTEM: E PHYSIOLOGICAL SYSTEMS AND ANATOMICAL REGIONS
OPERATION: Ø OTHER PROCEDURES: *(on multiple pages)* Methodologies which attempt to remediate or cure a disorder or disease

Body Region	Approach	Method	Qualifier
1 Nervous System	X External	Y Other Method	7 Examination
~~2 Circulatory System~~	~~3 Percutaneous~~ ~~X External~~	~~D Near Infrared Spectroscopy~~	~~Z No Qualifier~~
2 Circulatory System	3 Percutaneous	D Near Infrared Spectroscopy F Fiber Optic 3D Guided Procedure	Z No Qualifier
2 Circulatory System	X External	D Near Infrared Spectroscopy	Z No Qualifier
9 Head and Neck Region	Ø Open	C Robotic Assisted Procedure	Z No Qualifier
9 Head and Neck Region	Ø Open	E Fluorescence Guided Procedure	M Aminolevulinic Acid Z No Qualifier
9 Head and Neck Region	3 Percutaneous 4 Percutaneous Endoscopic 7 Via Natural or Artificial Opening 8 Via Natural or Artificial Opening Endoscopic	C Robotic Assisted Procedure E Fluorescence Guided Procedure	Z No Qualifier
9 Head and Neck Region	X External	B Computer Assisted Procedure	F With Fluoroscopy G With Computerized Tomography H With Magnetic Resonance Imaging Z No Qualifier
9 Head and Neck Region	X External	C Robotic Assisted Procedure	Z No Qualifier
9 Head and Neck Region	X External	Y Other Method	8 Suture Removal
H Integumentary System and Breast	3 Percutaneous	Ø Acupuncture	Ø Anesthesia Z No Qualifier
H Integumentary System and Breast	X External	6 Collection	2 Breast Milk ♀
H Integumentary System and Breast	X External	Y Other Method	9 Piercing
K Musculoskeletal System	X External	1 Therapeutic Massage	Z No Qualifier

Coding Clinic: 2Ø21, Q2, P2Ø – 8EØ9XBZ

SECTION: 8 OTHER PROCEDURES

BODY SYSTEM: E PHYSIOLOGICAL SYSTEMS AND ANATOMICAL REGIONS

OPERATION: Ø OTHER PROCEDURES: *(continued)*

Methodologies which attempt to remediate or cure a disorder or disease

Body Region	Approach	Method	Qualifier
K Musculoskeletal System	X External	Y Other Method	7 Examination
U Female Reproductive System	Ø Open 3 Percutaneous 4 Percutaneous Endoscopic 7 Via Natural or Artificial Opening 8 Via Natural or Artificial Opening Endoscopic	E Fluorescence Guided Procedure	N Pafolacianine
U Female Reproductive System	X External	Y Other Method	7 Examination
V Male Reproductive System ♂	X External	1 Therapeutic Massage	C Prostate D Rectum
V Male Reproductive System ♂	X External	6 Collection	3 Sperm
W Trunk Region	Ø Open 3 Percutaneous 4 Percutaneous Endoscopic 7 Via Natural or Artificial Opening 8 Via Natural or Artificial Opening Endoscopic	C Robotic Assisted Procedure	Z No Qualifier
W Trunk Region	Ø Open 3 Percutaneous 4 Percutaneous Endoscopic 7 Via Natural or Artificial Opening 8 Via Natural or Artificial Opening Endoscopic	E Fluorescence Guided Procedure	N Pafolacianine Z No Qualifier
W Trunk Region	X External	B Computer Assisted Procedure	F With Fluoroscopy G With Computerized Tomography H With Magnetic Resonance Imaging Z No Qualifier
W Trunk Region	X External	C Robotic Assisted Procedure	Z No Qualifier
W Trunk Region	X External	Y Other Method	8 Suture Removal
X Upper Extremity Y Lower Extremity	Ø Open 3 Percutaneous 4 Percutaneous Endoscopic	C Robotic Assisted Procedure E Fluorescence Guided Procedure	Z No Qualifier
X Upper Extremity Y Lower Extremity	X External	B Computer Assisted Procedure	F With Fluoroscopy G With Computerized Tomography H With Magnetic Resonance Imaging Z No Qualifier
X Upper Extremity Y Lower Extremity	X External	C Robotic Assisted Procedure	Z No Qualifier
X Upper Extremity Y Lower Extremity	X External	Y Other Method	8 Suture Removal
Z None	X External	Y Other Method	1 In Vitro Fertilization 4 Yoga Therapy 5 Meditation 6 Isolation

Coding Clinic: 2Ø19, Q1, P31; 2Ø15, Q1, P34 – 8EØW4CZ
Coding Clinic: 2Ø21, Q4, P5Ø – 8EØW3CZ

9 Chiropractic **585**
9W. Anatomical Regions 586
9WB. Manipulation 586

SECTION: 9 CHIROPRACTIC
BODY SYSTEM: W ANATOMICAL REGIONS
OPERATION: B MANIPULATION: Manual procedure that involves a directed thrust to move a joint past the physiological range of motion, without exceeding the anatomical limit

Body Region	Approach	Method	Qualifier
Ø Head 1 Cervical 2 Thoracic 3 Lumbar 4 Sacrum 5 Pelvis 6 Lower Extremities 7 Upper Extremities 8 Rib Cage 9 Abdomen	X External	B Non-Manual C Indirect Visceral D Extra-Articular F Direct Visceral G Long Lever Specific Contact H Short Lever Specific Contact J Long and Short Lever Specific Contact K Mechanically Assisted L Other Method	Z None

B Imaging 587
B0. Central Nervous System 589
B00. Plain Radiography 589
B01. Fluoroscopy 589
B02. Computerized Tomography (CT SCAN) 589
B03. Magnetic Resonance Imaging (MRI) 590
B04. Ultrasonography 590
B2. Heart 591
B20. Plain Radiography 591
B21. Fluoroscopy 591
B22. Computerized Tomography (CT SCAN) 592
B23. Magnetic Resonance Imaging (MRI) 592
B24. Ultrasonography 593
B3. Upper Arteries 594
B30. Plain Radiography 594
B31. Fluoroscopy 595
B32. Computerized Tomography (CT SCAN) 597
B33. Magnetic Resonance Imaging (MRI) 598
B34. Ultrasonography 598
B4. Lower Arteries 599
B40. Plain Radiography 599
B41. Fluoroscopy 600
B42. Computerized Tomography (CT SCAN) 601
B43. Magnetic Resonance Imaging (MRI) 601
B44. Ultrasonography 602
B5. Veins 603
B50. Plain Radiography 603
B51. Fluoroscopy 604
B52. Computerized Tomography (CT SCAN) 605
B53. Magnetic Resonance Imaging (MRI) 606
B54. Ultrasonography 607
B7. Lymphatic System 608
B70. Plain Radiography 608
B8. Eye 609
B80. Plain Radiography 609
B82. Computerized Tomography (CT SCAN) 609
B83. Magnetic Resonance Imaging (MRI) 610
B84. Ultrasonography 610
B9. Ear, Nose, Mouth, and Throat 611
B90. Plain Radiography 611
B91. Fluoroscopy 611
B92. Computerized Tomography (CT SCAN) 612
B93. Magnetic Resonance Imaging (MRI) 612
BB. Respiratory System 613
BB0. Plain Radiography 613
BB1. Fluoroscopy 613
BB2. Computerized Tomography (CT SCAN) 613
BB3. Magnetic Resonance Imaging (MRI) 614
BB4. Ultrasonography 614
BD. Gastrointestinal System 615
BD1. Fluoroscopy 615
BD2. Computerized Tomography (CT SCAN) 615
BD4. Ultrasonography 615
BF. Hepatobiliary System and Pancreas 616
BF0. Plain Radiography 616
BF1. Fluoroscopy 616
BF2. Computerized Tomography (CT SCAN) 616
BF3. Magnetic Resonance Imaging (MRI) 617
BF4. Ultrasonography 617
BF5. Other Imaging 617

BG. Endocrine System 618
BG2. Computerized Tomography (CT SCAN) 618
BG3. Magnetic Resonance Imaging (MRI) 618
BG4. Ultrasonography 618
BH. Skin, Subcutaneous Tissue and Breast 619
BHØ. Plain Radiography 619
BH3. Magnetic Resonance Imaging (MRI) 619
BH4. Ultrasonography 62Ø
BL. Connective Tissue 621
BL3. Magnetic Resonance Imaging (MRI) 621
BL4. Ultrasonography 621
BN. Skull and Facial Bones 622
BNØ. Plain Radiography 622
BN1. Fluoroscopy 622
BN2. Computerized Tomography (CT SCAN) 623
BN3. Magnetic Resonance Imaging (MRI) 623
BP. Non-Axial Upper Bones 624
BPØ. Plain Radiography 624
BP1. Fluoroscopy 625
BP2. Computerized Tomography (CT SCAN) 626
BP3. Magnetic Resonance Imaging (MRI) 627
BP4. Ultrasonography 627
BQ. Non-Axial Lower Bones 628
BQØ. Plain Radiography 628
BQ1. Fluoroscopy 629
BQ2. Computerized Tomography (CT SCAN) 63Ø
BQ3. Magnetic Resonance Imaging (MRI) 631
BQ4. Ultrasonography 632
BR. Axial Skeleton, Except Skull and Facial Bones 633
BRØ. Plain Radiography 633
BR1. Fluoroscopy 633
BR2. Computerized Tomography (CT SCAN) 634
BR3. Magnetic Resonance Imaging (MRI) 634
BR4. Ultrasonography 634
BT. Urinary System 635
BTØ. Plain Radiography 635
BT1. Fluoroscopy 635
BT2. Computerized Tomography (CT SCAN) 636
BT3. Magnetic Resonance Imaging (MRI) 636
BT4. Ultrasonography 637
BU. Female Reproductive System 638
BUØ. Plain Radiography 638
BU1. Fluoroscopy 638
BU3. Magnetic Resonance Imaging (MRI) 639
BU4. Ultrasonography 639
BV. Male Reproductive System 64Ø
BVØ. Plain Radiography 64Ø
BV1. Fluoroscopy 64Ø
BV2. Computerized Tomography (CT SCAN) 641
BV3. Magnetic Resonance Imaging (MRI) 641
BV4. Ultrasonography 641
BW. Anatomical Regions 642
BWØ. Plain Radiography 642
BW1. Fluoroscopy 642
BW2. Computerized Tomography (CT SCAN) 642
BW3. Magnetic Resonance Imaging (MRI) 643
BW4. Ultrasonography 643
BW5. Other Imaging 643
BY. Fetus and Obstetrical 644
BY3. Magnetic Resonance Imaging (MRI) 644
BY4. Ultrasonography 644

New/Revised Text in Green ~~deleted~~ Deleted ♀ Females Only ♂ Males Only Coding Clinic
Non-covered Limited Coverage Combination (See Appendix E) DRG Non-OR Non-OR Hospital-Acquired Condition

SECTION: B IMAGING
BODY SYSTEM: Ø CENTRAL NERVOUS SYSTEM
TYPE: Ø PLAIN RADIOGRAPHY: Planar display of an image developed from the capture of external ionizing radiation on photographic or photoconductive plate

Body Part	Contrast	Qualifier	Qualifier
B Spinal Cord	Ø High Osmolar 1 Low Osmolar Y Other Contrast Z None	Z None	Z None

SECTION: B IMAGING
BODY SYSTEM: Ø CENTRAL NERVOUS SYSTEM
TYPE: 1 FLUOROSCOPY: Single plane or bi-plane real-time display of an image developed from the capture of external ionizing radiation on a fluorescent screen. The image may also be stored by either digital or analog means.

Body Part	Contrast	Qualifier	Qualifier
B Spinal Cord	Ø High Osmolar 1 Low Osmolar Y Other Contrast Z None	Z None	Z None

SECTION: B IMAGING
BODY SYSTEM: Ø CENTRAL NERVOUS SYSTEM
TYPE: 2 COMPUTERIZED TOMOGRAPHY (CT SCAN): Computer-reformatted digital display of multiplanar images developed from the capture of multiple exposures of external ionizing radiation

Body Part	Contrast	Qualifier	Qualifier
Ø Brain 7 Cisterna 8 Cerebral Ventricle(s) 9 Sella Turcica/Pituitary Gland B Spinal Cord	Ø High Osmolar 1 Low Osmolar Y Other Contrast	Ø Unenhanced and Enhanced Z None	Z None
Ø Brain 7 Cisterna 8 Cerebral Ventricle(s) 9 Sella Turcica/Pituitary Gland B Spinal Cord	Z None	Z None	Z None

SECTION: B IMAGING
BODY SYSTEM: Ø CENTRAL NERVOUS SYSTEM
TYPE: 3 **MAGNETIC RESONANCE IMAGING (MRI):** Computer-reformatted digital display of multiplanar images developed from the capture of radiofrequency signals emitted by nuclei in a body site excited within a magnetic field

Body Part	Contrast	Qualifier	Qualifier
Ø Brain 9 Sella Turcica/Pituitary Gland B Spinal Cord C Acoustic Nerves	Y Other Contrast	Ø Unenhanced and Enhanced Z None	Z None
Ø Brain 9 Sella Turcica/Pituitary Gland B Spinal Cord C Acoustic Nerves	Z None	Z None	Z None

SECTION: B IMAGING
BODY SYSTEM: Ø CENTRAL NERVOUS SYSTEM
TYPE: 4 **ULTRASONOGRAPHY:** Real-time display of images of anatomy or flow information developed from the capture of reflected and attenuated high-frequency sound waves

Body Part	Contrast	Qualifier	Qualifier
Ø Brain B Spinal Cord	Z None	Z None	Z None

SECTION: B IMAGING
BODY SYSTEM: 2 HEART
TYPE: Ø PLAIN RADIOGRAPHY: Planar display of an image developed from the capture of external ionizing radiation on photographic or photoconductive plate

Body Part	Contrast	Qualifier	Qualifier
Ø Coronary Artery, Single 1 Coronary Arteries, Multiple 2 Coronary Artery Bypass Graft, Single 3 Coronary Artery Bypass Grafts, Multiple 4 Heart, Right 5 Heart, Left 6 Heart, Right and Left 7 Internal Mammary Bypass Graft, Right 8 Internal Mammary Bypass Graft, Left F Bypass Graft, Other	Ø High Osmolar 1 Low Osmolar Y Other Contrast	Z None	Z None

DRG Non-OR B2Ø[Ø1234578F][Ø1Y]ZZ

Coding Clinic: 2Ø18, Q1, P13 – B2151ZZ

SECTION: B IMAGING
BODY SYSTEM: 2 HEART
TYPE: 1 FLUOROSCOPY: Single plane or bi-plane real-time display of an image developed from the capture of external ionizing radiation on a fluorescent screen. The image may also be stored by either digital or analog means.

Body Part	Contrast	Qualifier	Qualifier
Ø Coronary Artery, Single 1 Coronary Arteries, Multiple 2 Coronary Artery Bypass Graft, Single 3 Coronary Artery Bypass Grafts, Multiple	Ø High Osmolar 1 Low Osmolar Y Other Contrast	1 Laser	Ø Intraoperative
Ø Coronary Artery, Single 1 Coronary Arteries, Multiple 2 Coronary Artery Bypass Graft, Single 3 Coronary Artery Bypass Grafts, Multiple	Ø High Osmolar 1 Low Osmolar Y Other Contrast	Z None	Z None
4 Heart, Right 5 Heart, Left 6 Heart, Right and Left 7 Internal Mammary Bypass Graft, Right 8 Internal Mammary Bypass Graft, Left F Bypass Graft, Other	Ø High Osmolar 1 Low Osmolar Y Other Contrast	Z None	Z None

DRG Non-OR B21[Ø123][Ø1Y]ZZ
DRG Non-OR B21[45678F][Ø1Y]ZZ

Coding Clinic: 2Ø16, Q3, P36 – B21

SECTION: B IMAGING

BODY SYSTEM: 2 HEART

TYPE: 2 COMPUTERIZED TOMOGRAPHY (CT SCAN): Computer-reformatted digital display of multiplanar images developed from the capture of multiple exposures of external ionizing radiation

Body Part	Contrast	Qualifier	Qualifier
1 Coronary Arteries, Multiple 3 Coronary Artery Bypass Grafts, Multiple 6 Heart, Right and Left	Ø High Osmolar 1 Low Osmolar Y Other Contrast	Ø Unenhanced and Enhanced Z None	Z None
1 Coronary Arteries, Multiple 3 Coronary Artery Bypass Grafts, Multiple 6 Heart, Right and Left	Z None	2 Intravascular Optical Coherence Z None	Z None

SECTION: B IMAGING

BODY SYSTEM: 2 HEART

TYPE: 3 MAGNETIC RESONANCE IMAGING (MRI): Computer-reformatted digital display of multiplanar images developed from the capture of radiofrequency signals emitted by nuclei in a body site excited within a magnetic field

Body Part	Contrast	Qualifier	Qualifier
1 Coronary Arteries, Multiple 3 Coronary Artery Bypass Grafts, Multiple 6 Heart, Right and Left	Y Other Contrast	Ø Unenhanced and Enhanced Z None	Z None
1 Coronary Arteries, Multiple 3 Coronary Artery Bypass Grafts, Multiple 6 Heart, Right and Left	Z None	Z None	Z None

B24

SECTION: B IMAGING
BODY SYSTEM: 2 HEART
TYPE: 4 ULTRASONOGRAPHY: Real-time display of images of anatomy or flow information developed from the capture of reflected and attenuated high-frequency sound waves

Body Part	Contrast	Qualifier	Qualifier
Ø Coronary Artery, Single 1 Coronary Arteries, Multiple 4 Heart, Right 5 Heart, Left 6 Heart, Right and Left B Heart with Aorta C Pericardium D Pediatric Heart	Y Other Contrast	Z None	Z None
Ø Coronary Artery, Single 1 Coronary Arteries, Multiple 4 Heart, Right 5 Heart, Left 6 Heart, Right and Left B Heart with Aorta C Pericardium D Pediatric Heart	Z None	Z None	3 Intravascular 4 Transesophageal Z None

SECTION: B IMAGING
BODY SYSTEM: 3 UPPER ARTERIES
TYPE: Ø PLAIN RADIOGRAPHY: Planar display of an image developed from the capture of external ionizing radiation on photographic or photoconductive plate

Body Part	Contrast	Qualifier	Qualifier
Ø Thoracic Aorta 1 Brachiocephalic-Subclavian Artery, Right 2 Subclavian Artery, Left 3 Common Carotid Artery, Right 4 Common Carotid Artery, Left 5 Common Carotid Arteries, Bilateral 6 Internal Carotid Artery, Right 7 Internal Carotid Artery, Left 8 Internal Carotid Arteries, Bilateral 9 External Carotid Artery, Right B External Carotid Artery, Left C External Carotid Arteries, Bilateral D Vertebral Artery, Right F Vertebral Artery, Left G Vertebral Arteries, Bilateral H Upper Extremity Arteries, Right J Upper Extremity Arteries, Left K Upper Extremity Arteries, Bilateral L Intercostal and Bronchial Arteries M Spinal Arteries N Upper Arteries, Other P Thoraco-Abdominal Aorta Q Cervico-Cerebral Arch R Intracranial Arteries S Pulmonary Artery, Right T Pulmonary Artery, Left	Ø High Osmolar 1 Low Osmolar Y Other Contrast Z None	Z None	Z None

New/Revised Text in Green ~~deleted~~ Deleted ♀ Females Only ♂ Males Only Coding Clinic
Non-covered Limited Coverage Combination (See Appendix E) DRG Non-OR Non-OR Hospital-Acquired Condition

SECTION: B IMAGING
BODY SYSTEM: 3 UPPER ARTERIES
TYPE: 1 FLUOROSCOPY: *(on multiple pages)*

Single plane or bi-plane real-time display of an image developed from the capture of external ionizing radiation on a fluorescent screen. The image may also be stored by either digital or analog means.

Body Part	Contrast	Qualifier	Qualifier
Ø Thoracic Aorta 1 Brachiocephalic-Subclavian Artery, Right 2 Subclavian Artery, Left 3 Common Carotid Artery, Right 4 Common Carotid Artery, Left 5 Common Carotid Arteries, Bilateral 6 Internal Carotid Artery, Right 7 Internal Carotid Artery, Left 8 Internal Carotid Arteries, Bilateral 9 External Carotid Artery, Right B External Carotid Artery, Left C External Carotid Arteries, Bilateral D Vertebral Artery, Right F Vertebral Artery, Left G Vertebral Arteries, Bilateral H Upper Extremity Arteries, Right J Upper Extremity Arteries, Left K Upper Extremity Arteries, Bilateral L Intercostal and Bronchial Arteries M Spinal Arteries N Upper Arteries, Other P Thoraco-Abdominal Aorta Q Cervico-Cerebral Arch R Intracranial Arteries S Pulmonary Artery, Right T Pulmonary Artery, Left U Pulmonary Trunk	Ø High Osmolar 1 Low Osmolar Y Other Contrast	1 Laser	Ø Intraoperative

SECTION: B IMAGING
BODY SYSTEM: 3 UPPER ARTERIES
TYPE: 1 FLUOROSCOPY: *(continued)*

Single plane or bi-plane real-time display of an image developed from the capture of external ionizing radiation on a fluorescent screen. The image may also be stored by either digital or analog means.

Body Part	Contrast	Qualifier	Qualifier
Ø Thoracic Aorta 1 Brachiocephalic-Subclavian Artery, Right 2 Subclavian Artery, Left 3 Common Carotid Artery, Right 4 Common Carotid Artery, Left 5 Common Carotid Arteries, Bilateral 6 Internal Carotid Artery, Right 7 Internal Carotid Artery, Left 8 Internal Carotid Arteries, Bilateral 9 External Carotid Artery, Right B External Carotid Artery, Left C External Carotid Arteries, Bilateral D Vertebral Artery, Right F Vertebral Artery, Left G Vertebral Arteries, Bilateral H Upper Extremity Arteries, Right J Upper Extremity Arteries, Left K Upper Extremity Arteries, Bilateral L Intercostal and Bronchial Arteries M Spinal Arteries N Upper Arteries, Other P Thoraco-Abdominal Aorta Q Cervico-Cerebral Arch R Intracranial Arteries S Pulmonary Artery, Right T Pulmonary Artery, Left U Pulmonary Trunk	Ø High Osmolar 1 Low Osmolar Y Other Contrast	Z None	Z None

SECTION: B IMAGING
BODY SYSTEM: 3 UPPER ARTERIES
TYPE: 1 FLUOROSCOPY: *(continued)*

Single plane or bi-plane real-time display of an image developed from the capture of external ionizing radiation on a fluorescent screen. The image may also be stored by either digital or analog means.

Body Part	Contrast	Qualifier	Qualifier
Ø Thoracic Aorta 1 Brachiocephalic-Subclavian Artery, Right 2 Subclavian Artery, Left 3 Common Carotid Artery, Right 4 Common Carotid Artery, Left 5 Common Carotid Arteries, Bilateral 6 Internal Carotid Artery, Right 7 Internal Carotid Artery, Left 8 Internal Carotid Arteries, Bilateral 9 External Carotid Artery, Right B External Carotid Artery, Left C External Carotid Arteries, Bilateral D Vertebral Artery, Right F Vertebral Artery, Left G Vertebral Arteries, Bilateral H Upper Extremity Arteries, Right J Upper Extremity Arteries, Left K Upper Extremity Arteries, Bilateral L Intercostal and Bronchial Arteries M Spinal Arteries N Upper Arteries, Other P Thoraco-Abdominal Aorta Q Cervico-Cerebral Arch R Intracranial Arteries S Pulmonary Artery, Right T Pulmonary Artery, Left U Pulmonary Trunk	Z None	Z None	Z None

SECTION: B IMAGING
BODY SYSTEM: 3 UPPER ARTERIES
TYPE: 2 COMPUTERIZED TOMOGRAPHY (CT SCAN): Computer-reformatted digital display of multiplanar images developed from the capture of multiple exposures of external ionizing radiation

Body Part	Contrast	Qualifier	Qualifier
Ø Thoracic Aorta 5 Common Carotid Arteries, Bilateral 8 Internal Carotid Arteries, Bilateral G Vertebral Arteries, Bilateral R Intracranial Arteries S Pulmonary Artery, Right T Pulmonary Artery, Left	Ø High Osmolar 1 Low Osmolar Y Other Contrast	Z None	Z None
Ø Thoracic Aorta 5 Common Carotid Arteries, Bilateral 8 Internal Carotid Arteries, Bilateral G Vertebral Arteries, Bilateral R Intracranial Arteries S Pulmonary Artery, Right T Pulmonary Artery, Left	Z None	2 Intravascular Optical Coherence Z None	Z None

SECTION: B IMAGING
BODY SYSTEM: 3 UPPER ARTERIES
TYPE: 3 **MAGNETIC RESONANCE IMAGING (MRI):** Computer-reformatted digital display of multiplanar images developed from the capture of radiofrequency signals emitted by nuclei in a body site excited within a magnetic field

Body Part	Contrast	Qualifier	Qualifier
Ø Thoracic Aorta 5 Common Carotid Arteries, Bilateral 8 Internal Carotid Arteries, Bilateral G Vertebral Arteries, Bilateral H Upper Extremity Arteries, Right J Upper Extremity Arteries, Left K Upper Extremity Arteries, Bilateral M Spinal Arteries Q Cervico-Cerebral Arch R Intracranial Arteries	Y Other Contrast	Ø Unenhanced and Enhanced Z None	Z None
Ø Thoracic Aorta 5 Common Carotid Arteries, Bilateral 8 Internal Carotid Arteries, Bilateral G Vertebral Arteries, Bilateral H Upper Extremity Arteries, Right J Upper Extremity Arteries, Left K Upper Extremity Arteries, Bilateral M Spinal Arteries Q Cervico-Cerebral Arch R Intracranial Arteries	Z None	Z None	Z None

SECTION: B IMAGING
BODY SYSTEM: 3 UPPER ARTERIES
TYPE: 4 **ULTRASONOGRAPHY:** Real-time display of images of anatomy or flow information developed from the capture of reflected and attenuated high-frequency sound waves

Body Part	Contrast	Qualifier	Qualifier
Ø Thoracic Aorta 1 Brachiocephalic-Subclavian Artery, Right 2 Subclavian Artery, Left 3 Common Carotid Artery, Right 4 Common Carotid Artery, Left 5 Common Carotid Arteries, Bilateral 6 Internal Carotid Artery, Right 7 Internal Carotid Artery, Left 8 Internal Carotid Arteries, Bilateral H Upper Extremity Arteries, Right J Upper Extremity Arteries, Left K Upper Extremity Arteries, Bilateral R Intracranial Arteries S Pulmonary Artery, Right T Pulmonary Artery, Left V Ophthalmic Arteries	Z None	Z None	3 Intravascular Z None

SECTION: B IMAGING
BODY SYSTEM: 4 LOWER ARTERIES
TYPE: Ø PLAIN RADIOGRAPHY: Planar display of an image developed from the capture of external ionizing radiation on photographic or photoconductive plate

Body Part	Contrast	Qualifier	Qualifier
Ø Abdominal Aorta 2 Hepatic Artery 3 Splenic Arteries 4 Superior Mesenteric Artery 5 Inferior Mesenteric Artery 6 Renal Artery, Right 7 Renal Artery, Left 8 Renal Arteries, Bilateral 9 Lumbar Arteries B Intra-Abdominal Arteries, Other C Pelvic Arteries D Aorta and Bilateral Lower Extremity Arteries F Lower Extremity Arteries, Right G Lower Extremity Arteries, Left J Lower Arteries, Other M Renal Artery Transplant	Ø High Osmolar 1 Low Osmolar Y Other Contrast	Z None	Z None

SECTION: B IMAGING
BODY SYSTEM: 4 LOWER ARTERIES
TYPE: 1 FLUOROSCOPY: Single plane or bi-plane real-time display of an image developed from the capture of external ionizing radiation on a fluorescent screen. The image may also be stored by either digital or analog means.

Body Part	Contrast	Qualifier	Qualifier
Ø Abdominal Aorta 2 Hepatic Artery 3 Splenic Arteries 4 Superior Mesenteric Artery 5 Inferior Mesenteric Artery 6 Renal Artery, Right 7 Renal Artery, Left 8 Renal Arteries, Bilateral 9 Lumbar Arteries B Intra-Abdominal Arteries, Other C Pelvic Arteries D Aorta and Bilateral Lower Extremity Arteries F Lower Extremity Arteries, Right G Lower Extremity Arteries, Left J Lower Arteries, Other	Ø High Osmolar 1 Low Osmolar Y Other Contrast	1 Laser	Ø Intraoperative
Ø Abdominal Aorta 2 Hepatic Artery 3 Splenic Arteries 4 Superior Mesenteric Artery 5 Inferior Mesenteric Artery 6 Renal Artery, Right 7 Renal Artery, Left 8 Renal Arteries, Bilateral 9 Lumbar Arteries B Intra-Abdominal Arteries, Other C Pelvic Arteries D Aorta and Bilateral Lower Extremity Arteries F Lower Extremity Arteries, Right G Lower Extremity Arteries, Left J Lower Arteries, Other	Ø High Osmolar 1 Low Osmolar Y Other Contrast	Z None	Z None
Ø Abdominal Aorta 2 Hepatic Artery 3 Splenic Arteries 4 Superior Mesenteric Artery 5 Inferior Mesenteric Artery 6 Renal Artery, Right 7 Renal Artery, Left 8 Renal Arteries, Bilateral 9 Lumbar Arteries B Intra-Abdominal Arteries, Other C Pelvic Arteries D Aorta and Bilateral Lower Extremity Arteries F Lower Extremity Arteries, Right G Lower Extremity Arteries, Left J Lower Arteries, Other	Z None	Z None	Z None

SECTION: B IMAGING
BODY SYSTEM: 4 LOWER ARTERIES
TYPE: 2 COMPUTERIZED TOMOGRAPHY (CT SCAN): Computer-reformatted digital display of multiplanar images developed from the capture of multiple exposures of external ionizing radiation

Body Part	Contrast	Qualifier	Qualifier
Ø Abdominal Aorta 1 Celiac Artery 4 Superior Mesenteric Artery 8 Renal Arteries, Bilateral C Pelvic Arteries F Lower Extremity Arteries, Right G Lower Extremity Arteries, Left H Lower Extremity Arteries, Bilateral M Renal Artery Transplant	Ø High Osmolar 1 Low Osmolar Y Other Contrast	Z None	Z None
Ø Abdominal Aorta 1 Celiac Artery 4 Superior Mesenteric Artery 8 Renal Arteries, Bilateral C Pelvic Arteries F Lower Extremity Arteries, Right G Lower Extremity Arteries, Left H Lower Extremity Arteries, Bilateral M Renal Artery Transplant	Z None	2 Intravascular Optical Coherence Z None	Z None

SECTION: B IMAGING
BODY SYSTEM: 4 LOWER ARTERIES
TYPE: 3 MAGNETIC RESONANCE IMAGING (MRI): Computer-reformatted digital display of multiplanar images developed from the capture of radiofrequency signals emitted by nuclei in a body site excited within a magnetic field

Body Part	Contrast	Qualifier	Qualifier
Ø Abdominal Aorta 1 Celiac Artery 4 Superior Mesenteric Artery 8 Renal Arteries, Bilateral C Pelvic Arteries F Lower Extremity Arteries, Right G Lower Extremity Arteries, Left H Lower Extremity Arteries, Bilateral	Y Other Contrast	Ø Unenhanced and Enhanced Z None	Z None
Ø Abdominal Aorta 1 Celiac Artery 4 Superior Mesenteric Artery 8 Renal Arteries, Bilateral C Pelvic Arteries F Lower Extremity Arteries, Right G Lower Extremity Arteries, Left H Lower Extremity Arteries, Bilateral	Z None	Z None	Z None

B44

SECTION: B IMAGING
BODY SYSTEM: 4 LOWER ARTERIES
TYPE: 4 ULTRASONOGRAPHY: Real-time display of images of anatomy or flow information developed from the capture of reflected and attenuated high-frequency sound waves

Body Part	Contrast	Qualifier	Qualifier
Ø Abdominal Aorta 4 Superior Mesenteric Artery 5 Inferior Mesenteric Artery 6 Renal Artery, Right 7 Renal Artery, Left 8 Renal Arteries, Bilateral B Intra-Abdominal Arteries, Other F Lower Extremity Arteries, Right G Lower Extremity Arteries, Left H Lower Extremity Arteries, Bilateral K Celiac and Mesenteric Arteries L Femoral Artery N Penile Arteries ♂	Z None	Z None	3 Intravascular Z None

SECTION: B IMAGING
BODY SYSTEM: 5 VEINS
TYPE: Ø PLAIN RADIOGRAPHY: Planar display of an image developed from the capture of external ionizing radiation on photographic or photoconductive plate

Body Part	Contrast	Qualifier	Qualifier
Ø Epidural Veins 1 Cerebral and Cerebellar Veins 2 Intracranial Sinuses 3 Jugular Veins, Right 4 Jugular Veins, Left 5 Jugular Veins, Bilateral 6 Subclavian Vein, Right 7 Subclavian Vein, Left 8 Superior Vena Cava 9 Inferior Vena Cava B Lower Extremity Veins, Right C Lower Extremity Veins, Left D Lower Extremity Veins, Bilateral F Pelvic (Iliac) Veins, Right G Pelvic (Iliac) Veins, Left H Pelvic (Iliac) Veins, Bilateral J Renal Vein, Right K Renal Vein, Left L Renal Veins, Bilateral M Upper Extremity Veins, Right N Upper Extremity Veins, Left P Upper Extremity Veins, Bilateral Q Pulmonary Vein, Right R Pulmonary Vein, Left S Pulmonary Veins, Bilateral T Portal and Splanchnic Veins V Veins, Other W Dialysis Shunt/Fistula	Ø High Osmolar 1 Low Osmolar Y Other Contrast	Z None	Z None

SECTION: B IMAGING
BODY SYSTEM: 5 VEINS
TYPE: 1 FLUOROSCOPY: Single plane or bi-plane real-time display of an image developed from the capture of external ionizing radiation on a fluorescent screen. The image may also be stored by either digital or analog means.

Body Part	Contrast	Qualifier	Qualifier
Ø Epidural Veins 1 Cerebral and Cerebellar Veins 2 Intracranial Sinuses 3 Jugular Veins, Right 4 Jugular Veins, Left 5 Jugular Veins, Bilateral 6 Subclavian Vein, Right 7 Subclavian Vein, Left 8 Superior Vena Cava 9 Inferior Vena Cava B Lower Extremity Veins, Right C Lower Extremity Veins, Left D Lower Extremity Veins, Bilateral F Pelvic (Iliac) Veins, Right G Pelvic (Iliac) Veins, Left H Pelvic (Iliac) Veins, Bilateral J Renal Vein, Right K Renal Vein, Left L Renal Veins, Bilateral M Upper Extremity Veins, Right N Upper Extremity Veins, Left P Upper Extremity Veins, Bilateral Q Pulmonary Vein, Right R Pulmonary Vein, Left S Pulmonary Veins, Bilateral T Portal and Splanchnic Veins V Veins, Other W Dialysis Shunt/Fistula	Ø High Osmolar 1 Low Osmolar Y Other Contrast Z None	Z None	A Guidance Z None

Coding Clinic: 2Ø15, Q4, P3Ø – B518ZZA

SECTION: B IMAGING
BODY SYSTEM: 5 VEINS
TYPE: 2 COMPUTERIZED TOMOGRAPHY (CT SCAN): Computer-reformatted digital display of multiplanar images developed from the capture of multiple exposures of external ionizing radiation

Body Part	Contrast	Qualifier	Qualifier
2 Intracranial Sinuses 8 Superior Vena Cava 9 Inferior Vena Cava F Pelvic (Iliac) Veins, Right G Pelvic (Iliac) Veins, Left H Pelvic (Iliac) Veins, Bilateral J Renal Vein, Right K Renal Vein, Left L Renal Veins, Bilateral Q Pulmonary Vein, Right R Pulmonary Vein, Left S Pulmonary Veins, Bilateral T Portal and Splanchnic Veins	Ø High Osmolar 1 Low Osmolar Y Other Contrast	Ø Unenhanced and Enhanced Z None	Z None
2 Intracranial Sinuses 8 Superior Vena Cava 9 Inferior Vena Cava F Pelvic (Iliac) Veins, Right G Pelvic (Iliac) Veins, Left H Pelvic (Iliac) Veins, Bilateral J Renal Vein, Right K Renal Vein, Left L Renal Veins, Bilateral Q Pulmonary Vein, Right R Pulmonary Vein, Left S Pulmonary Veins, Bilateral T Portal and Splanchnic Veins	Z None	2 Intravascular Optical Coherence Z None	Z None

SECTION: B IMAGING
BODY SYSTEM: 5 VEINS
TYPE: 3 MAGNETIC RESONANCE IMAGING (MRI): Computer-reformatted digital display of multiplanar images developed from the capture of radiofrequency signals emitted by nuclei in a body site excited within a magnetic field

Body Part	Contrast	Qualifier	Qualifier
1 Cerebral and Cerebellar Veins 2 Intracranial Sinuses 5 Jugular Veins, Bilateral 8 Superior Vena Cava 9 Inferior Vena Cava B Lower Extremity Veins, Right C Lower Extremity Veins, Left D Lower Extremity Veins, Bilateral H Pelvic (Iliac) Veins, Bilateral L Renal Veins, Bilateral M Upper Extremity Veins, Right N Upper Extremity Veins, Left P Upper Extremity Veins, Bilateral S Pulmonary Veins, Bilateral T Portal and Splanchnic Veins V Veins, Other	Y Other Contrast	Ø Unenhanced and Enhanced Z None	Z None
1 Cerebral and Cerebellar Veins 2 Intracranial Sinuses 5 Jugular Veins, Bilateral 8 Superior Vena Cava 9 Inferior Vena Cava B Lower Extremity Veins, Right C Lower Extremity Veins, Left D Lower Extremity Veins, Bilateral H Pelvic (Iliac) Veins, Bilateral L Renal Veins, Bilateral M Upper Extremity Veins, Right N Upper Extremity Veins, Left P Upper Extremity Veins, Bilateral S Pulmonary Veins, Bilateral T Portal and Splanchnic Veins V Veins, Other	Z None	Z None	Z None

SECTION: B IMAGING
BODY SYSTEM: 5 VEINS
TYPE: 4 ULTRASONOGRAPHY: Real-time display of images of anatomy or flow information developed from the capture of reflected and attenuated high-frequency sound waves

Body Part	Contrast	Qualifier	Qualifier
3 Jugular Veins, Right 4 Jugular Veins, Left 6 Subclavian Vein, Right 7 Subclavian Vein, Left 9 Inferior Vena Cava B Lower Extremity Veins, Right C Lower Extremity Veins, Left D Lower Extremity Veins, Bilateral J Renal Vein, Right K Renal Vein, Left L Renal Veins, Bilateral M Upper Extremity Veins, Right N Upper Extremity Veins, Left P Upper Extremity Veins, Bilateral T Portal and Splanchnic Veins	Z None	Z None	3 Intravascular A Guidance Z None

SECTION: B IMAGING

BODY SYSTEM: 7 LYMPHATIC SYSTEM

TYPE: Ø PLAIN RADIOGRAPHY: Planar display of an image developed from the capture of external ionizing radiation on photographic or photoconductive plate

Body Part	Contrast	Qualifier	Qualifier
Ø Abdominal/Retroperitoneal Lymphatics, Unilateral 1 Abdominal/Retroperitoneal Lymphatics, Bilateral 4 Lymphatics, Head and Neck 5 Upper Extremity Lymphatics, Right 6 Upper Extremity Lymphatics, Left 7 Upper Extremity Lymphatics, Bilateral 8 Lower Extremity Lymphatics, Right 9 Lower Extremity Lymphatics, Left B Lower Extremity Lymphatics, Bilateral C Lymphatics, Pelvic	Ø High Osmolar 1 Low Osmolar Y Other Contrast	Z None	Z None

B: IMAGING 7: LYMPHATIC SYSTEM Ø: PLAIN RADIOGRAPHY

SECTION: B IMAGING
BODY SYSTEM: 8 EYE
TYPE: Ø PLAIN RADIOGRAPHY: Planar display of an image developed from the capture of external ionizing radiation on photographic or photoconductive plate

Body Part	Contrast	Qualifier	Qualifier
Ø Lacrimal Duct, Right 1 Lacrimal Duct, Left 2 Lacrimal Ducts, Bilateral	Ø High Osmolar 1 Low Osmolar Y Other Contrast	Z None	Z None
3 Optic Foramina, Right 4 Optic Foramina, Left 5 Eye, Right 6 Eye, Left 7 Eyes, Bilateral	Z None	Z None	Z None

SECTION: B IMAGING
BODY SYSTEM: 8 EYE
TYPE: 2 COMPUTERIZED TOMOGRAPHY (CT SCAN): Computer-reformatted digital display of multiplanar images developed from the capture of multiple exposures of external ionizing radiation

Body Part	Contrast	Qualifier	Qualifier
5 Eye, Right 6 Eye, Left 7 Eyes, Bilateral	Ø High Osmolar 1 Low Osmolar Y Other Contrast	Ø Unenhanced and Enhanced Z None	Z None
5 Eye, Right 6 Eye, Left 7 Eyes, Bilateral	Z None	Z None	Z None

SECTION: B IMAGING
BODY SYSTEM: 8 EYE
TYPE: 3 MAGNETIC RESONANCE IMAGING (MRI): Computer-reformatted digital display of multiplanar images developed from the capture of radiofrequency signals emitted by nuclei in a body site excited within a magnetic field

Body Part	Contrast	Qualifier	Qualifier
5 Eye, Right 6 Eye, Left 7 Eyes, Bilateral	Y Other Contrast	Ø Unenhanced and Enhanced Z None	Z None
5 Eye, Right 6 Eye, Left 7 Eyes, Bilateral	Z None	Z None	Z None

SECTION: B IMAGING
BODY SYSTEM: 8 EYE
TYPE: 4 ULTRASONOGRAPHY: Real-time display of images of anatomy or flow information developed from the capture of reflected and attenuated high-frequency sound waves

Body Part	Contrast	Qualifier	Qualifier
5 Eye, Right 6 Eye, Left 7 Eyes, Bilateral	Z None	Z None	Z None

SECTION: B IMAGING
BODY SYSTEM: 9 EAR, NOSE, MOUTH, AND THROAT
TYPE: Ø PLAIN RADIOGRAPHY: Planar display of an image developed from the capture of external ionizing radiation on photographic or photoconductive plate

Body Part	Contrast	Qualifier	Qualifier
2 Paranasal Sinuses F Nasopharynx/Oropharynx H Mastoids	Z None	Z None	Z None
4 Parotid Gland, Right 5 Parotid Gland, Left 6 Parotid Glands, Bilateral 7 Submandibular Gland, Right 8 Submandibular Gland, Left 9 Submandibular Glands, Bilateral B Salivary Gland, Right C Salivary Gland, Left D Salivary Glands, Bilateral	Ø High Osmolar 1 Low Osmolar Y Other Contrast	Z None	Z None

SECTION: B IMAGING
BODY SYSTEM: 9 EAR, NOSE, MOUTH, AND THROAT
TYPE: 1 FLUOROSCOPY: Single plane or bi-plane real-time display of an image developed from the capture of external ionizing radiation on a fluorescent screen. The image may also be stored by either digital or analog means.

Body Part	Contrast	Qualifier	Qualifier
G Pharynx and Epiglottis J Larynx	Y Other Contrast Z None	Z None	Z None

SECTION: B IMAGING
BODY SYSTEM: 9 EAR, NOSE, MOUTH, AND THROAT
TYPE: 2 COMPUTERIZED TOMOGRAPHY (CT SCAN): Computer-reformatted digital display of multiplanar images developed from the capture of multiple exposures of external ionizing radiation

Body Part	Contrast	Qualifier	Qualifier
Ø Ear 2 Paranasal Sinuses 6 Parotid Glands, Bilateral 9 Submandibular Glands, Bilateral D Salivary Glands, Bilateral F Nasopharynx/Oropharynx J Larynx	Ø High Osmolar 1 Low Osmolar Y Other Contrast	Ø Unenhanced and Enhanced Z None	Z None
Ø Ear 2 Paranasal Sinuses 6 Parotid Glands, Bilateral 9 Submandibular Glands, Bilateral D Salivary Glands, Bilateral F Nasopharynx/Oropharynx J Larynx	Z None	Z None	Z None

SECTION: B IMAGING
BODY SYSTEM: 9 EAR, NOSE, MOUTH, AND THROAT
TYPE: 3 MAGNETIC RESONANCE IMAGING (MRI): Computer-reformatted digital display of multiplanar images developed from the capture of radiofrequency signals emitted by nuclei in a body site excited within a magnetic field

Body Part	Contrast	Qualifier	Qualifier
Ø Ear 2 Paranasal Sinuses 6 Parotid Glands, Bilateral 9 Submandibular Glands, Bilateral D Salivary Glands, Bilateral F Nasopharynx/Oropharynx J Larynx	Y Other Contrast	Ø Unenhanced and Enhanced Z None	Z None
Ø Ear 2 Paranasal Sinuses 6 Parotid Glands, Bilateral 9 Submandibular Glands, Bilateral D Salivary Glands, Bilateral F Nasopharynx/Oropharynx J Larynx	Z None	Z None	Z None

SECTION: B IMAGING
BODY SYSTEM: B RESPIRATORY SYSTEM
TYPE: Ø PLAIN RADIOGRAPHY: Planar display of an image developed from the capture of external ionizing radiation on photographic or photoconductive plate

Body Part	Contrast	Qualifier	Qualifier
7 Tracheobronchial Tree, Right 8 Tracheobronchial Tree, Left 9 Tracheobronchial Trees, Bilateral	Y Other Contrast	Z None	Z None
D Upper Airways	Z None	Z None	Z None

SECTION: B IMAGING
BODY SYSTEM: B RESPIRATORY SYSTEM
TYPE: 1 FLUOROSCOPY: Single plane or bi-plane real-time display of an image developed from the capture of external ionizing radiation on a fluorescent screen. The image may also be stored by either digital or analog means.

Body Part	Contrast	Qualifier	Qualifier
2 Lung, Right 3 Lung, Left 4 Lungs, Bilateral 6 Diaphragm C Mediastinum D Upper Airways	Z None	Z None	Z None
7 Tracheobronchial Tree, Right 8 Tracheobronchial Tree, Left 9 Tracheobronchial Trees, Bilateral	Y Other Contrast	Z None	Z None

SECTION: B IMAGING
BODY SYSTEM: B RESPIRATORY SYSTEM
TYPE: 2 COMPUTERIZED TOMOGRAPHY (CT SCAN): Computer-reformatted digital display of multiplanar images developed from the capture of multiple exposures of external ionizing radiation

Body Part	Contrast	Qualifier	Qualifier
4 Lungs, Bilateral 7 Tracheobronchial Tree, Right 8 Tracheobronchial Tree, Left 9 Tracheobronchial Trees, Bilateral F Trachea/Airways	Ø High Osmolar 1 Low Osmolar Y Other Contrast	Ø Unenhanced and Enhanced Z None	Z None
4 Lungs, Bilateral 7 Tracheobronchial Tree, Right 8 Tracheobronchial Tree, Left 9 Tracheobronchial Trees, Bilateral F Trachea/Airways	Z None	Z None	Z None

SECTION: B IMAGING
BODY SYSTEM: B RESPIRATORY SYSTEM
TYPE: 3 MAGNETIC RESONANCE IMAGING (MRI): Computer-reformatted digital display of multiplanar images developed from the capture of radiofrequency signals emitted by nuclei in a body site excited within a magnetic field

Body Part	Contrast	Qualifier	Qualifier
4 Lungs, Bilateral	Z None	3 Hyperpolarized Xenon 129(Xe-129)	Z None
G Lung Apices	Y Other Contrast	Ø Unenhanced and Enhanced Z None	Z None
G Lung Apices	Z None	Z None	Z None

SECTION: B IMAGING
BODY SYSTEM: B RESPIRATORY SYSTEM
TYPE: 4 ULTRASONOGRAPHY: Real-time display of images of anatomy or flow information developed from the capture of reflected and attenuated high-frequency sound waves

Body Part	Contrast	Qualifier	Qualifier
B Pleura C Mediastinum	Z None	Z None	Z None

SECTION: B IMAGING
BODY SYSTEM: D GASTROINTESTINAL SYSTEM
TYPE: 1 FLUOROSCOPY: Single plane or bi-plane real-time display of an image developed from the capture of external ionizing radiation on a fluorescent screen. The image may also be stored by either digital or analog means.

Body Part	Contrast	Qualifier	Qualifier
1 Esophagus 2 Stomach 3 Small Bowel 4 Colon 5 Upper GI 6 Upper GI and Small Bowel 9 Duodenum B Mouth/Oropharynx	Y Other Contrast Z None	Z None	Z None

SECTION: B IMAGING
BODY SYSTEM: D GASTROINTESTINAL SYSTEM
TYPE: 2 COMPUTERIZED TOMOGRAPHY (CT SCAN): Computer-reformatted digital display of multiplanar images developed from the capture of multiple exposures of external ionizing radiation

Body Part	Contrast	Qualifier	Qualifier
4 Colon	Ø High Osmolar 1 Low Osmolar Y Other Contrast	Ø Unenhanced and Enhanced Z None	Z None
4 Colon	Z None	Z None	Z None

SECTION: B IMAGING
BODY SYSTEM: D GASTROINTESTINAL SYSTEM
TYPE: 4 ULTRASONOGRAPHY: Real-time display of images of anatomy or flow information developed from the capture of reflected and attenuated high-frequency sound waves

Body Part	Contrast	Qualifier	Qualifier
1 Esophagus 2 Stomach 7 Gastrointestinal Tract 8 Appendix 9 Duodenum C Rectum	Z None	Z None	Z None

SECTION: B IMAGING
BODY SYSTEM: F HEPATOBILIARY SYSTEM AND PANCREAS
TYPE: Ø PLAIN RADIOGRAPHY: Planar display of an image developed from the capture of external ionizing radiation on photographic or photoconductive plate

Body Part	Contrast	Qualifier	Qualifier
Ø Bile Ducts 3 Gallbladder and Bile Ducts C Hepatobiliary System, All	Ø High Osmolar 1 Low Osmolar Y Other Contrast	Z None	Z None

Non-OR BFØ[3C][Ø1Y]ZZ

SECTION: B IMAGING
BODY SYSTEM: F HEPATOBILIARY SYSTEM AND PANCREAS
TYPE: 1 FLUOROSCOPY: Single plane or bi-plane real-time display of an image developed from the capture of external ionizing radiation on a fluorescent screen. The image may also be stored by either digital or analog means.

Body Part	Contrast	Qualifier	Qualifier
Ø Bile Ducts 1 Biliary and Pancreatic Ducts 2 Gallbladder 3 Gallbladder and Bile Ducts 4 Gallbladder, Bile Ducts, and Pancreatic Ducts 8 Pancreatic Ducts	Ø High Osmolar 1 Low Osmolar Y Other Contrast	Z None	Z None
5 Liver	Ø High Osmolar 1 Low Osmolar Y Other Contrast	Z None	Z None
5 Liver	Z None	Z None	A Guidance

SECTION: B IMAGING
BODY SYSTEM: F HEPATOBILIARY SYSTEM AND PANCREAS
TYPE: 2 COMPUTERIZED TOMOGRAPHY (CT SCAN): Computer-reformatted digital display of multiplanar images developed from the capture of multiple exposures of external ionizing radiation

Body Part	Contrast	Qualifier	Qualifier
5 Liver 6 Liver and Spleen 7 Pancreas C Hepatobiliary System, All	Ø High Osmolar 1 Low Osmolar Y Other Contrast	Ø Unenhanced and Enhanced Z None	Z None
5 Liver 6 Liver and Spleen 7 Pancreas C Hepatobiliary System, All	Z None	Z None	Z None

SECTION: B IMAGING
BODY SYSTEM: F HEPATOBILIARY SYSTEM AND PANCREAS
TYPE: 3 MAGNETIC RESONANCE IMAGING (MRI): Computer-reformatted digital display of multiplanar images developed from the capture of radiofrequency signals emitted by nuclei in a body site excited within a magnetic field

Body Part	Contrast	Qualifier	Qualifier
5 Liver 6 Liver and Spleen 7 Pancreas	Y Other Contrast	Ø Unenhanced and Enhanced Z None	Z None
5 Liver 6 Liver and Spleen 7 Pancreas	Z None	Z None	Z None

SECTION: B IMAGING
BODY SYSTEM: F HEPATOBILIARY SYSTEM AND PANCREAS
TYPE: 4 ULTRASONOGRAPHY: Real-time display of images of anatomy or flow information developed from the capture of reflected and attenuated high-frequency sound waves

Body Part	Contrast	Qualifier	Qualifier
Ø Bile Ducts 2 Gallbladder 3 Gallbladder and Bile Ducts 5 Liver 6 Liver and Spleen 7 Pancreas C Hepatobiliary System, All	Z None	Z None	Z None

SECTION: B IMAGING
BODY SYSTEM: F HEPATOBILIARY SYSTEM AND PANCREAS
TYPE: 5 OTHER IMAGING: Other specified modality for visualizing a body part

Body Part	Contrast	Qualifier	Qualifier
Ø Bile Ducts 2 Gallbladder 3 Gallbladder and Bile Ducts 5 Liver 6 Liver and Spleen 7 Pancreas C Hepatobiliary System, All	2 Fluorescing Agent	Ø Indocyanine Green Dye Z None	Ø Intraoperative Z None

SECTION: B IMAGING
BODY SYSTEM: G ENDOCRINE SYSTEM
TYPE: 2 COMPUTERIZED TOMOGRAPHY (CT SCAN): Computer-reformatted digital display of multiplanar images developed from the capture of multiple exposures of external ionizing radiation

Body Part	Contrast	Qualifier	Qualifier
2 Adrenal Glands, Bilateral 3 Parathyroid Glands 4 Thyroid Gland	Ø High Osmolar 1 Low Osmolar Y Other Contrast	Ø Unenhanced and Enhanced Z None	Z None
2 Adrenal Glands, Bilateral 3 Parathyroid Glands 4 Thyroid Gland	Z None	Z None	Z None

SECTION: B IMAGING
BODY SYSTEM: G ENDOCRINE SYSTEM
TYPE: 3 MAGNETIC RESONANCE IMAGING (MRI): Computer-reformatted digital display of multiplanar images developed from the capture of radiofrequency signals emitted by nuclei in a body site excited within a magnetic field

Body Part	Contrast	Qualifier	Qualifier
2 Adrenal Glands, Bilateral 3 Parathyroid Glands 4 Thyroid Gland	Y Other Contrast	Ø Unenhanced and Enhanced Z None	Z None
2 Adrenal Glands, Bilateral 3 Parathyroid Glands 4 Thyroid Gland	Z None	Z None	Z None

SECTION: B IMAGING
BODY SYSTEM: G ENDOCRINE SYSTEM
TYPE: 4 ULTRASONOGRAPHY: Real-time display of images of anatomy or flow information developed from the capture of reflected and attenuated high-frequency sound waves

Body Part	Contrast	Qualifier	Qualifier
Ø Adrenal Gland, Right 1 Adrenal Gland, Left 2 Adrenal Glands, Bilateral 3 Parathyroid Glands 4 Thyroid Gland	Z None	Z None	Z None

SECTION: B IMAGING
BODY SYSTEM: H SKIN, SUBCUTANEOUS TISSUE AND BREAST
TYPE: Ø PLAIN RADIOGRAPHY: Planar display of an image developed from the capture of external ionizing radiation on photographic or photoconductive plate

Body Part	Contrast	Qualifier	Qualifier
Ø Breast, Right 1 Breast, Left 2 Breasts, Bilateral	Z None	Z None	Z None
3 Single Mammary Duct, Right 4 Single Mammary Duct, Left 5 Multiple Mammary Ducts, Right 6 Multiple Mammary Ducts, Left	Ø High Osmolar 1 Low Osmolar Y Other Contrast Z None	Z None	Z None

SECTION: B IMAGING
BODY SYSTEM: H SKIN, SUBCUTANEOUS TISSUE AND BREAST
TYPE: 3 MAGNETIC RESONANCE IMAGING (MRI): Computer-reformatted digital display of multiplanar images developed from the capture of radiofrequency signals emitted by nuclei in a body site excited within a magnetic field

Body Part	Contrast	Qualifier	Qualifier
Ø Breast, Right 1 Breast, Left 2 Breasts, Bilateral D Subcutaneous Tissue, Head/Neck F Subcutaneous Tissue, Upper Extremity G Subcutaneous Tissue, Thorax H Subcutaneous Tissue, Abdomen and Pelvis J Subcutaneous Tissue, Lower Extremity	Y Other Contrast	Ø Unenhanced and Enhanced Z None	Z None
Ø Breast, Right 1 Breast, Left 2 Breasts, Bilateral D Subcutaneous Tissue, Head/Neck F Subcutaneous Tissue, Upper Extremity G Subcutaneous Tissue, Thorax H Subcutaneous Tissue, Abdomen and Pelvis J Subcutaneous Tissue, Lower Extremity	Z None	Z None	Z None

SECTION: B IMAGING

BODY SYSTEM: H SKIN, SUBCUTANEOUS TISSUE AND BREAST

TYPE: 4 ULTRASONOGRAPHY: Real-time display of images of anatomy or flow information developed from the capture of reflected and attenuated high-frequency sound waves

Body Part	Contrast	Qualifier	Qualifier
Ø Breast, Right 1 Breast, Left 2 Breasts, Bilateral 7 Extremity, Upper 8 Extremity, Lower 9 Abdominal Wall B Chest Wall C Head and Neck	Z None	Z None	Z None

SECTION: B IMAGING
BODY SYSTEM: L CONNECTIVE TISSUE
TYPE: 3 MAGNETIC RESONANCE IMAGING (MRI): Computer-reformatted digital display of multiplanar images developed from the capture of radiofrequency signals emitted by nuclei in a body site excited within a magnetic field

Body Part	Contrast	Qualifier	Qualifier
Ø Connective Tissue, Upper Extremity 1 Connective Tissue, Lower Extremity 2 Tendons, Upper Extremity 3 Tendons, Lower Extremity	Y Other Contrast	Ø Unenhanced and Enhanced Z None	Z None
Ø Connective Tissue, Upper Extremity 1 Connective Tissue, Lower Extremity 2 Tendons, Upper Extremity 3 Tendons, Lower Extremity	Z None	Z None	Z None

SECTION: B IMAGING
BODY SYSTEM: L CONNECTIVE TISSUE
TYPE: 4 ULTRASONOGRAPHY: Real-time display of images of anatomy or flow information developed from the capture of reflected and attenuated high-frequency sound waves

Body Part	Contrast	Qualifier	Qualifier
Ø Connective Tissue, Upper Extremity 1 Connective Tissue, Lower Extremity 2 Tendons, Upper Extremity 3 Tendons, Lower Extremity	Z None	Z None	Z None

SECTION: B IMAGING
BODY SYSTEM: N SKULL AND FACIAL BONES
TYPE: Ø PLAIN RADIOGRAPHY: Planar display of an image developed from the capture of external ionizing radiation on photographic or photoconductive plate

Body Part	Contrast	Qualifier	Qualifier
Ø Skull 1 Orbit, Right 2 Orbit, Left 3 Orbits, Bilateral 4 Nasal Bones 5 Facial Bones 6 Mandible B Zygomatic Arch, Right C Zygomatic Arch, Left D Zygomatic Arches, Bilateral G Tooth, Single H Teeth, Multiple J Teeth, All	Z None	Z None	Z None
7 Temporomandibular Joint, Right 8 Temporomandibular Joint, Left 9 Temporomandibular Joints, Bilateral	Ø High Osmolar 1 Low Osmolar Y Other Contrast Z None	Z None	Z None

SECTION: B IMAGING
BODY SYSTEM: N SKULL AND FACIAL BONES
TYPE: 1 FLUOROSCOPY: Single plane or bi-plane real-time display of an image developed from the capture of external ionizing radiation on a fluorescent screen. The image may also be stored by either digital or analog means.

Body Part	Contrast	Qualifier	Qualifier
7 Temporomandibular Joint, Right 8 Temporomandibular Joint, Left 9 Temporomandibular Joints, Bilateral	Ø High Osmolar 1 Low Osmolar Y Other Contrast Z None	Z None	Z None

SECTION: B IMAGING
BODY SYSTEM: N SKULL AND FACIAL BONES
TYPE: 2 COMPUTERIZED TOMOGRAPHY (CT SCAN): Computer-reformatted digital display of multiplanar images developed from the capture of multiple exposures of external ionizing radiation

Body Part	Contrast	Qualifier	Qualifier
Ø Skull 3 Orbits, Bilateral 5 Facial Bones 6 Mandible 9 Temporomandibular Joints, Bilateral F Temporal Bones	Ø High Osmolar 1 Low Osmolar Y Other Contrast Z None	Z None	Z None

SECTION: B IMAGING
BODY SYSTEM: N SKULL AND FACIAL BONES
TYPE: 3 MAGNETIC RESONANCE IMAGING (MRI): Computer-reformatted digital display of multiplanar images developed from the capture of radiofrequency signals emitted by nuclei in a body site excited within a magnetic field

Body Part	Contrast	Qualifier	Qualifier
9 Temporomandibular Joints, Bilateral	Y Other Contrast Z None	Z None	Z None

SECTION: B IMAGING
BODY SYSTEM: P NON-AXIAL UPPER BONES
TYPE: Ø PLAIN RADIOGRAPHY: Planar display of an image developed from the capture of external ionizing radiation on photographic or photoconductive plate

Body Part	Contrast	Qualifier	Qualifier
Ø Sternoclavicular Joint, Right 1 Sternoclavicular Joint, Left 2 Sternoclavicular Joints, Bilateral 3 Acromioclavicular Joints, Bilateral 4 Clavicle, Right 5 Clavicle, Left 6 Scapula, Right 7 Scapula, Left A Humerus, Right B Humerus, Left E Upper Arm, Right F Upper Arm, Left J Forearm, Right K Forearm, Left N Hand, Right P Hand, Left R Finger(s), Right S Finger(s), Left X Ribs, Right Y Ribs, Left	Z None	Z None	Z None
8 Shoulder, Right 9 Shoulder, Left C Hand/Finger Joint, Right D Hand/Finger Joint, Left G Elbow, Right H Elbow, Left L Wrist, Right M Wrist, Left	Ø High Osmolar 1 Low Osmolar Y Other Contrast Z None	Z None	Z None

SECTION: B IMAGING
BODY SYSTEM: P NON-AXIAL UPPER BONES
TYPE: 1 FLUOROSCOPY: Single plane or bi-plane real-time display of an image developed from the capture of external ionizing radiation on a fluorescent screen. The image may also be stored by either digital or analog means.

Body Part	Contrast	Qualifier	Qualifier
Ø Sternoclavicular Joint, Right 1 Sternoclavicular Joint, Left 2 Sternoclavicular Joints, Bilateral 3 Acromioclavicular Joints, Bilateral 4 Clavicle, Right 5 Clavicle, Left 6 Scapula, Right 7 Scapula, Left A Humerus, Right B Humerus, Left E Upper Arm, Right F Upper Arm, Left J Forearm, Right K Forearm, Left N Hand, Right P Hand, Left R Finger(s), Right S Finger(s), Left X Ribs, Right Y Ribs, Left	Z None	Z None	Z None
8 Shoulder, Right 9 Shoulder, Left L Wrist, Right M Wrist, Left	Ø High Osmolar 1 Low Osmolar Y Other Contrast Z None	Z None	Z None
C Hand/Finger Joint, Right D Hand/Finger Joint, Left G Elbow, Right H Elbow, Left	Ø High Osmolar 1 Low Osmolar Y Other Contrast	Z None	Z None

SECTION: B IMAGING
BODY SYSTEM: P NON-AXIAL UPPER BONES
TYPE: 2 COMPUTERIZED TOMOGRAPHY (CT SCAN): Computer-reformatted digital display of multiplanar images developed from the capture of multiple exposures of external ionizing radiation

Body Part	Contrast	Qualifier	Qualifier
Ø Sternoclavicular Joint, Right 1 Sternoclavicular Joint, Left W Thorax	Ø High Osmolar 1 Low Osmolar Y Other Contrast	Z None	Z None
2 Sternoclavicular Joints, Bilateral 3 Acromioclavicular Joints, Bilateral 4 Clavicle, Right 5 Clavicle, Left 6 Scapula, Right 7 Scapula, Left 8 Shoulder, Right 9 Shoulder, Left A Humerus, Right B Humerus, Left E Upper Arm, Right F Upper Arm, Left G Elbow, Right H Elbow, Left J Forearm, Right K Forearm, Left L Wrist, Right M Wrist, Left N Hand, Right P Hand, Left Q Hands and Wrists, Bilateral R Finger(s), Right S Finger(s), Left T Upper Extremity, Right U Upper Extremity, Left V Upper Extremities, Bilateral X Ribs, Right Y Ribs, Left	Ø High Osmolar 1 Low Osmolar Y Other Contrast Z None	Z None	Z None
C Hand/Finger Joint, Right D Hand/Finger Joint, Left	Z None	Z None	Z None

SECTION: B IMAGING
BODY SYSTEM: P NON-AXIAL UPPER BONES
TYPE: 3 MAGNETIC RESONANCE IMAGING (MRI): Computer-reformatted digital display of multiplanar images developed from the capture of radiofrequency signals emitted by nuclei in a body site excited within a magnetic field

Body Part	Contrast	Qualifier	Qualifier
8 Shoulder, Right 9 Shoulder, Left C Hand/Finger Joint, Right D Hand/Finger Joint, Left E Upper Arm, Right F Upper Arm, Left G Elbow, Right H Elbow, Left J Forearm, Right K Forearm, Left L Wrist, Right M Wrist, Left	Y Other Contrast	Ø Unenhanced and Enhanced Z None	Z None
8 Shoulder, Right 9 Shoulder, Left C Hand/Finger Joint, Right D Hand/Finger Joint, Left E Upper Arm, Right F Upper Arm, Left G Elbow, Right H Elbow, Left J Forearm, Right K Forearm, Left L Wrist, Right M Wrist, Left	Z None	Z None	Z None

SECTION: B IMAGING
BODY SYSTEM: P NON-AXIAL UPPER BONES
TYPE: 4 ULTRASONOGRAPHY: Real-time display of images of anatomy or flow information developed from the capture of reflected and attenuated high-frequency sound waves

Body Part	Contrast	Qualifier	Qualifier
8 Shoulder, Right 9 Shoulder, Left G Elbow, Right H Elbow, Left L Wrist, Right M Wrist, Left N Hand, Right P Hand, Left	Z None	Z None	1 Densitometry Z None

SECTION: B IMAGING
BODY SYSTEM: Q NON-AXIAL LOWER BONES
TYPE: Ø PLAIN RADIOGRAPHY: Planar display of an image developed from the capture of external ionizing radiation on photographic or photoconductive plate

Body Part	Contrast	Qualifier	Qualifier
Ø Hip, Right 1 Hip, Left	Ø High Osmolar 1 Low Osmolar Y Other Contrast	Z None	Z None
Ø Hip, Right 1 Hip, Left	Z None	Z None	1 Densitometry Z None
3 Femur, Right 4 Femur, Left	Z None	Z None	1 Densitometry Z None
7 Knee, Right 8 Knee, Left G Ankle, Right H Ankle, Left	Ø High Osmolar 1 Low Osmolar Y Other Contrast Z None	Z None	Z None
D Lower Leg, Right F Lower Leg, Left J Calcaneus, Right K Calcaneus, Left L Foot, Right M Foot, Left P Toe(s), Right Q Toe(s), Left V Patella, Right W Patella, Left	Z None	Z None	Z None
X Foot/Toe Joint, Right Y Foot/Toe Joint, Left	Ø High Osmolar 1 Low Osmolar Y Other Contrast	Z None	Z None

SECTION: B IMAGING
BODY SYSTEM: Q NON-AXIAL LOWER BONES
TYPE: 1 FLUOROSCOPY: Single plane or bi-plane real-time display of an image developed from the capture of external ionizing radiation on a fluorescent screen. The image may also be stored by either digital or analog means.

Body Part	Contrast	Qualifier	Qualifier
Ø Hip, Right 1 Hip, Left 7 Knee, Right 8 Knee, Left G Ankle, Right H Ankle, Left X Foot/Toe Joint, Right Y Foot/Toe Joint, Left	Ø High Osmolar 1 Low Osmolar Y Other Contrast Z None	Z None	Z None
3 Femur, Right 4 Femur, Left D Lower Leg, Right F Lower Leg, Left J Calcaneus, Right K Calcaneus, Left L Foot, Right M Foot, Left P Toe(s), Right Q Toe(s), Left V Patella, Right W Patella, Left	Z None	Z None	Z None

SECTION: B IMAGING
BODY SYSTEM: Q NON-AXIAL LOWER BONES
TYPE: 2 COMPUTERIZED TOMOGRAPHY (CT SCAN): Computer-reformatted digital display of multiplanar images developed from the capture of multiple exposures of external ionizing radiation

Body Part	Contrast	Qualifier	Qualifier
Ø Hip, Right 1 Hip, Left 3 Femur, Right 4 Femur, Left 7 Knee, Right 8 Knee, Left D Lower Leg, Right F Lower Leg, Left G Ankle, Right H Ankle, Left J Calcaneus, Right K Calcaneus, Left L Foot, Right M Foot, Left P Toe(s), Right Q Toe(s), Left R Lower Extremity, Right S Lower Extremity, Left V Patella, Right W Patella, Left X Foot/Toe Joint, Right Y Foot/Toe Joint, Left	Ø High Osmolar 1 Low Osmolar Y Other Contrast Z None	Z None	Z None
B Tibia/Fibula, Right C Tibia/Fibula, Left	Ø High Osmolar 1 Low Osmolar Y Other Contrast	Z None	Z None

SECTION: B IMAGING

BODY SYSTEM: Q NON-AXIAL LOWER BONES

TYPE: 3 MAGNETIC RESONANCE IMAGING (MRI): Computer-reformatted digital display of multiplanar images developed from the capture of radiofrequency signals emitted by nuclei in a body site excited within a magnetic field

Body Part	Contrast	Qualifier	Qualifier
Ø Hip, Right 1 Hip, Left 3 Femur, Right 4 Femur, Left 7 Knee, Right 8 Knee, Left D Lower Leg, Right F Lower Leg, Left G Ankle, Right H Ankle, Left J Calcaneus, Right K Calcaneus, Left L Foot, Right M Foot, Left P Toe(s), Right Q Toe(s), Left V Patella, Right W Patella, Left	Y Other Contrast	Ø Unenhanced and Enhanced Z None	Z None
Ø Hip, Right 1 Hip, Left 3 Femur, Right 4 Femur, Left 7 Knee, Right 8 Knee, Left D Lower Leg, Right F Lower Leg, Left G Ankle, Right H Ankle, Left J Calcaneus, Right K Calcaneus, Left L Foot, Right M Foot, Left P Toe(s), Right Q Toe(s), Left V Patella, Right W Patella, Left	Z None	Z None	Z None

SECTION: B IMAGING

BODY SYSTEM: Q NON-AXIAL LOWER BONES

TYPE: 4 ULTRASONOGRAPHY: Real-time display of images of anatomy or flow information developed from the capture of reflected and attenuated high-frequency sound waves

Body Part	Contrast	Qualifier	Qualifier
Ø Hip, Right 1 Hip, Left 2 Hips, Bilateral 7 Knee, Right 8 Knee, Left 9 Knees, Bilateral	Z None	Z None	Z None

SECTION: B IMAGING
BODY SYSTEM: R AXIAL SKELETON, EXCEPT SKULL AND FACIAL BONES
TYPE: Ø PLAIN RADIOGRAPHY: Planar display of an image developed from the capture of external ionizing radiation on photographic or photoconductive plate

Body Part	Contrast	Qualifier	Qualifier
Ø Cervical Spine 7 Thoracic Spine 9 Lumbar Spine G Whole Spine	Z None	Z None	1 Densitometry Z None
1 Cervical Disc(s) 2 Thoracic Disc(s) 3 Lumbar Disc(s) 4 Cervical Facet Joint(s) 5 Thoracic Facet Joint(s) 6 Lumbar Facet Joint(s) D Sacroiliac Joints	Ø High Osmolar 1 Low Osmolar Y Other Contrast Z None	Z None	Z None
8 Thoracolumbar Joint B Lumbosacral Joint C Pelvis F Sacrum and Coccyx H Sternum	Z None	Z None	Z None

SECTION: B IMAGING
BODY SYSTEM: R AXIAL SKELETON, EXCEPT SKULL AND FACIAL BONES
TYPE: 1 FLUOROSCOPY: Single plane or bi-plane real-time display of an image developed from the capture of external ionizing radiation on a fluorescent screen. The image may also be stored by either digital or analog means.

Body Part	Contrast	Qualifier	Qualifier
Ø Cervical Spine 1 Cervical Disc(s) 2 Thoracic Disc(s) 3 Lumbar Disc(s) 4 Cervical Facet Joint(s) 5 Thoracic Facet Joint(s) 6 Lumbar Facet Joint(s) 7 Thoracic Spine 8 Thoracolumbar Joint 9 Lumbar Spine B Lumbosacral Joint C Pelvis D Sacroiliac Joints F Sacrum and Coccyx G Whole Spine H Sternum	Ø High Osmolar 1 Low Osmolar Y Other Contrast Z None	Z None	Z None

SECTION: B IMAGING
BODY SYSTEM: R AXIAL SKELETON, EXCEPT SKULL AND FACIAL BONES
TYPE: 2 **COMPUTERIZED TOMOGRAPHY (CT SCAN):** Computer-reformatted digital display of multiplanar images developed from the capture of multiple exposures of external ionizing radiation

Body Part	Contrast	Qualifier	Qualifier
Ø Cervical Spine 7 Thoracic Spine 9 Lumbar Spine C Pelvis D Sacroiliac Joints F Sacrum and Coccyx	Ø High Osmolar 1 Low Osmolar Y Other Contrast Z None	Z None	Z None

SECTION: B IMAGING
BODY SYSTEM: R AXIAL SKELETON, EXCEPT SKULL AND FACIAL BONES
TYPE: 3 **MAGNETIC RESONANCE IMAGING (MRI):** Computer-reformatted digital display of multiplanar images developed from the capture of radiofrequency signals emitted by nuclei in a body site excited within a magnetic field

Body Part	Contrast	Qualifier	Qualifier
Ø Cervical Spine 1 Cervical Disc(s) 2 Thoracic Disc(s) 3 Lumbar Disc(s) 7 Thoracic Spine 9 Lumbar Spine C Pelvis F Sacrum and Coccyx	Y Other Contrast	Ø Unenhanced and Enhanced Z None	Z None
Ø Cervical Spine 1 Cervical Disc(s) 2 Thoracic Disc(s) 3 Lumbar Disc(s) 7 Thoracic Spine 9 Lumbar Spine C Pelvis F Sacrum and Coccyx	Z None	Z None	Z None

SECTION: B IMAGING
BODY SYSTEM: R AXIAL SKELETON, EXCEPT SKULL AND FACIAL BONES
TYPE: 4 **ULTRASONOGRAPHY:** Real-time display of images of anatomy or flow information developed from the capture of reflected and attenuated high-frequency sound waves

Body Part	Contrast	Qualifier	Qualifier
Ø Cervical Spine 7 Thoracic Spine 9 Lumbar Spine F Sacrum and Coccyx	Z None	Z None	Z None

SECTION: B IMAGING
BODY SYSTEM: T URINARY SYSTEM
TYPE: Ø PLAIN RADIOGRAPHY: Planar display of an image developed from the capture of external ionizing radiation on photographic or photoconductive plate

Body Part	Contrast	Qualifier	Qualifier
Ø Bladder 1 Kidney, Right 2 Kidney, Left 3 Kidneys, Bilateral 4 Kidneys, Ureters, and Bladder 5 Urethra 6 Ureter, Right 7 Ureter, Left 8 Ureters, Bilateral B Bladder and Urethra C Ileal Diversion Loop	Ø High Osmolar 1 Low Osmolar Y Other Contrast Z None	Z None	Z None

SECTION: B IMAGING
BODY SYSTEM: T URINARY SYSTEM
TYPE: 1 FLUOROSCOPY: Single plane or bi-plane real-time display of an image developed from the capture of external ionizing radiation on a fluorescent screen. The image may also be stored by either digital or analog means.

Body Part	Contrast	Qualifier	Qualifier
Ø Bladder 1 Kidney, Right 2 Kidney, Left 3 Kidneys, Bilateral 4 Kidneys, Ureters, and Bladder 5 Urethra 6 Ureter, Right 7 Ureter, Left B Bladder and Urethra C Ileal Diversion Loop D Kidney, Ureter, and Bladder, Right F Kidney, Ureter, and Bladder, Left G Ileal Loop, Ureters, and Kidneys	Ø High Osmolar 1 Low Osmolar Y Other Contrast Z None	Z None	Z None

SECTION: B IMAGING
BODY SYSTEM: T URINARY SYSTEM
TYPE: 2 COMPUTERIZED TOMOGRAPHY (CT SCAN): Computer-reformatted digital display of multiplanar images developed from the capture of multiple exposures of external ionizing radiation

Body Part	Contrast	Qualifier	Qualifier
Ø Bladder 1 Kidney, Right 2 Kidney, Left 3 Kidneys, Bilateral 9 Kidney Transplant	Ø High Osmolar 1 Low Osmolar Y Other Contrast	Ø Unenhanced and Enhanced Z None	Z None
Ø Bladder 1 Kidney, Right 2 Kidney, Left 3 Kidneys, Bilateral 9 Kidney Transplant	Z None	Z None	Z None

SECTION: B IMAGING
BODY SYSTEM: T URINARY SYSTEM
TYPE: 3 MAGNETIC RESONANCE IMAGING (MRI): Computer-reformatted digital display of multiplanar images developed from the capture of radiofrequency signals emitted by nuclei in a body site excited within a magnetic field

Body Part	Contrast	Qualifier	Qualifier
Ø Bladder 1 Kidney, Right 2 Kidney, Left 3 Kidneys, Bilateral 9 Kidney Transplant	Y Other Contrast	Ø Unenhanced and Enhanced Z None	Z None
Ø Bladder 1 Kidney, Right 2 Kidney, Left 3 Kidneys, Bilateral 9 Kidney Transplant	Z None	Z None	Z None

SECTION: B IMAGING
BODY SYSTEM: T URINARY SYSTEM
TYPE: 4 ULTRASONOGRAPHY: Real-time display of images of anatomy or flow information developed from the capture of reflected and attenuated high-frequency sound waves

Body Part	Contrast	Qualifier	Qualifier
Ø Bladder 1 Kidney, Right 2 Kidney, Left 3 Kidneys, Bilateral 5 Urethra 6 Ureter, Right 7 Ureter, Left 8 Ureters, Bilateral 9 Kidney Transplant J Kidneys and Bladder	Z None	Z None	Z None

SECTION: B IMAGING
BODY SYSTEM: U FEMALE REPRODUCTIVE SYSTEM
TYPE: Ø PLAIN RADIOGRAPHY: Planar display of an image developed from the capture of external ionizing radiation on photographic or photoconductive plate

Body Part	Contrast	Qualifier	Qualifier
Ø Fallopian Tube, Right ♀ 1 Fallopian Tube, Left ♀ 2 Fallopian Tubes, Bilateral ♀ 6 Uterus ♀ 8 Uterus and Fallopian Tubes ♀ 9 Vagina ♀	Ø High Osmolar 1 Low Osmolar Y Other Contrast	Z None	Z None

SECTION: B IMAGING
BODY SYSTEM: U FEMALE REPRODUCTIVE SYSTEM
TYPE: 1 FLUOROSCOPY: Single plane or bi-plane real-time display of an image developed from the capture of external ionizing radiation on a fluorescent screen. The image may also be stored by either digital or analog means.

Body Part	Contrast	Qualifier	Qualifier
Ø Fallopian Tube, Right ♀ 1 Fallopian Tube, Left ♀ 2 Fallopian Tubes, Bilateral ♀ 6 Uterus ♀ 8 Uterus and Fallopian Tubes ♀ 9 Vagina ♀	Ø High Osmolar 1 Low Osmolar Y Other Contrast Z None	Z None	Z None

SECTION: B IMAGING
BODY SYSTEM: U FEMALE REPRODUCTIVE SYSTEM
TYPE: 3 MAGNETIC RESONANCE IMAGING (MRI): Computer-reformatted digital display of multiplanar images developed from the capture of radiofrequency signals emitted by nuclei in a body site excited within a magnetic field

Body Part	Contrast	Qualifier	Qualifier
3 Ovary, Right ♀ 4 Ovary, Left ♀ 5 Ovaries, Bilateral ♀ 6 Uterus ♀ 9 Vagina ♀ B Pregnant Uterus ♀ C Uterus and Ovaries ♀	Y Other Contrast	Ø Unenhanced and Enhanced Z None	Z None
3 Ovary, Right ♀ 4 Ovary, Left ♀ 5 Ovaries, Bilateral ♀ 6 Uterus ♀ 9 Vagina ♀ B Pregnant Uterus ♀ C Uterus and Ovaries ♀	Z None	Z None	Z None

SECTION: B IMAGING
BODY SYSTEM: U FEMALE REPRODUCTIVE SYSTEM
TYPE: 4 ULTRASONOGRAPHY: Real-time display of images of anatomy or flow information developed from the capture of reflected and attenuated high-frequency sound waves

Body Part	Contrast	Qualifier	Qualifier
Ø Fallopian Tube, Right ♀ 1 Fallopian Tube, Left ♀ 2 Fallopian Tubes, Bilateral ♀ 3 Ovary, Right ♀ 4 Ovary, Left ♀ 5 Ovaries, Bilateral ♀ 6 Uterus ♀ C Uterus and Ovaries ♀	Y Other Contrast Z None	Z None	Z None

SECTION: B IMAGING
BODY SYSTEM: V MALE REPRODUCTIVE SYSTEM
TYPE: Ø **PLAIN RADIOGRAPHY:** Planar display of an image developed from the capture of external ionizing radiation on photographic or photoconductive plate

Body Part	Contrast	Qualifier	Qualifier
Ø Corpora Cavernosa ♂ 1 Epididymis, Right ♂ 2 Epididymis, Left ♂ 3 Prostate ♂ 5 Testicle, Right ♂ 6 Testicle, Left ♂ 8 Vasa Vasorum ♂	Ø High Osmolar 1 Low Osmolar Y Other Contrast	Z None	Z None

SECTION: B IMAGING
BODY SYSTEM: V MALE REPRODUCTIVE SYSTEM
TYPE: 1 **FLUOROSCOPY:** Single plane or bi-plane real-time display of an image developed from the capture of external ionizing radiation on a fluorescent screen. The image may also be stored by either digital or analog means.

Body Part	Contrast	Qualifier	Qualifier
Ø Corpora Cavernosa ♂ 8 Vasa Vasorum ♂	Ø High Osmolar 1 Low Osmolar Y Other Contrast Z None	Z None	Z None

SECTION: B IMAGING
BODY SYSTEM: V MALE REPRODUCTIVE SYSTEM
TYPE: 2 COMPUTERIZED TOMOGRAPHY (CT SCAN): Computer-reformatted digital display of multiplanar images developed from the capture of multiple exposures of external ionizing radiation

Body Part	Contrast	Qualifier	Qualifier
3 Prostate ♂	Ø High Osmolar 1 Low Osmolar Y Other Contrast	Ø Unenhanced and Enhanced Z None	Z None
3 Prostate ♂	Z None	Z None	Z None

SECTION: B IMAGING
BODY SYSTEM: V MALE REPRODUCTIVE SYSTEM
TYPE: 3 MAGNETIC RESONANCE IMAGING (MRI): Computer-reformatted digital display of multiplanar images developed from the capture of radiofrequency signals emitted by nuclei in a body site excited within a magnetic field

Body Part	Contrast	Qualifier	Qualifier
Ø Corpora Cavernosa ♂ 3 Prostate ♂ 4 Scrotum ♂ 5 Testicle, Right ♂ 6 Testicle, Left ♂ 7 Testicles, Bilateral ♂	Y Other Contrast	Ø Unenhanced and Enhanced Z None	Z None
Ø Corpora Cavernosa ♂ 3 Prostate ♂ 4 Scrotum ♂ 5 Testicle, Right ♂ 6 Testicle, Left ♂ 7 Testicles, Bilateral ♂	Z None	Z None	Z None

SECTION: B IMAGING
BODY SYSTEM: V MALE REPRODUCTIVE SYSTEM
TYPE: 4 ULTRASONOGRAPHY: Real-time display of images of anatomy or flow information developed from the capture of reflected and attenuated high-frequency sound waves

Body Part	Contrast	Qualifier	Qualifier
4 Scrotum ♂ 9 Prostate and Seminal Vesicles ♂ B Penis ♂	Z None	Z None	Z None

SECTION: B IMAGING
BODY SYSTEM: W ANATOMICAL REGIONS
TYPE: Ø PLAIN RADIOGRAPHY: Planar display of an image developed from the capture of external ionizing radiation on photographic or photoconductive plate

Body Part	Contrast	Qualifier	Qualifier
Ø Abdomen 1 Abdomen and Pelvis 3 Chest B Long Bones, All C Lower Extremity J Upper Extremity K Whole Body L Whole Skeleton M Whole Body, Infant	Z None	Z None	Z None

SECTION: B IMAGING
BODY SYSTEM: W ANATOMICAL REGIONS
TYPE: 1 FLUOROSCOPY: Single plane or bi-plane real-time display of an image developed from the capture of external ionizing radiation on a fluorescent screen. The image may also be stored by either digital or analog means.

Body Part	Contrast	Qualifier	Qualifier
1 Abdomen and Pelvis 9 Head and Neck C Lower Extremity J Upper Extremity	Ø High Osmolar 1 Low Osmolar Y Other Contrast Z None	Z None	Z None

SECTION: B IMAGING
BODY SYSTEM: W ANATOMICAL REGIONS
TYPE: 2 COMPUTERIZED TOMOGRAPHY (CT SCAN): Computer-reformatted digital display of multiplanar images developed from the capture of multiple exposures of external ionizing radiation

Body Part	Contrast	Qualifier	Qualifier
Ø Abdomen 1 Abdomen and Pelvis 4 Chest and Abdomen 5 Chest, Abdomen, and Pelvis 8 Head 9 Head and Neck F Neck G Pelvic Region	Ø High Osmolar 1 Low Osmolar Y Other Contrast	Ø Unenhanced and Enhanced Z None	Z None
Ø Abdomen 1 Abdomen and Pelvis 4 Chest and Abdomen 5 Chest, Abdomen, and Pelvis 8 Head 9 Head and Neck F Neck G Pelvic Region	Z None	Z None	Z None

SECTION: B IMAGING
BODY SYSTEM: W ANATOMICAL REGIONS
TYPE: 3 MAGNETIC RESONANCE IMAGING (MRI): Computer-reformatted digital display of multiplanar images developed from the capture of radiofrequency signals emitted by nuclei in a body site excited within a magnetic field

Body Part	Contrast	Qualifier	Qualifier
Ø Abdomen 8 Head F Neck G Pelvic Region H Retroperitoneum P Brachial Plexus	Y Other Contrast	Ø Unenhanced and Enhanced Z None	Z None
Ø Abdomen 8 Head F Neck G Pelvic Region H Retroperitoneum P Brachial Plexus	Z None	Z None	Z None
3 Chest	Y Other Contrast	Ø Unenhanced and Enhanced Z None	Z None

SECTION: B IMAGING
BODY SYSTEM: W ANATOMICAL REGIONS
TYPE: 4 ULTRASONOGRAPHY: Real-time display of images of anatomy or flow information developed from the capture of reflected and attenuated high-frequency sound waves

Body Part	Contrast	Qualifier	Qualifier
Ø Abdomen 1 Abdomen and Pelvis F Neck G Pelvic Region	Z None	Z None	Z None

SECTION: B IMAGING
BODY SYSTEM: W ANATOMICAL REGIONS
TYPE: 5 OTHER IMAGING: Other specified modality for visualizing a body part

Body Part	Contrast	Qualifier	Qualifier
2 Trunk 9 Head and Neck C Lower Extremity J Upper Extremity	Z None	1 Bacterial Autofluorescence	Z None

SECTION: B IMAGING
BODY SYSTEM: Y FETUS AND OBSTETRICAL
TYPE: 3 MAGNETIC RESONANCE IMAGING (MRI): Computer-reformatted digital display of multiplanar images developed from the capture of radiofrequency signals emitted by nuclei in a body site excited within a magnetic field

Body Part	Contrast	Qualifier	Qualifier
Ø Fetal Head ♀ 1 Fetal Heart ♀ 2 Fetal Thorax ♀ 3 Fetal Abdomen ♀ 4 Fetal Spine ♀ 5 Fetal Extremities ♀ 6 Whole Fetus ♀	Y Other Contrast	Ø Unenhanced and Enhanced Z None	Z None
Ø Fetal Head ♀ 1 Fetal Heart ♀ 2 Fetal Thorax ♀ 3 Fetal Abdomen ♀ 4 Fetal Spine ♀ 5 Fetal Extremities ♀ 6 Whole Fetus ♀	Z None	Z None	Z None

SECTION: B IMAGING
BODY SYSTEM: Y FETUS AND OBSTETRICAL
TYPE: 4 ULTRASONOGRAPHY: Real-time display of images of anatomy or flow information developed from the capture of reflected and attenuated high-frequency sound waves

Body Part	Contrast	Qualifier	Qualifier
7 Fetal Umbilical Cord ♀ 8 Placenta ♀ 9 First Trimester, Single Fetus ♀ B First Trimester, Multiple Gestation ♀ C Second Trimester, Single Fetus ♀ D Second Trimester, Multiple Gestation ♀ F Third Trimester, Single Fetus ♀ G Third Trimester, Multiple Gestation ♀	Z None	Z None	Z None

C Nuclear Medicine 645
C0. Central Nervous System 646
C01. Planar Nuclear Medicine Imaging 646
C02. Tomographic (TOMO) Nuclear Medicine Imaging 646
C03. Positron Emission Tomographic (PET) Imaging 647
C05. Nonimaging Nuclear Medicine Probe 647
C2. Heart 648
C21. Planar Nuclear Medicine Imaging 648
C22. Tomographic (TOMO) Nuclear Medicine Imaging 648
C23. Positron Emission Tomographic (PET) Imaging 649
C25. Nonimaging Nuclear Medicine Probe 649
C5. Veins 650
C51. Planar Nuclear Medicine Imaging 650
C7. Lymphatic and Hematologic System 651
C71. Planar Nuclear Medicine Imaging 651
C72. Tomographic (TOMO) Nuclear Medicine Imaging 651
C75. Nonimaging Nuclear Medicine Probe 652
C76. Nonimaging Nuclear Medicine Assay 652
C8. Eye 653
C81. Planar Nuclear Medicine Imaging 653
C9. Ear, Nose, Mouth, and Throat 654
C91. Planar Nuclear Medicine Imaging 654
CB. Respiratory System 655
CB1. Planar Nuclear Medicine Imaging 655
CB2. Tomographic (TOMO) Nuclear Medicine Imaging 655
CB3. Positron Emission Tomographic (PET) Imaging 655
CD. Gastrointestinal System 656
CD1. Planar Nuclear Medicine Imaging 656
CD2. Tomographic (TOMO) Nuclear Medicine Imaging 656
CF. Hepatobiliary System and Pancreas 657
CF1. Planar Nuclear Medicine Imaging 657
CF2. Tomographic (TOMO) Nuclear Medicine Imaging 657
CG. Endocrine System 658
CG1. Planar Nuclear Medicine Imaging 658
CG2. Tomographic (TOMO) Nuclear Medicine Imaging 658
CG4. Nonimaging Nuclear Medicine Uptake 658
CH. Skin, Subcutaneous Tissue and Breast 659
CH1. Planar Nuclear Medicine Imaging 659
CH2. Tomographic (TOMO) Nuclear Medicine Imaging 659
CP. Musculoskeletal System 660
CP1. Planar Nuclear Medicine Imaging 660
CP2. Tomographic (TOMO) Nuclear Medicine Imaging 660
CP5. Nonimaging Nuclear Medicine Probe 661
CT. Urinary System 662
CT1. Planar Nuclear Medicine Imaging 662
CT2. Tomographic (TOMO) Nuclear Medicine Imaging 662
CT6. Nonimaging Nuclear Medicine Assay 662
CV. Male Reproductive System 663
CV1. Planar Nuclear Medicine Imaging 663
CW. Anatomical Regions 664
CW1. Planar Nuclear Medicine Imaging 664
CW2. Tomographic (TOMO) Nuclear Medicine Imaging 664
CW3. Positron Emission Tomographic (PET) Imaging 665
CW5. Nonimaging Nuclear Medicine Probe 665
CW7. Systemic Nuclear Medicine Therapy 665

SECTION: C NUCLEAR MEDICINE
BODY SYSTEM: Ø CENTRAL NERVOUS SYSTEM
TYPE: 1 PLANAR NUCLEAR MEDICINE IMAGING: Introduction of radioactive materials into the body for single plane display of images developed from the capture of radioactive emissions

Body Part	Radionuclide	Qualifier	Qualifier
Ø Brain	1 Technetium 99m (Tc-99m) Y Other Radionuclide	Z None	Z None
5 Cerebrospinal Fluid	D Indium 111 (In-111) Y Other Radionuclide	Z None	Z None
Y Central Nervous System	Y Other Radionuclide	Z None	Z None

SECTION: C NUCLEAR MEDICINE
BODY SYSTEM: Ø CENTRAL NERVOUS SYSTEM
TYPE: 2 TOMOGRAPHIC (TOMO) NUCLEAR MEDICINE IMAGING: Introduction of radioactive materials into the body for three-dimensional display of images developed from the capture of radioactive emissions

Body Part	Radionuclide	Qualifier	Qualifier
Ø Brain	1 Technetium 99m (Tc-99m) F Iodine 123 (I-123) S Thallium 2Ø1 (Tl-2Ø1) Y Other Radionuclide	Z None	Z None
5 Cerebrospinal Fluid	D Indium 111 (In-111) Y Other Radionuclide	Z None	Z None
Y Central Nervous System	Y Other Radionuclide	Z None	Z None

SECTION: C NUCLEAR MEDICINE
BODY SYSTEM: Ø CENTRAL NERVOUS SYSTEM
TYPE: 3 POSITRON EMISSION TOMOGRAPHIC (PET) IMAGING: Introduction of radioactive materials into the body for three-dimensional display of images developed from the simultaneous capture, 180 degrees apart, of radioactive emissions

Body Part	Radionuclide	Qualifier	Qualifier
Ø Brain	B Carbon 11 (C-11) K Fluorine 18 (F-18) M Oxygen 15 (O-15) Y Other Radionuclide	Z None	Z None
Y Central Nervous System	Y Other Radionuclide	Z None	Z None

SECTION: C NUCLEAR MEDICINE
BODY SYSTEM: Ø CENTRAL NERVOUS SYSTEM
TYPE: 5 NONIMAGING NUCLEAR MEDICINE PROBE: Introduction of radioactive materials into the body for the study of distribution and fate of certain substances by the detection of radioactive emissions; or, alternatively, measurement of absorption of radioactive emissions from an external source

Body Part	Radionuclide	Qualifier	Qualifier
Ø Brain	V Xenon 133 (Xe-133) Y Other Radionuclide	Z None	Z None
Y Central Nervous System	Y Other Radionuclide	Z None	Z None

SECTION: C NUCLEAR MEDICINE
BODY SYSTEM: 2 HEART
TYPE: 1 PLANAR NUCLEAR MEDICINE IMAGING: Introduction of radioactive materials into the body for single plane display of images developed from the capture of radioactive emissions

Body Part	Radionuclide	Qualifier	Qualifier
6 Heart, Right and Left	1 Technetium 99m (Tc-99m) Y Other Radionuclide	Z None	Z None
G Myocardium	1 Technetium 99m (Tc-99m) D Indium 111 (In-111) S Thallium 201 (Tl-201) Y Other Radionuclide Z None	Z None	Z None
Y Heart	Y Other Radionuclide	Z None	Z None

SECTION: C NUCLEAR MEDICINE
BODY SYSTEM: 2 HEART
TYPE: 2 TOMOGRAPHIC (TOMO) NUCLEAR MEDICINE IMAGING: Introduction of radioactive materials into the body for three-dimensional display of images developed from the capture of radioactive emissions

Body Part	Radionuclide	Qualifier	Qualifier
6 Heart, Right and Left	1 Technetium 99m (Tc-99m) Y Other Radionuclide	Z None	Z None
G Myocardium	1 Technetium 99m (Tc-99m) D Indium 111 (In-111) K Fluorine 18 (F-18) S Thallium 201 (Tl-201) Y Other Radionuclide Z None	Z None	Z None
Y Heart	Y Other Radionuclide	Z None	Z None

SECTION: C NUCLEAR MEDICINE
BODY SYSTEM: 2 HEART
TYPE: 3 POSITRON EMISSION TOMOGRAPHIC (PET) IMAGING: Introduction of radioactive materials into the body for three-dimensional display of images developed from the simultaneous capture, 180 degrees apart, of radioactive emissions

Body Part	Radionuclide	Qualifier	Qualifier
G Myocardium	K Fluorine 18 (F-18) M Oxygen 15 (O-15) Q Rubidium 82 (Rb-82) R Nitrogen 13 (N-13) Y Other Radionuclide	Z None	Z None
Y Heart	Y Other Radionuclide	Z None	Z None

SECTION: C NUCLEAR MEDICINE
BODY SYSTEM: 2 HEART
TYPE: 5 NONIMAGING NUCLEAR MEDICINE PROBE: Introduction of radioactive materials into the body for the study of distribution and fate of certain substances by the detection of radioactive emissions; or, alternatively, measurement of absorption of radioactive emissions from an external source

Body Part	Radionuclide	Qualifier	Qualifier
6 Heart, Right and Left	1 Technetium 99m (Tc-99m) Y Other Radionuclide	Z None	Z None
Y Heart	Y Other Radionuclide	Z None	Z None

SECTION: C NUCLEAR MEDICINE

BODY SYSTEM: 5 VEINS

TYPE: 1 PLANAR NUCLEAR MEDICINE IMAGING: Introduction of radioactive materials into the body for single plane display of images developed from the capture of radioactive emissions

Body Part	Radionuclide	Qualifier	Qualifier
B Lower Extremity Veins, Right C Lower Extremity Veins, Left D Lower Extremity Veins, Bilateral N Upper Extremity Veins, Right P Upper Extremity Veins, Left Q Upper Extremity Veins, Bilateral R Central Veins	1 Technetium 99m (Tc-99m) Y Other Radionuclide	Z None	Z None
Y Veins	Y Other Radionuclide	Z None	Z None

SECTION: C NUCLEAR MEDICINE
BODY SYSTEM: 7 LYMPHATIC AND HEMATOLOGIC SYSTEM
TYPE: 1 PLANAR NUCLEAR MEDICINE IMAGING: Introduction of radioactive materials into the body for single plane display of images developed from the capture of radioactive emissions

Body Part	Radionuclide	Qualifier	Qualifier
Ø Bone Marrow	1 Technetium 99m (Tc-99m) D Indium 111 (In-111) Y Other Radionuclide	Z None	Z None
2 Spleen 5 Lymphatics, Head and Neck D Lymphatics, Pelvic J Lymphatics, Head K Lymphatics, Neck L Lymphatics, Upper Chest M Lymphatics, Trunk N Lymphatics, Upper Extremity P Lymphatics, Lower Extremity	1 Technetium 99m (Tc-99m) Y Other Radionuclide	Z None	Z None
3 Blood	D Indium 111 (In-111) Y Other Radionuclide	Z None	Z None
Y Lymphatic and Hematologic System	Y Other Radionuclide	Z None	Z None

SECTION: C NUCLEAR MEDICINE
BODY SYSTEM: 7 LYMPHATIC AND HEMATOLOGIC SYSTEM
TYPE: 2 TOMOGRAPHIC (TOMO) NUCLEAR MEDICINE IMAGING: Introduction of radioactive materials into the body for three-dimensional display of images developed from the capture of radioactive emissions

Body Part	Radionuclide	Qualifier	Qualifier
2 Spleen	1 Technetium 99m (Tc-99m) Y Other Radionuclide	Z None	Z None
Y Lymphatic and Hematologic System	Y Other Radionuclide	Z None	Z None

SECTION: C NUCLEAR MEDICINE
BODY SYSTEM: 7 LYMPHATIC AND HEMATOLOGIC SYSTEM
TYPE: 5 NONIMAGING NUCLEAR MEDICINE PROBE: Introduction of radioactive materials into the body for the study of distribution and fate of certain substances by the detection of radioactive emissions; or, alternatively, measurement of absorption of radioactive emissions from an external source

Body Part	Radionuclide	Qualifier	Qualifier
5 Lymphatics, Head and Neck D Lymphatics, Pelvic J Lymphatics, Head K Lymphatics, Neck L Lymphatics, Upper Chest M Lymphatics, Trunk N Lymphatics, Upper Extremity P Lymphatics, Lower Extremity	1 Technetium 99m (Tc-99m) Y Other Radionuclide	Z None	Z None
Y Lymphatic and Hematologic System	Y Other Radionuclide	Z None	Z None

SECTION: C NUCLEAR MEDICINE
BODY SYSTEM: 7 LYMPHATIC AND HEMATOLOGIC SYSTEM
TYPE: 6 NONIMAGING NUCLEAR MEDICINE ASSAY: Introduction of radioactive materials into the body for the study of body fluids and blood elements, by the detection of radioactive emissions

Body Part	Radionuclide	Qualifier	Qualifier
3 Blood	1 Technetium 99m (Tc-99m) 7 Cobalt 58 (Co-58) C Cobalt 57 (Co-57) D Indium 111 (In-111) H Iodine 125 (I-125) W Chromium (Cr-51) Y Other Radionuclide	Z None	Z None
Y Lymphatic and Hematologic System	Y Other Radionuclide	Z None	Z None

SECTION: C NUCLEAR MEDICINE
BODY SYSTEM: 8 EYE
TYPE: 1 PLANAR NUCLEAR MEDICINE IMAGING: Introduction of radioactive materials into the body for single plane display of images developed from the capture of radioactive emissions

Body Part	Radionuclide	Qualifier	Qualifier
9 Lacrimal Ducts, Bilateral	1 Technetium 99m (Tc-99m) Y Other Radionuclide	Z None	Z None
Y Eye	Y Other Radionuclide	Z None	Z None

SECTION: C NUCLEAR MEDICINE
BODY SYSTEM: 9 EAR, NOSE, MOUTH, AND THROAT
TYPE: 1 PLANAR NUCLEAR MEDICINE IMAGING: Introduction of radioactive materials into the body for single plane display of images developed from the capture of radioactive emissions

Body Part	Radionuclide	Qualifier	Qualifier
B Salivary Glands, Bilateral	1 Technetium 99m (Tc-99m) Y Other Radionuclide	Z None	Z None
Y Ear, Nose, Mouth, and Throat	Y Other Radionuclide	Z None	Z None

SECTION: C NUCLEAR MEDICINE
BODY SYSTEM: B RESPIRATORY SYSTEM
TYPE: 1 PLANAR NUCLEAR MEDICINE IMAGING: Introduction of radioactive materials into the body for single plane display of images developed from the capture of radioactive emissions

Body Part	Radionuclide	Qualifier	Qualifier
2 Lungs and Bronchi	1 Technetium 99m (Tc-99m) 9 Krypton (Kr-81m) T Xenon 127 (Xe-127) V Xenon 133 (Xe-133) Y Other Radionuclide	Z None	Z None
Y Respiratory System	Y Other Radionuclide	Z None	Z None

SECTION: C NUCLEAR MEDICINE
BODY SYSTEM: B RESPIRATORY SYSTEM
TYPE: 2 TOMOGRAPHIC (TOMO) NUCLEAR MEDICINE IMAGING: Introduction of radioactive materials into the body for three-dimensional display of images developed from the capture of radioactive emissions

Body Part	Radionuclide	Qualifier	Qualifier
2 Lungs and Bronchi	1 Technetium 99m (Tc-99m) 9 Krypton (Kr-81m) Y Other Radionuclide	Z None	Z None
Y Respiratory System	Y Other Radionuclide	Z None	Z None

SECTION: C NUCLEAR MEDICINE
BODY SYSTEM: B RESPIRATORY SYSTEM
TYPE: 3 POSITRON EMISSION TOMOGRAPHIC (PET) IMAGING: Introduction of radioactive materials into the body for three-dimensional display of images developed from the simultaneous capture, 180 degrees apart, of radioactive emissions

Body Part	Radionuclide	Qualifier	Qualifier
2 Lungs and Bronchi	K Fluorine 18 (F-18) Y Other Radionuclide	Z None	Z None
Y Respiratory System	Y Other Radionuclide	Z None	Z None

SECTION: C NUCLEAR MEDICINE
BODY SYSTEM: D GASTROINTESTINAL SYSTEM
TYPE: 1 PLANAR NUCLEAR MEDICINE IMAGING: Introduction of radioactive materials into the body for single plane display of images developed from the capture of radioactive emissions

Body Part	Radionuclide	Qualifier	Qualifier
5 Upper Gastrointestinal Tract 7 Gastrointestinal Tract	1 Technetium 99m (Tc-99m) D Indium 111 (In-111) Y Other Radionuclide	Z None	Z None
Y Digestive System	Y Other Radionuclide	Z None	Z None

SECTION: C NUCLEAR MEDICINE
BODY SYSTEM: D GASTROINTESTINAL SYSTEM
TYPE: 2 TOMOGRAPHIC (TOMO) NUCLEAR MEDICINE IMAGING: Introduction of radioactive materials into the body for three-dimensional display of images developed from the capture of radioactive emissions

Body Part	Radionuclide	Qualifier	Qualifier
7 Gastrointestinal Tract	1 Technetium 99m (Tc-99m) D Indium 111 (In-111) Y Other Radionuclide	Z None	Z None
Y Digestive System	Y Other Radionuclide	Z None	Z None

SECTION: C NUCLEAR MEDICINE
BODY SYSTEM: F HEPATOBILIARY SYSTEM AND PANCREAS
TYPE: 1 PLANAR NUCLEAR MEDICINE IMAGING: Introduction of radioactive materials into the body for single plane display of images developed from the capture of radioactive emissions

Body Part	Radionuclide	Qualifier	Qualifier
4 Gallbladder 5 Liver 6 Liver and Spleen C Hepatobiliary System, All	1 Technetium 99m (Tc-99m) Y Other Radionuclide	Z None	Z None
Y Hepatobiliary System and Pancreas	Y Other Radionuclide	Z None	Z None

SECTION: C NUCLEAR MEDICINE
BODY SYSTEM: F HEPATOBILIARY SYSTEM AND PANCREAS
TYPE: 2 TOMOGRAPHIC (TOMO) NUCLEAR MEDICINE IMAGING: Introduction of radioactive materials into the body for three-dimensional display of images developed from the capture of radioactive emissions

Body Part	Radionuclide	Qualifier	Qualifier
4 Gallbladder 5 Liver 6 Liver and Spleen	1 Technetium 99m (Tc-99m) Y Other Radionuclide	Z None	Z None
Y Hepatobiliary System and Pancreas	Y Other Radionuclide	Z None	Z None

SECTION: C NUCLEAR MEDICINE
BODY SYSTEM: G ENDOCRINE SYSTEM
TYPE: 1 PLANAR NUCLEAR MEDICINE IMAGING: Introduction of radioactive materials into the body for single plane display of images developed from the capture of radioactive emissions

Body Part	Radionuclide	Qualifier	Qualifier
1 Parathyroid Glands	1 Technetium 99m (Tc-99m) S Thallium 201 (Tl-201) Y Other Radionuclide	Z None	Z None
2 Thyroid Gland	1 Technetium 99m (Tc-99m) F Iodine 123 (I-123) G Iodine 131 (I-131) Y Other Radionuclide	Z None	Z None
4 Adrenal Glands, Bilateral	G Iodine 131 (I-131) Y Other Radionuclide	Z None	Z None
Y Endocrine System	Y Other Radionuclide	Z None	Z None

SECTION: C NUCLEAR MEDICINE
BODY SYSTEM: G ENDOCRINE SYSTEM
TYPE: 2 TOMOGRAPHIC (TOMO) NUCLEAR MEDICINE IMAGING: Introduction of radioactive materials into the body for three-dimensional display of images developed from the capture of radioactive emissions

Body Part	Radionuclide	Qualifier	Qualifier
1 Parathyroid Glands	1 Technetium 99m (Tc-99m) S Thallium 201 (Tl-201) Y Other Radionuclide	Z None	Z None
Y Endocrine System	Y Other Radionuclide	Z None	Z None

SECTION: C NUCLEAR MEDICINE
BODY SYSTEM: G ENDOCRINE SYSTEM
TYPE: 4 NONIMAGING NUCLEAR MEDICINE UPTAKE: Introduction of radioactive materials into the body for measurements of organ function, from the detection of radioactive emissions

Body Part	Radionuclide	Qualifier	Qualifier
2 Thyroid Gland	1 Technetium 99m (Tc-99m) F Iodine 123 (I-123) G Iodine 131 (I-131) Y Other Radionuclide	Z None	Z None
Y Endocrine System	Y Other Radionuclide	Z None	Z None

SECTION: C NUCLEAR MEDICINE
BODY SYSTEM: H SKIN, SUBCUTANEOUS TISSUE AND BREAST
TYPE: 1 PLANAR NUCLEAR MEDICINE IMAGING: Introduction of radioactive materials into the body for single plane display of images developed from the capture of radioactive emissions

Body Part	Radionuclide	Qualifier	Qualifier
Ø Breast, Right 1 Breast, Left 2 Breasts, Bilateral	1 Technetium 99m (Tc-99m) S Thallium 2Ø1 (Tl-2Ø1) Y Other Radionuclide	Z None	Z None
Y Skin, Subcutaneous Tissue, and Breast	Y Other Radionuclide	Z None	Z None

SECTION: C NUCLEAR MEDICINE
BODY SYSTEM: H SKIN, SUBCUTANEOUS TISSUE AND BREAST
TYPE: 2 TOMOGRAPHIC (TOMO) NUCLEAR MEDICINE IMAGING: Introduction of radioactive materials into the body for three-dimensional display of images developed from the capture of radioactive emissions

Body Part	Radionuclide	Qualifier	Qualifier
Ø Breast, Right 1 Breast, Left 2 Breasts, Bilateral	1 Technetium 99m (Tc-99m) S Thallium 2Ø1 (Tl-2Ø1) Y Other Radionuclide	Z None	Z None
Y Skin, Subcutaneous Tissue, and Breast	Y Other Radionuclide	Z None	Z None

SECTION: C NUCLEAR MEDICINE
BODY SYSTEM: P MUSCULOSKELETAL SYSTEM
TYPE: 1 **PLANAR NUCLEAR MEDICINE IMAGING:** Introduction of radioactive materials into the body for single plane display of images developed from the capture of radioactive emissions

Body Part	Radionuclide	Qualifier	Qualifier
1 Skull 4 Thorax 5 Spine 6 Pelvis 7 Spine and Pelvis 8 Upper Extremity, Right 9 Upper Extremity, Left B Upper Extremities, Bilateral C Lower Extremity, Right D Lower Extremity, Left F Lower Extremities, Bilateral Z Musculoskeletal System, All	1 Technetium 99m (Tc-99m) Y Other Radionuclide	Z None	Z None
Y Musculoskeletal System, Other	Y Other Radionuclide	Z None	Z None

SECTION: C NUCLEAR MEDICINE
BODY SYSTEM: P MUSCULOSKELETAL SYSTEM
TYPE: 2 **TOMOGRAPHIC (TOMO) NUCLEAR MEDICINE IMAGING:** Introduction of radioactive materials into the body for three-dimensional display of images developed from the capture of radioactive emissions

Body Part	Radionuclide	Qualifier	Qualifier
1 Skull 2 Cervical Spine 3 Skull and Cervical Spine 4 Thorax 6 Pelvis 7 Spine and Pelvis 8 Upper Extremity, Right 9 Upper Extremity, Left B Upper Extremities, Bilateral C Lower Extremity, Right D Lower Extremity, Left F Lower Extremities, Bilateral G Thoracic Spine H Lumbar Spine J Thoracolumbar Spine	1 Technetium 99m (Tc-99m) Y Other Radionuclide	Z None	Z None
Y Musculoskeletal System, Other	Y Other Radionuclide	Z None	Z None

SECTION: C NUCLEAR MEDICINE
BODY SYSTEM: P MUSCULOSKELETAL SYSTEM
TYPE: 5 NONIMAGING NUCLEAR MEDICINE PROBE: Introduction of radioactive materials into the body for the study of distribution and fate of certain substances by the detection of radioactive emissions; or, alternatively, measurement of absorption of radioactive emissions from an external source

Body Part	Radionuclide	Qualifier	Qualifier
5 Spine N Upper Extremities P Lower Extremities	Z None	Z None	Z None
Y Musculoskeletal System, Other	Y Other Radionuclide	Z None	Z None

SECTION: C NUCLEAR MEDICINE
BODY SYSTEM: T URINARY SYSTEM
TYPE: 1 PLANAR NUCLEAR MEDICINE IMAGING: Introduction of radioactive materials into the body for single plane display of images developed from the capture of radioactive emissions

Body Part	Radionuclide	Qualifier	Qualifier
3 Kidneys, Ureters, and Bladder	1 Technetium 99m (Tc-99m) F Iodine 123 (I-123) G Iodine 131 (I-131) Y Other Radionuclide	Z None	Z None
H Bladder and Ureters	1 Technetium 99m (Tc-99m) Y Other Radionuclide	Z None	Z None
Y Urinary System	Y Other Radionuclide	Z None	Z None

SECTION: C NUCLEAR MEDICINE
BODY SYSTEM: T URINARY SYSTEM
TYPE: 2 TOMOGRAPHIC (TOMO) NUCLEAR MEDICINE IMAGING: Introduction of radioactive materials into the body for three-dimensional display of images developed from the capture of radioactive emissions

Body Part	Radionuclide	Qualifier	Qualifier
3 Kidneys, Ureters, and Bladder	1 Technetium 99m (Tc-99m) Y Other Radionuclide	Z None	Z None
Y Urinary System	Y Other Radionuclide	Z None	Z None

SECTION: C NUCLEAR MEDICINE
BODY SYSTEM: T URINARY SYSTEM
TYPE: 6 NONIMAGING NUCLEAR MEDICINE ASSAY: Introduction of radioactive materials into the body for the study of body fluids and blood elements, by the detection of radioactive emissions

Body Part	Radionuclide	Qualifier	Qualifier
3 Kidneys, Ureters, and Bladder	1 Technetium 99m (Tc-99m) F Iodine 123 (I-123) G Iodine 131 (I-131) H Iodine 125 (I-125) Y Other Radionuclide	Z None	Z None
Y Urinary System	Y Other Radionuclide	Z None	Z None

CV1

SECTION: C NUCLEAR MEDICINE

BODY SYSTEM: V MALE REPRODUCTIVE SYSTEM

TYPE: 1 PLANAR NUCLEAR MEDICINE IMAGING: Introduction of radioactive materials into the body for single plane display of images developed from the capture of radioactive emissions

Body Part	Radionuclide	Qualifier	Qualifier
9 Testicles, Bilateral ♂	1 Technetium 99m (Tc-99m) Y Other Radionuclide	Z None	Z None
Y Male Reproductive System ♂	Y Other Radionuclide	Z None	Z None

SECTION: C NUCLEAR MEDICINE
BODY SYSTEM: W ANATOMICAL REGIONS
TYPE: 1 PLANAR NUCLEAR MEDICINE IMAGING: Introduction of radioactive materials into the body for single plane display of images developed from the capture of radioactive emissions

Body Part	Radionuclide	Qualifier	Qualifier
Ø Abdomen 1 Abdomen and Pelvis 4 Chest and Abdomen 6 Chest and Neck B Head and Neck D Lower Extremity J Pelvic Region M Upper Extremity N Whole Body	1 Technetium 99m (Tc-99m) D Indium 111 (In-111) F Iodine 123 (I-123) G Iodine 131 (I-131) L Gallium 67 (Ga-67) S Thallium 2Ø1 (Tl-2Ø1) Y Other Radionuclide	Z None	Z None
3 Chest	1 Technetium 99m (Tc-99m) D Indium 111 (In-111) F Iodine 123 (I-123) G Iodine 131 (I-131) K Fluorine 18 (F-18) L Gallium 67 (Ga-67) S Thallium 2Ø1 (Tl-2Ø1) Y Other Radionuclide	Z None	Z None
Y Anatomical Regions, Multiple	Y Other Radionuclide	Z None	Z None
Z Anatomical Region, Other	Z None	Z None	Z None

SECTION: C NUCLEAR MEDICINE
BODY SYSTEM: W ANATOMICAL REGIONS
TYPE: 2 TOMOGRAPHIC (TOMO) NUCLEAR MEDICINE IMAGING: Introduction of radioactive materials into the body for three-dimensional display of images developed from the capture of radioactive emissions

Body Part	Radionuclide	Qualifier	Qualifier
Ø Abdomen 1 Abdomen and Pelvis 3 Chest 4 Chest and Abdomen 6 Chest and Neck B Head and Neck D Lower Extremity J Pelvic Region M Upper Extremity	1 Technetium 99m (Tc-99m) D Indium 111 (In-111) F Iodine 123 (I-123) G Iodine 131 (I-131) K Fluorine 18 (F-18) L Gallium 67 (Ga-67) S Thallium 2Ø1 (Tl-2Ø1) Y Other Radionuclide	Z None	Z None
Y Anatomical Regions, Multiple	Y Other Radionuclide	Z None	Z None

SECTION: **C NUCLEAR MEDICINE**
BODY SYSTEM: W ANATOMICAL REGIONS
TYPE: 3 **POSITRON EMISSION TOMOGRAPHIC (PET) IMAGING:** Introduction of radioactive materials into the body for three-dimensional display of images developed from the simultaneous capture, 180 degrees apart, of radioactive emissions

Body Part	Radionuclide	Qualifier	Qualifier
N Whole Body	Y Other Radionuclide	Z None	Z None

SECTION: **C NUCLEAR MEDICINE**
BODY SYSTEM: W ANATOMICAL REGIONS
TYPE: 5 **NONIMAGING NUCLEAR MEDICINE PROBE:** Introduction of radioactive materials into the body for the study of distribution and fate of certain substances by the detection of radioactive emissions; or, alternatively, measurement of absorption of radioactive emissions from an external source

Body Part	Radionuclide	Qualifier	Qualifier
Ø Abdomen 1 Abdomen and Pelvis 3 Chest 4 Chest and Abdomen 6 Chest and Neck B Head and Neck D Lower Extremity J Pelvic Region M Upper Extremity	1 Technetium 99m (Tc-99m) D Indium 111 (In-111) Y Other Radionuclide	Z None	Z None

SECTION: **C NUCLEAR MEDICINE**
BODY SYSTEM: W ANATOMICAL REGIONS
TYPE: 7 **SYSTEMIC NUCLEAR MEDICINE THERAPY:** Introduction of unsealed radioactive materials into the body for treatment

Body Part	Radionuclide	Qualifier	Qualifier
Ø Abdomen 3 Chest	N Phosphorus 32 (P-32) Y Other Radionuclide	Z None	Z None
G Thyroid	G Iodine 131 (I-131) Y Other Radionuclide	Z None	Z None
N Whole Body	8 Samarium 153 (Sm-153) G Iodine 131 (I-131) N Phosphorus 32 (P-32) P Strontium 89 (Sr-89) Y Other Radionuclide	Z None	Z None
Y Anatomical Regions, Multiple	Y Other Radionuclide	Z None	Z None

D Radiation Therapy **666**
- DØ. Central and Peripheral Nervous System 668
  - DØØ. Beam Radiation 668
  - DØ1. Brachytherapy 668
  - DØ2. Stereotactic Radiosurgery 668
  - DØY. Other Radiation 668
- D7. Lymphatic and Hematologic System 669
  - D7Ø. Beam Radiation 669
  - D71. Brachytherapy 669
  - D72. Stereotactic Radiosurgery 670
  - D7Y. Other Radiation 670
- D8. Eye 671
  - D8Ø. Beam Radiation 671
  - D81. Brachytherapy 671
  - D82. Stereotactic Radiosurgery 671
  - D8Y. Other Radiation 671
- D9. Ear, Nose, Mouth, and Throat 672
  - D9Ø. Beam Radiation 672
  - D91. Brachytherapy 672
  - D92. Stereotactic Radiosurgery 673
  - D9Y. Other Radiation 673
- DB. Respiratory System 674
  - DBØ. Beam Radiation 674
  - DB1. Brachytherapy 674
  - DB2. Stereotactic Radiosurgery 675
  - DBY. Other Radiation 675
- DD. Gastrointestinal System 676
  - DDØ. Beam Radiation 676
  - DD1. Brachytherapy 676
  - DD2. Stereotactic Radiosurgery 677
  - DDY. Other Radiation 677
- DF. Hepatobiliary System and Pancreas 678
  - DFØ. Beam Radiation 678
  - DF1. Brachytherapy 678
  - DF2. Stereotactic Radiosurgery 678
  - DFY. Other Radiation 678
- DG. Endocrine System 679
  - DGØ. Beam Radiation 679
  - DG1. Brachytherapy 679
  - DG2. Stereotactic Radiosurgery 679
  - DGY. Other Radiation 679
- DH. Skin 680
  - DHØ. Beam Radiation 680
  - DHY. Other Radiation 680
- DM. Breast 681
  - DMØ. Beam Radiation 681
  - DM1. Brachytherapy 681
  - DM2. Stereotactic Radiosurgery 681
  - DMY. Other Radiation 681
- DP. Musculoskeletal System 682
  - DPØ. Beam Radiation 682
  - DPY. Other Radiation 682
- DT. Urinary System 683
  - DTØ. Beam Radiation 683
  - DT1. Brachytherapy 683
  - DT2. Stereotactic Radiosurgery 683
  - DTY. Other Radiation 683

DU. Female Reproductive System 684
DUØ. Beam Radiation 684
DU1. Brachytherapy 684
DU2. Stereotactic Radiosurgery 685
DUY. Other Radiation 685
DV. Male Reproductive System 686
DVØ. Beam Radiation 686
DV1. Brachytherapy 686
DV2. Stereotactic Radiosurgery 687
DVY. Other Radiation 687
DW. Anatomical Regions 688
DWØ. Beam Radiation 688
DW1. Brachytherapy 688
DW2. Stereotactic Radiosurgery 689
DWY. Other Radiation 689

SECTION: D RADIATION THERAPY
BODY SYSTEM: Ø CENTRAL AND PERIPHERAL NERVOUS SYSTEM
MODALITY: Ø BEAM RADIATION

Treatment Site	Modality Qualifier	Isotope	Qualifier
Ø Brain 1 Brain Stem 6 Spinal Cord 7 Peripheral Nerve	Ø Photons <1 MeV 1 Photons 1 - 1Ø MeV 2 Photons >1Ø MeV 4 Heavy Particles (Protons,Ions) 5 Neutrons 6 Neutron Capture	Z None	Z None
Ø Brain 1 Brain Stem 6 Spinal Cord 7 Peripheral Nerve	3 Electrons	Z None	Ø Intraoperative Z None

SECTION: D RADIATION THERAPY
BODY SYSTEM: Ø CENTRAL AND PERIPHERAL NERVOUS SYSTEM
MODALITY: 1 BRACHYTHERAPY

Treatment Site	Modality Qualifier	Isotope	Qualifier
Ø Brain 1 Brain Stem 6 Spinal Cord 7 Peripheral Nerve	9 High Dose Rate (HDR)	7 Cesium 137 (Cs-137) 8 Iridium 192 (Ir-192) 9 Iodine 125 (I-125) B Palladium 1Ø3 (Pd-1Ø3) C Californium 252 (Cf-252) Y Other Isotope	Z None
Ø Brain 1 Brain Stem 6 Spinal Cord 7 Peripheral Nerve	B Low Dose Rate (LDR)	6 Cesium 131 (Cs-131) 7 Cesium 137 (Cs-137) 8 Iridium 192 (Ir-192) 9 Iodine 125 (I-125) C Californium 252 (Cf-252) Y Other Isotope	Z None
Ø Brain 1 Brain Stem 6 Spinal Cord 7 Peripheral Nerve	B Low Dose Rate (LDR)	B Palladium 1Ø3 (Pd-1Ø3)	1 Unidirectional Source Z None

SECTION: D RADIATION THERAPY
BODY SYSTEM: Ø CENTRAL AND PERIPHERAL NERVOUS SYSTEM
MODALITY: 2 STEREOTACTIC RADIOSURGERY

Treatment Site	Modality Qualifier	Isotope	Qualifier
Ø Brain 1 Brain Stem 6 Spinal Cord 7 Peripheral Nerve	D Stereotactic Other Photon Radiosurgery H Stereotactic Particulate Radiosurgery J Stereotactic Gamma Beam Radiosurgery	Z None	Z None

DRG Non-OR DØ2[Ø167][DJ]ZZ

SECTION: D RADIATION THERAPY
BODY SYSTEM: Ø CENTRAL AND PERIPHERAL NERVOUS SYSTEM
MODALITY: Y OTHER RADIATION

Treatment Site	Modality Qualifier	Isotope	Qualifier
Ø Brain 1 Brain Stem 6 Spinal Cord 7 Peripheral Nerve	7 Contact Radiation 8 Hyperthermia C Intraoperative Radiation Therapy (IORT) F Plaque Radiation	Z None	Z None

SECTION: D RADIATION THERAPY
BODY SYSTEM: 7 LYMPHATIC AND HEMATOLOGIC SYSTEM
MODALITY: 0 BEAM RADIATION

Treatment Site	Modality Qualifier	Isotope	Qualifier
0 Bone Marrow 1 Thymus 2 Spleen 3 Lymphatics, Neck 4 Lymphatics, Axillary 5 Lymphatics, Thorax 6 Lymphatics, Abdomen 7 Lymphatics, Pelvis 8 Lymphatics, Inguinal	0 Photons <1 MeV 1 Photons 1 - 10 MeV 2 Photons >10 MeV 4 Heavy Particles (Protons, Ions) 5 Neutrons 6 Neutron Capture	Z None	Z None
0 Bone Marrow 1 Thymus 2 Spleen 3 Lymphatics, Neck 4 Lymphatics, Axillary 5 Lymphatics, Thorax 6 Lymphatics, Abdomen 7 Lymphatics, Pelvis 8 Lymphatics, Inguinal	3 Electrons	Z None	0 Intraoperative Z None

SECTION: D RADIATION THERAPY
BODY SYSTEM: 7 LYMPHATIC AND HEMATOLOGIC SYSTEM
MODALITY: 1 BRACHYTHERAPY

Treatment Site	Modality Qualifier	Isotope	Qualifier
0 Bone Marrow 1 Thymus 2 Spleen 3 Lymphatics, Neck 4 Lymphatics, Axillary 5 Lymphatics, Thorax 6 Lymphatics, Abdomen 7 Lymphatics, Pelvis 8 Lymphatics, Inguinal	9 High Dose Rate (HDR)	7 Cesium 137 (Cs-137) 8 Iridium 192 (Ir-192) 9 Iodine 125 (I-125) B Palladium 103 (Pd-103) C Californium 252 (Cf-252) Y Other Isotope	Z None
0 Bone Marrow 1 Thymus 2 Spleen 3 Lymphatics, Neck 4 Lymphatics, Axillary 5 Lymphatics, Thorax 6 Lymphatics, Abdomen 7 Lymphatics, Pelvis 8 Lymphatics, Inguinal	B Low Dose Rate (LDR)	6 Cesium 131 (Cs-131) 7 Cesium 137 (Cs-137) 8 Iridium 192 (Ir-192) 9 Iodine 125 (I-125) C Californium 252 (Cf-252) Y Other Isotope	Z None
0 Bone Marrow 1 Thymus 2 Spleen 3 Lymphatics, Neck 4 Lymphatics, Axillary 5 Lymphatics, Thorax 6 Lymphatics, Abdomen 7 Lymphatics, Pelvis 8 Lymphatics, Inguinal	B Low Dose Rate (LDR)	B Palladium 103 (Pd-103)	1 Unidirectional Source Z None

SECTION: D RADIATION THERAPY
BODY SYSTEM: 7 LYMPHATIC AND HEMATOLOGIC SYSTEM
MODALITY: 2 STEREOTACTIC RADIOSURGERY

Treatment Site	Modality Qualifier	Isotope	Qualifier
Ø Bone Marrow 1 Thymus 2 Spleen 3 Lymphatics, Neck 4 Lymphatics, Axillary 5 Lymphatics, Thorax 6 Lymphatics, Abdomen 7 Lymphatics, Pelvis 8 Lymphatics, Inguinal	D Stereotactic Other Photon Radiosurgery H Stereotactic Particulate Radiosurgery J Stereotactic Gamma Beam Radiosurgery	Z None	Z None

DRG Non-OR All Values

SECTION: D RADIATION THERAPY
BODY SYSTEM: 7 LYMPHATIC AND HEMATOLOGIC SYSTEM
MODALITY: Y OTHER RADIATION

Treatment Site	Modality Qualifier	Isotope	Qualifier
Ø Bone Marrow 1 Thymus 2 Spleen 3 Lymphatics, Neck 4 Lymphatics, Axillary 5 Lymphatics, Thorax 6 Lymphatics, Abdomen 7 Lymphatics, Pelvis 8 Lymphatics, Inguinal	8 Hyperthermia F Plaque Radiation	Z None	Z None

SECTION: D RADIATION THERAPY
BODY SYSTEM: 8 EYE
MODALITY: 0 BEAM RADIATION

Treatment Site	Modality Qualifier	Isotope	Qualifier
0 Eye	0 Photons <1 MeV 1 Photons 1 - 10 MeV 2 Photons >10 MeV 4 Heavy Particles (Protons, Ions) 5 Neutrons 6 Neutron Capture	Z None	Z None
0 Eye	3 Electrons	Z None	0 Intraoperative Z None

SECTION: D RADIATION THERAPY
BODY SYSTEM: 8 EYE
MODALITY: 1 BRACHYTHERAPY

Treatment Site	Modality Qualifier	Isotope	Qualifier
0 Eye	9 High Dose Rate (HDR)	7 Cesium 137 (Cs-137) 8 Iridium 192 (Ir-192) 9 Iodine 125 (I-125) B Palladium 103 (Pd-103) C Californium 252 (Cf-252) Y Other Isotope	Z None
0 Eye	B Low Dose Rate (LDR)	6 Cesium 131 (Cs-131) 7 Cesium 137 (Cs-137) 8 Iridium 192 (Ir-192) 9 Iodine 125 (I-125) C Californium 252 (Cf-252) Y Other Isotope	Z None
0 Eye	B Low Dose Rate (LDR)	B Palladium 103 (Pd-103)	1 Unidirectional Source Z None

SECTION: D RADIATION THERAPY
BODY SYSTEM: 8 EYE
MODALITY: 2 STEREOTACTIC RADIOSURGERY

Treatment Site	Modality Qualifier	Isotope	Qualifier
0 Eye	D Stereotactic Other Photon Radiosurgery H Stereotactic Particulate Radiosurgery J Stereotactic Gamma Beam Radiosurgery	Z None	Z None

DRG Non-OR All Values

SECTION: D RADIATION THERAPY
BODY SYSTEM: 8 EYE
MODALITY: Y OTHER RADIATION

Treatment Site	Modality Qualifier	Isotope	Qualifier
0 Eye	7 Contact Radiation 8 Hyperthermia F Plaque Radiation	Z None	Z None

SECTION: D RADIATION THERAPY
BODY SYSTEM: 9 EAR, NOSE, MOUTH, AND THROAT
MODALITY: Ø BEAM RADIATION

Treatment Site	Modality Qualifier	Isotope	Qualifier
Ø Ear 1 Nose 3 Hypopharynx 4 Mouth 5 Tongue 6 Salivary Glands 7 Sinuses 8 Hard Palate 9 Soft Palate B Larynx D Nasopharynx F Oropharynx	Ø Photons <1 MeV 1 Photons 1 - 1Ø MeV 2 Photons >1Ø MeV 4 Heavy Particles (Protons, Ions) 5 Neutrons 6 Neutron Capture	Z None	Z None
Ø Ear 1 Nose 3 Hypopharynx 4 Mouth 5 Tongue 6 Salivary Glands 7 Sinuses 8 Hard Palate 9 Soft Palate B Larynx D Nasopharynx F Oropharynx	3 Electrons	Z None	Ø Intraoperative Z None

SECTION: D RADIATION THERAPY
BODY SYSTEM: 9 EAR, NOSE, MOUTH, AND THROAT
MODALITY: 1 BRACHYTHERAPY *(on multiple pages)*

Treatment Site	Modality Qualifier	Isotope	Qualifier
Ø Ear 1 Nose 3 Hypopharynx 4 Mouth 5 Tongue 6 Salivary Glands 7 Sinuses 8 Hard Palate 9 Soft Palate B Larynx D Nasopharynx F Oropharynx	9 High Dose Rate (HDR)	7 Cesium 137 (Cs-137) 8 Iridium 192 (Ir-192) 9 Iodine 125 (I-125) B Palladium 1Ø3 (Pd-1Ø3) C Californium 252 (Cf-252) Y Other Isotope	Z None
Ø Ear 1 Nose 3 Hypopharynx 4 Mouth 5 Tongue 6 Salivary Glands 7 Sinuses 8 Hard Palate 9 Soft Palate B Larynx D Nasopharynx F Oropharynx	B Low Dose Rate (LDR)	6 Cesium 131 (Cs-131) 7 Cesium 137 (Cs-137) 8 Iridium 192 (Ir-192) 9 Iodine 125 (I-125) C Californium 252 (Cf-252) Y Other Isotope	Z None

SECTION: D RADIATION THERAPY
BODY SYSTEM: 9 EAR, NOSE, MOUTH, AND THROAT
MODALITY: 1 BRACHYTHERAPY *(continued)*

Treatment Site	Modality Qualifier	Isotope	Qualifier
Ø Ear 1 Nose 3 Hypopharynx 4 Mouth 5 Tongue 6 Salivary Glands 7 Sinuses 8 Hard Palate 9 Soft Palate B Larynx D Nasopharynx F Oropharynx	B Low Dose Rate (LDR)	B Palladium 1Ø3 (Pd-1Ø3)	1 Unidirectional Source Z None

SECTION: D RADIATION THERAPY
BODY SYSTEM: 9 EAR, NOSE, MOUTH, AND THROAT
MODALITY: 2 STEREOTACTIC RADIOSURGERY

Treatment Site	Modality Qualifier	Isotope	Qualifier
Ø Ear 1 Nose 4 Mouth 5 Tongue 6 Salivary Glands 7 Sinuses 8 Hard Palate 9 Soft Palate B Larynx C Pharynx D Nasopharynx	D Stereotactic Other Photon Radiosurgery H Stereotactic Particulate Radiosurgery J Stereotactic Gamma Beam Radiosurgery	Z None	Z None

DRG Non-OR All Values

SECTION: D RADIATION THERAPY
BODY SYSTEM: 9 EAR, NOSE, MOUTH, AND THROAT
MODALITY: Y OTHER RADIATION

Treatment Site	Modality Qualifier	Isotope	Qualifier
Ø Ear 1 Nose 5 Tongue 6 Salivary Glands 7 Sinuses 8 Hard Palate 9 Soft Palate	7 Contact Radiation 8 Hyperthermia F Plaque Radiation	Z None	Z None
3 Hypopharynx F Oropharynx	7 Contact Radiation 8 Hyperthermia	Z None	Z None
4 Mouth B Larynx D Nasopharynx	7 Contact Radiation 8 Hyperthermia C Intraoperative Radiation Therapy (IORT) F Plaque Radiation	Z None	Z None
C Pharynx	C Intraoperative Radiation Therapy (IORT) F Plaque Radiation	Z None	Z None

SECTION: D RADIATION THERAPY
BODY SYSTEM: B RESPIRATORY SYSTEM
MODALITY: 0 BEAM RADIATION

Treatment Site	Modality Qualifier	Isotope	Qualifier
Ø Trachea 1 Bronchus 2 Lung 5 Pleura 6 Mediastinum 7 Chest Wall 8 Diaphragm	Ø Photons <1 MeV 1 Photons 1 - 1Ø MeV 2 Photons >1Ø MeV 4 Heavy Particles (Protons, Ions) 5 Neutrons 6 Neutron Capture	Z None	Z None
Ø Trachea 1 Bronchus 2 Lung 5 Pleura 6 Mediastinum 7 Chest Wall 8 Diaphragm	3 Electrons	Z None	Ø Intraoperative Z None

SECTION: D RADIATION THERAPY
BODY SYSTEM: B RESPIRATORY SYSTEM
MODALITY: 1 BRACHYTHERAPY

Treatment Site	Modality Qualifier	Isotope	Qualifier
Ø Trachea 1 Bronchus 2 Lung 5 Pleura 6 Mediastinum 7 Chest Wall 8 Diaphragm	9 High Dose Rate (HDR)	7 Cesium 137 (Cs-137) 8 Iridium 192 (Ir-192) 9 Iodine 125 (I-125) B Palladium 1Ø3 (Pd-1Ø3) C Californium 252 (Cf-252) Y Other Isotope	Z None
Ø Trachea 1 Bronchus 2 Lung 5 Pleura 6 Mediastinum 7 Chest Wall 8 Diaphragm	B Low Dose Rate (LDR)	6 Cesium 131 (Cs-131) 7 Cesium 137 (Cs-137) 8 Iridium 192 (Ir-192) 9 Iodine 125 (I-125) C Californium 252 (Cf-252) Y Other Isotope	Z None
Ø Trachea 1 Bronchus 2 Lung 5 Pleura 6 Mediastinum 7 Chest Wall 8 Diaphragm	B Low Dose Rate (LDR)	B Palladium 1Ø3 (Pd-1Ø3)	1 Unidirectional Source Z None

SECTION: D RADIATION THERAPY
BODY SYSTEM: B RESPIRATORY SYSTEM
MODALITY: 2 STEREOTACTIC RADIOSURGERY

Treatment Site	Modality Qualifier	Isotope	Qualifier
Ø Trachea 1 Bronchus 2 Lung 5 Pleura 6 Mediastinum 7 Chest Wall 8 Diaphragm	D Stereotactic Other Photon Radiosurgery H Stereotactic Particulate Radiosurgery J Stereotactic Gamma Beam Radiosurgery	Z None	Z None

DRG Non-OR DB2[125678][DJ]ZZ

SECTION: D RADIATION THERAPY
BODY SYSTEM: B RESPIRATORY SYSTEM
MODALITY: Y OTHER RADIATION

Treatment Site	Modality Qualifier	Isotope	Qualifier
Ø Trachea 1 Bronchus 2 Lung 5 Pleura 6 Mediastinum 7 Chest Wall 8 Diaphragm	7 Contact Radiation 8 Hyperthermia F Plaque Radiation	Z None	Z None

SECTION: D RADIATION THERAPY
BODY SYSTEM: D GASTROINTESTINAL SYSTEM
MODALITY: Ø BEAM RADIATION

Treatment Site	Modality Qualifier	Isotope	Qualifier
Ø Esophagus 1 Stomach 2 Duodenum 3 Jejunum 4 Ileum 5 Colon 7 Rectum	Ø Photons <1 MeV 1 Photons 1 - 1Ø MeV 2 Photons >1Ø MeV 4 Heavy Particles (Protons, Ions) 5 Neutrons 6 Neutron Capture	Z None	Z None
Ø Esophagus 1 Stomach 2 Duodenum 3 Jejunum 4 Ileum 5 Colon 7 Rectum	3 Electrons	Z None	Ø Intraoperative Z None

SECTION: D RADIATION THERAPY
BODY SYSTEM: D GASTROINTESTINAL SYSTEM
MODALITY: 1 BRACHYTHERAPY

Treatment Site	Modality Qualifier	Isotope	Qualifier
Ø Esophagus 1 Stomach 2 Duodenum 3 Jejunum 4 Ileum 5 Colon 7 Rectum	9 High Dose Rate (HDR)	7 Cesium 137 (Cs-137) 8 Iridium 192 (Ir-192) 9 Iodine 125 (I-125) B Palladium 1Ø3 (Pd-1Ø3) C Californium 252 (Cf-252) Y Other Isotope	Z None
Ø Esophagus 1 Stomach 2 Duodenum 3 Jejunum 4 Ileum 5 Colon 7 Rectum	B Low Dose Rate (LDR)	6 Cesium 131 (Cs-131) 7 Cesium 137 (Cs-137) 8 Iridium 192 (Ir-192) 9 Iodine 125 (I-125) C Californium 252 (Cf-252) Y Other Isotope	Z None
Ø Esophagus 1 Stomach 2 Duodenum 3 Jejunum 4 Ileum 5 Colon 7 Rectum	B Low Dose Rate (LDR)	B Palladium 1Ø3 (Pd-1Ø3)	1 Unidirectional Source Z None

SECTION: D RADIATION THERAPY
BODY SYSTEM: D GASTROINTESTINAL SYSTEM
MODALITY: 2 STEREOTACTIC RADIOSURGERY

Treatment Site	Modality Qualifier	Isotope	Qualifier
Ø Esophagus 1 Stomach 2 Duodenum 3 Jejunum 4 Ileum 5 Colon 7 Rectum	D Stereotactic Other Photon Radiosurgery H Stereotactic Particulate Radiosurgery J Stereotactic Gamma Beam Radiosurgery	Z None	Z None

DRG Non-OR All Values

SECTION: D RADIATION THERAPY
BODY SYSTEM: D GASTROINTESTINAL SYSTEM
MODALITY: Y OTHER RADIATION

Treatment Site	Modality Qualifier	Isotope	Qualifier
Ø Esophagus	7 Contact Radiation 8 Hyperthermia F Plaque Radiation	Z None	Z None
1 Stomach 2 Duodenum 3 Jejunum 4 Ileum 5 Colon 7 Rectum	7 Contact Radiation 8 Hyperthermia C Intraoperative Radiation Therapy (IORT) F Plaque Radiation	Z None	Z None
8 Anus	C Intraoperative Radiation Therapy (IORT) F Plaque Radiation	Z None	Z None

SECTION: D RADIATION THERAPY
BODY SYSTEM: F HEPATOBILIARY SYSTEM AND PANCREAS
MODALITY: Ø BEAM RADIATION

Treatment Site	Modality Qualifier	Isotope	Qualifier
Ø Liver 1 Gallbladder 2 Bile Ducts 3 Pancreas	Ø Photons <1 MeV 1 Photons 1 - 1Ø MeV 2 Photons >1Ø MeV 4 Heavy Particles (Protons, Ions) 5 Neutrons 6 Neutron Capture	Z None	Z None
Ø Liver 1 Gallbladder 2 Bile Ducts 3 Pancreas	3 Electrons	Z None	Ø Intraoperative Z None

SECTION: D RADIATION THERAPY
BODY SYSTEM: F HEPATOBILIARY SYSTEM AND PANCREAS
MODALITY: 1 BRACHYTHERAPY

Treatment Site	Modality Qualifier	Isotope	Qualifier
Ø Liver 1 Gallbladder 2 Bile Ducts 3 Pancreas	9 High Dose Rate (HDR)	7 Cesium 137 (Cs-137) 8 Iridium 192 (Ir-192) 9 Iodine 125 (I-125) B Palladium 1Ø3 (Pd-1Ø3) C Californium 252 (Cf-252) Y Other Isotope	Z None
Ø Liver 1 Gallbladder 2 Bile Ducts 3 Pancreas	B Low Dose Rate (LDR)	6 Cesium 131 (Cs-131) 7 Cesium 137 (Cs-137) 8 Iridium 192 (Ir-192) 9 Iodine 125 (I-125) C Californium 252 (Cf-252) Y Other Isotope	Z None
Ø Liver 1 Gallbladder 2 Bile Ducts 3 Pancreas	B Low Dose Rate (LDR)	B Palladium 1Ø3 (Pd-1Ø3)	1 Unidirectional Source Z None

Coding Clinic: 2Ø22, Q2, P26 – DF1ØBYZ

SECTION: D RADIATION THERAPY
BODY SYSTEM: F HEPATOBILIARY SYSTEM AND PANCREAS
MODALITY: 2 STEREOTACTIC RADIOSURGERY

Treatment Site	Modality Qualifier	Isotope	Qualifier
Ø Liver 1 Gallbladder 2 Bile Ducts 3 Pancreas	D Stereotactic Other Photon Radiosurgery H Stereotactic Particulate Radiosurgery J Stereotactic Gamma Beam Radiosurgery	Z None	Z None

DRG Non-OR All Values

SECTION: D RADIATION THERAPY
BODY SYSTEM: F HEPATOBILIARY SYSTEM AND PANCREAS
MODALITY: Y OTHER RADIATION

Treatment Site	Modality Qualifier	Isotope	Qualifier
Ø Liver 1 Gallbladder 2 Bile Ducts 3 Pancreas	7 Contact Radiation 8 Hyperthermia C Intraoperative Radiation Therapy (IORT) F Plaque Radiation	Z None	Z None

SECTION: D RADIATION THERAPY
BODY SYSTEM: G ENDOCRINE SYSTEM
MODALITY: Ø BEAM RADIATION

Treatment Site	Modality Qualifier	Isotope	Qualifier
Ø Pituitary Gland 1 Pineal Body 2 Adrenal Glands 4 Parathyroid Glands 5 Thyroid	Ø Photons <1 MeV 1 Photons 1 - 1Ø MeV 2 Photons >1Ø MeV 5 Neutrons 6 Neutron Capture	Z None	Z None
Ø Pituitary Gland 1 Pineal Body 2 Adrenal Glands 4 Parathyroid Glands 5 Thyroid	3 Electrons	Z None	Ø Intraoperative Z None

SECTION: D RADIATION THERAPY
BODY SYSTEM: G ENDOCRINE SYSTEM
MODALITY: 1 BRACHYTHERAPY

Treatment Site	Modality Qualifier	Isotope	Qualifier
Ø Pituitary Gland 1 Pineal Body 2 Adrenal Glands 4 Parathyroid Glands 5 Thyroid	9 High Dose Rate (HDR)	7 Cesium 137 (Cs-137) 8 Iridium 192 (Ir-192) 9 Iodine 125 (I-125) B Palladium 1Ø3 (Pd-1Ø3) C Californium 252 (Cf-252) Y Other Isotope	Z None
Ø Pituitary Gland 1 Pineal Body 2 Adrenal Glands 4 Parathyroid Glands 5 Thyroid	B Low Dose Rate (LDR)	6 Cesium 131 (Cs-131) 7 Cesium 137 (Cs-137) 8 Iridium 192 (Ir-192) 9 Iodine 125 (I-125) C Californium 252 (Cf-252) Y Other Isotope	Z None
Ø Pituitary Gland 1 Pineal Body 2 Adrenal Glands 4 Parathyroid Glands 5 Thyroid	B Low Dose Rate (LDR)	B Palladium 1Ø3 (Pd-1Ø3)	1 Unidirectional Source Z None

SECTION: D RADIATION THERAPY
BODY SYSTEM: G ENDOCRINE SYSTEM
MODALITY: 2 STEREOTACTIC RADIOSURGERY

Treatment Site	Modality Qualifier	Isotope	Qualifier
Ø Pituitary Gland 1 Pineal Body 2 Adrenal Glands 4 Parathyroid Glands 5 Thyroid	D Stereotactic Other Photon Radiosurgery H Stereotactic Particulate Radiosurgery J Stereotactic Gamma Beam Radiosurgery	Z None	Z None

DRG Non-OR All Values

SECTION: D RADIATION THERAPY
BODY SYSTEM: G ENDOCRINE SYSTEM
MODALITY: Y OTHER RADIATION

Treatment Site	Modality Qualifier	Isotope	Qualifier
Ø Pituitary Gland 1 Pineal Body 2 Adrenal Glands 4 Parathyroid Glands 5 Thyroid	7 Contact Radiation 8 Hyperthermia F Plaque Radiation	Z None	Z None

SECTION: D RADIATION THERAPY
BODY SYSTEM: H SKIN
MODALITY: Ø BEAM RADIATION

Treatment Site	Modality Qualifier	Isotope	Qualifier
2 Skin, Face 3 Skin, Neck 4 Skin, Arm 6 Skin, Chest 7 Skin, Back 8 Skin, Abdomen 9 Skin, Buttock B Skin, Leg	Ø Photons <1 MeV 1 Photons 1 - 1Ø MeV 2 Photons >1Ø MeV 4 Heavy Particles (Protons, Ions) 5 Neutrons 6 Neutron Capture	Z None	Z None
2 Skin, Face 3 Skin, Neck 4 Skin, Arm 6 Skin, Chest 7 Skin, Back 8 Skin, Abdomen 9 Skin, Buttock B Skin, Leg	3 Electrons	Z None	Ø Intraoperative Z None

SECTION: D RADIATION THERAPY
BODY SYSTEM: H SKIN
MODALITY: Y OTHER RADIATION

Treatment Site	Modality Qualifier	Isotope	Qualifier
2 Skin, Face 3 Skin, Neck 4 Skin, Arm 6 Skin, Chest 7 Skin, Back 8 Skin, Abdomen 9 Skin, Buttock B Skin, Leg	7 Contact Radiation 8 Hyperthermia F Plaque Radiation	Z None	Z None
5 Skin, Hand C Skin, Foot	F Plaque Radiation	Z None	Z None

SECTION: D RADIATION THERAPY
BODY SYSTEM: M BREAST
MODALITY: Ø BEAM RADIATION

Treatment Site	Modality Qualifier	Isotope	Qualifier
Ø Breast, Left 1 Breast, Right	Ø Photons <1 MeV 1 Photons 1 - 1Ø MeV 2 Photons >1Ø MeV 4 Heavy Particles (Protons, Ions) 5 Neutrons 6 Neutron Capture	Z None	Z None
Ø Breast, Left 1 Breast, Right	3 Electrons	Z None	Ø Intraoperative Z None

SECTION: D RADIATION THERAPY
BODY SYSTEM: M BREAST
MODALITY: 1 BRACHYTHERAPY

Treatment Site	Modality Qualifier	Isotope	Qualifier
Ø Breast, Left 1 Breast, Right	9 High Dose Rate (HDR)	7 Cesium 137 (Cs-137) 8 Iridium 192 (Ir-192) 9 Iodine 125 (I-125) B Palladium 1Ø3 (Pd-1Ø3) C Californium 252 (Cf-252) Y Other Isotope	Z None
Ø Breast, Left 1 Breast, Right	B Low Dose Rate (LDR)	6 Cesium 131 (Cs-131) 7 Cesium 137 (Cs-137) 8 Iridium 192 (Ir-192) 9 Iodine 125 (I-125) C Californium 252 (Cf-252) Y Other Isotope	Z None
Ø Breast, Left 1 Breast, Right	B Low Dose Rate (LDR)	B Palladium 1Ø3 (Pd-1Ø3)	1 Unidirectional Source Z None

SECTION: D RADIATION THERAPY
BODY SYSTEM: M BREAST
MODALITY: 2 STEREOTACTIC RADIOSURGERY

Treatment Site	Modality Qualifier	Isotope	Qualifier
Ø Breast, Left 1 Breast, Right	D Stereotactic Other Photon Radiosurgery H Stereotactic Particulate Radiosurgery J Stereotactic Gamma Beam Radiosurgery	Z None	Z None

DRG Non-OR All Values

SECTION: D RADIATION THERAPY
BODY SYSTEM: M BREAST
MODALITY: Y OTHER RADIATION

Treatment Site	Modality Qualifier	Isotope	Qualifier
Ø Breast, Left 1 Breast, Right	7 Contact Radiation 8 Hyperthermia F Plaque Radiation	Z None	Z None

SECTION: D RADIATION THERAPY
BODY SYSTEM: P MUSCULOSKELETAL SYSTEM
MODALITY: Ø BEAM RADIATION

Treatment Site	Modality Qualifier	Isotope	Qualifier
Ø Skull 2 Maxilla 3 Mandible 4 Sternum 5 Rib(s) 6 Humerus 7 Radius/Ulna 8 Pelvic Bones 9 Femur B Tibia/Fibula C Other Bone	Ø Photons <1 MeV 1 Photons 1 - 1Ø MeV 2 Photons >1Ø MeV 4 Heavy Particles (Protons, Ions) 5 Neutrons 6 Neutron Capture	Z None	Z None
Ø Skull 2 Maxilla 3 Mandible 4 Sternum 5 Rib(s) 6 Humerus 7 Radius/Ulna 8 Pelvic Bones 9 Femur B Tibia/Fibula C Other Bone	3 Electrons	Z None	Ø Intraoperative Z None

SECTION: D RADIATION THERAPY
BODY SYSTEM: P MUSCULOSKELETAL SYSTEM
MODALITY: Y OTHER RADIATION

Treatment Site	Modality Qualifier	Isotope	Qualifier
Ø Skull 2 Maxilla 3 Mandible 4 Sternum 5 Rib(s) 6 Humerus 7 Radius/Ulna 8 Pelvic Bones 9 Femur B Tibia/Fibula C Other Bone	7 Contact Radiation 8 Hyperthermia F Plaque Radiation	Z None	Z None

SECTION: D RADIATION THERAPY
BODY SYSTEM: T URINARY SYSTEM
MODALITY: 0 BEAM RADIATION

Treatment Site	Modality Qualifier	Isotope	Qualifier
0 Kidney 1 Ureter 2 Bladder 3 Urethra	0 Photons <1 MeV 1 Photons 1 - 10 MeV 2 Photons >10 MeV 4 Heavy Particles (Protons, Ions) 5 Neutrons 6 Neutron Capture	Z None	Z None
0 Kidney 1 Ureter 2 Bladder 3 Urethra	3 Electrons	Z None	0 Intraoperative Z None

SECTION: D RADIATION THERAPY
BODY SYSTEM: T URINARY SYSTEM
MODALITY: 1 BRACHYTHERAPY

Treatment Site	Modality Qualifier	Isotope	Qualifier
0 Kidney 1 Ureter 2 Bladder 3 Urethra	9 High Dose Rate (HDR)	7 Cesium 137 (Cs-137) 8 Iridium 192 (Ir-192) 9 Iodine 125 (I-125) B Palladium 103 (Pd-103) C Californium 252 (Cf-252) Y Other Isotope	Z None
0 Kidney 1 Ureter 2 Bladder 3 Urethra	B Low Dose Rate (LDR)	6 Cesium 131 (Cs-131) 7 Cesium 137 (Cs-137) 8 Iridium 192 (Ir-192) 9 Iodine 125 (I-125) C Californium 252 (Cf-252) Y Other Isotope	Z None
0 Kidney 1 Ureter 2 Bladder 3 Urethra	B Low Dose Rate (LDR)	B Palladium 103 (Pd-103)	1 Unidirectional Source Z None

SECTION: D RADIATION THERAPY
BODY SYSTEM: T URINARY SYSTEM
MODALITY: 2 STEREOTACTIC RADIOSURGERY

Treatment Site	Modality Qualifier	Isotope	Qualifier
0 Kidney 1 Ureter 2 Bladder 3 Urethra	D Stereotactic Other Photon Radiosurgery H Stereotactic Particulate Radiosurgery J Stereotactic Gamma Beam Radiosurgery	Z None	Z None

DRG Non-OR All Values

SECTION: D RADIATION THERAPY
BODY SYSTEM: T URINARY SYSTEM
MODALITY: Y OTHER RADIATION

Treatment Site	Modality Qualifier	Isotope	Qualifier
0 Kidney 1 Ureter 2 Bladder 3 Urethra	7 Contact Radiation 8 Hyperthermia C Intraoperative Radiation Therapy (IORT) F Plaque Radiation	Z None	Z None

SECTION: D RADIATION THERAPY
BODY SYSTEM: U FEMALE REPRODUCTIVE SYSTEM
MODALITY: Ø BEAM RADIATION

Treatment Site	Modality Qualifier	Isotope	Qualifier
Ø Ovary ♀ 1 Cervix ♀ 2 Uterus ♀	Ø Photons <1 MeV 1 Photons 1 - 1Ø MeV 2 Photons >1Ø MeV 4 Heavy Particles (Protons, Ions) 5 Neutrons 6 Neutron Capture	Z None	Z None
Ø Ovary ♀ 1 Cervix ♀ 2 Uterus ♀	3 Electrons	Z None	Ø Intraoperative Z None

SECTION: D RADIATION THERAPY
BODY SYSTEM: U FEMALE REPRODUCTIVE SYSTEM
MODALITY: 1 BRACHYTHERAPY

Treatment Site	Modality Qualifier	Isotope	Qualifier
Ø Ovary ♀ 1 Cervix ♀ 2 Uterus ♀	9 High Dose Rate (HDR)	7 Cesium 137 (Cs-137) 8 Iridium 192 (Ir-192) 9 Iodine 125 (I-125) B Palladium 1Ø3 (Pd-1Ø3) C Californium 252 (Cf-252) Y Other Isotope	Z None
Ø Ovary ♀ 1 Cervix ♀ 2 Uterus ♀	B Low Dose Rate (LDR)	6 Cesium 131 (Cs-131) 7 Cesium 137 (Cs-137) 8 Iridium 192 (Ir-192) 9 Iodine 125 (I-125) C Californium 252 (Cf-252) Y Other Isotope	Z None
Ø Ovary ♀ 1 Cervix ♀ 2 Uterus ♀	B Low Dose Rate (LDR)	B Palladium 1Ø3 (Pd-1Ø3)	1 Unidirectional Source Z None

Coding Clinic: 2Ø17, Q4, P1Ø4 – DU11B7Z

SECTION: D RADIATION THERAPY
BODY SYSTEM: U FEMALE REPRODUCTIVE SYSTEM
MODALITY: 2 STEREOTACTIC RADIOSURGERY

Treatment Site	Modality Qualifier	Isotope	Qualifier
Ø Ovary♀ 1 Cervix♀ 2 Uterus♀	D Stereotactic Other Photon Radiosurgery H Stereotactic Particulate Radiosurgery J Stereotactic Gamma Beam Radiosurgery	Z None	Z None

DRG Non-OR All Values

SECTION: D RADIATION THERAPY
BODY SYSTEM: U FEMALE REPRODUCTIVE SYSTEM
MODALITY: Y OTHER RADIATION

Treatment Site	Modality Qualifier	Isotope	Qualifier
Ø Ovary♀ 1 Cervix♀ 2 Uterus♀	7 Contact Radiation 8 Hyperthermia C Intraoperative Radiation Therapy (IORT) F Plaque Radiation	Z None	Z None

SECTION: D RADIATION THERAPY
BODY SYSTEM: V MALE REPRODUCTIVE SYSTEM
MODALITY: 0 BEAM RADIATION

Treatment Site	Modality Qualifier	Isotope	Qualifier
Ø Prostate ♂ 1 Testis ♂	Ø Photons <1 MeV 1 Photons 1 - 1Ø MeV 2 Photons >1Ø MeV 4 Heavy Particles (Protons, Ions) 5 Neutrons 6 Neutron Capture	Z None	Z None
Ø Prostate ♂ 1 Testis ♂	3 Electrons	Z None	Ø Intraoperative Z None

SECTION: D RADIATION THERAPY
BODY SYSTEM: V MALE REPRODUCTIVE SYSTEM
MODALITY: 1 BRACHYTHERAPY

Treatment Site	Modality Qualifier	Isotope	Qualifier
Ø Prostate ♂ 1 Testis ♂	9 High Dose Rate (HDR)	7 Cesium 137 (Cs-137) 8 Iridium 192 (Ir-192) 9 Iodine 125 (I-125) B Palladium 1Ø3 (Pd-1Ø3) C Californium 252 (Cf-252) Y Other Isotope	Z None
Ø Prostate ♂ 1 Testis ♂	B Low Dose Rate (LDR)	6 Cesium 131 (Cs-131) 7 Cesium 137 (Cs-137) 8 Iridium 192 (Ir-192) 9 Iodine 125 (I-125) C Californium 252 (Cf-252) Y Other Isotope	Z None
Ø Prostate ♂ 1 Testis ♂	B Low Dose Rate (LDR)	B Palladium 1Ø3 (Pd-1Ø3)	1 Unidirectional Source Z None

SECTION: D RADIATION THERAPY
BODY SYSTEM: V MALE REPRODUCTIVE SYSTEM
MODALITY: 2 STEREOTACTIC RADIOSURGERY

Treatment Site	Modality Qualifier	Isotope	Qualifier
Ø Prostate ♂ 1 Testis ♂	D Stereotactic Other Photon Radiosurgery H Stereotactic Particulate Radiosurgery J Stereotactic Gamma Beam Radiosurgery	Z None	Z None

DRG Non-OR All Values

SECTION: D RADIATION THERAPY
BODY SYSTEM: V MALE REPRODUCTIVE SYSTEM
MODALITY: Y OTHER RADIATION

Treatment Site	Modality Qualifier	Isotope	Qualifier
Ø Prostate ♂	7 Contact Radiation 8 Hyperthermia C Intraoperative Radiation Therapy (IORT) F Plaque Radiation	Z None	Z None
1 Testis ♂	7 Contact Radiation 8 Hyperthermia F Plaque Radiation	Z None	Z None

SECTION: D RADIATION THERAPY
BODY SYSTEM: W ANATOMICAL REGIONS
MODALITY: Ø BEAM RADIATION

Treatment Site	Modality Qualifier	Isotope	Qualifier
1 Head and Neck 2 Chest 3 Abdomen 4 Hemibody 5 Whole Body 6 Pelvic Region	Ø Photons <1 MeV 1 Photons 1 - 1Ø MeV 2 Photons >1Ø MeV 4 Heavy Particles (Protons, Ions) 5 Neutrons 6 Neutron Capture	Z None	Z None
1 Head and Neck 2 Chest 3 Abdomen 4 Hemibody 5 Whole Body 6 Pelvic Region	3 Electrons	Z None	Ø Intraoperative Z None

SECTION: D RADIATION THERAPY
BODY SYSTEM: W ANATOMICAL REGIONS
MODALITY: 1 BRACHYTHERAPY

Treatment Site	Modality Qualifier	Isotope	Qualifier
Ø Cranial Cavity K Upper Back L Lower Back P Gastrointestinal Tract Q Respiratory Tract R Genitourinary Tract X Upper Extremity Y Lower Extremity	B Low Dose Rate (LDR)	B Palladium 1Ø3 (Pd-1Ø3)	1 Unidirectional Source Z None
1 Head and Neck 2 Chest 3 Abdomen 6 Pelvic Region	9 High Dose Rate (HDR)	7 Cesium 137 (Cs-137) 8 Iridium 192 (Ir-192) 9 Iodine 125 (I-125) B Palladium 1Ø3 (Pd-1Ø3) C Californium 252 (Cf-252) Y Other Isotope	Z None
1 Head and Neck 2 Chest 3 Abdomen 6 Pelvic Region	B Low Dose Rate (LDR)	6 Cesium 131 (Cs-131) 7 Cesium 137 (Cs-137) 8 Iridium 192 (Ir-192) 9 Iodine 125 (I-125) C Californium 252 (Cf-252) Y Other Isotope	Z None
1 Head and Neck 2 Chest 3 Abdomen 6 Pelvic Region	B Low Dose Rate (LDR)	B Palladium 1Ø3 (Pd-1Ø3)	1 Unidirectional Source Z None

Coding Clinic: 2Ø19, Q4, P44 – DW16BB1

SECTION: D RADIATION THERAPY
BODY SYSTEM: W ANATOMICAL REGIONS
MODALITY: 2 STEREOTACTIC RADIOSURGERY

Treatment Site	Modality Qualifier	Isotope	Qualifier
1 Head and Neck 2 Chest 3 Abdomen 6 Pelvic Region	D Stereotactic Other Photon Radiosurgery H Stereotactic Particulate Radiosurgery J Stereotactic Gamma Beam Radiosurgery	Z None	Z None

DRG Non-OR All Values

SECTION: D RADIATION THERAPY
BODY SYSTEM: W ANATOMICAL REGIONS
MODALITY: Y OTHER RADIATION

Treatment Site	Modality Qualifier	Isotope	Qualifier
1 Head and Neck 2 Chest 3 Abdomen 4 Hemibody 6 Pelvic Region	7 Contact Radiation 8 Hyperthermia F Plaque Radiation	Z None	Z None
5 Whole Body	7 Contact Radiation 8 Hyperthermia F Plaque Radiation	Z None	Z None
5 Whole Body	G Isotope Administration	D Iodine 131 (I-131) F Phosphorus 32 (P-32) G Strontium 89 (Sr-89) H Strontium 90 (Sr-90) Y Other Isotope	Z None

F Physical Rehabilitation and Diagnostic Audiology **690**
- FØ. Rehabilitation 691
  - FØØ. Speech Assessment 691
  - FØ1. Motor and/or Nerve Function Assessment 693
  - FØ2. Activities of Daily Living Assessment 695
  - FØ6. Speech Treatment 697
  - FØ7. Motor Treatment 699
  - FØ8. Activities of Daily Living Treatment 701
  - FØ9. Hearing Treatment 702
  - FØB. Cochlear Implant Treatment 702
  - FØC. Vestibular Treatment 703
  - FØD. Device Fitting 703
  - FØF. Caregiver Training 704
- F1. Diagnostic Audiology 705
  - F13. Hearing Assessment 705
  - F14. Hearing Aid Assessment 706
  - F15. Vestibular Assessment 707

New/Revised Text in Green ~~deleted~~ Deleted ♀ Females Only ♂ Males Only Coding Clinic
Non-covered Limited Coverage Combination (See Appendix E) DRG Non-OR Non-OR Hospital-Acquired Condition

SECTION: F PHYSICAL REHABILITATION AND DIAGNOSTIC AUDIOLOGY

SECTION QUALIFIER: Ø REHABILITATION

TYPE: Ø SPEECH ASSESSMENT: *(on multiple pages)*

Measurement of speech and related functions

Body System – Body Region	Type Qualifier	Equipment	Qualifier
3 Neurological System - Whole Body	G Communicative/Cognitive Integration Skills	K Audiovisual M Augmentative/Alternative Communication P Computer Y Other Equipment Z None	Z None
Z None	Ø Filtered Speech 3 Staggered Spondaic Word Q Performance Intensity Phonetically Balanced Speech Discrimination R Brief Tone Stimuli S Distorted Speech T Dichotic Stimuli V Temporal Ordering of Stimuli W Masking Patterns	1 Audiometer 2 Sound Field/Booth K Audiovisual Z None	Z None
Z None	1 Speech Threshold 2 Speech/Word Recognition	1 Audiometer 2 Sound Field/Booth 9 Cochlear Implant K Audiovisual Z None	Z None
Z None	4 Sensorineural Acuity Level	1 Audiometer 2 Sound Field/Booth Z None	Z None
Z None	5 Synthetic Sentence Identification	1 Audiometer 2 Sound Field/Booth 9 Cochlear Implant K Audiovisual	Z None
Z None	6 Speech and/or Language Screening 7 Nonspoken Language 8 Receptive/Expressive Language C Aphasia G Communicative/Cognitive Integration Skills L Augmentative/Alternative Communication System	K Audiovisual M Augmentative/Alternative Communication P Computer Y Other Equipment Z None	Z None
Z None	9 Articulation/Phonology	K Audiovisual P Computer Q Speech Analysis Y Other Equipment Z None	Z None
Z None	B Motor Speech	K Audiovisual N Biosensory Feedback P Computer Q Speech Analysis T Aerodynamic Function Y Other Equipment Z None	Z None

DRG Non-OR All Values

F: PHYSICAL REHABILITATION AND DIAGNOSTIC AUDIOLOGY Ø: REHABILITATION Ø: SPEECH ASSESSMENT

SECTION: F PHYSICAL REHABILITATION AND DIAGNOSTIC AUDIOLOGY

SECTION QUALIFIER: Ø REHABILITATION

TYPE: Ø SPEECH ASSESSMENT: *(continued)*

Measurement of speech and related functions

Body System – Body Region	Type Qualifier	Equipment	Qualifier
Z None	D Fluency	K Audiovisual N Biosensory Feedback P Computer Q Speech Analysis S Voice Analysis T Aerodynamic Function Y Other Equipment Z None	Z None
Z None	F Voice	K Audiovisual N Biosensory Feedback P Computer S Voice Analysis T Aerodynamic Function Y Other Equipment Z None	Z None
Z None	H Bedside Swallowing and Oral Function P Oral Peripheral Mechanism	Y Other Equipment Z None	Z None
Z None	J Instrumental Swallowing and Oral Function	T Aerodynamic Function W Swallowing Y Other Equipment	Z None
Z None	K Orofacial Myofunctional	K Audiovisual P Computer Y Other Equipment Z None	Z None
Z None	M Voice Prosthetic	K Audiovisual P Computer S Voice Analysis V Speech Prosthesis Y Other Equipment Z None	Z None
Z None	N Non-invasive Instrumental Status	N Biosensory Feedback P Computer Q Speech Analysis S Voice Analysis T Aerodynamic Function Y Other Equipment	Z None
Z None	X Other Specified Central Auditory Processing	Z None	Z None

DRG Non-OR All Values

SECTION: F PHYSICAL REHABILITATION AND DIAGNOSTIC AUDIOLOGY

SECTION QUALIFIER: 0 REHABILITATION

TYPE: 1 MOTOR AND/OR NERVE FUNCTION ASSESSMENT: *(on multiple pages)*

Measurement of motor, nerve, and related functions

Body System – Body Region	Type Qualifier	Equipment	Qualifier
0 Neurological System - Head and Neck 1 Neurological System - Upper Back/Upper Extremity 2 Neurological System - Lower Back/Lower Extremity 3 Neurological System - Whole Body	0 Muscle Performance	E Orthosis F Assistive, Adaptive, Supportive or Protective U Prosthesis Y Other Equipment Z None	Z None
0 Neurological System - Head and Neck 1 Neurological System - Upper Back/Upper Extremity 2 Neurological System - Lower Back/Lower Extremity 3 Neurological System - Whole Body	1 Integumentary Integrity 3 Coordination/Dexterity 4 Motor Function G Reflex Integrity	Z None	Z None
0 Neurological System - Head and Neck 1 Neurological System - Upper Back/Upper Extremity 2 Neurological System - Lower Back/Lower Extremity 3 Neurological System - Whole Body	5 Range of Motion and Joint Integrity 6 Sensory Awareness/ Processing/Integrity	Y Other Equipment Z None	Z None
D Integumentary System - Head and Neck F Integumentary System - Upper Back/Upper Extremity G Integumentary System - Lower Back/Lower Extremity H Integumentary System - Whole Body J Musculoskeletal System - Head and Neck K Musculoskeletal System - Upper Back/Upper Extremity L Musculoskeletal System - Lower Back/Lower Extremity M Musculoskeletal System - Whole Body	0 Muscle Performance	E Orthosis F Assistive, Adaptive, Supportive or Protective U Prosthesis Y Other Equipment Z None	Z None
D Integumentary System - Head and Neck F Integumentary System - Upper Back/Upper Extremity G Integumentary System - Lower Back/Lower Extremity H Integumentary System - Whole Body J Musculoskeletal System - Head and Neck K Musculoskeletal System - Upper Back/Upper Extremity L Musculoskeletal System - Lower Back/Lower Extremity M Musculoskeletal System - Whole Body	1 Integumentary Integrity	Z None	Z None
D Integumentary System - Head and Neck F Integumentary System - Upper Back/Upper Extremity G Integumentary System - Lower Back/Lower Extremity H Integumentary System - Whole Body J Musculoskeletal System - Head and Neck K Musculoskeletal System - Upper Back/Upper Extremity L Musculoskeletal System - Lower Back/Lower Extremity M Musculoskeletal System - Whole Body	5 Range of Motion and Joint Integrity 6 Sensory Awareness/ Processing/Integrity	Y Other Equipment Z None	Z None

DRG Non-OR All Values

SECTION: F **PHYSICAL REHABILITATION AND DIAGNOSTIC AUDIOLOGY**
SECTION QUALIFIER: Ø **REHABILITATION**
TYPE: 1 **MOTOR AND/OR NERVE FUNCTION ASSESSMENT:** *(continued)*
Measurement of motor, nerve, and related functions

Body System – Body Region	Type Qualifier	Equipment	Qualifier
N Genitourinary System	Ø Muscle Performance	E Orthosis F Assistive, Adaptive, Supportive or Protective U Prosthesis Y Other Equipment Z None	Z None
Z None	2 Visual Motor Integration	K Audiovisual M Augmentative/Alternative Communication N Biosensory Feedback P Computer Q Speech Analysis S Voice Analysis Y Other Equipment Z None	Z None
Z None	7 Facial Nerve Function	7 Electrophysiologic	Z None
Z None	9 Somatosensory Evoked Potentials	J Somatosensory	Z None
Z None	B Bed Mobility C Transfer F Wheelchair Mobility	E Orthosis F Assistive, Adaptive, Supportive or Protective U Prosthesis Z None	Z None
Z None	D Gait and/or Balance	E Orthosis F Assistive, Adaptive, Supportive or Protective U Prosthesis Y Other Equipment Z None	Z None

DRG Non-OR All Values

SECTION: F PHYSICAL REHABILITATION AND DIAGNOSTIC AUDIOLOGY

SECTION QUALIFIER: Ø REHABILITATION

TYPE: 2 ACTIVITIES OF DAILY LIVING ASSESSMENT: *(on multiple pages)*

Measurement of functional level for activities of daily living

Body System – Body Region	Type Qualifier	Equipment	Qualifier
Ø Neurological System - Head and Neck	9 Cranial Nerve Integrity D Neuromotor Development	Y Other Equipment Z None	Z None
1 Neurological System - Upper Back/Upper Extremity 2 Neurological System - Lower Back/Lower Extremity 3 Neurological System - Whole Body	D Neuromotor Development	Y Other Equipment Z None	Z None
4 Circulatory System - Head and Neck 5 Circulatory System - Upper Back/Upper Extremity 6 Circulatory System - Lower Back/Lower Extremity 8 Respiratory System - Head and Neck 9 Respiratory System - Upper Back/Upper Extremity B Respiratory System - Lower Back/Lower Extremity	G Ventilation, Respiration and Circulation	C Mechanical G Aerobic Endurance and Conditioning Y Other Equipment Z None	Z None
7 Circulatory System - Whole Body C Respiratory System - Whole Body	7 Aerobic Capacity and Endurance	E Orthosis G Aerobic Endurance and Conditioning U Prosthesis Y Other Equipment Z None	Z None
7 Circulatory System - Whole Body C Respiratory System - Whole Body	G Ventilation, Respiration and Circulation	C Mechanical G Aerobic Endurance and Conditioning Y Other Equipment Z None	Z None

DRG Non-OR All Values

SECTION: F PHYSICAL REHABILITATION AND DIAGNOSTIC AUDIOLOGY
SECTION QUALIFIER: Ø REHABILITATION
TYPE: 2 ACTIVITIES OF DAILY LIVING ASSESSMENT: *(continued)*

Measurement of functional level for activities of daily living

Body System – Body Region	Type Qualifier	Equipment	Qualifier
Z None	Ø Bathing/Showering 1 Dressing 3 Grooming/Personal Hygiene 4 Home Management	E Orthosis F Assistive, Adaptive, Supportive or Protective U Prosthesis Z None	Z None
Z None	2 Feeding/Eating 8 Anthropometric Characteristics F Pain	Y Other Equipment Z None	Z None
Z None	5 Perceptual Processing	K Audiovisual M Augmentative/Alternative Communication N Biosensory Feedback P Computer Q Speech Analysis S Voice Analysis Y Other Equipment Z None	Z None
Z None	6 Psychosocial Skills	Z None	Z None
Z None	B Environmental, Home and Work Barriers C Ergonomics and Body Mechanics	E Orthosis F Assistive, Adaptive, Supportive or Protective U Prosthesis Y Other Equipment Z None	Z None
Z None	H Vocational Activities and Functional Community or Work Reintegration Skills	E Orthosis F Assistive, Adaptive, Supportive or Protective G Aerobic Endurance and Conditioning U Prosthesis Y Other Equipment Z None	Z None

DRG Non-OR All Values

SECTION: F PHYSICAL REHABILITATION AND DIAGNOSTIC AUDIOLOGY

SECTION QUALIFIER: Ø REHABILITATION

TYPE: 6 SPEECH TREATMENT: *(on multiple pages)*

Application of techniques to improve, augment, or compensate for speech and related functional impairment

Body System – Body Region	Type Qualifier	Equipment	Qualifier
3 Neurological System - Whole Body	6 Communicative/Cognitive Integration Skills	K Audiovisual M Augmentative/Alternative Communication P Computer Y Other Equipment Z None	Z None
Z None	Ø Nonspoken Language 3 Aphasia 6 Communicative/Cognitive Integration Skills	K Audiovisual M Augmentative/Alternative Communication P Computer Y Other Equipment Z None	Z None
Z None	1 Speech-Language Pathology and Related Disorders Counseling 2 Speech-Language Pathology and Related Disorders Prevention	K Audiovisual Z None	Z None
Z None	4 Articulation/Phonology	K Audiovisual P Computer Q Speech Analysis T Aerodynamic Function Y Other Equipment Z None	Z None
Z None	5 Aural Rehabilitation	K Audiovisual L Assistive Listening M Augmentative/Alternative Communication N Biosensory Feedback P Computer Q Speech Analysis S Voice Analysis Y Other Equipment Z None	Z None
Z None	7 Fluency	4 Electroacoustic Immitance/ Acoustic Reflex K Audiovisual N Biosensory Feedback Q Speech Analysis S Voice Analysis T Aerodynamic Function Y Other Equipment Z None	Z None

DRG Non-OR All Values

SECTION: F PHYSICAL REHABILITATION AND DIAGNOSTIC AUDIOLOGY

SECTION QUALIFIER: Ø REHABILITATION

TYPE: 6 SPEECH TREATMENT: *(continued)*

Application of techniques to improve, augment, or compensate for speech and related functional impairment

Body System – Body Region	Type Qualifier	Equipment	Qualifier
Z None	8 Motor Speech	K Audiovisual N Biosensory Feedback P Computer Q Speech Analysis S Voice Analysis T Aerodynamic Function Y Other Equipment Z None	Z None
Z None	9 Orofacial Myofunctional	K Audiovisual P Computer Y Other Equipment Z None	Z None
Z None	B Receptive/Expressive Language	K Audiovisual L Assistive Listening M Augmentative/Alternative Communication P Computer Y Other Equipment Z None	Z None
Z None	C Voice	K Audiovisual N Biosensory Feedback P Computer S Voice Analysis T Aerodynamic Function V Speech Prosthesis Y Other Equipment Z None	Z None
Z None	D Swallowing Dysfunction	M Augmentative/Alternative Communication T Aerodynamic Function V Speech Prosthesis Y Other Equipment Z None	Z None

DRG Non-OR All Values

SECTION: F PHYSICAL REHABILITATION AND DIAGNOSTIC AUDIOLOGY

SECTION QUALIFIER: Ø REHABILITATION

TYPE: 7 MOTOR TREATMENT: *(on multiple pages)*

Exercise or activities to increase or facilitate motor function

Body System – Body Region	Type Qualifier	Equipment	Qualifier
Ø Neurological System - Head and Neck 1 Neurological System - Upper Back/Upper Extremity 2 Neurological System - Lower Back/Lower Extremity 3 Neurological System - Whole Body D Integumentary System - Head and Neck F Integumentary System - Upper Back/Upper Extremity G Integumentary System - Lower Back/Lower Extremity H Integumentary System - Whole Body J Musculoskeletal System - Head and Neck K Musculoskeletal System - Upper Back/Upper Extremity L Musculoskeletal System - Lower Back/Lower Extremity M Musculoskeletal System - Whole Body	Ø Range of Motion and Joint Mobility 1 Muscle Performance 2 Coordination/Dexterity 3 Motor Function	E Orthosis F Assistive, Adaptive, Supportive or Protective U Prosthesis Y Other Equipment Z None	Z None
Ø Neurological System - Head and Neck 1 Neurological System - Upper Back/Upper Extremity 2 Neurological System - Lower Back/Lower Extremity 3 Neurological System - Whole Body D Integumentary System - Head and Neck F Integumentary System - Upper Back/Upper Extremity G Integumentary System - Lower Back/Lower Extremity H Integumentary System - Whole Body J Musculoskeletal System - Head and Neck K Musculoskeletal System - Upper Back/Upper Extremity L Musculoskeletal System - Lower Back/Lower Extremity M Musculoskeletal System - Whole Body	6 Therapeutic Exercise	B Physical Agents C Mechanical D Electrotherapeutic E Orthosis F Assistive, Adaptive, Supportive or Protective G Aerobic Endurance and Conditioning H Mechanical or Electromechanical U Prosthesis Y Other Equipment Z None	Z None
Ø Neurological System - Head and Neck 1 Neurological System - Upper Back/Upper Extremity 2 Neurological System - Lower Back/Lower Extremity 3 Neurological System - Whole Body D Integumentary System - Head and Neck F Integumentary System - Upper Back/Upper Extremity G Integumentary System - Lower Back/Lower Extremity H Integumentary System - Whole Body J Musculoskeletal System - Head and Neck K Musculoskeletal System - Upper Back/Upper Extremity L Musculoskeletal System - Lower Back/Lower Extremity M Musculoskeletal System - Whole Body	7 Manual Therapy Techniques	Z None	Z None

DRG Non-OR All Values

SECTION: F PHYSICAL REHABILITATION AND DIAGNOSTIC AUDIOLOGY

SECTION QUALIFIER: Ø REHABILITATION

TYPE: 7 MOTOR TREATMENT: *(continued)*

Exercise or activities to increase or facilitate motor function

Body System – Body Region	Type Qualifier	Equipment	Qualifier
4 Circulatory System - Head and Neck 5 Circulatory System - Upper Back/Upper Extremity 6 Circulatory System - Lower Back/Lower Extremity 7 Circulatory System - Whole Body 8 Respiratory System - Head and Neck 9 Respiratory System - Upper Back/Upper Extremity B Respiratory System - Lower Back/Lower Extremity C Respiratory System - Whole Body	6 Therapeutic Exercise	B Physical Agents C Mechanical D Electrotherapeutic E Orthosis F Assistive, Adaptive, Supportive or Protective G Aerobic Endurance and Conditioning H Mechanical or Electromechanical U Prosthesis Y Other Equipment Z None	Z None
N Genitourinary System	1 Muscle Performance	E Orthosis F Assistive, Adaptive, Supportive or Protective U Prosthesis Y Other Equipment Z None	Z None
N Genitourinary System	6 Therapeutic Exercise	B Physical Agents C Mechanical D Electrotherapeutic E Orthosis F Assistive, Adaptive, Supportive or Protective G Aerobic Endurance and Conditioning H Mechanical or Electromechanical U Prosthesis Y Other Equipment Z None	Z None
Z None	4 Wheelchair Mobility	D Electrotherapeutic E Orthosis F Assistive, Adaptive, Supportive or Protective U Prosthesis Y Other Equipment Z None	Z None
Z None	5 Bed Mobility	C Mechanical E Orthosis F Assistive, Adaptive, Supportive or Protective U Prosthesis Y Other Equipment Z None	Z None
Z None	8 Transfer Training	C Mechanical D Electrotherapeutic E Orthosis F Assistive, Adaptive, Supportive or Protective U Prosthesis Y Other Equipment Z None	Z None
Z None	9 Gait Training/Functional Ambulation	C Mechanical D Electrotherapeutic E Orthosis F Assistive, Adaptive, Supportive or Protective G Aerobic Endurance and Conditioning U Prosthesis Y Other Equipment Z None	Z None

DRG Non-OR All Values

SECTION: F PHYSICAL REHABILITATION AND DIAGNOSTIC AUDIOLOGY

SECTION QUALIFIER: Ø REHABILITATION

TYPE: 8 ACTIVITIES OF DAILY LIVING TREATMENT: Exercise or activities to facilitate functional competence for activities of daily living

Body System – Body Region	Type Qualifier	Equipment	Qualifier
D Integumentary System - Head and Neck F Integumentary System - Upper Back/Upper Extremity G Integumentary System - Lower Back/Lower Extremity H Integumentary System - Whole Body J Musculoskeletal System - Head and Neck K Musculoskeletal System - Upper Back/Upper Extremity L Musculoskeletal System - Lower Back/Lower Extremity M Musculoskeletal System - Whole Body	5 Wound Management	B Physical Agents C Mechanical D Electrotherapeutic E Orthosis F Assistive, Adaptive, Supportive or Protective U Prosthesis Y Other Equipment Z None	Z None
Z None	Ø Bathing/Showering Techniques 1 Dressing Techniques 2 Grooming/Personal Hygiene	E Orthosis F Assistive, Adaptive, Supportive or Protective U Prosthesis Y Other Equipment Z None	Z None
Z None	3 Feeding/Eating	C Mechanical D Electrotherapeutic E Orthosis F Assistive, Adaptive, Supportive or Protective U Prosthesis Y Other Equipment Z None	Z None
Z None	4 Home Management	D Electrotherapeutic E Orthosis F Assistive, Adaptive, Supportive or Protective U Prosthesis Y Other Equipment Z None	Z None
Z None	6 Psychosocial Skills	Z None	Z None
Z None	7 Vocational Activities and Functional Community or Work Reintegration Skills	B Physical Agents C Mechanical D Electrotherapeutic E Orthosis F Assistive, Adaptive, Supportive or Protective G Aerobic Endurance and Conditioning U Prosthesis Y Other Equipment Z None	Z None

DRG Non-OR All Values

SECTION: F **PHYSICAL REHABILITATION AND DIAGNOSTIC AUDIOLOGY**
SECTION QUALIFIER: Ø **REHABILITATION**
TYPE: 9 **HEARING TREATMENT:** Application of techniques to improve, augment, or compensate for hearing and related functional impairment

Body System – Body Region	Type Qualifier	Equipment	Qualifier
Z None	Ø Hearing and Related Disorders Counseling 1 Hearing and Related Disorders Prevention	K Audiovisual Z None	Z None
Z None	2 Auditory Processing	K Audiovisual L Assistive Listening P Computer Y Other Equipment Z None	Z None
Z None	3 Cerumen Management	X Cerumen Management Z None	Z None

DRG Non-OR All Values

SECTION: F **PHYSICAL REHABILITATION AND DIAGNOSTIC AUDIOLOGY**
SECTION QUALIFIER: Ø **REHABILITATION**
TYPE: B **COCHLEAR IMPLANT TREATMENT:** Application of techniques to improve the communication abilities of individuals with cochlear implant

Body System – Body Region	Type Qualifier	Equipment	Qualifier
Z None	Ø Cochlear Implant Rehabilitation	1 Audiometer 2 Sound Field/Booth 9 Cochlear Implant K Audiovisual P Computer Y Other Equipment	Z None

DRG Non-OR All Values

SECTION: F PHYSICAL REHABILITATION AND DIAGNOSTIC AUDIOLOGY
SECTION QUALIFIER: Ø REHABILITATION
TYPE: C VESTIBULAR TREATMENT: Application of techniques to improve, augment, or compensate for vestibular and related functional impairment

Body System – Body Region	Type Qualifier	Equipment	Qualifier
3 Neurological System - Whole Body H Integumentary System - Whole Body M Musculoskeletal System - Whole Body	3 Postural Control	E Orthosis F Assistive, Adaptive, Supportive or Protective U Prosthesis Y Other Equipment Z None	Z None
Z None	Ø Vestibular	8 Vestibular/Balance Z None	Z None
Z None	1 Perceptual Processing 2 Visual Motor Integration	K Audiovisual L Assistive Listening N Biosensory Feedback P Computer Q Speech Analysis S Voice Analysis T Aerodynamic Function Y Other Equipment Z None	Z None

DRG Non-OR All Values

SECTION: F PHYSICAL REHABILITATION AND DIAGNOSTIC AUDIOLOGY
SECTION QUALIFIER: Ø REHABILITATION
TYPE: D DEVICE FITTING: Fitting of a device designed to facilitate or support achievement of a higher level of function

Body System – Body Region	Type Qualifier	Equipment	Qualifier
Z None	Ø Tinnitus Masker	5 Hearing Aid Selection/Fitting/Test Z None	Z None
Z None	1 Monaural Hearing Aid 2 Binaural Hearing Aid 5 Assistive Listening Device	1 Audiometer 2 Sound Field/Booth 5 Hearing Aid Selection/Fitting/Test K Audiovisual L Assistive Listening Z None	Z None
Z None	3 Augmentative/Alternative Communication System	M Augmentative/Alternative Communication	Z None
Z None	4 Voice Prosthetic	S Voice Analysis V Speech Prosthesis	Z None
Z None	6 Dynamic Orthosis 7 Static Orthosis 8 Prosthesis 9 Assistive, Adaptive, Supportive or Protective Devices	E Orthosis F Assistive, Adaptive, Supportive or Protective U Prosthesis Z None	Z None

DRG Non-OR FØDZØ[5Z]Z
DRG Non-OR FØDZ[125][125KLZ]Z
DRG Non-OR FØDZ3MZ
DRG Non-OR FØDZ4[SV]Z
DRG Non-OR FØDZ[67][EFUZ]Z
DRG Non-OR FØDZ8[EFU]Z

SECTION: F PHYSICAL REHABILITATION AND DIAGNOSTIC AUDIOLOGY

SECTION QUALIFIER: Ø REHABILITATION

TYPE: F CAREGIVER TRAINING: Training in activities to support patient's optimal level of function

Body System – Body Region	Type Qualifier	Equipment	Qualifier
Z None	Ø Bathing/Showering Technique 1 Dressing 2 Feeding and Eating 3 Grooming/Personal Hygiene 4 Bed Mobility 5 Transfer 6 Wheelchair Mobility 7 Therapeutic Exercise 8 Airway Clearance Techniques 9 Wound Management B Vocational Activities and Functional Community or Work Reintegration Skills C Gait Training/Functional Ambulation D Application, Proper Use and Care Devices F Application, Proper Use and Care of Orthoses G Application, Proper Use and Care of Prosthesis H Home Management	E Orthosis F Assistive, Adaptive, Supportive or Protective U Prosthesis Z None	Z None
Z None	J Communication Skills	K Audiovisual L Assistive Listening M Augmentative/Alternative Communication P Computer Z None	Z None

DRG Non-OR All Values

SECTION: F PHYSICAL REHABILITATION AND DIAGNOSTIC AUDIOLOGY

SECTION QUALIFIER: 1 DIAGNOSTIC AUDIOLOGY

TYPE: 3 HEARING ASSESSMENT: Measurement of hearing and related functions

Body System – Body Region	Type Qualifier	Equipment	Qualifier
Z None	Ø Hearing Screening	Ø Occupational Hearing 1 Audiometer 2 Sound Field/Booth 3 Tympanometer 8 Vestibular/Balance 9 Cochlear Implant Z None	Z None
Z None	1 Pure Tone Audiometry, Air 2 Pure Tone Audiometry, Air and Bone	Ø Occupational Hearing 1 Audiometer 2 Sound Field/Booth Z None	Z None
Z None	3 Bekesy Audiometry 6 Visual Reinforcement Audiometry 9 Short Increment Sensitivity Index B Stenger C Pure Tone Stenger	1 Audiometer 2 Sound Field/Booth Z None	Z None
Z None	4 Conditioned Play Audiometry 5 Select Picture Audiometry	1 Audiometer 2 Sound Field/Booth K Audiovisual Z None	Z None
Z None	7 Alternate Binaural or Monaural Loudness Balance	1 Audiometer K Audiovisual Z None	Z None
Z None	8 Tone Decay D Tympanometry F Eustachian Tube Function G Acoustic Reflex Patterns H Acoustic Reflex Threshold J Acoustic Reflex Decay	3 Tympanometer 4 Electroacoustic Immitance/ Acoustic Reflex Z None	Z None
Z None	K Electrocochleography L Auditory Evoked Potentials	7 Electrophysiologic Z None	Z None
Z None	M Evoked Otoacoustic Emissions, Screening N Evoked Otoacoustic Emissions, Diagnostic	6 Otoacoustic Emission (OAE) Z None	Z None
Z None	P Aural Rehabilitation Status	1 Audiometer 2 Sound Field/Booth 4 Electroacoustic Immitance/ Acoustic Reflex 9 Cochlear Implant K Audiovisual L Assistive Listening P Computer Z None	Z None
Z None	Q Auditory Processing	K Audiovisual P Computer Y Other Equipment Z None	Z None

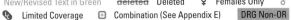

SECTION: F **PHYSICAL REHABILITATION AND DIAGNOSTIC AUDIOLOGY**

SECTION QUALIFIER: 1 **DIAGNOSTIC AUDIOLOGY**

TYPE: 4 **HEARING AID ASSESSMENT:** Measurement of the appropriateness and/or effectiveness of a hearing device

Body System – Body Region	Type Qualifier	Equipment	Qualifier
Z None	Ø Cochlear Implant	1 Audiometer 2 Sound Field/Booth 3 Tympanometer 4 Electroacoustic Immitance/ Acoustic Reflex 5 Hearing Aid Selection/ Fitting/Test 7 Electrophysiologic 9 Cochlear Implant K Audiovisual L Assistive Listening P Computer Y Other Equipment Z None	Z None
Z None	1 Ear Canal Probe Microphone 6 Binaural Electroacoustic Hearing Aid Check 8 Monaural Electroacoustic Hearing Aid Check	5 Hearing Aid Selection/ Fitting/Test Z None	Z None
Z None	2 Monaural Hearing Aid 3 Binaural Hearing Aid	1 Audiometer 2 Sound Field/Booth 3 Tympanometer 4 Electroacoustic Immitance/ Acoustic Reflex 5 Hearing Aid Selection/ Fitting/Test K Audiovisual L Assistive Listening P Computer Z None	Z None
Z None	4 Assistive Listening System/ Device Selection	1 Audiometer 2 Sound Field/Booth 3 Tympanometer 4 Electroacoustic Immitance/ Acoustic Reflex K Audiovisual L Assistive Listening Z None	Z None
Z None	5 Sensory Aids	1 Audiometer 2 Sound Field/Booth 3 Tympanometer 4 Electroacoustic Immitance/ Acoustic Reflex 5 Hearing Aid Selection/ Fitting/Test K Audiovisual L Assistive Listening Z None	Z None
Z None	7 Ear Protector Attentuation	Ø Occupational Hearing Z None	Z None

SECTION: F PHYSICAL REHABILITATION AND DIAGNOSTIC AUDIOLOGY

SECTION QUALIFIER: 1 DIAGNOSTIC AUDIOLOGY

TYPE: 5 VESTIBULAR ASSESSMENT: Measurement of the vestibular system and related functions

Body System – Body Region	Type Qualifier	Equipment	Qualifier
Z None	Ø Bithermal, Binaural Caloric Irrigation 1 Bithermal, Monaural Caloric Irrigation 2 Unithermal Binaural Screen 3 Oscillating Tracking 4 Sinusoidal Vertical Axis Rotational 5 Dix-Hallpike Dynamic 6 Computerized Dynamic Posturography	8 Vestibular/Balance Z None	Z None
Z None	7 Tinnitus Masker	5 Hearing Aid Selection/ Fitting/Test Z None	Z None

G Mental Health **7Ø8**
GZ1. Psychological Tests 7Ø9
GZ2. Crisis Intervention 7Ø9
GZ3. Medication Management 7Ø9
GZ5. Individual Psychotherapy 7Ø9
GZ6. Counseling 71Ø
GZ7. Family Psychotherapy 71Ø
GZB. Electroconvulsive Therapy 71Ø
GZC. Biofeedback 71Ø
GZF. Hypnosis 711
GZG. Narcosynthesis 711
GZH. Group Psychotherapy 711
GZJ. Light Therapy 711

SECTION: G MENTAL HEALTH
SECTION QUALIFIER: Z NONE
TYPE: 1 PSYCHOLOGICAL TESTS: The administration and interpretation of standardized psychological tests and measurement instruments for the assessment of psychological function

Qualifier	Qualifier	Qualifier	Qualifier
Ø Developmental 1 Personality and Behavioral 2 Intellectual and Psychoeducational 3 Neuropsychological 4 Neurobehavioral and Cognitive Status	Z None	Z None	Z None

SECTION: G MENTAL HEALTH
SECTION QUALIFIER: Z NONE
TYPE: 2 CRISIS INTERVENTION: Treatment of a traumatized, acutely disturbed or distressed individual for the purpose of short-term stabilization

Qualifier	Qualifier	Qualifier	Qualifier
Z None	Z None	Z None	Z None

SECTION: G MENTAL HEALTH
SECTION QUALIFIER: Z NONE
TYPE: 3 MEDICATION MANAGEMENT: Monitoring and adjusting the use of medications for the treatment of a mental health disorder

Qualifier	Qualifier	Qualifier	Qualifier
Z None	Z None	Z None	Z None

SECTION: G MENTAL HEALTH
SECTION QUALIFIER: Z NONE
TYPE: 5 INDIVIDUAL PSYCHOTHERAPY: Treatment of an individual with a mental health disorder by behavioral, cognitive, psychoanalytic, psychodynamic or psychophysiological means to improve functioning or well-being

Qualifier	Qualifier	Qualifier	Qualifier
Ø Interactive 1 Behavioral 2 Cognitive 3 Interpersonal 4 Psychoanalysis 5 Psychodynamic 6 Supportive 8 Cognitive-Behavioral 9 Psychophysiological	Z None	Z None	Z None

SECTION: G MENTAL HEALTH
SECTION QUALIFIER: Z NONE
TYPE: 6 **COUNSELING:** The application of psychological methods to treat an individual with normal developmental issues and psychological problems in order to increase function, improve well-being, alleviate distress, maladjustment or resolve crises

Qualifier	Qualifier	Qualifier	Qualifier
Ø Educational 1 Vocational 3 Other Counseling	Z None	Z None	Z None

SECTION: G MENTAL HEALTH
SECTION QUALIFIER: Z NONE
TYPE: 7 **FAMILY PSYCHOTHERAPY:** Treatment that includes one or more family members of an individual with a mental health disorder by behavioral, cognitive, psychoanalytic, psychodynamic or psychophysiological means to improve functioning or well-being

Qualifier	Qualifier	Qualifier	Qualifier
2 Other Family Psychotherapy	Z None	Z None	Z None

SECTION: G MENTAL HEALTH
SECTION QUALIFIER: Z NONE
TYPE: B **ELECTROCONVULSIVE THERAPY:** The application of controlled electrical voltages to treat a mental health disorder

Qualifier	Qualifier	Qualifier	Qualifier
Ø Unilateral-Single Seizure ~~1 Unilateral-Multiple Seizure~~ 2 Bilateral-Single Seizure ~~3 Bilateral-Multiple Seizure~~ 4 Other Electroconvulsive Therapy	Z None	Z None	Z None

SECTION: G MENTAL HEALTH
SECTION QUALIFIER: Z NONE
TYPE: C **BIOFEEDBACK:** Provision of information from the monitoring and regulating of physiological processes in conjunction with cognitive-behavioral techniques to improve patient functioning or well-being

Qualifier	Qualifier	Qualifier	Qualifier
9 Other Biofeedback	Z None	Z None	Z None

SECTION: G MENTAL HEALTH
SECTION QUALIFIER: Z NONE
TYPE: F **HYPNOSIS:** Induction of a state of heightened suggestibility by auditory, visual, and tactile techniques to elicit an emotional or behavioral response

Qualifier	Qualifier	Qualifier	Qualifier
Z None	Z None	Z None	Z None

SECTION: G MENTAL HEALTH
SECTION QUALIFIER: Z NONE
TYPE: G **NARCOSYNTHESIS:** Administration of intravenous barbiturates in order to release suppressed or repressed thoughts

Qualifier	Qualifier	Qualifier	Qualifier
Z None	Z None	Z None	Z None

SECTION: G MENTAL HEALTH
SECTION QUALIFIER: Z NONE
TYPE: H **GROUP PSYCHOTHERAPY:** Treatment of two or more individuals with a mental health disorder by behavioral, cognitive, psychoanalytic, psychodynamic, or psychophysiological means to improve functioning or well-being

Qualifier	Qualifier	Qualifier	Qualifier
Z None	Z None	Z None	Z None

SECTION: G MENTAL HEALTH
SECTION QUALIFIER: Z NONE
TYPE: J **LIGHT THERAPY:** Application of specialized light treatments to improve functioning or well-being

Qualifier	Qualifier	Qualifier	Qualifier
Z None	Z None	Z None	Z None

H Substance Abuse Treatment 712
HZ2. Detoxification Services 713
HZ3. Individual Counseling 713
HZ4. Group Counseling 713
HZ5. Individual Psychotherapy 714
HZ6. Family Counseling 714
HZ8. Medication Management 714
HZ9. Pharmacotherapy 715

SECTION: H **SUBSTANCE ABUSE TREATMENT**
SECTION QUALIFIER: Z **NONE**
TYPE: 2 **DETOXIFICATION SERVICES:** Detoxification from alcohol and/or drugs

Qualifier	Qualifier	Qualifier	Qualifier
Z None	Z None	Z None	Z None

Coding Clinic: 2020, Q1, P22 – HZ2ZZZZ

SECTION: H **SUBSTANCE ABUSE TREATMENT**
SECTION QUALIFIER: Z **NONE**
TYPE: 3 **INDIVIDUAL COUNSELING:** The application of psychological methods to treat an individual with addictive behavior

Qualifier	Qualifier	Qualifier	Qualifier
0 Cognitive 1 Behavioral 2 Cognitive-Behavioral 3 12-Step 4 Interpersonal 5 Vocational 6 Psychoeducation 7 Motivational Enhancement 8 Confrontational 9 Continuing Care B Spiritual C Pre/Post-Test Infectious Disease	Z None	Z None	Z None

DRG Non-OR HZ3[0123456789B]ZZZ

SECTION: H **SUBSTANCE ABUSE TREATMENT**
SECTION QUALIFIER: Z **NONE**
TYPE: 4 **GROUP COUNSELING:** The application of psychological methods to treat two or more individuals with addictive behavior

Qualifier	Qualifier	Qualifier	Qualifier
0 Cognitive 1 Behavioral 2 Cognitive-Behavioral 3 12-Step 4 Interpersonal 5 Vocational 6 Psychoeducation 7 Motivational Enhancement 8 Confrontational 9 Continuing Care B Spiritual C Pre/Post-Test Infectious Disease	Z None	Z None	Z None

DRG Non-OR HZ4[0123456789B]ZZZ

SECTION: H SUBSTANCE ABUSE TREATMENT
SECTION QUALIFIER: Z NONE
TYPE: 5 **INDIVIDUAL PSYCHOTHERAPY:** Treatment of an individual with addictive behavior by behavioral, cognitive, psychoanalytic, psychodynamic, or psychophysiological means

Qualifier	Qualifier	Qualifier	Qualifier
Ø Cognitive 1 Behavioral 2 Cognitive-Behavioral 3 12-Step 4 Interpersonal 5 Interactive 6 Psychoeducation 7 Motivational Enhancement 8 Confrontational 9 Supportive B Psychoanalysis C Psychodynamic D Psychophysiological	Z None	Z None	Z None

DRG Non-OR All Values

SECTION: H SUBSTANCE ABUSE TREATMENT
SECTION QUALIFIER: Z NONE
TYPE: 6 **FAMILY COUNSELING:** The application of psychological methods that includes one or more family members to treat an individual with addictive behavior

Qualifier	Qualifier	Qualifier	Qualifier
3 Other Family Counseling	Z None	Z None	Z None

SECTION: H SUBSTANCE ABUSE TREATMENT
SECTION QUALIFIER: Z NONE
TYPE: 8 **MEDICATION MANAGEMENT:** Monitoring and adjusting the use of replacement medications for the treatment of addiction

Qualifier	Qualifier	Qualifier	Qualifier
Ø Nicotine Replacement 1 Methadone Maintenance 2 Levo-alpha-acetyl-methadol (LAAM) 3 Antabuse 4 Naltrexone 5 Naloxone 6 Clonidine 7 Bupropion 8 Psychiatric Medication 9 Other Replacement Medication	Z None	Z None	Z None

SECTION: H SUBSTANCE ABUSE TREATMENT
SECTION QUALIFIER: Z NONE
TYPE: 9 PHARMACOTHERAPY: The use of replacement medications for the treatment of addiction

Qualifier	Qualifier	Qualifier	Qualifier
Ø Nicotine Replacement 1 Methadone Maintenance 2 Levo-alpha-acetyl-methadol (LAAM) 3 Antabuse 4 Naltrexone 5 Naloxone 6 Clonidine 7 Bupropion 8 Psychiatric Medication 9 Other Replacement Medication	Z None	Z None	Z None

X New Technology **716**
X0. Nervous System 718
X05. Destruction 718
X0H. Insertion 718
X0Z. Other Procedures 718
X2. Cardiovascular System 718
X27. Dilation 718
X28. Division 719
X2A. Assistance 719
X2C. Extirpation 719
X2H. Insertion 720
X2J. Inspection 720
X2K. Bypass 720
X2R. Replacement 721
X2U. Supplement 721
X2V. Restriction 721
XD. Gastrointestinal System 722
XD2. Monitoring 722
XDP. Irrigation 722
XF. Hepatobiliary System and Pancreas 722
XF5. Destruction 722
XFJ. Inspection 722
XH. Skin, Subcutaneous Tissue, Fascia and Breast 723
XHR. Replacement 723
XK. Muscles, Tendons, Bursae and Ligaments 723
XK0. Introduction 723
XKU. Supplement 723
XN. Bones 724
XNH. Insertion 724
XNR. Replacement 724
XNS. Reposition 724
XNU. Supplement 725
XR. Joints 725
XR2. Monitoring 725
XRG. Fusion 726
XRH. Insertion 728
XRR. Replacement 728
XT. Urinary System 728
XT2. Monitoring 728
XV. Male Reproductive System 729
XV5. Destruction 729
XW. Anatomical Regions 729
XW0. Introduction 729
XW1. Transfusion 735
XW2. Transfusion 735
XWH. Insertion 735
XX. Physiological Systems 736
XX2. Monitoring 736
XXA. Assistance 736
XXE. Measurement 737
XY. Extracorporeal 737
XY0. Introduction 737

ICD-10-PCS Coding Guidelines

New Technology Section Guidelines (section X)

D. New Technology Section

General guidelines

D1

Section X codes are standalone codes. They are not supplemental codes. Section X codes fully represent the specific procedure described in the code title, and do not require any additional codes from other sections of ICD-10-PCS. When section X contains a code title which describes a specific new technology procedure, only that X code is reported for the procedure. There is no need to report a broader, non-specific code in another section of ICD-10-PCS.

Example: XWØ4321 Introduction of Ceftazidime-Avibactam Anti-infective into Central Vein, Percutaneous Approach, New Technology Group 1, can be coded to indicate that Ceftazidime-Avibactam Anti-infective was administered via a central vein. A separate code from table 3EØ in the Administration section of ICD-10-PCS is not coded in addition to this code.

Selection of Principal Procedure

The following instructions should be applied in the selection of principal procedure and clarification on the importance of the relation to the principal diagnosis when more than one procedure is performed:

1. Procedure performed for definitive treatment of both principal diagnosis and secondary diagnosis
   a. Sequence procedure performed for definitive treatment most related to principal diagnosis as principal procedure.
2. Procedure performed for definitive treatment and diagnostic procedures performed for both principal diagnosis and secondary diagnosis
   a. Sequence procedure performed for definitive treatment most related to principal diagnosis as principal procedure.
3. A diagnostic procedure was performed for the principal diagnosis and a procedure is performed for definitive treatment of a secondary diagnosis
   a. Sequence diagnostic procedure as principal procedure, since the procedure most related to the principal diagnosis takes precedence.
4. No procedures performed that are related to principal diagnosis; procedures performed for definitive treatment and diagnostic procedures were performed for secondary diagnosis
   a. Sequence procedure performed for definitive treatment of secondary diagnosis as principal procedure, since there are no procedures (definitive or nondefinitive treatment) related to principal diagnosis.

SECTION: X NEW TECHNOLOGY
BODY SYSTEM: Ø NERVOUS SYSTEM
OPERATION: 5 **DESTRUCTION:** Physical eradication of all or a portion of a body part by the direct use of energy, force, or a destructive agent

Body Part	Approach	Device / Substance / Technology	Qualifier
1 Renal Sympathetic Nerve(s)	3 Percutaneous	2 Ultrasound Ablation	9 New Technology Group 9
1 Renal Sympathetic Nerve(s)	3 Percutaneous	3 Radiofrequency Ablation	A New Technology Group 9

SECTION: X NEW TECHNOLOGY
BODY SYSTEM: Ø NERVOUS SYSTEM
OPERATION: H **INSERTION:** Putting in a nonbiological appliance that monitors, assists, performs, or prevents a physiological function but does not physically take the place of a body part

Body Part	Approach	Device / Substance / Technology	Qualifier
K Sphenopalatine Ganglion	3 Percutaneous	Q Neurostimulator Lead	8 New Technology Group 8
Q Vagus Nerve ⊞	3 Percutaneous	R Neurostimulator Lead with Paired Stimulation System	8 New Technology Group 8

Non-OR XØHQ3R8 Non-OR XØHK3Q3 **Coding Clinic: 2022, Q4, P64 – XØHK3Q8**

SECTION: X NEW TECHNOLOGY
BODY SYSTEM: Ø NERVOUS SYSTEM
OPERATION: Z **OTHER PROCEDURES:** Methodologies which attempt to remediate or cure a disorder or disease

Body Part	Approach	Device / Substance / Technology	Qualifier
Ø Prefrontal Cortex	X External	1 Computer-assisted Transcranial Magnetic Stimulation	8 New Technology Group 8

SECTION: X NEW TECHNOLOGY
BODY SYSTEM: 2 CARDIOVASCULAR SYSTEM
OPERATION: 7 **DILATION:** Expanding an orifice or the lumen of a tubular body part

Body Part	Approach	Device / Substance / Technology	Qualifier
~~H Femoral Artery, Right~~ ~~J Femoral Artery, Left~~ ~~K Popliteal Artery, Proximal Right~~ ~~L Popliteal Artery, Proximal Left~~ ~~M Popliteal Artery, Distal Right~~ ~~N Popliteal Artery, Distal Left~~ P Anterior Tibial Artery, Right Q Anterior Tibial Artery, Left R Posterior Tibial Artery, Right S Posterior Tibial Artery, Left T Peroneal Artery, Right U Peroneal Artery, Left	3 Percutaneous	~~8 Intraluminal Device, Sustained Release Drug-eluting~~ ~~9 Intraluminal Device, Sustained Release Drug-eluting, Two~~ ~~B Intraluminal Device, Sustained Release Drug-eluting, Three~~ ~~C Intraluminal Device, Sustained Release Drug-eluting, Four or More~~ T Intraluminal Device, Everolimus-eluting Resorbable Scaffold(s)	~~5 New Technology Group 5~~ A New Technology Group 10

SECTION: X NEW TECHNOLOGY
BODY SYSTEM: 2 Cardiovascular Systems
OPERATION: 8 Division: Cutting into a body part, without draining fluids and/or gases from the body part, in order to separate or transect a body part

Body Part	Approach	Device / Substance / Technology	Qualifier
F Aortic Valve	3 Percutaneous	V Intraluminal Bioprosthetic Valve Leaflet Splitting Technology in Existing Valve	A New Technology Group 10

SECTION: X NEW TECHNOLOGY
BODY SYSTEM: 2 CARDIOVASCULAR SYSTEM
OPERATION: A ASSISTANCE: Taking over a portion of a physiological function by extracorporeal means

Body Part	Approach	Device / Substance / Technology	Qualifier
5 Innominate Artery and Left Common Carotid Artery	3 Percutaneous	1 Cerebral Embolic Filtration, Dual Filter	2 New Technology Group 2
6 Aortic Arch	3 Percutaneous	2 Cerebral Embolic Filtration, Single Deflection Filter	5 New Technology Group 5
7 Coronary Sinus	3 Percutaneous	5 Intermittent Coronary Sinus Occlusion	8 New Technology Group 8
H Common Carotid Artery, Right J Common Carotid Artery, Left	3 Percutaneous	3 Cerebral Embolic Filtration, Extracorporeal Flow Reversal Circuit	6 New Technology Group 6

Coding Clinic: 2016, Q4, P115 – X2A

Coding Clinic: 2021, Q1, P16-17 – X2A5312
Coding Clinic: 2023, Q3, P25 – X2A6325

DRG Non-OR X2A7358

SECTION: X NEW TECHNOLOGY
BODY SYSTEM: 2 CARDIOVASCULAR SYSTEM
OPERATION: C EXTIRPATION: Taking or cutting out solid matter from a body part

Body Part	Approach	Device / Substance / Technology	Qualifier
P Abdominal Aorta Q Upper Extremity Vein, Right R Upper Extremity Vein, Left S Lower Extremity Artery, Right T Lower Extremity Artery, Left U Lower Extremity Vein, Right V Lower Extremity Vein, Left Y Great Vessel	3 Percutaneous	7 Computer-aided Mechanical Aspiration	7 New Technology Group 7

SECTION: X NEW TECHNOLOGY
BODY SYSTEM: 2 CARDIOVASCULAR SYSTEM
OPERATION: H INSERTION: Putting in a nonbiological appliance that monitors, assists, performs, or prevents a physiological function but does not physically take the place of a body part

Body Part	Approach	Device / Substance / Technology	Qualifier
Ø Inferior Vena Cava 1 Superior Vena Cava	3 Percutaneous	R Intraluminal Device, Bioprosthetic Valve	9 New Technology Group 9
2 Femoral Vein, Right 3 Femoral Vein, Left	Ø Open	R Intraluminal Device, Bioprosthetic Valve	9 New Technology Group 9
6 Atrium, Right K Ventricle, Right	3 Percutaneous	V Intracardiac Pacemaker, Dual-Chamber	9 New Technology Group 9
L Axillary Artery, Right M Axillary Artery, Left X Thoracic Aorta, Ascending	Ø Open	F Conduit to Short-term External Heart Assist System	9 New Technology Group 9

Coding Clinic: 2Ø23, Q4, P6Ø – X2H3ØR9

SECTION: X NEW TECHNOLOGY
BODY SYSTEM: 2 CARDIOVASCULAR SYSTEM
OPERATION: J INSPECTION: Visually and/or manually exploring a body part

Body Part	Approach	Device / Substance / Technology	Qualifier
A Heart	X External	4 Transthoracic Echocardiography, Computer-aided Guidance	7 New Technology Group 7

SECTION: X NEW TECHNOLOGY
BODY SYSTEM: 2 CARDIOVASCULAR SYSTEM
OPERATION: K BYPASS: Altering the route of passage of the contents of a tubular body part

Body Part	Approach	Device / Substance / Technology	Qualifier
B Radial Artery, Right C Radial Artery, Left	3 Percutaneous	1 Thermal Resistance Energy	7 New Technology Group 7
H Femoral Artery, Right J Femoral Artery, Left	3 Percutaneous	D Conduit through Femoral Vein to Superficial Femoral Artery E Conduit through Femoral Vein to Popliteal Artery	9 New Technology Group 9

SECTION: X NEW TECHNOLOGY
BODY SYSTEM: 2 CARDIOVASCULAR SYSTEM
OPERATION: R REPLACEMENT: Putting in or on biological or synthetic material that physically takes the place and/or function of all or a portion of a body part

Body Part	Approach	Device / Substance / Technology	Qualifier
5 Upper Extremity Artery, Right 6 Upper Extremity Artery, Left 7 Lower Extremity Artery, Right 8 Lower Extremity Artery, Left	Ø Open	W Bioengineered Human Acellular Vessel	A New Technology Group 1Ø
J Tricuspid	3 Percutaneous	R Multi-plane Flex Technology Bioprosthetic Valve	A New Technology Group 1Ø
X Thoracic Aorta, Arch	Ø Open	N Branched Synthetic Substitute with Intraluminal Device	7 New Technology Group 7

Coding Clinic: 2Ø16, Q4, P116 – X2R

SECTION: X NEW TECHNOLOGY
BODY SYSTEM: 2 CARDIOVASCULAR SYSTEM
OPERATION: U SUPPLEMENT: Putting in or on biological or synthetic material that physically reinforces and/or augments the function of a portion of a body part

Body Part	Approach	Device / Substance / Technology	Qualifier
4 Coronary Artery/Arteries	Ø Open	7 Vein Graft Extraluminal Support Device(s)	9 New Technology Group 9
Q Upper Extremity Vein, Right R Upper Extremity Vein, Left	Ø Open	P Synthetic Substitute, Extraluminal Support Device	9 New Technology Group 9

SECTION: X NEW TECHNOLOGY
BODY SYSTEM: 2 CARDIOVASCULAR SYSTEM
OPERATION: V RESTRICTION: Partially closing an orifice or the lumen of a tubular body part

Body Part	Approach	Device / Substance / Technology	Qualifier
7 Coronary Sinus	3 Percutaneous	Q Reduction Device	7 New Technology Group 7
E Descending Thoracic Aorta and Abdominal Aorta	3 Percutaneous	S Branched Intraluminal Device, Manufactured Integrated System, Four or More Arteries	A New Technology Group 1Ø
W Thoracic Aorta, Descending	Ø Open	N Branched Synthetic Substitute with Intraluminal Device	7 New Technology Group 7

SECTION: X NEW TECHNOLOGY
BODY SYSTEM: D GASTROINTESTINAL SYSTEM
OPERATION: 2 **MONITORING:** Determining the level of a psysiological or physical function repetitively over a period of time

Body Part	Approach	Device / Substance / Technology	Qualifier
G Upper GI H Lower GI	4 Percutaneous Endoscopic 8 Via Natural or Artificial Opening Endoscopic	V Oxygen Saturation	7 New Technology Group 7

SECTION: X NEW TECHNOLOGY
BODY SYSTEM: D GASTROINTESTINAL SYSTEM
OPERATION: P **IRRIGATION:** Putting in or on a cleansing substance

Body Part	Approach	Device / Substance / Technology	Qualifier
H Lower GI	8 Via Natural or Artificial Opening Endoscopic	K Intraoperative Single-use Oversleeve	7 New Technology Group 7

SECTION: X NEW TECHNOLOGY
BODY SYSTEM: F HEPATOBILIARY SYSTEM AND PANCREAS
OPERATION: 5 **DESTRUCTION:** Physical eradication of all or a portion of a body part by the direct use of energy, force, or a destruction agent

Body Part	Approach	Device / Substance / Technology	Qualifier
Ø Liver 1 Liver, Right Lobe 2 Liver, Left Lobe	X External	Ø Ultrasound-guided Cavitation	8 New Technology Group 8

DRG Non-OR XF5[012]X08
Non-OR XF5[Ø12]XØ8

SECTION: X NEW TECHNOLOGY
BODY SYSTEM: F HEPATOBILIARY SYSTEM AND PANCREAS
OPERATION: J **INSPECTION:** Visually and/or manually exploring a body part

Body Part	Approach	Device / Substance / Technology	Qualifier
B Hepatobiliary Duct D Pancreatic Duck	8 Via Natural or Artificial Opening Endoscopic	A Single-use Duodenoscope	7 New Technology Group 7

SECTION: X NEW TECHNOLOGY
BODY SYSTEM: H SKIN, SUBCUTANEOUS TISSUE, FASCIA AND BREAST
OPERATION: R REPLACEMENT: Putting in or on biological or synthetic material that physically takes the place and/or function of all or a portion of a body part

Body Part	Approach	Device / Substance / Technology	Qualifier
Ø Skin, Head and Neck 1 Skin, Chest 2 Skin, Abdomen 3 Skin, Back 4 Skin, Right Upper Extremity 5 Skin, Left Upper Extremity 6 Skin, Right Lower Extremity 7 Skin, Left Lower Extremity	X External	G Prademagene Zamikeracel, Genetically Engineered Autologous Cell Therapy	A New Technology Group 1Ø
P Skin	X External	F Bioengineered Allogeneic Construct	7 New Technology Group 7

SECTION: X NEW TECHNOLOGY
BODY SYSTEM: K MUSCLES, TENDONS, BURSAE AND LIGAMENTS
OPERATION: Ø INTRODUCTION: Putting in or on a therapeutic, diagnostic, nutritional, physiological, or prophylactic substance except blood or blood products

Body Part	Approach	Device / Substance / Technology	Qualifier

SECTION: X NEW TECHNOLOGY
BODY SYSTEM: K MUSCLES, TENDONS, BURSAE AND LIGAMENTS
OPERATION: U SUPPLEMENT: Putting in or on biological or synthetic material that physically reinforces and/or augments the function of a portion of a body part

Body Part	Approach	Device / Substance / Technology	Qualifier
C Upper Spine Bursa and Ligament D Lower Spine Bursa and Ligament	Ø Open	6 Posterior Vertebral Tether	8 New Technology Group 8

Non-OR XKU[CD]Ø68

SECTION: X NEW TECHNOLOGY
BODY SYSTEM: N BONES
OPERATION: H INSERTION: Putting in a nonbiological appliance that monitors, assists, performs, or prevents a physiological function by does not physically take the place of a body part

Body Part	Approach	Device / Substance / Technology	Qualifier
6 Pelvic Bone, Right 7 Pelvic Bone, Left	Ø Open 3 Percutaneous	5 Internal Fixation Device with Tulip Connector	8 New Technology Group 8
G Tibia, Right H Tibia, Left	Ø Open	F Tibial Extension with Motion Sensors	9 New Technology Group 9

Non-OR XNH[67][Ø3]58

SECTION: X NEW TECHNOLOGY
BODY SYSTEM: N BONES
OPERATION: R REPLACEMENT: Putting in or on biological or synthetic material that physically takes the place and/or function of all or a portion of a body part

Body Part	Approach	Device / Substance / Technology	Qualifier
8 Skull	Ø Open	D Synthetic Substitute, Ultrasound Penetrable	9 New Technology Group 9
L Tarsal, Right M Tarsal, Left	Ø Open	9 Synthetic Substitute, Talar Prosthesis	9 New Technology Group 9

SECTION: X NEW TECHNOLOGY
BODY SYSTEM: N BONES
OPERATION: S REPOSITION: *(on multiple pages)* Moving to its normal location, or other suitable location, all or a portion of a body part

Body Part	Approach	Device / Substance / Technology	Qualifier
Ø Lumbar Vertebra	Ø Open	3 Magnetically Controlled Growth Rod(s)	2 New Technology Group 2
Ø Lumbar Vertebra	Ø Open	C Posterior (Dynamic) Distraction Device	7 New Technology Group 7
Ø Lumbar Vertebra	3 Percutaneous	3 Magnetically Controlled Growth Rod(s)	2 New Technology Group 2
Ø Lumbar Vertebra	3 Percutaneous	C Posterior (Dynamic) Distraction Device	7 New Technology Group 7
3 Cervical Vertebra	Ø Open 3 Percutaneous	3 Magnetically Controlled Growth Rod(s)	2 New Technology Group 2

SECTION: **X NEW TECHNOLOGY**
BODY SYSTEM: N BONES
OPERATION: S **REPOSITION:** *(continued)*
Moving to its normal location, or other suitable location, all or a portion of a body part

4 Thoracic Vertebra	Ø Open	3 Magnetically Controlled Growth Rod(s)	2 New Technology Group 2
4 Thoracic Vertebra	Ø Open	C Posterior (Dynamic) Distraction Device	7 New Technology Group 7
4 Thoracic Vertebra	3 Percutaneous	3 Magnetically Controlled Growth Rod(s)	2 New Technology Group 2
4 Thoracic Vertebra	3 Percutaneous	C Posterior (Dynamic) Distraction Device	7 New Technology Group 7

Coding Clinic: 2016, Q4, P117 – XNS

Coding Clinic: 2017, Q4, P75 – XNSØØ32

SECTION: **X NEW TECHNOLOGY**
BODY SYSTEM: N BONES
OPERATION: U **SUPPLEMENT:** Putting in or on biological or synthetic material that physically reinforces and/or augments the function of a portion of a body part

Body Part	Approach	Device / Substance / Technology	Qualifier
Ø Lumbar Vertebra 4 Thoracic Vertebra	3 Percutaneous	5 Synthetic Substitute, Mechanically Expandable (Paired)	6 New Technology Group 6

SECTION: **X NEW TECHNOLOGY**
BODY SYSTEM: R JOINTS
OPERATION: 2 **MONITORING:** Determining the level of a physiological or physical function repetitively over a period of time

Body Part	Approach	Device / Substance / Technology	Qualifier

SECTION: X NEW TECHNOLOGY
BODY SYSTEM: R JOINTS
OPERATION: G FUSION: *(on multiple pages)*

Joining together portions of an articular body part rendering the articular body part immobile

Body Part	Approach	Device / Substance / Technology	Qualifier
Ø Occipital-cervical Joint	Ø Open	9 Interbody Fusion Device, Nanotextured Surface	2 New Technology Group 2
Ø Occipital-cervical Joint	Ø Open	F Interbody Fusion Device, Radiolucent Porous	3 New Technology Group 3
1 Cervical Vertebral Joint	Ø Open	9 Interbody Fusion Device, Nanotextured Surface	2 New Technology Group 2
1 Cervical Vertebral Joint	Ø Open	F Interbody Fusion Device, Radiolucent Porous	3 New Technology Group 3
2 Cervical Vertebral Joints, 2 or more	Ø Open	9 Interbody Fusion Device, Nanotextured Surface	2 New Technology Group 2
2 Cervical Vertebral Joints, 2 or more	Ø Open	F Interbody Fusion Device, Radiolucent Porous	3 New Technology Group 3
4 Cervicothoracic Vertebral Joint	Ø Open	9 Interbody Fusion Device, Nanotextured Surface	2 New Technology Group 2
4 Cervicothoracic Vertebral Joint	Ø Open	F Interbody Fusion Device, Radiolucent Porous	3 New Technology Group 3
6 Thoracic Vertebral Joint	Ø Open	9 Interbody Fusion Device, Nanotextured Surface	2 New Technology Group 2
6 Thoracic Vertebral Joint	Ø Open	F Interbody Fusion Device, Radiolucent Porous	3 New Technology Group 3
7 Thoracic Vertebral Joints, 2 to 7	Ø Open	9 Interbody Fusion Device, Nanotextured Surface	2 New Technology Group 2
7 Thoracic Vertebral Joints, 2 to 7	Ø Open	F Interbody Fusion Device, Radiolucent Porous	3 New Technology Group 3
8 Thoracic Vertebral Joints, 8 or more	Ø Open	9 Interbody Fusion Device, Nanotextured Surface	2 New Technology Group 2
8 Thoracic Vertebral Joints, 8 or more	Ø Open	F Interbody Fusion Device, Radiolucent Porous	3 New Technology Group 3
A Thoracolumbar Vertebral Joint	Ø Open	9 Interbody Fusion Device, Nanotextured Surface	2 New Technology Group 2
A Thoracolumbar Vertebral Joint	Ø Open	E Facet Joint Fusion Device, Paired Titanium Cages	A New Technology Group 1Ø
A Thoracolumbar Vertebral Joint	Ø Open	F Interbody Fusion Device, Radiolucent Porous	3 New Technology Group 3
A Thoracolumbar Vertebral Joint ~~B Lumbar Vertebral Joint~~ ~~C Lumbar Vertebral Joints, 2 or more~~ ~~D Lumbosacral Joint~~	Ø Open 3 Percutaneous 4 Percutaneous Endoscopic	R Interbody Fusion Device, ~~Customizable~~ Custom-Made Anatomically Designed	7 New Technology Group 7
B Lumbar Vertebral Joint	Ø Open	9 Interbody Fusion Device, Nanotextured Surface	2 New Technology Group 2
B Lumbar Vertebral Joint	Ø Open	E Facet Joint Fusion Device, Paired Titanium Cages	A New Technology Group 1Ø
B Lumbar Vertebral Joint	Ø Open	F Interbody Fusion Device, Radiolucent Porous	3 New Technology Group 3
B Lumbar Vertebral Joint	Ø Open 3 Percutaneous 4 Percutaneous Endoscopic	R Interbody Fusion Device, ~~Customizable~~ Custom-Made Anatomically Designed	7 New Technology Group 7
C Lumbar Vertebral, Joints, 2 or more	Ø Open	9 Interbody Fusion Device, Nanotextured Surface	2 New Technology Group 2
C Lumbar Vertebral Joints, 2 or more	Ø Open	E Facet Joint Fusion Device, Paired Titanium Cages	A New Technology Group 1Ø

⊟ XRGC[Ø34]R7

- XRGAØR7 when reported with Secondary Diagnosis K68.11, T81.4ØXA-T81.49XA, or T82.7XXA
- XRGA3R7 when reported with Secondary Diagnosis K68.11, T81.4ØXA-T81.49XA, or T82.7XXA
- XRGA4R7 when reported with Secondary Diagnosis K68.11, T81.4ØXA-T81.49XA, or T82.7XXA
- XRGBØR7 when reported with Secondary Diagnosis K68.11, T81.4ØXA-T81.49XA, or T82.7XXA
- XRGB3R7 when reported with Secondary Diagnosis K68.11, T81.4ØXA-T81.49XA, or T82.7XXA
- XRGB4R7 when reported with Secondary Diagnosis K68.11, T81.4ØXA-T81.49XA, or T82.7XXA
- XRGCØR7 when reported with Secondary Diagnosis K68.11, T81.4ØXA-T81.49XA, or T82.7XXA
- XRGC3R7 when reported with Secondary Diagnosis K68.11, T81.4ØXA-T81.49XA, or T82.7XXA
- XRGC4R7 when reported with Secondary Diagnosis K68.11, T81.4ØXA-T81.49XA, or T82.7XXA

SECTION: X NEW TECHNOLOGY
BODY SYSTEM: R JOINTS
OPERATION: G FUSION: *(continued)*

Joining together portions of an articular body part rendering the articular body part immobile

Body Part	Approach	Device / Substance / Technology	Qualifier
C Lumbar Vertebral Joints, 2 or more	Ø Open	F Interbody Fusion Device, Radiolucent Porous	3 New Technology Group 3
C Lumbar Vertebral Joints, 2 or more ⊞	Ø Open 3 Percutaneous 4 Percutaneous Endoscopic	R Interbody Fusion Device, ~~Customizable~~ Custom-Made Anatomically Designed	7 New Technology Group 7
D Lumbosacral Joint	Ø Open	9 Interbody Fusion Device, Nanotextured Surface	2 New Technology Group 2
D Lumbosacral Joint	Ø Open	E Facet Joint Fusion Device, Paired Titanium Cages	A New Technology Group 1Ø
D Lumbosacral Joint	Ø Open	F Interbody Fusion Device, Radiolucent Porous	3 New Technology Group 3
D Lumbosacral Joint	Ø Open 3 Percutaneous 4 Percutaneous Endoscopic	R Interbody Fusion Device, ~~Customizable~~ Custom-Made Anatomically Designed	7 New Technology Group 7
E Sacroiliac Joint, Right F Sacroiliac Joint, Left	Ø Open 3 Percutaneous	5 Internal Fixation Device with Tulip Connector	8 New Technology Group 8
~~J Ankle Joint, Right~~ ~~K Ankle Joint, Left~~ ~~L Tarsal Joint, Right~~ ~~M Tarsal Joint, Left~~	~~Ø Open~~	~~B Internal Fixation Device, Open-truss Design~~	~~9 New Technology Group 9~~
J Ankle Joint, Right	Ø Open	B Internal Fixation Device, Open-truss Design	9 New Technology Group 9
J Ankle Joint, Right	Ø Open	C Internal Fixation Device, Gyroid-Sheet Lattice Design	A New Technology Group 1Ø
K Ankle Joint, Left	Ø Open	B Internal Fixation Device, Open-truss Design	9 New Technology Group 9
K Ankle Joint, Left	Ø Open	C Internal Fixation Device, Gyroid-Sheet Lattice Design	A New Technology Group 1Ø
L Tarsal Joint, Right	Ø Open	B Internal Fixation Device, Open-truss Design	9 New Technology Group 9
L Tarsal Joint, Right	Ø Open	C Internal Fixation Device, Gyroid-Sheet Lattice Design	A New Technology Group 1Ø
M Tarsal Joint, Left	Ø Open	B Internal Fixation Device, Open-truss Design	9 New Technology Group 9
M Tarsal Joint, Left	Ø Open	C Internal Fixation Device, Gyroid-Sheet Lattice Design	A New Technology Group 1Ø

XRGCØ92 when reported with Secondary Diagnosis K68.11, T81.4ØXA-T81.49XA, or T82.7XXA

XRGDØ92 when reported with Secondary Diagnosis K68.11, T81.4ØXA-T81.49XA, or T82.7XXA

XRGDØR7 when reported with Secondary Diagnosis K68.11, T81.4ØXA-T81.49XA, or T82.7XXA

XRGD3R7 when reported with Secondary Diagnosis K68.11, T81.4ØXA-T81.49XA, or T82.7XXA

XRGD4R7 when reported with Secondary Diagnosis K68.11, T81.4ØXA-T81.49XA, or T82.7XXA

Non-OR XRG[EF][Ø3]58

Coding Clinic: 2Ø17, Q4, P76 – XRG[BD]F3

SECTION: X NEW TECHNOLOGY
BODY SYSTEM: R JOINTS
OPERATION: H INSERTION: Putting in a nonbiological appliance that monitors, assists, performs, or prevents a physiological function but does not physically take the place of a body part

Body Part	Approach	Device / Substance / Technology	Qualifier
~~B Lumbar Vertebral Joint~~ ~~D Lumbosacral Joint~~	~~Ø Open~~	~~1 Posterior Spinal Motion Preservation Device~~	~~8 New Technology Group 8~~
6 Thoracic Vertebral Joint 7 Thoracic Vertebral Joints, 2 to 7 8 Thoracic Vertebral Joints, 8 or more A Thoracolumbar Vertebral Joint	Ø Open 3 Percutaneous 4 Percutaneous Endoscopic	F Carbon/PEEK Spinal Stabilization Device, Pedicle Based	A New Technology Group 1Ø
B Lumbar Vertebral Joint	Ø Open	1 Posterior Spina Motion Preservation Device	8 New Technology Group 8
B Lumbar Vertebral Joint C Lumbar Vertebral Joints, 2 or more	Ø Open 3 Percutaneous 4 Percutaneous Endoscopic	F Carbon/PEEK Spinal Stabilization Device, Pedicle Based	A New Technology Group 1Ø
D Lumbosacral Joint	Ø Open	1 Posterior Spina Motion Preservation Device	8 New Technology Group 8
D Lumbosacral Joint	Ø Open 3 Percutaneous 4 Percutaneous Endoscopic	F Carbon/PEEK Spinal Stabilization Device, Pedicle Based	A New Technology Group 1Ø

Non-OR XRH[BD]Ø18

SECTION: X NEW TECHNOLOGY
BODY SYSTEM: R JOINTS
OPERATION: R REPLACEMENT: Putting in or on biological or synthetic material that physically takes the place and/or function of all or a portion of a body part

Body Part	Approach	Device / Substance / Technology	Qualifier
G Knee Joint, Right ⊞ ⊗ H Knee Joint, Left ⊞ ⊗	Ø Open	L Synthetic Substitute, Lateral Meniscus M Synthetic Substitute, Medial Meniscus	8 New Technology Group 8

⊞ XRR[GH]Ø[LM]8

Non-OR XRR[GH]Ø[LM]8

⊗ XRR[GH]Ø[LM]8 when reported with Secondary Diagnosis from I26.Ø2-I26.Ø9, I26.92-I26.99, or I82.4Ø1-I82.4Z9

SECTION: X NEW TECHNOLOGY
BODY SYSTEM: T URINARY SYSTEM
OPERATION: 2 MONITORING: Determining the level of a physiological or physical function repetitively over a period of time

Body Part	Approach	Device / Substance / Technology	Qualifier
5 Kidney	X External	E Fluorescent Pyrazine	5 New Technology Group 5

SECTION: X NEW TECHNOLOGY
BODY SYSTEM: V MALE REPRODUCTIVE SYSTEM
OPERATION: 5 DESTRUCTION: Physical eradication of all or a portion of a body part by the direct use of energy, force, or a destructive agent

Body Part	Approach	Device / Substance / Technology	Qualifier

SECTION: X NEW TECHNOLOGY
BODY SYSTEM: W ANATOMICAL REGIONS
OPERATION: Ø INTRODUCTION: *(on multiple pages)*
Putting in or on a therapeutic, diagnostic, nutritional, physiological, or prophylactic substance except blood or blood products

Body Part	Approach	Device / Substance / Technology	Qualifier
Ø Skin	X External	2 Anacaulase-bcdb	7 New Technology Group 7
1 Subcutaneous Tissue	3 Percutaneous	1 Daratumumab and Hyaluronidase-fihj ~~4 Teclistamab Antineoplastic~~	8 New Technology Group 8
1 Subcutaneous Tissue	3 Percutaneous	2 Talquetamab Antineoplastic	9 New Technology Group 9
1 Subcutaneous Tissue	3 Percutaneous	4 Teclistamab Antineoplastic	8 New Technology Group 8
1 Subcutaneous Tissue	3 Percutaneous	6 Dasiglucagon	A New Technology Group 1Ø
1 Subcutaneous Tissue	3 Percutaneous	9 Satralizumab-mwge	7 New Technology Group 7
1 Subcutaneous Tissue	3 Percutaneous	F Other New Technology Therapeutic Substance	5 New Technology Group 5
1 Subcutaneous Tissue	3 Percutaneous	G REGN-COV2 Monoclonal Antibody H Other New Technology Monoclonal Antibody K Leronlimab Monoclonal Antibody	6 New Technology Group 6
1 Subcutaneous Tissue	3 Percutaneous	L Elranatamab Antineoplastic	9 New Technology Group 9
1 Subcutaneous Tissue	3 Percutaneous	S COVID-19 Vaccine Dose 1	6 New Technology Group 6
1 Subcutaneous Tissue	3 Percutaneous	S Epcoritamab Monoclonal Antibody	9 New Technology Group 9
1 Subcutaneous Tissue	3 Percutaneous	T COVID-19 Vaccine Dose 2 U COVID-19 Vaccine	6 New Technology Group 6
1 Subcutaneous Tissue	3 Percutaneous	V COVID-19 Vaccine Dose 3	7 New Technology Group 7
1 Subcutaneous Tissue	3 Percutaneous	W Caplacizumab	5 New Technology Group 5
1 Subcutaneous Tissue	3 Percutaneous	W COVID-19 Vaccine Booster	7 New Technology Group 7
1 Subcutaneous Tissue	X External	2 Anacaulase-bcdb	7 New Technology Group 7
2 Muscle	Ø Open	D Engineered Allogeneic Thymus Tissue	8 New Technology Group 8
2 Muscle	3 Percutaneous	S COVID-19 Vaccine Dose 1 T COVID-19 Vaccine Dose 2 U COVID-19 Vaccine Dose	6 New Technology Group 6
2 Muscle	3 Percutaneous	V COVID-19 Vaccine Dose 3 W COVID-19 Vaccine Booster X Tixagevimab and Cilgavimab Monoclonal Antibody Y Other New Technology Monoclonal Antibody	7 New Technology Group 7
3 Peripheral Vein	3 Percutaneous	Ø Brexanolone	6 New Technology Group 6
3 Peripheral Vein	3 Percutaneous	Ø Spesolimab Monoclonal Antibody	8 New Technology Group 8
3 Peripheral Vein	3 Percutaneous	2 Nerinitide 3 Durvalumab Antineoplastic	6 New Technology Group 6
3 Peripheral Vein	3 Percutaneous	3 Bentracimab, Ticagrelor Reversal Agent 4 Cefepime-taniborbactam Anti-infective	A New Technology Group 1Ø

SECTION: X NEW TECHNOLOGY
BODY SYSTEM: W ANATOMICAL REGIONS
OPERATION: Ø INTRODUCTION: *(continued)*
Putting in or on a therapeutic, diagnostic, nutritional, physiological, or prophylactic substance except blood or blood products

Body Part	Approach	Device / Substance / Technology	Qualifier
3 Peripheral Vein	3 Percutaneous	5 Narsoplimab Monoclonal Antibody	7 New Technology Group 7
3 Peripheral Vein	3 Percutaneous	5 Mosunetuzumab Antineoplastic	8 New Technology Group 8
3 Peripheral Vein	3 Percutaneous	5 Ceftobiprole Medocaril Anti-infective	A New Technology Group 1Ø
3 Peripheral Vein	3 Percutaneous	6 Lefamulin Anti-infective	6 New Technology Group 6
3 Peripheral Vein	3 Percutaneous	6 Terlipressin	7 New Technology Group 7
3 Peripheral Vein	3 Percutaneous	6 Afamitresgene Autoleucel Immunotherapy	8 New Technology Group 8
3 Peripheral Vein	3 Percutaneous	7 Coagulation Factor Xa, Inactivated	2 New Technology Group 2
3 Peripheral Vein	3 Percutaneous	7 Trilaciclib	7 New Technology Group 7
3 Peripheral Vein	3 Percutaneous	7 Tabelecleucel Immunotherapy	8 New Technology Group 8
3 Peripheral Vein	3 Percutaneous	8 Lurbinectedin	7 New Technology Group 7
3 Peripheral Vein	3 Percutaneous	8 Treosulfan	8 New Technology Group 8
3 Peripheral Vein	3 Percutaneous	8 Obecabtagene Autoleucel	A New Technology Group 1Ø
3 Peripheral Vein	3 Percutaneous	9 Ceftolozane/Tazobactam Anti-infective	6 New Technology Group 6
3 Peripheral Vein	3 Percutaneous	9 Inebilzumab-cdon	8 New Technology Group 8
3 Peripheral Vein	3 Percutaneous	9 Odronextamab Antineoplastic	A New Technology Group 1Ø
3 Peripheral Vein	3 Percutaneous	A Cefiderocol Anti-infective	6 New Technology Group 6
3 Peripheral Vein	3 Percutaneous	A Ciltacabtagene Autoleucel	7 New Technology Group 7
3 Peripheral Vein	3 Percutaneous	B Cytarabine and Daunorubicin Liposome Antineoplastic	3 New Technology Group 3
3 Peripheral Vein	3 Percutaneous	B Omadacycline Anti-infective	6 New Technology Group 6
3 Peripheral Vein	3 Percutaneous	B Amivantamab Monoclonal Antibody	7 New Technology Group 7
3 Peripheral Vein	3 Percutaneous	B Orca-T Allogeneic T-cell Immunotherapy	A New Technology Group 1Ø
3 Peripheral Vein	3 Percutaneous	C Eculizumab	6 New Technology Group 6
3 Peripheral Vein	3 Percutaneous	C Engineered Chimeric Antigen Receptor T-cell Immunotherapy, Autologous	7 New Technology Group 7
3 Peripheral Vein	3 Percutaneous	C Zanidatamab Antineoplastic	A New Technology Group 1Ø
3 Peripheral Vein	3 Percutaneous	D Atezolizumab Antineoplastic	6 New Technology Group 6
3 Peripheral Vein	3 Percutaneous	D Donislecel-jujn Allogeneic Pancreatic Islet Cellular Suspension	A New Technology Group 1Ø
3 Peripheral Vein	3 Percutaneous	E Remdesivir Anti-infective	5 New Technology Group 5
3 Peripheral Vein	3 Percutaneous	E Etesevimab Monoclonal Antibody	6 New Technology Group 6
3 Peripheral Vein	3 Percutaneous	F Other New Technology Therapeutic Substance	3 New Technology Group 3
3 Peripheral Vein	3 Percutaneous	F Other New Technology Therapeutic Substance	5 New Technology Group 5
3 Peripheral Vein	3 Percutaneous	F Bamlanivimab Monoclonal Antibody	6 New Technology Group 6
3 Peripheral Vein	3 Percutaneous	F Non-Chimeric Antigen Receptor T-cell Immune Effector Cell Therapy	A New Technology Group 1Ø

DRG Non-OR XW0[34]3C3
DRG Non-OR XW033[6AGHJK][78]

Coding Clinic: 2Ø15, Q4, P13, P15 – XWØ4331, XWØ4351
Coding Clinic: 2Ø21, Q4, P111 – XWØ33F5

SECTION: **X NEW TECHNOLOGY**
BODY SYSTEM: **W ANATOMICAL REGIONS**
OPERATION: **Ø INTRODUCTION:** *(continued)*
Putting in or on a therapeutic, diagnostic, nutritional, physiological, or prophylactic substance except blood or blood products

Body Part	Approach	Device / Substance / Technology	Qualifier
~~3 Peripheral Vein~~	~~3 Percutaneous~~	~~G Plazomicin Anti-infective~~	~~4 New Technology Group 4~~
3 Peripheral Vein	3 Percutaneous	G Sarilumab	5 New Technology Group 5
3 Peripheral Vein	3 Percutaneous	G REGN-COV2 Monoclonal Antibody	6 New Technology Group 6
3 Peripheral Vein	3 Percutaneous	G Engineered Chimeric Antigen Receptor T-cell Immunotherapy, Allogeneic	7 New Technology Group 7
~~3 Peripheral Vein~~	~~3 Percutaneous~~	~~H Synthetic Human Angiotensin II~~	~~4 New Technology Group 4~~
3 Peripheral Vein	3 Percutaneous	H Tocilizumab	5 New Technology Group 5
3 Peripheral Vein	3 Percutaneous	H Other New Technology Monoclonal Antibody	6 New Technology Group 6
3 Peripheral Vein	3 Percutaneous	H Axicabtagene Ciloleucel Immunotherapy J Tisagenlecleucel Immunotherapy K Idecabtagene Vicleucel Immunotherapy	7 New Technology Group 7
~~3 Peripheral Vein~~	~~3 Percutaneous~~	~~K Fosfomycin Anti-infective~~	~~5 New Technology Group 5~~
~~3 Peripheral Vein~~	~~3 Percutaneous~~	~~K Idecabtagene Vicleucel Immunotherapy~~	~~7 New Technology Group 7~~
3 Peripheral Vein	3 Percutaneous	K Sulbactam-Durlobactam	9 New Technology Group 9
3 Peripheral Vein	3 Percutaneous	L CD24Fc Immunomodulator	6 New Technology Group 6
3 Peripheral Vein	3 Percutaneous	L Lifileucel Immunotherapy M Brexucabtagene Autoleucel Immunotherapy N Lisocabtagene Maraleucel Immuntherapy	7 New Technology Group 7
~~3 Peripheral Vein~~	~~3 Percutaneous~~	~~N Meropenem-vaborbactam Anti-infective~~	~~5 New Technology Group 5~~
~~3 Peripheral Vein~~	~~3 Percutaneous~~	~~N Lisocabtagene Maraleucel Immuntherapy~~	~~7 New Technology Group 7~~
3 Peripheral Vein	3 Percutaneous	P Glofitamab Antineoplastic	9 New Technology Group 9
3 Peripheral Vein	3 Percutaneous	Q Tagraxofusp-erzs Antineoplastic	5 New Technology Group 5
3 Peripheral Vein	3 Percutaneous	Q Posoleucel R Rezafungin	9 New Technology Group 9
3 Peripheral Vein	3 Percutaneous	S Iobenguane I-131 Antineoplastic ~~U Imipenem-cilastatin-relebactam Anti-infective~~ W Caplacizumab	5 New Technology Group 5
4 Central Vein	3 Percutaneous	Ø Brexanolone	6 New Technology Group 6
4 Central Vein	3 Percutaneous	Ø Spesolimab Monoclonal Antibody	8 New Technology Group 8
~~4 Central Vein~~	~~3 Percutaneous~~	~~Ø Brexanolone~~	~~6 New Technology Group 6~~
4 Central Vein	3 Percutaneous	2 Nerinitide 3 Durvalumab Antineoplastic	6 New Technology Group 6
4 Central Vein	3 Percutaneous	3 Bentracimab, Ticagrelor Reversal Agent 4 Cefepime-taniborbactam Anti-infective	A New Technology Group 1Ø
4 Central Vein	3 Percutaneous	5 Narsoplimab Monoclonal Antibody	7 New Technology Group 7
4 Central Vein	3 Percutaneous	5 Mosunetuzumab Antineoplastic	0 New Technology Group 8
4 Central Vein	3 Percutaneous	5 Ceftobiprole Medocaril Anti-infective	A New Technology Group 1Ø
4 Central Vein	3 Percutaneous	6 Lefamulin Anti-infective	6 New Technology Group 6
4 Central Vein	3 Percutaneous	6 Terlipressin	7 New Technology Group 7
4 Central Vein	3 Percutaneous	6 Afamitresgene Autoleucel Immunotherapy	8 New Technology Group 8
4 Central Vein	3 Percutaneous	7 Coagulation Factor Xa, Inactivated	2 New Technology Group 2
4 Central Vein	3 Percutaneous	7 Trilaciclib	7 New Technology Group 7

SECTION: X **NEW TECHNOLOGY**
BODY SYSTEM: W **ANATOMICAL REGIONS**
OPERATION: Ø **INTRODUCTION:** *(continued)*
Putting in or on a therapeutic, diagnostic, nutritional, physiological, or prophylactic substance except blood or blood products

Body Part	Approach	Device / Substance / Technology	Qualifier
4 Central Vein	3 Percutaneous	7 Tabelecleuce Immunotherapy	8 New Technology Group 8
4 Central Vein	3 Percutaneous	8 Lurbinectedin	7 New Technology Group 7
4 Central Vein	3 Percutaneous	8 Treosulfan	8 New Technology Group 8
4 Central Vein	3 Percutaneous	8 Obecabtagene Autoleucel	A New Technology Group 1Ø
4 Central Vein	3 Percutaneous	9 Ceftolozane/Tazobactam Anti-infective	6 New Technology Group 6
4 Central Vein	3 Percutaneous	9 Inebilizumab-cdon	8 New Technology Group 8
4 Central Vein	3 Percutaneous	9 Odronextamab Antineoplastic	A New Technology Group 1Ø
4 Central Vein	3 Percutaneous	A Cefiderocol Anti-infective	6 New Technology Group 6
4 Central Vein	3 Percutaneous	A Ciltacabtagene Autoleucel	7 New Technology Group 7
4 Central Vein	3 Percutaneous	B Cytarabine and Daunorubicin Liposome Antineoplastic	3 New Technology Group 3
4 Central Vein	3 Percutaneous	B Omadacycline Anti-infective	6 New Technology Group 6
4 Central Vein	3 Percutaneous	B Amivantamab Monoclonal Antibody	7 New Technology Group 7
4 Central Vein	3 Percutaneous	B Orca-T Allogeneic T-cell Immunotherapy	A New Technology Group 1Ø
4 Central Vein	3 Percutaneous	C Eculizumab	6 New Technology Group 6
4 Central Vein	3 Percutaneous	C Engineered Autologous Chimeric Antigen Receptor T-cell Immunotherapy, Autologous	7 New Technology Group 7
4 Central Vein	3 Percutaneous	C Zanidatamab Antineoplastic	A New Technology Group 1Ø
4 Central Vein	3 Percutaneous	D Atezolizumab Antineoplastic	6 New Technology Group 6
4 Central Vein	3 Percutaneous	E Remdesivir Anti-infective	5 New Technology Group 5
4 Central Vein	3 Percutaneous	E Etesevimab Monoclonal Antibody	6 New Technology Group 6
4 Central Vein	3 Percutaneous	F Other New Technology Therapeutic Substance	3 New Technology Group 3
4 Central Vein	3 Percutaneous	F Other New Technology Therapeutic Substance	5 New Technology Group 5
4 Central Vein	3 Percutaneous	F Bamlanivimab Monoclonal Antibody	6 New Technology Group 6
4 Central Vein	3 Percutaneous	F Non-Chimeric Antigen Receptor T-cell Immune Effector Cell Therapy	A New Technology Group 1Ø
~~4 Central Vein~~	~~3 Percutaneous~~	~~G Plazomicin Anti-infective~~	~~4 New Technology Group 4~~
4 Central Vein	3 Percutaneous	G Sarilumab	5 New Technology Group 5
4 Central Vein	3 Percutaneous	G REGN-COV2 Monoclonal Antibody	6 New Technology Group 6
4 Central Vein	3 Percutaneous	G Engineered Chimeric Antigen Receptor T-cell Immunotherapy, Allogeneic	7 New Technology Group 7
~~4 Central Vein~~	~~3 Percutaneous~~	~~H Synthetic Human Angiotensin II~~	~~4 New Technology Group 4~~
4 Central Vein	3 Percutaneous	H Tocilizumab	5 New Technology Group 5
4 Central Vein	3 Percutaneous	H Other New Technology Monoclonal Antibody	6 New Technology Group 6
4 Central Vein	3 Percutaneous	H Axicabtagene Ciloleucel Immunotherapy J Tisagenlecleucel Immunotherapy K Idecabtagene Vicleucel Immunotherapy	7 New Technology Group 7
4 Central Vein	3 Percutaneous	K Fosfomycin Anti-infective	5 New Technology Group 5
~~4 Central Vein~~	~~3 Percutaneous~~	~~K Idecabtagene Vicleucel Immunotherapy~~	~~7 New Technology Group 7~~

DRG Non-OR XWØ43[567ACGHJKLMN][7]

Coding Clinic: 2021, Q4, P111 – XWØ43F5

SECTION: X **NEW TECHNOLOGY**
BODY SYSTEM: W **ANATOMICAL REGIONS**
OPERATION: Ø **INTRODUCTION:** *(continued)*
Putting in or on a therapeutic, diagnostic, nutritional, physiological, or prophylactic substance except blood or blood products

Body Part	Approach	Device / Substance / Technology	Qualifier
4 Central Vein	3 Percutaneous	K Sulbactam-Durlobactam	9 New Technology Group 9
4 Central Vein	3 Percutaneous	L CD24Fc Immunomodulator	6 New Technology Group 6
4 Central Vein	3 Percutaneous	L Lifileucel Immunotherapy M Brexucabtagene Autoleucel Immunotherapy N Lisocabtagene Maraleucel Immuntherapy	7 New Technology Group 7
~~4 Central Vein~~	~~3 Percutaneous~~	~~N Meropenem-vaborbactam Anti-infective~~	~~5 New Technology Group 5~~
~~4 Central Vein~~	~~3 Percutaneous~~	~~N Lisocabtagene Maraleucel Immuntherapy~~	~~7 New Technology Group 7~~
4 Central Vein	3 Percutaneous	P Glofitamab Antineoplastic	9 New Technology Group 9
4 Central Vein	3 Percutaneous	Q Tagraxofusp-erzs Antineoplastic	5 New Technology Group 5
4 Central Vein	3 Percutaneous	Q Posoleucel R Rezafungin	9 New Technology Group 9
4 Central Vein	3 Percutaneous	S Iobenguane I-131 Antineoplastic ~~U Imipenem-cilastatin-relebactam Anti-infective~~ W Caplacizumab	5 New Technology Group 5
5 Peripheral Artery	3 Percutaneous	T Melphalan Hydrochloride Antineoplastic	9 New Technology Group 9
~~9 Nose~~	~~7 Via Natural or Artificial Opening~~	~~M Esketamine Hydrochloride~~	~~5 New Technology Group 5~~
D Mouth and Pharynx	X External	3 Maribavir Anti-infective	8 New Technology Group 8
D Mouth and Pharynx	X External	6 Lefamulin Anti-infective	6 New Technology Group 6
D Mouth and Pharynx	X External	8 Uridine Triacetate	2 New Technology Group 2
D Mouth and Pharynx	X External	F Other New Technology Therapeutic Substance ~~J Apalutamide Antineoplastic~~	5 New Technology Group 5
D Mouth and Pharynx	X External	J Quizartinib Antineoplastic	9 New Technology Group 9
D Mouth and Pharynx	X External	K Sabizabulin	8 New Technology Group 8
~~D Mouth and Pharynx~~	~~X External~~	~~L Erdafitinib Antineoplastic~~	~~5 New Technology Group 5~~
D Mouth and Pharynx	X External	M Baricitinib	6 New Technology Group 6
D Mouth and Pharynx	X External	N SER-1Ø9	9 New Technology Group 9
~~D Mouth and Pharynx~~	~~X External~~	~~R Venetoclax Antineoplastic~~	~~5 New Technology Group 5~~
D Mouth and Pharynx	X External	R Fostamatinib	7 New Technology Group 7
~~D Mouth and Pharynx~~	~~X External~~	~~T Ruxolitinib~~ ~~V Gilteritinib Antineoplastic~~	~~5 New Technology Group 5~~
G Upper GI	7 Via Natural or Artificial Opening	3 Maribavir Anti-infective K Sabizabulin	8 New Technology Group 8
G Upper GI	7 Via Natural or Artificial Opening	M Baricitinib	6 New Technology Group 6
G Upper GI	7 Via Natural or Artificial Opening	R Fostamatinib	7 New Technology Group 7
G Upper GI	8 Via Natural or Artificial Opening Endoscopic	8 Mineral-based Topical Hemostatic Agent	6 New Technology Group 6
H Lower GI	7 Via Natural or Artificial Opening	3 Maribavir Anti-infective K Sabizabulin	8 New Technology Group 8
H Lower GI	7 Via Natural or Artificial Opening	M Baricitinib	6 New Technology Group 6

SECTION: X **NEW TECHNOLOGY**
BODY SYSTEM: W **ANATOMICAL REGIONS**
OPERATION: Ø **INTRODUCTION:** *(continued)*
Putting in or on a therapeutic, diagnostic, nutritional, physiological, or prophylactic substance except blood or blood products

Body Part	Approach	Device / Substance / Technology	Qualifier
H Lower GI	7 Via Natural or Artificial Opening	R Fostamatinib	7 New Technology Group 7
H Lower GI	7 Via Natural or Artificial Opening	X Broad Consortium Microbiota-based Live Biotherapeutic Suspension	8 New Technology Group 8
H Lower GI	8 Via Natural or Artificial Opening Endoscopic	8 Mineral-based Topical Hemostatic Agent	6 New Technology Group 6
J Coronary Artery, One Artery K Coronary Artery, Two Arteries L Coronary Artery, Three Arteries M Coronary Artery, Four or More Arteries	3 Percutaneous	H Paclitaxel-Coated Balloon Technology, One Balloon J Paclitaxel-Coated Balloon Technology, Two Balloons K Paclitaxel-Coated Balloon Technology, Three Balloons L Paclitaxel-Coated Balloon Technology, Four or More Balloons	A New Technology Group 1Ø
Q Cranial Cavity and Brain	3 Percutaneous	1 Eladocagene exuparvovec	6 New Technology Group 6
V Bones	Ø Open	P Antibiotic-eluting Bone Void Filler	7 New Technology Group 7
U Joints	Ø Open	G Vancomycin Hydrochloride and Tobramycin Sulfate Anti-Infective, Temporary Irrigation Spacer System	A New Technology Group 1Ø
V Bones	Ø Open	P Antibiotic-eluting Bone Void Filler	7 New Technology Group 7
V Bone	3 Percutaneous	W AGN1 Bone Void Filler	A New Technology Group 1Ø

Coding Clinic: 2Ø21, Q4, P111 – XWØDXF5
Coding Clinic: 2Ø23, Q3, P7; 2Ø23, Q2, P27 – XWØG886

SECTION: X NEW TECHNOLOGY
BODY SYSTEM: W ANATOMICAL REGIONS
OPERATION: 1 TRANSFUSION: Putting in blood or blood products

Body Part	Approach	Device / Substance / Technology	Qualifier
3 Peripheral Vein	3 Percutaneous	2 Plasma, Convalescent (Nonautologous)	5 New Technology Group 5
3 Peripheral Vein	3 Percutaneous	7 Marnetegragene Autotemcel	A New Technology Group 10
3 Peripheral Vein	3 Percutaneous	B Betibeglogene Autotemcel C Omidubicel	8 New Technology Group 8
3 Peripheral Vein	3 Percutaneous	D High-Dose Intravenous Immune Globulin E Hyperinmmune Globulin	7 New Technology Group 7
3 Peripheral Vein	3 Percutaneous	F OTL-103 G OTL-200	8 New Technology Group 8
3 Peripheral Vein	3 Percutaneous	H Lovotibeglogene Autotemcel	9 New Technology Group 9
3 Peripheral Vein	3 Percutaneous	J Exagamglogene Autotemcel	8 New Technology Group 8
4 Central Vein	3 Percutaneous	2 Plasma, Convalescent (Nonautologous)	5 New Technology Group 5
4 Central Vein	3 Percutaneous	7 Marnetegragene Autotemcel	A New Technology Group 10
4 Central Vein	3 Percutaneous	B Betibeglogene Autotemcel C Omidubicel	8 New Technology Group 8
4 Central Vein	3 Percutaneous	D High-Dose Intravenous Immune Globulin E Hyperinmmune Globulin	7 New Technology Group 7
4 Central Vein	3 Percutaneous	F OTL-103 G OTL-200	8 New Technology Group 8
4 Central Vein	3 Percutaneous	H Lovotibeglogene Autotemcel	9 New Technology Group 9
4 Central Vein	3 Percutaneous	J Exagamglogene Autotemcel	8 New Technology Group 8

DRG Non-OR XW1[34]3[BCFG]8

SECTION: X NEW TECHNOLOGY
BODY SYSTEM: W ANATOMICAL REGIONS
OPERATION: 2 TRANSFUSION: Putting in blood or blood products

Body Part	Approach	Device / Substance / Technology	Qualifier

SECTION: X NEW TECHNOLOGY
BODY SYSTEM: W ANATOMICAL REGIONS
OPERATION: H INSERTION: Putting in a nonbiological appliance that monitors, assists, performs, or prevents a physiological function but does not physically take the place of a body part

Body Part	Approach	Device / Substance / Technology	Qualifier
D Mouth and Pharynx	7 Via Natural or Artificial Opening	Q Neurostimulator Lead	7 New Technology Group 7

SECTION: X NEW TECHNOLOGY
BODY SYSTEM: X PHYSIOLOGICAL SYSTEMS
OPERATION: 2 MONITORING: Determining the level of a physiological or physical function repetitively over a period of time

Body Part	Approach	Device / Substance / Technology	Qualifier
Ø Central Nervous	X External	8 Brain Electrical Activity, Computer-aided Detection and Notification	9 New Technology Group 9
5 Circulatory	X External	Ø Blood Flow, Adhesive Ultrasound Patch Technology	A New Technology Group 1Ø
F Musculoskeletal	3 Percutaneous	W Muscle Compartment Pressure, Micro-Electro-Mechanical System	9 New Technology Group 9
K Subcutaneous Tissue	X External	P Interstitial Fluid Volume, Sub-Epidermal Moisture using Electrical Biocapacitance	9 New Technology Group 9

SECTION: X NEW TECHNOLOGY
BODY SYSTEM: X PHYSIOLOGICAL SYSTEMS
OPERATION: A ASSISTANCE: Taking over a portion of a physiological function by extracorporeal means

Body Part	Approach	Device / Substance / Technology	Qualifier
5 Circulatory	3 Percutaneous	6 Filtration, Blood Pathogens	A New Technology Group 1Ø

SECTION: X NEW TECHNOLOGY
BODY SYSTEM: X PHYSIOLOGICAL SYSTEMS
OPERATION: E MEASUREMENT: Determining the level of a physiological or physical function at a point in time

Body Part	Approach	Device / Substance / Technology	Qualifier
Ø Central Nervous	X External	Ø Intracranial Vascular Activity, Computer-aided Assessment	7 New Technology Group 7
Ø Central Nervous	X External	1 Intracranial Cerebrospinal Fluid Flow, Computer-aided Triage and Notification	A New Technology Group 1Ø
Ø Central Nervous	X External	4 Brain Electrical Activity, Computer-aided Semiologic Analysis	8 New Technology Group 8
2 Cardiac	X External	1 Output, Computer-aided Assessment	9 New Technology Group 9
3 Arterial	X External	2 Pulmonary Artery Flow, Computer-aided Triage and Notification	7 New Technology Group 7
3 Arterial	X External	5 Coronary Artery Flow, Quantitative Flow Ratio Analysis 6 Coronary Artery Flow, Computer-aided Valve Modeling and Notification	8 New Technology Group 8
5 Circulatory	X External	2 Infection, Phenotypic Fully Automated Rapid Susceptibility Technology with Controlled Inoculum	A New Technology Group 1Ø
5 Circulatory	X External	3 Infection, Whole Blood Reverse Transcription and Quantitative Real-time Polymerase Chain Reaction	8 New Technology Group 8
5 Circulatory	X External	4 Infection, Positive Blood Culture Small Molecule Sensor Array Technology	A New Technology Group 1Ø
~~5 Circulatory~~	~~X External~~	~~M Infection, Whole Blood Nucleic Acid-base Microbial Detection~~	~~5 New Technology Group 5~~
5 Circulatory	X External	N Infection, Positive Blood Culture Fluorescence Hybridization for Organism Identification, Concentration and Susceptibility	6 New Technology Group 6
5 Circulatory	X External	R Infection, Mechanical Initial Specimen Diversion Technique Using Active Negative Pressure T Intracranial Arterial Flow, Whole Blood mRNA V Infection, Serum/Plasma Nanoparticle Fluorescence SARS-CoV-2 Antibody Detection	7 New Technology Group 7
5 Circulatory	X External	Y Infection, Other Positive Blood/Isolated Colonies Bimodal Phenotypic Susceptibility Technology	9 New Technology Group 9
9 Nose	7 Via Natural or Artificial Opening	U Infection, Nasopharyngeal Fluid SARS-CoV-2 Polymerase Chain Reaction	7 New Technology Group 7
B Respiratory	X External	Q Infection, Lower Respiratory Fluid Nucleic Acid-base Microbial Detection	6 New Technology Group 6

SECTION: X NEW TECHNOLOGY
BODY SYSTEM: Y EXTRACORPOREAL
OPERATION: Ø INTRODUCTION: Putting in or on a therapeutic, diagnostic, nutritional, physiological, or prophylactic substance except blood or blood products

Body Part	Approach	Device / Substance / Technology	Qualifier
V Vein Graft	X External	8 Endothelial Damage Inhibitor	3 New Technology Group 3
Y Extracorporeal	X External	2 Taurolidine Anti-infective and Heparin Anticoagulant	8 New Technology Group 8
Y Extracorporeal	X External	3 Nafamostat Anticoagulant	7 New Technology Group 7

INDEX

INDEX TO PROCEDURES

3

3f (Aortic) Bioprosthesis valve *use* Zooplastic Tissue in Heart and Great Vessels

A

Abdominal aortic plexus *use* Abdominal Sympathetic Nerve
Abdominal cavity *use* Peritoneal Cavity
Abdominal esophagus *use* Esophagus, Lower
Abdominohysterectomy *see* Resection, Uterus ØUT9
Abdominoplasty
  see Alteration, Abdominal Wall, ØWØF
  see Repair, Abdominal Wall, ØWQF
  see Supplement, Abdominal Wall, ØWUF
Abductor hallucis muscle
  use Foot Muscle, Right
  use Foot Muscle, Left
ABECMA® *use* Idecabtagene Vicleucel Immunotherapy
AbioCor® Total Replacement Heart *use* Synthetic Substitute
Ablation
  see Control bleeding in
  see Destruction
Abortion
  Products of Conception 1ØAØ
  Abortifacient 1ØAØ7ZX
  Laminaria 1ØAØ7ZW
  Vacuum 1ØAØ7Z6
Abrasion *see* Extraction
Absolute Pro Vascular (OTW) Self-Expanding Stent System *use* Intraluminal Device
Accelerate PhenoTest™ BC XXE5XN6
Accessory cephalic vein
  use Cephalic Vein, Right
  use Cephalic Vein, Left
Accessory obturator nerve *use* Lumbar Plexus
Accessory phrenic nerve *use* Phrenic Nerve
Accessory spleen *use* Spleen
Acculink (RX) Carotid Stent System *use* Intraluminal Device
Acellular Hydrated Dermis *use* Nonautologous Tissue Substitute
Acetabular cup *use* Liner in Lower Joints
Acetabulectomy
  see Excision, Lower Bones ØQB
  see Resection, Lower Bones ØQT
Acetabulofemoral joint
  use Hip Joint, Right
  use Hip Joint, Left
Acetabuloplasty
  see Repair, Lower Bones ØQQ
  see Replacement, Lower Bones ØQR
  see Supplement, Lower Bones ØQU
Achilles tendon
  use Lower Leg Tendon, Right
  use Lower Leg Tendon, Left
Achillorrhaphy *use* Repair, Tendons ØLQ
Achillotenotomy, achillotomy
  see Division, Tendons ØL8
  see Drainage, Tendons ØL9
Acoustic Pulse Thrombolysis *see* Fragmentation, Artery
Acromioclavicular ligament
  use Shoulder Bursa and Ligament, Right
  use Shoulder Bursa and Ligament, Left
Acromion (process)
  use Scapula, Right
  use Scapula, Left
Acromionectomy
  see Excision, Upper Joints ØRB
  see Resection, Upper Joints ØRT
Acromioplasty
  see Repair, Upper Joints ØRQ
  see Replacement, Upper Joints ØRR
  see Supplement, Upper Joints ØRU
ACTEMRA® *use* Tocilzumab
Activa PC neurostimulator *use* Stimulator Generator, Multiple Array in ØJH
Activa RC neurostimulator *use* Stimulator Generator, Multiple Array Rechargeable in ØJH
Activa SC neurostimulator *use* Stimulator Generator, Single Array in ØJH
Activities of Daily Living Assessment FØ2
Activities of Daily Living Treatment FØ8
ACUITY™ Steerable Lead
  use Cardiac Lead, Pacemaker in Ø2H
  use Cardiac Lead, Defibrillator in O2H
Acupuncture
  Breast
    Anesthesia 8EØH3ØØ
    No Qualifier 8EØH3ØZ
  Integumentary System
    Anesthesia 8EØH3ØØ
    No Qualifier 8EØH3ØZ
Adductor brevis muscle
  use Upper Leg Muscle, Right
  use Upper Leg Muscle, Left
Adductor hallucis muscle
  use Foot Muscle, Right
  use Foot Muscle, Left
Adductor longus muscle
  use Upper Leg Muscle, Right
  use Upper Leg Muscle, Left
Adductor magnus muscle
  use Upper Leg Muscle, Right
  use Upper Leg Muscle, Left
▶**Adductor pollicis muscle**
  ▶*use* Hand Muscle, Right
  ▶*use* Hand Muscle, Left
Adenohypophysis *use* Pituitary Gland
Adenoidectomy
  see Excision, Adenoids ØCBQ
  see Resection, Adenoids ØCTQ
Adenoidotomy *see* Drainage, Adenoids ØC9Q
Adhesiolysis *see* Release
▶**Adhesive Ultrasound Patch Technology, Blood Flow** XX25XØA
Administration
  Blood products *see* Transfusion
  Other substance *see* Introduction of substance in or on
Adrenalectomy
  see Excision, Endocrine System ØGB
  see Resection, Endocrine System ØGT
Adrenalorrhaphy *see* Repair, Endocrine System ØGQ
Adrenalotomy *see* Drainage, Endocrine System ØG9
Advancement
  see Reposition
  see Transfer
Advisa (MRI) *use* Pacemaker, Dual Chamber in ØJH
afami-cel *use* Afamitresgene Autoleucel Immunotherapy
Afamitresgene Autoleucel Immunotherapy XWØ
AFX® Endovascular AAA System *use* Intraluminal Device
▶**AGENT™ Paclitaxel-Coated Balloon** *see* New Technology, Anatomical Regions XWØ
▶**AGN1 Bone Void Filler** XWØV3WA
Aidoc briefcase for PE (pulmonary embolism) XXE3X27
AIGISRx Antibacterial Envelope *use* Anti-Infective Envelope
Alar ligament of axis *use* Head and Neck Bursa and Ligament
Alfapump® system *use* Other Device
Alimentation *see* Introduction of substance in or on
ALPPS (Associating liver partition and portal vein ligation)
  see Division, Hepatobiliary System and Pancreas ØF8
  see Resection, Hepatobiliary System and Pancreas ØFT
Alteration
  Abdominal Wall ØWØF
  Ankle Region
    Left ØYØL
    Right ØYØK
  Arm
    Lower
      Left ØXØF
      Right ØXØD
    Upper
      Left ØXØ9
      Right ØXØ8
  Axilla
    Left ØXØ5
    Right ØXØ4
  Back
    Lower ØWØL
    Upper ØWØK
  Breast
    Bilateral ØHØV
    Left ØHØU
    Right ØHØT
  Buttock
    Left ØYØ1
    Right ØYØØ
  Chest Wall ØWØ8
  Ear
    Bilateral Ø9Ø2
    Left Ø9Ø1
    Right Ø9ØØ
  Elbow Region
    Left ØXØC
    Right ØXØB
  Extremity
    Lower
      Left ØYØB
      Right ØYØ9
    Upper
      Left ØXØ7
      Right ØXØ6
  Eyelid
    Lower
      Left Ø8ØR
      Right Ø8ØQ
    Upper
      Left Ø8ØP
      Right Ø8ØN
  Face ØWØ2
  Head ØWØØ
  Jaw
    Lower ØWØ5
    Upper ØWØ4
  Knee Region
    Left ØYØG
    Right ØYØF
  Leg
    Lower
      Left ØYØJ
      Right ØYØH
    Upper
      Left ØYØD
      Right ØYØC
  Lip
    Lower ØCØ1X
    Upper ØCØØX
  Nasal Mucosa and Soft Tissue Ø9ØK
  Neck ØWØ6
  Perineum
    Female ØWØN
    Male ØWØM
  Shoulder Region
    Left ØXØ3
    Right ØXØ2

3

▶ New ➠ Revised ~~deleted~~ Deleted

Alteration *(Continued)*
Subcutaneous Tissue and Fascia
Abdomen ØJØ8
Back ØJØ7
Buttock ØJØ9
Chest ØJØ6
Face ØJØ1
Lower Arm
Left ØJØH
Right ØJØG
Lower Leg
Left ØJØP
Right ØJØN
Neck
Left ØJØ5
Right ØJØ4
Upper Arm
Left ØJØF
Right ØJØD
Upper Leg
Left ØJØM
Right ØJØL
Alteration
Wrist Region
Left ØXØH
Right ØXØG
Alveolar process of mandible *use* Maxilla
Alveolar process of maxilla
use Maxilla, Right
use Maxilla, Left
Alveolectomy
see Excision, Head and Facial Bones ØNB
see Resection, Head and Facial Bones ØNT
Alveoloplasty
see Repair, Head and Facial Bones ØNQ
see Replacement, Head and Facial Bones ØNR
see Supplement, Head and Facial Bones ØNU
Alveolotomy
see Division, Head and Facial Bones ØN8
see Drainage, Head and Facial Bones ØN9
Ambulatory cardiac monitoring 4A12X45
Amivantamab monoclonal antibody XWØ
Amniocentesis *see* Drainage, Products of Conception 1Ø9Ø
Amnioinfusion *see* Introduction of substance in or on, Products of Conception 3EØE
Amnioscopy 1ØJØ8ZZ
Amniotomy *see* Drainage, Products of Conception 1Ø9Ø
AMPLATZER® Muscular VSD Occluder *use* Synthetic Substitute
Amputation *see* Detachment
AMS 8ØØ® Urinary Control System *use* Artificial Sphincter in Urinary System
▶ **AMTAGVI™** *use* Lifileucel Immunotherapy
Anacaulase-bcdb XWØ
Anal orifice *use* Anus
Analog radiography *see* Plain Radiography
Analog radiology *see* Plain Radiography
Anastomosis *see* Bypass
Anatomical snuffbox
use Lower Arm and Wrist Muscle, Right
use Lower Arm and Wrist Muscle, Left
▶ **Anconeus muscle**
▶ *use* Lower Arm and Wrist Muscle, Right
▶ *use* Lower Arm and Wrist Muscle, Left
Andexanet Alfa, Factor Xa Inhibitor Reversal Agent *use* Coagulation Factor Xa, Inactivated
Andexxa *use* Coagulation Factor Xa, Inactivated
AneuRx® AAA Advantage® *use* Intraluminal Device
Angiectomy
see Excision, Heart and Great Vessels Ø2B
see Excision, Upper Arteries Ø3B
see Excision, Lower Arteries Ø4B
see Excision, Upper Veins Ø5B
see Excision, Lower Veins Ø6B
Angiocardiography
Combined right and left heart *see* Fluoroscopy, Heart, Right and Left B216
Left Heart *see* Fluoroscopy, Heart, Left B215
Right Heart *see* Fluoroscopy, Heart, Right B214
SPY system intravascular fluorescence *see* Monitoring, Physiological Systems 4A1
Angiography
see Computerized Tomography (CT Scan), Artery
see Fluoroscopy, Artery
see Magnetic Resonance Imaging (MRI), Artery
see Plain Radiography, Artery
Angioplasty
see Dilation, Heart and Great Vessels Ø27
see Repair, Heart and Great Vessels Ø2Q
see Replacement, Heart and Great Vessels Ø2R
see Supplement, Heart and Great Vessels Ø2U
see Dilation, Upper Arteries Ø37
see Repair, Upper Arteries Ø3Q
see Replacement, Upper Arteries Ø3R
see Supplement, Upper Arteries Ø3U
see Dilation, Lower Arteries Ø47
see Repair, Lower Arteries Ø4Q
see Replacement, Lower Arteries Ø4R
see Supplement, Lower Arteries Ø4U
Angiorrhaphy
see Repair, Heart and Great Vessels Ø2Q
see Repair, Upper Arteries Ø3Q
see Repair, Lower Arteries Ø4Q
Angioscopy
Ø2JY4ZZ
Ø3JY4ZZ
Ø4JY4ZZ
Angiotensin II *use* Vasopressor
Angiotripsy
see Occlusion, Upper Arteries Ø3L
see Occlusion, Lower Arteries Ø4L
▶ **Angio Vac System, for extracorporeal filtration during percutaneous thrombectomy** 5AØ5AØL
Angular artery *use* Face Artery
Angular vein
use Face Vein, Right
use Face Vein, Left
Ankle Truss System™ (ATS) *use* Internal Fixation Device, Open-truss Design in New Technology
▶ **Annalise Enterprise CTB Triage software** (Measurement of Intracranial Cerebrospinal Fluid Flow) XXEØX1A
Annular ligament
use Elbow Bursa and Ligament, Right
use Elbow Bursa and Ligament, Left
Annuloplasty
see Repair, Heart and Great Vessels Ø2Q
▶ *see* Restriction, Heart and Great Vessels Ø2V
see Supplement, Heart and Great Vessels Ø2U
Annuloplasty ring *use* Synthetic Substitute
Anoplasty
see Repair, Anus ØDQQ
see Supplement, Anus ØDUQ
Anorectal junction *use* Rectum
Anoscopy ØDJD8ZZ
Ansa cervicalis *use* Cervical Plexus
Antabuse therapy HZ93ZZZ
Antebrachial fascia
use Subcutaneous Tissue and Fascia, Right Lower Arm
use Subcutaneous Tissue and Fascia, Left Lower Arm
Anterior (pectoral) lymph node
use Lymphatic, Right Axillary
use Lymphatic, Left Axillary
Anterior cerebral artery *use* Intracranial Artery
Anterior cerebral vein *use* Intracranial Vein
Anterior choroidal artery *use* Intracranial Artery
Anterior circumflex humeral artery
use Axillary Artery, Right
use Axillary Artery, Left
Anterior communicating artery *use* Intracranial Artery
Anterior cruciate ligament (ACL)
use Knee Bursa and Ligament, Right
use Knee Bursa and Ligament, Left
Anterior crural nerve *use* Femoral Nerve
Anterior facial vein
use Face Vein, Right
use Face Vein, Left
Anterior intercostal artery
use Internal Mammary Artery, Right
use Internal Mammary Artery, Left
Anterior interosseous nerve *use* Median Nerve
Anterior lateral malleolar artery
use Anterior Tibial Artery, Right
use Anterior Tibial Artery, Left
Anterior lingual gland *use* Minor Salivary Gland
Anterior medial malleolar artery
use Anterior Tibial Artery, Right
use Anterior Tibial Artery, Left
Anterior spinal artery
use Vertebral Artery, Right
use Vertebral Artery, Left
Anterior tibial recurrent artery
use Anterior Tibial Artery, Right
use Anterior Tibial Artery, Left
Anterior ulnar recurrent artery
use Ulnar Artery, Right
use Ulnar Artery, Left
Anterior vagal trunk *use* Vagus Nerve
Anterior vertebral muscle
use Neck Muscle, Right
use Neck Muscle, Left
Antibacterial Envelope (TYRX) (AIGISRx) *use* Anti-Infective Envelope
Antibiotic-eluting bone void filler XWØVØP7
Antigen-free air conditioning *see* Atmospheric Control, Physiological Systems 6AØ
Antihelix
use External Ear, Right
use External Ear, Left
use External Ear, Bilateral
Antimicrobial envelope *use* Anti-Infective Envelope
Anti-SARS-CoV-2 hyperimmune globulin *use* Hyperimmune Globulin
Antitragus
use External Ear, Right
use External Ear, Left
use External Ear, Bilateral
Antrostomy *see* Drainage, Ear, Nose, Sinus Ø99
Antrotomy *see* Drainage, Ear, Nose, Sinus Ø99
Antrum of Highmore
use Maxillary Sinus, Right
use Maxillary Sinus, Left
Aortic annulus *use* Aortic Valve
Aortic arch *use* Thoracic Aorta, Ascending/Arch
Aortic intercostal artery *use* Upper Artery
▶ **Aortic isthmus** *use* Thoracic Aorta, Ascending/Arch
Aortix™ System *use* Short-term External Heart Assist System in Heart and Great Vessels
Aortography
see Plain Radiography, Upper Arteries B3Ø
see Fluoroscopy, Upper Arteries B31
see Plain Radiography, Lower Arteries B4Ø
see Fluoroscopy, Lower Arteries B41
Aortoplasty
see Repair, Aorta, Thoracic, Descending Ø2QW
see Repair, Aorta, Thoracic, Ascending/Arch Ø2QX
see Replacement, Aorta, Thoracic, Descending Ø2RW
see Replacement, Aorta, Thoracic, Ascending/Arch Ø2RX

▶ New ➠ Revised ~~deleted~~ Deleted

Aortoplasty *(Continued)*
see Supplement, Aorta, Thoracic, Descending Ø2UW
see Supplement, Aorta, Thoracic, Ascending/Arch Ø2UX
see Repair, Aorta, Abdominal Ø4QØ
see Replacement, Aorta, Abdominal Ø4RØ
see Supplement, Aorta, Abdominal Ø4UØ
➠ **Apalutamide Antineoplastic** *use* Other Antineoplastic
Apical (subclavicular) lymph node
use Lymphatic, Axillary, Right
use Lymphatic, Axillary, Left
ApiFix® Minimally Invasive Deformity Correction (MID-C) system *use* Posterior (Dynamic)Distraction Device in New Technology
Apneustic center *use* Pons
Appendectomy
see Excision, Appendix ØDBJ
see Resection, Appendix ØDTJ
Appendiceal orifice *use* Appendix
Appendicolysis *see* Release, Appendix ØDNJ
Appendicotomy *see* Drainage, Appendix ØD9J
Application *see* Introduction of substance in or on
Aprevo™ *use* Interbody Fusion Device, Custom-Made Anatomically Designed in New Technology
Aquablation therapy, prostate ØV5Ø8ZZ
Aquapheresis 6A55ØZ3
Aqueduct of Sylvius *use* Cerebral Ventricle
Aqueous humour
use Anterior Chamber, Right
use Anterior Chamber, Left
Arachnoid mater, intracranial *use* Cerebral Meninges
Arachnoid mater, spinal *use* Spinal Meninges
Arcuate artery
use Foot Artery, Right
use Foot Artery, Left
Areola
use Nipple, Right
use Nipple, Left
AROM (artificial rupture of membranes) 1Ø9Ø7ZC
Arterial canal (duct) *use* Pulmonary Artery, Left
Arterial pulse tracing *see* Measurement, Arterial 4AØ3
Arteriectomy
see Excision, Heart and Great Vessels Ø2B
see Excision, Upper Arteries Ø3B
see Excision, Lower Arteries Ø4B
Arteriography
see Plain Radiography, Heart B2Ø
see Fluoroscopy, Heart B21
see Plain Radiography, Upper Arteries B3Ø
see Fluoroscopy, Upper Arteries B31
see Plain Radiography, Lower Arteries B4Ø
see Fluoroscopy, Lower Arteries B41
Arterioplasty
see Repair, Heart and Great Vessels Ø2Q
see Replacement, Heart and Great Vessels Ø2R
see Supplement, Heart and Great Vessels Ø2U
see Repair, Upper Arteries Ø3Q
see Replacement, Upper Arteries Ø3R
see Supplement, Upper Arteries Ø3U
see Repair, Lower Arteries Ø4Q
see Replacement, Lower Arteries Ø4R
see Supplement, Lower Arteries Ø4U
Arteriorrhaphy
see Repair, Heart and Great Vessels Ø2Q
see Repair, Upper Arteries Ø3Q
see Repair, Lower Arteries Ø4Q
Arterioscopy
see Inspection, Great Vessel Ø2JY
see Inspection, Artery, Upper Ø3JY
see Inspection, Artery, Lower Ø4JY
Arteriovenous Fistula, Extraluminal Support Device, Supplement X2U
Arthrectomy
see Excision, Upper Joints ØRB
see Resection, Upper Joints ØRT
see Excision, Lower Joints ØSB
see Resection, Lower Joints ØST
Arthrocentesis
see Drainage, Upper Joints ØR9
see Drainage, Lower Joints ØS9
Arthrodesis
see Fusion, Upper Joints ØRG
see Fusion, Lower Joints ØSG
Arthrography
see Plain Radiography, Skull and Facial Bones BNØ
see Plain Radiography, Non-Axial Upper Bones BPØ
see Plain Radiography, Non-Axial Lower Bones BQØ
Arthrolysis
see Release, Upper Joints ØRN
see Release, Lower Joints ØSN
Arthropexy
see Repair, Upper Joints ØRQ
see Reposition, Upper Joints ØRS
see Repair, Lower Joints ØSQ
see Reposition, Lower Joints ØSS
Arthroplasty
see Repair, Upper Joints ØRQ
see Replacement, Upper Joints ØRR
see Supplement, Upper Joints ØRU
see Repair, Lower Joints ØSQ
see Replacement, Lower Joints ØSR
see Supplement, Lower Joints ØSU
Arthroplasty, radial head
see Replacement, Radius, Right ØPRH
see Replacement, Radius, Left ØPRJ
Arthroscopy
see Inspection, Upper Joints ØRJ
see Inspection, Lower Joints ØSJ
see Drainage, Upper Joints ØR9
see Drainage, Lower Joints ØS9
Articulating Spacer (Antibiotic) *use* Articulating Spacer in Lower Joints
Artificial anal sphincter (AAS) *use* Artificial Sphincter in Gastrointestinal System
Artificial bowel sphincter (neosphincter) *use* Artificial Sphincter in Gastrointestinal System
Artificial Sphincter
Insertion of device in
Anus ØDHQ
Bladder ØTHB
Bladder Neck ØTHC
Urethra ØTHD
Removal of device from
Anus ØDPQ
Bladder ØTPB
Urethra ØTPD
Revision of device in
Anus ØDWQ
Bladder ØTWB
Urethra ØTWD
Artificial urinary sphincter (AUS) *use* Artificial Sphincter in Urinary System
Aryepiglottic fold *use* Larynx
Arytenoid cartilage *use* Larynx
Arytenoid muscle
use Neck Muscle, Right
use Neck Muscle, Left
Arytenoidectomy *see* Excision, Larynx ØCBS
Arytenoidopexy *see* Repair, Larynx ØCQS
Ascenda Intrathecal Catheter *use* Infusion Device
Ascending aorta *use* Thoracic Aorta, Ascending/Arch
Ascending palatine artery *use* Face Artery
Ascending pharyngeal artery
use External Carotid Artery, Right
use External Carotid Artery, Left
aScope™ Duodeno *see* New Technology, Hepatobiliary System and Pancreas XFJ
Aspiration, fine needle
Fluid or gas *see* Drainage
Tissue biopsy
see Extraction
see Excision
Assessment
Activities of daily living *see* Activities of Daily Living Assessment, Rehabilitation FØ2
Hearing *see* Hearing Assessment, Diagnostic Audiology F13
Hearing aid *see* Hearing Aid Assessment, Diagnostic Audiology F14
Intravascular perfusion, using indocyanine green (ICG) dye *see* Monitoring, Physiological Systems 4A1
Motor function *see* Motor Function Assessment, Rehabilitation FØ1
Nerve function *see* Motor Function Assessment, Rehabilitation FØ1
Speech *see* Speech Assessment, Rehabilitation FØØ
Vestibular *see* Vestibular Assessment, Diagnostic Audiology F15
Vocational *see* Activities of Daily Living Treatment, Rehabilitation FØ8
Assistance
Cardiac
Continuous
Output
Balloon Pump 5AØ221Ø
Impeller Pump 5AØ221D
Other Pump 5AØ2216
Pulsatile Compression 5AØ2215
Oxygenation, Supersaturated 5AØ222C
Intermittent
Balloon Pump 5AØ211Ø
Impeller Pump 5AØ211D
Other Pump 5AØ2116
Pulsatile Compression 5AØ2115
Circulatory
▶ Intraoperative, Filtration, Peripheral Veno-venous 5AØ5AØL
Continuous, Oxygenation, Hyperbaric 5AØ5221
Intermittent, Oxygenation, Hyperbaric 5AØ5121
Respiratory
8-24 Consecutive Hours, Ventilation, Intubated Prone Positioning 5AØ9C5K
24-96 Consecutive Hours
Continuous Negative Airway Pressure 5AØ9459
Continuous Positive Airway Pressure 5AØ9457
~~High Nasal Flow/Velocity 5AØ945A~~
▶ High Flow/Velocity Cannula 5AØ945A
Intermittent Negative Airway Pressure 5AØ945B
Intermittent Positive Airway Pressure 5AØ9458
No Qualifier 5AØ945Z
Continuous, Filtration 5AØ92ØZ
Greater than 24 Consecutive Hours, Ventilation, Intubated Prone Positioning 5AØ9D5K
Greater than 96 Consecutive Hours
Continuous Negative Airway Pressure 5AØ9559
Continuous Positive Airway Pressure 5AØ9557
~~High Nasal Flow/Velocity 5AØ955A~~
▶ High Flow/Velocity Cannula 5AØ945A
Intermittent Negative Airway Pressure 5AØ955B
Intermittent Positive Airway Pressure 5AØ9558
No Qualifier 5AØ955Z

A

▶ New ➠ Revised ~~deleted~~ Deleted

Assistance *(Continued)*
Cardiac *(Continued)*
Less than 8 Consecutive Hours, Ventilation, Intubated Prone Positioning 5AØ9B5K
Less than 24 Consecutive Hours
Continuous Negative Airway Pressure 5AØ9359
Continuous Positive Airway Pressure 5AØ9357
~~High Nasal Flow/Velocity 5AØ935A~~
▶High Flow/Velocity Cannula 5AØ945A
Intermittent Negative Airway Pressure 5AØ935B
Intermittent Positive Airway Pressure 5AØ9358
No Qualifier 5AØ935Z
Associating liver partition and portal vein ligation (ALPPS)
see Division, Hepatobiliary System and Pancreas ØF8
see Resection, Hepatobiliary System and Pancreas ØFT
Assurant (Cobalt) stent *use* Intraluminal Device
▶**ASTar®** XXE5X2A
Atezolizumab Antineoplastic XWØ
Atherectomy
see Extirpation, Heart and Great Vessels Ø2C
see Extirpation, Upper Arteries Ø3C
see Extirpation, Lower Arteries Ø4C
Atlantoaxial joint *use* Cervical Vertebral Joint
Atmospheric Control 6AØZ
AtriClip LAA Exclusion System *use* Extraluminal Device **Atrioseptoplasty**
see Repair, Heart and Great Vessels Ø2Q
see Replacement, Heart and Great Vessels Ø2R
see Supplement, Heart and Great Vessels Ø2U
Atrioventricular node *use* Conduction Mechanism
Atrium dextrum cordis *use* Atrium, Right
Atrium pulmonale *use* Atrium, Left
Attain Ability® lead
use Cardiac Lead, Pacemaker in Ø2H
use Cardiac Lead, Defibrillator in Ø2H
Attain StarFix® (OTW) lead
use Cardiac Lead, Pacemaker in Ø2H
use Cardiac Lead, Defibrillator in O2H
Audiology, diagnostic
see Hearing Assessment, Diagnostic Audiology F13
see Hearing Aid Assessment, Diagnostic Audiology F14
see Vestibular Assessment, Diagnostic Audiology F15
Audiometry *see* Hearing Assessment, Diagnostic Audiology F13
Auditory tube
use Eustachian Tube, Right
use Eustachian Tube, Left
Auerbach's (myenteric) plexus *use* Nerve, Abdominal Sympathetic
Auricle
use External Ear, Right
use External Ear, Left
use External Ear, Bilateral
Auricularis muscle *use* Head Muscle
Autograft *use* Autologous Tissue Substitute
AutoLITT® System *see* Destruction
Autologous artery graft
use Autologous Arterial Tissue in Heart and Great Vessels
use Autologous Arterial Tissue in Upper Arteries
use Autologous Arterial Tissue in Lower Arteries
use Autologous Arterial Tissue in Upper Veins
use Autologous Arterial Tissue in Lower Veins
Autologous vein graft
use Autologous Venous Tissue in Heart and Great Vessels
use Autologous Venous Tissue in Upper Arteries
use Autologous Venous Tissue in Lower Arteries
use Autologous Venous Tissue in Upper Veins
use Autologous Venous Tissue in Lower Veins
Automated chest compression (ACC) 5A1221J
AutoPulse® resuscitation system 5A1221J
Autotransfusion *see* Transfusion
Autotransplant
Adrenal tissue *see* Reposition, Endocrine System ØGS
Kidney
see Reposition, Urinary System ØTS
Pancreatic tissue *see* Reposition, Pancreas ØFSG
Parathyroid tissue *see* Reposition, Endocrine System ØGS
Thyroid tissue *see* Reposition, Endocrine System ØGS
Tooth *see* Reattachment, Mouth and Throat ØCM
Aveir™ AR, as dual chamber *use* Intracardiac Pacemaker, Dual-Chamber in New Technology
Aveir™ DR, dual chamber *use* Intracardiac Pacemaker, Dual-Chamber in New Technology
Aveir™ VR, as single chamber *use* Intracardiac Pacemaker in Heart and Great Vessels
Avulsion *see* Extraction
AVYCAZ® (ceftazidime-avibactam) *use* Other Anti-infective
Axial Lumbar Interbody Fusion System *use* Interbody Fusion Device in Lower Joints
AxiaLIF® System *use* Interbody Fusion Device in Lower Joints
Axicabtagene Ciloleucel *use* Axicabtagene Ciloleucel Immunotherapy
Axicabtagene Ciloleucel Immunotherapy XWØ
Axillary fascia
use Subcutaneous Tissue and Fascia, Right Upper Arm
use Subcutaneous Tissue and Fascia, Left Upper Arm
Axillary nerve *use* Brachial Plexus
AZEDRA *use* Iobenguane I-131 Antineoplastic

A

B

BAK/C® Interbody Cervical Fusion System
use Interbody Fusion Device in Upper Joints
BAL (bronchial alveolar lavage), diagnostic *see* Drainage, Respiratory System 0B9
Balanoplasty
see Repair, Penis 0VQS
see Supplement, Penis 0VUS
Balloon atrial septostomy (BAS) 02163Z7
Balloon Pump
Continuous, Output 5A02210
Intermittent, Output 5A02110
▶ **Balversa™** (Erdafitinib Antineoplastic) *use* Other Antineoplastic
Bamlanivimab monoclonal antibody XW0
Bandage, Elastic *see* Compression
Banding
see Occlusion
see Restriction
Banding, esophageal varices *see* Occlusion, Vein, Esophageal 06L3
Banding, laparoscopic (adjustable) gastric
Surgical correction *see* Revision of device in, Stomach 0DW6
Initial procedure 0DV64CZ
Bard® Composix® (E/X) (LP) mesh *use* Synthetic Substitute
Bard® Composix® Kugel® patch *use* Synthetic Substitute
Bard® Dulex™ mesh *use* Synthetic Substitute
Bard® Ventralex™ hernia patch *use* Synthetic Substitute
Baricitinib XW0
Barium swallow *see* Fluoroscopy, Gastrointestinal System BD1
Baroreflex Activation Therapy® (BAT®)
use Stimulator Generator in Subcutaneous Tissue and Fascia
use Stimulator Lead in Upper Arteries
Barricaid® Annular Closure Device (ACD) *use* Synthetic Substitute
Bartholin's (greater vestibular) gland *use* Vestibular Gland
Basal (internal) cerebral vein *use* Intracranial Vein
Basal metabolic rate (BMR) *see* Measurement, Physiological Systems 4A0Z
Basal nuclei *use* Basal Ganglia
Base of Tongue *use* Pharynx
Basilar artery *use* Intracranial Artery
Basis pontis *use* Pons
Beam Radiation
Abdomen DW03
Intraoperative DW033Z0
Adrenal Gland DG02
Intraoperative DG023Z0
Bile Ducts DF02
Intraoperative DF023Z0
Bladder DT02
Intraoperative DT023Z0
Bone
Other DP0C
Intraoperative DP0C3Z0
Bone Marrow D700
Intraoperative D7003Z0
Brain D000
Intraoperative D0003Z0
Brain Stem D001
Intraoperative D0013Z0
Breast
Left DM00
Intraoperative DM003Z0
Right DM01
Intraoperative DM013Z0
Bronchus DB01
Intraoperative DB013Z0
Cervix DU01
Intraoperative DU013Z0

Beam Radiation *(Continued)*
Chest DW02
Intraoperative DW023Z0
Chest Wall DB07
Intraoperative DB073Z0
Colon DD05
Intraoperative DD053Z0
Diaphragm DB08
Intraoperative DB083Z0
Duodenum DD02
Intraoperative DD023Z0
Ear D900
Intraoperative D9003Z0
Esophagus DD00
Intraoperative DD003Z0
Eye D800
Intraoperative D8003Z0
Femur DP09
Intraoperative DP093Z0
Fibula DP0B
Intraoperative DP0B3Z0
Gallbladder DF01
Intraoperative DF013Z0
Gland
Adrenal DG02
Intraoperative DG023Z0
Parathyroid DG04
Intraoperative DG043Z0
Pituitary DG00
Intraoperative DG003Z0
Thyroid DG05
Intraoperative DG053Z0
Glands
Salivary D906
Intraoperative D9063Z0
Head and Neck DW01
Intraoperative DW013Z0
Hemibody DW04
Intraoperative DW043Z0
Humerus DP06
Intraoperative DP063Z0
Hypopharynx D903
Intraoperative D9033Z0
Ileum DD04
Intraoperative DD043Z0
Jejunum DD03
Intraoperative DD033Z0
Kidney DT00
Intraoperative DT003Z0
Larynx D90B
Intraoperative D90B3Z0
Liver DF00
Intraoperative DF003Z0
Lung DB02
Intraoperative DB023Z0
Lymphatics
Abdomen D706
Intraoperative D7063Z0
Axillary D704
Intraoperative D7043Z0
Inguinal D708
Intraoperative D7083Z0
Neck D703
Intraoperative D7033Z0
Pelvis D707
Intraoperative D7073Z0
Thorax D705
Intraoperative D7053Z0
Mandible DP03
Intraoperative DP033Z0
Maxilla DP02
Intraoperative DP023Z0
Mediastinum DB06
Intraoperative DB063Z0
Mouth D904
Intraoperative D9043Z0
Nasopharynx D90D
Intraoperative D90D3Z0
Neck and Head DW01
Intraoperative DW013Z0

Beam Radiation *(Continued)*
Nerve
Peripheral D007
Intraoperative D0073Z0
Nose D901
Intraoperative D9013Z0
Oropharynx D90F
Intraoperative D90F3Z0
Ovary DU00
Intraoperative DU003Z0
Palate
Hard D908
Intraoperative D9083Z0
Soft D909
Intraoperative D9093Z0
Pancreas DF03
Intraoperative DF033Z0
Parathyroid Gland DG04
Intraoperative DG043Z0
Pelvic Bones DP08
Intraoperative DP083Z0
Pelvic Region DW06
Intraoperative DW063Z0
Pineal Body DG01
Intraoperative DG013Z0
Pituitary Gland DG00
Intraoperative DG003Z0
Pleura DB05
Intraoperative DB053Z0
Prostate DV00
Intraoperative DV003Z0
Radius DP07
Intraoperative DP073Z0
Rectum DD07
Intraoperative DD073Z0
Rib DP05
Intraoperative DP053Z0
Sinuses D907
Intraoperative D9073Z0
Skin
Abdomen DH08
Intraoperative DH083Z0
Arm DH04
Intraoperative DH043Z0
Back DH07
Intraoperative DH073Z0
Buttock DH09
Intraoperative DH093Z0
Chest DH06
Intraoperative DH063Z0
Face DH02
Intraoperative DH023Z0
Leg DH0B
Intraoperative DH0B3Z0
Neck DH03
Intraoperative DH033Z0
Skull DP00
Intraoperative DP003Z0
Spinal Cord D006
Intraoperative D0063Z0
Spleen D702
Intraoperative D7023Z0
Sternum DP04
Intraoperative DP043Z0
Stomach DD01
Intraoperative DD013Z0
Testis DV01
Intraoperative DV013Z0
Thymus D701
Intraoperative D7013Z0
Thyroid Gland DG05
Intraoperative DG053Z0
Tibia DP0B
Intraoperative DP0B3Z0
Tongue D905
Intraoperative D9053Z0
Trachea DB00
Intraoperative DB003Z0

Beam Radiation *(Continued)*
Ulna DP07
Intraoperative DP073Z0
Ureter DT01
Intraoperative DT013Z0
Urethra DT03
Intraoperative DT033Z0
Uterus DU02
Intraoperative DU023Z0
Whole Body DW05
Intraoperative DW053Z0
Bedside swallow F00ZJWZ
Bentracimab, Ticagrelor Reversal Agent XW0
Berlin Heart Ventricular Assist Device *use* Implantable Heart Assist System in Heart and Great Vessels
beti-cel *use* Betibeglogene Autotemcel
Betibeglogene Autotemcel XW1
Bezlotoxumab infusion *see* Introduction with qualifier Other Therapeutic Monoclonal Antibody
Biceps brachii muscle
use Upper Arm Muscle, Right
use Upper Arm Muscle, Left
Biceps femoris muscle
use Upper Leg Muscle, Right
use Upper Leg Muscle, Left
Bicipital aponeurosis
use Subcutaneous Tissue and Fascia, Right Lower Arm
use Subcutaneous Tissue and Fascia, Left Lower Arm
Bicuspid valve *use* Mitral Valve
Bill light therapy *see* Phototherapy, Skin 6A60
Bioactive embolization coil(s) *use* Intraluminal Device, Bioactive in Upper Arteries
Bioengineered allogeneic construct, skin XHRPXF7
▶ **Bioengineered Human Acellular Vessel** X2R
Biofeedback GZC9ZZZ
BioFire® Film Array® Pneumonia Panel XXEBXQ6
Biopsy
see Drainage with qualifier Diagnostic
see Excision with qualifier Diagnostic
see Extraction with qualifier Diagnostic
BiPAP *see* Assistance, Respiratory 5A09
Bisection *see* Division
Biventricular external heart assist system *use* Short-term External Heart Assist System in Heart and Great Vessels
▶ **BlackArmor® Carbon/PEEK fixation system** *use* Carbon/PEEK Spinal Stabilization Device, Pedicle Based in New Technology
Blepharectomy
see Excision, Eye 08B
see Resection, Eye 08T
Blepharoplasty
see Repair, Eye 08Q
see Replacement, Eye 08R
see Reposition, Eye 08S
see Supplement, Eye 08U
Blepharorrhaphy *see* Repair, Eye 08Q
Blepharotomy *see* Drainage, Eye 089
Blinatumomab *use* Other Antineoplastic
BLINCYTO® (blinatumomab) *use* Other Antineoplastic
Block, Nerve, anesthetic injection 3E0T3BZ
Blood glucose monitoring system *use* Monitoring Device
Blood pressure *see* Measurement, Arterial 4A03
BMR (basal metabolic rate) *see* Measurement, Physiological Systems 4A0Z
Body of femur
use Femoral Shaft, Right
use Femoral Shaft, Left
Body of fibula
use Fibula, Right
use Fibula, Left
Bone anchored hearing device
use Hearing Device, Bone Conduction in 09H
use Hearing Device, in Head and Facial Bones
Bone bank bone graft *use* Nonautologous Tissue Substitute
Bone Growth Stimulator
Insertion of device in
Bone
Facial 0NHW
Lower 0QHY
Nasal 0NHB
Upper 0PHY
Skull 0NH0
Removal of device from
Bone
Facial 0NPW
Lower 0QPY
Nasal 0NPB
Upper 0PPY
Skull 0NP0
Revision of device in
Bone
Facial 0NWW
Lower 0QWY
Nasal 0NWB
Upper 0PWY
Skull 0NW0
Bone marrow transplant *see* Transfusion, Circulatory 302
Bone morphogenetic protein 2 (BMP 2) *use* Recombinant Bone Morphogenetic Protein
Bone screw (interlocking) (lag) (pedicle) (recessed)
use Internal Fixation Device in Head and Facial Bones
use Internal Fixation Device in Upper Bones
use Internal Fixation Device in Lower Bones
Bony labyrinth
use Inner Ear, Right
use Inner Ear, Left
Bony orbit
use Orbit, Right
use Orbit, Left
Bony vestibule
use Inner Ear, Right
use Inner Ear, Left
Botallo's duct *use* Pulmonary Artery, Left
Bovine pericardial valve *use* Zooplastic Tissue in Heart and Great Vessels
Bovine pericardium graft *use* Zooplastic Tissue in Heart and Great Vessels
BP (blood pressure) *see* Measurement, Arterial 4A03
Brachial (lateral) lymph node
use Lymphatic, Axillary Right
use Lymphatic, Axillary Left
Brachialis muscle
use Upper Arm Muscle, Right
use Upper Arm Muscle, Left
Brachiocephalic artery *use* Innominate Artery
Brachiocephalic trunk *use* Innominate Artery
Brachiocephalic vein
use Innominate Vein, Right
use Innominate Vein, Left
Brachioradialis muscle
use Lower Arm and Wrist Muscle, Right
use Lower Arm and Wrist Muscle, Left
Brachytherapy
Abdomen DW13
Adrenal Gland DG12
Back
Lower DW1LBB
Upper DW1KBB
Bile Ducts DF12
Bladder DT12
Bone Marrow D710
Brain D010
Brain Stem D011
Breast
Left DM10
Right DM11
Bronchus DB11
Cervix DU11
Chest DW12
Brachytherapy *(Continued)*
Chest Wall DB17
Colon DD15
Cranial Cavity DW10BB
Diaphragm DB18
Duodenum DD12
Ear D910
Esophagus DD10
Extremity
Lower DW1YBB
Upper DW1XBB
Eye D810
Gallbladder DF11
Gastrointestinal Tract DW1PBB
Genitourinary Tract DW1RBB
Gland
Adrenal DG12
Parathyroid DG14
Pituitary DG10
Thyroid DG15
Glands, Salivary D916
Head and Neck DW11
Hypopharynx D913
Ileum DD14
Jejunum DD13
Kidney DT10
Larynx D91B
Liver DF10
Lung DB12
Lymphatics
Abdomen D716
Axillary D714
Inguinal D718
Neck D713
Pelvis D717
Thorax D715
Mediastinum DB16
Mouth D914
Nasopharynx D91D
Neck and Head DW11
Nerve, Peripheral D017
Nose D911
Oropharynx D91F
Ovary DU10
Palate
Hard D918
Soft D919
Pancreas DF13
Parathyroid Gland DG14
Pelvic Region DW16
Pineal Body DG11
Pituitary Gland DG10
Pleura DB15
Prostate DV10
Rectum DD17
Respiratory Tract DW1QBB
Sinuses D917
Spinal Cord D016
Spleen D712
Stomach DD11
Testis DV11
Thymus D711
Thyroid Gland DG15
Tongue D915
Trachea DB10
Ureter DT11
Urethra DT13
Uterus DU12
Brachytherapy, CivaSheet®
see Brachytherapy with qualifier Unidirectional Source
see Insertion with device Radioactive Element
Brachytherapy seeds *use* Radioactive Element
▶ **Brain Connectomic Analysis Mapping** 00K0XZ1
Brain Electrical Activity
Computer-aided Detection and Notification XX20X89
Computer-aided Semiologic Analysis XXE0X48

▶**Branched Intraluminal Device, Manufactured Integrated System, Four or More Arteries, Aorta,Thoracodominal** X2VE3SA
Broad Consortium Microbiota-based Live Biotherapeutic Suspension XW0H7X8
Breast procedures, skin only *use* Skin, Chest
Brexanolone XW0
Brexucabtagene Autoleucel *use* Brexucabtagene Autoleucel Immunotherapy
Brexucabtagene Autoleucel Immunotherapy XW0
Broad ligament *use* Uterine Supporting Structure
Bromelain-enriched proteolytic enzyme *use* Anacaulase-bcdb
Bronchial artery *use* Upper Artery
Bronchography
see Plain Radiography, Respiratory System BB0
see Fluoroscopy, Respiratory System BB1
Bronchoplasty
see Repair, Respiratory System 0BQ
see Supplement, Respiratory System 0BU
Bronchorrhaphy *see* Repair, Respiratory System 0BQ
Bronchoscopy 0BJ08ZZ
Bronchotomy *see* Drainage, Respiratory System 0B9
Bronchus Intermedius *use* Main Bronchus, Right
BRYAN® Cervical Disc System *use* Synthetic Substitute
Buccal gland *use* Buccal Mucosa
Buccinator lymph node *use* Lymphatic, Head
Buccinator muscle *use* Facial Muscle
Buckling, scleral with implant *see* Supplement, Eye 08U
Bulbospongiosus muscle *use* Perineum Muscle
Bulbourethral (Cowper's) gland *use* Urethra
Bundle of His *use* Conduction Mechanism
Bundle of Kent *use* Conduction Mechanism
Bunionectomy *see* Excision, Lower Bones 0QB
Bursectomy
see Excision, Bursae and Ligaments 0MB
see Resection, Bursae and Ligaments 0MT
Bursocentesis *see* Drainage, Bursae and Ligaments 0M9
Bursography
see Plain Radiography, Non-Axial Upper Bones BP0
see Plain Radiography, Non-Axial Lower Bones BQ0
Bursotomy
see Division, Bursae and Ligaments 0M8
see Drainage, Bursae and Ligaments 0M9
BVS 5000 Ventricular Assist Device *use* Short-term External Heart Assist System in Heart and Great Vessels
Bypass
Anterior Chamber
Left 08133
Right 08123
Aorta
Abdominal 0410
Thoracic
Ascending/Arch 021X
Descending 021W
Artery
Anterior Tibial
Left 041Q
Right 041P
Axillary
Left 03160
Right 03150
Brachial
Left 0318
Right 0317
Common Carotid
Left 031J0
Right 031H0
Common Iliac
Left 041D
Right 041C

Bypass *(Continued)*
Artery *(Continued)*
Coronary
Four or More Arteries 0213
One Artery 0210
Three Arteries 0212
Two Arteries 0211
External Carotid
Left 031N0
Right 031M0
External Iliac
Left 041J
Right 041H
Femoral
Left 041L
Right 041K
Foot
Left 041W
Right 041V
Hepatic 0413
Innominate 03120
Internal Carotid
Left 031L0
Right 031K0
Internal Iliac
Left 041F
Right 041E
Intracranial 031G0
Peroneal
Left 041U
Right 041T
Popliteal
Left 041N
Right 041M
Posterior Tibial
Left 041S
Right 041R
Pulmonary
Left 021R
Right 021Q
Pulmonary Trunk 021P
Radial
Left 031C
Right 031B
Splenic 0414
Subclavian
Left 03140
Right 03130
Temporal
Left 031T0
Right 031S0
Ulnar
Left 031A
Right 0319
Atrium
Left 0217
Right 0216
Bladder 0T1B
Cavity, Cranial 0W110J
Cecum 0D1H
Cerebral Ventricle 0016
▶Cisterna Chyli 071L
Colon
Ascending 0D1K
Descending 0D1M
Sigmoid 0D1N
Transverse 0D1L
Conduit through Femoral Vein to Popliteal Artery X2K
Conduit through Femoral Vein to Superficial Femoral Artery X2K
Duct
Common Bile 0F19
Cystic 0F18
Hepatic
Common 0F17
Left 0F16
Right 0F15
Lacrimal
Left 081Y
Right 081X
Pancreatic 0F1D
Accessory 0F1F

Bypass *(Continued)*
Duodenum 0D19
Ear
Left 091E0
Right 091D0
Esophagus 0D15
Lower 0D13
Middle 0D12
Upper 0D11
Fallopian Tube
Left 0U16
Right 0U15
Gallbladder 0F14
Ileum 0D1B
Intestine
Large 0D1E
Small 0D1E
Jejunum 0D1A
Kidney Pelvis
Left 0T14
Right 0T13
▶Lymphatic
▶Aortic 071D
▶Axillary
▶Left 0716
▶Right 0715
▶Head 0710
▶Inguinal
▶Left 071J
▶Right 071H
▶Internal Mammary
▶Left 0719
▶Right 0718
▶Lower Extremity
▶Left 071G
▶Right 071F
▶Mesenteric 071B
▶Neck
▶Left 0712
▶Right 0711
▶Pelvis 071C
▶Thoracic Duct 071K
▶Thorax 0717
▶Upper Extremity
▶Left 0714
▶Right 0713
Pancreas 0F1G
Pelvic Cavity 0W1J
Peritoneal Cavity 0W1G
Pleural Cavity
Left 0W1B
Right 0W19
Spinal Canal 001U
Stomach 0D16
Trachea 0B11
Ureter
Left 0T17
Right 0T16
Vein Ureters, Bilateral 0T18
Vas Deferens
Bilateral 0V1Q
Left 0V1P
Right 0V1N
Axillary
Left 0518
Right 0517
Azygos 0510
Basilic
Left 051C
Right 051B
Brachial
Left 051A
Right 0519
Cephalic
Left 051F
Right 051D
Colic 0617
Common Iliac
Left 061D
Right 061C
Esophageal 0613

▶ New ➠ Revised ~~deleted~~ Deleted

B

Bypass *(Continued)*
Vas Deferens *(Continued)*
External Iliac
Left Ø61G
Right Ø61F
External Jugular
Left Ø51Q
Right Ø51P
Face
Left Ø51V
Right Ø51T
Femoral
Left Ø61N
Right Ø61M
Foot
Left Ø61V
Right Ø61T
Gastric Ø612
Hand
Left Ø51H
Right Ø51G

Bypass *(Continued)*
Vas Deferens *(Continued)*
Hemiazygos Ø511
Hepatic Ø614
Hypogastric
Left Ø61J
Right Ø61H
Inferior Mesenteric Ø616
Innominate
Left Ø514
Right Ø513
Internal Jugular
Left Ø51N
Right Ø51M
Intracranial Ø51L
Portal Ø618
Renal
Left Ø61B
Right Ø619

Bypass *(Continued)*
Vas Deferens *(Continued)*
Saphenous
Left Ø61Q
Right Ø61P
Splenic Ø611
Subclavian
Left Ø516
Right Ø515
Superior Mesenteric Ø615
Vertebral
Left Ø51S
Right Ø51R
Vena Cava
Inferior Ø61Ø
Superior Ø21V
Ventricle
Left Ø21L
Right Ø21K
Bypass, cardiopulmonary 5A1221Z

B

C

Caesarean section *see* Extraction, Products of Conception 10DØ
Calcaneocuboid joint
use Tarsal Joint, Right
use Tarsal Joint, Left
Calcaneocuboid ligament
use Foot Bursa and Ligament, Right
use Foot Bursa and Ligament, Left
Calcaneofibular ligament
use Ankle Bursa and Ligament, Right
use Ankle Bursa and Ligament, Left
Calcaneus
use Tarsal, Right
use Tarsal, Left
Cannulation
see Bypass
see Dilation
see Drainage
see Irrigation
Canthorrhaphy *see* Repair, Eye Ø8Q
Canthotomy *see* Release, Eye Ø8N
Canturio™ te (Tibial Extension) *use* Tibial Extension with Motion Sensors in New Technology
Capitate bone
use Carpal, Right
use Carpal, Left
Caplacizumab XWØ
Capsulectomy, lens *see* Excision, Eye Ø8B
Capsulorrhaphy, joint
see Repair, Upper Joints ØRQ
see Repair, Lower Joints ØSQ
Caption guidance system X2JAX47
▶**Carbon/PEEK Spinal Stabilization Device, Pedicle Based**
▶Lumbar Vertebral XRHB
▶2 or more XRHC
▶Lumbosacral XRHD
▶Thoracic Vertebral XRH6
▶2 to 7 XRH7
▶8 or more XRH8
▶Thoracolumbar Vertebral XRHA
Cardia *use* Esophagogastric Junction
Cardiac contractility modulation lead *use* Cardiac Lead in Heart and Great Vessels
Cardiac event recorder *use* Monitoring Device
Cardiac Lead
Defibrillator
Atrium
Left Ø2H7
Right Ø2H6
Pericardium Ø2HN
Vein, Coronary Ø2H4
Ventricle
Left Ø2HL
Right Ø2HK
Insertion of device in
Atrium
Left Ø2H7
Right Ø2H6
Pericardium Ø2HN
Vein, Coronary Ø2H4
Ventricle
Left Ø2HL
Right Ø2HK
Pacemaker
Atrium
Left Ø2H7
Right Ø2H6
Pericardium Ø2HN
Vein, Coronary Ø2H4
Ventricle
Left Ø2HL
Right Ø2HK
Removal of device from, Heart Ø2PA
Revision of device in, Heart Ø2WA
Cardiac plexus *use* Nerve, Thoracic Sympathetic
Cardiac Resynchronization Defibrillator Pulse Generator
Abdomen ØJH8
Chest ØJH6
Cardiac Resynchronization Pacemaker Pulse Generator
Abdomen ØJH8
Chest ØJH6
Cardiac resynchronization therapy (CRT) lead
use Cardiac Lead, Pacemaker in O2H
use Cardiac Lead, Defibrillator in Ø2H
Cardiac Rhythm Related Device
Insertion of device in
Abdomen ØJH8
Chest ØJH6
Removal of device from, Subcutaneous Tissue and Fascia, Trunk ØJPT
Revision of device in, Subcutaneous Tissue and Fascia, Trunk ØJWT
Cardiocentesis *see* Drainage, Pericardial Cavity ØW9D
Cardioesophageal junction *use* Esophagogastric Junction
Cardiolysis *see* Release, Heart and Great Vessels Ø2N
CardioMEMS® pressure sensor *use* Monitoring Device, Pressure Sensor in Ø2H
Cardiomyotomy *see* Division, Esophagogastric Junction ØD84
Cardioplegia *see* Introduction of substance in or on, Heart 3EØ8
Cardiorrhaphy *see* Repair, Heart and Great Vessels Ø2Q
Cardioversion 5A22Ø4Z
Caregiver Training FØFZ
Carmat total artificial heart (TAH) *use* Biologic with Synthetic Substitute, Autoregulated Electrohydraulic in Ø2R
Caroticotympanic artery
use Internal Carotid Artery, Right
use Internal Carotid Artery, Left
Carotid (artery) sinus (baroreceptor) lead *use* Stimulator Lead in Upper Arteries
Carotid glomus
use Carotid Body, Left
use Carotid Body, Right
use Carotid Bodies, Bilateral
Carotid sinus
use Internal Carotid Artery, Right
use Internal Carotid Artery, Left
Carotid sinus nerve *use* Glossopharyngeal Nerve
Carotid WALLSTENT® Monorail® Endoprosthesis *use* Intraluminal Device
Carpectomy
see Excision, Upper Bones ØPB
see Resection, Upper Bones ØPT
Carpometacarpal ligament
use Hand Bursa and Ligament, Right
use Hand Bursa and Ligament, Left
CARVYKTI™ *use* Ciltacabtagene Autoleucel
▶**CASGEVY™** *use* Exagamglogene Autotemcel
Casirivimab (REGN1Ø933) and Imdevimab (REGN1Ø987) *use* REGN-COV2 Monoclonal Antibody
Casting *see* Immobilization
CAT scan *see* Computerized Tomography (CT Scan)
Catheterization
see Dilation
see Drainage
see Insertion of device in
see Irrigation
Heart *see* Measurement, Cardiac 4AØ2
Umbilical vein, for infusion Ø6HØ33T
Cauda equina *use* Lumbar Spinal Cord
Cauterization
see Destruction
see Repair
Cavernous plexus *use* Head and Neck Sympathetic Nerve
Cavoatrial junction *use* Superior Vena Cava
CBMA (Concentrated Bone Marrow Aspirate) *use* Other Substance
CBMA (Concentrated Bone Marrow Aspirate) injection *see* Introduction of substance in or on, Muscle 3EØ2
CD24Fc Immunomodulator XWØ
Cecectomy
see Excision, Cecum ØDBH
see Resection, Cecum ØDTH
Cecocolostomy
see Bypass, Gastrointestinal System ØD1
see Drainage, Gastrointestinal System ØD9
Cecopexy
see Repair, Cecum ØDQH
see Reposition, Cecum ØDSH
Cecoplication *see* Restriction, Cecum ØDVH
Cecorrhaphy *see* Repair, Cecum ØDQH
Cecostomy
see Bypass, Cecum ØD1H
see Drainage, Cecum ØD9H
Cecotomy *see* Drainage, Cecum ØD9H
▶**Cefepime-taniborbactam Anti-infective** XWØ
Cefiderocol Anti-infective XWØ
Ceftazidime-avibactam *use* Other Anti-infective
▶**Ceftobiprole Medocaril Anti-infective** XWØ
Ceftolozane/Tazobactam Anti-infective XWØ
Celiac (solar) plexus *use* Abdominal Sympathetic Nerve
Celiac ganglion *use* Abdominal Sympathetic Nerve
Celiac lymph node *use* Lymphatic, Aortic
Celiac trunk *use* Celiac Artery
Central axillary lymph node
use Lymphatic, Right Axillary
use Lymphatic, Left Axillary
Central venous pressure *see* Measurement, Venous 4AØ4
Centrimag® Blood Pump *use* Short-term External Heart Assist System in Heart and Great Vessels
Cephalogram BNØØZZZ
CERAMENT® G *use* Antibiotic-eluting Bone Void Filler
Ceramic on ceramic bearing surface *use* Synthetic Substitute, Ceramic in ØSR
Cerclage *see* Restriction
Cerebral aqueduct (Sylvius) *use* Cerebral Ventricle
Cerebral Embolic Filtration
Duel Filter X2A5312
Extracorporeal Flow Reversal Circuit X2A
Single Deflection Filter X2A6325
Cerebrum *use* Brain
Ceribell® Monitor XX2ØX89
Cervical esophagus *use* Esophagus, Upper
Cervical facet joint
use Cervical Vertebral Joint
use Cervical Vertebral Joint, 2 or more
Cervical ganglion *use* Head and Neck Sympathetic Nerve
Cervical interspinous ligament *use* Head and Neck Bursa and Ligament
Cervical intertransverse ligament *use* Head and Neck Bursa and Ligament
Cervical ligamentum flavum *use* Head and Neck Bursa and Ligament
Cervical lymph node
use Lymphatic, Right Neck
use Lymphatic, Left Neck
Cervicectomy
see Excision, Cervix ØUBC
see Resection, Cervix ØUTC
Cervicothoracic facet joint *use* Cervicothoracic Vertebral Joint
Cesarean section *see* Extraction, Products of Conception 1ØDØ
Cesium-131 Collagen Implant *use* Radioactive Element, Cesium-131 Collagen Implant in ØØH
Change device in
Abdominal Wall ØW2FX
Back
Lower ØW2LX

Upper ØW2KX
Bladder ØT2BX
Bone
Facial ØN2WX
Lower ØQ2YX
Nasal ØN2BX
Upper ØP2YX
Bone Marrow Ø72TX
Brain ØØ2ØX
Breast
Left ØH2UX
Right ØH2TX
Bursa and Ligament
Lower ØM2YX
Upper ØM2XX
Cavity, Cranial ØW21X
Chest Wall ØW28X
Cisterna Chyli Ø72LX
Diaphragm ØB2TX
Duct
Hepatobiliary ØF2BX
Pancreatic ØF2DX
Ear
Left Ø92JX
Right Ø92HX
Epididymis and Spermatic Cord ØV2MX
Extremity
Lower
Left ØY2BX
Right ØY29X
Upper
Left ØX27X
Right ØX26X
Eye
Left Ø821X
Right Ø82ØX
Face ØW22X
Fallopian Tube ØU28X
Gallbladder ØF24X
Gland
Adrenal ØG25X
Endocrine ØG2SX
Pituitary ØG2ØX
Salivary ØC2AX
Head ØW2ØX
Intestinal Tract
Lower Intestinal Tract ØD2DXUZ
Upper Intestinal Tract ØD2ØXUZ
Jaw
Lower ØW25X
Upper ØW24X
Joint
Lower ØS2YX
Upper ØR2YX
Kidney ØT25X
Larynx ØC2SX
Liver ØF2ØX
Lung
Left ØB2LX
Right ØB2KX
Lymphatic Ø72NX
Thoracic Duct Ø72KX
Mediastinum ØW2CX
Mesentery ØD2VX
Mouth and Throat ØC2YX
Muscle
Lower ØK2YX
Upper ØK2XX
Nasal Mucosa and Soft Tissue Ø92KX
Neck ØW26X
Nerve
Cranial ØØ2EX
Peripheral Ø12YX
Omentum ØD2UX
Ovary ØU23X
Pancreas ØF2GX
Parathyroid Gland ØG2RX
Pelvic Cavity ØW2JX
Penis ØV2SX
Pericardial Cavity ØW2DX
Perineum
Female ØW2NX
Male ØW2MX
Peritoneal Cavity ØW2GX
Peritoneum ØD2WX
Pineal Body ØG21X
Pleura ØB2QX
Pleural Cavity
Left ØW2BX
Right ØW29X
Products of Conception 1Ø2Ø7
Prostate and Seminal Vesicles ØV24X
Retroperitoneum ØW2HX
Scrotum and Tunica Vaginalis ØV28X
Sinus Ø92YX
Skin ØH2PX
Skull ØN2ØX
Spinal Canal ØØ2UX
Spleen Ø72PX
Subcutaneous Tissue and Fascia
Head and Neck ØJ2SX
Lower Extremity ØJ2WX
Trunk ØJ2TX
Upper Extremity ØJ2VX
Tendon
Lower ØL2YX
Upper ØL2XX
Testis ØV2DX
Thymus Ø72MX
Thyroid Gland ØG2KX
Trachea ØB21
Tracheobronchial Tree ØB2ØX
Ureter ØT29X
Urethra ØT2DX
Uterus and Cervix ØU2DXHZ
Vagina and Cul-de-sac ØU2HXGZ
Vas Deferens ØV2RX
Vulva ØU2MX
Change device in or on
Abdominal Wall 2WØ3X
Anorectal 2YØ3X5Z
Arm
Lower
Left 2WØDX
Right 2WØCX
Upper
Left 2WØBX
Right 2WØAX
Back 2WØ5X
Chest Wall 2WØ4X
Ear 2YØ2X5Z
Extremity
Lower
Left 2WØMX
Right 2WØLX
Upper
Left 2WØ9X
Right 2WØ8X
Face 2WØ1X
Finger
Left 2WØKX
Right 2WØJX
Foot
Left 2WØTX
Right 2WØSX
Genital Tract, Female 2YØ4X5Z
Hand
Left 2WØFX
Right 2WØEX
Head 2WØØX
Inguinal Region
Left 2WØ7X
Right 2WØ6X
Leg
Lower
Left 2WØRX
Right 2WØQX
Upper
Left 2WØPX
Right 2WØNX
Mouth and Pharynx 2YØØX5Z
Nasal 2YØ1X5Z
Neck 2WØ2X
Thumb
Left 2WØHX
Right 2WØGX
Toe
Left 2WØVX
Right 2WØUX
Urethra 2YØ5X5Z
Chemoembolization *see* Introduction of substance in or on
Chemosurgery, Skin 3EØØXTZ
Chemothalamectomy *see* Destruction, Thalamus ØØ59
Chemotherapy, Infusion for cancer *see* Introduction of substance in or on
Chest compression (CPR), external
Manual 5A12Ø12
Mechanical 5A1221J
Chest x-ray *see* Plain Radiography, Chest BWØ3
Chin *use* Subcutaneous Tissue and Fascia, Face
Chiropractic Manipulation
Abdomen 9WB9X
Cervical 9WB1X
Extremities
Lower 9WB6X
Upper 9WB7X
Head 9WBØX
Lumbar 9WB3X
Pelvis 9WB5X
Rib Cage 9WB8X
Sacrum 9WB4X
Thoracic 9WB2X
Choana *use* Nasopharynx
Cholangiogram
see Plain Radiography, Hepatobiliary System and Pancreas BFØ
see Fluoroscopy, Hepatobiliary System and Pancreas BF1
Cholecystectomy
see Excision, Gallbladder ØFB4
see Resection, Gallbladder ØFT4
Cholecystojejunostomy
see Bypass, Hepatobiliary System and Pancreas ØF1
see Drainage, Hepatobiliary System and Pancreas ØF9
Cholecystopexy
see Repair, Gallbladder ØFQ4
see Reposition, Gallbladder ØFS4
Cholecystoscopy ØFJ44ZZ
Cholecystostomy
see Bypass, Gallbladder ØF14
see Drainage, Gallbladder ØF94
Cholecystotomy *see* Drainage, Gallbladder ØF94
Choledochectomy
see Excision, Hepatobiliary System and Pancreas ØFB
see Resection, Hepatobiliary System and Pancreas ØFT
Choledocholithotomy *see* Extirpation, Duct, Common Bile ØFC9
Choledochoplasty
see Repair, Hepatobiliary System and Pancreas ØFQ
see Replacement, Hepatobiliary System and Pancreas ØFR
see Supplement, Hepatobiliary System and Pancreas ØFU
Choledochoscopy ØFJB8ZZ
Choledochotomy *see* Drainage, Hepatobiliary System and Pancreas ØF9
Cholelithotomy *see* Extirpation, Hepatobiliary System and Pancreas ØFC
Chondrectomy
see Excision, Upper Joints ØRB
see Excision, Lower Joints ØSB
Knee *see* Excision, Lower Joints ØSB
Semilunar cartilage *see* Excision, Lower Joints ØSB

Chondroglossus muscle *use* Tongue, Palate, Pharynx Muscle
Chorda tympani *use* Facial Nerve
Chordotomy *see* Division, Central Nervous System and Cranial Nerves 008
Choroid plexus *use* Cerebral Ventricle
Choroidectomy
see Excision, Eye 08B
see Resection, Eye 08T
Ciliary body
use Eye, Right
use Eye, Left
Ciliary ganglion *use* Head and Neck Sympathetic Nerve
Cilta-cel *use* Ciltacabtagene Autoleucel
Ciltacabtagene autoleucel XW0
Circle of Willis *use* Intracranial Artery
Circumcision 0VTTXZZ
Circumflex iliac artery
use Femoral Artery, Right
use Femoral Artery, Left
CivaSheet® *use* Radioactive Element
CivaSheet® Bradytherapy
see Bradytherapy with qualifier Unidirectional Source
see Insertion with device Radioactive Element
Clamp and rod internal fixation system (CRIF)
use Internal Fixation Device in Upper Bones
use Internal Fixation Device in Lower Bones
Clamping *see* Occlusion
Claustrum *use* Basal Ganglia
Claviculectomy
see Excision, Upper Bones 0PB
see Resection, Upper Bones 0PT
Claviculotomy
see Division, Upper Bones 0P8
see Drainage, Upper Bones 0P9
Clipping, aneurysm
see Occlusion using Extraluminal Device
see Restriction using Extraluminal Device
Clitorectomy, clitoridectomy
see Excision, Clitoris 0UBJ
see Resection, Clitoris 0UTJ
Clolar *use* Clofarabine
Closure
see Occlusion
see Repair
Clysis *see* Introduction of substance in or on
Coagulation *see* Destruction
Coagulation Factor Xa, Inactivated XW0
Coagulation Factor Xa, (Recombinant) Inactivated
use Coagulation Factor Xa, Inactivated
COALESCE® radiolucent interbody fusion device
use Interbody Fusion Device in Upper Joints
use Interbody Fusion Device in Lower Joints
CoAxia NeuroFlo catheter *use* Intraluminal Device
Cobalt/chromium head and polyethylene socket *use* Synthetic Substitute, Metal on Polyethylene in 0SR
Cobalt/chromium head and socket *use* Synthetic Substitute, Metal in 0SR
Coccygeal body *use* Coccygeal Glomus
Coccygeus muscle
use Trunk Muscle, Right
use Trunk Muscle, Left
Cochlea
use Inner Ear, Right
use Inner Ear, Left
Cochlear implant (CI), multiple channel (electrode) *use* Hearing Device, Multiple Channel Cochlear Prosthesis in 09H
Cochlear implant (CI), single channel (electrode) *use* Hearing Device, Single Channel Cochlear Prosthesis in 09H
Cochlear Implant Treatment F0BZ0
Cochlear nerve *use* Acoustic Nerve
COGNIS® CRT-D *use* Cardiac Resynchronization Defibrillator Pulse Generator in 0JH
COHERE® radiolucent interbody fusion device
use Interbody Fusion Device in Upper Joints
use Interbody Fusion Device in Lower Joints
Colectomy
see Excision, Gastrointestinal System 0DB
see Resection, Gastrointestinal System 0DT
Collapse *see* Occlusion
Collection from
Breast, Breast Milk 8E0HX62
Indwelling Device
Circulatory System
Blood 8C02X6K
Other Fluid 8C02X6L
Nervous System
Cerebrospinal Fluid 8C01X6J
Other Fluid 8C01X6L
Integumentary System, Breast Milk 8E0HX62
Reproductive System, Male, Sperm 8E0VX63
Colocentesis *see* Drainage, Gastrointestinal System 0D9
Colofixation
see Repair, Gastrointestinal System 0DQ
see Reposition, Gastrointestinal System 0DS
Cololysis *see* Release, Gastrointestinal System 0DN
Colonic Z-Stent® *use* Intraluminal Device
Colonoscopy 0DJD8ZZ
Colopexy
see Repair, Gastrointestinal System 0DQ
see Reposition, Gastrointestinal System 0DS
Coloplication *see* Restriction, Gastrointestinal System 0DV
Coloproctectomy
see Excision, Gastrointestinal System 0DB
see Resection, Gastrointestinal System 0DT
Coloproctostomy
see Bypass, Gastrointestinal System 0D1
see Drainage, Gastrointestinal System 0D9
Colopuncture *see* Drainage, Gastrointestinal System 0D9
Colorrhaphy *see* Repair, Gastrointestinal System 0DQ
Colostomy
see Bypass, Gastrointestinal System 0D1
see Drainage, Gastrointestinal System 0D9
Colpectomy
see Excision, Vagina 0UBG
see Resection, Vagina 0UTG
Colpocentesis *see* Drainage, Vagina 0U9G
Colpopexy
see Repair, Vagina 0UQG
see Reposition, Vagina 0USG
Colpoplasty
see Repair, Vagina 0UQG
see Supplement, Vagina 0UUG
Colporrhaphy *see* Repair, Vagina 0UQG
Colposcopy 0UJH8ZZ
Columella *use* Nasal Mucosa and Soft Tissue
▶ **Columvi™** *use* Glofitamab Antineoplastic
COMIRNATY®
use COVID-19 Vaccine Dose 1
use COVID-19 Vaccine Dose 2
use COVID-19 Vaccine
use COVID-19 Vaccine Dose 3
use COVID-19 Vaccine Booster
Common digital vein
use Foot Vein, Right
use Foot Vein, Left
Common facial vein
use Face Vein, Right
use Face Vein, Left
Common fibular nerve *use* Peroneal Nerve
Common hepatic artery *use* Hepatic Artery
Common iliac (subaortic) lymph node *use* Lymphatic, Pelvis
Common interosseous artery
use Ulnar Artery, Right
use Ulnar Artery, Left
Common peroneal nerve *use* Peroneal Nerve
Complete (SE) stent *use* Intraluminal Device
Compression *see* Restriction
Abdominal Wall 2W13X
Arm
Lower
Left 2W1DX
Right 2W1CX
Upper
Left 2W1BX
Right 2W1AX
Back 2W15X
Chest Wall 2W14X
Extremity
Lower
Left 2W1MX
Right 2W1LX
Upper
Left 2W19X
Right 2W18X
Face 2W11X
Finger
Left 2W1KX
Right 2W1JX
Foot
Left 2W1TX
Right 2W1SX
Hand
Left 2W1FX
Right 2W1EX
Head 2W10X
Inguinal Region
Left 2W17X
Right 2W16X
Leg
Lower
Left 2W1RX
Right 2W1QX
Upper
Left 2W1PX
Right 2W1NX
Neck 2W12X
Thumb
Left 2W1HX
Right 2W1GX
Toe
Left 2W1VX
Right 2W1UX
Computer-aided Assessment
Cardiac Output XXE2X19
Intracranial Vascular Activity XXE0X07
Computer-aided guidance, transthoracic echocardiography X2JAX47
Computer-aided mechanical aspiration X2C
Computer-aided triage and notification, pulmonary artery flow XXE3X27
Computer-aided Valve Modeling and Notification, Coronary Artery Flow XXE3X68
Computer-assisted intermittent aspiration see new technology, cardiovascular system X2C
Computer Assisted Procedure
Extremity
Lower
No Qualifier 8E0YXBZ
With Computerized Tomography 8E0YXBG
With Fluoroscopy 8E0YXBF
With Magnetic Resonance Imaging 8E0YXBH
Upper
No Qualifier 8E0XXBZ
With Computerized Tomography 8E0XXBG
With Fluoroscopy 8E0XXBF
With Magnetic Resonance Imaging 8E0XXBH

C

▶ New ➠ Revised ~~deleted~~ Deleted

Computer Assisted Procedure *(Continued)*
Head and Neck Region
No Qualifier 8E09XBZ
With Computerized Tomography 8E09XBG
With Fluoroscopy 8E09XBF
With Magnetic Resonance Imaging 8E09XBH
Trunk Region
No Qualifier 8E0WXBZ
With Computerized Tomography 8E0WXBG
With Fluoroscopy 8E0WXBF
With Magnetic Resonance Imaging 8E0WXBH
Computer-assisted Transcranial Magnetic Stimulation X0Z0X18
Computerized Tomography (CT Scan)
Abdomen BW20
Chest and Pelvis BW25
Abdomen and Chest BW24
Abdomen and Pelvis BW21
Airway, Trachea BB2F
Ankle
Left BQ2H
Right BQ2G
Aorta
Abdominal B420
Intravascular Optical Coherence B420Z2Z
Thoracic B320
Intravascular Optical Coherence B320Z2Z
Arm
Left BP2F
Right BP2E
Artery
Celiac B421
Intravascular Optical Coherence B421Z2Z
Common Carotid
Bilateral B325
Intravascular Optical Coherence B325Z2Z
Coronary
Bypass Graft
Multiple B223
Intravascular Optical Coherence B223Z2Z
Multiple B221
Intravascular Optical Coherence B221Z2Z
Internal Carotid
Bilateral B328
Intravascular Optical Coherence B328Z2Z
Intracranial B32R
Intravascular Optical Coherence B32RZ2Z
Lower Extremity
Bilateral B42H
Intravascular Optical Coherence B42HZ2Z
Left B42G
Intravascular Optical Coherence B42GZ2Z
Right B42F
Intravascular Optical Coherence B42FZ2Z
Pelvic B42C
Intravascular Optical Coherence B42CZ2Z
Pulmonary
Left B32T
Intravascular Optical Coherence B32TZ2Z
Right B32S
Intravascular Optical Coherence B32SZ2Z

Computerized Tomography (CT Scan) *(Continued)*
Artery *(Continued)*
Renal
Bilateral B428
Intravascular Optical Coherence B428Z2Z
Transplant B42M
Intravascular Optical Coherence B42MZ2Z
Superior Mesenteric B424
Intravascular Optical Coherence B424Z2Z
Vertebral
Bilateral B32G
Intravascular Optical Coherence B32GZ2Z
Bladder BT20
Bone
Facial BN25
Temporal BN2F
Brain B020
Calcaneus
Left BQ2K
Right BQ2J
Cerebral Ventricle B028
Chest, Abdomen and Pelvis BW25
Chest and Abdomen BW24
Cisterna B027
Clavicle
Left BP25
Right BP24
Coccyx BR2F
Colon BD24
Ear B920
Elbow
Left BP2H
Right BP2G
Extremity
Lower
Left BQ2S
Right BQ2R
Upper
Bilateral BP2V
Left BP2U
Right BP2T
Eye
Bilateral B827
Left B826
Right B825
Femur
Left BQ24
Right BQ23
Fibula
Left BQ2C
Right BQ2B
Finger
Left BP2S
Right BP2R
Foot
Left BQ2M
Right BQ2L
Forearm
Left BP2K
Right BP2J
Gland
Adrenal, Bilateral BG22
Parathyroid BG23
Parotid, Bilateral B926
Salivary, Bilateral B92D
Submandibular, Bilateral B929
Thyroid BG24
Hand
Left BP2P
Right BP2N
Hands and Wrists, Bilateral BP2Q
Head BW28
Head and Neck BW29

Computerized Tomography (CT Scan) *(Continued)*
Heart
Right and Left B226
Intravascular Optical Coherence B226Z2Z
Hepatobiliary System, All BF2C
Hip
Left BQ21
Right BQ20
Humerus
Left BP2B
Right BP2A
Intracranial Sinus B522
Intravascular Optical Coherence B522Z2Z
Joint
Acromioclavicular, Bilateral BP23
Finger
Left BP2DZZZ
Right BP2CZZZ
Foot
Left BQ2Y
Right BQ2X
Hand
Left BP2DZZZ
Right BP2CZZZ
Sacroiliac BR2D
Sternoclavicular
Bilateral BP22
Left BP21
Right BP20
Temporomandibular, Bilateral BN29
Toe
Left BQ2Y
Right BQ2X
Kidney
Bilateral BT23
Left BT22
Right BT21
Transplant BT29
Knee
Left BQ28
Right BQ27
Larynx B92J
Leg
Left BQ2F
Right BQ2D
Liver BF25
Liver and Spleen BF26
Lung, Bilateral BB24
Mandible BN26
Nasopharynx B92F
Neck BW2F
Neck and Head BW29
Orbit, Bilateral BN23
Oropharynx B92F
Pancreas BF27
Patella
Left BQ2W
Right BQ2V
Pelvic Region BW2G
Pelvis BR2C
Chest and Abdomen BW25
Pelvis and Abdomen BW21
Pituitary Gland B029
Prostate BV23
Ribs
Left BP2Y
Right BP2X
Sacrum BR2F
Scapula
Left BP27
Right BP26
Sella Turcica B029
Shoulder
Left BP29
Right BP28
Sinus
Intracranial B522
Intravascular Optical Coherence B522Z2Z
Paranasal B922
Skull BN20

Computerized Tomography (CT Scan) *(Continued)*
Spinal Cord BØ2B
Spine
Cervical BR2Ø
Lumbar BR29
Thoracic BR27
Spleen and Liver BF26
Thorax BP2W
Tibia
Left BQ2C
Right BQ2B
Toe
Left BQ2Q
Right BQ2P
Trachea BB2F
Tracheobronchial Tree
Bilateral BB29
Left BB28
Right BB27
Vein
Pelvic (Iliac)
Left B52G
Intravascular Optical Coherence B52GZ2Z
Right B52F
Intravascular Optical Coherence B52FZ2Z
Pelvic (Iliac) Bilateral B52H
Intravascular Optical Coherence B52HZ2Z
Portal B52T
Intravascular Optical Coherence B52TZ2Z
Pulmonary
Bilateral B52S
Intravascular Optical Coherence B52SZ2Z
Left B52R
Intravascular Optical Coherence B52RZ2Z
Right B52Q
Intravascular Optical Coherence B52QZ2Z
Renal
Bilateral B52L
Intravascular Optical Coherence B52LZ2Z
Left B52K
Intravascular Optical Coherence B52KZ2Z
Right B52J
Intravascular Optical Coherence B52JZ2Z
~~Spanchnic B52T~~
~~Intravascular Optical Coherence B52TZ2Z~~
▶Splanchnic B52T
▶Intravascular Optical Coherence B52TZ2Z
Vena Cava
Inferior B529
Intravascular Optical Coherence B529Z2Z
Superior B528
Intravascular Optical Coherence B528Z2Z
Ventricle, Cerebral BØ28
Wrist
Left BP2M
Right BP2L
Concerto II CRT-D *use* Cardiac Resynchronization Defibrillator Pulse Generator in ØJH
Conduit through Femoral Vein to Popliteal Artery, Bypass X2K
Conduit through Femoral Vein to Superficial Femoral Artery, Bypass X2K
Conduit to Short-term External Heart Assist System, Insertion X2H
Condylectomy
see Excision, Head and Facial Bones ØNB
see Excision, Upper Bones ØPB
see Excision, Lower Bones ØQB
Condyloid process
use Mandible, Left
use Mandible, Right
Condylotomy
see Division, Head and Facial Bones ØN8
see Drainage, Head and Facial Bones ØN9
see Division, Upper Bones ØP8
see Drainage, Upper Bones ØP9
see Division, Lower Bones ØQ8
see Drainage, Lower Bones ØQ9
Condylysis
see Release, Head and Facial Bones ØNN
see Release, Upper Bones ØPN
see Release, Lower Bones ØQN
Conization, cervix *see* Excision, Cervix ØUBC
Conjunctivoplasty
see Repair, Eye Ø8Q
see Replacement, Eye Ø8R
▶**Connectomic Analysis (Brain) Mapping** ØØKØXZ1
CONSERVE® PLUS Total Resurfacing Hip System *use* Resurfacing Device in Lower Joints
Construction
Auricle, ear *see* Replacement, Ear, Nose, Sinus Ø9R
Ileal conduit *see* Bypass, Urinary System ØT1
Consulta CRT-D *use* Cardiac Resynchronization Defibrillator Pulse Generator in ØJH
Consulta CRT-P *use* Cardiac Resynchronization Pacemaker Pulse Generator in ØJH
Contact Radiation
Abdomen DWY37ZZ
Adrenal Gland DGY27ZZ
Bile Ducts DFY27ZZ
Bladder DTY27ZZ
Bone, Other DPYC7ZZ
Brain DØYØ7ZZ
Brain Stem DØY17ZZ
Breast
Left DMYØ7ZZ
Right DMY17ZZ
Bronchus DBY17ZZ
Cervix DUY17ZZ
Chest DWY27ZZ
Chest Wall DBY77ZZ
Colon DDY57ZZ
Diaphragm DBY87ZZ
Duodenum DDY27ZZ
Ear D9YØ7ZZ
Esophagus DDYØ7ZZ
Eye D8YØ7ZZ
Femur DPY97ZZ
Fibula DPYB7ZZ
Gallbladder DFY17ZZ
Gland
Adrenal DGY27ZZ
Parathyroid DGY47ZZ
Pituitary DGYØ7ZZ
Thyroid DGY57ZZ
Glands, Salivary D9Y67ZZ
Head and Neck DWY17ZZ
Hemibody DWY47ZZ
Humerus DPY67ZZ
Hypopharynx D9Y37ZZ
Ileum DDY47ZZ
Jejunum DDY37ZZ
Kidney DTYØ7ZZ
Larynx D9YB7ZZ
Liver DFYØ7ZZ
Lung DBY27ZZ
Mandible DPY37ZZ
Contact Radiation *(Continued)*
Maxilla DPY27ZZ
Mediastinum DBY67ZZ
Mouth D9Y47ZZ
Nasopharynx D9YD7ZZ
Neck and Head DWY17ZZ
Nerve, Peripheral DØY77ZZ
Nose D9Y17ZZ
Oropharynx D9YF7ZZ
Ovary DUYØ7ZZ
Palate
Hard D9Y87ZZ
Soft D9Y97ZZ
Pancreas DFY37ZZ
Parathyroid Gland DGY47ZZ
Pelvic Bones DPY87ZZ
Pelvic Region DWY67ZZ
Pineal Body DGY17ZZ
Pituitary Gland DGYØ7ZZ
Pleura DBY57ZZ
Prostate DVYØ7ZZ
Radius DPY77ZZ
Rectum DDY77ZZ
Rib DPY57ZZ
Sinuses D9Y77ZZ
Skin
Abdomen DHY87ZZ
Arm DHY47ZZ
Back DHY77ZZ
Buttock DHY97ZZ
Chest DHY67ZZ
Face DHY27ZZ
Leg DHYB7ZZ
Neck DHY37ZZ
Skull DPYØ7ZZ
Spinal Cord DØY67ZZ
Sternum DPY47ZZ
Stomach DDY17ZZ
Testis DVY17ZZ
Thyroid Gland DGY57ZZ
Tibia DPYB7ZZ
Tongue D9Y57ZZ
Trachea DBYØ7ZZ
Ulna DPY77ZZ
Ureter DTY17ZZ
Urethra DTY37ZZ
Uterus DUY27ZZ
Whole Body DWY57ZZ
ContaCT software (Measurement of intracranial arterial flow) 4AØ3X5D
CONTAK RENEWAL® 3 RF (HE) CRT-D *use* Cardiac Resynchronization Defibrillator Pulse Generator in ØJH
Contegra Pulmonary Valved Conduit *use* Zooplastic Tissue in Heart and Great Vessels
~~CONTEPO™ use Fosfomycin Anti-infective~~
▶**CONTEPO™** (Fosfomycin Anti-infective) *use* Other Anti-infective
Continent ileostomy see Bypass, Ileum ØD1B
Continuous Glucose Monitoring (CGM) device *use* Monitoring Device
Continuous Negative Airway Pressure
24-96 Consecutive Hours, Ventilation 5AØ9459
Greater than 96 Consecutive Hours, Ventilation 5AØ9559
Less than 24 Consecutive Hours, Ventilation 5AØ9359
Continuous Positive Airway Pressure
24-96 Consecutive Hours, Ventilation 5AØ9457
Greater than 96 Consecutive Hours, Ventilation 5AØ9557
Less than 24 Consecutive Hours, Ventilation 5AØ9357
Continuous renal replacement therapy (CRRT) 5A1D9ØZ

Contraceptive Device
Change device in, Uterus and Cervix ØU2DXHZ
Insertion of device in
Cervix ØUHC
Subcutaneous Tissue and Fascia
Abdomen ØJH8
Chest ØJH6
Lower Arm
Left ØJHH
Right ØJHG
Lower Leg
Left ØJHP
Right ØJHN
Upper Arm
Left ØJHF
Right ØJHD
Upper Leg
Left ØJHM
Right ØJHL
Uterus ØUH9
Removal of device from
Subcutaneous Tissue and Fascia
Lower Extremity ØJPW
Trunk ØJPT
Upper Extremity ØJPV
Uterus and Cervix ØUPD
Revision of device in
Subcutaneous Tissue and Fascia
Lower Extremity ØJWW
Trunk ØJWT
Upper Extremity ØJWV
Uterus and Cervix ØUWD
Contractility Modulation Device
Abdomen ØJH8
Chest ØJH6
Control, Epistaxis *see* Control bleeding in, Nasal Mucosa and Soft Tissue Ø93K
Control bleeding in
Abdominal Wall ØW3F
Ankle Region
Left ØY3L
Right ØY3K
Arm
Lower
Left ØX3F
Right ØX3D
Upper
Left ØX39
Right ØX38
Axilla
Left ØX35
Right ØX34
Back
Lower ØW3L
Upper ØW3K
Buttock
Left ØY31
Right ØY3Ø
Cavity, Cranial ØW31
Chest Wall ØW38
Elbow Region
Left ØX3C
Right ØX3B
Extremity
Lower
Left ØY3B
Right ØY39
Upper
Left ØX37
Right ØX36
Face ØW32
Femoral Region
Left ØY38
Right ØY37
Foot
Left ØY3N
Right ØY3M
Control bleeding in *(Continued)*
Gastrointestinal Tract ØW3P
Genitourinary Tract ØW3R
Hand
Left ØX3K
Right ØX3J
Head ØW3Ø
Inguinal Region
Left ØY36
Right ØY35
Jaw
Lower ØW35
Upper ØW34
Knee Region
Left ØY3G
Right ØY3F
Leg
Lower
Left ØY3J
Right ØY3H
Upper
Left ØY3D
Right ØY3C
Mediastinum ØW3C
Nasal Mucosa and Soft Tissue Ø93K
Neck ØW36
Oral Cavity and Throat ØW33
Pelvic Cavity ØW3J
Pericardial Cavity ØW3D
Perineum
Female ØW3N
Male ØW3M
Peritoneal Cavity ØW3G
Pleural Cavity
Left ØW3B
Right ØW39
Respiratory Tract ØW3Q
Retroperitoneum ØW3H
Shoulder Region
Left ØX33
Right ØX32
Wrist Region
Left ØX3H
Right ØX3G
Control bleeding using tourniquet, external *see* Compression, Anatomical Regions 2W1
Conus arteriosus *use* Ventricle, Right
Conus medullaris *use* Spinal Cord, Lumbar
Convalescent plasma (nonautologous) *see* New Technology, Anatomical Regions XW1
Conversion
Cardiac rhythm 5A22Ø4Z
Gastrostomy to jejunostomy feeding device *see* Insertion of device in, Jejunum ØDHA
Cook Biodesign® Fistula Plug(s) *use* Nonautologous Tissue Substitute
Cook Biodesign® Hernia Graft(s) *use* Nonautologous Tissue Substitute
Cook Biodesign® Layered Graft(s) *use* Nonautologous Tissue Substitute
Cook Zenapro™ Layered Graft(s) *use* Nonautologous Tissue Substitute
Cook Zenith AAA Endovascular Graft
use Intraluminal Device
Cook Zenith® Fenestrated AAA Endovascular Graft
use Intraluminal Device, Branched or Fenestrated, One or Two Arteries in Ø4V
use Intraluminal Device, Branched or Fenestrated, Three or More Arteries in Ø4V
Coracoacromial ligament
use Shoulder Bursa and Ligament, Right
use Shoulder Bursa and Ligament, Left
Coracobrachialis muscle
use Upper Arm Muscle, Right
use Upper Arm Muscle, Left
Coracoclavicular ligament
use Shoulder Bursa and Ligament, Right
use Shoulder Bursa and Ligament, Left
Coracohumeral ligament
use Shoulder Bursa and Ligament, Right
use Shoulder Bursa and Ligament, Left
Coracoid process
use Scapula, Right
use Scapula, Left
Cordotomy *see* Division, Central Nervous System and Cranial Nerves ØØ8
Core needle biopsy *see* Biopsy
CoreValve transcatheter aortic valve *use* Zooplastic Tissue in Heart and Great Vessels
Cormet Hip Resurfacing System *use* Resurfacing Device in Lower Joints
Corniculate cartilage *use* Larynx
CoRoent® XL *use* Interbody Fusion Device in Lower Joints
Coronary arteriography
see Plain Radiography, Heart B2Ø
see Fluoroscopy, Heart B21
Corox (OTW) Bipolar Lead
use Cardiac Lead, Pacemaker in Ø2H
use Cardiac Lead, Defibrillator in Ø2H
Corpus callosum *use* Brain
Corpus cavernosum *use* Penis
Corpus spongiosum *use* Penis
Corpus striatum *use* Basal Ganglia
Corrugator supercilii muscle *use* Facial Muscle
Cortical strip neurostimulator lead *use* Neurostimulator Lead in Central Nervous System and Cranial Nerves
COSELA™ *use* Trilaciclib
Costatectomy
see Excision, Upper Bones ØPB
see Resection, Upper Bones ØPT
Costectomy
see Excision, Upper Bones ØPB
see Resection, Upper Bones ØPT
Costocervical trunk
use Subclavian Artery, Right
use Subclavian Artery, Left
Costochondrectomy
see Excision, Upper Bones ØPB
see Resection, Upper Bones ØPT
Costoclavicular ligament
use Shoulder Bursa and Ligament, Right
use Shoulder Bursa and Ligament, Left
Costosternoplasty
see Repair, Upper Bones ØPQ
see Replacement, Upper Bones ØPR
see Supplement, Upper Bones ØPU
Costotomy
see Division, Upper Bones ØP8
see Drainage, Upper Bones ØP9
Costotransverse joint *use* Thoracic Vertebral Joint
Costotransverse ligament *use* Rib(s) Bursa and Ligament
Costovertebral joint *use* Thoracic Vertebral Joint
Costoxiphoid ligament *use* Sternum Bursa and Ligament
Counseling
Family, for substance abuse, Other Family Counseling HZ63ZZZ
Group
12-Step HZ43ZZZ
Behavioral HZ41ZZZ
Cognitive HZ4ØZZZ
Cognitive-Behavioral HZ42ZZZ
Confrontational HZ48ZZZ
Continuing Care HZ49ZZZ
Infectious Disease
Post-Test HZ4CZZZ
Pre-Test HZ4CZZZ
Interpersonal HZ44ZZZ
Motivational Enhancement HZ47ZZZ
Psychoeducation HZ46ZZZ
Spiritual HZ4BZZZ
Vocational HZ45ZZZ

C

Counseling *(Continued)*
Individual
12-Step HZ33ZZZ
Behavioral HZ31ZZZ
Cognitive HZ30ZZZ
Cognitive-Behavioral HZ32ZZZ
Confrontational HZ38ZZZ
Continuing Care HZ39ZZZ
Infectious Disease
Post-Test HZ3CZZZ
Pre-Test HZ3CZZZ
Interpersonal HZ34ZZZ
Motivational Enhancement HZ37ZZZ
Psychoeducation HZ36ZZZ
Spiritual HZ3BZZZ
Vocational HZ35ZZZ
Mental Health Services
Educational GZ60ZZZ
Other Counseling GZ63ZZZ
Vocational GZ61ZZZ
Countershock, cardiac 5A2204Z
Corvia IASD® *use* Synthetic Substitute
COVID-19 XW0
COVID-19 Vaccine Dose 1 XW0
COVID-19 Vaccine Dose 2 XW0
Cowper's (bulbourethral) gland *use* Urethra
CPAP (continuous positive airway pressure) *see* Assistance, Respiratory 5A09
Craniectomy
see Excision, Head and Facial Bones 0NB
see Resection, Head and Facial Bones 0NT
Cranioplasty
see Repair, Head and Facial Bones 0NQ
see Replacement, Head and Facial Bones 0NR
see Supplement, Head and Facial Bones 0NU
Craniotomy
see Drainage, Central Nervous System and Cranial Nerves 009
see Division, Head and Facial Bones 0N8
see Drainage, Head and Facial Bones 0N9
Creation
Perineum
Female 0W4N0
Male 0W4M0
Valve
Aortic 024F0
Mitral 024G0
Tricuspid 024J0
Cremaster muscle *use* Perineum Muscle
CRESEMBA® (isavuconazonium sulfate) *use* Other Anti-infective
Cribriform plate
use Ethmoid Bone, Right
use Ethmoid Bone, Left
Cricoid cartilage *use* Trachea
Cricoidectomy *see* Excision, Larynx 0CBS
Cricothyroid artery
use Thyroid Artery, Right
use Thyroid Artery, Left
Cricothyroid muscle
use Neck Muscle, Right
use Neck Muscle, Left
Crisis Intervention GZ2ZZZZ
CRRT (Continuous renal replacement therapy) 5A1D90Z
Crural fascia
use Subcutaneous Tissue and Fascia, Right Upper Leg
use Subcutaneous Tissue and Fascia, Left Upper Leg
Crushing, nerve
Cranial *see* Destruction, Central Nervous System and Cranial Nerves 005
Peripheral *see* Destruction, Peripheral Nervous System 015
Cryoablation *see* Destruction
▶ **Cryoanalgesia** *see* Destruction, Peripheral Nervous System 015
▶ **CryoICE® cryo-ablation probe (Cryo2)**
▶ *see* Destruction, Peripheral Nervous System 015
▶ *see* Destruction, Conduction Mechanism 0258
▶ **CryoICE® CryoSPHERE(R) cryoablation probe (CryoS, CryoS-L)** *see* Destruction, Peripheral Nervous System 015
Cryotherapy *see* Destruction
Cryptorchidectomy
see Excision, Male Reproductive System 0VB
see Resection, Male Reproductive System 0VT
Cryptorchiectomy
see Excision, Male Reproductive System 0VB
see Resection, Male Reproductive System 0VT
Cryptotomy
see Division, Gastrointestinal System 0D8
see Drainage, Gastrointestinal System 0D9
CT scan *see* Computerized Tomography (CT Scan)
CT sialogram *see* Computerized Tomography (CT Scan), Ear, Nose, Mouth and Throat B92
CTX001™ *use* Exagamglogene Autotemcel
Cubital lymph node
use Lymphatic, Right Upper Extremity
use Lymphatic, Left Upper Extremity
Cubital nerve *use* Ulnar Nerve
Cuboid bone
use Tarsal, Right
use Tarsal, Left
Cuboideonavicular joint
use Tarsal Joint, Right
use Tarsal Joint, Left
Culdocentesis *see* Drainage, Cul-de-sac 0U9F
Culdoplasty
see Repair, Cul-de-sac 0UQF
see Supplement, Cul-de-sac 0UUF
Culdoscopy 0UJH8ZZ
Culdotomy *see* Drainage, Cul-de-sac 0U9F
Culmen *use* Cerebellum
Cultured epidermal cell autograft *use* Autologous Tissue Substitute
Cuneiform cartilage *use* Larynx
Cuneonavicular joint
use Tarsal Joint, Right
use Tarsal Joint, Left
Cuneonavicular ligament
use Foot Bursa and Ligament, Right
use Foot Bursa and Ligament, Left
Curettage
see Excision
see Extraction
Cutaneous (transverse) cervical nerve *use* Nerve, Cervical Plexus
CVP (central venous pressure) *see* Measurement, Venous 4A04
Cyclodiathermy *see* Destruction, Eye 085
Cyclophotocoagulation *see* Destruction, Eye 085
CYPHER® Stent *use* Intraluminal Device, Drug-eluting in Heart and Great Vessels
Cystectomy
see Excision, Bladder 0TBB
see Resection, Bladder 0TTB
Cystocele repair *see* Repair, Subcutaneous Tissue and Fascia, Pelvic Region 0JQC
Cystography
see Plain Radiography, Urinary System BT0
see Fluoroscopy, Urinary System BT1
Cystolithotomy *see* Extirpation, Bladder 0TCB
Cystopexy
see Repair, Bladder 0TQB
see Reposition, Bladder 0TSB
Cystoplasty
see Repair, Bladder 0TQB
see Replacement, Bladder 0TRB
see Supplement, Bladder 0TUB
Cystorrhaphy *see* Repair, Bladder 0TQB
Cystoscopy 0TJB8ZZ
Cystostomy *see* Bypass, Bladder 0T1B
Cystostomy tube *use* Drainage Device
Cystotomy *see* Drainage, Bladder 0T9B
Cystourethrography
see Plain Radiography, Urinary System BT0
see Fluoroscopy, Urinary System BT1
Cystourethroplasty
see Repair, Urinary System 0TQ
see Replacement, Urinary System 0TR
see Supplement, Urinary System 0TU
CYTALUX® (Pafolacianine), in Fluorescence Guided Procedure *see* Fluorescence Guided Procedure
Cytarabine and Daunorubicin Liposome Antineoplastic XW0

C

▶ New ➡ Revised ~~deleted~~ Deleted

D

DBS lead *use* Neurostimulator Lead in Central Nervous System and Cranial Nerves
Daratumumab and Hyaluronidase-fihj XWØ1318
Darzalex Faspro® *use* Daratumumab and Hyaluronidase-fihj
Dasiglucagon XWØ136A
DeBakey Left Ventricular Assist Device *use* Implantable Heart Assist System in Heart and Great Vessels
Debridement
Excisional *see* Excision
Non-excisional *see* Extraction
Debris collection circuit, during percutaneous thrombectomy 5AØ5AØL
Decompression, Circulatory 6A15
Decortication, lung
see Extirpation, Respiratory System ØBC
see Release, Respiratory System ØBN
Deep brain neurostimulator lead *use* Neurostimulator Lead in Central Nervous System and Cranial Nerves
Deep cervical fascia
use Subcutaneous Tissue and Fascia, Right Neck
use Subcutaneous Tissue and Fascia, Left Neck
Deep cervical vein
use Vertebral Vein, Right
use Vertebral Vein, Left
Deep circumflex iliac artery
use External Iliac Artery, Right
use External Iliac Artery, Left
Deep facial vein
use Face Vein, Right
use Face Vein, Left
Deep femoral (profunda femoris) vein
use Femoral Vein, Right
use Femoral Vein, Left
Deep femoral artery
use Femoral Artery, Right
use Femoral Artery, Left
Deep Inferior Epigastric Artery Perforator Flap
Replacement
Bilateral ØHRVØ77
Left ØHRUØ77
Right ØHRTØ77
Transfer
Left ØKXG
Right ØKXF
Deep palmar arch
use Hand Artery, Right
use Hand Artery, Left
Deep transverse perineal muscle *use* Perineum Muscle
DefenCath™ *use* Taurolidine Anti-infective and Heparin Anticoagulant
Deferential artery
use Internal Iliac Artery, Right
use Internal Iliac Artery, Left
Defibrillator Generator
Abdomen ØJH8
Chest ØJH6
Defibrillator Lead
Insertion of device in, Mediastinum ØWHC
Removal of device from, Mediastinum ØWPC
Revision of device in, Mediastinum ØWWC
Defibtech Automated Chest Compression (ACC) device 5A1221J
Defitelio *use* Other Substance
Defitelio® infusion *see* Introduction of substance in or on, Physiological Systems and Anatomical Regions 3EØ
Delivery
Cesarean *see* Extraction, Products of Conception 1ØDØ
Forceps *see* Extraction, Products of Conception 1ØDØ
Manually assisted 1ØEØXZZ
Products of Conception 1ØEØXZZ
Vacuum assisted *see* Extraction, Products of Conception 1ØDØ
Delta frame external fixator
use External Fixation Device, Hybrid in ØPH
use External Fixation Device, Hybrid in ØPS
use External Fixation Device, Hybrid in ØQH
use External Fixation Device, Hybrid in ØQS
Delta III Reverse shoulder prosthesis *use* Synthetic Substitute, Reverse Ball and Socket in ØRR
Deltoid fascia
use Subcutaneous Tissue and Fascia, Right Upper Arm
use Subcutaneous Tissue and Fascia, Left Upper Arm
Deltoid ligament
use Ankle Bursa and Ligament, Right
use Ankle Bursa and Ligament, Left
Deltoid muscle
use Shoulder Muscle, Right
use Shoulder Muscle, Left
Deltopectoral (infraclavicular) lymph node
use Lymphatic, Right Upper Extremity
use Lymphatic, Left Upper Extremity
Denervation
Cranial nerve *see* Destruction, Central Nervous System and Cranial Nerves ØØ5
Peripheral nerve *see* Destruction, Peripheral Nervous System Ø15
Dens *use* Cervical Vertebra
Densitometry
Plain Radiography
Femur
Left BQØ4ZZ1
Right BQØ3ZZ1
Hip
Left BQØ1ZZ1
Right BQØØZZ1
Spine
Cervical BRØØZZ1
Lumbar BRØ9ZZ1
Thoracic BRØ7ZZ1
Whole BRØGZZ1
Ultrasonography
Elbow
Left BP4HZZ1
Right BP4GZZ1
Hand
Left BP4PZZ1
Right BP4NZZ1
Shoulder
Left BP49ZZ1
Right BP48ZZ1
Wrist
Left BP4MZZ1
Right BP4LZZ1
Denticulate (dentate) ligament *use* Spinal Meninges
Depressor anguli oris muscle *use* Facial Muscle
Depressor labii inferioris muscle *use* Facial Muscle
Depressor septi nasi muscle *use* Facial Muscle
Depressor supercilii muscle *use* Facial Muscle
Dermabrasion *see* Extraction, Skin and Breast ØHD
Dermis *see* Skin
Descending genicular artery
use Femoral Artery, Right
use Femoral Artery, Left
Destruction
Acetabulum
Left ØQ55
Right ØQ54
Adenoids ØC5Q
Ampulla of Vater ØF5C
Anal Sphincter ØD5R
Anterior Chamber
Left Ø8533ZZ
Right Ø8523ZZ
Anus ØD5Q
Aorta
Abdominal Ø45Ø
Thoracic
Destruction *(Continued)*
Aorta *(Continued)*
Ascending/Arch Ø25X
Descending Ø25W
Aortic Body ØG5D
Appendix ØD5J
Artery
Anterior Tibial
Left Ø45Q
Right Ø45P
Axillary
Left Ø356
Right Ø355
Brachial
Left Ø358
Right Ø357
Celiac Ø451
Colic
Left Ø457
Middle Ø458
Right Ø456
Common Carotid
Left Ø35J
Right Ø35H
Common Iliac
Left Ø45D
Right Ø45C
External Carotid
Left Ø35N
Right Ø35M
External Iliac
Left Ø45J
Right Ø45H
Face Ø35R
Femoral
Left Ø45L
Right Ø45K
Foot
Left Ø45W
Right Ø45V
Gastric Ø452
Hand
Left Ø35F
Right Ø35D
Hepatic Ø453
Inferior Mesenteric Ø45B
Innominate Ø352
Internal Carotid
Left Ø35L
Right Ø35K
Internal Iliac
Left Ø45F
Right Ø45E
Internal Mammary
Left Ø351
Right Ø35Ø
Intracranial Ø35G
Lower Ø45Y
Peroneal
Left Ø45U
Right Ø45T
Popliteal
Left Ø45N
Right Ø45M
Posterior Tibial
Left Ø45S
Right Ø45R
Pulmonary
Left Ø25R
Right Ø25Q
Pulmonary Trunk Ø25P
Radial
Left Ø35C
Right Ø35B
Renal
Left Ø45A
Right Ø459
Splenic Ø454
Subclavian
Left Ø354
Right Ø353

D

- Destruction *(Continued)*
  - Artery *(Continued)*
    - Superior Mesenteric Ø455
    - Temporal
      - Left Ø35T
      - Right Ø35S
    - Thyroid
      - Left Ø35V
      - Right Ø35U
    - Ulnar
      - Left Ø35A
      - Right Ø359
    - Upper Ø35Y
    - Vertebral
      - Left Ø35Q
      - Right Ø35P
  - Atrium
    - Left Ø257
    - Right Ø256
  - Auditory Ossicle
    - Left Ø95A
    - Right Ø959
  - Basal Ganglia ØØ58
  - Bladder ØT5B
  - Bladder Neck ØT5C
  - Bone
    - Ethmoid
      - Left ØN5G
      - Right ØN5F
    - Frontal ØN51
    - Hyoid ØN5X
    - Lacrimal
      - Left ØN5J
      - Right ØN5H
    - Nasal ØN5B
    - Occipital ØN57
    - Palatine
      - Left ØN5L
      - Right ØN5K
    - Parietal
      - Left ØN54
      - Right ØN53
    - Pelvic
      - Left ØQ53
      - Right ØQ52
    - Sphenoid ØN5C
    - Temporal
      - Left ØN56
      - Right ØN55
    - Zygomatic
      - Left ØN5N
      - Right ØN5M
  - Brain ØØ5Ø
    - ▶Stereoelectroencephalographic Radiofrequency Ablation ØØ5Ø3Z4
  - Breast
    - Bilateral ØH5V
    - Left ØH5U
    - Right ØH5T
  - Bronchus
    - Lingula ØB59
    - Lower Lobe
      - Left ØB5B
      - Right ØB56
    - Main
      - Left ØB57
      - Right ØB53
    - Middle Lobe, Right ØB55
    - Upper Lobe
      - Left ØB58
      - Right ØB54
  - Buccal Mucosa ØC54
  - Bursa and Ligament
    - Abdomen
      - Left ØM5J
      - Right ØM5H
    - Ankle
      - Left ØM5R
      - Right ØM5Q
    - Elbow
      - Left ØM54
      - Right ØM53

- Destruction *(Continued)*
  - Bursa and Ligament *(Continued)*
    - Foot
      - Left ØM5T
      - Right ØM5S
    - Hand
      - Left ØM58
      - Right ØM57
    - Head and Neck ØM5Ø
    - Hip
      - Left ØM5M
      - Right ØM5L
    - Knee
      - Left ØM5P
      - Right ØM5N
    - Lower Extremity
      - Left ØM5W
      - Right ØM5V
    - Perineum ØM5K
    - Rib(s) ØM5G
    - Shoulder
      - Left ØM52
      - Right ØM51
    - Spine
      - Lower ØM5D
      - Upper ØM5C
    - Sternum ØM5F
    - Upper Extremity
      - Left ØM5B
      - Right ØM59
    - Wrist
      - Left ØM56
      - Right ØM55
  - Carina ØB52
  - Carotid Bodies, Bilateral ØG58
  - Carotid Body
    - Left ØG56
    - Right ØG57
  - Carpal
    - Left ØP5N
    - Right ØP5M
  - Cecum ØD5H
  - Cerebellum ØØ5C
  - Cerebral Hemisphere ØØ57
  - Cerebral Meninges ØØ51
  - Cerebral Ventricle ØØ56
  - Cervix ØU5C
  - Chordae Tendineae Ø259
  - Choroid
    - Left Ø85B
    - Right Ø85A
  - Cisterna Chyli Ø75L
  - Clavicle
    - Left ØP5B
    - Right ØP59
  - Clitoris ØU5J
  - Coccygeal Glomus ØG5B
  - Coccyx ØQ5S
  - Colon
    - Ascending ØD5K
    - Descending ØD5M
    - Sigmoid ØD5N
    - Transverse ØD5L
  - Conduction Mechanism Ø258
  - Conjunctiva
    - Left Ø85TXZZ
    - Right Ø85SXZZ
  - Cord
    - Bilateral ØV5H
    - Left ØV5G
    - Right ØV5F
  - Cornea
    - Left Ø859XZZ
    - Right Ø858XZZ
  - Cul-de-sac ØU5F
  - Diaphragm ØB5T
  - Disc
    - Cervical Vertebral ØR53
    - Cervicothoracic Vertebral ØR55
    - Lumbar Vertebral ØS52
    - Lumbosacral ØS54
    - Thoracic Vertebral ØR59
    - Thoracolumbar Vertebral ØR5B

- Destruction *(Continued)*
  - Duct
    - Common Bile ØF59
    - Cystic ØF58
    - Hepatic
      - Common ØF57
      - Left ØF56
      - Right ØF55
    - Lacrimal
      - Left Ø85Y
      - Right Ø85X
    - Pancreatic ØF5D
      - Accessory ØF5F
    - Parotid
      - Left ØC5C
      - Right ØC5B
    - Thoracic Ø75K
  - Duodenum ØD59
  - Dura Mater ØØ52
  - Ear
    - External
      - Left Ø951
      - Right Ø95Ø
    - External Auditory Canal
      - Left Ø954
      - Right Ø953
    - Inner
      - Left Ø95E
      - Right Ø95D
    - Middle
      - Left Ø956
      - Right Ø955
  - Endometrium ØU5B
  - Epididymis
    - Bilateral ØV5L
    - Left ØV5K
    - Right ØV5J
  - Epiglottis ØC5R
  - Esophagogastric Junction ØD54
  - Esophagus ØD55
    - Lower ØD53
    - Middle ØD52
    - Upper ØD51
  - Eustachian Tube
    - Left Ø95G
    - Right Ø95F
  - Eye
    - Left Ø851XZZ
    - Right Ø85ØXZZ
  - Eyelid
    - Lower
      - Left Ø85R
      - Right Ø85Q
    - Upper
      - Left Ø85P
      - Right Ø85N
  - Fallopian Tube
    - Left ØU56
    - Right ØU55
  - Fallopian Tubes, Bilateral ØU57
  - Femoral Shaft
    - Left ØQ59
    - Right ØQ58
  - Femur
    - Lower
      - Left ØQ5C
      - Right ØQ5B
    - Upper
      - Left ØQ57
      - Right ØQ56
  - Fibula
    - Left ØQ5K
    - Right ØQ5J
  - Finger Nail ØH5QXZZ
  - Gallbladder ØF54
  - Gingiva
    - Lower ØC56
    - Upper ØC55
  - Gland
    - Adrenal
      - Bilateral ØG54
      - Left ØG52
      - Right ØG53

▶ New ➡ Revised ~~deleted~~ Deleted

Destruction (Continued)
Gland (Continued)
Lacrimal
Left Ø85W
Right Ø85V
Minor Salivary ØC5J
Parotid
Left ØC59
Right ØC58
Pituitary ØG5Ø
Sublingual
Left ØC5F
Right ØC5D
Submaxillary
Left ØC5H
Right ØC5G
Vestibular ØU5L
Glenoid Cavity
Left ØP58
Right ØP57
Glomus Jugulare ØG5C
Humeral Head
Left ØP5D
Right ØP5C
Humeral Shaft
Left ØP5G
Right ØP5F
Hymen ØU5K
Hypothalamus ØØ5A
Ileocecal Valve ØD5C
Ileum ØD5B
Intestine
Large ØD5E
Left ØD5G
Right ØD5F
Small ØD58
Iris
Left Ø85D3ZZ
Right Ø85C3ZZ
Jejunum ØD5A
Joint
Acromioclavicular
Left ØR5H
Right ØR5G
Ankle
Left ØS5G
Right ØS5F
Carpal
Left ØR5R
Right ØR5Q
Carpometacarpal
Left ØR5T
Right ØR5S
Cervical Vertebral ØR51
Cervicothoracic Vertebral ØR54
Coccygeal ØS56
Elbow
Left ØR5M
Right ØR5L
Finger Phalangeal
Left ØR5X
Right ØR5W
Hip
Left ØS5B
Right ØS59
Knee
Left ØS5D
Right ØS5C
Lumbar Vertebral ØS5Ø
Lumbosacral ØS53
Metacarpophalangeal
Left ØR5V
Right ØR5U
Metatarsal-Phalangeal
Left ØS5N
Right ØS5M
Occipital-cervical ØR5Ø
Sacrococcygeal ØS55
Sacroiliac
Left ØS58
Right ØS57

Destruction (Continued)
Joint (Continued)
Shoulder
Left ØR5K
Right ØR5J
Sternoclavicular
Left ØR5F
Right ØR5E
Tarsal
Left ØS5J
Right ØS5H
Tarsometatarsal
Left ØS5L
Right ØS5K
Temporomandibular
Left ØR5D
Right ØR5C
Thoracic Vertebral ØR56
Thoracolumbar Vertebral ØR5A
Toe Phalangeal
Left ØS5Q
Right ØS5P
Wrist
Left ØR5P
Right ØR5N
Kidney
Left ØT51
Right ØT5Ø
Kidney Pelvis
Left ØT54
Right ØT53
Larynx ØC5S
Lens
Left Ø85K3ZZ
Right Ø85J3ZZ
Lip
Lower ØC51
Upper ØC5Ø
Liver ØF5Ø
Left Lobe ØF52
Right Lobe ØF51
Ultrasound-guided Cavitation XF5
Lung
Bilateral ØB5M
Left ØB5L
Lower Lobe
Left ØB5J
Right ØB5F
Middle Lobe, Right ØB5D
Right ØB5K
Upper Lobe
Left ØB5G
Right ØB5C
Lung Lingula ØB5H
Lymphatic
Aortic Ø75D
Axillary
Left Ø756
Right Ø755
Head Ø75Ø
Inguinal
Left Ø75J
Right Ø75H
Internal Mammary
Left Ø759
Right Ø758
Lower Extremity
Left Ø75G
Right Ø75F
Mesenteric Ø75B
Neck
Left Ø752
Right Ø751
Pelvis Ø75C
Thorax Ø757
Upper Extremity
Left Ø754
Right Ø753
Mandible
Left ØN5V
Right ØN5T

Destruction (Continued)
Maxilla ØN5R
Medulla Oblongata ØØ5D
Mesentery ØD5V
Metacarpal
Left ØP5Q
Right ØP5P
Metatarsal
Left ØQ5P
Right ØQ5N
Muscle
Abdomen
Left ØK5L
Right ØK5K
Extraocular
Left Ø85M
Right Ø85L
Facial ØK51
Foot
Left ØK5W
Right ØK5V
Hand
Left ØK5D
Right ØK5C
Head ØK5Ø
Hip
Left ØK5P
Right ØK5N
Lower Arm and Wrist
Left ØK5B
Right ØK59
Lower Leg
Left ØK5T
Right ØK5S
Neck
Left ØK53
Right ØK52
Papillary Ø25D
Perineum ØK5M
Shoulder
Left ØK56
Right ØK55
Thorax
Left ØK5J
Right ØK5H
Tongue, Palate, Pharynx ØK54
Trunk
Left ØK5G
Right ØK5F
Upper Arm
Left ØK58
Right ØK57
Upper Leg
Left ØK5R
Right ØK5Q
Nasal Mucosa and Soft Tissue Ø95K
Nasopharynx Ø95N
Nerve
Abdominal Sympathetic Ø15M
Abducens ØØ5L
Accessory ØØ5R
Acoustic ØØ5N
Brachial Plexus Ø153
Cervical Ø151
Cervical Plexus Ø153
Facial ØØ5M
Femoral Ø15D
Glossopharyngeal ØØ5P
Head and Neck Sympathetic Ø15K
Hypoglossal ØØ5S
Lumbar Ø15B
Lumbar Plexus Ø159
Lumbar Sympathetic Ø15N
Lumbosacral Plexus Ø15A
Median Ø155
Oculomotor ØØ5H
Olfactory ØØ5F
Optic ØØ5G
Peroneal Ø15H
Phrenic Ø152
Pudendal Ø15C
Radial Ø156

- **Destruction** *(Continued)*
  - Nerve *(Continued)*
    - Sacral Ø15R
    - Sacral Plexus Ø15Q
    - Sacral Sympathetic Ø15P
    - Sciatic Ø15F
    - Thoracic Ø158
    - Thoracic Sympathetic Ø15L
    - Tibial Ø15G
    - Trigeminal ØØ5K
    - Trochlear ØØ5J
    - Ulnar Ø154
    - Vagus ØØ5Q
  - Nipple
    - Left ØH5X
    - Right ØH5W
  - Omentum ØD5U
  - Orbit
    - Left ØN5Q
    - Right ØN5P
  - Ovary
    - Bilateral ØU52
    - Left ØU51
    - Right ØU5Ø
  - Palate
    - Hard ØC52
    - Soft ØC53
  - Pancreas ØF5G
  - Para-aortic Body ØG59
  - Paraganglion Extremity ØG5F
  - Parathyroid Gland ØG5R
    - Inferior
      - Left ØG5P
      - Right ØG5N
    - Multiple ØG5Q
    - Superior
      - Left ØG5M
      - Right ØG5L
  - Patella
    - Left ØQ5F
    - Right ØQ5D
  - Penis ØV5S
  - Pericardium Ø25N
  - Peritoneum ØD5W
  - Phalanx
    - Finger
      - Left ØP5V
      - Right ØP5T
    - Thumb
      - Left ØP5S
      - Right ØP5R
    - Toe
      - Left ØQ5R
      - Right ØQ5Q
  - Pharynx ØC5M
  - Pineal Body ØG51
  - Pleura
    - Left ØB5P
    - Right ØB5N
  - Pons ØØ5B
  - Prepuce ØV5T
  - Prostate ØV5Ø
  - Radius
    - Left ØP5J
    - Right ØP5H
  - Rectum ØD5P
  - ~~Renal Sympathetic Nerve(s), Ultrasound Ablation XØ51329~~
  - ▶Renal Sympathetic Nerve(s)
    - ▶Radiofrequency Ablation XØ5133A
    - ▶Ultrasound Ablation XØ51329
  - Retina
    - Left Ø85F3ZZ
    - Right Ø85E3ZZ
  - Retinal Vessel
    - Left Ø85H3ZZ
    - Right Ø85G3ZZ
  - Ribs
    - 1 to 2 ØP51
    - 3 or More ØP52
  - Sacrum ØQ51

- **Destruction** *(Continued)*
  - Scapula
    - Left ØP56
    - Right ØP55
  - Sclera
    - Left Ø857XZZ
    - Right Ø856XZZ
  - Scrotum ØV55
  - Septum
    - Atrial Ø255
    - Nasal Ø95M
    - Ventricular Ø25M
  - Sinus
    - Accessory Ø95P
    - Ethmoid
      - Left Ø95V
      - Right Ø95U
    - Frontal
      - Left Ø95T
      - Right Ø95S
    - Mastoid
      - Left Ø95C
      - Right Ø95B
    - Maxillary
      - Left Ø95R
      - Right Ø95Q
    - Sphenoid
      - Left Ø95X
      - Right Ø95W
  - Skin
    - Abdomen ØH57XZ
    - Back ØH56XZ
    - Buttock ØH58XZ
    - Chest ØH55XZ
    - Ear
      - Left ØH53XZ
      - Right ØH52XZ
    - Face ØH51XZ
    - Foot
      - Left ØH5NXZ
      - Right ØH5MXZ
    - Hand
      - Left ØH5GXZ
      - Right ØH5FXZ
    - Inguinal ØH5AXZ
    - Lower Arm
      - Left ØH5EXZ
      - Right ØH5DXZ
    - Lower Leg
      - Left ØH5LXZ
      - Right ØH5KXZ
    - Neck ØH54XZ
    - Perineum ØH59XZ
    - Scalp ØH5ØXZ
    - Upper Arm
      - Left ØH5CXZ
      - Right ØH5BXZ
    - Upper Leg
      - Left ØH5JXZ
      - Right ØH5HXZ
  - Skull ØN5Ø
  - Spinal Cord
    - Cervical ØØ5W
    - Lumbar ØØ5Y
    - Thoracic ØØ5X
  - Spinal Meninges ØØ5T
  - Spleen Ø75P
  - Sternum ØP5Ø
  - Stomach ØD56
    - Pylorus ØD57
  - Subcutaneous Tissue and Fascia
    - Abdomen ØJ58
    - Back ØJ57
    - Buttock ØJ59
    - Chest ØJ56
    - Face ØJ51
    - Foot
      - Left ØJ5R
      - Right ØJ5Q
    - Hand
      - Left ØJ5K
      - Right ØJ5J

- **Destruction** *(Continued)*
  - Subcutaneous Tissue and Fascia *(Continued)*
    - Lower Arm
      - Left ØJ5H
      - Right ØJ5G
    - Lower Leg
      - Left ØJ5P
      - Right ØJ5N
    - Neck
      - Left ØJ55
      - Right ØJ54
    - Pelvic Region ØJ5C
    - Perineum ØJ5B
    - Scalp ØJ5Ø
    - Upper Arm
      - Left ØJ5F
      - Right ØJ5D
    - Upper Leg
      - Left ØJ5M
      - Right ØJ5L
  - Tarsal
    - Left ØQ5M
    - Right ØQ5L
  - Tendon
    - Abdomen
      - Left ØL5G
      - Right ØL5F
    - Ankle
      - Left ØL5T
      - Right ØL5S
    - Foot
      - Left ØL5W
      - Right ØL5V
    - Hand
      - Left ØL58
      - Right ØL57
    - Head and Neck ØL5Ø
    - Hip
      - Left ØL5K
      - Right ØL5J
    - Knee
      - Left ØL5R
      - Right ØL5Q
    - Lower Arm and Wrist
      - Left ØL56
      - Right ØL55
    - Lower Leg
      - Left ØL5P
      - Right ØL5N
    - Perineum ØL5H
    - Shoulder
      - Left ØL52
      - Right ØL51
    - Thorax
      - Left ØL5D
      - Right ØL5C
    - Trunk
      - Left ØL5B
      - Right ØL59
    - Upper Arm
      - Left ØL54
      - Right ØL53
    - Upper Leg
      - Left ØL5M
      - Right ØL5L
  - Testis
    - Bilateral ØV5C
    - Left ØV5B
    - Right ØV59
  - Thalamus ØØ59
  - Thymus Ø75M
  - Thyroid Gland
    - Left Lobe ØG5G
    - Right Lobe ØG5H
  - Tibia
    - Left ØQ5H
    - Right ØQ5G
  - Toe Nail ØH5RXZZ
  - Tongue ØC57
  - Tonsils ØC5P

Destruction *(Continued)*
Tooth
Lower ØC5X
Upper ØC5W
Trachea ØB51
Tunica Vaginalis
Left ØV57
Right ØV56
Turbinate, Nasal Ø95L
Tympanic Membrane
Left Ø958
Right Ø959
Ulna
Left ØP5L
Right ØP5K
Ureter
Left ØT57
Right ØT56
Urethra ØT5D
Uterine Supporting Structure ØU54
Uterus ØU59
Uvula ØC5N
Vagina ØU5G
Valve
Aortic Ø25F
Mitral Ø25G
Pulmonary Ø25H
Tricuspid Ø25J
Vas Deferens
Bilateral ØV5Q
Left ØV5P
Right ØV5N
Vein
Axillary
Left Ø558
Right Ø557
Azygos Ø550
Basilic
Left Ø55C
Right Ø55B
Brachial
Left Ø55A
Right Ø559
Cephalic
Left Ø55F
Right Ø55D
Colic Ø657
Common Iliac
Left Ø65D
Right Ø65C
Coronary Ø254
Esophageal Ø653
External Iliac
Left Ø65G
Right Ø65F
External Jugular
Left Ø55Q
Right Ø55P
Face
Left Ø55V
Right Ø55T
Femoral
Left Ø65N
Right Ø65M
Foot
Left Ø65V
Right Ø65T
Gastric Ø652
Hand
Left Ø55H
Right Ø55G
Hemiazygos Ø551
Hepatic Ø654
Hypogastric
Left Ø65J
Right Ø65H
Inferior Mesenteric Ø656
Innominate
Left Ø554
Right Ø553

Destruction *(Continued)*
Vein *(Continued)*
Internal Jugular
Left Ø55N
Right Ø55M
Intracranial Ø55L
Lower Ø65Y
Portal Ø658
Pulmonary
Left Ø25T
Right Ø25S
Renal
Left Ø65B
Right Ø659
Saphenous
Left Ø65Q
Right Ø65P
Splenic Ø651
Subclavian
Left Ø556
Right Ø555
Superior Mesenteric Ø655
Upper Ø55Y
Vertebral
Left Ø55S
Right Ø55R
Vena Cava
Inferior Ø650
Superior Ø25V
Ventricle
Left Ø25L
Right Ø25K
Vertebra
Cervical ØP53
Lumbar ØQ50
Thoracic ØP54
Vesicle
Bilateral ØV53
Left ØV52
Right ØV51
Vitreous
Left Ø8553ZZ
Right Ø8543ZZ
Vocal Cord
Left ØC5V
Right ØC5T
Vulva ØU5M
Detachment
Arm
Lower
Left ØX6FØZ
Right ØX6DØZ
Upper
Left ØX69ØZ
Right ØX68ØZ
Elbow Region
Left ØX6CØZZ
Right ØX6BØZZ
Femoral Region
Left ØY68ØZZ
Right ØY67ØZZ
Finger
Index
Left ØX6PØZ
Right ØX6NØZ
Little
Left ØX6WØZ
Right ØX6VØZ
Middle
Left ØX6RØZ
Right ØX6QØZ
Ring
Left ØX6TØZ
Right ØX6SØZ
Foot
Left ØY6NØZ
Right ØY6MØZ
Forequarter
Left ØX61ØZZ
Right ØX60ØZZ

Detachment *(Continued)*
Hand
Left ØX6KØZ
Right ØX6JØZ
Hindquarter
Bilateral ØY64ØZZ
Left ØY63ØZZ
Right ØY62ØZZ
Knee Region
Left ØY6GØZZ
Right ØY6FØZZ
Leg
Lower
Left ØY6JØZ
Right ØY6HØZ
Upper
Left ØY6DØZ
Right ØY6CØZ
Shoulder Region
Left ØX63ØZZ
Right ØX62ØZZ
Thumb
Left ØX6MØZ
Right ØX6LØZ
Toe
1st
Left ØY6QØZ
Right ØY6PØZ
2nd
Left ØY6SØZ
Right ØY6RØZ
3rd
Left ØY6UØZ
Right ØY6TØZ
4th
Left ØY6WØZ
Right ØY6VØZ
5th
Left ØY6YØZ
Right ØY6XØZ
Determination, Mental status GZ14ZZZ
Detorsion
see Release
see Reposition
DETOUR® System
use Conduit through Femoral Vein to Superficial Femoral Artery in New Technology
use Conduit through Femoral Vein to Popliteal Artery in New Technology
Detoxification Services, for substance abuse HZ2ZZZZ
Device Fitting FØDZ
Diagnostic Audiology *see* Audiology, Diagnostic
Diagnostic imaging *see* Imaging, Diagnostic
Diagnostic radiology *see* Imaging, Diagnostic
Dialysis
Hemodialysis *see* Performance, Urinary 5A1D
Peritoneal 3E1M39Z
Diaphragma sellae *use* Dura Mater
Diaphragmatic pacemaker generator *use* Stimulator Generator in Subcutaneous Tissue and Fascia
Diaphragmatic Pacemaker Lead
Insertion of device in, Diaphragm ØBHT
Removal of device from, Diaphragm ØBPT
Revision of device in, Diaphragm ØBWT
Digital radiography, plain *see* Plain Radiography
Dilation
Ampulla of Vater ØF7C
Anus ØD7Q
Aorta
Abdominal Ø470
Thoracic
Ascending/Arch Ø27X
Descending Ø27W

Dilation *(Continued)*
  Artery
    Anterior Tibial
      Left Ø47Q
        ▶Intraluminal Device, Everolimus-eluting Resorbable Scaffold(s) X27Q3TA
        ~~Sustained Release Drug-eluting Intraluminal Device X27Q385~~
          ~~Four or More X27Q3C5~~
          ~~Three X27Q3B5~~
          ~~Two X27Q395~~
      Right Ø47P
        ▶Intraluminal Device, Everolimus-eluting Resorbable Scaffold(s) X27P3TA
        ~~Sustained Release Drug-eluting Intraluminal Device X27P385~~
          ~~Four or More X27P3C5~~
          ~~Three X27P3B5~~
          ~~Two X27P395~~
    Axillary
      Left Ø376
      Right Ø375
    Brachial
      Left Ø378
      Right Ø377
    Celiac Ø471
    Colic
      Left Ø477
      Middle Ø478
      Right Ø476
    Common Carotid
      Left Ø37J
      Right Ø37H
    Common Iliac
      Left Ø47D
      Right Ø47C
    Coronary
      Four or More Arteries Ø273
      One Artery Ø27Ø
      Three Arteries Ø272
      Two Arteries Ø271
    External Carotid
      Left Ø37N
      Right Ø37M
    External Iliac
      Left Ø47J
      Right Ø47H
    Face Ø37R
    Femoral
      Left Ø47L
        ~~Sustained Release Drug-eluting Intraluminal Device X27J385~~
          ~~Four or More X27J3C5~~
          ~~Three X27J3B5~~
          ~~Two X27J395~~
      Right Ø47K
        ~~Sustained Release Drug-eluting Intraluminal Device X27H385~~
          ~~Four or More X27H3C5~~
          ~~Three X27H3B5~~
          ~~Two X27H395~~
    Foot
      Left Ø47W
      Right Ø47V
    Gastric Ø472
    Hand
      Left Ø37F
      Right Ø37D
    Hepatic Ø473
    Inferior Mesenteric Ø47B
    Innominate Ø372
    Internal Carotid
      Left Ø37L
      Right Ø37K
    Internal Iliac
      Left Ø47F
      Right Ø47E
    Internal Mammary
      Left Ø371
      Right Ø37Ø

Dilation *(Continued)*
  Artery *(Continued)*
    Intracranial Ø37G
    Lower Ø47Y
    Peroneal
      Left Ø47U
        ▶Intraluminal Device, Everolimus-eluting Resorbable Scaffold(s) X27U3TA
        ~~Sustained Release Drug-eluting Intraluminal Device X27U385~~
          ~~Four or More X27U3C5~~
          ~~Three X27U3B5~~
          ~~Two X27U395~~
      Right Ø47T
        ▶Intraluminal Device, Everolimus-eluting Resorbable Scaffold(s) X27T3TA
        ~~Sustained Release Drug-eluting Intraluminal Device X27T385~~
          ~~Four or More X27T3C5~~
          ~~Three X27T3B5~~
          ~~Two X27T395~~
    Popliteal
      Left Ø47N
      Left Distal
        ~~Sustained Release Drug-eluting Intraluminal Device X27N385~~
          ~~Four or More X27N3C5~~
          ~~Three X27N3B5~~
          ~~Two X27N395~~
      Left Proximal
        ~~Sustained Release Drug-eluting Intraluminal Device X27L385~~
          ~~Four or More X27L3C5~~
          ~~Three X27L3B5~~
          ~~Two X27L395~~
      Right Ø47M
      Right Distal
        ~~Sustained Release Drug-eluting Intraluminal Device X27M385~~
          ~~Four or More X27M3C5~~
          ~~Three X27M3B5~~
          ~~Two X27M395~~
      Right Proximal
        ~~Sustained Release Drug-eluting Intraluminal Device X27K385~~
          ~~Four or More X27K3C5~~
          ~~Three X27K3B5~~
          ~~Two X27K395~~
    Posterior Tibial
      Left Ø47S
        ▶Intraluminal Device, Everolimus-eluting Resorbable Scaffold(s) X27S3TA
        ~~Sustained Release Drug-eluting Intraluminal Device X27S385~~
          ~~Four or More X27S3C5~~
          ~~Three X27S3B5~~
          ~~Two X27S395~~
      Right Ø47R
        ▶Intraluminal Device, Everolimus-eluting Resorbable Scaffold(s) X27R3TA
        ~~Sustained Release Drug-eluting Intraluminal Device X27R385~~
          ~~Four or More X27R3C5~~
          ~~Three X27R3B5~~
          ~~Two X27R395~~
    Pulmonary
      Left Ø27R
      Right Ø27Q
    Pulmonary Trunk Ø27P
    Radial
      Left Ø37C
      Right Ø37B
    Renal
      Left Ø47A
      Right Ø479

Dilation *(Continued)*
  Artery *(Continued)*
    Splenic Ø474
    Subclavian
      Left Ø374
      Right Ø373
    Superior Mesenteric Ø475
    Temporal
      Left Ø37T
      Right Ø37S
    Thyroid
      Left Ø37V
      Right Ø37U
    Ulnar
      Left Ø37A
      Right Ø379
    Upper Ø37Y
    Vertebral
      Left Ø37Q
      Right Ø37P
  Bladder ØT7B
  Bladder Neck ØT7C
  Bronchus
    Lingula ØB79
    Lower Lobe
      Left ØB7B
      Right ØB76
    Main
      Left ØB77
      Right ØB73
    Middle Lobe, Right ØB75
    Upper Lobe
      Left ØB78
      Right ØB74
  Carina ØB72
  Cecum ØD7H
  Cerebral Ventricle ØØ76
  Cervix ØU7C
  Colon
    Ascending ØD7K
    Descending ØD7M
    Sigmoid ØD7N
    Transverse ØD7L
  Duct
    Common Bile ØF79
    Cystic ØF78
    Hepatic
      Common ØF77
      Left ØF76
      Right ØF75
    Lacrimal
      Left Ø87Y
      Right Ø87X
    Pancreatic ØF7D
      Accessory ØF7F
    Parotid
      Left ØC7C
      Right ØC7B
  Duodenum ØD79
  Esophagogastric Junction ØD74
  Esophagus ØD75
    Lower ØD73
    Middle ØD72
    Upper ØD71
  Eustachian Tube
    Left Ø97G
    Right Ø97F
  Fallopian Tube
    Left ØU76
    Right ØU75
  Fallopian Tubes, Bilateral ØU77
  Hymen ØU7K
  Ileocecal Valve ØD7C
  Ileum ØD7B
  Intestine
    Large ØD7E
      Left ØD7G
      Right ØD7F
    Small ØD78
  Jejunum ØD7A

▶ New ➡ Revised ~~deleted~~ Deleted

Dilation *(Continued)*
Kidney Pelvis
Left 0T74
Right 0T73
Larynx 0C7S
▶Nasopharynx 097N
Pharynx 0C7M
Rectum 0D7P
Stomach 0D76 Pylorus 0D77
Trachea 0B71
Ureter
Left 0T77
Right 0T76
Ureters, Bilateral 0T78
Urethra 0T7D
Uterus 0U79
Vagina 0U7G
Valve
Aortic 027F
Ileocecal 0D7C
Mitral 027G
Pulmonary 027H
Tricuspid 027J
Vas Deferens
Bilateral 0V7Q
Left 0V7P
Right 0V7N
Vein
Axillary
Left 0578
Right 0577
Azygos 0570
Basilic
Left 057C
Right 057B
Brachial
Left 057A
Right 0579
Cephalic
Left 057F
Right 057D
Colic 0677
Common Iliac
Left 067D
Right 067C
Esophageal 0673
External Iliac
Left 067G
Right 067F
External Jugular
Left 057Q
Right 057P
Face
Left 057V
Right 057T
Femoral
Left 067N
Right 067M
Foot
Left 067V
Right 067T
Gastric 0672
Hand
Left 057H
Right 057G
Hemiazygos 0571
Hepatic 0674
Hypogastric
Left 067J
Right 067H
Inferior Mesenteric 0676
Innominate
Left 0574
Right 0573
Internal Jugular
Left 057N
Right 057M
Intracranial 057L
Lower 067Y
Portal 0678

Dilation *(Continued)*
Vein *(Continued)*
Pulmonary
Left 027T
Right 027S
Renal
Left 067B
Right 0679
Saphenous
Left 067Q
Right 067P
Splenic 0671
Subclavian
Left 0576
Right 0575
Superior Mesenteric 0675
Upper 057Y
Vertebral
Left 057S
Right 057R
Vena Cava
Inferior 0670
Superior 027V
Ventricle
Left 027L
Right 027K
Direct Lateral Interbody Fusion (DLIF) device
use Interbody Fusion Device in Lower Joints
Disarticulation *see* Detachment
Discectomy, diskectomy
see Excision, Upper Joints 0RB
see Resection, Upper Joints 0RT
see Excision, Lower Joints 0SB
see Resection, Lower Joints 0ST
Discography
see Plain Radiography, Axial Skeleton, Except Skull and Facial Bones BR0
see Fluoroscopy, Axial Skeleton, Except Skull and Facial Bones BR1
Dismembered pyeloplasty *see* Repair, Kidney Pelvis
Distal humerus
use Humeral Shaft, Right
use Humeral Shaft, Left
Distal humerus, involving joint
use Elbow Joint, Right
use Elbow Joint, Left
Distal radioulnar joint
use Wrist Joint, Right
use Wrist Joint, Left
Diversion *see* Bypass
Diverticulectomy *see* Excision, Gastrointestinal System 0DB
Division
Acetabulum
Left 0Q85
Right 0Q84
Anal Sphincter 0D8R
Basal Ganglia 0088
Bladder Neck 0T8C
Bone
Ethmoid
Left 0N8G
Right 0N8F
Frontal 0N81
Hyoid 0N8X
Lacrimal
Left 0N8J
Right 0N8H
Nasal 0N8B
Occipital 0N87
Palatine
Left 0N8L
Right 0N8K
Parietal
Left 0N84
Right 0N83
Pelvic
Left 0Q83
Right 0Q82

Division *(Continued)*
Bone *(Continued)*
Sphenoid 0N8C
Temporal
Left 0N86
Right 0N85
Zygomatic
Left 0N8N
Right 0N8M
Brain 0080
Bursa and Ligament
Abdomen
Left 0M8J
Right 0M8H
Ankle
Left 0M8R
Right 0M8Q
Elbow
Left 0M84
Right 0M83
Foot
Left 0M8T
Right 0M8S
Hand
Left 0M88
Right 0M87
Head and Neck 0M80
Hip
Left 0M8M
Right 0M8L
Knee
Left 0M8P
Right 0M8N
Lower Extremity
Left 0M8W
Right 0M8V
Perineum 0M8K
Rib(s) 0M8G
Shoulder
Left 0M82
Right 0M81
Spine
Lower 0M8D
Upper 0M8C
Sternum 0M8F
Upper Extremity
Left 0M8B
Right 0M89
Wrist
Left 0M86
Right 0M85
Carpal
Left 0P8N
Right 0P8M
Cerebral Hemisphere 0087
Chordae Tendineae 0289
Clavicle
Left 0P8B
Right 0P89
Coccyx 0Q8S
Conduction Mechanism 0288
Esophagogastric Junction 0D84
Femoral Shaft
Left 0Q89
Right 0Q88
Femur
Lower
Left 0Q8C
Right 0Q8B
Upper
Left 0Q87
Right 0Q86
Fibula
Left 0Q8K
Right 0Q8J
Gland, Pituitary 0G80
Glenoid Cavity
Left 0P88
Right 0P87

- Division *(Continued)*
  - Humeral Head
    - Left ØP8D
    - Right ØP8C
  - Humeral Shaft
    - Left ØP8G
    - Right ØP8F
  - Hymen ØU8K
  - ▶Intraluminal Bioprosthetic Valve Leaflet Splitting Technology in Existing Valve X28F3VA
  - Kidneys, Bilateral ØT82
  - Liver ØF8Ø
    - Left Lobe ØF82
    - Right Lobe ØF81
  - Mandible
    - Left ØN8V
    - Right ØN8T
  - Maxilla ØN8R
  - Metacarpal
    - Left ØP8Q
    - Right ØP8P
  - Metatarsal
    - Left ØQ8P
    - Right ØQ8N
  - Muscle
    - Abdomen
      - Left ØK8L
      - Right ØK8K
    - Facial ØK81
    - Foot
      - Left ØK8W
      - Right ØK8V
    - Hand
      - Left ØK8D
      - Right ØK8C
    - Head ØK8Ø
    - Hip
      - Left ØK8P
      - Right ØK8N
    - Lower Arm and Wrist
      - Left ØK8B
      - Right ØK89
    - Lower Leg
      - Left ØK8T
      - Right ØK8S
    - Neck
      - Left ØK83
      - Right ØK82
    - Papillary Ø28D
    - Perineum ØK8M
    - Shoulder
      - Left ØK86
      - Right ØK85
    - Thorax
      - Left ØK8J
      - Right ØK8H
    - Tongue, Palate, Pharynx ØK84
    - Trunk
      - Left ØK8G
      - Right ØK8F
    - Upper Arm
      - Left ØK88
      - Right ØK87
    - Upper Leg
      - Left ØK8R
      - Right ØK8Q
  - Nerve
    - Abdominal Sympathetic Ø18M
    - Abducens ØØ8L
    - Accessory ØØ8R
    - Acoustic ØØ8N
    - Brachial Plexus Ø183
    - Cervical Ø181
    - Cervical Plexus Ø18Ø
    - Facial ØØ8M
    - Femoral Ø18D
    - Glossopharyngeal ØØ8P
    - Head and Neck Sympathetic Ø18K
    - Hypoglossal ØØ8S
    - Lumbar Ø18B
    - Lumbar Plexus Ø189

- Division *(Continued)*
  - Nerve *(Continued)*
    - Lumbar Sympathetic Ø18N
    - Lumbosacral Plexus Ø18A
    - Median Ø185
    - Oculomotor ØØ8H
    - Olfactory ØØ8F
    - Optic ØØ8G
    - Peroneal Ø18H
    - Phrenic Ø182
    - Pudendal Ø18C
    - Radial Ø186
    - Sacral Ø18R
    - Sacral Plexus Ø18Q
    - Sacral Sympathetic Ø18P
    - Sciatic Ø18F
    - Thoracic Ø188
    - Thoracic Sympathetic Ø18L
    - Tibial Ø18G
    - Trigeminal ØØ8K
    - Trochlear ØØ8J
    - Ulnar Ø184
    - Vagus ØØ8Q
  - Orbit
    - Left ØN8Q
    - Right ØN8P
  - Ovary
    - Bilateral ØU82
    - Left ØU81
    - Right ØU8Ø
  - Pancreas ØF8G
  - Patella
    - Left ØQ8F
    - Right ØQ8D
  - Perineum, Female ØW8NXZZ
  - Phalanx
    - Finger
      - Left ØP8V
      - Right ØP8T
    - Thumb
      - Left ØP8S
      - Right ØP8R
    - Toe
      - Left ØQ8R
      - Right ØQ8Q
  - Radius
    - Left ØP8J
    - Right ØP8H
  - Ribs
    - 1 to 2 ØP81
    - 3 or More ØP82
  - Sacrum ØQ81
  - Scapula
    - Left ØP86
    - Right ØP85
  - Skin
    - Abdomen ØH87XZZ
    - Back ØH86XZZ
    - Buttock ØH88XZZ
    - Chest ØH85XZZ
    - Ear
      - Left ØH83XZZ
      - Right ØH82XZZ
    - Face ØH81XZZ
    - Foot
      - Left ØH8NXZZ
      - Right ØH8MXZZ
    - Hand
      - Left ØH8GXZZ
      - Right ØH8FXZZ
    - Inguinal ØH8AXZZ
    - Lower Arm
      - Left ØH8EXZZ
      - Right ØH8DXZZ
    - Lower Leg
      - Left ØH8LXZZ
      - Right ØH8KXZZ
    - Neck ØH84XZZ
    - Perineum ØH89XZZ
    - Scalp ØH8ØXZZ

- Division *(Continued)*
  - Skin *(Continued)*
    - Upper Arm
      - Left ØH8CXZZ
      - Right ØH8BXZZ
    - Upper Leg
      - Left ØH8JXZZ
      - Right ØH8HXZZ
  - Skull ØN8Ø
  - Spinal Cord
    - Cervical ØØ8W
    - Lumbar ØØ8Y
    - Thoracic ØØ8X
  - Sternum ØP8Ø
  - Stomach, Pylorus ØD87
  - Subcutaneous Tissue and Fascia
    - Abdomen ØJ88
    - Back ØJ87
    - Buttock ØJ89
    - Chest ØJ86
    - Face ØJ81
    - Foot
      - Left ØJ8R
      - Right ØJ8Q
    - Hand
      - Left ØJ8K
      - Right ØJ8J
    - Head and Neck ØJ8S
    - Lower Arm
      - Left ØJ8H
      - Right ØJ8G
    - Lower Extremity ØJ8W
    - Lower Leg
      - Left ØJ8P
      - Right ØJ8N
    - Neck
      - Left ØJ85
      - Right ØJ84
    - Pelvic Region ØJ8C
    - Perineum ØJ8B
    - Scalp ØJ8Ø
    - Trunk ØJ8T
    - Upper Arm
      - Left ØJ8F
      - Right ØJ8D
    - Upper Extremity ØJ8V
    - Upper Leg
      - Left ØJ8M
      - Right ØJ8L
  - Tarsal
    - Left ØQ8M
    - Right ØQ8L
  - Tendon
    - Abdomen
      - Left ØL8G
      - Right ØL8F
    - Ankle
      - Left ØL8T
      - Right ØL8S
    - Foot
      - Left ØL8W
      - Right ØL8V
    - Hand
      - Left ØL88
      - Right ØL87
    - Head and Neck ØL8Ø
    - Hip
      - Left ØL8K
      - Right ØL8J
    - Knee
      - Left ØL8R
      - Right ØL8Q
    - Lower Arm and Wrist
      - Left ØL86
      - Right ØL85
    - Lower Leg
      - Left ØL8P
      - Right ØL8N
    - Perineum ØL8H
    - Shoulder
      - Left ØL82
      - Right ØL81

Division *(Continued)*
Tendon *(Continued)*
Thorax
Left ØL8D
Right ØL8C
Trunk
Left ØL8B
Right ØL89
Upper Arm
Left ØL84
Right ØL83
Upper Leg
Left ØL8M
Right ØL8L
Thyroid Gland Isthmus ØG8J
Tibia
Left ØQ8H
Right ØQ8G
Turbinate, Nasal Ø98L
Ulna
Left ØP8L
Right ØP8K
Uterine Supporting Structure ØU84
Vertebra
Cervical ØP83
Lumbar ØQ8Ø
Thoracic ØP84
~~Dnase (Deoxyribonuclease) use Other Substance~~
Dnase (Deoxyribonuclease) *use* Other Substance
Donislecel-jujn Allogeneic Pancreatic Islet Cellular Suspension XWØ33DA
Doppler study *see* Ultrasonography
Dorsal digital nerve *use* Radial Nerve
Dorsal metacarpal vein
use Hand Vein, Right
use Hand Vein, Left
Dorsal metatarsal artery
use Foot Artery, Right
use Foot Artery, Left
Dorsal metatarsal vein
use Foot Vein, Right
use Foot Vein, Left
Dorsal root ganglion
use Spinal Cord
use Cervical Spinal Cord
use Thoracic Spinal Cord
use Lumbar Spinal Cord
Dorsal scapular artery
use Subclavian Artery, Right
use Subclavian Artery, Left
Dorsal scapular nerve *use* Brachial Plexus
Dorsal venous arch
use Foot Vein, Right
use Foot Vein, Left
Dorsalis pedis artery
use Anterior Tibial Artery, Right
use Anterior Tibial Artery, Left
DownStream® System
5AØ512C
5AØ522C
Drainage
Abdominal Wall ØW9F
Acetabulum
Left ØQ95
Right ØQ94
Adenoids ØC9Q
Ampulla of Vater ØF9C
Anal Sphincter ØD9R
Ankle Region
Left ØY9L
Right ØY9K
Anterior Chamber
Left Ø893
Right Ø892
Anus ØD9Q
Aorta, Abdominal Ø49Ø
Aortic Body ØG9D
Appendix ØD9J

Drainage *(Continued)*
Arm
Lower
Left ØX9F
Right ØX9D
Upper
Left ØX99
Right ØX98
Artery
Anterior Tibial
Left Ø49Q
Right Ø49P
Axillary
Left Ø396
Right Ø395
Brachial
Left Ø398
Right Ø397
Celiac Ø491
Colic
Left Ø497
Middle Ø498
Right Ø496
Common Carotid
Left Ø39J
Right Ø39H
Common Iliac
Left Ø49D
Right Ø49C
External Carotid
Left Ø39N
Right Ø39M
External Iliac
Left Ø49J
Right Ø49H
Face Ø39R
Femoral
Left Ø49L
Right Ø49K
Foot
Left Ø49W
Right Ø49V
Gastric Ø492
Hand
Left Ø39F
Right Ø39D
Hepatic Ø493
Inferior Mesenteric Ø49B
Innominate Ø392
Internal Carotid
Left Ø39L
Right Ø39K
Internal Iliac
Left Ø49F
Right Ø49E
Internal Mammary
Left Ø391
Right Ø39Ø
Intracranial Ø39G
Lower Ø49Y
Peroneal
Left Ø49U
Right Ø49T
Popliteal
Left Ø49N
Right Ø49M
Posterior Tibial
Left Ø49S
Right Ø49R
Radial
Left Ø39C
Right Ø39B
Renal
Left Ø49A
Right Ø499
Splenic Ø494
Subclavian
Left Ø394
Right Ø393
Superior Mesenteric Ø495

Drainage *(Continued)*
Artery *(Continued)*
Temporal
Left Ø39T
Right Ø39S
Thyroid
Left Ø39V
Right Ø39U
Ulnar
Left Ø39A
Right Ø399
Upper Ø39Y
Vertebral
Left Ø39Q
Right Ø39P
Auditory Ossicle
Left Ø99A
Right Ø999
Axilla
Left ØX95
Right ØX94
Back
Lower ØW9L
Upper ØW9K
Basal Ganglia ØØ98
Bladder ØT9B
Bladder Neck ØT9C
Bone
Ethmoid
Left ØN9G
Right ØN9F
Frontal ØN91
Hyoid ØN9X
Lacrimal
Left ØN9J
Right ØN9H
Nasal ØN9B
Occipital ØN97
Palatine
Left ØN9L
Right ØN9K
Parietal
Left ØN94
Right ØN93
Pelvic
Left ØQ93
Right ØQ92
Sphenoid ØN9C
Temporal
Left ØN96
Right ØN95
Zygomatic
Left ØN9N
Right ØN9M
Bone Marrow Ø79T
Brain ØØ9Ø
Breast Bilateral ØH9V
Left ØH9U
Right ØH9T
Bronchus
Lingula ØB99
Lower Lobe
Left ØB9B
Right ØB96
Main
Left ØB97
Right ØB93
Middle Lobe, Right ØB95
Upper Lobe
Left ØB98
Right ØB94
Buccal Mucosa ØC94
Bursa and Ligament
Abdomen
Left ØM9J
Right ØM9H
Ankle
Left ØM9R
Right ØM9Q
Elbow
Left ØM94
Right ØM93

D

New Revised ~~deleted~~ Deleted

Drainage *(Continued)*
  Bursa and Ligament *(Continued)*
    Foot
      Left ØM9T
      Right ØM9S
    Hand
      Left ØM98
      Right ØM97
    Head and Neck ØM9Ø
    Hip
      Left ØM9M
      Right ØM9L
    Knee
      Left ØM9P
      Right ØM9N
    Lower Extremity
      Left ØM9W
      Right ØM9V
    Perineum ØM9K
    Rib(s) ØM9G
    Shoulder
      Left ØM92
      Right ØM91
    Spine
      Lower ØM9D
      Upper ØM9C
    Sternum ØM9F
    Upper Extremity
      Left ØM9B
      Right ØM99
    Wrist
      Left ØM96
      Right ØM95
  Buttock
    Left ØY91
    Right ØY9Ø
  Carina ØB92
  Carotid Bodies, Bilateral ØG98
  Carotid Body
    Left ØG96
    Right ØG97
  Carpal
    Left ØP9N
    Right ØP9M
  Cavity, Cranial ØW91
  Cecum ØD9H
  Cerebellum ØØ9C
  Cerebral Hemisphere ØØ97
  Cerebral Meninges ØØ91
  Cerebral Ventricle ØØ96
  Cervix ØU9C
  Chest Wall ØW98
  Choroid
    Left Ø89B
    Right Ø89A
  Cisterna Chyli Ø79L
  Clavicle
    Left ØP9B
    Right ØP99
  Clitoris ØU9J
  Coccygeal Glomus ØG9B
  Coccyx ØQ9S
  Colon
    Ascending ØD9K
    Descending ØD9M
    Sigmoid ØD9N
    Transverse ØD9L
  Conjunctiva
    Left Ø89T
    Right Ø89S
  Cord
    Bilateral ØV9H
    Left ØV9G
    Right ØV9F
  Cornea
    Left Ø899
    Right Ø898
  Cul-de-sac ØU9F
  Diaphragm ØB9T
  Disc
    Cervical Vertebral ØR93
    Cervicothoracic Vertebral ØR95

Drainage *(Continued)*
  Disc *(Continued)*
    Lumbar Vertebral ØS92
    Lumbosacral ØS94
    Thoracic Vertebral ØR99
    Thoracolumbar Vertebral ØR9B
  Duct
    Common Bile ØF99
    Cystic ØF98
    Hepatic
      Common ØF97
      Left ØF96
      Right ØF95
    Lacrimal
      Left Ø89Y
      Right Ø89X
    Pancreatic ØF9D
      Accessory ØF9F
    Parotid
      Left ØC9C
      Right ØC9B
  Duodenum ØD99
  Dura Mater ØØ92
  Ear
    External
      Left Ø991
      Right Ø99Ø
    External Auditory Canal
      Left Ø994
      Right Ø993
    Inner
      Left Ø99E
      Right Ø99D
    Middle
      Left Ø996
      Right Ø995
  Elbow Region
    Left ØX9C
    Right ØX9B
  Epididymis
    Bilateral ØV9L
    Left ØV9K
    Right ØV9J
  Epidural Space, Intracranial ØØ93
  Epiglottis ØC9R
  Esophagogastric Junction ØD94
  Esophagus ØD95
    Lower ØD93
    Middle ØD92
    Upper ØD91
  Eustachian Tube
    Left Ø99G
    Right Ø99F
  Extremity
    Lower
      Left ØY9B
      Right ØY99
    Upper
      Left ØX97
      Right ØX96
  Eye
    Left Ø891
    Right Ø89Ø
  Eyelid
    Lower
      Left Ø89R
      Right Ø89Q
    Upper
      Left Ø89P
      Right Ø89N
  Face ØW92
  Fallopian Tube
    Left ØU96
    Right ØU95
  Fallopian Tubes, Bilateral ØU97
  Femoral Region
    Left ØY98
    Right ØY97
  Femoral Shaft
    Left ØQ99
    Right ØQ98

Drainage *(Continued)*
  Femur
    Lower
      Left ØQ9C
      Right ØQ9B
    Upper
      Left ØQ97
      Right ØQ96
  Fibula
    Left ØQ9K
    Right ØQ9J
  Finger Nail ØH9Q
  Foot
    Left ØY9N
    Right ØY9M
  Gallbladder ØF94
  Gingiva
    Lower ØC96
    Upper ØC95
  Gland
    Adrenal
      Bilateral ØG94
      Left ØG92
      Right ØG93
    Lacrimal
      Left Ø89W
      Right Ø89V
    Minor Salivary ØC9J
    Parotid
      Left ØC99
      Right ØC98
    Pituitary ØG9Ø
    Sublingual
      Left ØC9F
      Right ØC9D
    Submaxillary
      Left ØC9H
      Right ØC9G
    Vestibular ØU9L
  Glenoid Cavity
    Left ØP98
    Right ØP97
  Glomus Jugulare ØG9C
  Hand
    Left ØX9K
    Right ØX9J
  Head ØW9Ø
  Humeral Head
    Left ØP9D
    Right ØP9C
  Humeral Shaft
    Left ØP9G
    Right ØP9F
  Hymen ØU9K
  Hypothalamus ØØ9A
  Ileocecal Valve ØD9C
  Ileum ØD9B
  Inguinal Region
    Left ØY96
    Right ØY95
  Intestine
    Large ØD9E
      Left ØD9G
      Right ØD9F
    Small ØD98
  Iris
    Left Ø89D
    Right Ø89C
  Jaw
    Lower ØW95
    Upper ØW94
  Jejunum ØD9A
  Joint
    Acromioclavicular
      Left ØR9H
      Right ØR9G
    Ankle
      Left ØS9G
      Right ØS9F
    Carpal
      Left ØR9R
      Right ØR9Q

D

- Drainage *(Continued)*
  - Joint *(Continued)*
    - Carpometacarpal
      - Left ØR9T
      - Right ØR9S
    - Cervical Vertebral ØR91
    - Cervicothoracic Vertebral ØR94
    - Coccygeal ØS96
    - Elbow
      - Left ØR9M
      - Right ØR9L
    - Finger Phalangeal
      - Left ØR9X
      - Right ØR9W
    - Hip
      - Left ØS9B
      - Right ØS99
    - Knee
      - Left ØS9D
      - Right ØS9C
    - Lumbar Vertebral ØS9Ø
    - Lumbosacral ØS93
    - Metacarpophalangeal
      - Left ØR9V
      - Right ØR9U
    - Metatarsal-Phalangeal
      - Left ØS9N
      - Right ØS9M
    - Occipital-cervical ØR9Ø
    - Sacrococcygeal ØS95
    - Sacroiliac
      - Left ØS98
      - Right ØS97
    - Shoulder
      - Left ØR9K
      - Right ØR9J
    - Sternoclavicular
      - Left ØR9F
      - Right ØR9E
    - Tarsal
      - Left ØS9J
      - Right ØS9H
    - Tarsometatarsal
      - Left ØS9L
      - Right ØS9K
    - Temporomandibular
      - Left ØR9D
      - Right ØR9C
    - Thoracic Vertebral ØR96
    - Thoracolumbar Vertebral ØR9A
    - Toe Phalangeal
      - Left ØS9Q
      - Right ØS9P
    - Wrist
      - Left ØR9P
      - Right ØR9N
  - Kidney
    - Left ØT91
    - Right ØT9Ø
  - Kidney Pelvis
    - Left ØT94
    - Right ØT93
  - Knee Region
    - Left ØY9G
    - Right ØY9F
  - Larynx ØC9S
  - Leg
    - Lower
      - Left ØY9J
      - Right ØY9H
    - Upper
      - Left ØY9D
      - Right ØY9C
  - Lens
    - Left Ø89K
    - Right Ø89J
  - Lip
    - Lower ØC91
    - Upper ØC9Ø
  - Liver ØF9Ø
    - Left Lobe ØF92
    - Right Lobe ØF91

- Drainage *(Continued)*
  - Lung
    - Bilateral ØB9M
    - Left ØB9L
    - Lower Lobe
      - Left ØB9J
      - Right ØB9F
    - Middle Lobe, Right ØB9D
    - Right ØB9K
    - Upper Lobe
      - Left ØB9G
      - Right ØB9C
  - Lung Lingula ØB9H
  - Lymphatic
    - Aortic Ø79D
    - Axillary
      - Left Ø796
      - Right Ø795
    - Head Ø79Ø
    - Inguinal
      - Left Ø79J
      - Right Ø79H
    - Internal Mammary
      - Left Ø799
      - Right Ø798
    - Lower Extremity
      - Left Ø79G
      - Right Ø79F
    - Mesenteric Ø79B
    - Neck
      - Left Ø792
      - Right Ø791
    - Pelvis Ø79C
    - Thoracic Duct Ø79K
    - Thorax Ø797
    - Upper Extremity
      - Left Ø794
      - Right Ø793
  - Mandible
    - Left ØN9V
    - Right ØN9T
  - Maxilla ØN9R
  - Mediastinum ØW9C
  - Medulla Oblongata ØØ9D
  - Mesentery ØD9V
  - Metacarpal
    - Left ØP9Q
    - Right ØP9P
  - Metatarsal
    - Left ØQ9P
    - Right ØQ9N
  - Muscle
    - Abdomen
      - Left ØK9L
      - Right ØK9K
    - Extraocular
      - Left Ø89M
      - Right Ø89L
    - Facial ØK91
    - Foot
      - Left ØK9W
      - Right ØK9V
    - Hand
      - Left ØK9D
      - Right ØK9C
    - Head ØK9Ø
    - Hip
      - Left ØK9P
      - Right ØK9N
    - Lower Arm and Wrist
      - Left ØK9B
      - Right ØK99
    - Lower Leg
      - Left ØK9T
      - Right ØK9S
    - Neck
      - Left ØK93
      - Right ØK92
    - Perineum ØK9M
    - Shoulder
      - Left ØK96
      - Right ØK95

- Drainage *(Continued)*
  - Muscle *(Continued)*
    - Thorax
      - Left ØK9J
      - Right ØK9H
    - Tongue, Palate, Pharynx ØK94
    - Trunk
      - Left ØK9G
      - Right ØK9F
    - Upper Arm
      - Left ØK98
      - Right ØK97
    - Upper Leg
      - Left ØK9R
      - Right ØK9Q
  - Nasal Mucosa and Soft Tissue Ø99K
  - Nasopharynx Ø99N
  - Neck ØW96
  - Nerve
    - Abdominal Sympathetic Ø19M
    - Abducens ØØ9L
    - Accessory ØØ9R
    - Acoustic ØØ9N
    - Brachial Plexus Ø193
    - Cervical Ø191
    - Cervical Plexus Ø19Ø
    - Facial ØØ9M
    - Femoral Ø19D
    - Glossopharyngeal ØØ9P
    - Head and Neck Sympathetic Ø19K
    - Hypoglossal ØØ9S
    - Lumbar Ø19B
    - Lumbar Plexus Ø199
    - Lumbar Sympathetic Ø19N
    - Lumbosacral Plexus Ø19A
    - Median Ø195
    - Oculomotor ØØ9H
    - Olfactory ØØ9F
    - Optic ØØ9G
    - Peroneal Ø19H
    - Phrenic Ø192
    - Pudendal Ø19C
    - Radial Ø196
    - Sacral Ø19R
    - Sacral Sympathetic Ø19P
    - Sciatic Ø19F
    - Thoracic Ø198
    - Thoracic Sympathetic Ø19L
    - Tibial Ø19G
    - Trigeminal ØØ9K
    - Trochlear ØØ9J
    - Ulnar Ø194
    - Vagus ØØ9Q
  - Nipple
    - Left ØH9X
    - Right ØH9W
  - Omentum ØD9U
  - Oral Cavity and Throat ØW93
  - Orbit
    - Left ØN9Q
    - Right ØN9P
  - Ovary
    - Bilateral ØU92
    - Left ØU91
    - Right ØU9Ø
  - Palate
    - Hard ØC92
    - Soft ØC93
  - Pancreas ØF9G
  - Para-aortic Body ØG99
  - Paraganglion Extremity ØG9F
  - Parathyroid Gland ØG9R
    - Inferior
      - Left ØG9P
      - Right ØG9N
    - Multiple ØG9Q
    - Superior
      - Left ØG9P
      - Right ØG9L
  - Patella
    - Left ØQ9F
    - Right ØQ9D

D

Drainage *(Continued)*
- Pelvic Cavity 0W9J
- Penis 0V9S
- Pericardial Cavity 0W9D
- Perineum
  - Female 0W9N
  - Male 0W9M
- Peritoneal Cavity 0W9G
- Peritoneum 0D9W
- Phalanx
  - Finger
    - Left 0P9V
    - Right 0P9T
  - Thumb
    - Left 0P9S
    - Right 0P9R
  - Toe
    - Left 0Q9R
    - Right 0Q9Q
- Pharynx 0C9M
- Pineal Body 0G91
- Pleura
  - Left 0B9P
  - Right 0B9N
- Pleural Cavity
  - Left 0W9B
  - Right 0W99
- Pons 009B
- Prepuce 0V9T
- Products of Conception
  - Amniotic Fluid
    - Diagnostic 1090
    - Therapeutic 1090
  - Fetal Blood 1090
  - Fetal Cerebrospinal Fluid 1090
  - Fetal Fluid, Other 1090
  - Fluid, Other 1090
- Prostate 0V90
- Radius
  - Left 0P9J
  - Right 0P9H
- Rectum 0D9P
- Retina
  - Left 089F
  - Right 089E
- Retinal Vessel
  - Left 089H
  - Right 089G
- Retroperitoneum 0W9H
- Ribs
  - 1 to 2 0P91
  - 3 or More 0P92
- Sacrum 0Q91
- Scapula
  - Left 0P96
  - Right 0P95
- Sclera
  - Left 0897
  - Right 0896
- Scrotum 0V95
- Septum, Nasal 099M
- Shoulder Region
  - Left 0X93
  - Right 0X92
- Sinus
  - Accessory 099P
  - Ethmoid
    - Left 099V
    - Right 099U
  - Frontal
    - Left 099T
    - Right 099S
  - Mastoid
    - Left 099C
    - Right 099B
  - Maxillary
    - Left 099R
    - Right 099Q
  - Sphenoid
    - Left 099X
    - Right 099W

Drainage *(Continued)*
- Skin
  - Abdomen 0H97
  - Back 0H96
  - Buttock 0H98
  - Chest 0H95
  - Ear
    - Left 0H93
    - Right 0H92
  - Face 0H91
  - Foot
    - Left 0H9N
    - Right 0H9M
  - Hand
    - Left 0H9G
    - Right 0H9F
  - Inguinal 0H9A
  - Lower Arm
    - Left 0H9E
    - Right 0H9D
  - Lower Leg
    - Left 0H9L
    - Right 0H9K
  - Neck 0H94
  - Perineum 0H99
  - Scalp 0H90
  - Upper Arm
    - Left 0H9C
    - Right 0H9B
  - Upper Leg
    - Left 0H9J
    - Right 0H9H
- Skull 0N90
- Spinal Canal 009U
- Spinal Cord
  - Cervical 009W
  - Lumbar 009Y
  - Thoracic 009X
- Spinal Meninges 009T
- Spleen 079P
- Sternum 0P90
- Stomach 0D96
  - Pylorus 0D97
- Subarachnoid Space, Intracranial 0095
- Subcutaneous Tissue and Fascia
  - Abdomen 0J98
  - Back 0J97
  - Buttock 0J99
  - Chest 0J96
  - Face 0J91
  - Foot
    - Left 0J9R
    - Right 0J9Q
  - Hand
    - Left 0J9K
    - Right 0J9J
  - Lower Arm
    - Left 0J9H
    - Right 0J9G
  - Lower Leg
    - Left 0J9P
    - Right 0J9N
  - Neck
    - Left 0J95
    - Right 0J94
  - Pelvic Region 0J9C
  - Perineum 0J9B
  - Scalp 0J90
  - Upper Arm
    - Left 0J9F
    - Right 0J9D
  - Upper Leg
    - Left 0J9M
    - Right 0J9L
- Subdural Space, Intracranial 0094
- Tarsal
  - Left 0Q9M
  - Right 0Q9L
- Tendon
  - Abdomen
    - Left 0L9G
    - Right 0L9F

Drainage *(Continued)*
- Tendon *(Continued)*
  - Ankle
    - Left 0L9T
    - Right 0L9S
  - Foot
    - Left 0L9W
    - Right 0L9V
  - Hand
    - Left 0L98
    - Right 0L97
  - Head and Neck 0L90
  - Hip
    - Left 0L9K
    - Right 0L9J
  - Knee
    - Left 0L9R
    - Right 0L9Q
  - Lower Arm and Wrist
    - Left 0L96
    - Right 0L95
  - Lower Leg
    - Left 0L9P
    - Right 0L9N
  - Perineum 0L9H
  - Shoulder
    - Left 0L92
    - Right 0L91
  - Thorax
    - Left 0L9D
    - Right 0L9C
  - Trunk
    - Left 0L9B
    - Right 0L99
  - Upper Arm
    - Left 0L94
    - Right 0L93
  - Upper Leg
    - Left 0L9M
    - Right 0L9L
- Testis
  - Bilateral 0V9C
  - Left 0V9B
  - Right 0V99
- Thalamus 0099
- Thymus 079M
- Thyroid Gland 0G9K
  - Left Lobe 0G9G
  - Right Lobe 0G9H
- Tibia
  - Left 0Q9H
  - Right 0Q9G
- Toe Nail 0H9R
- Tongue 0C97
- Tonsils 0C9P
- Tooth
  - Lower 0C9X
  - Upper 0C9W
- Trachea 0B91
- Tunica Vaginalis
  - Left 0V97
  - Right 0V96
- Turbinate, Nasal 099L
- Tympanic Membrane
  - Left 0998
  - Right 0997
- Ulna
  - Left 0P9L
  - Right 0P9K
- Ureter
  - Left 0T97
  - Right 0T96
- Ureters, Bilateral 0T98
- Urethra 0T9D
- Uterine Supporting Structure 0U94
- Uterus 0U99
- Uvula 0C9N
- Vagina 0U9G
- Vas Deferens
  - Bilateral 0V9Q
  - Left 0V9P
  - Right 0V9N

Drainage *(Continued)*
Vein
Axillary
Left Ø598
Right Ø597
Azygos Ø59Ø
Basilic
Left Ø59C
Right Ø59B
Brachial
Left Ø59A
Right Ø599
Cephalic
Left Ø59F
Right Ø59D
Colic Ø697
Common Iliac
Left Ø69D
Right Ø69C
Esophageal Ø693
External Iliac
Left Ø69G
Right Ø69F
External Jugular
Left Ø59Q
Right Ø59P
Face
Left Ø59V
Right Ø59T
Femoral
Left Ø69N
Right Ø69M
Foot
Left Ø69V
Right Ø69T
Gastric Ø692
Hand
Left Ø59H
Right Ø59G
Hemiazygos Ø591
Hepatic Ø694
Hypogastric
Left Ø69J
Right Ø69H
Inferior Mesenteric Ø696
Innominate
Left Ø594
Right Ø593
Internal Jugular
Left Ø59N
Right Ø59M
Intracranial Ø59L
Lower Ø69Y
Portal Ø698
Renal
Left Ø69B
Right Ø699
Saphenous
Left Ø69Q
Right Ø69P
Splenic Ø691
Subclavian
Left Ø596
Right Ø595
Superior Mesenteric Ø695
Upper Ø59Y
Vertebral
Left Ø59S
Right Ø59R
Vena Cava, Inferior Ø69Ø

Drainage *(Continued)*
Vertebra
Cervical ØP93
Lumbar ØQ9Ø
Thoracic ØP94
Vesicle
Bilateral ØV93
Left ØV92
Right ØV91
Vitreous
Left Ø895
Right Ø894
Vocal Cord
Left ØC9V
Right ØC9T
Vulva ØU9M
Wrist Region
Left ØX9H
Right ØX9G
Dressing
Abdominal Wall 2W23X4Z
Arm
Lower
Left 2W2DX4Z
Right 2W2CX4Z
Upper
Left 2W2BX4Z
Right 2W2AX4Z
Back 2W25X4Z
Chest Wall 2W24X4Z
Extremity
Lower
Left 2W2MX4Z
Right 2W2LX4Z
Upper
Left 2W29X4Z
Right 2W28X4Z
Face 2W21X4Z
Finger
Left 2W2KX4Z
Right 2W2JX4Z
Foot
Left 2W2TX4Z
Right 2W2SX4Z
Hand
Left 2W2FX4Z
Right 2W2EX4Z
Head 2W2ØX4Z
Inguinal Region
Left 2W27X4Z
Right 2W26X4Z
Leg
Lower
Left 2W2RX4Z
Right 2W2QX4Z
Upper
Left 2W2PX4Z
Right 2W2NX4Z
Neck 2W22X4Z
Thumb
Left 2W2HX4Z
Right 2W2GX4Z
Toe
Left 2W2VX4Z
Right 2W2UX4Z
Driver stent (RX) (OTW) *use* Intraluminal Device
Drotrecogin alfa, Infusion *see* Introduction of Recombinant Human-activated Protein C

▶**Drug-eluting resorbable scaffold intraluminal device** *use* Intraluminal Device, Everolimus-eluting Resorbable Scaffold(s) in New Technology
Duct of Santorini *use* Duct, Pancreatic, Accessory
Duct of Wirsung *use* Duct, Pancreatic
Ductogram, mammary *see* Plain Radiography, Skin, Subcutaneous Tissue and Breast BHØ
Ductography, mammary *see* Plain Radiography, Skin, Subcutaneous Tissue and Breast BHØ
Ductus deferens
use Vas Deferens, Right
use Vas Deferens, Left
use Vas Deferens, Bilateral
use Vas Deferens
Duodenal ampulla *use* Ampulla of Vater
Duodenectomy
see Excision, Duodenum ØDB9
see Resection, Duodenum ØDT9
Duodenocholedochotomy *see* Drainage, Gallbladder ØF94
Duodenocystostomy
see Bypass, Gallbladder ØF14
see Drainage, Gallbladder ØF94
Duodenoenterostomy
see Bypass, Gastrointestinal System ØD1
see Drainage, Gastrointestinal System ØD9
Duodenojejunal flexure *use* Jejunum
Duodenolysis *see* Release, Duodenum ØDN9
Duodenorrhaphy *see* Repair, Duodenum ØDQ9
Duodenoscopy, single-use (aScope™ Duodeno) (EXALT™ Model D) *see* New Technology, Hepatobiliary System and Pancreas XFJ
Duodenostomy
see Bypass, Duodenum ØD19
see Drainage, Duodenum ØD99
Duodenotomy *see* Drainage, Duodenum ØD99
DuraGraft® Endothelial Damage Inhibitor *use* Endothelial Damage Inhibitor
DuraHeart Left Ventricular Assist System *use* Implantable Heart Assist System in Heart and Great Vessels
Dural venous sinus *use* Vein, Intracranial
Dura mater, intracranial *use* Dura Mater
Dura mater, spinal *use* Spinal Meninges
Durata® Defibrillation Lead *use* Cardiac Lead, Defibrillator in Ø2H
Durvalumab Antineoplastic XWØ
~~DynaClip® (Forte)~~
~~use Internal Fixation Device, Sustained Compression in ØRG~~
~~use Internal Fixation Device, Sustained Compression in ØSG~~
▶**DynaClip® (Delta)(Forte)(Quattro)**
▶*use* Internal Fixation Device, Sustained Compression in ØRG
▶*use* Internal Fixation Device, Sustained Compression in ØSG
DynaNail® (Helix) (Hybrid) (Mini)
use Internal Fixation Device, Sustained Compression in ØRG
use Internal Fixation Device, Sustained Compression in ØSG
Dynesys® Dynamic Stabilization System
use Spinal Stabilization Device, Pedicle-Based in ØRH
use Spinal Stabilization Device, Pedicle-Based in ØSH

E

E-Luminexx™ (Biliary) (Vascular) Stent *use* Intraluminal Device
Earlobe
  use External Ear, Right
  use External Ear, Left
  use External Ear, Bilateral
▶**EB-1Ø1 gene-corrected autologous cell therapy** *use* Prademagene Zamikeracel, Genetically Engineered Autologous Cell Therapy in New Technology
▶**EB-1Ø1 gene-corrected keratinocyte sheets** *use* Prademagene Zamikeracel, Genetically Engineered Autologous Cell Therapy in New Technology
▶**EBVALLO™** *use* Tabelecleucel Immunotherapy
ECCO2R (Extracorporeal Carbon Dioxide Removal) 5AØ92ØZ
Echocardiogram *see* Ultrasonography, Heart B24
EchoGo Heart Failure 1.Ø software XXE2X19
Echography *see* Ultrasonography
EchoTip® Insight™ Portosystemic Pressure Gradient Measurement System 4AØ44B2
ECMO *see* Performance, Circulatory 5A15
ECMO, intraoperative *see* Performance, Circulatory 5A15A
Eculizumab XWØ
▶**Edwards EVOQUE tricuspid valve replacement system** *use* Multi-plane Flex Technology Bioprosthetic Valve in New Technology
EDWARDS INTUITY Elite valve system (rapid deployment technique) *see* Replacement, Valve, Aortic Ø2RF
EEG (electroencephalogram) *see* Measurement, Central Nervous 4AØØ
EGD (esophagogastroduodenoscopy) ØDJØ8ZZ
Eighth cranial nerve *use* Acoustic Nerve
Ejaculatory duct
  use Vas Deferens, Right
  use Vas Deferens, Left
  use Vas Deferens, Bilateral
  use Vas Deferens
EKG (electrocardiogram) *see* Measurement, Cardiac 4AØ2
EKOS™ EkoSonic® Endovascular System *see* Fragmentation, Artery
Eladocagene exuparvovec XWØQ316
Electrical bone growth stimulator (EBGS)
  use Bone Growth Stimulator in Head and Facial Bones
  use Bone Growth Stimulator in Upper Bones
  use Bone Growth Stimulator in Lower Bones
Electrical muscle stimulation (EMS) lead *use* Stimulator Lead in Muscles
Electrocautery
  Destruction *see* Destruction
  Repair *see* Repair
Electroconvulsive Therapy
  ~~Bilateral-Multiple Seizure GZB3ZZZ~~
  Bilateral-Single Seizure GZB2ZZZ
  Electroconvulsive Therapy, Other GZB4ZZZ
  ~~Unilateral-Multiple Seizure GZB1ZZZ~~
  Unilateral-Single Seizure GZBØZZZ
Electroencephalogram (EEG) *see* Measurement, Central Nervous 4AØØ
Electromagnetic Therapy
  Central Nervous 6A22
  Urinary 6A21
Electronic muscle stimulator lead *use* Stimulator Lead in Muscles
Electrophysiologic stimulation (EPS) *see* Measurement, Cardiac 4AØ2
Electroshock therapy *see* Electroconvulsive Therapy
Elevation, bone fragments, skull *see* Reposition, Head and Facial Bones ØNS
Eleventh cranial nerve *use* Accessory Nerve
Ellipsys® vascular access system *see* New Technology, Cardiovascular System X2K
Elranatamab Antineoplastic XWØ13L9
▶**ELREXFIO™** *use* Elranatamab Antineoplastic
Eluvia™ Drug-Eluting Vascular Stent System
  ~~use Intraluminal Device, Sustained Release Drug-eluting in New Technology~~
  ~~use Intraluminal Device, Sustained Release Drug-eluting, Two in New Technology~~
  ~~use Intraluminal Device, Sustained Release Drug-eluting, Three in New Technology~~
  ~~use Intraluminal Device, Sustained Release Drug-eluting, Four or More in New Technology~~
  ▶*use* Intraluminal Device, Drug-eluting in Lower Arteries
  ▶*use* Intraluminal Device, Drug-eluting, Two in Lower Arteries
  ▶*use* Intraluminal Device, Drug-eluting, Three in Lower Arteries
  ▶*use* Intraluminal Device, Drug-eluting, Four or More in Lower Arteries
ELZONRIS™
  use Tagraxofusp-erzs Antineoplastic
Embolectomy *see* Extirpation
▶**Emboli trap circuit, during percutaneous thrombectomy** 5AØ5AØL
Embolization
  see Occlusion
  see Restriction
Embolization coil(s) *use* Intraluminal Device
EMG (electromyogram) *see* Measurement, Musculoskeletal 4AØF
Encephalon *use* Brain
Endarterectomy
  see Extirpation, Upper Arteries Ø3C
  see Extirpation, Lower Arteries Ø4C
Endeavor® (III) (IV) (Sprint) Zotarolimus-eluting Coronary Stent System *use* Intraluminal Device, Drug-eluting in Heart and Great Vessels
EndoAVF procedure, using magnetic-guided radiofrequency *see* Bypass, Upper Arteries Ø31
EndoAVF procedure, using thermal resistance energy *see* New Technology, Cardiovascular System X2K
Endologix AFX® Endovascular AAA System use Intraluminal Device
EndoSure® sensor *use* Monitoring Device, Pressure Sensor in Ø2H
ENDOTAK RELIANCE® (G) Defibrillation Lead *use* Cardiac Lead, Defibrillator in Ø2H
Endothelial damage inhibitor, applied to vein graft XYØVX83
Endotracheal tube (cuffed) (double-lumen) *use* Intraluminal Device, Endotracheal Airway in Respiratory System
Endovascular fistula creation, using magnetic-guided radiofrequency *see* Bypass, Upper Arteries Ø31
Endovascular fistula creation, using thermal resistance energy *see* New Technology, Cardiovascular System X2K
Endurant® Endovascular Stent Graft *use* Intraluminal Device
Endurant® II AAA stent graft system *use* Intraluminal Device
Engineered Allogeneic Thymus Tissue XWØ2ØD8
Engineered chimeric antigen receptor T-cell immunotherapy
  Allogeneic XWØ
  Autologous XWØ
Enlargement
  see Dilation
  see Repair
ENROUTE® Transcarotid Neuroprotection System *see* New Technology, Cardiovascular System X2A
EnRhythm *use* Pacemaker, Dual Chamber in ØJH
ENSPRYNG™ *use* Satralizumab-mwge
Enterorrhaphy *see* Repair, Gastrointestinal System ØDQ
Enterra gastric neurostimulator *use* Stimulator Generator, Multiple Array in ØJH
Enucleation
  Eyeball *see* Resection, Eye Ø8T
  Eyeball with prosthetic implant *see* Replacement, Eye Ø8R
Epcoritamab Monoclonal Antibody XWØ13S9
Ependyma *use* Cerebral Ventricle
Epic™ Stented Tissue Valve (aortic) *use* Zooplastic Tissue in Heart and Great Vessels
Epicel® cultured epidermal autograft *use* Autologous Tissue Substitute
Epidermis *use* Skin
Epididymectomy
  see Excision, Male Reproductive System ØVB
  see Resection, Male Reproductive System ØVT
Epididymoplasty
  see Repair, Male Reproductive System ØVQ
  see Supplement, Male Reproductive System ØVU
Epididymorrhaphy *see* Repair, Male Reproductive System ØVQ
Epididymotomy *see* Drainage, Male Reproductive System ØV9
Epidural space, spinal use Spinal Canal
Epiphysiodesis
  see Insertion of device in, Upper Bones ØPH
  see Repair, Upper Bones ØPQ
  see Insertion of device in, Lower Bones ØQH
  see Repair, Lower Bones ØQQ
Epiploic foramen *use* Peritoneum
Epiretinal Visual Prosthesis
  Left Ø8H1Ø5Z
  Right Ø8HØØ5Z
Episiorrhaphy *see* Repair, Perineum, Female ØWQN
Episiotomy *see* Division, Perineum, Female ØW8N
Epithalamus *use* Thalamus
Epitroclear lymph node
  use Lymphatic, Right Upper Extremity
  use Lymphatic, Left Upper Extremity
▶**EPKINLY™** *use* Epcoritamab Monoclonal Antibody
EPS (electrophysiologic stimulation) *see* Measurement, Cardiac 4AØ2
Eptifibatide, infusion *see* Introduction of Platelet Inhibitor
ERCP (endoscopic retrograde cholangiopancreatography) *see* Fluoroscopy, Hepatobiliary System and Pancreas BF1
Erector spinae muscle
  use Trunk Muscle, Right
  use Trunk Muscle, Left
➠**Erdafitinib Antineoplastic** ~~XWØDXL5~~ *use* Other Antineoplastic
~~ERLEADA™ use Apalutamide Antineoplastic~~
▶**ERLEADA™** (Apalutamide Antineoplastic) use Other Antineoplastic
➠**Esketamine Hydrochloride** ~~XWØ97M5~~ *use* Other Substance
Esophageal artery *use* Upper Artery
Esophageal obturator airway (EOA) *use* Intraluminal Device, Airway in Gastrointestinal System
Esophageal plexus *use* Thoracic Sympathetic Nerve
Esophagectomy
  see Excision, Gastrointestinal System ØDB
  see Resection, Gastrointestinal System ØDT
Esophagocoloplasty
  see Repair, Gastrointestinal System ØDQ
  see Supplement, Gastrointestinal System ØDU
Esophagoenterostomy
  see Bypass, Gastrointestinal System ØD1
  see Drainage, Gastrointestinal System ØD9

▶ New ➠ Revised ~~deleted~~ Deleted

Esophagoesophagostomy
see Bypass, Gastrointestinal System ØD1
see Drainage, Gastrointestinal System ØD9
Esophagogastrectomy
see Excision, Gastrointestinal System ØDB
see Resection, Gastrointestinal System ØDT
Esophagogastroduodenoscopy (EGD) ØDJØ8ZZ
Esophagogastroplasty
see Repair, Gastrointestinal System ØDQ
see Supplement, Gastrointestinal System ØDU
Esophagogastroscopy ØDJ68ZZ
Esophagogastrostomy
see Bypass, Gastrointestinal System ØD1
see Drainage, Gastrointestinal System ØD9
Esophagojejunoplasty *see* Supplement, Gastrointestinal System ØDU
Esophagojejunostomy
see Bypass, Gastrointestinal System ØD1
see Drainage, Gastrointestinal System ØD9
Esophagomyotomy *see* Division, Esophagogastric Junction ØD84
Esophagoplasty
see Repair, Gastrointestinal System ØDQ
see Replacement, Esophagus ØDR5
see Supplement, Gastrointestinal System ØDU
Esophagoplication *see* Restriction, Gastrointestinal System ØDV
Esophagorrhaphy *see* Repair, Gastrointestinal System ØDQ
Esophagoscopy ØDJØ8ZZ
Esophagotomy *see* Drainage, Gastrointestinal System ØD9
Esprit™ BTK (scaffold) (stent) *use* Intraluminal Device, Everolimus-eluting Resorbable Scaffold(s) in New Technology
Esteem® implantable hearing system *use* Hearing Device in Ear, Nose, Sinus
ESWL (extracorporeal shock wave lithotripsy) *see* Fragmentation
Etesevimab monoclonal antibody XWØ
Ethmoidal air cell
use Ethmoid Sinus, Right
use Ethmoid Sinus, Left
Ethmoidectomy
see Excision, Ear, Nose, Sinus Ø9B
see Resection, Ear, Nose, Sinus Ø9T
see Excision, Head and Facial Bones ØNB
see Resection, Head and Facial Bones ØNT
Ethmoidotomy *see* Drainage, Ear, Nose, Sinus Ø99
Evacuation
Hematoma *see* Extirpation
Other Fluid *see* Drainage
Evera (XT)(S)(DR/VR) *use* Defibrillator Generator in ØJH
Everolimus-eluting coronary stent *use* Intraluminal Device, Drug-eluting in Heart and Great Vessels
Everolimus Eluting Resorbable Scaffold System *use* Intraluminal Device, Everolimus-eluting Resorbable Scaffold(s) in New Technology
EV ICD System (Extravascular implantable defibrillator lead) *use* Defibrillator Lead in AnatomicalRegions, General
Evisceration
Eyeball *see* Resection, Eye Ø8T
Eyeball with prosthetic implant *see* Replacement, Eye Ø8R
Evo® sEEG-RF probes (for radiofrequency ablation of brain tissue) ØØ5Ø3Z4
Ex-PRESS™ mini glaucoma shunt *use* Synthetic Substitute
Exagamglogene Autotemcel XW1
EXALT™ Model D Single-Use Duodenoscope *see* New Technology, Hepatobiliary System and Pancreas XFJ
Examination *see* Inspection
Exchange *see* Change device in

Excision
Abdominal Wall ØWBF
Acetabulum
Left ØQB5
Right ØQB4
Adenoids ØCBQ
Ampulla of Vater ØFBC
Anal Sphincter ØDBR
Ankle Region
Left ØYBL
Right ØYBK
Anus ØDBQ
Aorta
Abdominal Ø4BØ
Thoracic
Ascending/Arch Ø2BX
Descending Ø2BW
Aortic Body ØGBD
Appendix ØDBJ
Arm
Lower
Left ØXBF
Right ØXBD
Upper
Left ØXB9
Right ØXB8
Artery
Anterior Tibial
Left Ø4BQ
Right Ø4BP
Axillary
Left Ø3B6
Right Ø3B5
Brachial
Left Ø3B8
Right Ø3B7
Celiac Ø4B1
Colic
Left Ø4B7
Middle Ø4B8
Right Ø4B6
Common Carotid
Left Ø3BJ
Right Ø3BH
Common Iliac
Left Ø4BD
Right Ø4BC
External Carotid
Left Ø3BN
Right Ø3BM
External Iliac
Left Ø4BJ
Right Ø4BH
Face Ø3BR
Femoral
Left Ø4BL
Right Ø4BK
Foot
Left Ø4BW
Right Ø4BV
Gastric Ø4B2
Hand
Left Ø3BF
Right Ø3BD
Hepatic Ø4B3
Inferior Mesenteric Ø4BB
Innominate Ø3B2
Internal Carotid
Left Ø3BL
Right Ø3BK
Internal Iliac
Left Ø4BF
Right Ø4BE
Internal Mammary
Left Ø3B1
Right Ø3BØ
Intracranial Ø3BG
Lower Ø4BY
Peroneal
Left Ø4BU
Right Ø4BT

Excision *(Continued)*
Artery *(Continued)*
Popliteal
Left Ø4BN
Right Ø4BM
Posterior Tibial
Left Ø4BS
Right Ø4BR
Pulmonary
Left Ø2BR
Right Ø2BQ
Pulmonary Trunk Ø2BP
Radial
Left Ø3BC
Right Ø3BB
Renal
Left Ø4BA
Right Ø4B9
Splenic Ø4B4
Subclavian
Left Ø3B4
Right Ø3B3
Superior Mesenteric Ø4B5
Temporal
Left Ø3BT
Right Ø3BS
Thyroid
Left Ø3BV
Right Ø3BU
Ulnar
Left Ø3BA
Right Ø3B9
Upper Ø3BY
Vertebral
Left Ø3BQ
Right Ø3BP
Atrium
Left Ø2B7
Right Ø2B6
Auditory Ossicle
Left Ø9BA
Right Ø9B9
Axilla
Left ØXB5
Right ØXB4
Back
Lower ØWBL
Upper ØWBK
Basal Ganglia ØØB8
Bladder ØTBB
Bladder Neck ØTBC
Bone
Ethmoid
Left ØNBG
Right ØNBF
Frontal ØNB1
Hyoid ØNBX
Lacrimal
Left ØNBJ
Right ØNBH
Nasal ØNBB
Occipital ØNB7
Palatine
Left ØNBL
Right ØNBK
Parietal
Left ØNB4
Right ØNB3
Pelvic
Left ØQB3
Right ØQB2
Sphenoid ØNBC
Temporal
Left ØNB6
Right ØNB5
Zygomatic
Left ØNBN
Right ØNBM
Brain ØØBØ
Breast
Bilateral ØHBV
Left ØHBU

Excision *(Continued)*
Breast *(Continued)*
Right ØHBT
Supernumerary ØHBY
Bronchus
Lingula ØBB9
Lower Lobe
Left ØBBB
Right ØBB6
Main
Left ØBB7
Right ØBB3
Middle Lobe, Right ØBB5
Upper Lobe
Left ØBB8
Right ØBB4
Buccal Mucosa ØCB4
Bursa and Ligament
Abdomen
Left ØMBJ
Right ØMBH
Ankle
Left ØMBR
Right ØMBQ
Elbow
Left ØMB4
Right ØMB3
Foot
Left ØMBT
Right ØMBS
Hand
Left ØMB8
Right ØMB7
Head and Neck ØMBØ
Hip
Left ØMBM
Right ØMBL
Knee
Left ØMBP
Right ØMBN
Lower Extremity
Left ØMBW
Right ØMBV
Perineum ØMBK
Rib(s) ØMBG
Shoulder
Left ØMB2
Right ØMB1
Spine
Lower ØMBD
Upper ØMBC
Sternum ØMBF
Upper Extremity
Left ØMBB
Right ØMB9
Wrist
Left ØMB6
Right ØMB5
Buttock
Left ØYB1
Right ØYBØ
Carina ØBB2
Carotid Bodies, Bilateral ØGB8
Carotid Body
Left ØGB6
Right ØGB7
Carpal
Left ØPBN
Right ØPBM
Cecum ØDBH
Cerebellum ØØBC
Cerebral Hemisphere ØØB7
Cerebral Meninges ØØB1
Cerebral Ventricle ØØB6
Cervix ØUBC
Chest Wall ØWB8
Chordae Tendineae Ø2B9
Choroid
Left Ø8BB
Right Ø8BA

Excision *(Continued)*
Cisterna Chyli Ø7BL
Clavicle
Left ØPBB
Right ØPB9
Clitoris ØUBJ
Coccygeal Glomus ØGBB
Coccyx ØQBS
Colon
Ascending ØDBK
Descending ØDBM
Sigmoid ØDBN
Transverse ØDBL
Conduction Mechanism Ø2B8
Conjunctiva
Left Ø8BTXZ
Right Ø8BSXZ
Cord
Bilateral ØVBH
Left ØVBG
Right ØVBF
Cornea
Left Ø8B9XZ
Right Ø8B8XZ
Cul-de-sac ØUBF
Diaphragm ØBBT
Disc
Cervical Vertebral ØRB3
Cervicothoracic Vertebral ØRB5
Lumbar Vertebral ØSB2
Lumbosacral ØSB4
Thoracic Vertebral ØRB9
Thoracolumbar Vertebral ØRBB
Duct
Common Bile ØFB9
Cystic ØFB8
Hepatic
Common ØFB7
Left ØFB6
Right ØFB5
Lacrimal
Left Ø8BY
Right Ø8BX
Pancreatic ØFBD
Accessory ØFBF
Parotid
Left ØCBC
Right ØCBB
Duodenum ØDB9
Dura Mater ØØB2
Ear
External
Left Ø9B1
Right Ø9BØ
External Auditory Canal
Left Ø9B4
Right Ø9B3
Inner
Left Ø9BE
Right Ø9BD
Middle
Left Ø9B6
Right Ø9B5
Elbow Region
Left ØXBC
Right ØXBB
Epididymis
Bilateral ØVBL
Left ØVBK
Right ØVBJ
Epiglottis ØCBR
Esophagogastric Junction ØDB4
Esophagus ØDB5
Lower ØDB3
Middle ØDB2
Upper ØDB1
Eustachian Tube
Left Ø9BG
Right Ø9BF

Excision *(Continued)*
Extremity
Lower
Left ØYBB
Right ØYB9
Upper
Left ØXB7
Right ØXB6
Eye
Left Ø8B1
Right Ø8BØ
Eyelid
Lower
Left Ø8BR
Right Ø8BQ
Upper
Left Ø8BP
Right Ø8BN
Face ØWB2
Fallopian Tube
Left ØUB6
Right ØUB5
Fallopian Tubes, Bilateral ØUB7
Femoral Region
Left ØYB8
Right ØYB7
Femoral Shaft
Left ØQB9
Right ØQB8
Femur
Lower
Left ØQBC
Right ØQBB
Upper
Left ØQB7
Right ØQB6
Fibula
Left ØQBK
Right ØQBJ
Finger Nail ØHBQXZ
Floor of mouth *see* Excision, Oral Cavity and Throat ØWB3
Foot
Left ØYBN
Right ØYBM
Gallbladder ØFB4
Gingiva
Lower ØCB6
Upper ØCB5
Gland
Adrenal
Bilateral ØGB4
Left ØGB2
Right ØGB3
Lacrimal
Left Ø8BW
Right Ø8BV
Minor Salivary ØCBJ
Parotid
Left ØCB9
Right ØCB8
Pituitary ØGBØ
Sublingual
Left ØCBF
Right ØCBD
Submaxillary
Left ØCBH
Right ØCBG
Vestibular ØUBL
Glenoid Cavity
Left ØPB8
Right ØPB7
Glomus Jugulare ØGBC
Hand
Left ØXBK
Right ØXBJ
Head ØWBØ
Humeral Head
Left ØPBD
Right ØPBC

E

- Excision *(Continued)*
  - Humeral Shaft
    - Left ØPBG
    - Right ØPBF
  - Hymen ØUBK
  - Hypothalamus ØØBA
  - Ileocecal Valve ØDBC
  - Ileum ØDBB
  - Inguinal Region
    - Left ØYB6
    - Right ØYB5
  - Intestine
    - Large ØDBE
      - Left ØDBG
      - Right ØDBF
    - Small ØDB8
  - Iris
    - Left Ø8BD3Z
    - Right Ø8BC3Z
  - Jaw
    - Lower ØWB5
    - Upper ØWB4
  - Jejunum ØDBA
  - Joint
    - Acromioclavicular
      - Left ØRBH
      - Right ØRBG
    - Ankle
      - Left ØSBG
      - Right ØSBF
    - Carpal
      - Left ØRBR
      - Right ØRBQ
    - Carpometacarpal
      - Left ØRBT
      - Right ØRBS
    - Cervical Vertebral ØRB1
    - Cervicothoracic Vertebral ØRB4
    - Coccygeal ØSB6
    - Elbow
      - Left ØRBM
      - Right ØRBL
    - Finger Phalangeal
      - Left ØRBX
      - Right ØRBW
    - Hip
      - Left ØSBB
      - Right ØSB9
    - Knee
      - Left ØSBD
      - Right ØSBC
    - Lumbar Vertebral ØSBØ
    - Lumbosacral ØSB3
    - Metacarpophalangeal
      - Left ØRBV
      - Right ØRBU
    - Metatarsal-Phalangeal
      - Left ØSBN
      - Right ØSBM
    - Occipital-cervical ØRBØ
    - Sacrococcygeal ØSB5
    - Sacroiliac
      - Left ØSB8
      - Right ØSB7
    - Shoulder
      - Left ØRBK
      - Right ØRBJ
    - Sternoclavicular
      - Left ØRBF
      - Right ØRBE
    - Tarsal
      - Left ØSBJ
      - Right ØSBH
    - Tarsometatarsal
      - Left ØSBL
      - Right ØSBK
    - Temporomandibular
      - Left ØRBD
      - Right ØRBC
    - Thoracic Vertebral ØRB6
    - Thoracolumbar Vertebral ØRBA

- Excision *(Continued)*
  - Joint *(Continued)*
    - Toe Phalangeal
      - Left ØSBQ
      - Right ØSBP
    - Wrist
      - Left ØRBP
      - Right ØRBN
  - Kidney
    - Left ØTB1
    - Right ØTBØ
  - Kidney Pelvis
    - Left ØTB4
    - Right ØTB3
  - Knee Region
    - Left ØYBG
    - Right ØYBF
  - Larynx ØCBS
  - Leg
    - Lower
      - Left ØYBJ
      - Right ØYBH
    - Upper
      - Left ØYBD
      - Right ØYBC
  - Lens
    - Left Ø8BK3Z
    - Right Ø8BJ3Z
  - Lip
    - Lower ØCB1
    - Upper ØCBØ
  - Liver ØFBØ
    - Left Lobe ØFB2
    - Right Lobe ØFB1
  - Lung
    - Bilateral ØBBM
    - Left ØBBL
    - Lower Lobe
      - Left ØBBJ
      - Right ØBBF
    - Middle Lobe, Right ØBBD
    - Right ØBBK
    - Upper Lobe
      - Left ØBBG
      - Right ØBBC
  - Lung Lingula ØBBH
  - Lymphatic
    - Aortic Ø7BD
    - Axillary
      - Left Ø7B6
      - Right Ø7B5
    - Head Ø7BØ
    - Inguinal
      - Left Ø7BJ
      - Right Ø7BH
    - Internal Mammary
      - Left Ø7B9
      - Right Ø7B8
    - Lower Extremity
      - Left Ø7BG
      - Right Ø7BF
    - Mesenteric Ø7BB
    - Neck
      - Left Ø7B2
      - Right Ø7B1
    - Pelvis Ø7BC
    - Thoracic Duct Ø7BK
    - Thorax Ø7B7
    - Upper Extremity
      - Left Ø7B4
      - Right Ø7B3
  - Mandible
    - Left ØNBV
    - Right ØNBT
  - Maxilla ØNBR
  - Mediastinum ØWBC
  - Medulla Oblongata ØØBD
  - Mesentery ØDBV
  - Metacarpal
    - Left ØPBQ
    - Right ØPBP

- Excision *(Continued)*
  - Metatarsal
    - Left ØQBP
    - Right ØQBN
  - Muscle
    - Abdomen
      - Left ØKBL
      - Right ØKBK
    - Extraocular
      - Left Ø8BM
      - Right Ø8BL
    - Facial ØKB1
    - Foot
      - Left ØKBW
      - Right ØKBV
    - Hand
      - Left ØKBD
      - Right ØKBC
    - Head ØKBØ
    - Hip
      - Left ØKBP
      - Right ØKBN
    - Lower Arm and Wrist
      - Left ØKBB
      - Right ØKB9
    - Lower Leg
      - Left ØKBT
      - Right ØKBS
    - Neck
      - Left ØKB3
      - Right ØKB2
    - Papillary Ø2BD
    - Perineum ØKBM
    - Shoulder
      - Left ØKB6
      - Right ØKB5
    - Thorax
      - Left ØKBJ
      - Right ØKBH
    - Tongue, Palate, Pharynx ØKB4
    - Trunk
      - Left ØKBG
      - Right ØKBF
    - Upper Arm
      - Left ØKB8
      - Right ØKB7
    - Upper Leg
      - Left ØKBR
      - Right ØKBQ
  - Nasal Mucosa and Soft Tissue Ø9BK
  - Nasopharynx Ø9BN
  - Neck ØWB6
  - Nerve
    - Abdominal Sympathetic Ø1BM
    - Abducens ØØBL
    - Accessory ØØBR
    - Acoustic ØØBN
    - Brachial Plexus Ø1B3
    - Cervical Ø1B1
    - Cervical Plexus Ø1BØ
    - Facial ØØBM
    - Femoral Ø1BD
    - Glossopharyngeal ØØBP
    - Head and Neck Sympathetic Ø1BK
    - Hypoglossal ØØBS
    - Lumbar Ø1BB
    - Lumbar Plexus Ø1B9
    - Lumbar Sympathetic Ø1BN
    - Lumbosacral Plexus Ø1BA
    - Median Ø1B5
    - Oculomotor ØØBH
    - Olfactory ØØBF
    - Optic ØØBG
    - Peroneal Ø1BH
    - Phrenic Ø1B2
    - Pudendal Ø1BC
    - Radial Ø1B6
    - Sacral Ø1BR
    - Sacral Plexus Ø1BQ
    - Sacral Sympathetic Ø1BP
    - Sciatic Ø1BF

E

Excision (Continued)
Nerve (Continued)
Thoracic Ø1B8
Thoracic Sympathetic Ø1BL
Tibial Ø1BG
Trigeminal ØØBK
Trochlear ØØBJ
Ulnar Ø1B4
Vagus ØØBQ
Nipple
Left ØHBX
Right ØHBW
Omentum ØDBU
Oral Cavity and Throat ØWB3
Orbit
Left ØNBQ
Right ØNBP
Ovary
Bilateral ØUB2
Left ØUB1
Right ØUBØ
Palate
Hard ØCB2
Soft ØCB3
Pancreas ØFBG
Para-aortic Body ØGB9
Paraganglion Extremity ØGBF
Parathyroid Gland ØGBR
Inferior
Left ØGBP
Right ØGBN
Multiple ØGBQ
Superior
Left ØGBM
Right ØGBL
Patella
Left ØQBF
Right ØQBD
Penis ØVBS
Pericardium Ø2BN
Perineum
Female ØWBN
Male ØWBM
Peritoneum ØDBW
Phalanx
Finger
Left ØPBV
Right ØPBT
Thumb
Left ØPBS
Right ØPBR
Toe
Left ØQBR
Right ØQBQ
Pharynx ØCBM
Pineal Body ØGB1
Pleura
Left ØBBP
Right ØBBN
Pons ØØBB
Prepuce ØVBT
Prostate ØVBØ
Radius
Left ØPBJ
Right ØPBH
Rectum ØDBP
Retina
Left Ø8BF3Z
Right Ø8BE3Z
Retroperitoneum ØWBH
Ribs
1 to 2 ØPB1
3 or More ØPB2
Sacrum ØQB1
Scapula
Left ØPB6
Right ØPB5
Sclera
Left Ø8B7XZ
Right Ø8B6XZ

Excision (Continued)
Scrotum ØVB5
Septum
Atrial Ø2B5
Nasal Ø9BM
Ventricular Ø2BM
Shoulder Region
Left ØXB3
Right ØXB2
Sinus
Accessory Ø9BP
Ethmoid
Left Ø9BV
Right Ø9BU
Frontal
Left Ø9BT
Right Ø9BS
Mastoid
Left Ø9BC
Right Ø9BB
Maxillary
Left Ø9BR
Right Ø9BQ
Sphenoid
Left Ø9BX
Right Ø9BW
Skin
Abdomen ØHB7XZ
Back ØHB6XZ
Buttock ØHB8XZ
Chest ØHB5XZ
Ear
Left ØHB3XZ
Right ØHB2XZ
Face ØHB1XZ
Foot
Left ØHBNXZ
Right ØHBMXZ
Hand
Left ØHBGXZ
Right ØHBFXZ
Inguinal ØHBAXZ
Lower Arm
Left ØHBEXZ
Right ØHBDXZ
Lower Leg
Left ØHBLXZ
Right ØHBKXZ
Neck ØHB4XZ
Perineum ØHB9XZ
Scalp ØHBØXZ
Upper Arm
Left ØHBCXZ
Right ØHBBXZ
Upper Leg
Left ØHBJXZ
Right ØHBHXZ
Skull ØNBØ
Spinal Cord
Cervical ØØBW
Lumbar ØØBY
Thoracic ØØBX
Spinal Meninges ØØBT
Spleen Ø7BP
Sternum ØPBØ
Stomach ØDB6
Pylorus ØDB7
Subcutaneous Tissue and Fascia
Abdomen ØJB8
Back ØJB7
Buttock ØJB9
Chest ØJB6
Face ØJB1
Foot
Left ØJBR
Right ØJBQ
Hand
Left ØJBK
Right ØJBJ

Excision (Continued)
Subcutaneous Tissue and Fascia (Continued)
Lower Arm
Left ØJBH
Right ØJBG
Lower Leg
Left ØJBP
Right ØJBN
Neck
Left Ø6B5
Right Ø6B4
Pelvic Region ØJBC
Perineum ØJBB
Scalp ØJBØ
Upper Arm
Left ØJBF
Right ØJBD
Upper Leg
Left ØJBM
Right ØJBL
Tarsal
Left ØQBM
Right ØQBL
Tendon
Abdomen
Left ØLBG
Right ØLBF
Ankle
Left ØLBT
Right ØLBS
Foot
Left ØLBW
Right ØLBV
Hand
Left ØLB8
Right ØLB7
Head and Neck ØLBØ
Hip
Left ØLBK
Right ØLBJ
Knee
Left ØLBR
Right ØLBQ
Lower Arm and Wrist
Left ØLB6
Right ØLB5
Lower Leg
Left ØLBP
Right ØLBN
Perineum ØLBH
Shoulder
Left ØLB2
Right ØLB1
Thorax
Left ØLBD
Right ØLBC
Trunk
Left ØLBB
Right ØLB9
Upper Arm
Left ØLB4
Right ØLB3
Upper Leg
Left ØLBM
Right ØLBL
Testis
Bilateral ØVBC
Left ØVBB
Right ØVB9
Thalamus ØØB9
Thymus Ø7BM
Thyroid Gland
Left Lobe ØGBG
Right Lobe ØGBH
Thyroid Gland Isthmus ØGBJ
Tibia
Left ØQBH
Right ØQBG
Toe Nail ØHBRXZ
Tongue ØCB7

E

Excision *(Continued)*
Tonsils ØCBP
Tooth
Lower ØCBX
Upper ØCBW
Trachea ØBB1
Tunica Vaginalis
Left ØVB7
Right ØVB6
Turbinate, Nasal Ø9BL
Tympanic Membrane
Left Ø9B8
Right Ø9B7
Ulna
Left ØPBL
Right ØPBK
Ureter
Left ØTB7
Right ØTB6
Urethra ØTBD
Uterine Supporting Structure ØUB4
Uterus ØUB9
Uvula ØCBN
Vagina ØUBG
Valve
Aortic Ø2BF
Mitral Ø2BG
Pulmonary Ø2BH
Tricuspid Ø2BJ
Vas Deferens
Bilateral ØVBQ
Left ØVBP
Right ØVBN
Vein
Axillary
Left Ø5B8
Right Ø5B7
Azygos Ø5BØ
Basilic
Left Ø5BC
Right Ø5BB
Brachial
Left Ø5BA
Right Ø5B9
Cephalic
Left Ø5BF
Right Ø5BD
Colic Ø6B7
Common Iliac
Left Ø6BD
Right Ø6BC
Coronary Ø2B4
Esophageal Ø6B3
External Iliac
Left Ø6BG
Right Ø6BF
External Jugular
Left Ø5BQ
Right Ø5BP
Face
Left Ø5BV
Right Ø5BT
Femoral
Left Ø6BN
Right Ø6BM
Foot
Left Ø6BV
Right Ø6BT
Gastric Ø6B2
Hand
Left Ø5BH
Right Ø5BG
Hemiazygos Ø5B1
Hepatic Ø6B4
Hypogastric
Left Ø6BJ
Right Ø6BH
Inferior Mesenteric Ø6B6

Excision *(Continued)*
Vein *(Continued)*
Innominate
Left Ø5B4
Right Ø5B3
Internal Jugular
Left Ø5BN
Right Ø5BM
Intracranial Ø5BL
Lower Ø6BY
Portal Ø6B8
Pulmonary
Left Ø2BT
Right Ø2BS
Renal
Left Ø6BB
Right Ø6B9
Saphenous
Left Ø6BQ
Right Ø6BP
Splenic Ø6B1
Subclavian
Left Ø5B6
Right Ø5B5
Superior Mesenteric Ø6B5
Upper Ø5BY
Vertebral
Left Ø5BS
Right Ø5BR
Vena Cava
Inferior Ø6BØ
Superior Ø2BV
Ventricle
Left Ø2BL
Right Ø2BK
Vertebra
Cervical ØPB3
Lumbar ØQBØ
Thoracic ØPB4
Vesicle
Bilateral ØVB3
Left ØVB2
Right ØVB1
Vitreous
Left Ø8B53Z
Right Ø8B43Z
Vocal Cord
Left ØCBV
Right ØCBT
Vulva ØUBM
Wrist Region
Left ØXBH
Right ØXBG
EXCLUDER® AAA Endoprosthesis
use Intraluminal Device, Branched or Fenestrated, One or Two Arteries in Ø4V
use Intraluminal Device, Branched or Fenestrated, Three or More Arteries in Ø4V
use Intraluminal Device
EXCLUDER® IBE Endoprosthesis use Intraluminal Device, Branched or Fenestrated, One or Two Arteries in Ø4V
Exclusion, Left atrial appendage (LAA) *see* Occlusion, Atrium, Left Ø2L7
Exercise, rehabilitation *see* Motor Treatment, Rehabilitation FØ7
Exploration *see* Inspection
▶**Exploratory**
▶*see* Inspection, Anatomical Regions, General ØWJ
▶*see* Laparotomy
▶*see* Thoracotomy
Express® (LD) Premounted Stent System *use* Intraluminal Device
Express® Biliary SD Monorail® Premounted Stent System *use* Intraluminal Device
Express® SD Renal Monorail® Premounted Stent System *use* Intraluminal Device
Extensor carpi radialis muscle
use Lower Arm and Wrist Muscle, Right
use Lower Arm and Wrist Muscle, Left

Extensor carpi ulnaris muscle
use Lower Arm and Wrist Muscle, Right
use Lower Arm and Wrist Muscle, Left
Extensor digitorum brevis muscle
use Foot Muscle, Right
use Foot Muscle, Left
Extensor digitorum longus muscle
use Lower Leg Muscle, Right
use Lower Leg Muscle, Left
Extensor hallucis brevis muscle
use Foot Muscle, Right
use Foot Muscle, Left
Extensor hallucis longus muscle
use Lower Leg Muscle, Right
use Lower Leg Muscle, Left
External anal sphincter *use* Anal Sphincter
External auditory meatus
use External Auditory Canal, Right
use External Auditory Canal, Left
External fixator
use External Fixation Device in Head and Facial Bones
use External Fixation Device in Upper Bones
use External Fixation Device in Lower Bones
use External Fixation Device in Upper Joints
use External Fixation Device in Lower Joints
External maxillary artery *use* Face Artery
External naris *use* Nasal Mucosa and Soft Tissue
External oblique aponeurosis *use* Subcutaneous Tissue and Fascia, Trunk
External oblique muscle
use Abdomen Muscle, Right
use Abdomen Muscle, Left
External popliteal nerve *use* Peroneal Nerve
External pudendal artery
use Femoral Artery, Right
use Femoral Artery, Left
External pudendal vein
use Saphenous Vein, Right
use Saphenous Vein, Left
External urethral sphincter *use* Urethra
Extirpation
Acetabulum
Left ØQC5
Right ØQC4
Adenoids ØCCQ
Ampulla of Vater ØFCC
Anal Sphincter ØDCR
Anterior Chamber
Left Ø8C3
Right Ø8C2
Anus ØDCQ
Aorta
Abdominal Ø4CØ
Thoracic
Ascending/Arch Ø2CX
Descending Ø2CW
Aortic Body ØGCD
Appendix ØDCJ
Artery
Anterior Tibial
Left Ø4CQ
Right Ø4CP
Axillary
Left Ø3C6
Right Ø3C5
Brachial
Left Ø3C8
Right Ø3C7
Celiac Ø4C1
Colic
Left Ø4C7
Middle Ø4C8
Right Ø4C6
Common Carotid
Left Ø3CJ
Right Ø3CH
Common Iliac
Left Ø4CD
Right Ø4CC

E

- Extirpation *(Continued)*
  - Artery *(Continued)*
    - Coronary
      - Four or More Arteries Ø2C3
      - One Artery Ø2CØ
      - Three Arteries Ø2C2
      - Two Arteries Ø2C1
    - External Carotid
      - Left Ø3CN
      - Right Ø3CM
    - External Iliac
      - Left Ø4CJ
      - Right Ø4CH
    - Face Ø3CR
    - Femoral
      - Left Ø4CL
      - Right Ø4CK
    - Foot
      - Left Ø4CW
      - Right Ø4CV
    - Gastric Ø4C2
    - Hand
      - Left Ø3CF
      - Right Ø3CD
    - Hepatic Ø4C3
    - Inferior Mesenteric Ø4CB
    - Innominate Ø3C2
    - Internal Carotid
      - Left Ø3CL
      - Right Ø3CK
    - Internal Iliac
      - Left Ø4CF
      - Right Ø4CE
    - Internal Mammary
      - Left Ø3C1
      - Right Ø3CØ
    - Intracranial Ø3CG
    - Jaw
      - Lower ØWC5
      - Upper ØWC4
    - Lower Ø4CY
    - Peroneal
      - Left Ø4CU
      - Right Ø4CT
    - Popliteal
      - Left Ø4CN
      - Right Ø4CM
    - Posterior Tibial
      - Left Ø4CS
      - Right Ø4CR
    - Pulmonary
      - Left Ø2CR
      - Right Ø2CQ
    - Pulmonary Trunk Ø2CP
    - Radial
      - Left Ø3CC
      - Right Ø3CB
    - Renal
      - Left Ø4CA
      - Right Ø4C9
    - Splenic Ø4C4
    - Subclavian
      - Left Ø3C4
      - Right Ø3C3
    - Superior Mesenteric Ø4C5
    - Temporal
      - Left Ø3CT
      - Right Ø3CS
    - Thyroid
      - Left Ø3CV
      - Right Ø3CU
    - Ulnar
      - Left Ø3CA
      - Right Ø3C9
    - Upper Ø3CY
    - Vertebral
      - Left Ø3CQ
      - Right Ø3CP
  - Atrium
    - Left Ø2C7
    - Right Ø2C6

- Extirpation *(Continued)*
  - Auditory Ossicle
    - Left Ø9CA
    - Right Ø9C9
  - Basal Ganglia ØØC8
  - Bladder ØTCB
  - Bladder Neck ØTCC
  - Bone
    - Ethmoid
      - Left ØNCG
      - Right ØNCF
    - Frontal ØNC1
    - Hyoid ØNCX
    - Lacrimal
      - Left ØNCJ
      - Right ØNCH
    - Nasal ØNCB
    - Occipital ØNC7
    - Palatine
      - Left ØNCL
      - Right ØNCK
    - Parietal
      - Left ØNC4
      - Right ØNC3
    - Pelvic
      - Left ØQC3
      - Right ØQC2
    - Sphenoid ØNCC
    - Temporal
      - Left ØNC6
      - Right ØNC5
    - Zygomatic
      - Left ØNCN
      - Right ØNCM
  - Brain ØØCØ
  - Breast
    - Bilateral ØHCV
    - Left ØHCU
    - Right ØHCT
  - Bronchus
    - Lingula ØBC9
    - Lower Lobe
      - Left ØBCB
      - Right ØBC6
    - Main
      - Left ØBC7
      - Right ØBC3
    - Middle Lobe, Right ØBC5
    - Upper Lobe
      - Left ØBC8
      - Right ØBC4
  - Buccal Mucosa ØCC4
  - Bursa and Ligament
    - Abdomen
      - Left ØMCJ
      - Right ØMCH
    - Ankle
      - Left ØMCR
      - Right ØMCQ
    - Elbow
      - Left ØMC4
      - Right ØMC3
    - Foot
      - Left ØMCT
      - Right ØMCS
    - Hand
      - Left ØMC8
      - Right ØMC7
    - Head and Neck ØMCØ
    - Hip
      - Left ØMCM
      - Right ØMCL
    - Knee
      - Left ØMCP
      - Right ØMCN
    - Lower Extremity
      - Left ØMCW
      - Right ØMCV
    - Perineum ØMCK
    - Rib(s) ØMCG

- Extirpation *(Continued)*
  - Bursa and Ligament *(Continued)*
    - Shoulder
      - Left ØMC2
      - Right ØMC1
    - Spine
      - Lower ØMCD
      - Upper ØMCC
    - Sternum ØMCF
    - Upper Extremity
      - Left ØMCB
      - Right ØMC9
    - Wrist
      - Left ØMC6
      - Right ØMC5
  - Carina ØBC2
  - Carotid Bodies, Bilateral ØGC8
  - Carotid Body
    - Left ØGC6
    - Right ØGC7
  - Carpal
    - Left ØPCN
    - Right ØPCM
  - Cavity, Cranial ØWC1
  - Cecum ØDCH
  - Cerebellum ØØCC
  - Cerebral Hemisphere ØØC7
  - Cerebral Meninges ØØC1
  - Cerebral Ventricle ØØC6
  - Cervix ØUCC
  - Chordae Tendineae Ø2C9
  - Choroid
    - Left Ø8CB
    - Right Ø8CA
  - Cisterna Chyli Ø7CL
  - Clavicle
    - Left ØPCB
    - Right ØPC9
  - Clitoris ØUCJ
  - Coccygeal Glomus ØGCB
  - Coccyx ØQCS
  - Colon
    - Ascending ØDCK
    - Descending ØDCM
    - Sigmoid ØDCN
    - Transverse ØDCL
  - Computer-aided Mechanical Aspiration X2C
  - Conduction Mechanism Ø2C8
  - Conjunctiva
    - Left Ø8CTXZZ
    - Right Ø8CSXZZ
  - Cord
    - Bilateral ØVCH
    - Left ØVCG
    - Right ØVCF
  - Cornea
    - Left Ø8C9XZZ
    - Right Ø8C8XZZ
  - Cul-de-sac ØUCF
  - Diaphragm ØBCT
  - Disc
    - Cervical Vertebral ØRC3
    - Cervicothoracic Vertebral ØRC5
    - Lumbar Vertebral ØSC2
    - Lumbosacral ØSC4
    - Thoracic Vertebral ØRC9
    - Thoracolumbar Vertebral ØRCB
  - Duct
    - Common Bile ØFC9
    - Cystic ØFC8
    - Hepatic
      - Common ØFC7
      - Left ØFC6
      - Right ØFC5
    - Lacrimal
      - Left Ø8CY
      - Right Ø8CX
    - Pancreatic ØFCD
      - Accessory ØFCF
    - Parotid
      - Left ØCCC
      - Right ØCCB

E

- Extirpation *(Continued)*
  - Duodenum ØDC9
  - Dura Mater ØØC2
  - Ear
    - External
      - Left Ø9C1
      - Right Ø9CØ
    - External Auditory Canal
      - Left Ø9C4
      - Right Ø9C3
    - Inner
      - Left Ø9CE
      - Right Ø9CD
    - Middle
      - Left Ø9C6
      - Right Ø9C5
  - Endometrium ØUCB
  - Epididymis
    - Bilateral ØVCL
    - Left ØVCK
    - Right ØVCJ
  - Epidural Space, Intracranial ØØC3
  - Epiglottis ØCCR
  - Esophagogastric Junction ØDC4
  - Esophagus ØDC5
    - Lower ØDC3
    - Middle ØDC2
    - Upper ØDC1
  - Eustachian Tube
    - Left Ø9CG
    - Right Ø9CF
  - Eye
    - Left Ø8C1XZZ
    - Right Ø8CØXZZ
  - Eyelid
    - Lower
      - Left Ø8CR
      - Right Ø8CQ
    - Upper
      - Left Ø8CP
      - Right Ø8CN
  - Fallopian Tube
    - Left ØUC6
    - Right ØUC5
  - Fallopian Tubes, Bilateral ØUC7
  - Femoral Shaft
    - Left ØQC9
    - Right ØQC8
  - Femur
    - Lower
      - Left ØQCC
      - Right ØQCB
    - Upper
      - Left ØQC7
      - Right ØQC6
  - Fibula
    - Left ØQCK
    - Right ØQCJ
  - Finger Nail ØHCQXZZ
  - Gallbladder ØFC4
  - Gastrointestinal Tract ØWCP
  - Genitourinary Tract ØWCR
  - Gingiva
    - Lower ØCC6
    - Upper ØCC5
  - Gland
    - Adrenal
      - Bilateral ØGC4
      - Left ØGC2
      - Right ØGC3
    - Lacrimal
      - Left Ø8CW
      - Right Ø8CV
    - Minor Salivary ØCCJ
    - Parotid
      - Left ØCC9
      - Right ØCC8
    - Pituitary ØGCØ
    - Sublingual
      - Left ØCCF
      - Right ØCCD

- Extirpation *(Continued)*
  - Gland *(Continued)*
    - Submaxillary
      - Left ØCCH
      - Right ØCCG
    - Vestibular ØUCL
  - Glenoid Cavity
    - Left ØPC8
    - Right ØPC7
  - Glomus Jugulare ØGCC
  - Humeral Head
    - Left ØPCD
    - Right ØPCC
  - Humeral Shaft
    - Left ØPCG
    - Right ØPCF
  - Hymen ØUCK
  - Hypothalamus ØØCA
  - Ileocecal Valve ØDCC
  - Ileum ØDCB
  - Intestine
    - Large ØDCE
      - Left ØDCG
      - Right ØDCF
    - Small ØDC8
  - Iris
    - Left Ø8CD
    - Right Ø8CC
  - Jejunum ØDCA
  - Joint
    - Acromioclavicular
      - Left ØRCH
      - Right ØRCG
    - Ankle
      - Left ØSCG
      - Right ØSCF
    - Carpal
      - Left ØRCR
      - Right ØRCQ
    - Carpometacarpal
      - Left ØRCT
      - Right ØRCS
    - Cervical Vertebral ØRC1
    - Cervicothoracic Vertebral ØRC4
    - Coccygeal ØSC6
    - Elbow
      - Left ØRCM
      - Right ØRCL
    - Finger Phalangeal
      - Left ØRCX
      - Right ØRCW
    - Hip
      - Left ØSCB
      - Right ØSC9
    - Knee
      - Left ØSCD
      - Right ØSCC
    - Lumbar Vertebral ØSCØ
    - Lumbosacral ØSC3
    - Metacarpophalangeal
      - Left ØRCV
      - Right ØRCU
    - Metatarsal-Phalangeal
      - Left ØSCN
      - Right ØSCM
    - Occipital-cervical ØRCØ
    - Sacrococcygeal ØSC5
    - Sacroiliac
      - Left ØSC8
      - Right ØSC7
    - Shoulder
      - Left ØRCK
      - Right ØRCJ
    - Sternoclavicular
      - Left ØRCF
      - Right ØRCE
    - Tarsal
      - Left ØSCJ
      - Right ØSCH

- Extirpation *(Continued)*
  - Joint *(Continued)*
    - Tarsometatarsal
      - Left ØSCL
      - Right ØSCK
    - Temporomandibular
      - Left ØRCD
      - Right ØRCC
    - Thoracic Vertebral ØRC6
    - Thoracolumbar Vertebral ØRCA
    - Toe Phalangeal
      - Left ØSCQ
      - Right ØSCP
    - Wrist
      - Left ØRCP
      - Right ØRCN
  - Kidney
    - Left ØTC1
    - Right ØTCØ
  - Kidney Pelvis
    - Left ØTC4
    - Right ØTC3
  - Larynx ØCCS
  - Lens
    - Left Ø8CK
    - Right Ø8CJ
  - Lip
    - Lower ØCC1
    - Upper ØCCØ
  - Liver ØFCØ
    - Left Lobe ØFC2
    - Right Lobe ØFC1
  - Lung
    - Bilateral ØBCM
    - Left ØBCL
    - Lower Lobe
      - Left ØBCJ
      - Right ØBCF
    - Middle Lobe, Right ØBCD
    - Right ØBCK
    - Upper Lobe
      - Left ØBCG
      - Right ØBCC
  - Lung Lingula ØBCH
  - Lymphatic
    - Aortic Ø7CD
    - Axillary
      - Left Ø7C6
      - Right Ø7C5
    - Head Ø7CØ
    - Inguinal
      - Left Ø7CJ
      - Right Ø7CH
    - Internal Mammary
      - Left Ø7C9
      - Right Ø7C8
    - Lower Extremity
      - Left Ø7CG
      - Right Ø7CF
    - Mesenteric Ø7CB
    - Neck
      - Left Ø7C2
      - Right Ø7C1
    - Pelvis Ø7CC
    - Thoracic Duct Ø7CK
    - Thorax Ø7C7
    - Upper Extremity
      - Left Ø7C4
      - Right Ø7C3
  - Mandible
    - Left ØNCV
    - Right ØNCT
  - Maxilla ØNCR
  - Mediastinum ØWCC
  - Medulla Oblongata ØØCD
  - Mesentery ØDCV
  - Metacarpal
    - Left ØPCQ
    - Right ØPCP

E

Extirpation (Continued)
Joint (Continued)
Metatarsal
Left ØQCP
Right ØQCN
Muscle
Abdomen
Left ØKCL
Right ØKCK
Extraocular
Left Ø8CM
Right Ø8CL
Facial ØKC1
Foot
Left ØKCW
Right ØKCV
Hand
Left ØKCD
Right ØKCC
Head ØKCØ
Hip
Left ØKCP
Right ØKCN
Lower Arm and Wrist
Left ØKCB
Right ØKC9
Lower Leg
Left ØKCT
Right ØKCS
Neck
Left ØKC3
Right ØKC2
Papillary Ø2CD
Perineum ØKCM
Shoulder
Left ØKC6
Right ØKC5
Thorax
Left ØKCJ
Right ØKCH
Tongue, Palate, Pharynx ØKC4
Trunk
Left ØKCG
Right ØKCF
Upper Arm
Left ØKC8
Right ØKC7
Upper Leg
Left ØKCR
Right ØKCQ
Nasal Mucosa and Soft Tissue Ø9CK
Nasopharynx Ø9CN
Nerve
Abdominal Sympathetic Ø1CM
Abducens ØØCL
Accessory ØØCR
Acoustic ØØCN
Brachial Plexus Ø1C3
Cervical Ø1C1
Cervical Plexus Ø1CØ
Facial ØØCM
Femoral Ø1CD
Glossopharyngeal ØØCP
Head and Neck Sympathetic Ø1CK
Hypoglossal ØØCS
Lumbar Ø1CB
Lumbar Plexus Ø1C9
Lumbar Sympathetic Ø1CN
Lumbosacral Plexus Ø1CA
Median Ø1C5
Oculomotor ØØCH
Olfactory ØØCF
Optic ØØCG
Peroneal Ø1CH
Phrenic Ø1C2
Pudendal Ø1CC
Radial Ø1C6
Sacral Ø1CR
Sacral Plexus Ø1CQ
Sacral Sympathetic Ø1CP
Sciatic Ø1CF

Extirpation (Continued)
Nerve (Continued)
Thoracic Ø1C8
Thoracic Sympathetic Ø1CL
Tibial Ø1CG
Trigeminal ØØCK
Trochlear ØØCJ
Ulnar Ø1C4
Vagus ØØCQ
Nipple
Left ØHCX
Right ØHCW
Omentum ØDCU
Oral Cavity and Throat ØWC3
Orbit
Left ØNCQ
Right ØNCP
Orbital Atherectomy see Extirpation, Heart and Great Vessels Ø2C
Ovary
Bilateral ØUC2
Left ØUC1
Right ØUCØ
Palate
Hard ØCC2
Soft ØCC3
Pancreas ØFCG
Para-aortic Body ØGC9
Paraganglion Extremity ØGCF
Parathyroid Gland ØGCR
Inferior
Left ØGCP
Right ØGCN
Multiple ØGCQ
Superior
Left ØGCM
Right ØGCL
Patella
Left ØQCF
Right ØQCD
Pelvic Cavity ØWCJ
Penis ØVCS
Pericardial Cavity ØWCD
Pericardium Ø2CN
Peritoneal Cavity ØWCG
Peritoneum ØDCW
Phalanx
Finger
Left ØPCV
Right ØPCT
Thumb
Left ØPCS
Right ØPCR
Toe
Left ØQCR
Right ØQCQ
Pharynx ØCCM
Pineal Body ØGC1
Pleura
Left ØBCP
Right ØBCN
Pleural Cavity
Left ØWCB
Right ØWC9
Pons ØØCB
Prepuce ØVCT
Prostate ØVCØ
Radius
Left ØPCJ
Right ØPCH
Rectum ØDCP
Respiratory Tract ØWCQ
Retina
Left Ø8CF
Right Ø8CE
Retinal Vessel
Left Ø8CH
Right Ø8CG
Retroperitoneum ØWCH

Extirpation (Continued)
Ribs
1 to 2 ØPC1
3 or More ØPC2
Sacrum ØQC1
Scapula
Left ØPC6
Right ØPC5
Sclera
Left Ø8C7XZZ
Right Ø8C6XZZ
Scrotum ØVC5
Septum
Atrial Ø2C5
Nasal Ø9CM
Ventricular Ø2CM
Sinus
Accessory Ø9CP
Ethmoid
Left Ø9CV
Right Ø9CU
Frontal
Left Ø9CT
Right Ø9CS
Mastoid
Left Ø9CC
Right Ø9CB
Maxillary
Left Ø9CR
Right Ø9CQ
Sphenoid
Left Ø9CX
Right Ø9CW
Skin
Abdomen ØHC7XZZ
Back ØHC6XZZ
Buttock ØHC8XZZ
Chest ØHC5XZZ
Ear
Left ØHC3XZZ
Right ØHC2XZZ
Face ØHC1XZZ
Foot
Left ØHCNXZZ
Right ØHCMXZZ
Hand
Left ØHCGXZZ
Right ØHCFXZZ
Inguinal ØHCAXZZ
Lower Arm
Left ØHCEXZZ
Right ØHCDXZZ
Lower Leg
Left ØHCLXZZ
Right ØHCKXZZ
Neck ØHC4XZZ
Perineum ØHC9XZZ
Scalp ØHCØXZZ
Upper Arm
Left ØHCCXZZ
Right ØHCBXZZ
Upper Leg
Left ØHCJXZZ
Right ØHCHXZZ
Spinal Canal ØØCU
Spinal Cord
Cervical ØØCW
Lumbar ØØCY
Thoracic ØØCX
Spinal Meninges ØØCT
Spleen Ø7CP
Sternum ØPCØ
Stomach ØDC6
Pylorus ØDC7
Subarachnoid Space, Intracranial ØØC5
Subcutaneous Tissue and Fascia
Abdomen ØJC8
Back ØJC7
Buttock ØJC9
Chest ØJC6
Face ØJC1

E

Extirpation (Continued)
Subcutaneous Tissue and Fascia (Continued)
Foot
Left ØJCR
Right ØJCQ
Hand
Left ØJCK
Right ØJCJ
Lower Arm
Left ØJCH
Right ØJCG
Lower Leg
Left ØJCP
Right ØJCN
Neck
Left ØJC5
Right ØJC4
Pelvic Region ØJCC
Perineum ØJCB
Scalp ØJCØ
Upper Arm
Left ØJCF
Right ØJCD
Upper Leg
Left ØJCM
Right ØJCL
Subdural Space, Intracranial ØØC4
Tarsal
Left ØQCM
Right ØQCL
Tendon
Abdomen
Left ØLCG
Right ØLCF
Ankle
Left ØLCT
Right ØLCS
Foot
Left ØLCW
Right ØLCV
Hand
Left ØLC8
Right ØLC7
Head and Neck ØLCØ
Hip
Left ØLCK
Right ØLCJ
Knee
Left ØLCR
Right ØLCQ
Lower Arm and Wrist
Left ØLC6
Right ØLC5
Lower Leg
Left ØLCP
Right ØLCN
Perineum ØLCH
Shoulder
Left ØLC2
Right ØLC1
Thorax
Left ØLCD
Right ØLCC
Trunk
Left ØLCB
Right ØLC9
Upper Arm
Left ØLC4
Right ØLC3
Upper Leg
Left ØLCM
Right ØLCL
Testis
Bilateral ØVCC
Left ØVCB
Right ØVC9
Thalamus ØØC9
Thymus Ø7CM
Thyroid Gland ØGCK
Left Lobe ØGCG
Right Lobe ØGCH

Extirpation (Continued)
Tibia
Left ØQCH
Right ØQCG
Toe Nail ØHCRXZZ
Tongue ØCC7
Tonsils ØCCP
Tooth
Lower ØCCX
Upper ØCCW
Trachea ØBC1
Tunica Vaginalis
Left ØVC7
Right ØVC6
Turbinate, Nasal Ø9CL
Tympanic Membrane
Left Ø9C8
Right Ø9C7
Ulna
Left ØPCL
Right ØPCK
Ureter
Left ØTC7
Right ØTC6
Urethra ØTCD
Uterine Supporting Structure ØUC4
Uterus ØUC9
Uvula ØCCN
Vagina ØUCG
Valve
Aortic Ø2CF
Mitral Ø2CG
Pulmonary Ø2CH
Tricuspid Ø2CJ
Vas Deferens
Bilateral ØVCQ
Left ØVCP
Right ØVCN
Vein
Axillary
Left Ø5C8
Right Ø5C7
Azygos Ø5CØ
Basilic
Left Ø5CC
Right Ø5CB
Brachial
Left Ø5CA
Right Ø5C9
Cephalic
Left Ø5CF
Right Ø5CD
Colic Ø6C7
Common Iliac
Left Ø6CD
Right Ø6CC
Coronary Ø2C4
Esophageal Ø6C3
External Iliac
Left Ø6CG
Right Ø6CF
External Jugular
Left Ø5CQ
Right Ø5CP
Face
Left Ø5CV
Right Ø5CT
Femoral
Left Ø6CN
Right Ø6CM
Foot
Left Ø6CV
Right Ø6CT
Gastric Ø6C2
Hand
Left Ø5CH
Right Ø5CG
Hemiazygos Ø5C1
Hepatic Ø6C4

Extirpation (Continued)
Vein (Continued)
Hypogastric
Left Ø6CJ
Right Ø6CH
Inferior Mesenteric Ø6C6
Innominate
Left Ø5C4
Right Ø5C3
Internal Jugular
Left Ø5CN
Right Ø5CM
Intracranial Ø5CL
Lower Ø6CY
Portal Ø6C8
Pulmonary
Left Ø2CT
Right Ø2CS
Renal
Left Ø6CB
Right Ø6C9
Saphenous
Left Ø6CQ
Right Ø6CP
Splenic Ø6C1
Subclavian
Left Ø5C6
Right Ø5C5
Superior Mesenteric Ø6C5
Upper Ø5CY
Vertebral
Left Ø5CS
Right Ø5CR
Vena Cava
Inferior Ø6CØ
Superior Ø2CV
Ventricle
Left Ø2CL
Right Ø2CK
Vertebra
Cervical ØPC3
Lumbar ØQCØ
Thoracic ØPC4
Vesicle
Bilateral ØVC3
Left ØVC2
Right ØVC1
Vitreous
Left Ø8C5
Right Ø8C4
Vocal Cord
Left ØCCV
Right ØCCT
Vulva ØUCM
Extracorporeal Carbon Dioxide Removal (ECCO2R) 5AØ92ØZ
▶ Extracorporeal filter circuit, during percutaneous thrombectomy 5AØ5AØL
▶ Extracorporeal Pathogen Removal Procedure XXA536A
▶ Extracorporeal return, during percutaneous thrombectomy 5AØ5AØL
Extracorporeal shock wave lithotripsy *see* Fragmentation
Extracranial-intracranial bypass (EC-IC) *see* Bypass, Upper Arteries Ø31
Extraction
Acetabulum
Left ØQD5ØZZ
Right ØQD4ØZZ
Ampulla of Vater ØFDC
Anus ØDDQ
Appendix ØDDJ
Auditory Ossicle
Left Ø9DAØZZ
Right Ø9D9ØZZ
Bone
Ethmoid
Left ØNDGØZZ
Right ØNDFØZZ

Extraction (Continued)
Bone (Continued)
Frontal ØND1ØZZ
Hyoid ØNDXØZZ
Lacrimal
Left ØNDJØZZ
Right ØNDHØZZ
Nasal ØNDBØZZ
Occipital ØND7ØZZ
Palatine
Left ØNDLØZZ
Right ØNDKØZZ
Parietal
Left ØND4ØZZ
Right ØND3ØZZ
Pelvic
Left ØQD3ØZZ
Right ØQD2ØZZ
Sphenoid ØNDCØZZ
Temporal
Left ØND6ØZZ
Right ØND5ØZZ
Zygomatic
Left ØNDNØZZ
Right ØNDMØZZ
Bone Marrow Ø7DT
Iliac Ø7DR
Sternum Ø7DQ
Vertebral Ø7DS
Brain ØØDØ
Breast
Bilateral ØHDVØZZ
Left ØHDUØZZ
Right ØHDTØZZ
Supernumerary ØHDYØZXZ
Bronchus
Lingula ØBD9
Lower Lobe
Left ØBDB
Right ØBD6
Main
Left ØBD7
Right ØBD3
Middle Lobe, Right ØBD5
Upper Lobe
Left ØBD8
Right ØBD4
Bursa and Ligament
Abdomen
Left ØMDJ
Right ØMDH
Ankle
Left ØMDR
Right ØMDQ
Elbow
Left ØMD4
Right ØMD3
Foot
Left ØMDT
Right ØMDS
Hand
Left ØMD8
Right ØMD7
Head and Neck ØMDØ
Hip
Left ØMDM
Right ØMDL
Knee
Left ØMDP
Right ØMDN
Lower Extremity
Left ØMDW
Right ØMDV
Perineum ØMDK
Rib(s) ØMDG
Shoulder
Left ØMD2
Right ØMD1
Spine
Lower ØMDD
Upper ØMDC

Extraction (Continued)
Bursa and Ligament (Continued)
Sternum ØMDF
Upper Extremity
Left ØMDB
Right ØMD9
Wrist
Left ØMD6
Right ØMD5
Carina ØBD2
Carpal
Left ØPDNØZZ
Right ØPDMØZZ
Cecum ØDDH
Cerebellum ØØDC
Cerebral Hemisphere ØØD7
Cerebral Meninges ØØD1
Cisterna Chyli Ø7DL
Clavicle
Left ØPDBØZZ
Right ØPD9ØZZ
Coccyx ØQDSØZZ
Colon
Ascending ØDDK
Descending ØDDM
Sigmoid ØDDN
Transverse ØDDL
Cornea
Left Ø8D9XZ
Right Ø8D8XZ
Duct
Common Bile ØFD9
Cystic ØFD8
Hepatic
Common ØFD7
Left ØFD6
Right ØFD5
Pancreatic ØFDD
Accessory ØFDF
Duodenum ØDD9
Dura Mater ØØD2
Endometrium ØUDB
Esophagogastric Junction ØDD4
Esophagus ØDD5
Lower ØDD3
Middle ØDD2
Upper ØDD1
Femoral Shaft
Left ØQD9ØZZ
Right ØQD8ØZZ
Femur
Lower
Left ØQDCØZZ
Right ØQDBØZZ
Upper
Left ØQD7ØZZ
Right ØQD6ØZZ
Fibula
Left ØQDKØZZ
Right ØQDJØZZ
Finger Nail ØHDQXZZ
Gallbladder ØFD4
Glenoid Cavity
Left ØPD8ØZZ
Right ØPD7ØZZ
Hair ØHDSXZZ
Humeral Head
Left ØPDDØZZ
Right ØPDCØZZ
Humeral Shaft
Left ØPDGØZZ
Right ØPDFØZZ
Ileocecal Valve ØDDC
Ileum ØDDB
Intestine
Large ØDDE
Left ØDDG
Right ØDDF
Small ØDD8
Jejunum ØDDA

Extraction (Continued)
Kidney
Left ØTD1
Right ØTDØ
Lens
Left Ø8DK3ZZ
Right Ø8DJ3ZZ
Liver ØFDØ
Left Lobe ØFD2
Right Lobe ØFD1
Lung
Bilateral ØBDM
Left ØBDL
Lower Lobe
Left ØBDJ
Right ØBDF
Middle Lobe, Right ØBDD
Right ØBDK
Upper Lobe
Left ØBDG
Right ØBDC
Lung Lingula ØBDH
Lymphatic
Aortic Ø7DD
Axillary
Left Ø7D6
Right Ø7D5
Head Ø7DØ
Inguinal
Left Ø7DJ
Right Ø7DH
Internal Mammary
Left Ø7D9
Right Ø7D8
Lower Extremity
Left Ø7DG
Right Ø7DF
Mesenteric Ø7DB
Neck
Left Ø7D2
Right Ø7D1
Pelvis Ø7DC
Thoracic Duct Ø7DK
Thorax Ø7D7
Upper Extremity
Left Ø7D4
Right Ø7D3
Mandible
Left ØNDVØZZ
Right ØNDTØZZ
Maxilla ØNDRØZZ
Metacarpal
Left ØPDQØZZ
Right ØPDPØZZ
Metatarsal
Left ØQDPØZZ
Right ØQDNØZZ
Muscle
Abdomen
Left ØKDLØZZ
Right ØKDKØZZ
Facial ØKD1ØZZ
Foot
Left ØKDWØZZ
Right ØKDVØZZ
Hand
Left ØKDDØZZ
Right ØKDCØZZ
Head ØKDØØZZ
Hip
Left ØKDPØZZ
Right ØKDNØZZ
Lower Arm and Wrist
Left ØKDBØZZ
Right ØKD9ØZZ
Lower Leg
Left ØKDTØZZ
Right ØKDSØZZ

E

▶ New ➠ Revised ~~deleted~~ Deleted

Extraction *(Continued)*
Muscle *(Continued)*
Neck
Left ØKD3ØZZ
Right ØKD2ØZZ
Perineum ØKDMØZZ
Shoulder
Left ØKD6ØZZ
Right ØKD5ØZZ
Thorax
Left ØKDJØZZ
Right ØKDHØZZ
Tongue, Palate, Pharynx ØKD4ØZZ
Trunk
Left ØKDGØZZ
Right ØKDFØZZ
Upper Arm
Left ØKD8ØZZ
Right ØKD7ØZZ
Upper Leg
Left ØKDRØZZ
Right ØKDQØZZ
Nerve
Abdominal Sympathetic Ø1DM
Abducens ØØDL
Accessory ØØDR
Acoustic ØØDN
Brachial Plexus Ø1D3
Cervical Ø1D1
Cervical Plexus Ø1DØ
Facial ØØDM
Femoral Ø1DD
Glossopharyngeal ØØDP
Head and Neck Sympathetic Ø1DK
Hypoglossal ØØDS
Lumbar Ø1DB
Lumbar Plexus Ø1D9
Lumbar Sympathetic Ø1DN
Lumbosacral Plexus Ø1DA
Median Ø1D5
Oculomotor ØØDH
Olfactory ØØDF
Optic ØØDG
Peroneal Ø1DH
Phrenic Ø1D2
Pudendal Ø1DC
Radial Ø1D6
Sacral Ø1DR
Sacral Plexus Ø1DQ
Sacral Sympathetic Ø1DP
Sciatic Ø1DF
Thoracic Ø1D8
Thoracic Sympathetic Ø1DL
Tibial Ø1DG
Trigeminal ØØDK
Trochlear ØØDJ
Ulnar Ø1D4
Vagus ØØDQ
Orbit
Left ØNDQØZZ
Right ØNDPØZZ
Pancreas ØFDG
Patella
Left ØQDFØZZ
Right ØQDDØZZ
Phalanx
Finger
Left ØPDVØZZ
Right ØPDTØZZ
Thumb
Left ØPDSØZZ
Right ØPDRØZZ
Toe
Left ØQDRØZZ
Right ØQDQØZZ
Ova ØUDN
Pleura
Left ØBDP
Right ØBDN

Extraction *(Continued)*
Products of Conception
Ectopic 1ØD2
Extraperitoneal 1ØDØØZ2
High 1ØDØØZØ
High Forceps 1ØDØ7Z5
Internal Version 1ØDØ7Z7
Low 1ØDØØZ1
Low Forceps 1ØDØ7Z3
Mid Forceps 1ØDØ7Z4
Other 1ØDØ7Z8
Retained 1ØD1
Vacuum 1ØDØ7Z6
Radius
Left ØPDJØZZ
Right ØPDHØZZ
Rectum ØDDP
Ribs
1 to 2 ØPD1ØZZ
3 or More ØPD2ØZZ
Sacrum ØQD1ØZZ
Scapula
Left ØPD6ØZZ
Right ØPD5ØZZ
Septum, Nasal Ø9DM
Sinus
Accessory Ø9DP
Ethmoid
Left Ø9DV
Right Ø9DU
Frontal
Left Ø9DT
Right Ø9DS
Mastoid
Left Ø9DC
Right Ø9DB
Maxillary
Left Ø9DR
Right Ø9DQ
Sphenoid
Left Ø9DX
Right Ø9DW
Skin
Abdomen ØHD7XZZ
Back ØHD6XZZ
Buttock ØHD8XZZ
Chest ØHD5XZZ
Ear
Left ØHD3XZZ
Right ØHD2XZZ
Face ØHD1XZZ
Foot
Left ØHDNXZZ
Right ØHDMXZZ
Hand
Left ØHDGXZZ
Right ØHDFXZZ
Inguinal ØHDAXZZ
Lower Arm
Left ØHDEXZZ
Right ØHDDXZZ
Lower Leg
Left ØHDLXZZ
Right ØHDKXZZ
Neck ØHD4XZZ
Perineum ØHD9XZZ
Scalp ØHDØXZZ
Upper Arm
Left ØHDCXZZ
Right ØHDBXZZ
Upper Leg
Left ØHDJXZZ
Right ØHDHXZZ
Skull ØNDØØZZ
Spinal Meninges ØØDT
Spleen Ø7DP
Sternum ØPDØØZZ
Stomach ØDD6
Pylorus ØDD7

Extraction *(Continued)*
Subcutaneous Tissue and Fascia
Abdomen ØJD8
Back ØJD7
Buttock ØJD9
Chest ØJD6
Face ØJD1
Foot
Left ØJDR
Right ØJDQ
Hand
Left ØJDK
Right ØJDJ
Lower Arm
Left ØJDH
Right ØJDG
Lower Leg
Left ØJDP
Right ØJDN
Neck
Left ØJD5
Right ØJD4
Pelvic Region ØJDC
Perineum ØJDB
Scalp ØJDØ
Upper Arm
Left ØJDF
Right ØJDD
Upper Leg
Left ØJDM
Right ØJDL
Tarsal
Left ØQDMØZZ
Right ØQDLØZZ
Tendon
Abdomen
Left ØLDGØZZ
Right ØLDFØZZ
Ankle
Left ØLDTØZZ
Right ØLDSØZZ
Foot
Left ØLDWØZZ
Right ØLDVØZZ
Hand
Left ØLD8ØZZ
Right ØLD7ØZZ
Head and Neck ØLDØØZZ
Hip
Left ØLDKØZZ
Right ØLDJØZZ
Knee
Left ØLDRØZZ
Right ØLDQØZZ
Lower Arm and Wrist
Left ØLD6ØZZ
Right ØLD5ØZZ
Lower Leg
Left ØLDPØZZ
Right ØLDNØZZ
Perineum ØLDHØZZ
Shoulder
Left ØLD2ØZZ
Right ØLD1ØZZ
Thorax
Left ØLDDØZZ
Right ØLDCØZZ
Trunk
Left ØLDBØZZ
Right ØLD9ØZZ
Upper Arm
Left ØLD4ØZZ
Right ØLD3ØZZ
Upper Leg
Left ØLDMØZZ
Right ØLDLØZZ
Thymus Ø7DM
Tibia
Left ØQDHØZZ
Right ØQDGØZZ

E

Extraction *(Continued)*
- Toe Nail ØHDRXZZ
- Tooth
  - Lower ØCDXXZ
  - Upper ØCDWXZ
- Trachea ØBD1
- Turbinate, Nasal Ø9DL
- Tympanic Membrane
  - Left Ø9D8
  - Right Ø9D7
- Ulna
  - Left ØPDLØZZ
  - Right ØPDKØZZ
- Vein
  - Basilic
    - Left Ø5DC
    - Right Ø5DB
  - Brachial
    - Left Ø5DA
    - Right Ø5D9
  - Cephalic
    - Left Ø5DF
    - Right Ø5DD
  - Femoral
    - Left Ø6DN
    - Right Ø6DM
  - Foot
    - Left Ø6DV
    - Right Ø6DT
  - Hand
    - Left Ø5DH
    - Right Ø5DG
  - Lower Ø6DY
  - Saphenous
    - Left Ø6DQ
    - Right Ø6DP
  - Upper Ø5DY
- Vertebra
  - Cervical ØPD3ØZZ
  - Lumbar ØQDØØZZ
  - Thoracic ØPD4ØZZ
- Vocal Cord
  - Left ØCDV
  - Right ØCDT

Extradural space, intracranial *use* Epidural Space, Intracranial

Extradural space, spinal *use* Spinal Canal

EXtreme Lateral Interbody Fusion (XLIF) device *use* Interbody Fusion Device in Lower Joints

F

Face lift *see* Alteration, Face ØWØ2
Facet FiXation implant *use* Facet Joint Fusion Device, Paired Titanium Cages in New Technology
Facet Joint Fusion Device, Paired Titanium Cages
 Lumbar Vertebral XRGBØEA
  2 or more XRGCØEA
 Lumbosacral XRGDØEA
 Thoracolumbar Vertebral XRGAØEA
Facet replacement spinal stabilization device
 use Spinal Stabilization Device, Facet Replacement in ØRH
 use Spinal Stabilization Device, Facet Replacement in ØSH
Facial artery *use* Face Artery
Factor Xa Inhibitor Reversal Agent, Andexanet Alfa *use* Coagulation Factor Xa, Inactivated
False vocal cord *use* Larynx
Falx cerebri *use* Dura Mater
Fascia lata
 use Subcutaneous Tissue and Fascia, Right Upper Leg
 use Subcutaneous Tissue and Fascia, Left Upper Leg
Fasciaplasty, fascioplasty
 see Repair, Subcutaneous Tissue and Fascia ØJQ
 see Replacement, Subcutaneous Tissue and Fascia ØJR
Fasciectomy
 see Excision, Subcutaneous Tissue and Fascia ØJB
Fasciorrhaphy *see* Repair, Subcutaneous Tissue and Fascia ØJQ
Fasciotomy
 see Division, Subcutaneous Tissue and Fascia ØJ8
 see Drainage, Subcutaneous Tissue and Fascia ØJ9
 see Release
Feeding Device
 Change device in
  Lower Intestinal Tract ØD2DXUZ
  Upper Intestinal Tract ØD2ØXUZ
 Insertion of device in
  Duodenum ØDH9
  Esophagus ØDH5
  Ileum ØDHB
  Intestine, Small ØDH8
  Jejunum ØDHA
  Stomach ØDH6
 Removal of device from
  Esophagus ØDP5
  Intestinal Tract
   Lower Intestinal Tract ØDPD
   Upper Intestinal Tract ØDPØ
  Stomach ØDP6
 Revision of device in
  Intestinal Tract
   Lower Intestinal Tract ØDWD
   Upper Intestinal Tract ØDWØ
  Stomach ØDW6
Femoral head
 use Upper Femur, Right
 use Upper Femur, Left
Femoral lymph node
 use Lymphatic, Right Lower Extremity
 use Lymphatic, Left Lower Extremity
Femoropatellar joint
 use Knee Joint, Right
 use Knee Joint, Left
 use Knee Joint, Femoral Surface, Right
 use Knee Joint, Femoral Surface, Left
Femorotibial joint
 use Knee Joint, Right
 use Knee Joint, Left
 use Knee Joint, Tibial Surface, Right
 use Knee Joint, Tibial Surface, Left
FETROJA® *use* Cefiderocol Anti-infective
FFX® (Facet FiXation) implant *use* Facet Joint Fusion Device, Paired Titanium Cages in NewTechnology
FGS (fluorescence-guided surgery)
 see Fluorescence Guided Procedure
Fiber Optic 3D Guided Procedure, Circulatory System 8EØ23FZ
Fibular artery
 use Peroneal Artery, Right
 use Peroneal Artery, Left
Fibular sesamoid
 use Metatarsal, Right
 use Metatarsal, Left
Fibularis brevis muscle
 use Lower Leg Muscle, Right
 use Lower Leg Muscle, Left
Fibularis longus muscle
 use Lower Leg Muscle, Right
 use Lower Leg Muscle, Left
Fifth cranial nerve *use* Trigeminal Nerve
Filtration, Blood Pathogens XXA536A
Filtration circuit, during percutaneous thrombectomy 5AØ5AØL
Filum terminale *use* Spinal Meninges
Fimbriectomy
 see Excision, Female Reproductive System ØUB
 see Resection, Female Reproductive System ØUT
Fine needle aspiration
 Fluid or gas *see* Drainage
 Tissue biopsy
  see Extraction
  see Excision
First cranial nerve *use* Olfactory Nerve
First intercostal nerve *use* Brachial Plexus
Fish skin *use* Nonautologous Tissue Substitute
Fistulization
 see Bypass
 see Drainage
 see Repair
Fistulization, Tracheoesophageal ØB11ØD6
Fitting
 Arch bars, for fracture reduction *see* Reposition, Mouth and Throat ØCS
 Arch bars, for immobilization *see* Immobilization, Face 2W31
 Artificial limb *see* Device Fitting, Rehabilitation FØD
 Hearing aid *see* Device Fitting, Rehabilitation FØD
 Ocular prosthesis FØDZ8UZ
 Prosthesis, limb *see* Device Fitting, Rehabilitation FØD
 Prosthesis, ocular FØDZ8UZ
Fixation, bone
 External, with fracture reduction *see* Reposition
 External, without fracture reduction *see* Insertion
 Internal, with fracture reduction *see* Reposition
 Internal, without fracture reduction *see* Insertion
FLAIR® Endovascular Stent Graft *use* Intraluminal Device
Flexible Composite Mesh *use* Synthetic Substitute
Flexor carpi radialis muscle
 use Lower Arm and Wrist Muscle, Right
 use Lower Arm and Wrist Muscle, Left
Flexor carpi ulnaris muscle
 use Lower Arm and Wrist Muscle, Right
 use Lower Arm and Wrist Muscle, Left
Flexor digitorum brevis muscle
 use Foot Muscle, Right
 use Foot Muscle, Left
Flexor digitorum longus muscle
 use Lower Leg Muscle, Right
 use Lower Leg Muscle, Left
Flexor hallucis brevis muscle
 use Foot Muscle, Right
 use Foot Muscle, Left
Flexor hallucis longus muscle
 use Lower Leg Muscle, Right
 use Lower Leg Muscle, Left
Flexor pollicis longus muscle
 use Lower Arm and Wrist Muscle, Right
 use Lower Arm and Wrist Muscle, Left
FloPatch FP12Ø XX25XØA
Flourish® Pediatric Esophageal Atresia Device
 use Magnetic Lengthening Device in Gastrointestinal System
Flow Diverter embolization device
 use Intraluminal Device, Flow Diverter in Ø3V
FlowSense Noninvasive Thermal Sensor 4BØØXWØ
Fluorescence Guided Procedure
 Extremity
  Lower 8EØY
  Upper 8EØX
 Head and Neck Region 8EØ9
  Aminolevulinic Acid 8EØ9ØEM
  No Qualifier 8EØ9ØEZ
 Reproductive System, Female, Pafolacianine (CYTALUX®) 8EØU
 Trunk Region
  No Qualifier 8EØW
  Pafolacianine (CYTALUX®) 8EØW
Fluorescent Pyrazine, Kidney XT25XE5
Fluoroscopy
 Abdomen and Pelvis BW11
 Airway, Upper BB1DZZZ
 Ankle
  Left BQ1H
  Right BQ1G
 Aorta
  Abdominal B41Ø
   Laser, Intraoperative B41Ø
  Thoracic B31Ø
   Laser, Intraoperative B31Ø
  Thoraco-Abdominal B31P
   Laser, Intraoperative B31P
 Aorta and Bilateral Lower Extremity Arteries B41D
  Laser, Intraoperative B41D
 Arm
  Left BP1FZZZ
  Right BP1EZZZ
 Artery
  Brachiocephalic-Subclavian
   Right B311
   Laser, Intraoperative B311
  Bronchial B31L
   Laser, Intraoperative B31L
  Bypass Graft, Other B21F
  Cervico-Cerebral Arch B31Q
   Laser, Intraoperative B31Q
  Common Carotid
   Bilateral B315
    Laser, Intraoperative B315
   Left B314
    Laser, Intraoperative B314
   Right B313
    Laser, Intraoperative B313
  Coronary
   Bypass Graft
    Multiple B213
     Laser, Intraoperative B213
    Single B212
     Laser, Intraoperative B212
   Multiple B211
    Laser, Intraoperative B211
   Single B21Ø
    Laser, Intraoperative B21Ø
  External Carotid
   Bilateral B31C
    Laser, Intraoperative B31C
   Left B31B
    Laser, Intraoperative B31B

F

- Fluoroscopy *(Continued)*
  - Artery *(Continued)*
    - External Carotid *(Continued)*
      - Right B319
        - Laser, Intraoperative B319
    - Hepatic B412
      - Laser, Intraoperative B412
    - Inferior Mesenteric B415
      - Laser, Intraoperative B415
    - Intercostal B31L
      - Laser, Intraoperative B31L
    - Internal Carotid
      - Bilateral B318
        - Laser, Intraoperative B318
      - Left B317
        - Laser, Intraoperative B317
      - Right B316
        - Laser, Intraoperative B316
    - Internal Mammary Bypass Graft
      - Left B218
      - Right B217
    - Intra-Abdominal
      - Other B41B
      - Laser, Intraoperative B41B
    - Intracranial B31R
      - Laser, Intraoperative B31R
    - Liver BF15
    - Lower
      - Other B41J
      - Laser, Intraoperative B41J
    - Lower Extremity
      - Bilateral and Aorta B41D
        - Laser, Intraoperative B41D
      - Left B41G
        - Laser, Intraoperative B41G
      - Right B41F
        - Laser, Intraoperative B41F
    - Lumbar B419
      - Laser, Intraoperative B419
    - Pelvic B41C
      - Laser, Intraoperative B41C
    - Pulmonary
      - Left B31T
        - Laser, Intraoperative B31T
      - Right B31S
        - Laser, Intraoperative B31S
    - Pulmonary Trunk B31U
      - Laser, Intraoperative B31U
    - Renal
      - Bilateral B418
        - Laser, Intraoperative B418
      - Left B417
        - Laser, Intraoperative B417
      - Right B416
        - Laser, Intraoperative B416
    - Spinal B31M
      - Laser, Intraoperative B31M
    - Splenic B413
      - Laser, Intraoperative B413
    - Subclavian, Left B312
      - Left B312
      - Laser, Intraoperative B312
    - Superior Mesenteric B414
      - Laser, Intraoperative B414
    - Upper
      - Other B31N
      - Laser, Intraoperative B31N
    - Upper Extremity
      - Bilateral B31K
        - Laser, Intraoperative B31K
      - Left B31J
        - Laser, Intraoperative B31J
      - Right B31H
        - Laser, Intraoperative B31H
    - Vertebral
      - Bilateral B31G
        - Laser, Intraoperative B31G
      - Left B31F
        - Laser, Intraoperative B31F
      - Right B31D
        - Laser, Intraoperative B31D

- Fluoroscopy *(Continued)*
  - Bile Duct BF1Ø
    - Pancreatic Duct and Gallbladder BF14
  - Bile Duct and Gallbladder BF13
  - Biliary Duct BF11
  - Bladder BT1Ø
    - Kidney and Ureter BT14
      - Left BT1F
      - Right BT1D
  - Bladder and Urethra BT1B
  - Bowel, Small BD1
  - Calcaneus
    - Left BQ1KZZZ
    - Right BQ1JZZZ
  - Clavicle
    - Left BP15ZZZ
    - Right BP14ZZZ
  - Coccyx BR1F
  - Colon BD14
  - Corpora Cavernosa BV1Ø
  - Dialysis Fistula B51W
  - Dialysis Shunt B51W
  - Diaphragm BB16ZZZ
  - Disc
    - Cervical BR11
    - Lumbar BR13
    - Thoracic BR12
  - Duodenum BD19
  - Elbow
    - Left BP1H
    - Right BP1G
  - Epiglottis B91G
  - Esophagus BD11
  - Extremity
    - Lower BW1C
    - Upper BW1J
  - Facet Joint
    - Cervical BR14
    - Lumbar BR16
    - Thoracic BR15
  - Fallopian Tube
    - Bilateral BU12
    - Left BU11
    - Right BU1Ø
  - Fallopian Tube and Uterus BU18
  - Femur
    - Left BQ14ZZZ
    - Right BQ13ZZZ
  - Finger
    - Left BP1SZZZ
    - Right BP1RZZZ
  - Foot
    - Left BQ1MZZZ
    - Right BQ1LZZZ
  - Forearm
    - Left BP1KZZZ
    - Right BP1JZZZ
  - Gallbladder BF12
    - Bile Duct and Pancreatic Duct BF14
  - Gallbladder and Bile Duct BF13
  - Gastrointestinal, Upper BD1
  - Hand
    - Left BP1PZZZ
    - Right BP1NZZZ
  - Head and Neck BW19
  - Heart
    - Left B215
    - Right B214
    - Right and Left B216
  - Hip
    - Left BQ11
    - Right BQ1Ø
  - Humerus
    - Left BP1BZZZ
    - Right BP1AZZZ
  - Ileal Diversion Loop BT1C
  - Ileal Loop, Ureters and Kidney BT1G
  - Intracranial Sinus B512

- Fluoroscopy *(Continued)*
  - Joint
    - Acromioclavicular, Bilateral BP13ZZZ
    - Finger
      - Left BP1D
      - Right BP1C
    - Foot
      - Left BQ1Y
      - Right BQ1X
    - Hand
      - Left BP1D
      - Right BP1C
    - Lumbosacral BR1B
    - Sacroiliac BR1D
    - Sternoclavicular
      - Bilateral BP12ZZZ
      - Left BP11ZZZ
      - Right BP1ØZZZ
    - Temporomandibular
      - Bilateral BN19
      - Left BN18
      - Right BN17
    - Thoracolumbar BR18
    - Toe
      - Left BQ1Y
      - Right BQ1X
  - Kidney
    - Bilateral BT13
    - Ileal Loop and Ureter BT1G
    - Left BT12
    - Right BT11
    - Ureter and Bladder BT14
      - Left BT1F
      - Right BT1D
  - Knee
    - Left BQ18
    - Right BQ17
  - Larynx B91J
  - Leg
    - Left BQ1FZZZ
    - Right BQ1DZZZ
  - Lung
    - Bilateral BB14ZZZ
    - Left BB13ZZZ
    - Right BB12ZZZ
  - Mediastinum BB1CZZZ
  - Mouth BD1B
  - Neck and Head BW19
  - Oropharynx BD1B
  - Pancreatic Duct BF1
    - ~~Gallbladder and Bile Duct BF14~~
    - ▶Gallbladder and Bile Duct BF14
  - Patella
    - Left BQ1WZZZ
    - Right BQ1VZZZ
  - Pelvis BR1C
  - Pelvis and Abdomen BW11
  - ~~Pharynx B91G~~
  - ▶Pharynx B91G
  - Ribs
    - Left BP1YZZZ
    - Right BP1XZZZ
  - Sacrum BR1F
  - Scapula
    - Left BP17ZZZ
    - Right BP16ZZZ
  - Shoulder
    - Left BP19
    - Right BP18
  - Sinus, Intracranial B512
  - Spinal Cord BØ1B
  - Spine
    - Cervical BR1Ø
    - Lumbar BR19
    - Thoracic BR17
    - Whole BR1G
  - Sternum BR1H
  - Stomach BD12
  - Toe
    - Left BQ1QZZZ
    - Right BQ1PZZZ

Fluoroscopy *(Continued)*
  Tracheobronchial Tree
    Bilateral BB19YZZ
    Left BB18YZZ
    Right BB17YZZ
  Ureter
    Ileal Loop and Kidney BT1G
    Kidney and Bladder BT14
      Left BT1F
      Right BT1D
    Left BT17
    Right BT16
  Urethra BT15
  Urethra and Bladder BT1B
  Uterus BU16
  Uterus and Fallopian Tube BU18
  Vagina BU19
  Vasa Vasorum BV18
  Vein
    Cerebellar B511
    Cerebral B511
    Epidural B51Ø
    Jugular
      Bilateral B515
      Left B514
      Right B513
    Lower Extremity
      Bilateral B51D
      Left B51C
      Right B51B
    Other B51V
    Pelvic (Iliac)
      Left B51G
      Right B51F
    Pelvic (Iliac) Bilateral B51H
    Portal B51T
    Pulmonary
      Bilateral B51S
      Left B51R
      Right B51Q
    Renal
      Bilateral B51L
      Left B51K
      Right B51J
    ~~Spanchnic B51T~~
    ▶Splanchnic B51T
    Subclavian
      Left B517
      Right B516
    Upper Extremity
      Bilateral B51P
      Left B51N
      Right B51M
  Vena Cava
    Inferior B519
    Superior B518
  Wrist
    Left BP1M
    Right BP1L
Fluoroscopy, laser intraoperative
  see Fluoroscopy, Heart B21
  see Fluoroscopy, Upper Arteries B31
  see Fluoroscopy, Lower Arteries B41
Flushing *see* Irrigation
Foley catheter *use* Drainage Device
Fontan completion procedure Stage II *see* Bypass, Vena Cava, Inferior Ø61Ø
Foramen magnum *use* Occipital Bone
Foramen of Monro (intraventricular) *use* Cerebral Ventricle
Foreskin *use* Prepuce
Formula™ Balloon-Expandable Renal Stent System *use* Intraluminal Device
➡**Fosfomycin Anti-infective** ~~XWØ~~ *use* Other Anti-infective
~~Fosfomycin injection use Fosfomycin Anti-infective~~
Fossa of Rosenmuller *use* Nasopharynx
Fourth cranial nerve *use* Nerve, Trochlear
Fourth ventricle *use* Cerebral Ventricle
Fovea
  use Retina, Right
  use Retina, Left
Fragmentation
  Ampulla of Vater ØFFC
  Anus ØDFQ
  Appendix ØDFJ
  Artery
    Anterior Tibial
      Left Ø4FQ3Z
      Right Ø4FP3Z
    Axillary
      Left Ø3F63Z
      Right Ø3F53Z
    Brachial
      Left Ø3F83Z
      Right Ø3F73Z
    Common Iliac
      Left Ø4FD3Z
      Right Ø4FC3Z
    Coronary
      Four or More Arteries Ø2F33ZZ
      One Artery Ø2FØ3ZZ
      Three Arteries Ø2F23ZZ
      Two Arteries Ø2F13ZZ
    External Iliac
      Left Ø4FD3Z
      Right Ø4FH3Z
    Femoral
      Left Ø4FL3Z
      Right Ø4FK3Z
    Innominate Ø3F23Z
    Internal Iliac
      Left Ø4FF3Z
      Right Ø4FE3Z
    Intracranial Ø3FG3Z
    Lower Ø4FY3Z
    Peroneal
      Left Ø4FU3Z
      Right Ø4FT3Z
    Popliteal
      Left Ø4FN3Z
      Right Ø4FM3Z
    Posterior Tibial
      Left Ø4FN3Z
      Right Ø4FM3Z
    Pulmonary
      Left Ø2FR3Z
      Right Ø2FQ3Z
    Pulmonary Trunk Ø2FP3Z
    Radial
      Left Ø3FC3Z
      Right Ø3FB3Z
    Subclavian
      Left Ø3F43Z
      Right Ø3F33Z
    Ulnar
      Left Ø3FA3Z
      Right Ø3F93Z
  Bladder ØTFB
  Bladder Neck ØTFC
  Bronchus
    Lingula ØBF9
    Lower Lobe
      Left ØBFB
      Right ØBF6
    Main
      Left ØBF7
      Right ØBF3
    Middle Lobe, Right ØBF5
    Upper Lobe
      Left ØBF8
      Right ØBF4
  Carina ØBF2
  Cavity, Cranial ØWF1
  Cecum ØDFH
  Cerebral Ventricle ØØF6
  Colon
    Ascending ØDFK
    Descending ØDFM
Fragmentation *(Continued)*
  Colon *(Continued)*
    Sigmoid ØDFN
    Transverse ØDFL
  Duct
    Common Bile ØFF9
    Cystic ØFF8
    Hepatic
      Common ØFF7
      Left ØFF6
      Right ØFF5
    Pancreatic ØFFD
      Accessory ØFFF
    Parotid
      Left ØCFC
      Right ØCFB
  Duodenum ØDF9
  Epidural Space, Intracranial ØØF3
  Esophagus ØDF5
  Fallopian Tube
    Left ØUF6
    Right ØUF5
  Fallopian Tubes, Bilateral ØUF7
  Gallbladder ØFF4
  Gastrointestinal Tract ØWFP
  Genitourinary Tract ØWFR
  Ileum ØDFB
  Intestine
    Large ØDFE
      Left ØDFG
      Right ØDFF
    Small ØDF8
  Jejunum ØDFA
  Kidney Pelvis
    Left ØTF4
    Right ØTF3
  Mediastinum ØWFC
  Oral Cavity and Throat ØWF3
  Pelvic Cavity ØWFJ
  Pericardial Cavity ØWFD
  Pericardium Ø2FN
  Peritoneal Cavity ØWFG
  Pleural Cavity
    Left ØWFB
    Right ØWF9
  Rectum ØDFP
  Respiratory Tract ØWFQ
  Spinal Canal ØØFU
  Stomach ØDF6
  Subarachnoid Space, Intracranial ØØF5
  Subdural Space, Intracranial ØØF4
  Trachea ØBF1
  Ureter
    Left ØTF7
    Right ØTF6
  Urethra ØTFD
  Uterus ØUF9
  Vein
    Axillary
      Left Ø5F83Z
      Right Ø5F73Z
    Basilic
      Left Ø5FC3Z
      Right Ø5F73Z
    Brachial
      Left Ø5FC3Z
      Right Ø5FB3Z
    Cephalic
      Left Ø5FF3Z
      Right Ø5 FD3Z
    Common Iliac
      Left Ø6FD3Z
      Right Ø6FC3Z
    External Iliac
      Left Ø6FG3Z
      Right Ø6FF3Z
    Femoral
      Left Ø6FN3Z
      Right Ø6FM3Z

F

Fragmentation *(Continued)*
Vein *(Continued)*
Hypogastric
Left Ø6FJ3Z
Right Ø6FH3Z
Innominate
Left Ø5F43Z
Right Ø5F33Z
Lower Ø6FY3Z
Pulmonary
Left Ø2FT3Z
Right Ø2FS3Z
Saphenous
Left Ø6FQ3Z
Right Ø5F53Z
Upper
Vitreous
Left Ø8F5
Right Ø8F4
Fragmentation, Ultrasonic *see* Fragmentation, Artery
Freestyle (Stentless) Aortic Root Bioprosthesis *use* Zooplastic Tissue in Heart and Great Vessels
Frenectomy
see Excision, Mouth and Throat ØCB
see Resection, Mouth and Throat ØCT
Frenoplasty, frenuloplasty
see Repair, Mouth and Throat ØCQ
see Replacement, Mouth and Throat ØCR
see Supplement, Mouth and Throat ØCU
Frenotomy
see Drainage, Mouth and Throat ØC9
see Release, Mouth and Throat ØCN
Frenulotomy
see Drainage, Mouth and Throat ØC9
see Release, Mouth and Throat ØCN
Frenulum labii inferioris *use* Lower Lip
Frenulum labii superioris *use* Upper Lip
Frenulum linguae *use* Tongue
Frenulumectomy
see Excision, Mouth and Throat ØCB
see Resection, Mouth and Throat ØCT
Frontal lobe *use* Cerebral Hemisphere
Frontal vein
use Face Vein, Right
use Face Vein, Left
Frozen elephant trunk (FET) technique, aortic arch replacement
see Replacement, Heart and Great Vessels Ø2R
see New Technology, Cardiovascular System X2R
Frozen elephant trunk (FET) technique, thoracic aorta restriction
see Restriction, Heart and Great Vessels Ø2V
see New Technology, Cardiovascular System X2V
FUJIFILM EP-7ØØØX system for oxygen saturation endoscopic imaging (OXEI) *see* New Technology, Gastrointestinal System XD2
Fulguration *see* Destruction
Fundoplication, gastroesophageal *see* Restriction, Esophagogastric Junction ØDV4
Fundus uteri *use* Uterus
Fusion
Acromioclavicular
Left ØRGH
Right ØRGG
Ankle
Left ØSGG
▶Gyroid-Sheet Lattice Design Internal Fixation Device XRGKØCA
Open-truss Design Internal Fixation Device XRGKØB9
Right ØSGF
▶Gyroid-Sheet Lattice Design Internal Fixation Device XRGJØCA
Open-truss Design Internal Fixation Device XRGJØB9
Carpal
Left ØRGR
Right ØRGQ
Carpometacarpal
Left ØRGT
Right ØRGS
Cervical Vertebral ØRG1
2 or more ØRG2
Cervicothoracic Vertebral ØRG4
Coccygeal ØSG6
Elbow
Left ØRGM
Right ØRGL
Finger Phalangeal
Left ØRGX
Right ØRGW
Hip
Left ØSGB
Right ØSG9
Knee
Left ØSGD
Right ØSGC
Lumbar Vertebral ØSGØ
2 or more ØSG1
▶Facet Joint Fusion Device, Paired Titanium Cages XRGCØEA
Interbody Fusion Device, Custom-Made Anatomically Designed XRGC
▶Facet Joint Fusion Device, Paired Titanium Cages XRGBØEA
Interbody Fusion Device, Custom-Made Anatomically Designed XRGB
Fusion *(Continued)*
Lumbosacral ØSG3
▶Facet Joint Fusion Device, Paired Titanium Cages XRGDØEA
Interbody Fusion Device, Custom-Made Anatomically Designed XRGD
Metacarpophalangeal
Left ØRGV
Right ØRGU
Metatarsal-Phalangeal
Left ØSGN
Right ØSGM
Occipital-cervical ØRGØ
Sacrococcygeal ØSG5
Sacroiliac
Internal Fixation Device with Tulip Connector XRG
Left ØSG8
Right ØSG7
Shoulder
Left ØRGK
Right ØRGJ
Sternoclavicular
Left ØRGF
Right ØRGE
Tarsal
Left ØSGJ
▶Gyroid-Sheet Lattice Design Internal Fixation Device XRGMØCA
Open-truss Design Internal Fixation Device XRGMØB9
Right ØSGH
▶Gyroid-Sheet Lattice Design Internal Fixation Device XRGLØCA
Open-truss Design Internal Fixation Device XRGLØB9
Tarsometatarsal
Left ØSGL
Right ØSGK
Temporomandibular
Left ØRGD
Right ØRGC
Thoracic Vertebral ØRG6
2 to 7 ØRG7
8 or more ØRG8
Thoracolumbar Vertebral ØRGA
▶Facet Joint Fusion Device, Paired Titanium Cages XRGAØEA
Interbody Fusion Device, Custom-Made Anatomically Designed XRGA
Toe Phalangeal
Left ØSGQ
Right ØSGP
Wrist
Left ØRGP
Right ØRGN
Fusion screw (compression) (lag) (locking)
use Internal Fixation Device in Upper Joints
use Internal Fixation Device in Lower Joints

F

G

Gait training *see* Motor Treatment, Rehabilitation FØ7
Galea aponeurotica *use* Subcutaneous Tissue and Fascia, Scalp
Gammaglobulin *use* Globulin
GammaTile™ ~~*use* Radioactive Element, Cesium-131 Collagen Implant in ØØH~~
▶ *use* Radioactive Element, Cesium-131 Collagen Implant in ØØH
▶ *use* Radioactive Element, Palladium-1Ø3 Collagen Implant in ØØH
GAMUNEX-C, for COVID-19 treatment *use* High-Dose Intravenous Immune Globulin
Ganglion impar (ganglion of Walther) *use* Sacral Sympathetic Nerve
Ganglionectomy
 Destruction of lesion *see* Destruction
 Excision of lesion *see* Excision
Gasserian ganglion *use* Trigeminal Nerve
Gastrectomy
 Partial *see* Excision, Stomach ØDB6
 Total *see* Resection, Stomach ØDT6
 Vertical (sleeve) *see* Excision, Stomach ØDB6
Gastric electrical stimulation (GES) lead *use* Stimulator Lead in Gastrointestinal System
Gastric lymph node *use* Lymphatic, Aortic
Gastric pacemaker lead *use* Stimulator Lead in Gastrointestinal System
Gastric plexus *see* Abdominal Sympathetic Nerve
Gastrocnemius muscle
 use Lower Leg Muscle, Right
 use Lower Leg Muscle, Left
Gastrocolic ligament *use* Omentum
Gastrocolic omentum *use* Omentum
Gastrocolostomy
 see Bypass, Gastrointestinal System ØD1
 see Drainage, Gastrointestinal System ØD9
Gastroduodenal artery *use* Hepatic Artery
Gastroduodenectomy
 see Excision, Gastrointestinal System ØDB
 see Resection, Gastrointestinal System ØDT
Gastroduodenoscopy ØDJØ8ZZ
Gastroenteroplasty
 see Repair, Gastrointestinal System ØDQ
 see Supplement, Gastrointestinal System ØDU
Gastroenterostomy
 see Bypass, Gastrointestinal System ØD1
 see Drainage, Gastrointestinal System ØD9
Gastroesophageal (GE) junction *use* Esophagogastric Junction
Gastrogastrostomy
 see Bypass, Stomach ØD16
 see Drainage, Stomach ØD96
Gastrohepatic omentum *use* Omentum
Gastrojejunostomy
 see Bypass, Stomach ØD16
 see Drainage, Stomach ØD96
Gastrolysis *see* Release, Stomach ØDN6
Gastropexy
 see Repair, Stomach ØDQ6
 see Reposition, Stomach ØDS6
Gastrophrenic ligament *use* Omentum
Gastroplasty
 see Repair, Stomach ØDQ6
 see Supplement, Stomach ØDU6
Gastroplication *see* Restriction, Stomach ØDV6
Gastropylorectomy *see* Excision, Gastrointestinal System ØDB
Gastrorrhaphy *see* Repair, Stomach ØDQ6
Gastroscopy ØDJ68ZZ
Gastrosplenic ligament *use* Omentum
Gastrostomy
 see Bypass, Stomach ØD16
 see Drainage, Stomach ØD96
Gastrotomy *see* Drainage, Stomach ØD96
Gemellus muscle
 use Hip Muscle, Right
 use Hip Muscle, Left
Geniculate ganglion *use* Facial Nerve
Geniculate nucleus *use* Thalamus
Genioglossus muscle *use* Tongue, Palate, Pharynx Muscle
Genioplasty *see* Alteration, Jaw, Lower ØWØ5
Genitofemoral nerve *use* Lumbar Plexus
GIAPREZA™ *use* Vasopressor
~~Gilteritinib Antineoplastic XWØDXV5~~
▶ **Gilteritinib** *use* Other Antineoplastic
Gingivectomy *see* Excision, Mouth and Throat ØCB
Gingivoplasty
 see Repair, Mouth and Throat ØCQ
 see Replacement, Mouth and Throat ØCR
 see Supplement, Mouth and Throat ØCU
Glans penis *use* Prepuce
Glenohumeral joint
 use Shoulder Joint, Right
 use Shoulder Joint, Left
Glenohumeral ligament
 use Shoulder Bursa and Ligament, Right
 use Shoulder Bursa and Ligament, Left
Glenoid fossa (of scapula)
 use Glenoid Cavity, Right
 use Glenoid Cavity, Left
Glenoid ligament (labrum)
 use Shoulder Joint, Right
 use Shoulder Joint, Left
Globus pallidus *use* Basal Ganglia
Glofitamab Antineoplastic XWØ
Glomectomy
 see Excision, Endocrine System ØGB
 see Resection, Endocrine System ØGT
Glossectomy
 see Excision, Tongue ØCB7
 see Resection, Tongue ØCT7
Glossoepiglottic fold *use* Epiglottis
Glossopexy
 see Repair, Tongue ØCQ7
 see Reposition, Tongue ØCS7
Glossoplasty
 see Repair, Tongue ØCQ7
 see Replacement, Tongue ØCR7
 see Supplement, Tongue ØCU7
Glossorrhaphy *see* Repair, Tongue ØCQ7
Glossotomy *see* Drainage, Tongue ØC97
Glottis *use* Larynx
Gluteal Artery Perforator Flap
 Replacement
  Bilateral ØHRVØ79
  Left ØHRUØ79
  Right ØHRTØ79
 Transfer
  Left ØKXG
  Right ØKXF
Gluteal lymph node *use* Lymphatic, Pelvis
Gluteal vein
 use Hypogastric Vein, Right
 use Hypogastric Vein, Left
Gluteus maximus muscle
 use Hip Muscle, Right
 use Hip Muscle, Left
Gluteus medius muscle
 use Hip Muscle, Right
 use Hip Muscle, Left
Gluteus minimus muscle
 use Hip Muscle, Right
 use Hip Muscle, Left
GORE EXCLUDER® AAA Endoprosthesis
 use Intraluminal Device, Branched or Fenestrated, One or Two Arteries in Ø4V
 use Intraluminal Device, Branched or Fenestrated, Three or More Arteries in Ø4V
 use Intraluminal Device
GORE EXCLUDER® IBE Endoprosthesis *use* Intraluminal Device, Branched or Fenestrated, One or Two Arteries in Ø4V
▶ **GORE® EXCLUDER® TAMBE Device (Thoracoabdominal Branch Endoprosthesis)** *use* Branched Intraluminal Device, Manufactured Integrated System, Four or More Arteries in New Technology
GORE TAG® Thoracic Endoprosthesis *use* Intraluminal Device
GORE® DUALMESH® *use* Synthetic Substitute
Gracilis muscle
 use Upper Leg Muscle, Right
 use Upper Leg Muscle, Left
Graft
 see Replacement
 see Supplement
Great auricular nerve *use* Lumbar Plexus
Great cerebral vein *use* Intracranial Vein
Great(er) saphenous vein
 use Saphenous Vein, Right
 use Saphenous Vein, Left
Greater alar cartilage *use* Nasal Mucosa and Soft Tissue
Greater occipital nerve *use* Cervical Nerve
Greater Omentum *use* Omentum
Greater splanchnic nerve *use* Thoracic Sympathetic Nerve
Greater superficial petrosal nerve *use* Facial Nerve
Greater trochanter
 use Upper Femur, Right
 use Upper Femur, Left
Greater tuberosity
 use Humeral Head, Right
 use Humeral Head, Left
Greater vestibular (Bartholin's) gland *use* Vestibular Gland
Greater wing *use* Sphenoid Bone
GS-5734 *use* Remdesivir Anti-infective
Guedel airway *use* Intraluminal Device, Airway in Mouth and Throat
Guidance, catheter placement
 EKG *see* Measurement, Physiological Systems 4AØ
 Fluoroscopy *see* Fluoroscopy, Veins B51
 Ultrasound *see* Ultrasonography, Veins B54
▶ **Gyroid-Sheet Lattice Design Internal Fixation Device**
 ▶ Ankle
  ▶ Left XRGKØCA
  ▶ Right XRGJØCA
 ▶ Tarsal
  ▶ Left XRGMØCA
  ▶ Right XRGLØCA

H

Hallux
use Toe, 1st, Right
use Toe, 1st, Left
Hamate bone
use Carpal, Right
use Carpal, Left
Hamstring muscle
use Upper Leg Muscle, Right
use Upper Leg Muscle, Left
Hancock Bioprosthesis (aortic) (mitral) valve *use* Zooplastic Tissue in Heart and Great Vessels
Hancock Bioprosthetic Valved Conduit *use* Zooplastic Tissue in Heart and Great Vessels
Harmony™ transcatheter pulmonary valve (TPV) placement 02RH38M
Harvesting, stem cells *see* Pheresis, Circulatory 6A55
HAV™ (Human Acellular Vessel) *use* Bioengineered Human Acellular Vessel in New Technology
hdIVIG (high-dose intravenous immunoglobulin), for COVID-19 treatment *use* High-Dose Intravenous Immune Globulin
Head of fibula
use Fibula, Right
use Fibula, Left
Hearing Aid Assessment F14Z
Hearing Assessment F13Z
Hearing Device
Bone Conduction
Left 09HE
Right 09HD
Insertion of device in
Left 0NH6[034]SZ
Right 0NH5[034]SZ
Multiple Channel Cochlear Prosthesis
Left 09HE
Right 09HD
Removal of device from, Skull 0NP0
Revision of device in, Skull 0NW0
Single Channel Cochlear Prosthesis
Left 09HE
Right 09HD
Hearing Treatment F09Z
Heart Assist System
Implantable
Insertion of device in, Heart 02HA
Removal of device from, Heart 02PA
Revision of device in, Heart 02WA
Short-term External
Insertion of device in
Aorta, Thoracic, Descending 02HW3RZ
Heart 02HA
Removal of device from
Aorta, Thoracic, Descending 02PW3RZ
Heart 02PA
Revision of device in
Aorta, Thoracic, Descending 02WW3RZ
Heart 02WA
HeartMate 3™ LVAS *use* Implantable Heart Assist System in Heart and Great Vessels
HeartMate II® Left Ventricular Assist Device (LVAD) *use* Implantable Heart Assist System in Heart and Great Vessels
HeartMate XVE® Left Ventricular Assist Device (LVAD) *use* Implantable Heart Assist System in Heart and Great Vessels
HeartMate® implantable heart assist system *see* Insertion of device in, Heart 02HA
Helix
use External Ear, Right
use External Ear, Left
use External Ear, Bilateral
Hematopoietic cell transplant (HCT) *see* Transfusion, Circulatory 302
Hemicolectomy *see* Resection, Gastrointestinal System 0DT
Hemicystectomy *see* Excision, Urinary System 0TB
Hemigastrectomy *see* Excision, Gastrointestinal System 0DB
Hemiglossectomy *see* Excision, Mouth and Throat 0CB
Hemilaminectomy
see Excision, Upper Bones 0PB
see Excision, Lower Bones 0QB
Hemilaminotomy
see Release, Central Nervous System 00N
see Release, Peripheral Nervous System 01N
see Drainage, Upper Bones 0P9
see Excision, Upper Bones 0PB
see Release, Upper Bones 0PN
see Drainage, Lower Bones 0Q9
see Excision, Lower Bones 0QB
see Release, Lower Bones 0QN
Hemilaryngectomy *see* Excision, Larynx 0CBS
Hemimandibulectomy *see* Excision, Head and Facial Bones 0NB
Hemimaxillectomy *see* Excision, Head and Facial Bones 0NB
Hemipylorectomy *see* Excision, Gastrointestinal System 0DB
Hemispherectomy
see Excision, Central Nervous System and Cranial Nerves 00B
see Resection, Central Nervous System and Cranial Nerves 00T
Hemithyroidectomy
see Excision, Endocrine System 0GB
see Resection, Endocrine System 0GT
Hemodialysis *see* Performance, Urinary 5A1D
Hemolung® Respiratory Assist System (RAS) 5A0920Z
Hemospray® Endoscopic Hemostat *use* Mineral-based Topical Hemostatic Agent
Hepatectomy
see Excision, Hepatobiliary System and Pancreas 0FB
see Resection, Hepatobiliary System and Pancreas 0FT
Hepatic artery proper *use* Hepatic Artery
Hepatic flexure *use* Transverse Colon
Hepatic lymph node *use* Aortic Lymphatic
Hepatic plexus *use* Abdominal Sympathetic Nerve
Hepatic portal vein *use* Portal Vein
Hepaticoduodenostomy
see Bypass, Hepatobiliary System and Pancreas 0F1
see Drainage, Hepatobiliary System and Pancreas 0F9
Hepaticotomy *see* Drainage, Hepatobiliary System and Pancreas 0F9
Hepatocholedochostomy *see* Drainage, Duct, Common Bile 0F99
Hepatogastric ligament *use* Omentum
Hepatopancreatic ampulla *use* Ampulla of Vater
Hepatopexy
see Repair, Hepatobiliary System and Pancreas 0FQ
see Reposition, Hepatobiliary System and Pancreas 0FS
Hepatorrhaphy *see* Repair, Hepatobiliary System and Pancreas 0FQ
Hepatotomy *see* Drainage, Hepatobiliary System and Pancreas 0F9
HEPZATO™ KIT (melphalan hydrochloride Hepatic Delivery System) *use* MelphalanHydrochloride Antineoplastic
Herculink (RX) Elite Renal Stent System *use* Intraluminal Device
Herniorrhaphy
see Repair, Anatomical Regions, General 0WQ
see Repair, Anatomical Regions, Lower Extremities 0YQ
Herniorrhaphy *(Continued)*
With synthetic substitute
see Supplement, Anatomical Regions, General 0WU
see Supplement, Anatomical Regions, Lower Extremities 0YU
HIG (hyperimmune globulin), for COVID-19 treatment *use* Hyperimmune Globulin
High-dose intravenous immune globulin, for COVID-19 treatment XW1
High-dose intravenous immunoglobulin (hdIVIG), for COVID-19 treatment *use* High-Dose Intravenous Immune Globulin
Hip (joint) liner *use* Liner in Lower Joints
HIPEC (hyperthermic intraperitoneal chemotherapy) 3E0M30Y
HistoSonics® System *see* New Technology, Hepatobiliary System and Pancreas XF5
Histotripsy, liver *see* New Technology, Hepatobiliary System and Pancreas XF5
hIVIG (hyperimmune intravenous immunoglobulin), for COVID-19 treatment *use* Hyperimmune Globulin
Holter monitoring 4A12X45
Holter valve ventricular shunt *use* Synthetic Substitute
Human Acellular Vessel™ (HAV) *use* Bioengineered Human Acellular Vessel in New Technology
Human angiotensin II, synthetic *use* Vasopressor
Humeroradial joint
use Elbow Joint, Right
use Elbow Joint, Left
Humeroulnar joint
use Elbow Joint, Right
use Elbow Joint, Left
Humerus, distal
use Humeral Shaft, Right
use Humeral Shaft, Left
Hydrocelectomy *see* Excision, Male Reproductive System 0VB
Hydrotherapy
Assisted exercise in pool *see* Motor Treatment, Rehabilitation F07
Whirlpool *see* Activities of Daily Living Treatment, Rehabilitation F08
Hymenectomy
see Excision, Hymen 0UBK
see Resection, Hymen 0UTK
Hymenoplasty
see Repair, Hymen 0UQK
see Supplement, Hymen 0UUK
Hymenorrhaphy *see* Repair, Hymen 0UQK
Hymenotomy
see Division, Hymen 0U8K
see Drainage, Hymen 0U9K
Hyoglossus muscle *use* Tongue, Palate, Pharynx Muscle
Hyoid artery
use Thyroid Artery, Right
use Thyroid Artery, Left
Hyperalimentation *see* Introduction of substance in or on
Hyperbaric oxygenation
Decompression sickness treatment *see* Decompression, Circulatory 6A15
Other treatment see Assistance, Circulatory 5A05
Hyperimmune globulin *use* Globulin
Hyperimmune globulin, for COVID-19 treatment XW1
Hyperimmune intravenous immunoglobulin (hIVIG), for COVID-19 treatment *use* Hyperimmune Globulin
Hyperthermia
Radiation Therapy
Abdomen DWY38ZZ
Adrenal Gland DGY28ZZ
Bile Ducts DFY28ZZ

▶ New ➠ Revised ~~deleted~~ Deleted

Hyperthermia *(Continued)*
- Radiation Therapy *(Continued)*
  - Bladder DTY28ZZ
  - Bone, Other DPYC8ZZ
  - Bone Marrow D7Y08ZZ
  - Brain D0Y08ZZ
  - Brain Stem D0Y18ZZ
  - Breast
    - Left DMY08ZZ
    - Right DMY18ZZ
  - Bronchus DBY18ZZ
  - Cervix DUY18ZZ
  - Chest DWY28ZZ
  - Chest Wall DBY78ZZ
  - Colon DDY58ZZ
  - Diaphragm DBY88ZZ
  - Duodenum DDY28ZZ
  - Ear D9Y08ZZ
  - Esophagus DDY08ZZ
  - Eye D8Y08ZZ
  - Femur DPY98ZZ
  - Fibula DPYB8ZZ
  - Gallbladder DFY18ZZ
  - Gland
    - Adrenal DGY28ZZ
    - Parathyroid DGY48ZZ
    - Pituitary DGY08ZZ
    - Thyroid DGY58ZZ
  - Glands, Salivary D9Y68ZZ
  - Head and Neck DWY18ZZ
  - Hemibody DWY48ZZ
  - Humerus DPY68ZZ
  - Hypopharynx D9Y38ZZ
  - Ileum DDY48ZZ
  - Jejunum DDY38ZZ
  - Kidney DTY08ZZ
  - Larynx D9YB8ZZ
  - Liver DFY08ZZ
  - Lung DBY28ZZ
  - Lymphatics
    - Abdomen D7Y68ZZ
    - Axillary D7Y48ZZ
    - Inguinal D7Y88ZZ
    - Neck D7Y38ZZ
    - Pelvis D7Y78ZZ
    - Thorax D7Y58ZZ
  - Mandible DPY38ZZ

Hyperthermia *(Continued)*
- Radiation Therapy *(Continued)*
  - Maxilla DPY28ZZ
  - Mediastinum DBY68ZZ
  - Mouth D9Y48ZZ
  - Nasopharynx D9YD8ZZ
  - Neck and Head DWY18ZZ
  - Nerve, Peripheral D0Y78ZZ
  - Nose D9Y18ZZ
  - Oropharynx D9YF8ZZ
  - Ovary DUY08ZZ
  - Palate
    - Hard D9Y88ZZ
    - Soft D9Y98ZZ
  - Pancreas DFY38ZZ
  - Parathyroid Gland DGY48ZZ
  - Pelvic Bones DPY88ZZ
  - Pelvic Region DWY68ZZ
  - Pineal Body DGY18ZZ
  - Pituitary Gland DGY08ZZ
  - Pleura DBY58ZZ
  - Prostate DVY08ZZ
  - Radius DPY78ZZ
  - Rectum DDY78ZZ
  - Rib DPY58ZZ
  - Sinuses D9Y78ZZ
  - Skin
    - Abdomen DHY88ZZ
    - Arm DHY48ZZ
    - Back DHY78ZZ
    - Buttock DHY98ZZ
    - Chest DHY68ZZ
    - Face DHY28ZZ
    - Leg DHYB8ZZ
    - Neck DHY38ZZ
  - Skull DPY08ZZ
  - Spinal Cord D0Y68ZZ
  - Spleen D7Y28ZZ
  - Sternum DPY48ZZ
  - Stomach DDY18ZZ
  - Testis DVY18ZZ
  - Thymus D7Y18ZZ
  - Thyroid Gland DGY58ZZ
  - Tibia DPYB8ZZ
  - Tongue D9Y58ZZ
  - Trachea DBY08ZZ

Hyperthermia *(Continued)*
- Radiation Therapy *(Continued)*
  - Ulna DPY78ZZ
  - Ureter DTY18ZZ
  - Urethra DTY38ZZ
  - Uterus DUY28ZZ
  - Whole Body DWY58ZZ
- Whole Body 6A3Z

Hyperthermic intraperitoneal chemotherapy (HIPEC) 3E0M30Y

Hypnosis GZFZZZZ

Hypogastric artery
- *use* Internal Iliac Artery, Right
- *use* Internal Iliac Artery, Left

Hypopharynx *use* Pharynx

Hypophysectomy
- *see* Excision, Gland, Pituitary 0GB0
- *see* Resection, Gland, Pituitary 0GT0

Hypophysis *use* Gland, Pituitary

Hypothalamotomy *see* Destruction, Thalamus 0059

Hypothenar muscle
- *use* Hand Muscle, Right
- *use* Hand Muscle, Left

Hypothermia, Whole Body 6A4Z

Hysterectomy
- Supracervical *see* Resection, Uterus 0UT9
- Total *see* Resection, Uterus 0UT9

Hysterolysis *see* Release, Uterus 0UN9

Hysteropexy
- *see* Repair, Uterus 0UQ9
- *see* Reposition, Uterus 0US9

Hysteroplasty
- *see* Repair, Uterus 0UQ9

Hysterorrhaphy *see* Repair, Uterus 0UQ9

Hysteroscopy 0UJD8ZZ

Hysterotomy
- *see* Drainage, Uterus 0U99

Hysterotrachelectomy
- *see* Resection, Uterus 0UT9
- *see* Resection, Cervix 0UTC

Hysterotracheloplasty
- *see* Repair, Uterus 0UQ9

Hysterotrachelorrhaphy *see* Repair, Uterus 0UQ9

I

IABP (Intra-aortic balloon pump) *see* Assistance, Cardiac 5A02
IAEMT (Intraoperative anesthetic effect monitoring and titration) *see* Monitoring, Central Nervous 4A10
IASD® (InterAtrial Shunt Device), Corvia *use* Synthetic Substitute
Idarucizumab, Pradaxa® (dabigatran) reversal agent *use* Other Therapeutic Substance
Ide-cel *use* Idecabtagene Vicleucel Immunotherapy
Idecabtagene vicleucel *use* Idecabtagene Vicleucel Immunotherapy
Idecabtagene vicleucel immunotherapy XW0
iFuse Bedrock™ Granite Implant System *use* Internal Fixation Device with Tulip Connector in New Technology
IGIV-C, for COVID-19 treatment *use* Hyperimmune Globulin
IHD (Intermittent hemodialysis) 5A1D70Z
Ileal artery *use* Superior Mesenteric Artery
Ileectomy
see Excision, Ileum 0DBB
see Resection, Ileum 0DTB
Ileocolic artery *use* Superior Mesenteric Artery
Ileocolic vein *use* Colic Vein
Ileopexy
see Repair, Ileum 0DQB
see Reposition, Ileum 0DSB
Ileorrhaphy *see* Repair, Ileum 0DQB
Ileoscopy 0DJD8ZZ
Ileostomy
see Bypass, Ileum 0D1B
see Drainage, Ileum 0D9B
Ileotomy *see* Drainage, Ileum 0D9B
Ileoureterostomy *see* Bypass, Bladder 0T1B
Iliac crest
use Pelvic Bone, Right
use Pelvic Bone, Left
Iliac fascia
use Subcutaneous Tissue and Fascia, Right Upper Leg
use Subcutaneous Tissue and Fascia, Left Upper Leg
Iliac lymph node *use* Lymphatic, Pelvis
Iliacus muscle
use Hip Muscle, Right
use Hip Muscle, Left
Iliofemoral ligament
use Hip Bursa and Ligament, Right
use Hip Bursa and Ligament, Left
Iliohypogastric nerve *use* Lumbar Plexus
Ilioinguinal nerve *use* Lumbar Plexus
Iliolumbar artery
use Internal Iliac Artery, Right
use Internal Iliac Artery, Left
Iliolumbar ligament *use* Lower Spine Bursa and Ligament
▶ **Iliopsoas muscle**
▶ *use* Hip Muscle, Right
▶ *use* Hip Muscle, Left
Iliotibial tract (band)
use Subcutaneous Tissue and Fascia, Right Upper Leg
use Subcutaneous Tissue and Fascia, Left Upper Leg
Ilium
use Pelvic Bone, Right
use Pelvic Bone, Left
Ilizarov external fixator
use External Fixation Device, Ring in 0PH
use External Fixation Device, Ring in 0PS
use External Fixation Device, Ring in 0QH
use External Fixation Device, Ring in 0QS
Ilizarov-Vecklich device
use External Fixation Device, Limb Lengthening in 0PH
use External Fixation Device, Limb Lengthening in 0QH
Imaging, diagnostic
see Plain Radiography
see Fluoroscopy
see Computerized Tomography (CT Scan)
see Magnetic Resonance Imaging (MRI)
see Ultrasonography
Imdevimab (REGN10987) and casirivimab (REGN10933) *use* REGN-COV2 Monoclonal Antibody
IMFINZI® *use* Durvalumab Antineoplastic
IMI/REL
use Other Anti-infective ~~Imipenem-cilastatin-relebactam Anti-infective~~
Imipenem-cilastatin-relebactam Anti-infective *use* Other Anti-infective ~~XW0~~
Immobilization
Abdominal Wall 2W33X
Arm
Lower
Left 2W3DX
Right 2W3CX
Upper
Left 2W3BX
Right 2W3AX
Back 2W35X
Chest Wall 2W34X
Extremity
Lower
Left 2W3MX
Right 2W3LX
Upper
Left 2W39X
Right 2W38X
Face 2W31X
Finger
Left 2W3KX
Right 2W3JX
Foot
Left 2W3TX
Right 2W3SX
Hand
Left 2W3FX
Right 2W3EX
Head 2W30X
Inguinal Region
Left 2W37X
Right 2W36X
Leg
Lower
Left 2W3RX
Right 2W3QX
Upper
Left 2W3PX
Right 2W3NX
Neck 2W32X
Thumb
Left 2W3HX
Right 2W3GX
Toe
Left 2W3VX
Right 2W3UX
Immunization *see* Introduction of Serum, Toxoid, and Vaccine
Immunoglobulin *use* Globulin
Immunotherapy *see* Introduction of Immunotherapeutic Substance
Immunotherapy, antineoplastic
Interferon *see* Introduction of Low-dose Interleukin-2
Interleukin-2 of high-dose *see* Introduction, High-dose Interleukin-2
Interleukin-2, low-dose *see* Introduction of Low-dose Interleukin-2
Monoclonal antibody *see* Introduction of Monoclonal Antibody
Proleukin, high-dose *see* Introduction of High-dose Interleukin-2
Proleukin, low-dose *see* Introduction of Low-dose Interleukin-2
Impella® 5.5 with SmartAssist® System *use* Conduit to Short-term External Heart Assist System in New Technology
Impella® heart pump *use* Short-term External Heart Assist System in Heart and Great Vessels
Impeller Pump
Continuous, Output 5A0221D
Intermittent, Output 5A0211D
Implantable cardioverter-defibrillator (ICD) *use* Defibrillator Generator in 0JH
Implantable drug infusion pump (anti-spasmodic) (chemotherapy) (pain) *use* Infusion Device, Pump in Subcutaneous Tissue and Fascia
Implantable glucose monitoring device *use* Monitoring Device
Implantable hemodynamic monitor (IHM) *use* Monitoring Device, Hemodynamic in 0JH
Implantable hemodynamic monitoring system (IHMS) *use* Monitoring Device, Hemodynamic in 0JH
Implantable Miniature Telescope™ (IMT) use Synthetic Substitute, Intraocular Telescope in 08R
Implantation
see Replacement
see Insertion
Implanted (venous) (access) port *use* Vascular Access Device, Totally Implantable in Subcutaneous Tissue and Fascia
IMV (intermittent mandatory ventilation) *see* Assistance, Respiratory 5A09
In Vitro Fertilization 8E0ZXY1
Incision, abscess *see* Drainage
Incudectomy
see Excision, Ear, Nose, Sinus 09B
see Resection, Ear, Nose, Sinus 09T
Incudopexy
see Repair, Ear, Nose, Sinus 09Q
see Reposition, Ear, Nose, Sinus 09S
Incus
use Ossicle, Auditory, Right
use Ossicle, Auditory, Left
Induction of labor
Artificial rupture of membranes *see* Drainage, Pregnancy 109
Oxytocin *see* Introduction of Hormone
InDura, intrathecal catheter (1P) (spinal) *use* Infusion Device
Inebilizumab-cdon XW0
Inferior cardiac nerve *use* Thoracic Sympathetic Nerve
Inferior cerebellar vein *use* Intracranial Vein
Inferior cerebral vein *use* Intracranial Vein
Inferior epigastric artery
use External Iliac Artery, Right
use External Iliac Artery, Left
Inferior epigastric lymph node *use* Lymphatic, Pelvis
Inferior genicular artery
use Popliteal Artery, Right
use Popliteal Artery, Left
Inferior gluteal artery
use Internal Iliac Artery, Right
use Internal Iliac Artery, Left
Inferior gluteal nerve *use* Sacral Plexus Nerve
Inferior hypogastric plexus *use* Abdominal Sympathetic Nerve
Inferior labial artery *use* Face Artery
Inferior longitudinal muscle *use* Tongue, Palate, Pharynx Muscle
Inferior mesenteric ganglion *use* Abdominal Sympathetic Nerve
Inferior mesenteric lymph node *use* Mesenteric Lymphatic
Inferior mesenteric plexus *use* Abdominal Sympathetic Nerve
Inferior oblique muscle
use Extraocular Muscle, Right
use Extraocular Muscle, Left

Inferior pancreaticoduodenal artery *use* Superior Mesenteric Artery
Inferior phrenic artery *use* Abdominal Aorta
Inferior rectus muscle
use Extraocular Muscle, Right
use Extraocular Muscle, Left
Inferior suprarenal artery
use Renal Artery, Right
use Renal Artery, Left
Inferior tarsal plate
use Lower Eyelid, Right
use Lower Eyelid, Left
Inferior thyroid vein
use Innominate Vein, Right
use Innominate Vein, Left
Inferior tibiofibular joint
use Ankle Joint, Right
use Ankle Joint, Left
Inferior turbinate *use* Nasal Turbinate
Inferior ulnar collateral artery
use Brachial Artery, Right
use Brachial Artery, Left
Inferior vesical artery
use Internal Iliac Artery, Right
use Internal Iliac Artery, Left
Infraauricular lymph node *use* Lymphatic, Head
Infraclavicular (deltopectoral) lymph node
use Lymphatic, Right Upper Extremity
use Lymphatic, Left Upper Extremity
Infrahyoid muscle
use Neck Muscle, Right
use Neck Muscle, Left
Infraparotid lymph node *use* Lymphatic, Head
Infraspinatus fascia
use Subcutaneous Tissue and Fascia, Right Upper Arm
use Subcutaneous Tissue and Fascia, Left Upper Arm
Infraspinatus muscle
use Shoulder Muscle, Right
use Shoulder Muscle, Left
Infundibulopelvic ligament *use* Uterine Supporting Structure
Infusion *see* Introduction of substance in or on
Infusion Device, Pump
Insertion of device in
Abdomen ØJH8
Back ØJH7
Chest ØJH6
Lower Arm
Left ØJHH
Right ØJHG
Lower Leg
Left ØJHP
Right ØJHN
Trunk ØJHT
Upper Arm
Left ØJHF
Right ØJHD
Upper Leg
Left ØJHM
Right ØJHL
Removal of device from
Lower Extremity ØJPW
Trunk ØJPT
Upper Extremity ØJPV
Revision of device in
Lower Extremity ØJWW
Trunk ØJWT
Upper Extremity ØJWV
Infusion, glucarpidase
Central vein 3EØ43GQ
Peripheral vein 3EØ33GQ
Inguinal canal
use Inguinal Region, Right
use Inguinal Region, Left
use Inguinal Region, Bilateral
Inguinal triangle
see Inguinal Region, Right
see Inguinal Region, Left
see Inguinal Region, Bilateral
Injection *see* Introduction of substance in or on
Injection reservoir, port *use* Vascular Access Device, Reservoir in Subcutaneous Tissue and Fascia
Injection reservoir, pump *use* Infusion Device, Pump in Subcutaneous Tissue and Fascia
▶ **Innova™ stent** *use* Intraluminal Device
Insemination, artificial 3EØP7LZ
Insertion
Antimicrobial envelope *see* Introduction of Anti-infective
Aqueous drainage shunt
see Bypass, Eye Ø81
see Drainage, Eye Ø89
Bone, Pelvic, Internal Fixation Device with Tulip Connector XNH
Conduit to Short-term External Heart Assist System X2H
Intracardiac Pacemaker, Dual-Chamber X2H
Intraluminal Device, Bioprosthetic Valve X2H
Joint
~~Lumbar Vertebral, Posterior Spinal Motion Preservation Device XRHBØ18~~
~~Lumbosacral, Posterior Spinal Motion Preservation Device XRHDØ18~~
▶ Lumbar Vertebral
▶ 2 or more, Carbon/PEEK Spinal Stabilization Device, Pedicle Based XRHC
▶ Carbon/PEEK Spinal Stabilization Device, Pedicle Based XRHB
▶ Posterior Spinal Motion Preservation Device XRHBØ18
▶ Lumbosacral
▶ Carbon/PEEK Spinal Stabilization Device, Pedicle Based XRHD
▶ Posterior Spinal Motion Preservation Device XRHDØ18
▶ Thoracic Vertebral
▶ 2 to 7, Carbon/PEEK Spinal Stabilization Device, Pedicle Based XRH7
▶ 8 or more, Carbon/PEEK Spinal Stabilization Device, Pedicle Based XRH8
▶ Carbon/PEEK Spinal Stabilization Device, Pedicle Based XRH6
▶ Thoracolumbar Vertebral, Carbon/PEEK Spinal Stabilization Device, Pedicle Based XRHA
Neurostimulator Lead, Sphenopalatine Ganglion XØHK3Q8
Neurostimulator Lead with Paired Stimulation System XØHQ3R8
Products of Conception 1ØHØ
Spinal Stabilization Device
see Insertion of device in, Upper Joints ØRH
see Insertion of device in, Lower Joints ØSH
Tibial Extension with Motion Sensors XNH
Insertion of device in
Abdominal Wall ØWHF
Acetabulum
Left ØQH5
Right ØQH4
Anal Sphincter ØDHR
Ankle Region
Left ØYHL
Right ØYHK
Anus ØDHQ
Aorta
Abdominal Ø4HØ
Thoracic
Ascending/Arch Ø2HX
Descending Ø2HW
Arm
Lower
Left ØXHF
Right ØXHD
Upper
Left ØXH9
Right ØXH8
Insertion of device in *(Continued)*
Artery
Anterior Tibial
Left Ø4HQ
Right Ø4HP
Axillary
Left Ø3H6
Right Ø3H5
Brachial
Left Ø3H8
Right Ø3H7
Celiac Ø4H1
Colic
Left Ø4H7
Middle Ø4H8
Right Ø4H6
Common Carotid
Left Ø3HJ
Right Ø3HH
Common Iliac
Left Ø4HD
Right Ø4HC
Coronary
Four or More Arteries Ø2H3
One Artery Ø2HØ
Three Arteries Ø2H2
Two Arteries Ø2H1
External Carotid
Left Ø3HN
Right Ø3HM
External Iliac
Left Ø4HJ
Right Ø4HH
Face Ø3HR
Femoral
Left Ø4HL
Right Ø4HK
Foot
Left Ø4HW
Right Ø4HV
Gastric Ø4H2
Hand
Left Ø3HF
Right Ø3HD
Hepatic Ø4H3
Inferior Mesenteric Ø4HB
Innominate Ø3H2
Internal Carotid
Left Ø3HL
Right Ø3HK
Internal Iliac
Left Ø4HF
Right Ø4HE
Internal Mammary
Left Ø3H1
Right Ø3HØ
Intracranial Ø3HG
Lower Ø4HY
Peroneal
Left Ø4HU
Right Ø4HT
Popliteal
Left Ø4HN
Right Ø4HM
Posterior Tibial
Left Ø4HS
Right Ø4HR
Pulmonary
Left Ø2HR
Right Ø2HQ
Pulmonary Trunk Ø2HP
Radial
Left Ø3HC
Right Ø3HB
Renal
Left Ø4HA
Right Ø4H9
Splenic Ø4H4
Subclavian
Left Ø3H4
Right Ø3H3

Insertion of device in (Continued)
Artery (Continued)
Superior Mesenteric Ø4H5
Temporal
Left Ø3HT
Right Ø3HS
Thyroid
Left Ø3HV
Right Ø3HU
Ulnar
Left Ø3HA
Right Ø3H9
Upper Ø3HY
Vertebral
Left Ø3HQ
Right Ø3HP
Atrium
Left Ø2H7
Right Ø2H6
Axilla
Left ØXH5
Right ØXH4
Back
Lower ØWHL
Upper ØWHK
Bladder ØTHB
Bladder Neck ØTHC
Bone
Ethmoid
Left ØNHG
Right ØNHF
Facial ØNHW
Frontal ØNH1
Hyoid ØNHX
Lacrimal
Left ØNHJ
Right ØNHH
Lower ØQHY
Nasal ØNHB
Occipital ØNH7
Palatine
Left ØNHL
Right ØNHK
Parietal
Left ØNH4
Right ØNH3
Pelvic
Left ØQH3
Right ØQH2
Sphenoid ØNHC
Temporal
Left ØNH6
Right ØNH5
Upper ØPHY
Zygomatic
Left ØNHN
Right ØNHM
Bone Marrow Ø7HT
Brain ØØHØ
Breast
Bilateral ØHHV
Left ØHHU
Right ØHHT
Bronchus
Lingula ØBH9
Lower Lobe
Left ØBHB
Right ØBH6
Main
Left ØBH7
Right ØBH3
Middle Lobe, Right ØBH5
Upper Lobe
Left ØBH8
Right ØBH4
Bursa and Ligament
Lower ØMHY
Upper ØMHX

Insertion of device in (Continued)
Buttock
Left ØYH1
Right ØYHØ
Carpal
Left ØPHN
Right ØPHM
Cavity, Cranial ØWH1
Cerebral Ventricle ØØH6
Cervix ØUHC
Chest Wall ØWH8
Cisterna Chyli Ø7HL
Clavicle
Left ØPHB
Right ØPH9
Coccyx ØQHS
Cul-de-sac ØUHF
Diaphragm ØBHT
Disc
Cervical Vertebral ØRH3
Cervicothoracic Vertebral ØRH5
Lumbar Vertebral ØSH2
Lumbosacral ØSH4
Thoracic Vertebral ØRH9
Thoracolumbar Vertebral ØRHB
Duct
Hepatobiliary ØFHB
Pancreatic ØFHD
Duodenum ØDH9
Ear
Inner
Left Ø9HE
Right Ø9HD
Left Ø9HJ
Right Ø9HH
Elbow Region
Left ØXHC
Right ØXHB
Epididymis and Spermatic Cord ØVHM
Esophagus ØDH5
Lower, Magnetic Lengthening Device ØDH37JZ
Middle, Magnetic Lengthening Device ØDH27JZ
Upper, Magnetic Lengthening Device ØDH17JZ
Extremity
Lower
Left ØYHB
Right ØYH9
Upper
Left ØXH7
Right ØXH6
Eye
Left Ø8H1
Right Ø8HØ
Face ØWH2
Fallopian Tube ØUH8
Femoral Region
Left ØYH8
Right ØYH7
Femoral Shaft
Left ØQH9
Right ØQH8
Femur
Lower
Left ØQHC
Right ØQHB
Upper
Left ØQH7
Right ØQH6
Fibula
Left ØQHK
Right ØQHJ
Foot
Left ØYHN
Right ØYHM
Gallbladder ØFH4
Gastrointestinal Tract ØWHP
Genitourinary Tract ØWHR

Insertion of device in (Continued)
Gland
Endocrine ØGHS
Salivary ØCHA
Glenoid Cavity
Left ØPH8
Right ØPH7
Hand
Left ØXHK
Right ØXHJ
Head ØWHØ
Heart Ø2HA
Humeral Head
Left ØPHD
Right ØPHC
Humeral Shaft
Left ØPHG
Right ØPHF
Ileum ØDHB
Inguinal Region
Left ØYH6
Right ØYH5
Intestinal Tract
Lower Intestinal Tract ØDHD
Upper Intestinal Tract ØDHØ
Intestine
Large ØDHE
Small ØDH8
Jaw
Lower ØWH5
Upper ØWH4
Jejunum ØDHA
Joint
Acromioclavicular
Left ØRHH
Right ØRHG
Ankle
Left ØSHG
Right ØSHF
Carpal
Left ØRHR
Right ØRHQ
Carpometacarpal
Left ØRHT
Right ØRHS
Cervical Vertebral ØRH1
Cervicothoracic Vertebral ØRH4
Coccygeal ØSH6
Elbow
Left ØRHM
Right ØRHL
Finger Phalangeal
Left ØRHX
Right ØRHW
Hip
Left ØSHB
Right ØSH9
Knee
Left ØSHD
Right ØSHC
Lumbar Vertebral ØSHØ
Lumbosacral ØSH3
Metacarpophalangeal
Left ØRHV
Right ØRHU
Metatarsal-Phalangeal
Left ØSHN
Right ØSHM
Occipital-cervical ØRHØ
Sacrococcygeal ØSH5
Sacroiliac
Left ØSH8
Right ØSH7
Shoulder
Left ØRHK
Right ØRHJ
Sternoclavicular
Left ØRHF
Right ØRHE
Tarsal
Left ØSHJ
Right ØSHH

Insertion of device in *(Continued)*
Joint *(Continued)*
Tarsometatarsal
Left ØSHL
Right ØSHK
Temporomandibular
Left ØRHD
Right ØRHC
Thoracic Vertebral ØRH6
Thoracolumbar Vertebral ØRHA
Toe Phalangeal
Left ØSHQ
Right ØSHP
Wrist
Left ØRHP
Right ØRHN
Kidney ØTH5
Knee Region
Left ØYHG
Right ØYHF
Larynx ØCHS
Leg
Lower
Left ØYHJ
Right ØYHH
Upper
Left ØYHD
Right ØYHC
Liver ØFHØ
Left Lobe ØFH2
Right Lobe ØFH1
Lung
Left ØBHL
Right ØBHK
Lymphatic Ø7HN
Thoracic Duct Ø7HK
Mandible
Left ØNHV
Right ØNHT
Maxilla ØNHR
Mediastinum ØWHC
Metacarpal
Left ØPHQ
Right ØPHP
Metatarsal
Left ØQHP
Right ØQHN
Mouth and Throat ØCHY
Muscle
Lower ØKHY
Upper ØKHX
Nasal Mucosa and Soft Tissue Ø9HK
Nasopharynx Ø9HN
Neck ØWH6
Nerve
Cranial ØØHE
Peripheral Ø1HY
Nipple
Left ØHHX
Right ØHHW
Oral Cavity and Throat ØWH3
Orbit
Left ØNHQ
Right ØNHP
Ovary ØUH3
Pancreas ØFHG
Patella
Left ØQHF
Right ØQHD
Pelvic Cavity ØWHJ
Penis ØVHS
Pericardial Cavity ØWHD
Pericardium Ø2HN
Perineum
Female ØWHN
Male ØWHM
Peritoneal Cavity ØWHG
Phalanx
Finger
Left ØPHV
Right ØPHT

Insertion of device in *(Continued)*
Phalanx *(Continued)*
Finger *(Continued)*
Thumb
Left ØPHS
Right ØPHR
Toe
Left ØQHR
Right ØQHQ
Pleura ØBHQ
Pleural Cavity
Left ØWHB
Right ØWH9
Prostate ØVHØ
Prostate and Seminal Vesicles ØVH4
Radius
Left ØPHJ
Right ØPHH
Rectum ØDHP
Respiratory Tract ØWHQ
Retroperitoneum ØWHH
Ribs
1 to 2 ØPH1
3 or More ØPH2
Sacrum ØQH1
Scapula
Left ØPH6
Right ØPH5
Scrotum and Tunica Vaginalis ØVH8
Shoulder Region
Left ØXH3
Right ØXH2
Sinus Ø9HY
Skin ØHHPXYZ
Skull ØNHØ
Spinal Canal ØØHU
Spinal Cord ØØHV
Spleen Ø7HP
Sternum ØPHØ
Stomach ØDH6
Subcutaneous Tissue and Fascia
Abdomen ØJH8
Back ØJH7
Buttock ØJH9
Chest ØJH6
Face ØJH1
Foot
Left ØJHR
Right ØJHQ
Hand
Left ØJHK
Right ØJHJ
Head and Neck ØJHS
Lower Arm
Left ØJHH
Right ØJHG
Lower Extremity ØJHW
Lower Leg
Left ØJHP
Right ØJHN
Neck
Left ØJH5
Right ØJH4
Pelvic Region ØJHC
Perineum ØJHB
Scalp ØJHØ
Trunk ØJHT
Upper Arm
Left ØJHF
Right ØJHD
Upper Extremity ØJHV
Upper Leg
Left ØJHM
Right ØJHL
Tarsal
Left ØQHM
Right ØQHL
Tendon
Lower ØLHY
Upper ØLHX
Testis ØVHD

Insertion of device in *(Continued)*
Thymus Ø7HM
Tibia
Left ØQHH
Right ØQHG
Tongue ØCH7
Trachea ØBH1
Tracheobronchial Tree ØBHØ
Ulna
Left ØPHL
Right ØPHK
Ureter ØTH9
Urethra ØTHD
Uterus ØUH9
Uterus and Cervix ØUHD
Vagina ØUHG
Vagina and Cul-de-sac ØUHH
Vas Deferens ØVHR
Vein
Axillary
Left Ø5H8
Right Ø5H7
Azygos Ø5HØ
Basilic
Left Ø5HC
Right Ø5HB
Brachial
Left Ø5HA
Right Ø5H9
Cephalic
Left Ø5HF
Right Ø5HD
Colic Ø6H7
Common Iliac
Left Ø6HD
Right Ø6HC
Coronary Ø2H4
Esophageal Ø6H3
External Iliac
Left Ø6HG
Right Ø6HF
External Jugular
Left Ø5HQ
Right Ø5HP
Face
Left Ø5HV
Right Ø5HT
Femoral
Left Ø6HN
Right Ø6HM
Foot
Left Ø6HV
Right Ø6HT
Gastric Ø6H2
Hand
Left Ø5HH
Right Ø5HG
Hemiazygos Ø5H1
Hepatic Ø6H4
Hypogastric
Left Ø6HJ
Right Ø6HH
Inferior Mesenteric Ø6H6
Innominate
Left Ø5H4
Right Ø5H3
Internal Jugular
Left Ø5HN
Right Ø5HM
Intracranial Ø5HL
Lower Ø6HY
Portal Ø6H8
Pulmonary
Left Ø2HT
Right Ø2HS
Renal
Left Ø6HB
Right Ø6H9
Saphenous
Left Ø6HQ
Right Ø6HP

Insertion of device in *(Continued)*
Vein *(Continued)*
Splenic Ø6H1
Subclavian
Left Ø5H6
Right Ø5H5
Superior Mesenteric Ø6H5
Upper Ø5HY
Vertebral
Left Ø5HS
Right Ø5HR
Vena Cava
Inferior Ø6HØ
Superior Ø2HV
Ventricle
Left Ø2HL
Right Ø2HK
Vertebra
Cervical ØPH3
Lumbar ØQHØ
Thoracic ØPH4
Wrist Region
Left ØXHH
Right ØXHG
Inspection
Abdominal Wall ØWJF
Ankle Region
Left ØYJL
Right ØYJK
Arm
Lower
Left ØXJF
Right ØXJD
Upper
Left ØXJ9
Right ØXJ8
Artery
Lower Ø4JY
Upper Ø3JY
Axilla
Left ØXJ5
Right ØXJ4
Back
Lower ØWJL
Upper ØWJK
Bladder ØTJB
Bone
Facial ØNJW
Lower ØQJY
Nasal ØNJB
Upper ØPJY
Bone Marrow Ø7JT
Brain ØØJØ
Breast
Left ØHJU
Right ØHJT
Bursa and Ligament
Lower ØMJY
Upper ØMJX
Buttock
Left ØYJ1
Right ØYJØ
Cavity, Cranial ØWJ1
Chest Wall ØWJ8
Cisterna Chyli Ø7JL
Diaphragm ØBJT
Disc
Cervical Vertebral ØRJ3
Cervicothoracic Vertebral ØRJ5
Lumbar Vertebral ØSJ2
Lumbosacral ØSJ4
Thoracic Vertebral ØRJ9
Thoracolumbar Vertebral ØRJB
Duct
Hepatobiliary ØFJB
Pancreatic ØFJD
Ear
Inner
Left Ø9JE
Right Ø9JD
Left Ø9JJ
Right Ø9JH

Inspection *(Continued)*
Elbow Region
Left ØXJC
Right ØXJB
Epididymis and Spermatic Cord ØVJM
Extremity
Lower
Left ØYJB
Right ØYJ9
Upper
Left ØXJ7
Right ØXJ6
Eye
Left Ø8J1XZZ
Right Ø8JØXZZ
Face ØWJ2
Fallopian Tube ØUJ8
Femoral Region
Bilateral ØYJE
Left ØYJ8
Right ØYJ7
Finger Nail ØHJQXZZ
Foot
Left ØYJN
Right ØYJM
Gallbladder ØFJ4
Gastrointestinal Tract ØWJP
Genitourinary Tract ØWJR
Gland
Adrenal ØGJ5
Endocrine ØGJS
Pituitary ØGJØ
Salivary ØCJA
Great Vessel Ø2JY
Hand
Left ØXJK
Right ØXJJ
Head ØWJØ
Heart Ø2JA
Inguinal Region
Bilateral ØYJA
Left ØYJ6
Right ØYJ5
Intestinal Tract
Lower Intestinal Tract ØDJD
Upper Intestinal Tract ØDJØ
Jaw
Lower ØWJ5
Upper ØWJ4
Joint
Acromioclavicular
Left ØRJH
Right ØRJG
Ankle
Left ØSJG
Right ØSJF
Carpal
Left ØRJR
Right ØRJQ
Carpometacarpal
Left ØRJT
Right ØRJS
Cervical Vertebral ØRJ1
Cervicothoracic Vertebral ØRJ4
Coccygeal ØSJ6
Elbow
Left ØRJM
Right ØRJL
Finger Phalangeal
Left ØRJX
Right ØRJW
Hip
Left ØSJB
Right ØSJ9
Knee
Left ØSJD
Right ØSJC
Lumbar Vertebral ØSJØ
Lumbosacral ØSJ3
Metacarpophalangeal
Left ØRJV
Right ØRJU

Inspection *(Continued)*
Joint *(Continued)*
Metatarsal-Phalangeal
Left ØSJN
Right ØSJM
Occipital-cervical ØRJØ
Sacrococcygeal ØSJ5
Sacroiliac
Left ØSJ8
Right ØSJ7
Shoulder
Left ØRJK
Right ØRJJ
Sternoclavicular
Left ØRJF
Right ØRJE
Tarsal
Left ØSJJ
Right ØSJH
Tarsometatarsal
Left ØSJL
Right ØSJK
Temporomandibular
Left ØRJD
Right ØRJC
Thoracic Vertebral ØRJ6
Thoracolumbar Vertebral ØRJA
Toe Phalangeal
Left ØSJQ
Right ØSJP
Wrist
Left ØRJP
Right ØRJN
Kidney ØTJ5
Knee Region
Left ØYJG
Right ØYJF
Larynx ØCJS
Leg
Lower
Left ØYJJ
Right ØYJH
Upper
Left ØYJD
Right ØYJC
Lens
Left Ø8JKXZZ
Right Ø8JJXZZ
Liver ØFJØ
Lung
Left ØBJL
Right ØBJK
Lymphatic Ø7JN
Thoracic Duct Ø7JK
Mediastinum ØWJC
Mesentery ØDJV
Mouth and Throat ØCJY
Muscle
Extraocular
Left Ø8JM
Right Ø8JL
Lower ØKJY
Upper ØKJX
Nasal Mucosa and Soft Tissue Ø9JK
Neck ØWJ6
Nerve
Cranial ØØJE
Peripheral Ø1JY
Omentum ØDJU
Oral Cavity and Throat ØWJ3
Ovary ØUJ3
Pancreas ØFJG
Parathyroid Gland ØGJR
Pelvic Cavity ØWJD
Penis ØVJS
Pericardial Cavity ØWJD
Perineum
Female ØWJN
Male ØWJM
Peritoneal Cavity ØWJG
Peritoneum ØDJW
Pineal Body ØGJ1

Inspection *(Continued)*
Pleura ØBJQ
Pleural Cavity
Left ØWJB
Right ØWJ9
Products of Conception 10JØ
Ectopic 10J2
Retained 10J1
Prostate and Seminal Vesicles ØVJ4
Respiratory Tract ØWJQ
Retroperitoneum ØWJH
Scrotum and Tunica Vaginalis ØVJ8
Shoulder Region
Left ØXJ3
Right ØXJ2
Sinus Ø9JY
Skin ØHJPXZZ
Skull ØNJØ
Spinal Canal ØØJU
Spinal Cord ØØJV
Spleen Ø7JP
Stomach ØDJ6
Subcutaneous Tissue and Fascia
Head and Neck ØJJS
Lower Extremity ØJJW
Trunk ØJJT
Upper Extremity ØJJV
Tendon
Lower ØLJY
Upper ØLJX
Testis ØVJD
Thymus Ø7JM
Thyroid Gland ØGJK
Toe Nail ØHJRXZZ
Trachea ØBJ1
Tracheobronchial Tree ØBJØ
Tympanic Membrane
Left Ø9J8
Right Ø9J7
Ureter ØTJ9
Urethra ØTJD
Uterus and Cervix ØUJD
Vagina and Cul-de-sac ØUJH
Vas Deferens ØVJR
Vein
Lower Ø6JY
Upper Ø5JY
Vulva ØUJM
Wall
Abdominal ØWJF
Chest ØWJ8
Wrist Region
Left ØXJH
Right ØXJG
Inspiris Resilia valve *use* Zooplastic Tissue in Heart and Great Vessels
Instillation *see* Introduction of substance in or on
Insufflation *see* Introduction of substance in or on
Intellis™ neurostimulator *use* Stimulator Generator, Multiple Array Rechargeable in ØJH
Interatrial septum *use* Atrial Septum
InterAtrial Shunt Device IASD®, Corvia *use* Synthetic Substitute
Interbody fusion (spine) cage
use Interbody Fusion Device in Upper Joints
use Interbody Fusion Device in Lower Joints
Interbody Fusion Device
Interbody Fusion Device, Custom-Made Anatomically Designed
Lumbar Vertebral XRGB
2 or more XRGC
Lumbosacral XRGD
Thoracolumbar Vertebral XRGA
Intercarpal joint
use Carpal Joint, Right
use Carpal Joint, Left
Intercarpal ligament
use Hand Bursa and Ligament, Right
use Hand Bursa and Ligament, Left
INTERCEPT Blood System for Plasma Pathogen Reduced Cryoprecipitated Fibrinogen Complex *use* Pathogen Reduced Cryoprecipitated Fibrinogen Complex
INTERCEPT Fibrinogen Complex *use* Pathogen Reduced Cryoprecipitated Fibrinogen Complex
Interclavicular ligament
use Shoulder Bursa and Ligament, Right
use Shoulder Bursa and Ligament, Left
Intercostal lymph node *use* Lymphatic, Thorax
Intercostal muscle
use Thorax Muscle, Right
use Thorax Muscle, Left
Intercostal nerve *use* Thoracic Nerve
Intercostobrachial nerve *use* Thoracic Nerve
Intercuneiform joint
use Tarsal Joint, Right
use Tarsal Joint, Left
Intercuneiform ligament
use Foot Bursa and Ligament, Right
use Foot Bursa and Ligament, Left
Intermediate bronchus *use* Main Bronchus, Right
Intermittent Coronary Sinus Occlusion X2A7358
Intermediate cuneiform bone
use Tarsal, Right
use Tarsal, Left
Intermittent hemodialysis (IHD) 5A1D70Z
Intermittent mandatory ventilation *see* Assistance, Respiratory 5AØ9
Intermittent Negative Airway Pressure
24-96 Consecutive Hours, Ventilation 5AØ945B
Greater than 96 Consecutive Hours, Ventilation 5AØ955B
Less than 24 Consecutive Hours, Ventilation 5AØ935B
Intermittent Positive Airway Pressure
24-96 Consecutive Hours, Ventilation 5AØ9458
Greater than 96 Consecutive Hours, Ventilation 5AØ9558
Less than 24 Consecutive Hours, Ventilation 5AØ9358
Intermittent positive pressure breathing *see* Assistance, Respiratory 5AØ9
Internal (basal) cerebral vein *use* Intracranial Vein
Internal anal sphincter *use* Anal Sphincter
Internal carotid artery, intracranial portion *use* Intracranial Artery
Internal carotid plexus *use* Head and Neck Sympathetic Nerve
Internal Fixation Device with Tulip Connector
Fusion, Joint, Sacroiliac XRG
Insertion, Bone, Pelvic XNH
Internal iliac vein
use Hypogastric Vein, Right
use Hypogastric Vein, Left
Internal maxillary artery
use External Carotid Artery, Right
use External Carotid Artery, Left
Internal naris *use* Nasal Mucosa and Soft Tissue
Internal oblique muscle
use Abdomen Muscle, Right
use Abdomen Muscle, Left
Internal pudendal artery
use Internal Iliac Artery, Right
use Internal Iliac Artery, Left
Internal pudendal vein
use Hypogastric Vein, Right
use Hypogastric Vein, Left
Internal thoracic artery
use Internal Mammary Artery, Right
use Internal Mammary Artery, Left
use Subclavian Artery, Right
use Subclavian Artery, Left
Internal urethral sphincter *use* Urethra
Interphalangeal (IP) joint
use Finger Phalangeal Joint, Right
use Finger Phalangeal Joint, Left
use Toe Phalangeal Joint, Right
use Toe Phalangeal Joint, Left
Interphalangeal ligament
use Hand Bursa and Ligament, Right
use Hand Bursa and Ligament, Left
use Foot Bursa and Ligament, Right
use Foot Bursa and Ligament, Left
Interrogation, cardiac rhythm related device
Interrogation only *see* Measurement, Cardiac 4BØ2
With cardiac function testing *see* Measurement, Cardiac 4AØ2
Interruption *see* Occlusion
Interspinalis muscle
use Trunk Muscle, Right
use Trunk Muscle, Left
Interspinous ligament, cervical *use* Head and Neck Bursa and Ligament
Interspinous ligament, lumbar *use* Lower Spine Bursa and Ligament
Interspinous ligament, thoracic *use* Upper Spine Bursa and Ligament
Interspinous process spinal stabilization device
use Spinal Stabilization Device, Interspinous Process in ØRH
use Spinal Stabilization Device, Interspinous Process in ØSH
InterStim® Therapy lead *use* Neurostimulator Lead in Peripheral Nervous System
InterStim™ II Therapy neurostimulator *use* Stimulator Generator, Single Array in ØJH
InterStim™ Micro Therapy neurostimulator *use* Stimulator Generator, Single Array Rechargeable in ØJH
Interstitial Fluid Volume, Sub-Epidermal Moisture using Electrical Biocapacitance XX2KXP9
Intertransversarius muscle
use Trunk Muscle, Right
use Trunk Muscle, Left
Intertransverse ligament, cervical *use* Head and Neck Bursa and Ligament
Intertransverse ligament, lumbar *use* Lower Spine Bursa and Ligament
Intertransverse ligament, thoracic *use* Upper Spine Bursa and Ligament
Interventricular foramen (Monro) *use* Cerebral Ventricle
Interventricular septum *use* Ventricular Septum
Intestinal lymphatic trunk *use* Cisterna Chyli
Intra.OX 8EØ2XDZ
Intracardiac Pacemaker, Dual-Chamber, Insertion X2H
Intracranial arterial flow, whole blood mRNA XXE5XT7
Intracranial Cerebrospinal Fluid Flow, Computer-aided Triage and Notification XXEØX1A
Intraluminal Bioprosthetic Valve Leaflet Splitting Technology in Existing Valve, Division X28F3VA
Intraluminal Device
Airway
Esophagus ØDH5
Mouth and Throat ØCHY
Nasopharynx Ø9HN
Bioactive
Occlusion
Common Carotid
Left Ø3LJ
Right Ø3LH
External Carotid
Left Ø3LN
Right Ø3LM
Internal Carotid
Left Ø3LL
Right Ø3LK

- Intraluminal Device *(Continued)*
  - Bioactive *(Continued)*
    - Occlusion *(Continued)*
      - Intracranial Ø3LG
      - Vertebral
        - Left Ø3LQ
        - Right Ø3LP
    - Restriction
      - Common Carotid
        - Left Ø3VJ
        - Right Ø3VH
      - External Carotid
        - Left Ø3VN
        - Right Ø3VM
      - Internal Carotid
        - Left Ø3VL
        - Right Ø3VK
      - Intracranial Ø3VG
      - Vertebral
        - Left Ø3VQ
        - Right Ø3VP
  - Bioprosthetic Valve, Insertion X2H
  - Endobronchial Valve
    - Lingula ØBH9
    - Lower Lobe
      - Left ØBHB
      - Right ØBH6
    - Main
      - Left ØBH7
      - Right ØBH3
    - Middle Lobe, Right ØBH5
    - Upper Lobe
      - Left ØBH8
      - Right ØBH4
  - Endotracheal Airway
    - Change device in, Trachea ØB21XEZ
    - Insertion of device in, Trachea ØBH1
  - ▶Everolimus-eluting Resorbable Scaffold(s)
    - ▶Anterior Tibial
      - ▶Left X27Q3TA
      - ▶Right X27P3TA
    - ▶Peroneal
      - ▶Left X27U3TA
      - ▶Right X27T3TA
    - ▶Posterior Tibial
      - ▶Left X27S3TA
      - ▶Right X27R3TA
  - Pessary
    - Change device in, Vagina and Cul-de-sac ØU2HXGZ
    - Insertion of device in
      - Cul-de-sac ØUHF
      - Vagina ØUHG
- Intramedullary (IM) rod (nail)
  - *use* Internal Fixation Device, Intramedullary in Upper Bones
  - *use* Internal Fixation Device, Intramedullary in Lower Bones
- Intramedullary skeletal kinetic distractor (ISKD)
  - *use* Internal Fixation Device, Intramedullary in Upper Bones
  - *use* Internal Fixation Device, Intramedullary in Lower Bones
- Intraocular Telescope
  - Left Ø8RK3ØZ
  - Right Ø8RJ3ØZ
- Intraoperative Radiation Therapy (IORT)
  - Anus DDY8CZZ
  - Bile Ducts DFY2CZZ
  - Bladder DTY2CZZ
  - Brain DØYØCZZ
  - Brain Stem DØY1CZZ
  - Cervix DUY1CZZ
  - Colon DDY5CZZ
  - Duodenum DDY2CZZ
  - Gallbladder DFY1CZZ
  - Ileum DDY4CZZ
  - Jejunum DDY3CZZ
  - Kidney DTYØCZZ
  - Larynx D9YBCZZ
  - Liver DFYØCZZ
- Intraoperative Radiation Therapy (IORT) *(Continued)*
  - Mouth D9Y4CZZ
  - Nasopharynx D9YDCZZ
  - Nerve, Peripheral DØY7CZZ
  - Ovary DUYØCZZ
  - Pancreas DFY3CZZ
  - Pharynx D9YCCZZ
  - Prostate DVYØCZZ
  - Rectum DDY7CZZ
  - Spinal Cord DØY6CZZ
  - Stomach DDY1CZZ
  - Ureter DTY1CZZ
  - Urethra DTY3CZZ
  - Uterus DUY2CZZ
- Intrauterine device (IUD) *use* Contraceptive Device in Female Reproductive System
- Intravascular fluorescence angiography (IFA) *see* Monitoring, Physiological Systems 4A1
- Intravascular Lithotripsy (IVL) *see* Fragmentation
- Intravascular ultrasound assisted thrombolysis *see* Fragmentation, Artery
- Introduction of substance in or on
  - Artery
    - Central 3EØ6
      - Analgesics 3EØ6
      - Anesthetic, Intracirculatory 3EØ6
      - Anti-infective 3EØ6
      - Anti-inflammatory 3EØ6
      - Antiarrhythmic 3EØ6
      - Antineoplastic 3EØ6
      - Destructive Agent 3EØ6
      - Diagnostic Substance, Other 3EØ6
      - Electrolytic Substance 3EØ6
      - Hormone 3EØ6
      - Hypnotics 3EØ6
      - Immunotherapeutic 3EØ6
      - Nutritional Substance 3EØ6
      - Platelet Inhibitor 3EØ6
      - Radioactive Substance 3EØ6
      - Sedatives 3EØ6
      - Serum 3EØ6
      - Thrombolytic 3EØ6
      - Toxoid 3EØ6
      - Vaccine 3EØ6
      - Vasopressor 3EØ6
      - Water Balance Substance 3EØ6
    - Coronary 3EØ7
      - Diagnostic Substance, Other 3EØ7
      - Platelet Inhibitor 3EØ7
      - Thrombolytic 3EØ7
    - Peripheral 3EØ5
      - Analgesics 3EØ5
      - Anesthetic, Intracirculatory 3EØ5
      - Anti-infective 3EØ5
      - Anti-inflammatory 3EØ5
      - Antiarrhythmic 3EØ5
      - Antineoplastic 3EØ5
      - Destructive Agent 3EØ5
      - Diagnostic Substance, Other 3EØ5
      - Electrolytic Substance 3EØ5
      - Hormone 3EØ5
      - Hypnotics 3EØ5
      - Immunotherapeutic 3EØ5
      - Nutritional Substance 3EØ5
      - Platelet Inhibitor 3EØ5
      - Radioactive Substance 3EØ5
      - Sedatives 3EØ5
      - Serum 3EØ5
      - Thrombolytic 3EØ5
      - Toxoid 3EØ5
      - Vaccine 3EØ5
      - Vasopressor 3EØ5
      - Water Balance Substance 3EØ5
  - Biliary Tract 3EØJ
    - Analgesics 3EØJ
    - Anesthetic Agent 3EØJ
    - Anti-infective 3EØJ
    - Anti-inflammatory 3EØJ
    - Antineoplastic 3EØJ
    - Destructive Agent 3EØJ
- Introduction of substance in or on *(Continued)*
  - Biliary Tract *(Continued)*
    - Diagnostic Substance, Other 3EØJ
    - Electrolytic Substance 3EØJ
    - Gas 3EØJ
    - Hypnotics 3EØJ
    - Islet Cells, Pancreatic 3EØJ
    - Nutritional Substance 3EØJ
    - Radioactive Substance 3EØJ
    - Sedatives 3EØJ
    - Water Balance Substance 3EØJ
  - Bone 3EØV3G
    - Analgesics 3EØV3NZ
    - Anesthetic Agent 3EØV3BZ
    - Anti-infective 3EØV32
    - Anti-inflammatory 3EØV33Z
    - Antineoplastic 3EØV3Ø
    - Destructive Agent 3EØV3TZ
    - Diagnostic Substance, Other 3EØV3KZ
    - Electrolytic Substance 3EØV37Z
    - Hypnotics 3EØV3NZ
    - Nutritional Substance 3EØV36Z
    - Radioactive Substance 3EØV3HZ
    - Sedatives 3EØV3NZ
    - Water Balance Substance 3EØV37Z
  - Bone Marrow 3EØA3GC
    - Antineoplastic 3EØA3Ø
  - Brain 3EØQ
    - Analgesics 3EØQ
    - Anesthetic Agent 3EØQ
    - Anti-infective 3EØQ
    - Anti-inflammatory 3EØQ
    - Antineoplastic 3EØQ
    - Destructive Agent 3EØQ
    - Diagnostic Substance, Other 3EØQ
    - Electrolytic Substance 3EØQ
    - Gas 3EØQ
    - Hypnotics 3EØQ
    - Nutritional Substance 3EØQ
    - Radioactive Substance 3EØQ
    - Sedatives 3EØQ
    - Stem Cells
      - Embryonic 3EØQ
      - Somatic 3EØQ
    - Water Balance Substance 3EØQ
  - Cranial Cavity 3EØQ
    - Analgesics 3EØQ
    - Anesthetic Agent 3EØQ
    - Anti-infective 3EØQ
    - Anti-inflammatory 3EØQ
    - Antineoplastic 3EØQ
    - Destructive Agent 3EØQ
    - Diagnostic Substance, Other 3EØQ
    - Electrolytic Substance 3EØQ
    - Gas 3EØQ
    - Hypnotics 3EØQ
    - Nutritional Substance 3EØQ
    - Radioactive Substance 3EØQ
    - Sedatives 3EØQ
    - Stem Cells
      - Embryonic 3EØQ
      - Somatic 3EØQ
    - Water Balance Substance 3EØQ
  - Ear 3EØB
    - Analgesics 3EØB
    - Anesthetic Agent 3EØB
    - Anti-infective 3EØB
    - Anti-inflammatory 3EØB
    - Antineoplastic 3EØB
    - Destructive Agent 3EØB
    - Diagnostic Substance, Other 3EØB
    - Hypnotics 3EØB
    - Radioactive Substance 3EØB
    - Sedatives 3EØB
  - Epidural Space 3EØS3GC
    - Analgesics 3EØS3NZ
    - Anesthetic Agent 3EØS3BZ
    - Anti-infective 3EØS32
    - Anti-inflammatory 3EØS33Z
    - Antineoplastic 3EØS3Ø
    - Destructive Agent 3EØS3TZ
    - Diagnostic Substance, Other 3EØS3KZ

▶ New ➠ Revised ~~deleted~~ Deleted

- Introduction of substance in or on *(Continued)*
  - Epidural Space *(Continued)*
    - Electrolytic Substance 3EØS37Z
    - Gas 3EØS
    - Hypnotics 3EØS3NZ
    - Nutritional Substance 3EØS36Z
    - Radioactive Substance 3EØS3HZ
    - Sedatives 3EØS3NZ
    - Water Balance Substance 3EØS37Z
  - Eye 3EØC
    - Analgesics 3EØC
    - Anesthetic Agent 3EØC
    - Anti-infective 3EØC
    - Anti-inflammatory 3EØC
    - Antineoplastic 3EØC
    - Destructive Agent 3EØC
    - Diagnostic Substance, Other 3EØC
    - Gas 3EØC
    - Hypnotics 3EØC
    - Pigment 3EØC
    - Radioactive Substance 3EØC
    - Sedatives 3EØC
  - Gastrointestinal Tract
    - Lower 3EØH
      - Analgesics 3EØH
      - Anesthetic Agent 3EØH
      - Anti-infective 3EØH
      - Anti-inflammatory 3EØH
      - Antineoplastic 3EØH
      - Destructive Agent 3EØH
      - Diagnostic Substance, Other 3EØH
      - Electrolytic Substance 3EØH
      - Gas 3EØH
      - Hypnotics 3EØH
      - Nutritional Substance 3EØH
      - Radioactive Substance 3EØH
      - Sedatives 3EØH
      - Water Balance Substance 3EØH
    - Upper 3EØG
      - Analgesics 3EØG
      - Anesthetic Agent 3EØG
      - Anti-infective 3EØG
      - Anti-inflammatory 3EØG
      - Antineoplastic 3EØG
      - Destructive Agent 3EØG
      - Diagnostic Substance, Other 3EØG
      - Electrolytic Substance 3EØG
      - Gas 3EØG
      - Hypnotics 3EØG
      - Nutritional Substance 3EØG
      - Radioactive Substance 3EØG
      - Sedatives 3EØG
      - Water Balance Substance 3EØG
  - Genitourinary Tract 3EØK
    - Analgesics 3EØK
    - Anesthetic Agent 3EØK
    - Anti-infective 3EØK
    - Anti-inflammatory 3EØK
    - Antineoplastic 3EØK
    - Destructive Agent 3EØK
    - Diagnostic Substance, Other 3EØK
    - Electrolytic Substance 3EØK
    - Gas 3EØK
    - Hypnotics 3EØK
    - Nutritional Substance 3EØK
    - Radioactive Substance 3EØK
    - Sedatives 3EØK
    - Water Balance Substance 3EØK
  - Heart 3EØ8
    - Diagnostic Substance, Other 3EØ8
    - Platelet Inhibitor 3EØ8
    - Thrombolytic 3EØ8
  - Joint 3EØU
    - Analgesics 3EØU3NZ
    - Anesthetic Agent 3EØU3BZ
    - Anti-infective 3EØU
    - Anti-inflammatory 3EØU33Z
    - Antineoplastic 3EØU3Ø
    - Destructive Agent 3EØU3TZ
    - Diagnostic Substance, Other 3EØU3KZ
    - Electrolytic Substance 3EØU37Z
    - Gas 3EØU3SF
- Introduction of substance in or on *(Continued)*
  - Joint *(Continued)*
    - Hypnotics 3EØU3NZ
    - Nutritional Substance 3EØU36Z
    - Radioactive Substance 3EØU3HZ
    - Sedatives 3EØU3NZ
    - Water Balance Substance 3EØU37Z
  - Lymphatic 3EØW3GC
    - Analgesics 3EØW3NZ
    - Anesthetic Agent 3EØW3BZ
    - Anti-infective 3EØW32
    - Anti-inflammatory 3EØW33Z
    - Antineoplastic 3EØW3Ø
    - Destructive Agent 3EØW3TZ
    - Diagnostic Substance, Other 3EØW3KZ
    - Electrolytic Substance 3EØW37Z
    - Hypnotics 3EØW3NZ
    - Nutritional Substance 3EØW36Z
    - Radioactive Substance 3EØW3HZ
    - Sedatives 3EØW3NZ
    - Water Balance Substance 3EØW37Z
  - Mouth 3EØD
    - Analgesics 3EØD
    - Anesthetic Agent 3EØD
    - Anti-infective 3EØD
    - Anti-inflammatory 3EØD
    - Antiarrhythmic 3EØD
    - Antineoplastic 3EØD
    - Destructive Agent 3EØD
    - Diagnostic Substance, Other 3EØD
    - Electrolytic Substance 3EØD
    - Hypnotics 3EØD
    - Nutritional Substance 3EØD
    - Radioactive Substance 3EØD
    - Sedatives 3EØD
    - Serum 3EØD
    - Toxoid 3EØD
    - Vaccine 3EØD
    - Water Balance Substance 3EØD
  - Mucous Membrane 3EØØXGC
    - Analgesics 3EØØXNZ
    - Anesthetic Agent 3EØØXBZ
    - Anti-infective 3EØØX2
    - Anti-inflammatory 3EØØX3Z
    - Antineoplastic 3EØØXØ
    - Destructive Agent 3EØØXTZ
    - Diagnostic Substance, Other 3EØØXKZ
    - Hypnotics 3EØØXNZ
    - Pigment 3EØØXMZ
    - Sedatives 3EØØXNZ
    - Serum 3EØØX4Z
    - Toxoid 3EØØX4Z
    - Vaccine 3EØØX4Z
  - Muscle 3EØ23GC
    - Analgesics 3EØ23NZ
    - Anesthetic Agent 3EØ23BZ
    - Anti-infective 3EØ232
    - Anti-inflammatory 3EØ233Z
    - Antineoplastic 3EØ23Ø
    - Destructive Agent 3EØ23TZ
    - Diagnostic Substance, Other 3EØ23KZ
    - Electrolytic Substance 3EØ237Z
    - Hypnotics 3EØ23NZ
    - Nutritional Substance 3EØ236Z
    - Radioactive Substance 3EØ23HZ
    - Sedatives 3EØ23NZ
    - Serum 3EØ234Z
    - Toxoid 3EØ234Z
    - Vaccine 3EØ234Z
    - Water Balance Substance 3EØ237Z
  - Nerve
    - Cranial 3EØX3GC
      - Anesthetic Agent 3EØX3BZ
      - Anti-inflammatory 3EØX33Z
      - Destructive Agent 3EØX3TZ
    - Peripheral 3EØT3GC
      - Anesthetic Agent 3EØT3BZ
      - Anti-inflammatory 3EØT33Z
      - Destructive Agent 3EØT3TZ
- Introduction of substance in or on *(Continued)*
  - Nerve *(Continued)*
    - Plexus 3EØT3GC
      - Anesthetic Agent 3EØT3BZ
      - Anti-inflammatory 3EØT33Z
      - Destructive Agent 3EØT3TZ
  - Nose 3EØ9
    - Analgesics 3EØ9
    - Anesthetic Agent 3EØ9
    - Anti-infective 3EØ9
    - Anti-inflammatory 3EØ9
    - Antineoplastic 3EØ9
    - Destructive Agent 3EØ9
    - Diagnostic Substance, Other 3EØ9
    - Hypnotics 3EØ9
    - Radioactive Substance 3EØ9
    - Sedatives 3EØ9
    - Serum 3EØ9
    - Toxoid 3EØ9
    - Vaccine 3EØ9
  - Pancreatic Tract 3EØJ
    - Analgesics 3EØJ
    - Anesthetic Agent 3EØJ
    - Anti-infective 3EØJ
    - Anti-inflammatory 3EØJ
    - Antineoplastic 3EØJ
    - Destructive Agent 3EØJ
    - Diagnostic Substance, Other 3EØJ
    - Electrolytic Substance 3EØJ
    - Gas 3EØJ
    - Hypnotics 3EØJ
    - Islet Cells, Pancreatic 3EØJ
    - Nutritional Substance 3EØJ
    - Radioactive Substance 3EØJ
    - Sedatives 3EØJ
    - Water Balance Substance 3EØJ
  - Pericardial Cavity 3EØY
    - Analgesics 3EØY3NZ
    - Anesthetic Agent 3EØY3BZ
    - Anti-infective 3EØY32
    - Anti-inflammatory 3EØY33Z
    - Antineoplastic 3EØY
    - Destructive Agent 3EØY3TZ
    - Diagnostic Substance, Other 3EØY3KZ
    - Electrolytic Substance 3EØY37Z
    - Gas 3EØY
    - Hypnotics 3EØY3NZ
    - Nutritional Substance 3EØY36Z
    - Radioactive Substance 3EØY3HZ
    - Sedatives 3EØY3NZ
    - Water Balance Substance 3EØY37Z
  - Peritoneal Cavity 3EØM
    - Adhesion Barrier 3EØM
    - Analgesics 3EØM3NZ
    - Anesthetic Agent 3EØM3BZ
    - Anti-infective 3EØM32
    - Anti-inflammatory 3EØM33Z
    - Antineoplastic 3EØM
    - Destructive Agent 3EØM3TZ
    - Diagnostic Substance, Other 3EØM3KZ
    - Electrolytic Substance 3EØM37Z
    - Gas 3EØM
    - Hypnotics 3EØM3NZ
    - Nutritional Substance 3EØM36Z
    - Radioactive Substance 3EØM3HZ
    - Sedatives 3EØM3NZ
    - Water Balance Substance 3EØM37Z
  - Pharynx 3EØD
    - Analgesics 3EØD
    - Anesthetic Agent 3EØD
    - Anti-infective 3EØD
    - Anti-inflammatory 3EØD
    - Antiarrhythmic 3EØD
    - Antineoplastic 3EØD
    - Destructive Agent 3EØD
    - Diagnostic Substance, Other 3EØD
    - Electrolytic Substance 3EØD
    - Hypnotics 3EØD
    - Nutritional Substance 3EØD
    - Radioactive Substance 3EØD
    - Sedatives 3EØD
    - Serum 3EØD

Introduction of substance in or on *(Continued)*
Pharynx *(Continued)*
Toxoid 3EØD
Vaccine 3EØD
Water Balance Substance 3EØD
Pleural Cavity 3EØL
Adhesion Barrier 3EØL
Analgesics 3EØL3NZ
Anesthetic Agent 3EØL3BZ
Anti-infective 3EØL32
Anti-inflammatory 3EØL33Z
Antineoplastic 3EØL
Destructive Agent 3EØL3TZ
Diagnostic Substance, Other 3EØL3KZ
Electrolytic Substance 3EØL37Z
Gas 3EØL
Hypnotics 3EØL3NZ
Nutritional Substance 3EØL36Z
Radioactive Substance 3EØL3HZ
Sedatives 3EØL3NZ
▶Thrombolytic 3EØL317
Water Balance Substance 3EØL37Z
Products of Conception 3EØE
Analgesics 3EØE
Anesthetic Agent 3EØE
Anti-infective 3EØE
Anti-inflammatory 3EØE
Antineoplastic 3EØE
Destructive Agent 3EØE
Diagnostic Substance, Other 3EØE
Electrolytic Substance 3EØE
Gas 3EØE
Hypnotics 3EØE
Nutritional Substance 3EØE
Radioactive Substance 3EØE
Sedatives 3EØE
Water Balance Substance 3EØE
Reproductive
Female 3EØP
Adhesion Barrier 3EØP
Analgesics 3EØP
Anesthetic Agent 3EØP
Anti-infective 3EØP
Anti-inflammatory 3EØP
Antineoplastic 3EØP
Destructive Agent 3EØP
Diagnostic Substance, Other 3EØP
Electrolytic Substance 3EØP
Gas 3EØP
Hormone 3EØP
Hypnotics 3EØP
Nutritional Substance 3EØP
Ovum, Fertilized 3EØP
Radioactive Substance 3EØP
Sedatives 3EØP
Sperm 3EØP
Water Balance Substance 3EØP
Male 3EØN
Analgesics 3EØN
Anesthetic Agent 3EØN
Anti-infective 3EØN
Anti-inflammatory 3EØN
Antineoplastic 3EØN
Destructive Agent 3EØN
Diagnostic Substance, Other 3EØN
Electrolytic Substance 3EØN
Gas 3EØN
Hypnotics 3EØN
Nutritional Substance 3EØN
Radioactive Substance 3EØN
Sedatives 3EØN
Water Balance Substance 3EØN
Respiratory Tract 3EØF
Analgesics 3EØF
Anesthetic Agent 3EØF
Anti-infective 3EØF
Anti-inflammatory 3EØF
Antineoplastic 3EØF
Destructive Agent 3EØF
Diagnostic Substance, Other 3EØF
Electrolytic Substance 3EØF
Gas 3EØF

Introduction of substance in or on *(Continued)*
Respiratory Tract *(Continued)*
Hypnotics 3EØF
Nutritional Substance 3EØF
Radioactive Substance 3EØF
Sedatives 3EØF
Water Balance Substance 3EØF
Skin 3EØØXGC
Analgesics 3EØØXNZ
Anesthetic Agent 3EØØXBZ
Anti-infective 3EØØX2
Anti-inflammatory 3EØØX3Z
Antineoplastic 3EØØXØ
Destructive Agent 3EØØXTZ
Diagnostic Substance, Other 3EØØXKZ
Hypnotics 3EØØXNZ
Pigment 3EØØXMZ
Sedatives 3EØØXNZ
Serum 3EØØX4Z
Toxoid 3EØØX4Z
Vaccine 3EØØX4Z
Spinal Canal 3EØR3GC
Analgesics 3EØR3NZ
Anesthetic Agent 3EØR3BZ
Anti-infective 3EØR32
Anti-inflammatory 3EØR33Z
Antineoplastic 3EØR3Ø
Destructive Agent 3EØR3TZ
Diagnostic Substance, Other 3EØR3KZ
Electrolytic Substance 3EØR37Z
Gas 3EØR
Hypnotics 3EØR3NZ
Nutritional Substance 3EØR36Z
Radioactive Substance 3EØR3HZ
Sedatives 3EØR3NZ
Stem Cells
Embryonic 3EØR
Somatic 3EØR
Water Balance Substance 3EØR37Z
Subcutaneous Tissue 3EØ13GC
Analgesics 3EØ13NZ
Anesthetic Agent 3EØ13BZ
Anti-infective 3EØ1
Anti-inflammatory 3EØ133Z
Antineoplastic 3EØ13Ø
Destructive Agent 3EØ13TZ
Diagnostic Substance, Other 3EØ13KZ
Electrolytic Substance 3EØ137Z
Hormone 3EØ13V
Hypnotics 3EØ13NZ
Nutritional Substance 3EØ136Z
Radioactive Substance 3EØ13HZ
Sedatives 3EØ13NZ
Serum 3EØ134Z
Toxoid 3EØ134Z
Vaccine 3EØ134Z
Water Balance Substance 3EØ137Z
Vein
Central 3EØ4
Analgesics 3EØ4
Anesthetic, Intracirculatory 3EØ4
Anti-infective 3EØ4
Anti-inflammatory 3EØ4
Antiarrhythmic 3EØ4
Antineoplastic 3EØ4
Destructive Agent 3EØ4
Diagnostic Substance, Other 3EØ4
Electrolytic Substance 3EØ4
Hormone 3EØ4
Hypnotics 3EØ4
Immunotherapeutic 3EØ4
Nutritional Substance 3EØ4
Platelet Inhibitor 3EØ4
Radioactive Substance 3EØ4
Sedatives 3EØ4
Serum 3EØ4
Thrombolytic 3EØ4
Toxoid 3EØ4
Vaccine 3EØ4
Vasopressor 3EØ4
Water Balance Substance 3EØ4

Introduction of substance in or on *(Continued)*
Vein *(Continued)*
Peripheral 3EØ3
Analgesics 3EØ3
Anesthetic, Intracirculatory 3EØ3
Anti-infective 3EØ3
Anti-inflammatory 3EØ3
Antiarrhythmic 3EØ3
Antineoplastic 3EØ3
Destructive Agent 3EØ3
Diagnostic Substance, Other 3EØ3
Electrolytic Substance 3EØ3
Hormone 3EØ3
Hypnotics 3EØ3
Immunotherapeutic 3EØ3
Islet Cells, Pancreatic 3EØ3
Nutritional Substance 3EØ3
Platelet Inhibitor 3EØ3
Radioactive Substance 3EØ3
Sedatives 3EØ3
Serum 3EØ3
Thrombolytic 3EØ3
Toxoid 3EØ3
Vaccine 3EØ3
Vasopressor 3EØ3
Water Balance Substance 3EØ3
Intubated prone positioning *see* Assistance, Respiratory 5AØ9
Intubation
Airway
see Insertion of device in, Trachea ØBH1
see Insertion of device in, Mouth and Throat ØCHY
see Insertion of device in, Esophagus ØDH5
Drainage device *see* Drainage
Feeding Device *see* Insertion of device in, Gastrointestinal System ØDH
INTUITY Elite valve system, EDWARDS (rapid deployment technique) *see* Replacement, Valve, Aortic Ø2RF
Iobenguane 1-131 Antineoplastic XWØ
Iobenguane 1-131, High Specific Activity (HSA) *use* Iobenguane 1-131Antineoplastic
IPPB (intermittent positive pressure breathing) *see* Assistance, Respiratory 5AØ9
Iridectomy
see Excision, Eye Ø8B
see Resection, Eye Ø8T
Iridoplasty
see Repair, Eye Ø8Q
see Replacement, Eye Ø8R
see Supplement, Eye Ø8U
Iridotomy *see* Drainage, Eye Ø89
▶**Irreversible Electroporation (IRE)**
▶*see* Destruction, Heart and Great Vessels Ø25
▶*see* Destruction, Hepatobiliary System and Pancreas ØF5
Irrigation
Biliary Tract, Irrigating Substance 3E1J
Brain, Irrigating Substance 3E1Q38Z
Cranial Cavity, Irrigating Substance 3E1Q38Z
Ear, Irrigating Substance 3E1B
Epidural Space, Irrigating Substance 3E1S38Z
Eye, Irrigating Substance 3E1C
Gastrointestinal Tract
Lower, Irrigating Substance 3E1H
Upper, Irrigating Substance 3E1G
Genitourinary Tract, Irrigating Substance 3E1K
Irrigating Substance 3C1ZX8Z
Joint, Irrigating Substance 3E1U
Mucous Membrane, Irrigating Substance 3E1Ø
Nose, Irrigating Substance 3E19
Pancreatic Tract, Irrigating Substance 3E1J
Pericardial Cavity, Irrigating Substance 3E1Y38Z
Peritoneal Cavity
Dialysate 3E1M39Z
Irrigating Substance 3E1M
Pleural Cavity, Irrigating Substance 3E1L38Z

Irrigation *(Continued)*
Reproductive
Female, Irrigating Substance 3E1P
Male, Irrigating Substance 3E1N
Respiratory Tract, Irrigating Substance 3E1F
Skin, Irrigating Substance 3E10
Spinal Canal, Irrigating Substance 3E1R38Z
Isavuconazole (isavuconazonium sulfate) *use* Other Anti-infective
ISC-REST kit
ISCDx XXE5XT7
QIAGEN Access Anti-SARS-CoV-2 Total Test XXE5XV7
QIAstat-Dx Respiratory SARS-CoV-2 Panel XXE97U7
Ischemic Stroke System (ISS500) *use* Neurostimulator Lead in New Technology
Ischiatic nerve *use* Sciatic Nerve
Ischiocavernosus muscle *use* Perineum Muscle
Ischiofemoral ligament
use Hip Bursa and Ligament, Right
use Hip Bursa and Ligament, Left
Ischium
use Pelvic Bone, Right
use Pelvic Bone, Left
Isolation 8E0ZXY6
Isotope administration, other radiation, whole body DWY5G
ISS500 (Ischemic Stroke System) *use* Neurostimulator Lead in New Technology
Itrel (3) (4) neurostimulator *use* Stimulator Generator, Single Array in 0JH

J

~~Jakafi® use Ruxolitinib~~
▶**JAKAFI®** (Ruxolitinib) *use* Other Substance
Jejunal artery *use* Superior Mesenteric Artery
Jejunectomy
see Excision, Jejunum 0DBA
see Resection, Jejunum 0DTA
Jejunocolostomy
see Bypass, Gastrointestinal System 0D1
see Drainage, Gastrointestinal System 0D9
Jejunopexy
see Repair, Jejunum 0DQA
see Reposition, Jejunum 0DSA
Jejunostomy
see Bypass, Jejunum 0D1A
see Drainage, Jejunum 0D9A
Jejunotomy *see* Drainage, Jejunum 0D9A
Joint fixation plate
use Internal Fixation Device in Upper Joints
use Internal Fixation Device in Lower Joints
Joint liner (insert) *use* Liner in Lower Joints
Joint spacer (antibiotic)
use Spacer in Upper Joints
use Spacer in Lower Joints
Jugular body *use* Glomus Jugulare
Jugular lymph node
use Lymphatic, Right Neck
use Lymphatic, Left Neck
▶**Juxtaductal aorta** *use* Thoracic Aorta, Ascending/Arch

K

Kappa *use* Pacemaker, Dual Chamber in 0JH
Kcentra *use* 4-Factor Prothrombin Complex Concentrate
Keratectomy, kerectomy
see Excision, Eye 08B
see Resection, Eye 08T
Keratocentesis *see* Drainage, Eye 089
Keratoplasty
see Repair, Eye 08Q
see Replacement, Eye 08R
see Supplement, Eye 08U
Keratotomy
see Drainage, Eye 089
see Repair, Eye 08Q
▶**Kerecis®** (GraftGuide) (MariGen) (SurgiBind) (SurgiClose) *use* Nonautologous Tissue Substitute
KEVZARA® *use* Sarilumab
Keystone Heart TriGuard 3™ CEPD (cerebral embolic protection device) X2A6325
Kirschner wire (K-wire)
use Internal Fixation Device in Head and Facial Bones
use Internal Fixation Device in Upper Bones
use Internal Fixation Device in Lower Bones
use Internal Fixation Device in Upper Joints
use Internal Fixation Device in Lower Joints
Knee (implant) insert *use* Liner in Lower Joints
KUB x-ray *see* Plain Radiography, Kidney, Ureter and Bladder BT04
Kuntscher nail
use Internal Fixation Device, Intramedullary in Upper Bones
use Internal Fixation Device, Intramedullary in Lower Bones
KYMRIAH® *use* Tisagenlecleucel Immunotherapy

L

Labia majora *use* Vulva
Labia minora *use* Vulva
Labial gland
use Upper Lip
use Lower Lip
Labiectomy
see Excision, Female Reproductive System ØUB
see Resection, Female Reproductive System ØUT
Lacrimal canaliculus
use Lacrimal Duct, Right
use Lacrimal Duct, Left
Lacrimal punctum
use Lacrimal Duct, Right
use Lacrimal Duct, Left
Lacrimal sac
use Lacrimal Duct, Right
use Lacrimal Duct, Left
LAGB (laparoscopic adjustable gastric banding)
Initial procedure ØDV64CZ
Surgical correction *use* Revision of device in, Stomach ØDW6
Laminectomy
see Release, Central Nervous System and Cranial Nerves ØØN
see Release, Peripheral Nervous System Ø1N
see Excision, Upper Bones ØPB
see Excision, Lower Bones ØQB
Laminotomy
see Release, Central Nervous System ØØN
see Release, Peripheral Nervous System Ø1N
see Drainage, Upper Bones ØP9
see Excision, Upper Bones ØPB
see Release, Upper Bones ØPN
see Drainage, Lower Bones ØQ9
see Excision, Lower Bones ØQB
see Release, Lower Bones ØQN
▶**Lantidra™** *use* Donislecel-jujn Allogeneic Pancreatic Islet Cellular Suspension
LAP-BAND® adjustable gastric banding system *use* Extraluminal Device
Laparoscopic-assisted transanal pull-through
see Excision, Gastrointestinal System ØDB
see Resection, Gastrointestinal System ØDT
Laparoscopy *see* Inspection
Laparotomy
Drainage *see* Drainage, Peritoneal Cavity ØW9G
Exploratory *see* Inspection, Peritoneal *use* Nerve, Lumbar Plexus ØWJG
Laryngectomy
see Excision, Larynx ØCBS
see Resection, Larynx ØCTS
Laryngocentesis *see* Drainage, Larynx ØC9S
Laryngogram *see* Fluoroscopy, Larynx B91J
Laryngopexy
see Repair, Larynx ØCQS
Laryngopharynx *use* Pharynx
Laryngoplasty
see Repair, Larynx ØCQS
see Replacement, Larynx ØCRS
see Supplement, Larynx ØCUS
Laryngorrhaphy *see* Repair, Larynx ØCQS
Laryngoscopy ØCJS8ZZ
Laryngotomy *see* Drainage, Larynx ØC9S
Laser Interstitial Thermal Therapy
Ampulla of Vater ØF5C
Anus ØD5Q
Aortic Body ØG5D
Appendix ØD5J
Brain ØØ5Ø
Breast
Bilateral ØH5V
Left ØH5U
Right ØH5T
Laser Interstitial Thermal Therapy *(Continued)*
Carotid Bodies, Bilateral ØG58
Carotid Body
Left ØG56
Right ØG57
Cecum ØD5H
Coccygeal Glomus ØG5B
Colon
Ascending ØD5K
Descending ØD5M
Sigmoid ØD5N
Transverse ØD5L
Duct
Common Bile ØF59
Cystic ØF58
Hepatic
Common ØF57
Left ØF56
Right ØF55
Pancreatic ØF5D
Accessory ØF5F
Duodenum ØD59
Esophagogastric Junction ØD54
Esophagus ØD55
Lower ØD53
Middle ØD52
Upper ØD51
Gallbladder ØF54
Gland
Adrenal
Bilateral ØG54
Left ØG52
Right ØG53
Pituitary ØG5Ø
Glomus Jugulare ØG5C
Ileocecal Valve ØD5C
Ileum ØD5B
Intestine
Large ØD5E
Left ØD5G
Right ØD5F
Small ØD58
Jejunum ØD5A
Liver ØF5Ø
Left Lobe ØF52
Right Lobe ØF51
Lung
Bilateral ØB5M
Left ØB5L
Lower Lobe
Left ØB5J
Right ØB5F
Middle Lobe, Right ØB5D
Right ØB5K
Upper Lobe
Left ØB5G
Right ØB5C
Lung Lingula ØB5H
Pancreas ØF5G
Para-aortic Body ØG59
Paraganglion Extremity ØG5F
Parathyroid Gland ØG5R
Inferior
Left ØG5P
Right ØG5N
Multiple ØG5Q
Superior
Left ØG5M
Right ØG5L
Pineal Body ØG51
Prostate ØV5Ø
Rectum ØD5P
Sacrum ØQ51
Spinal Cord
Cervical ØØ5W
Lumbar ØØ5Y
Thoracic ØØ5X
Stomach ØD56
Pylorus ØD57
Laser Interstitial Thermal Therapy *(Continued)*
Thyroid Gland ØG5K
Left Lobe ØG5G
Right Lobe ØG5H
Vertebra
Cervical ØP53
Lumbar ØQ5Ø
Thoracic ØP54
Lateral (brachial) lymph node
use Lymphatic, Right Axillary
use Lymphatic, Left Axillary
Lateral canthus
use Upper Eyelid, Right
use Upper Eyelid, Left
Lateral collateral ligament (LCL)
use Knee Bursa and Ligament, Right
use Knee Bursa and Ligament, Left
Lateral condyle of femur
use Lower Femur, Right
use Lower Femur, Left
Lateral condyle of tibia
use Tibia, Right
use Tibia, Left
Lateral cuneiform bone
use Tarsal, Right
use Tarsal, Left
Lateral epicondyle of femur
use Lower Femur, Right
use Lower Femur, Left
Lateral epicondyle of humerus
use Humeral Shaft, Right
use Humeral Shaft, Left
Lateral femoral cutaneous nerve *use* Lumbar Plexus
Lateral malleolus
use Fibula, Right
use Fibula, Left
Lateral meniscus
use Knee Joint, Right
use Knee Joint, Left
Lateral nasal cartilage *use* Nasal Mucosa and Soft Tissue
Lateral plantar artery
use Foot Artery, Right
use Foot Artery, Left
Lateral plantar nerve *use* Tibial Nerve
Lateral rectus muscle
use Extraocular Muscle, Right
use Extraocular Muscle, Left
Lateral sacral artery
use Internal Iliac Artery, Right
use Internal Iliac Artery, Left
Lateral sacral vein
use Hypogastric Vein, Right
use Hypogastric Vein, Left
Lateral sural cutaneous nerve *use* Peroneal Nerve
Lateral tarsal artery
use Foot Artery, Right
use Foot Artery, Left
Lateral temporomandibular ligament *use* Head and Neck Bursa and Ligament
Lateral thoracic artery
use Axillary Artery, Right
use Axillary Artery, Left
Latissimus dorsi muscle
use Trunk Muscle, Right
use Trunk Muscle, Left
Latissimus Dorsi Myocutaneous Flap
Replacement
Bilateral ØHRVØ75
Left ØHRUØ75
Right ØHRTØ75
Transfer
Left ØKXG
Right ØKXF
Lavage
see Irrigation
Bronchial alveolar, diagnostic *see* Drainage, Respiratory System ØB9

L

▶ New ➡ Revised ~~deleted~~ Deleted

▶**Leaflet laceration/division/modification/ splitting device, used during transcatheter aortic valve replacement (TAVR) procedure** X28F3VA
Least splanchnic nerve *use* Thoracic Sympathetic Nerve
Lefamulin Anti-infective XWØ
Left ascending lumbar vein *use* Hemiazygos Vein
Left atrioventricular valve *use* Mitral Valve
Left auricular appendix *use* Atrium, Left
Left colic vein *use* Colic Vein
Left coronary sulcus *use* Heart, Left
Left gastric artery *use* Gastric Artery
Left gastroepiploic artery *use* Splenic Artery
Left gastroepiploic vein *use* Splenic Vein
Left inferior phrenic vein *use* Renal Vein, Left
Left inferior pulmonary vein *use* Pulmonary Vein, Left
Left jugular trunk *use* Thoracic Duct
Left lateral ventricle *use* Cerebral Ventricle
Left ovarian vein *use* Renal Vein, Left
Left second lumbar vein *use* Renal Vein, Left
Left subclavian trunk *use* Thoracic Duct
Left subcostal vein *use* Hemiazygos Vein
Left superior pulmonary vein *use* Pulmonary Vein, Left
Left suprarenal vein *use* Renal Vein, Left
Left testicular vein *use* Renal Vein, Left
Lengthening
  Bone, with device *see* Insertion of Limb Lengthening Device
  Muscle, by incision *see* Division, Muscles ØK8
  Tendon, by incision *see* Division, Tendons ØL8
Leptomeninges, intracranial *use* Cerebral Meninges
Leptomeninges, spinal *use* Spinal Meninges
Leronlimab monoclonal antibody XWØ13K6
Lesser alar cartilage *use* Nasal Mucosa and Soft Tissue
Lesser occipital nerve *use* Cervical Plexus
Lesser Omentum *use* Omentum
Lesser saphenous vein
  use Saphenous Vein, Right
  use Saphenous Vein, Left
Lesser splanchnic nerve *use* Thoracic Sympathetic Nerve
Lesser trochanter
  use Upper Femur, Right
  use Upper Femur, Left
Lesser tuberosity
  use Humeral Head, Right
  use Humeral Head, Left
Lesser wing *use* Sphenoid Bone
Leukopheresis, therapeutic *see* Pheresis, Circulatory 6A55
Levator anguli oris muscle *use* Facial Muscle
Levator ani muscle *use* Perineum Muscle
Levator labii superioris alaeque nasi muscle *use* Facial Muscle
Levator labii superioris muscle *use* Facial Muscle
Levator palpebrae superioris muscle
  use Upper Eyelid, Right
  use Upper Eyelid, Left
Levator scapulae muscle
  use Neck Muscle, Right
  use Neck Muscle, Left
Levator veli palatini muscle *use* Tongue, Palate, Pharynx Muscle
Levatores costarum muscle
  use Thorax Muscle, Right
  use Thorax Muscle, Left
Lifeline ARM Automated Chest Compression (ACC) device 5A1221J
LifeStent® (Flexstar) (XL) Vascular Stent System *use* Intraluminal Device
Lifileucel *use* Lifileucel Immunotherapy
Lifileucel immunotherapy XWØ
Ligament of head of fibula
  use Knee Bursa and Ligament, Right
  use Knee Bursa and Ligament, Left
Ligament of the lateral malleolus
  use Ankle Bursa and Ligament, Right
  use Ankle Bursa and Ligament, Left
Ligamentum flavum, cervical *use* Head and Neck Bursa and Ligament
Ligamentum flavum, lumbar *use* Lower Spine Bursa and Ligament
Ligamentum flavum, thoracic *use* Upper Spine Bursa and Ligament
Ligation *see* Occlusion
Ligation, hemorrhoid *see* Occlusion, Lower Veins, Hemorrhoidal Plexus
Light Therapy GZJZZZZ
LigaPASS 2.Ø™ PJK Prevention System *use* Posterior Vertebral Tether in New Technology
▶**LimFlow™ TADV (Transcatheter Arterialization of the Deep Veins) Procedure** *see* Bypass, Lower Arteries Ø41
▶**LimFlow™ Transcatheter Arterialization of the Deep Veins (TADV) System** *use* Synthetic Substitute
Liner
  Removal of device from
    Hip
      Left ØSPBØ9Z
      Right ØSP9Ø9Z
    Knee
      Left ØSPDØ9Z
      Right ØSPCØ9Z
  Revision of device in
    Hip
      Left ØSWBØ9Z
      Right ØSW9Ø9Z
    Knee
      Left ØSWDØ9Z
      Right ØSWCØ9Z
  Supplement
    Hip
      Left ØSUBØ9Z
        Acetabular Surface ØSUEØ9Z
        Femoral Surface ØSUSØ9Z
      Right ØSU9Ø9Z
        Acetabular Surface ØSUAØ9Z
        Femoral Surface ØSURØ9Z
    Knee
      Left ØSUDØ9
        Femoral Surface ØSUUØ9Z
        Tibial Surface ØSUWØ9Z
      Right ØSUCØ9
        Femoral Surface ØSUTØ9Z
        Tibial Surface ØSUVØ9Z
Lingual artery
  use Artery, External Carotid, Right
  use Artery, External Carotid, Left
Lingual tonsil *use* Pharynx
Lingulectomy, lung
  see Excision, Lung Lingula ØBBH
  see Resection, Lung Lingula ØBTH
Lisocabtagene Maraleucel *use* Lisocabtagene Maraleucel Immunotherapy
Lisocabtagene Maraleucel Immunotherapy XWØ
Lithoplasty *see* Fragmentatio
Lithotripsy
  see Fragmentation
  With removal of fragments *see* Extirpation
LITT (laser interstitial thermal therapy)
  see Laser Interstitial Thermal Therapy
  see Destruction
LIVIAN™ CRT-D *use* Cardiac Resynchronization Defibrillator Pulse Generator in ØJH
LIVTENCITY™ *use* Maribavir Anti-infective
Lobectomy
  see Excision, Central Nervous System and Cranial Nerves ØØB
  see Excision, Respiratory System ØBB
Lobectomy *(Continued)*
  see Resection, Respiratory System ØBT
  see Excision, Hepatobiliary System and Pancreas ØFB
  see Resection, Hepatobiliary System and Pancreas ØFT
  see Excision, Endocrine System ØGB
  see Resection, Endocrine System ØGT
Lobotomy *see* Division, Brain ØØ8Ø
Localization
  see Map
  see Imaging
Locus ceruleus *use* Pons
Longeviti ClearFit® Cranial Implant *use* Synthetic Substitute, Ultrasound Penetrable in New Technology
▶**LOEP® (Local Osteo-Enhancement Procedure)** XWØV3WA
Longeviti ClearFit® OTS Cranial Implant *use* Synthetic Substitute, Ultrasound Penetrable in New Technology
Long thoracic nerve *use* Brachial Plexus
Loop ileostomy *see* Bypass, Ileum ØD1B
Loop recorder, implantable *use* Monitoring Device
Lovotibeglogene Autotemcel XW1
Lower GI series *see* Fluoroscopy, Colon BD14
Lower Respiratory Fluid Nucleic Acid-base Microbial Detection XXEBXQ6
LTX regional anticoagulant *use* Nafamostat Anticoagulant
LUCAS® chest compression system 5A1221J
Lumbar artery *use* Abdominal Aorta
▶**Lumbar Artery Perforator Flap**
  ▶Bilateral ØHRVØ7B
  ▶Left ØHRUØ7B
  ▶Right ØHRTØ7B
Lumbar facet joint *use* Lumbar Vertebral Joint
Lumbar ganglion *use* Lumbar Sympathetic Nerve
Lumbar lymph node *use* Lymphatic, Aortic
Lumbar lymphatic trunk *use* Cisterna Chyli
Lumbar splanchnic nerve *use* Lumbar Sympathetic Nerve
Lumbosacral facet joint *use* Lumbosacral Joint
Lumbosacral trunk *use* Lumbar Nerve
▶**LumiGuide** (Fiber optic 3D guidance for endovascular procedures) 8EØ23FZ
Lumpectomy
  see Excision
Lunate bone
  use Carpal, Right
  use Carpal, Left
Lunotriquetral ligament
  use Hand Bursa and Ligament, Right
  use Hand Bursa and Ligament, Left
LUNSUMIO™ *use* Mosunetuzumab Antineoplastic
Lurbinectedin XWØ
▶**LVA (Lymphovenous Anastomosis)** *see* Bypass, Lymphatic and Hemic Systems Ø71
▶**LVB (Lymphovenous Bypass)** *see* Bypass, Lymphatic and Hemic Systems Ø71
▶**LYFGENIA™** *use* Lovotibeglogene Autotemcel
Lymphadenectomy
  see Excision, Lymphatic and Hemic Systems Ø7B
  see Resection, Lymphatic and Hemic Systems Ø7T
Lymphadenotomy *see* Drainage, Lymphatic and Hemic Systems Ø79
Lymphangiectomy
  see Excision, Lymphatic and Hemic Systems Ø7B
  see Resection, Lymphatic and Hemic Systems Ø7T

Lymphangiogram *see* Plain Radiography, Lymphatic System B7Ø
Lymphangioplasty
see Repair, Lymphatic and Hemic Systems Ø7Q
see Supplement, Lymphatic and Hemic Systems Ø7U
Lymphangiorrhaphy *see* Repair, Lymphatic and Hemic Systems Ø7Q
Lymphangiotomy *see* Drainage, Lymphatic and Hemic Systems Ø79
▶**LVB (Lymphovenous Bypass)** *see* Bypass, Lymphatic and Hemic Systems Ø71
▶**LYFGENIA™** *use* Lovotibeglogene Autotemcel
▶**Lymphaticovenular Anastomosis** *see* Bypass, Lymphatic and Hemic Systems Ø71
▶**Lymphovenous Anastomosis (LVA)** *see* Bypass, Lymphatic and Hemic Systems Ø71
▶**Lymphovenous Bypass (LVB)** *see* Bypass, Lymphatic and Hemic Systems Ø71
▶**Lymphovenous Shunt** *see* Bypass, Lymphatic and Hemic Systems Ø71
Lysis *see* Release
▶**LZRSE-COL7A1 engineered autologous epidermal sheets** *use* Prademagene Zamikeracel,Genetically Engineered Autologous Cell Therapy in New Technology

L

▶ New ➠ Revised ~~deleted~~ Deleted

M

- **Macula**
  - *use* Retina, Right
  - *use* Retina, Left
- **MAGEC® Spinal Bracing and Distraction System** *use* Magnetically Controlled Growth Rod(s) in New Technology
- **Magnet extraction, ocular foreign body** *see* Extirpation, Eye Ø8C
- **Magnetic-guided radiofrequency endovascular fistula**
  - Radial Artery, Left Ø31C3ZF
  - Radial Artery, Right Ø31B3ZF
  - Ulnar Artery, Left Ø31A3ZF
  - Ulnar Artery, Right Ø3193ZF
- **Magnetic Resonance Imaging (MRI)**
  - Abdomen BW3Ø
  - Ankle
    - Left BQ3H
    - Right BQ3G
  - Aorta
    - Abdominal B43Ø
    - Thoracic B33Ø
  - Arm
    - Left BP3F
    - Right BP3E
  - Artery
    - Celiac B431
    - Cervico-Cerebral Arch B33Q
    - Common Carotid, Bilateral B335
    - Coronary
      - Bypass Graft, Multiple B233
      - Multiple B231
    - Internal Carotid, Bilateral B338
    - Intracranial B33R
    - Lower Extremity
      - Bilateral B43H
      - Left B43G
      - Right B43F
    - Pelvic B43C
    - Renal, Bilateral B438
    - Spinal B33M
    - Superior Mesenteric B434
    - Upper Extremity
      - Bilateral B33K
      - Left B33J
      - Right B33H
    - Vertebral, Bilateral B33G
  - Bladder BT3Ø
  - Brachial Plexus BW3P
  - Brain BØ3Ø
  - Breast
    - Bilateral BH32
    - Left BH31
    - Right BH3Ø
  - Calcaneus
    - Left BQ3K
    - Right BQ3J
  - Chest BW33Y
  - Coccyx BR3F
  - Connective Tissue
    - Lower Extremity BL31
    - Upper Extremity BL3Ø
  - Corpora Cavernosa BV3Ø
  - Disc
    - Cervical BR31
    - Lumbar BR33
    - Thoracic BR32
  - Ear B93Ø
  - Elbow
    - Left BP3H
    - Right BP3G
  - Eye
    - Bilateral B837
    - Left B836
    - Right B835
  - Femur
    - Left BQ34
    - Right BQ33
  - Fetal Abdomen BY33

- **Magnetic Resonance Imaging (MRI)** *(Continued)*
  - Fetal Extremity BY35
  - Fetal Head BY3Ø
  - Fetal Heart BY31
  - Fetal Spine BY34
  - Fetal Thorax BY32
  - Fetus, Whole BY36
  - Foot
    - Left BQ3M
    - Right BQ3L
  - Forearm
    - Left BP3K
    - Right BP3J
  - Gland
    - Adrenal, Bilateral BG32
    - Parathyroid BG33
    - Parotid, Bilateral B936
    - Salivary, Bilateral B93D
    - Submandibular, Bilateral B939
    - Thyroid BG34
  - Head BW38
  - Heart, Right and Left B236
  - Hip
    - Left BQ31
    - Right BQ3Ø
  - Intracranial Sinus B532
  - Joint
    - Finger
      - Left BP3D
      - Right BP3C
    - Hand
      - Left BP3D
      - Right BP3C
    - Temporomandibular, Bilateral BN39
  - Kidney
    - Bilateral BT33
    - Left BT32
    - Right BT31
    - Transplant BT39
  - Knee
    - Left BQ38
    - Right BQ37
  - Larynx B93J
  - Leg
    - Left BQ3F
    - Right BQ3D
  - Liver BF35
  - Liver and Spleen BF36
  - Lung Apices BB3G
  - Lung, Bilateral, Hyperpolarized Xenon 129 (Xe-129) BB34Z3Z
  - Nasopharynx B93F
  - Neck BW3F
  - Nerve
    - Acoustic BØ3C
    - Brachial Plexus BW3P
  - Oropharynx B93F
  - Ovary
    - Bilateral BU35
    - Left BU34
    - Right BU33
  - Ovary and Uterus BU3C
  - Pancreas BF37
  - Patella
    - Left BQ3W
    - Right BQ3V
  - Pelvic Region BW3G
  - Pelvis BR3C
  - Pituitary Gland BØ39
  - Plexus, Brachial BW3P
  - Prostate BV33
  - Retroperitoneum BW3H
  - Sacrum BR3F
  - Scrotum BV34
  - Sella Turcica BØ39
  - Shoulder
    - Left BP39
    - Right BP38
  - Sinus
    - Intracranial B532
    - Paranasal B932

- **Magnetic Resonance Imaging (MRI)** *(Continued)*
  - Spinal Cord BØ3B
  - Spine
    - Cervical BR3Ø
    - Lumbar BR39
    - Thoracic BR37
  - Spleen and Liver BF36
  - Subcutaneous Tissue
    - Abdomen BH3H
    - Extremity
      - Lower BH3J
      - Upper BH3F
    - Head BH3D
    - Neck BH3D
    - Pelvis BH3H
    - Thorax BH3G
  - Tendon
    - Lower Extremity BL33
    - Upper Extremity BL32
  - Testicle
    - Bilateral BV37
    - Left BV36
    - Right BV35
  - Toe
    - Left BQ3Q
    - Right BQ3P
  - Uterus BU36
    - Pregnant BU3B
  - Uterus and Ovary BU3C
  - Vagina BU39
  - Vein
    - Cerebellar B531
    - Cerebral B531
    - Jugular, Bilateral B535
    - Lower Extremity
      - Bilateral B53D
      - Left B53C
      - Right B53B
    - Other B53V
    - Pelvic (Iliac) Bilateral B53H
    - Portal B53T
    - Pulmonary, Bilateral B53S
    - Renal, Bilateral B53L
    - ~~Spanchnic B53T~~
    - ▶Splanchnic B53T
    - Upper Extremity
      - Bilateral B53P
      - Left B53N
      - Right B53M
  - Vena Cava
    - Inferior B539
    - Superior B538
  - Wrist
    - Left BP3M
    - Right BP3L
- **Magnetically Controlled Growth Rod(s)**
  - Cervical XNS3
  - Lumbar XNSØ
  - Thoracic XNS4
- **Magnus Neuromodulation System (MNS)** XØZØX18
- **Malleotomy** *see* Drainage, Ear, Nose, Sinus Ø99
- **Malleus**
  - *use* Auditory Ossicle, Right
  - *use* Auditory Ossicle, Left
- **Mammaplasty, mammoplasty**
  - *see* Alteration, Skin and Breast ØHØ
  - *see* Repair, Skin and Breast ØHQ
  - *see* Replacement, Skin and Breast ØHR
  - *see* Supplement, Skin and Breast ØHU
- **Mammary duct**
  - *use* Breast, Right
  - *use* Breast, Left
  - *use* Breast, Bilateral
- **Mammary gland**
  - *use* Breast, Right
  - *use* Breast, Left
  - *use* Breast, Bilateral
- **Mammectomy**
  - *see* Excision, Skin and Breast ØHB
  - *see* Resection, Skin and Breast ØHT

M

Mammillary body *use* Hypothalamus
Mammography *see* Plain Radiography, Skin, Subcutaneous Tissue and Breast BH0
Mammotomy *see* Drainage, Skin and Breast 0H9
Mandibular nerve *use* Trigeminal Nerve
Mandibular notch
use Mandible, Right
use Mandible, Left
Mandibulectomy
see Excision, Head and Facial Bones 0NB
see Resection, Head and Facial Bones 0NT
Manipulation
Adhesions *see* Release
Chiropractic *see* Chiropractic Manipulation
Manual removal, retained placenta *see* Extraction, Products of Conception, Retained 10D1
Manubrium *use* Sternum
Map
Basal Ganglia 00K8
Brain 00K0
▶Connectomic Analysis 00K0XZ1
Cerebellum 00KC
Cerebral Hemisphere 00K7
Conduction Mechanism 02K8
Hypothalamus 00KA
Medulla Oblongata 00KD
Pons 00KB
Thalamus 00K9
Mapping
▶Connectomic Analysis (Brain) 00K0XZ1
Doppler ultrasound *see* Ultrasonography
Electrocardiogram only *see* Measurement, Cardiac 4A02
Maribavir Anti-infective XW0
Mark IV Breathing Pacemaker System *use* Stimulator Generator in Subcutaneous Tissue and Fascia
▶**Marnetegragene Autotemcel** XW1
MarrowStim™ PAD Kit for CBMA (Concentrated Bone Marrow Aspirate) *use* Other Substance
MarrowStim™ PAD Kit, for injection of concentrated bone marrow aspirate *see* Introduction of substance in or on, Muscle 3E02
Marsupialization
see Drainage
see Excision
Massage, cardiac
External 5A12012
Open 02QA0ZZ
Masseter muscle *use* Head Muscle
Masseteric fascia *use* Subcutaneous Tissue and Fascia, Face
Mastectomy
see Excision, Skin and Breast 0HB
see Resection, Skin and Breast 0HT
Mastoid (postauricular) lymph node
use Lymphatic, Right Neck
use Lymphatic, Left Neck
Mastoid air cells
use Mastoid Sinus, Right
use Mastoid Sinus, Left
Mastoid process
use Temporal Bone, Right
use Temporal Bone, Left
Mastoidectomy
see Excision, Ear, Nose, Sinus 09B
see Resection, Ear, Nose, Sinus 09T
Mastoidotomy *see* Drainage, Ear, Nose, Sinus 099
Mastopexy
see Reposition, Skin and Breast 0HS
see Repair, Skin and Breast 0HQ
Mastorrhaphy *see* Repair, Skin and Breast 0HQ
Mastotomy *see* Drainage, Skin and Breast 0H9
Maxillary artery
use External Carotid Artery, Right
use External Carotid Artery, Left
Maxillary nerve *use* Trigeminal Nerve
Maximo II DR (VR) *use* Defibrillator Generator in 0JH
Maximo II DR CRT-D *use* Cardiac Resynchronization Defibrillator Pulse Generator in 0JH
Measurement
Arterial
Flow
Coronary 4A03
Intracranial 4A03X5D
Peripheral 4A03
Pulmonary 4A03
Pressure
Coronary 4A03
Peripheral 4A03
Pulmonary 4A03
Thoracic, Other 4A03
Pulse
Coronary 4A03
Peripheral 4A03
Pulmonary 4A03
Saturation, Peripheral 4A03
Sound, Peripheral 4A03
Biliary
Flow 4A0C
Pressure 4A0C
Cardiac
Action Currents 4A02
Defibrillator 4B02XTZ
Electrical Activity 4A02
Guidance 4A02X4A
No Qualifier 4A02X4Z
Output 4A02
Pacemaker 4B02XSZ
Rate 4A02
Rhythm 4A02
Sampling and Pressure
Bilateral 4A02
Left Heart 4A02
Right Heart 4A02
Sound 4A02
Total Activity, Stress 4A02XM4
Central Nervous
Cerebrospinal Fluid Shunt, Wireless Sensor 4B00XW0
Conductivity 4A00
Electrical Activity 4A00
Pressure 4A000BZ
Intracranial 4A00
Saturation, Intracranial 4A00
Stimulator 4B00XVZ
Temperature, Intracranial 4A00
Circulatory, Volume 4A05XLZ
Gastrointestinal
Motility 4A0B
Pressure 4A0B
Secretion 4A0B
▶Intracranial Cerebrospinal Fluid Flow, Computer-aided Triage and Notification XXE0X1A
Lower Respiratory Fluid Nucleic Acid-base Microbial Detection XXEBXQ6
Lymphatic
Flow 4A06
Pressure 4A06
Metabolism 4A0Z
Musculoskeletal
Contractility 4A0F
Pressure 4A0F3BE
Stimulator 4B0FXVZ
Olfactory, Acuity 4A08X0Z
Peripheral Nervous
Conductivity
Motor 4A01
Sensory 4A01
Electrical Activity 4A01
Stimulator 4B01XVZ
▶Phenotypic Fully Automated Rapid Susceptibility Technology with Controlled Inoculum XXE5X2A
Measurement *(Continued)*
Positive Blood Culture Fluorescence Hybridization for Organism Identification, Concentration and Susceptibility XXE5XN6
▶Positive Blood Culture Small Molecule Sensor Array Technology XXE5X4A
Products of Conception
Cardiac
Electrical Activity 4A0H
Rate 4A0H
Rhythm 4A0H
Sound 4A0H
Nervous
Conductivity 4A0J
Electrical Activity 4A0J
Pressure 4A0J
Respiratory
Capacity 4A09
Flow 4A09
Pacemaker 4B09XSZ
Rate 4A09
Resistance 4A09
Total Activity 4A09
Volume 4A09
Sleep 4A0ZXQZ
Temperature 4A0Z
Urinary
Contractility 4A0D
Flow 4A0D
Pressure 4A0D
Resistance 4A0D
Volume 4A0D
Venous
Flow
Central 4A04
Peripheral 4A04
Portal 4A04
Pulmonary 4A04
Pressure
Central 4A04
Peripheral 4A04
Portal 4A04
Pulmonary 4A04
Pulse
Central 4A04
Peripheral 4A04
Portal 4A04
Pulmonary 4A04
Saturation, Peripheral 4A04
Visual
Acuity 4A07X0Z
Mobility 4A07X7Z
Pressure 4A07XBZ
~~Whole Blood Nucleic Acid-base Microbial Detection XXE5XM5~~
Meatoplasty, urethra *see* Repair, Urethra 0TQD
Meatotomy *see* Drainage, Urinary System 0T9
Mechanical chest compression (mCPR) 5A1221J
Mechanical initial specimen diversion technique using active negative pressure (blood collection) XXE5XR7
Mechanical ventilation *see* Performance, Respiratory 5A19
Medial canthus
use Lower Eyelid, Right
use Lower Eyelid, Left
Medial collateral ligament (MCL)
use Knee Bursa and Ligament, Right
use Knee Bursa and Ligament, Left
Medial condyle of femur
use Lower Femur, Right
use Lower Femur, Left
Medial condyle of tibia
use Tibia, Right
use Tibia, Left
Medial cuneiform bone
use Tarsal, Right
use Tarsal, Left

M

Medial epicondyle of femur
- *use* Lower Femur, Right
- *use* Lower Femur, Left

Medial epicondyle of humerus
- *use* Humeral Shaft, Right
- *use* Humeral Shaft, Left

Medial malleolus
- *use* Tibia, Right
- *use* Tibia, Left

Medial meniscus
- *use* Knee Joint, Right
- *use* Knee Joint, Left

Medial plantar artery
- *use* Foot Artery, Right
- *use* Foot Artery, Left

Medial plantar nerve *use* Tibial Nerve

Medial popliteal nerve *use* Tibial Nerve

Medial rectus muscle
- *use* Extraocular Muscle, Right
- *use* Extraocular Muscle, Left

Medial sural cutaneous nerve *use* Tibial Nerve

Median antebrachial vein
- *use* Basilic Vein, Right
- *use* Basilic Vein, Left

Median cubital vein
- *use* Basilic Vein, Right
- *use* Basilic Vein, Left

Median sacral artery *use* Abdominal Aorta

Mediastinal cavity *use* Mediastinum

Mediastinal lymph node *use* Lymphatic, Thorax

Mediastinal space *use* Mediastinum

Mediastinoscopy ØWJC4ZZ

Medication Management GZ3ZZZZ
- for substance abuse
  - Antabuse HZ83ZZZ
  - Bupropion HZ87ZZZ
  - Clonidine HZ86ZZZ
  - Levo-alpha-acetyl-methadol (LAAM) HZ82ZZZ
  - Methadone Maintenance HZ81ZZZ
  - Naloxone HZ85ZZZ
  - Naltrexone HZ84ZZZ
  - Nicotine Replacement HZ8ØZZZ
  - Other Replacement Medication HZ89ZZZ
  - Psychiatric Medication HZ88ZZZ

Meditation 8EØZXY5

Medtronic Endurant® II AAA stent graft system *use* Intraluminal Device

Meissner's (submucous) plexus *use* Abdominal Sympathetic Nerve

Melody® transcatheter pulmonary valve *use* Zooplastic Tissue in Heart and Great Vessels

Melphalan Hydrochloride Antineoplastic XWØ53T9

Membranous urethra *use* Urethra

Meningeorrhaphy
- *see* Repair, Cerebral Meninges ØØQ1
- *see* Repair, Spinal Meninges ØØQT

Meniscectomy, knee
- *see* Excision, Joint, Knee, Right ØSBC
- *see* Excision, Joint, Knee, Left ØSBD

Mental foramen
- *use* Mandible, Right
- *use* Mandible, Left

Mentalis muscle *use* Facial Muscle

Mentoplasty *see* Alteration, Jaw, Lower ØWØ5

▶ **Meropenem-vaborbactam Anti-infective** *use* Other Anti-infective

Mesenterectomy *see* Excision, Mesentery ØDBV

Mesenteriorrhaphy, mesenterorrhaphy *see* Repair, Mesentery ØDQV

Mesenteriplication *see* Repair, Mesentery ØDQV

Mesoappendix *use* Mesentery

Mesocolon *use* Mesentery

Metacarpal ligament
- *use* Hand Bursa and Ligament, Right
- *use* Hand Bursa and Ligament, Left

Metacarpophalangeal ligament
- *use* Hand Bursa and Ligament, Right
- *use* Hand Bursa and Ligament, Left

Metal on metal bearing surface *use* Synthetic Substitute, Metal in ØSR

Metatarsal ligament
- *use* Foot Bursa and Ligament, Right
- *use* Foot Bursa and Ligament, Left

Metatarsectomy
- *see* Excision, Lower Bones ØQB
- *see* Resection, Lower Bones ØQT

Metatarsophalangeal (MTP) joint
- *use* Metatarsal-Phalangeal Joint, Right
- *use* Metatarsal-Phalangeal Joint, Left

Metatarsophalangeal ligament
- *use* Foot Bursa and Ligament, Right
- *use* Foot Bursa and Ligament, Left

Metathalamus *use* Thalamus

Micro-Driver stent (RX) (OTW) *use* Intraluminal Device

MicroMed HeartAssist *use* Implantable Heart Assist System in Heart and Great Vessels

▶ **Microsurgical Lymph Bypass** *see* Bypass, Lymphatic and Hemic Systems Ø71

Micrus CERECYTE microcoil *use* Intraluminal Device, Bioactive in Upper Arteries

Midcarpal joint
- *use* Carpal Joint, Right
- *use* Carpal Joint, Left

Middle cardiac nerve *use* Thoracic Sympathetic Nerve

Middle cerebral artery *use* Intracranial Artery

Middle cerebral vein *use* Intracranial Vein

Middle colic vein *use* Colic Vein

Middle genicular artery
- *use* Popliteal Artery, Right
- *use* Popliteal Artery, Left

Middle hemorrhoidal vein
- *use* Hypogastric Vein, Right
- *use* Hypogastric Vein, Left

Middle meningeal artery, intracranial portion *use* Intracranial Artery

Middle rectal artery
- *use* Internal Iliac Artery, Right
- *use* Internal Iliac Artery, Left

Middle suprarenal artery *use* Abdominal Aorta

Middle temporal artery
- *use* Temporal Artery, Right
- *use* Temporal Artery, Left

Middle turbinate *use* Nasal Turbinate

Mineral-based Topical Hemostatic Agent XWØ

MIRODERM™ Biologic Wound Matrix *use* Nonautologous Tissue Substitute

MIRODERM™ skin graft *see* Replacement, Skin and Breast ØHR

MitraClip valve repair system *use* Synthetic Substitute

Mitral annulus *use* Mitral Valve

Mitroflow® Aortic Pericardial Heart Valve *use* Zooplastic Tissue in Heart and Great Vessels

MNS (Magnus Neuromodulation System) XØZØX18

Mobilization, adhesions *see* Release

Molar gland *use* Buccal Mucosa

MoleculLight i:X® wound imaging *see* Other Imaging, Anatomical Regions BW5

Monitoring
- ▶ Adhesive Ultrasound Patch Technology, Blood Flow XX25XØA
- Arterial
  - Flow
    - Coronary 4A13
    - Peripheral 4A13
    - Pulmonary 4A13
  - Pressure
    - Coronary 4A13
    - Peripheral 4A13
    - Pulmonary 4A13
  - Pulse
    - Coronary 4A13
    - Peripheral 4A13
    - Pulmonary 4A13
  - Saturation, Peripheral 4A13
  - Sound, Peripheral 4A13
- Brain Electrical Activity, Computer-aided Detection and Notification XX2ØX89
- Cardiac
  - Electrical Activity 4A12
    - Ambulatory 4A12X45
    - No Qualifier 4A12X4Z
  - Output 4A12
  - Rate 4A12
  - Rhythm 4A12
  - Sound 4A12
  - Total Activity, Stress 4A12XM4
  - Vascular Perfusion, Indocyanine Green Dye 4A12XSH
- Central Nervous
  - Conductivity 4A1Ø
  - Electrical Activity
    - Intraoperative 4A1Ø
    - No Qualifier 4A1Ø
  - Pressure 4A1ØØBZ
    - Intracranial 4A1Ø
  - Saturation, Intracranial 4A1Ø
  - Temperature, Intracranial 4A1Ø
- Gastrointestinal
  - Motility 4A1B
  - Pressure 4A1B
  - Secretion 4A1B
  - Vascular Perfusion, Indocyanine Green Dye 4A1BXSH
- ▶ Interstitial Fluid Volume, Sub-Epidermal Moisture using Electrical Biocapacitance XX2KXP9
- Kidney, Fluorescent Pyrazine XT25XE5
- Lymphatic
  - Flow
  - Indocyanine Green Dye 4A16
  - No Qualifier 4A16
  - Pressure 4A16
- Muscle Compartment Pressure, Micro-Electro-Mechanical System XX2F3W9
- Oxygen Saturation Endoscopic Imaging (OXEI) XD2
- Peripheral Nervous
  - Conductivity
    - Motor 4A11
    - Sensory 4A11
  - Electrical Activity Intraoperative 4A11
  - No Qualifier 4A11
- Products of Conception
  - Cardiac
    - Electrical Activity 4A1H
    - Rate 4A1H
    - Rhythm 4A1H
    - Sound 4A1H
  - Nervous
    - Conductivity 4A1J
    - Electrical Activity 4A1J
    - Pressure 4A1J
- Respiratory
  - Capacity 4A19
  - Flow 4A19
  - Rate 4A19
  - Resistance 4A19
  - Volume 4A19
- Skin and Breast, Vascular Perfusion, Indocyanine Green Dye 4A1GXSH
- Sleep 4A1ZXQZ
- Temperature 4A1Z
- Urinary
  - Contractility 4A1D
  - Flow 4A1D
  - Pressure 4A1D
  - Resistance 4A1D
  - Volume 4A1D

Monitoring *(Continued)*
Venous
Flow
Central 4A14
Peripheral 4A14
Portal 4A14
Pulmonary 4A14
Pressure
Central 4A14
Peripheral 4A14
Portal 4A14
Pulmonary 4A14
Pulse
Central 4A14
Peripheral 4A14
Portal 4A14
Pulmonary 4A14
Saturation
Central 4A14
Portal 4A14
Pulmonary 4A14
Monitoring Device, Hemodynamic
Abdomen ØJH8
Chest ØJH6
Mosaic Bioprosthesis (aortic) (mitral) valve *use* Zooplastic Tissue in Heart and Great Vessels
Mosunetuzumab Antineoplastic XWØ
Motor Function Assessment FØ1
Motor Treatment FØ7
MR Angiography
see Magnetic Resonance Imaging (MRI), Heart B23
see Magnetic Resonance Imaging (MRI), Upper Arteries B33
see Magnetic Resonance Imaging (MRI), Lower Arteries B43
MULTI-LINK (VISION)(MINI-VISION) (ULTRA) Coronary Stent System *use* Intraluminal Device
▶**Multi-plane Flex Technology Bioprosthetic Valve** X2RJ3RA
Multiple sleep latency test 4AØZXQZ
Muscle Compartment Pressure, Micro-Electro-Mechanical System XX2F3W9
Musculocutaneous nerve *use* Brachial Plexus Nerve
Musculopexy
see Repair, Muscles ØKQ
see Reposition, Muscles ØKS
Musculophrenic artery
use Internal Mammary Artery, Right
use Internal Mammary Artery, Left
Musculoplasty
see Repair, Muscles ØKQ
see Supplement, Muscles ØKU
Musculorrhaphy *see* Repair, Muscles ØKQ
Musculospiral nerve *use* Radial Nerve
MYØ1 Continuous Compartmental Pressure Monitor XX2F3W9
Myectomy
see Excision, Muscles ØKB
see Resection, Muscles ØKT
Myelencephalon *use* Medulla Oblongata
Myelogram
CT *see* Computerized Tomography (CT Scan), Central Nervous System BØ2
MRI *see* Magnetic Resonance Imaging (MRI), Central Nervous System BØ3
Myenteric (Auerbach's) plexus *use* Abdominal Sympathetic Nerve
Myocardial Bridge Release *see* Release, Artery, Coronary
Myomectomy *see* Excision, Female Reproductive System ØUB
Myometrium *use* Uterus
Myopexy
see Repair, Muscles ØKQ
see Reposition, Muscles ØKS
Myoplasty
see Repair, Muscles ØKQ
see Supplement, Muscles ØKU
Myorrhaphy *see* Repair, Muscles ØKQ
Myoscopy *see* Inspection, Muscles ØKJ
Myotomy
see Division, Muscles ØK8
see Drainage, Muscles ØK9
Myringectomy
see Excision, Ear, Nose, Sinus Ø9B
see Resection, Ear, Nose, Sinus Ø9T
Myringoplasty
see Repair, Ear, Nose, Sinus Ø9Q
see Replacement, Ear, Nose, Sinus Ø9R
see Supplement, Ear, Nose, Sinus Ø9U
Myringostomy *see* Drainage, Ear, Nose, Sinus Ø99
Myringotomy *see* Drainage, Ear, Nose, Sinus Ø99

M

N

NA-1 (Nerinitide) *use* Nerinitide
Nafamostat anticoagulant XYØYX37
Nail bed
  use Finger Nail
  use Toe Nail
Nail plate
  use Finger Nail
  use Toe Nail
nanoLOCK™ interbody fusion device
  use Interbody Fusion Device in Upper Joints
  use Interbody Fusion Device in Lower Joints
Narcosynthesis GZGZZZZ
Narsoplimab monoclonal antibody XWØ
Nasal cavity *use* Nasal Mucosa and Soft Tissue
Nasal concha *use* Nasal Turbinate
Nasalis muscle *use* Facial Muscle
Nasolacrimal duct
  use Lacrimal Duct, Right
  use Lacrimal Duct, Left
Nasopharyngeal airway (NPA) *use* Intraluminal Device, Airway in Ear, Nose, Sinus
Navicular bone
  use Tarsal, Right
  use Tarsal, Left
Near Infrared Spectroscopy, Circulatory System 8EØ2
Neck of femur
  use Upper Femur, Right
  use Upper Femur, Left
Neck of humerus (anatomical)(surgical)
  use Humeral Head, Right
  use Humeral Head, Left
Nelli® Seizure Monitoring System XXEØX48
Neovasc Reducer™ *use* Reduction Device in New Technology
Nephrectomy
  see Excision, Urinary System ØTB
  see Resection, Urinary System ØTT
Nephrolithotomy *see* Extirpation, Urinary System ØTC
Nephrolysis *see* Release, Urinary System ØTN
Nephropexy
  see Repair, Urinary System ØTQ
  see Reposition, Urinary System ØTS
Nephroplasty
  see Repair, Urinary System ØTQ
  see Supplement, Urinary System ØTU
Nephropyeloureterostomy
  see Bypass, Urinary System ØT1
  see Drainage, Urinary System ØT9
Nephrorrhaphy *see* Repair, Urinary System ØTQ
Nephroscopy, transurethral ØTJ58ZZ
Nephrostomy
  see Bypass, Urinary System ØT1
  see Drainage, Urinary System ØT9
Nephrotomography
  see Plain Radiography, Urinary System BTØ
  see Fluoroscopy, Urinary System BT1
Nephrotomy
  see Division, Urinary System ØT8
  see Drainage, Urinary System ØT9
Nerinitide XWØ
Nerve conduction study
  see Measurement, Central Nervous 4AØØ
  see Measurement, Peripheral Nervous 4AØ1
Nerve Function Assessment FØ1
Nerve to the stapedius *use* Facial Nerve
Nesiritide *use* Human B-type Natriuretic Peptide
Neurectomy
  see Excision, Central Nervous System and Cranial Nerves ØØB
  see Excision, Peripheral Nervous System Ø1B
Neurexeresis
  see Extraction, Central Nervous System and Cranial Nerves ØØD
  see Extraction, Peripheral Nervous System Ø1D
NeuroBlate™ System *see* Destruction
Neurohypophysis *use* Gland, Pituitary
Neurolysis
  see Release, Central Nervous System and Cranial Nerves ØØN
  see Release, Peripheral Nervous System Ø1N
Neuromuscular electrical stimulation (NEMS) lead *use* Stimulator Lead in Muscles
Neurophysiologic monitoring *see* Monitoring, Central Nervous 4A1Ø
Neuroplasty
  see Repair, Central Nervous System and Cranial Nerves ØØQ
  see Supplement, Central Nervous System and Cranial Nerves ØØU
  see Repair, Peripheral Nervous System Ø1Q
  see Supplement, Peripheral Nervous System Ø1U
Neurorrhaphy
  see Repair, Central Nervous System and Cranial Nerves ØØQ
  see Repair, Peripheral Nervous System Ø1Q
Neurostimulator Generator
  Insertion of device in, Skull ØNHØØNZ
  Removal of device from, Skull ØNPØØNZ
  Revision of device in, Skull ØNWØØNZ
Neurostimulator generator, multiple channel *use* Stimulator Generator, Multiple Array in ØJH
Neurostimulator generator, multiple channel rechargeable *use* Stimulator Generator, Multiple Array Rechargeable in ØJH
Neurostimulator generator, single channel *use* Stimulator Generator, Single Array in ØJH
Neurostimulator generator, single channel rechargeable *use* Stimulator Generator, Single Array Rechargeable in ØJH
Neurostimulator Lead
  Insertion of device in
    Brain ØØHØ
    Canal, Spinal ØØHU
    Cerebral Ventricle ØØH6
    Nerve
      Cranial ØØHE
      Peripheral Ø1HY
    Spinal Canal ØØHU
    Spinal Cord ØØHV
    Vein
      Azygos Ø5HØ
      Innominate
        Left Ø5H4
        Right Ø5H3
  Removal of device from
    Brain ØØPØ
    Cerebral Ventricle ØØP6
    Nerve
      Cranial ØØPE
      Peripheral Ø1PY
    Spinal Canal ØØPU
    Spinal Cord ØØPV
    Vein
      Azygos Ø5PØ
      Innominate
        Left Ø5P4
        Right Ø5P3
  Revision of device in
    Brain ØØWØ
    Cerebral Ventricle ØØW6
    Nerve
      Cranial ØØWE
      Peripheral Ø1WY
    Spinal Canal ØØWU
    Spinal Cord ØØWV
    Vein
      Azygos Ø5WØ
      Innominate
        Left Ø5W4
        Right Ø5W3
  Sphenopalatine Ganglion, Insertion XØHK3Q8
Neurostimulator Lead with Paired Stimulation System, Insertion XØHQ3R8
Neurostimulator Lead in Oropharynx XWHD7Q7
Neurotomy
  see Division, Central Nervous System and Cranial Nerves ØØ8
  see Division, Peripheral Nervous System Ø18
Neurotripsy
  see Destruction, Central Nervous System and Cranial Nerves ØØ5
  see Destruction, Peripheral Nervous System Ø15
Neutralization plate
  use Internal Fixation Device in Head and Facial Bones
  use Internal Fixation Device in Upper Bones
  use Internal Fixation Device in Lower Bones
New Technology
  ▶ Adhesive Ultrasound Patch Technology, Blood Flow XX25XØA
  Afamitresgene Autoleucel Immunotherapy XWØ
  ▶ AGN1 Bone Void Filler XWØV3WA
  Amivantamab Monoclonal Antibody XWØ
  Anacaulase-bcdb XWØ
  Antibiotic-eluting Bone Void Filler XWØVØP7
  Aorta
    Thoracic Arch using Branched Synthetic Substitute with Intraluminal Device X2RXØN7
    Thoracic Descending using Branched Synthetic Substitute with Intraluminal Device X2VWØN7
    ▶ Thoracodominal, Branched Intraluminal Device, Manufactured Integrated System, Four or More Arteries X2VE3SA
  ~~Apalutamide Antineoplastic XWØDXJ5~~
  Atezolizumab Antineoplastic XWØ
  Axicabtagene Ciloleucel Immunotherapy XWØ
  Bamlanivimab Monoclonal Antibody XWØ
  Baricitinib XWØ
  ▶ Bentracimab, Ticagrelor Reversal Agent XWØ
  Betibeglogene Autotemcel XW1
  Bioengineered Allogeneic Construct, Skin XHRPXF7
  ▶ Bioengineered Human Acellular Vessel X2R
  Brain Electrical Activity
    Computer-aided Detection and Notification XX2ØX89
    Computer-aided Semiologic Analysis XXEØX48
  Brexanolone XWØ
  Brexucabtagene Autoleucel Immunotherapy XWØ
  Broad Consortium Microbiota-based Live Biotherapeutic Suspension XWØH7X8
  Bypass
    Conduit through Femoral Vein to Popliteal Artery X2K
    Conduit through Femoral Vein to Superficial Femoral Artery X2K
  Caplacizumab XWØ
  ▶ Cefepime-taniborbactam Anti-infective XWØ
  Cefiderocol Anti-infective XWØ
  ▶ Ceftobiprole Medocaril Anti-infective XWØ
  Ceftolozane/Tazobactam Anti-infective XWØ
  Cerebral Embolic Filtration
    Duel Filter X2A5312
    Extracorporeal Flow Reversal Circuit X2A
    Single Deflection Filter X2A6325
  CD24Fc Immunomodulator XWØ
  Ciltacabtagene Autoleucel XWØ
  Coagulation Factor Xa, Inactivated XWØ
  Computer-aided Assessment
    Cardiac Output XXE2X19
    Intracranial Vascular Activity XXEØXØ7
  Computer-aided Guidance, Transthoracic Echocardiography X2JAX47

New Technology *(Continued)*
Computer-aided Mechanical Aspiration X2C
Computer-aided Triage and Notification, Pulmonary Artery Flow XXE3X27
Computer-aided Valve Modeling and Notification, Coronary Artery Flow XXE3X68
Computer-assisted Transcranial Magnetic Stimulation XØZØX18
Coronary Sinus, Reduction Device X2V73Q7
Covid-19 Vaccine XWØ
Covid-19 Vaccine Dose 1 XWØ
Covid-19 Vaccine Dose 2 XWØ
Cytarabine and Daunorubicin Liposome Antineoplastic XWØ
Daratumumab and Hyaluronidase-fihj XWØ1318
▶Dasiglucagon XWØ136A
Destruction
Liver, Ultrasound-guided Cavitation XF5
Renal Sympathetic Nerve(s), Ultrasound Ablation XØ51329
Dilation
Anterior Tibial
~~Left~~
~~Sustained Release Drug-eluting Intraluminal Device X27Q385~~
~~Four or More X27Q3C5~~
~~Three X27Q3B5~~
~~Two X27Q395~~
~~Right~~
~~Sustained Release Drug-eluting Intraluminal Device X27P385~~
~~Four or More X27P3C5~~
~~Three X27P3B5~~
~~Two X27P395~~
▶Left, Intraluminal Device, Everolimus-eluting Resorbable Scaffold(s) X27Q3TA
▶Right, Intraluminal Device, Everolimus-eluting Resorbable Scaffold(s) X27P3TA
~~Femoral~~
~~Left~~
~~Sustained Release Drug-eluting Intraluminal Device X27J385~~
~~Four or More X27J3C5~~
~~Three X27J3B5~~
~~Two X27J395~~
~~Right~~
~~Sustained Release Drug-eluting Intraluminal Device X27H385~~
~~Four or More X27H3C5~~
~~Three X27H3B5~~
~~Two X27H395~~
Peroneal
~~Left~~
~~Sustained Release Drug-eluting Intraluminal Device X27U385~~
~~Four or More X27U3C5~~
~~Three X27U3B5~~
~~Two X27U395~~
~~Right~~
~~Sustained Release Drug-eluting Intraluminal Device X27T385~~
~~Four or More X27T3C5~~
~~Three X27T3B5~~
~~Two X27T395~~
▶Left, Intraluminal Device, Everolimus-eluting Resorbable Scaffold(s) X27U3TA
▶Right, Intraluminal Device, Everolimus-eluting Resorbable Scaffold(s) X27T3TA
~~Popliteal~~
~~Left Distal~~
~~Sustained Release Drug-eluting Intraluminal Device X27N385~~
~~Four or More X27N3C5~~
~~Three X27N3B5~~
~~Two X27N395~~

New Technology *(Continued)*
Dilation *(Continued)*
Popliteal *(Continued)*
~~Left Proximal~~
~~Sustained Release Drug-eluting Intraluminal Device X27L385~~
~~Four or More X27L3C5~~
~~Three X27L3B5~~
~~Two X27L395~~
~~Right Distal~~
~~Sustained Release Drug-eluting Intraluminal Device X27M385~~
~~Four or More X27M3C5~~
~~Three X27M3B5~~
~~Two X27M395~~
~~Right Proximal~~
~~Sustained Release Drug-eluting Intraluminal Device X27K385~~
~~Four or More X27K3C5~~
~~Three X27K3B5~~
~~Two X27K395~~
~~Posterior Tibial~~
~~Left~~
~~Sustained Release Drug-eluting Intraluminal Device X27S385~~
~~Four or More X27S3C5~~
~~Three X27S3B5~~
~~Two X27S395~~
~~Right~~
~~Sustained Release Drug-eluting Intraluminal Device X27R385~~
~~Four or More X27R3C5~~
~~Three X27R3B5~~
~~Two X27R395~~
▶Left, Intraluminal Device, Everolimus-eluting Resorbable Scaffold(s) X27S3TA
▶Right, Intraluminal Device, Everolimus-eluting Resorbable Scaffold(s) X27R3TA
▶Division, Intraluminal Bioprosthetic Valve Leaflet Splitting Technology in Existing Valve X28F3VA
▶Donislecel-jujn Allogeneic Pancreatic Islet Cellular Suspension XWØ33DA
Durvalumab Antineoplastic XWØ
Eculizumab XWØ
Eladocagene exuparvovec XWØQ316
Elranatamab Antineoplastic XWØ13L9
Endothelial Damage Inhibitor XYØVX83
Engineered Allogeneic Thymus Tissue XWØ2ØD8
Engineered Chimeric Antigen Receptor T-cell Immunotherapy
Allogeneic XWØ
Autologous XWØ
Epcoritamab Monoclonal Antibody XWØ13S9
~~Erdafitinib Antineoplastic XWØDXL5~~
~~Esketamine Hydrochloride XWØ97M5~~
Etesevimab Monoclonal Antibody XWØ
Exagamglogene Autotemcel XW1
▶Filtration, Blood Pathogens XXA536A
~~Fosfomycin Antineoplatic XWØ~~
Fusion
Ankle
~~Left, Open-truss Design Internal Fixation Device XRGKØB9~~
~~Right, Open-truss Design Internal Fixation Device XRGJØB9~~
▶Left
▶Gyroid-Sheet Lattice Design Internal Fixation Device XRGKØCA
▶Open-truss Design Internal Fixation Device XRGKØB9
▶Right
▶Gyroid-Sheet Lattice Design Internal Fixation Device XRGJØCA
▶Open-truss Design Internal Fixation Device XRGJØB9

New Technology *(Continued)*
Fusion *(Continued)*
Lumbar Vertebral
~~2 or more, Interbody Fusion Device, Custom-Made Anatomically Designed XRGC~~
▶2 or more
▶Facet Joint Fusion Device, Paired Titanium Cages XRGCØEA
▶Interbody Fusion Device, Custom-Made Anatomically Designed XRGC
▶Facet Joint Fusion Device, Paired Titanium Cages XRGBØEA
Interbody Fusion Device, Custom-Made Anatomically Designed XRGB
~~Lumbosacral, Interbody Fusion Device, Custom-Made Anatomically Designed XRGD~~
▶Lumbosacral
▶Facet Joint Fusion Device, Paired Titanium Cages XRGDØEA
▶Interbody Fusion Device, Custom-Made Anatomically Designed XRGD
Sacroiliac, Internal Fixation Device with Tulip Connector XRG
Tarsal
~~Left, Open-truss Design Internal Fixation Device XRGMØB9~~
~~Right, Open-truss Design Internal Fixation Device XRGLØB9~~
▶Left
▶Gyroid-Sheet Lattice Design Internal Fixation Device XRGMØCA
▶Open-truss Design Internal Fixation Device XRGMØB9
▶Right
▶Gyroid-Sheet Lattice Design Internal Fixation Device XRGLØCA
▶Open-truss Design Internal Fixation Device XRGLØB9
~~Thoracolumbar Vertebral, Interbody Fusion Device, Custom-Made AnatomicallyDesigned XRGA~~
▶Thoracolumbar Vertebral
▶Facet Joint Fusion Device, Paired Titanium Cages XRGAØEA
▶Interbody Fusion Device, Custom-Made Anatomically Designed XRGA
~~Gilteritinib Antineoplastic XWØDXV5~~
Glofitamab Antineoplastic XWØ
High-Dose Intravenous Immune Globulin, for COVID-19 treatment XW1
Hyperimmune Globulin, for COVID-19 treatment XW1
Idecabtagene Vicleucel Immunotherapy XWØ
~~Imipenem-cilastatin-relebactam Anti-infective XWØ~~
Inebilizumab-cdon XWØ
Insertion
Bone, Pelvic, Internal Fixation Device with Tulip Connector XNH
Conduit to Short-term External Heart Assist System X2H
Intracardiac Pacemaker, Dual-Chamber X2H
Intraluminal Device, Bioprosthetic Valve X2H
Joint
~~Lumbar Vertebral, Posterior Spinal Motion Preservation Device XRHBØ18~~
~~Lumbosacral, Posterior Spinal Motion Preservation Device XRHDØ18~~

N

▶ New ➠ Revised ~~deleted~~ Deleted

New Technology (Continued)
Insertion (Continued)
Joint (Continued)
▶Lumbar Vertebral
▶2 or more, Carbon/PEEK Spinal Stabilization Device, Pedicle Based XRHC
▶Carbon/PEEK Spinal Stabilization Device, Pedicle Based XRHB
▶Posterior Spinal Motion Preservation Device XRHB018
▶Lumbosacral
▶Carbon/PEEK Spinal Stabilization Device, Pedicle Based XRHD
▶Posterior Spinal Motion Preservation Device XRHD018
▶Thoracic Vertebral
▶2 to 7, Carbon/PEEK Spinal Stabilization Device, Pedicle Based XRH7
▶8 or more, Carbon/PEEK Spinal Stabilization Device, Pedicle Based XRH8
▶Carbon/PEEK Spinal Stabilization Device, Pedicle Based XRH6
▶Thoracolumbar Vertebral, Carbon/PEEK Spinal Stabilization Device, Pedicle Based XRHA
Neurostimulator Lead, Sphenopalatine Ganglion X0HK3Q8
Neurostimulator Lead with Paired Stimulation System X0HQ3R8
Tibial Extension with Motion Sensors XNH
Intermittent Coronary Sinus Occlusion X2A7358
▶Interstitial Fluid Volume, Sub-Epidermal Moisture using Electrical Biocapacitance XX2KXP9
Intracranial Arterial Flow, Whole Blood mRNA XXE5XT7
▶Intracranial Cerebrospinal Fluid Flow, Computer-aided Triage and Notification XXE0X1A
Iobenguane I-131 Antineoplastic XW0
Kidney, Fluorescent Pyrazine XT25XE5
Lefamulin Anti-infective XW0
Leronlimab Monoclonal Antibody XW013K6
Lifileucel Immunotherapy XW0
Lisocabtagene Maraleucel Immunotherapy XW0
Lovotibeglogene Autotemcel XW1
Lower Respiratory Fluid Nucleic Acid-base Microbial Detection XXEBXQ6
Lurbinectedin XW0
Maribavir Anti-infective XW0
▶Marnetegragene Autotemcel XW1
Mechanical Initial Specimen Diversion Technique Using Active Negative Pressure (blood collection) XXE5XR7
Melphalan Hydrochloride Antineoplastic XW053T9
~~Meropenem-vaborbactam Anti-infective XW0~~
Mineral-based Topical Hemostatic Agent XW0
Mosunetuzumab Antineoplastic XW0
▶Multi-plane Flex Technology Bioprosthetic Valve X2RJ3RA
Muscle Compartment Pressure, Micro-Electro-Mechanical System XX2F3W9
Nafamostat Anticoagulant XY0YX37
Narsoplimab Monoclonal Antibody XW0
Nerinitide XW0
Neurostimulator Lead in Oropharynx XWHD7Q7
▶Non-Chimeric Antigen Receptor T-cell Immune Effector Cell Therapy XW0
▶Obecabtagene Autoleucel XW0
▶Odronextamab Antineoplastic XW0
Omadacycline Anti-infective XW0
Omidubicel XW1
▶Orca-T Allogeneic T-cell Immunotherapy XW0

New Technology (Continued)
Other New Technology Therapeutic Substance XW0
Other Positive Blood/Isolated Colonies Bimodal Phenotypic Susceptibility Technology XXE5XY9
OTL-103 XW1
OTL-200 XW1
Quantitative Flow Ratio Analysis, Coronary Artery Flow XXE3X58
Oxygen Saturation Endoscopic Imaging (OXEI) XD2
▶Paclitaxel-Coated Balloon Technology XW0
▶Phenotypic Fully Automated Rapid Susceptibility Technology with Controlled Inoculum XXE5X2A
Plasma, Convalescent (Nonautologous) XW1
Positive Blood Culture Fluorescence Hybridization for Organism Identification, Concentration and Susceptibility XXE5XN6
▶Positive Blood Culture Small Molecule Sensor Array Technology XXE5X4A
Posoleucel XW0
Quizartinib Antineoplastic XW0DXJ9
Radial artery arteriovenous fistula, using Thermal Resistance Energy X2K
REGN-COV2 Monoclonal Antibody XW0
Remdesivir Anti-infection XW0
▶Renal Sympathetic Nerve(s), Radiofrequency Ablation X05133A
Replacement
Lateral Meniscus Synthetic Substitute XRR
Medial Meniscus Synthetic Substitute XRR
Reposition
Cervical, Magnetically Controlled Growth Rod(s) XNS3
Lumbar
Magnetically Controlled Growth Rod(s) XNS0
Posterior (Dynamic) Distraction Device XNS0
Thoracic
Magnetically Controlled Growth Rod(s) XNS4
Posterior (Dynamic) Distraction Device XNS4
~~Ruxolitinib XW0DXT5~~
Rezafungin XW0
Sabizabulin XW0
Sarilumab XW0
SARS-CoV-2 Antibody Detection, Serum/Plasma Nanoparticle Fluorescence XXE5XV7
SARS-CoV-2 Polymerase Chain Reaction, Nasopharyngeal Fluid XXE97U7
Satralizumab-mwge XW01397
SER-109 XW0DXN9
Single-use Duodenoscope XFJ
Single-use Oversleeve with Intraoperative Colonic Irrigation XDPH8K7
▶Skin
▶Abdomen, Prademagene Zamikeracel, Genetically Engineered Autologous Cell Therapy XHR2XGA
▶Back, Prademagene Zamikeracel, Genetically Engineered Autologous Cell TherapyXHR3XGA
▶Chest, Prademagene Zamikeracel, Genetically Engineered Autologous Cell TherapyXHR1XGA
▶Head and Neck, Prademagene Zamikeracel, Genetically Engineered Autologous Cell Therapy XHR0XGA
▶Lower Extremity
▶Left, Prademagene Zamikeracel, Genetically Engineered Autologous Cell TherapyXHR7XGA
▶Right, Prademagene Zamikeracel, Genetically Engineered Autologous Cell TherapyXHR6XGA

New Technology (Continued)
Skin (Continued)
▶Upper Extremity
▶Left, Prademagene Zamikeracel, Genetically Engineered Autologous Cell TherapyXHR5XGA
▶Right, Prademagene Zamikeracel, Genetically Engineered Autologous Cell TherapyXHR4XGA
▶Vancomycin Hydrochloride and Tobramycin Sulfate Anti-Infective, Temporary Irrigation Spacer System XW0U0GA
▶Zanidatamab Antineoplastic XW0
Spesolimab Monoclonal Antibody XW0
Sulbactam-Durlobactam XW0
Supplement
Arteriovenous Fistula, Extraluminal Support Device X2U
Bursa and Ligament, Spine, Posterior Vertebral Tether XKU
Coronary Artery/Arteries, Vein Graft Extraluminal Support Device(s) X2U4079
Vertebra
Lumbar, Mechanically Expandable (Paired) Synthetic Substitute XNU0356
Thoracic, Mechanically Expandable (Paired) Synthetic Substitute XNU4356
Tabelecleucel Immunotherapy XW0
Tagraxofusp-erzs Antineoplastic XW0
Talar Prosthesis Synthetic Substitute XNR
▶Talquetamab Antineoplastic XW01329
Taurolidine Anti-infective and Heparin Anticoagulant XY0YX28
Teclistamab Antineoplastic XW01348
Terlipressin XW0
Tisagenlecleucel Immunotherapy XW0
Tocilizumab XW0
Treosulfan XW0
Trilaciclib XW0
Ultrasound Penetrable Synthetic Substitute, Skull XNR80D9
Uridine Triacetate XW0DX82
~~Venetoclax Antineoplastic XW0DXR5~~
~~Whole Blood Nucleic Acid-base Microbial Detection XXE5XM5~~
Whole Blood Reverse Transcription and Quantitative Real-time Polymerase Chain Reaction XXE5X38
NexoBrid™ *use* Anacaulase-bcdb
Ninth cranial nerve *use* Glossopharyngeal Nerve
NIRS (Near Infrared Spectroscopy) *see* Physiological Systems and Anatomical Regions
Nitinol framed polymer mesh *use* Synthetic Substitute
Niyad™ *use* Nafamostat Anticoagulant
▶**Non-Chimeric Antigen Receptor T-cell Immune Effector Cell Therapy** XW0
Non-tunneled central venous catheter *use* Infusion Device
Nonimaging Nuclear Medicine Assay
Bladder, Kidneys and Ureters CT63
Blood C763
Kidneys, Ureters and Bladder CT63
Lymphatics and Hematologic System C76YYZZ
Ureters, Kidneys and Bladder CT63
Urinary System CT6YYZZ
Nonimaging Nuclear Medicine Probe
Abdomen CW50
Abdomen and Chest CW54
Abdomen and Pelvis CW51
Brain C050
Central Nervous System C05YYZZ
Chest CW53
Chest and Abdomen CW54

Nonimaging Nuclear Medicine Probe *(Continued)*
Chest and Neck CW56
Extremity
Lower CP5PZZZ
Upper CP5NZZZ
Head and Neck CW5B
Heart C25YYZZ
Right and Left C256
Lymphatics
Head C75J
Head and Neck C755
Lower Extremity C75P
Neck C75K
Pelvic C75D
Trunk C75M
Upper Chest C75L
Upper Extremity C75N Lymphatics and Hematologic System C75YYZZ
Musculoskeletal System, Other CP5YYZZ
Neck and Chest CW56
Neck and Head CW5B
Pelvic Region CW5J
Pelvis and Abdomen CW51
Spine CP55ZZZ
Nonimaging Nuclear Medicine Uptake
Endocrine System CG4YYZZ
Gland, Thyroid CG42
Nostril *use* Nasal Mucosa and Soft Tissue
Novacor Left Ventricular Assist Device *use* Implantable Heart Assist System in Heart and Great Vessels
Novation® Ceramic AHS® (Articulation Hip System) *use* Synthetic Substitute, Ceramic in ØSR
Nuclear medicine
see Planar Nuclear Medicine Imaging
see Tomographic (Tomo) Nuclear Medicine Imaging
see Positron Emission Tomographic (PET) Imaging
see Nonimaging Nuclear Medicine Uptake
see Nonimaging Nuclear Medicine Probe
see Nonimaging Nuclear Medicine Assay
see Systemic Nuclear Medicine Therapy
Nuclear scintigraphy *see* Nuclear Medicine
NUsurface® Meniscus Implant
use Synthetic Substitute, Lateral Meniscus in New Technology
use Synthetic Substitute, Medial Meniscus in New Technology
Nutrition, concentrated substances
Enteral infusion 3EØG36Z
Parenteral (peripheral) infusion *see* Introduction of Nutritional Substance
NUZYRA™ *use* Omadacycline Anti-infective

N

O

obe-cel *use* Obecabtagene Autoleucel
Obecabtagene Autoleucel XWØ
Obliteration *see* Destruction
Obturator artery
  use Internal Iliac Artery, Right
  use Internal Iliac Artery, Left
Obturator lymph node *use* Lymphatic, Pelvis
Obturator muscle
  use Hip Muscle, Right
  use Hip Muscle, Left
Obturator nerve *use* Lumbar Plexus
Obturator vein
  use Hypogastric Vein, Right
  use Hypogastric Vein, Left
Obtuse margin *use* Heart, Left
Occipital artery
  use External Carotid Artery, Right
  use External Carotid Artery, Left
Occipital lobe *use* Cerebral Hemisphere
Occipital lymph node
  use Lymphatic, Right Neck
  use Lymphatic, Left Neck
Occipitofrontalis muscle *use* Facial Muscle
Occlusion
  Ampulla of Vater ØFLC
  Anus ØDLQ
  Aorta
    Abdominal Ø4LØ
    Thoracic, Descending Ø2LW
  Artery
    Anterior Tibial
      Left Ø4LQ
      Right Ø4LP
    Axillary
      Left Ø3L6
      Right Ø3L5
    Brachial
      Left Ø3L8
      Right Ø3L7
    Celiac Ø4L1
    Colic
      Left Ø4L7
      Middle Ø4L8
      Right Ø4L6
    Common Carotid
      Left Ø3LJ
      Right Ø3LH
    Common Iliac
      Left Ø4LD
      Right Ø4LC
    External Carotid
      Left Ø3LN
      Right Ø3LM
    External Iliac
      Left Ø4LJ
      Right Ø4LH
    Face Ø3LR
    Femoral
      Left Ø4LL
      Right Ø4LK
    Foot
      Left Ø4LW
      Right Ø4LV
    Gastric Ø4L2
    Hand
      Left Ø3LF
      Right Ø3LD
    Hepatic Ø4L3
    Inferior Mesenteric Ø4LB
    Innominate Ø3L2
    Internal Carotid
      Left Ø3LL
      Right Ø3LK
    Internal Iliac
      Left Ø4LF
      Right Ø4LE

Occlusion *(Continued)*
  Artery *(Continued)*
    Internal Mammary
      Left Ø3L1
      Right Ø3LØ
    Intracranial Ø3LG
  Artery
    Lower Ø4LY
    Peroneal
      Left Ø4LU
      Right Ø4LT
    Popliteal
      Left Ø4LN
      Right Ø4LM
    Posterior Tibial
      Left Ø4LS
      Right Ø4LR
    Pulmonary
      Left Ø2LR
      Right Ø2LQ
    Pulmonary Trunk Ø2LP
    Radial
      Left Ø3LC
      Right Ø3LB
    Renal
      Left Ø4LA
      Right Ø4L9
    Splenic Ø4L4
    Subclavian
      Left Ø3L4
      Right Ø3L3
    Superior Mesenteric Ø4L5
    Temporal
      Left Ø3LT
      Right Ø3LS
    Thyroid
      Left Ø3LV
      Right Ø3LU
    Ulnar
      Left Ø3LA
      Right Ø3L9
    Upper Ø3LY
    Vertebral
      Left Ø3LQ
      Right Ø3LP
  Atrium, Left Ø2L7
  Bladder ØTLB
  Bladder Neck ØTLC
  Bronchus
    Lingula ØBL9
    Lower Lobe
      Left ØBLB
      Right ØBL6
    Main
      Left ØBL7
      Right ØBL3
    Middle Lobe, Right ØBL5
    Upper Lobe
      Left ØBL8
      Right ØBL4
  Carina ØBL2
  Cecum ØDLH
  Cisterna Chyli Ø7LL
  Colon
    Ascending ØDLK
    Descending ØDLM
    Sigmoid ØDLN
    Transverse ØDLL
  Cord
    Bilateral ØVLH
    Left ØVLG
    Right ØVLF
  Cul-de-sac ØULF
  Duct
    Common Bile ØFL9
    Cystic ØFL8
    Hepatic
      Common ØFL7
      Left ØFL6
      Right ØFL5

Occlusion *(Continued)*
  Duct *(Continued)*
    Lacrimal
      Left Ø8LY
      Right Ø8LX
    Pancreatic ØFLD
      Accessory ØFLF
  Duct
    Parotid
      Left ØCLC
      Right ØCLB
  Duodenum ØDL9
  Esophagogastric Junction ØDL4
  Esophagus ØDL5
    Lower ØDL3
    Middle ØDL2
    Upper ØDL1
  Fallopian Tube
    Left ØUL6
    Right ØUL5
  Fallopian Tubes, Bilateral ØUL7
  Ileocecal Valve ØDLC
  Ileum ØDLB
  Intestine
    Large ØDLE
      Left ØDLG
      Right ØDLF
    Small ØDL8
  Jejunum ØDLA
  Kidney Pelvis
    Left ØTL4
    Right ØTL3
  Left atrial appendage (LAA) *see* Occlusion, Atrium, Left Ø2L7
  Lymphatic
    Aortic Ø7LD
    Axillary
      Left Ø7L6
      Right Ø7L5
    Head Ø7LØ
    Inguinal
      Left Ø7LJ
      Right Ø7LH
    Internal Mammary
      Left Ø7L9
      Right Ø7L8
    Lower Extremity
      Left Ø7LG
      Right Ø7LF
    Mesenteric Ø7LB
    Neck
      Left Ø7L2
      Right Ø7L1
    Pelvis Ø7LC
    Thoracic Duct Ø7LK
    Thorax Ø7L7
    Upper Extremity
      Left Ø7L4
      Right Ø7L3
  Rectum ØDLP
  Stomach ØDL6
    Pylorus ØDL7
  Trachea ØBL1
  Ureter
    Left ØTL7
    Right ØTL6
  Urethra ØTLD
  Vagina ØULG
  Valve, Pulmonary Ø2LH
  Vas Deferens
    Bilateral ØVLQ
    Left ØVLP
    Right ØVLN
  Vein
    Axillary
      Left Ø5L8
      Right Ø5L7
    Azygos Ø5LØ
    Basilic
      Left Ø5LC
      Right Ø5LB

O

Occlusion (Continued)
Vein (Continued)
Brachial
Left Ø5LA
Right Ø5L9
Cephalic
Left Ø5LF
Right Ø5LD
Vein
Colic Ø6L7
Common Iliac
Left Ø6LD
Right Ø6LC
Esophageal Ø6L3
External Iliac
Left Ø6LG
Right Ø6LF
External Jugular
Left Ø5LQ
Right Ø5LP
Face
Left Ø5LV
Right Ø5LT
Femoral
Left Ø6LN
Right Ø6LM
Foot
Left Ø6LV
Right Ø6LT
Gastric Ø6L2
Hand
Left Ø5LH
Right Ø5LG
Hemiazygos Ø5L1
Hepatic Ø6L4
Hypogastric
Left Ø6LJ
Right Ø6LH
Inferior Mesenteric Ø6L6
Innominate
Left Ø5L4
Right Ø5L3
Internal Jugular
Left Ø5LN
Right Ø5LM
Intracranial Ø5LL
Lower Ø6LY
Portal Ø6L8
Pulmonary
Left Ø2LT
Right Ø2LS
Renal
Left Ø6LB
Right Ø6L9
Saphenous
Left Ø6LQ
Right Ø6LP
Splenic Ø6L1
Subclavian
Left Ø5L6
Right Ø5L5
Superior Mesenteric Ø6L5
Upper Ø5LY
Vertebral
Left Ø5LS
Right Ø5LR
Vena Cava
Inferior Ø6LØ
Superior Ø2LV
Occlusion, REBOA (resuscitative endovascular balloon occlusion of the aorta)
Ø2LW3DJ
Ø4LØ3DJ
Occupational therapy *see* Activities of Daily Living Treatment, Rehabilitation FØ8
Octagam 10%, for COVID-19 treatment *use* High-Dose Intravenous Immune Globulin
Odentectomy
see Excision, Mouth and Throat ØCB
see Resection, Mouth and Throat ØCT
Odontoid process *use* Cervical Vertebra
▶ Odronextamab Antineoplastic XWØ
Olecranon bursa
use Elbow Bursa and Ligament, Right
use Elbow Bursa and Ligament, Left
Olecranon process
use Ulna, Right
use Ulna, Left
Olfactory bulb *use* Olfactory Nerve
Olumiant® *use* Baricitinib
Omadacycline Anti-infective XWØ
Omentectomy, omentumectomy
see Excision, Gastrointestinal System ØDB
see Resection, Gastrointestinal System ØDT
Omentofixation *see* Repair, Gastrointestinal System ØDQ
Omentoplasty
see Repair, Gastrointestinal System ØDQ
see Replacement, Gastrointestinal System ØDR
see Supplement, Gastrointestinal System ØDU
▶ Omentoplasty, pedicled *see* Transfer, Omentum ØDXU
Omentorrhaphy *see* Repair, Gastrointestinal System ØDQ
Omentotomy *see* Drainage, Gastrointestinal System ØD9
Omidubicel XW1
▶ Omisirge® *use* Omidubicel
Omnilink Elite Vascular Balloon Expandable Stent System *use* Intraluminal Device
▶ OneRF™ Ablation System ØØ5Ø3Z4
Onychectomy
see Excision, Skin and Breast ØHB
see Resection, Skin and Breast ØHT
Onychoplasty
see Repair, Skin and Breast ØHQ
see Replacement, Skin and Breast ØHR
Onychotomy *see* Drainage, Skin and Breast ØH9
Oophorectomy
see Excision, Female Reproductive System ØUB
see Resection, Female Reproductive System ØUT
Oophoropexy
see Repair, Female Reproductive System ØUQ
see Reposition, Female Reproductive System ØUS
Oophoroplasty
see Repair, Female Reproductive System ØUQ
see Supplement, Female Reproductive System ØUU
Oophororrhaphy *see* Repair, Female Reproductive System ØUQ
Oophorostomy *see* Drainage, Female Reproductive System ØU9
Oophorotomy
see Division, Female Reproductive System ØU8
see Drainage, Female Reproductive System ØU9
Oophorrhaphy *see* Repair, Female Reproductive System ØUQ
Open Pivot (mechanical) valve *use* Synthetic Substitute
Open Pivot Aortic Valve Graft (AVG) *use* Synthetic Substitute
Open-truss Design Internal Fixation Device
Ankle
Left XRGKØB9
Right XRGJØB9
Tarsal
Left XRGMØB9
Right XRGLØB9
Ophthalmic artery *use* Intracranial Artery
Ophthalmic nerve *use* Trigeminal Nerve
Ophthalmic vein *use* Intracranial Vein
Opponensplasty
Tendon replacement *see* Replacement, Tendons ØLR
Tendon transfer *see* Transfer, Tendons ØLX
Optic chiasma *use* Optic Nerve
Optic disc
use Retina, Right
use Retina, Left
Optic foramen *use* Sphenoid Bone
Optical coherence tomography, intravascular *see* Computerized Tomography (CT Scan)
Optimizer™ III implantable pulse generator *use* Contractility Modulation Device in ØJH
Orbicularis oculi muscle
use Upper Eyelid, Right
use Upper Eyelid, Left
Orbicularis oris muscle *use* Facial Muscle
Orbital atherectomy *see* Extirpation, Heart and Great Vessels Ø2C
Orbital fascia *use* Subcutaneous Tissue and Fascia, Face
Orbital portion of ethmoid bone
use Orbit, Right
use Orbit, Left
Orbital portion of frontal bone
use Orbit, Right
use Orbit, Left
Orbital portion of lacrimal bone
use Orbit, Right
use Orbit, Left
Orbital portion of maxilla
use Orbit, Right
use Orbit, Left
Orbital portion of palatine bone
use Orbit, Right
use Orbit, Left
Orbital portion of sphenoid bone
use Orbit, Right
use Orbit, Left
Orbital portion of zygomatic bone
use Orbit, Right
use Orbit, Left
▶ Orca-T Allogeneic T-cell Immunotherapy XWØ
Orchectomy, orchidectomy, orchiectomy
see Excision, Male Reproductive System ØVB
see Resection, Male Reproductive System ØVT
Orchidoplasty, orchioplasty
see Repair, Male Reproductive System ØVQ
see Replacement, Male Reproductive System ØVR
see Supplement, Male Reproductive System ØVU
Orchidorrhaphy, orchiorrhaphy *see* Repair, Male Reproductive System ØVQ
Orchidotomy, orchiotomy, orchotomy *see* Drainage, Male Reproductive System ØV9
Orchiopexy
see Repair, Male Reproductive System ØVQ
see Reposition, Male Reproductive System ØVS
Oropharyngeal airway (OPA) *use* Intraluminal Device, Airway in Mouth and Throat
Oropharynx *use* Pharynx
Ossiculectomy
see Excision, Ear, Nose, Sinus Ø9B
see Resection, Ear, Nose, Sinus Ø9T
Ossiculotomy *see* Drainage, Ear, Nose, Sinus Ø99
▶ OSSURE® XWØV3WA
▶ OSSURE™ implant material *use* AGN1 Bone Void Filler
Ostectomy
see Excision, Head and Facial Bones ØNB
see Resection, Head and Facial Bones ØNT
see Excision, Upper Bones ØPB
see Resection, Upper Bones ØPT
see Excision, Lower Bones ØQB
see Resection, Lower Bones ØQT
Osteoclasis
see Division, Head and Facial Bones ØN8
see Division, Upper Bones ØP8
see Division, Lower Bones ØQ8

O

▶ New ➠ Revised ~~deleted~~ Deleted

Osteolysis
see Release, Head and Facial Bones ØNN
see Release, Upper Bones ØPN
see Release, Lower Bones ØQN
Osteopathic Treatment
Abdomen 7WØ9X
Cervical 7WØ1X
Extremity
Lower 7WØ6X
Upper 7WØ7X
Head 7WØØX
Lumbar 7WØ3X
Pelvis 7WØ5X
Rib Cage 7WØ8X
Sacrum 7WØ4X
Thoracic 7WØ2X
Osteopexy
see Repair, Head and Facial Bones ØNQ
see Reposition, Head and Facial Bones ØNS
see Repair, Upper Bones ØPQ
see Reposition, Upper Bones ØPS
see Repair, Lower Bones ØQQ
see Reposition, Lower Bones ØQS
Osteoplasty
see Repair, Head and Facial Bones ØNQ
see Replacement, Head and Facial Bones ØNR
see Supplement, Head and Facial Bones ØNU
see Repair, Upper Bones ØPQ
see Replacement, Upper Bones ØPR
see Supplement, Upper Bones ØPU
see Repair, Lower Bones ØQQ
see Replacement, Lower Bones ØQR
see Supplement, Lower Bones ØQU
Osteorrhaphy
see Repair, Head and Facial Bones ØNQ
see Repair, Upper Bones ØPQ
see Repair, Lower Bones ØQQ
Osteotomy, ostotomy
see Division, Head and Facial Bones ØN8
see Drainage, Head and Facial Bones ØN9
see Division, Upper Bones ØP8
see Drainage, Upper Bones ØP9
see Division, Lower Bones ØQ8
see Drainage, Lower Bones ØQ9
Other Imaging
Bile Duct, Indocyanine Green Dye, Intraoperative BF5Ø2ØØ
Bile Duct and Gallbladder, Indocyanine Green Dye, Intraoperative BF532ØØ
Extremity
Lower BW5CZ1Z
Upper BW5JZ1Z
Gallbladder, Indocyanine Green Dye, Intraoperative BF522ØØ
Gallbladder and Bile Duct, Indocyanine Green Dye, Intraoperative BF532ØØ
Head and Neck BW59Z1Z
Hepatobiliary System, All, Indocyanine Green Dye, Intraoperative BF5C2ØØ
Liver, Indocyanine Green Dye, Intraoperative BF552ØØ
Liver and Spleen, Indocyanine Green Dye, Intraoperative BF5C2ØØ
Neck and Head BW59Z1Z
Pancreas, Indocyanine Green Dye, Intraoperative BF572ØØ
Spleen and liver, Indocyanine Green Dye, Intraoperative BF562ØØ
Trunk BW52Z1Z
Other new technology monoclonal antibody XWØ
Other New Technology Therapeutic Substance XWØ
Other Positive Blood/Isolated Colonies Bimodal Phenotypic Susceptibility Technology XXE5XY9
Otic ganglion *use* Head and Neck Sympathetic Nerve
OTL-1Ø1 *use* Hematopoietic Stem/Progenitor Cells, Genetically Modified
OTL-2ØØ XW1
OTL-1Ø3 XW1
Otoplasty
see Repair, Ear, Nose, Sinus Ø9Q
see Replacement, Ear, Nose, Sinus Ø9R
see Supplement, Ear, Nose, Sinus Ø9U
Otoscopy *see* Inspection, Ear, Nose, Sinus Ø9J
Oval window
use Middle Ear, Right
use Middle Ear, Left
Ovarian artery *use* Abdominal Aorta
Ovarian ligament *use* Uterine Supporting Structure
Ovariectomy
see Excision, Female Reproductive System ØUB
Ovariectomy
see Resection, Female Reproductive System ØUT
Ovariocentesis *see* Drainage, Female Reproductive System ØU9
Ovariopexy
see Repair, Female Reproductive System ØUQ
see Reposition, Female Reproductive System ØUS
Ovariotomy
see Division, Female Reproductive System ØU8
see Drainage, Female Reproductive System ØU9
Ovatio™ CRT-D *use* Cardiac Resynchronization Defibrillator Pulse Generator in ØJH
Oversewing
Gastrointestinal ulcer *see* Repair, Gastrointestinal System ØDQ
Pleural bleb *see* Repair, Respiratory System ØBQ
Oviduct
use Fallopian Tube, Right
use Fallopian Tube, Left
Oximetry, Fetal pulse 1ØHØ73Z
OXINIUM *use* Synthetic Substitute, Oxidized Zirconium on Polyethylene in ØSR
Oxygen saturation endoscopic imaging (OXEI) XD2
Oxygenation
Extracorporeal membrane (ECMO) *see* Performance, Circulatory 5A15
Hyperbaric *see* Assistance, Circulatory 5AØ5
Supersaturated *see* Assistance, Circulatory 5AØ2

O

P

Pacemaker
  Dual Chamber
    Abdomen 0JH8
    Chest 0JH6
  Intracardiac
    Insertion of device in
      Atrium
        Left 02H7
        Right 02H6
      Vein, Coronary 02H4
      Ventricle
        Left 02HL
        Right 02HK
    Removal of device from, Heart 02PA
    Revision of device in, Heart 02WA
  Single Chamber
    Abdomen 0JH8
    Chest 0JH6
  Single Chamber Rate Responsive
    Abdomen 0JH8
    Chest 0JH6
Packing
  Abdominal Wall 2W43X5Z
  Anorectal 2Y43X5Z
  Arm
    Lower
      Left 2W4DX5Z
      Right 2W4CX5Z
    Upper
      Left 2W4BX5Z
      Right 2W4AX5Z
  Back 2W45X5Z
  Chest Wall 2W44X5Z
  Ear 2Y42X5Z
  Extremity
    Lower
      Left 2W4MX5Z
      Right 2W4LX5Z
    Upper
      Left 2W49X5Z
      Right 2W48X5Z
  Face 2W41X5Z
  Finger
    Left 2W4KX5Z
    Right 2W4JX5Z
  Foot
    Left 2W4TX5Z
    Right 2W4SX5Z
  Genital Tract, Female 2Y44X5Z
  Hand
    Left 2W4FX5Z
    Right 2W4EX5Z
  Head 2W40X5Z
  Inguinal Region
    Left 2W47X5Z
    Right 2W46X5Z
  Leg
    Lower
      Left 2W4RX5Z
      Right 2W4QX5Z
    Upper
      Left 2W4PX5Z
      Right 2W4NX5Z
  Mouth and Pharynx 2Y40X5Z
  Nasal 2Y41X5Z
  Neck 2W42X5Z
  Thumb
    Left 2W4HX5Z
    Right 2W4GX5Z
  Toe
    Left 2W4VX5Z
    Right 2W4UX5Z
  Urethra 2Y45X5Z
▶ **Paclitaxel-Coated Balloon Technology** XW0
Paclitaxel-eluting coronary stent *use* Intraluminal Device, Drug-eluting in Heart and Great Vessels
Paclitaxel-eluting peripheral stent
  use Intraluminal Device, Drug-eluting in Upper Arteries
  use Intraluminal Device, Drug-eluting in Lower Arteries
Palatine gland *use* Buccal Mucosa
Palatine tonsil *use* Tonsils
Palatine uvula *use* Uvula
Palatoglossal muscle *use* Tongue, Palate, Pharynx Muscle
Palatopharyngeal muscle *use* Tongue, Palate, Pharynx Muscle
Palatoplasty
  see Repair, Mouth and Throat 0CQ
  see Replacement, Mouth and Throat 0CR
  see Supplement, Mouth and Throat 0CU
Palatorrhaphy *see* Repair, Mouth and Throat 0CQ
▶ **Palladium-103 Collagen Implant** *use* Radioactive Element, Palladium-103 Collagen Implant in00H
Palmar (volar) digital vein
  use Hand Vein, Right
  use Hand Vein, Left
Palmar (volar) metacarpal vein
  use Hand Vein, Right
  use Hand Vein, Left
Palmar cutaneous nerve
  use Radial Nerve
  use Median Nerve
Palmar fascia (aponeurosis)
  use Subcutaneous Tissue and Fascia, Right Hand
  use Subcutaneous Tissue and Fascia, Left Hand
Palmar interosseous muscle
  use Hand Muscle, Right
  use Hand Muscle, Left
Palmar ulnocarpal ligament
  use Wrist Bursa and Ligament, Right
  use Wrist Bursa and Ligament, Left
Palmaris longus muscle
  use Lower Arm and Wrist Muscle, Right
  use Lower Arm and Wrist Muscle, Left
Pancreatectomy
  see Excision, Pancreas 0FBG
  see Resection, Pancreas 0FTG
Pancreatic artery *use* Splenic Artery
Pancreatic plexus *use* Abdominal Sympathetic Nerve
Pancreatic vein *use* Splenic Vein
Pancreaticoduodenostomy *see* Bypass, Hepatobiliary System and Pancreas 0F1
Pancreaticosplenic lymph node *use* Lymphatic, Aortic
Pancreatogram, endoscopic retrograde *see* Fluoroscopy, Pancreatic Duct BF18
Pancreatolithotomy *see* Extirpation, Pancreas 0FCG
Pancreatotomy
  see Division, Pancreas 0F8G
  see Drainage, Pancreas 0F9G
Panniculectomy
  see Excision, Skin, Abdomen 0HB7
  see Excision, Subcutaneous Tissue and Fascia, Abdomen 0JB8
Paraaortic lymph node *use* Lymphatic, Aortic
Paracentesis
  Eye *see* Drainage, Eye 089
  Peritoneal Cavity *see* Drainage, Peritoneal Cavity 0W9G
  Tympanum *see* Drainage, Ear, Nose, Sinus 099
Paradise™ Ultrasound Renal Denervation System X051329
Parapharyngeal space *use* Neck
Pararectal lymph node *use* Lymphatic, Mesenteric
Parasternal lymph node *use* Lymphatic, Thorax
Parathyroidectomy
  see Excision, Endocrine System 0GB
  see Resection, Endocrine System 0GT
Paratracheal lymph node *use* Lymphatic, Thorax
Paraurethral (Skene's) gland *use* Vestibular Gland
Parenteral nutrition, total *see* Introduction of Nutritional Substance
Parietal lobe *use* Cerebral Hemisphere
Parotid lymph node *use* Lymphatic, Head
Parotid plexus *use* Facial Nerve
Parotidectomy
  see Excision, Mouth and Throat 0CB
  see Resection, Mouth and Throat 0CT
Pars flaccida
  use Tympanic Membrane, Right
  use Tympanic Membrane, Left
Partial joint replacement
  Hip *see* Replacement, Lower Joints 0SR
  Knee *see* Replacement, Lower Joints 0SR
  Shoulder *see* Replacement, Upper Joints 0RR
Partially absorbable mesh *use* Synthetic Substitute
Patch, blood, spinal 3E0R3GC
Patellapexy
  see Repair, Lower Bones 0QQ
  see Reposition, Lower Bones 0QS
Patellaplasty
  see Repair, Lower Bones 0QQ
  see Replacement, Lower Bones 0QR
  see Supplement, Lower Bones 0QU
Patellar ligament
  use Knee Bursa and Ligament, Right
  use Knee Bursa and Ligament, Left
Patellar tendon
  use Knee Tendon, Right
  use Knee Tendon, Left
Patellectomy
  see Excision, Lower Bones 0QB
  see Resection, Lower Bones 0QT
Patellofemoral joint
  use Knee Joint, Right
  use Knee Joint, Left
  use Knee Joint, Femoral Surface, Right
  use Knee Joint, Femoral Surface, Left
pAVF (percutaneous arteriovenous fistula), using magnetic-guided radiofrequency *see* Bypass, Upper Arteries 031
pAVF (percutaneous arteriovenous fistula), using thermal resistance energy *see* New Technology, Cardiovascular System X2K
Pectineus muscle
  use Upper Leg Muscle, Right
  use Upper Leg Muscle, Left
Pectoral (anterior) lymph node
  use Lymphatic, Right Axillary
  use Lymphatic, Left Axillary
Pectoral fascia *use* Subcutaneous Tissue and Fascia, Chest
Pectoralis major muscle
  use Thorax Muscle, Right
  use Thorax Muscle, Left
Pectoralis minor muscle
  use Thorax Muscle, Right
  use Thorax Muscle, Left
Pedicle-based dynamic stabilization device
  use Spinal Stabilization Device, Pedicle-Based in 0RH
  use Spinal Stabilization Device, Pedicle-Based in 0SH
PEEP (positive end expiratory pressure) *see* Assistance, Respiratory 5A09
PEG (percutaneous endoscopic gastrostomy) 0DH63UZ
PEJ (percutaneous endoscopic jejunostomy) 0DHA3UZ
Pelvic splanchnic nerve
  use Abdominal Sympathetic Nerve
  use Sacral Sympathetic Nerve
Penectomy
  see Excision, Male Reproductive System 0VB
  see Resection, Male Reproductive System 0VT
Penumbra Indigo® aspiration system *see* New Technology, Cardiovascular System X2C
Penile urethra *use* Urethra

P

▶ New ➠ Revised ~~deleted~~ Deleted

PERCEPT™ PC neurostimulator *use* Stimulator Generator, Multiple Array in ØJH
Perceval sutureless valve (rapid deployment technique) *see* Replacement, Valve, Aortic Ø2RF
Perianal skin *use* Skin, Perineum
Percutaneous endoscopic gastrojejunostomy (PEG/J) tube *use* Feeding Device in Gastrointestinal System
Percutaneous endoscopic gastrostomy (PEG) tube *use* Feeding Device in Gastrointestinal System
Percutaneous nephrostomy catheter *use* Drainage Device
Percutaneous transluminal coronary angioplasty (PTCA) *see* Dilation, Heart and Great Vessels Ø27
▶Percutaneous tricuspid valve replacement
▶EVOQUE valve/system (Edwards) X2RJ3RA
▶Other valve/system Ø2RJ38Z
Performance
Biliary
Multiple, Filtration 5A1C6ØZ
Single, Filtration 5A1CØØZ
Cardiac
Continuous
Output 5A1221Z
Pacing 5A1223Z
Intermittent, Pacing 5A1213Z
Single, Output, Manual 5A12Ø12
Circulatory
Continuous
Central Membrane 5A1522F
Peripheral Veno-arterial Membrane 5A1522G
Peripheral Veno-venous Membrane 5A1522H
Intraoperative
Central Membrane 5A15A2F
Peripheral Veno-arterial Membrane 5A15A2G
Peripheral Veno-venous Membrane 5A15A2H
Respiratory
24-96 Consecutive Hours, Ventilation 5A1945Z
Greater than 96 Consecutive Hours, Ventilation 5A1955Z
Less than 24 Consecutive Hours, Ventilation 5A1935Z
Single, Ventilation, Nonmechanical 5A19Ø54
Urinary
Continuous, Greater than 18 hours per day, Filtration 5A1D9ØZ
Intermittent, Less than 6 Hours Per Day, Filtration 5A1D7ØZ
Prolonged Intermittent, 6-18 hours per day, Filtration 5A1D8ØZ
Perfusion *see* Introduction of substance in or on
Perfusion, donor organ
Heart 6AB5ØBZ
Kidney(s) 6ABTØBZ
Liver 6ABFØBZ
Lung(s) 6ABBØBZ
Pericardiectomy
see Excision, Pericardium Ø2BN
see Resection, Pericardium Ø2TN
Pericardiocentesis
see Drainage, Cavity, Pericardial ØW9D
Pericardiolysis *see* Release, Pericardium Ø2NN
Pericardiophrenic artery
use Internal Mammary Artery, Right
use Internal Mammary Artery, Left
Pericardioplasty
see Repair, Pericardium Ø2QN
see Replacement, Pericardium Ø2RN
see Supplement, Pericardium Ø2UN
Pericardiorrhaphy *see* Repair, Pericardium Ø2QN
Pericardiostomy *see* Drainage, Cavity, Pericardial ØW9D
Pericardiotomy *see* Drainage, Cavity, Pericardial ØW9D
Perimetrium *use* Uterus
Peripheral Intravascular Lithotripsy (Peripheral IVL) see Fragmentation
Peripheral parenteral nutrition *see* Introduction of Nutritional Substance
Peripherally inserted central catheter (PICC) *use* Infusion Device
Peritoneal dialysis 3E1M39Z
Peritoneocentesis
see Drainage, Peritoneum ØD9W
see Drainage, Cavity, Peritoneal ØW9G
Peritoneoplasty
see Repair, Peritoneum ØDQW
see Replacement, Peritoneum ØDRW
see Supplement, Peritoneum ØDUW
Peritoneoscopy ØDJW4ZZ
Peritoneotomy *see* Drainage, Peritoneum ØD9W
Peritoneumectomy
see Excision, Peritoneum ØDBW
Peroneus brevis muscle
use Lower Leg Muscle, Right
use Lower Leg Muscle, Left
Peroneus longus muscle
use Lower Leg Muscle, Right
use Lower Leg Muscle, Left
Pessary ring *use* Intraluminal Device, Pessary in Female Reproductive System
▶Petrous part of temporal bone
▶*use* Temporal Bone, Right
▶*use* Temporal Bone, Left
PET scan *see* Positron Emission Tomographic (PET) Imaging
~~Petrous part of temporal bone~~
~~use Temporal Bone, Right~~
~~use Temporal Bone, Left~~
Phacoemulsification, lens
With IOL implant *see* Replacement, Eye Ø8R
Without IOL implant *see* Extraction, Eye Ø8D
Phagenyx® system XWHD7Q7
Phalangectomy
see Excision, Upper Bones ØPB
see Resection, Upper Bones ØPT
see Excision, Lower Bones ØQB
see Resection, Lower Bones ØQT
Phallectomy
see Excision, Penis ØVBS
see Resection, Penis ØVTS
Phalloplasty
see Repair, Penis ØVQS
see Supplement, Penis ØVUS
Phallotomy *see* Drainage, Penis ØV9S
Pharmacotherapy, for substance abuse
Antabuse HZ93ZZZ
Bupropion HZ97ZZZ
Clonidine HZ96ZZZ
Levo-alpha-acetyl-methadol (LAAM) HZ92ZZZ
Methadone Maintenance HZ91ZZZ
Naloxone HZ95ZZZ
Naltrexone HZ94ZZZ
Nicotine Replacement HZ90ZZZ
Psychiatric Medication HZ98ZZZ
Replacement Medication, Other HZ99ZZZ
Pharyngeal constrictor muscle *use* Tongue, Palate, Pharynx Muscle
Pharyngeal plexus *use* Vagus Nerve
Pharyngeal recess *use* Nasopharynx
Pharyngeal tonsil *use* Adenoids
Pharyngogram *see* Fluoroscopy, Pharynx B91G
Pharyngoplasty
see Repair, Mouth and Throat ØCQ
see Replacement, Mouth and Throat ØCR
see Supplement, Mouth and Throat ØCU
Pharyngorrhaphy *see* Repair, Mouth and Throat ØCQ
Pharyngotomy *see* Drainage, Mouth and Throat ØC9
Pharyngotympanic tube
use Eustachian Tube, Right
use Eustachian Tube, Left
▶Phenotypic Fully Automated Rapid Susceptibility Technology with Controlled Inoculum XXE5X2A
Pheresis
Erythrocytes 6A55
Leukocytes 6A55
Plasma 6A55
Platelets 6A55
Stem Cells
Cord Blood 6A55
Hematopoietic 6A55
Phlebectomy
see Excision, Upper Veins Ø5B
see Extraction, Upper Veins Ø5D
see Excision, Lower Veins Ø6B
see Extraction, Lower Veins Ø6D
Phlebography
see Plain Radiography, Veins B5Ø
Impedance 4AØ4X51
Phleborrhaphy
see Repair, Upper Veins Ø5Q
see Repair, Lower Veins Ø6Q
Phlebotomy
see Drainage, Upper Veins Ø59
see Drainage, Lower Veins Ø69
Photocoagulation
For Destruction *see* Destruction
For Repair *see* Repair
Photopheresis, therapeutic *see* Phototherapy, Circulatory 6A65
Phototherapy
Circulatory 6A65
Skin 6A6Ø
Ultraviolet light see Ultraviolet Light Therapy, Physiological Systems 6A8
Phrenectomy, phrenoneurectomy *see* Excision, Nerve, Phrenic Ø1B2
Phrenemphraxis *see* Destruction, Nerve, Phrenic Ø152
Phrenic nerve stimulator generator *use* Stimulator Generator in Subcutaneous Tissue and Fascia
Phrenic nerve stimulator lead *use* Diaphragmatic Pacemaker Lead in Respiratory System
Phreniclasis *see* Destruction, Nerve, Phrenic Ø152
Phrenicoexeresis *see* Extraction, Nerve, Phrenic Ø1D2
Phrenicotomy *see* Division, Nerve, Phrenic Ø182
Phrenicotripsy *see* Destruction, Nerve, Phrenic Ø152
Phrenoplasty
see Repair, Respiratory System ØBQ
see Supplement, Respiratory System ØBU
Phrenotomy *see* Drainage, Respiratory System ØB9
Physiatry *see* Motor Treatment, Rehabilitation FØ7
Physical medicine *see* Motor Treatment, Rehabilitation FØ7
Physical therapy *see* Motor Treatment, Rehabilitation FØ7
PHYSIOMESH™ Flexible Composite Mesh *use* Synthetic Substitute
Pia mater, intracranial *use* Cerebral Meninges
Pia mater, spinal *use* Spinal Meninges
PiCSO® Impulse System X2A7358
Pinealectomy
see Excision, Pineal Body ØGB1
see Resection, Pineal Body ØGT1
Pinealoscopy ØGJ14ZZ
Pinealotomy *see* Drainage, Pineal Body ØG91
Pinna
use External Ear, Right
use External Ear, Left
use External Ear, Bilateral
Pipeline™ (flex) embolization device *use* Intraluminal Device, Flow Diverter in Ø3V
Piriform recess (sinus) *use* Pharynx

P

▶ New ➠ Revised ~~deleted~~ Deleted

Piriformis muscle
use Hip Muscle, Right
use Hip Muscle, Left
PIRRT (Prolonged intermittent renal replacement therapy) 5A1D80Z
▶**Piscine skin** use Nonautologous Tissue Substitute
Pisiform bone
use Carpal, Right
use Carpal, Left
Pisohamate ligament
use Hand Bursa and Ligament, Right
use Hand Bursa and Ligament, Left
Pisometacarpal ligament
use Hand Bursa and Ligament, Right
use Hand Bursa and Ligament, Left
Pituitectomy
see Excision, Gland, Pituitary ØGBØ
see Resection, Gland, Pituitary ØGTØ
Plain film radiology *see* Plain Radiography
Plain Radiography
Abdomen BWØØZZZ
Abdomen and Pelvis BWØ1ZZZ
Abdominal Lymphatic
Bilateral B7Ø1
Unilateral B7ØØ
Airway, Upper BBØDZZZ
Ankle
Left BQØH
Right BQØG
Aorta
Abdominal B4ØØ
Thoracic B3ØØ
Thoraco-Abdominal B3ØP
Aorta and Bilateral Lower Extremity Arteries B4ØD
Arch
Bilateral BNØDZZZ
Left BNØCZZZ
Right BNØBZZZ
Arm
Left BPØFZZZ
Right BPØEZZZ
Artery
Brachiocephalic-Subclavian, Right B3Ø1
Bronchial B3ØL
Bypass Graft, Other B2ØF
Cervico-Cerebral Arch B3ØQ
Common Carotid
Bilateral B3Ø5
Left B3Ø4
Right B3Ø3
Coronary
Bypass Graft
Multiple B2Ø3
Single B2Ø2
Multiple B2Ø1
Single B2ØØ
External Carotid
Bilateral B3ØC
Left B3ØB
Right B3Ø9
Hepatic B4Ø2
Inferior Mesenteric B4Ø5
Intercostal B3ØL
Internal Carotid
Bilateral B3Ø8
Left B3Ø7
Right B3Ø6
Internal Mammary Bypass Graft
Left B2Ø8
Right B2Ø7
Intra-Abdominal, Other B4ØB
Intracranial B3ØR
Lower, Other B4ØJ
Lower Extremity
Bilateral and Aorta B4ØD
Left B4ØG
Right B4ØF
Lumbar B4Ø9
Pelvic B4ØC

Plain Radiography *(Continued)*
Artery *(Continued)*
Pulmonary
Left B3ØT
Right B3ØS
Renal
Bilateral B4Ø8
Left B4Ø7
Right B4Ø6
Transplant B4ØM
Spinal B3ØM
Splenic B4Ø3
Subclavian, Left B3Ø2
Superior Mesenteric B4Ø4
Upper, Other B3ØN
Upper Extremity
Bilateral B3ØK
Left B3ØJ
Right B3ØH
Vertebral
Bilateral B3ØG
Left B3ØF
Right B3ØD
Bile Duct BFØØ
Bile Duct and Gallbladder BFØ3
Bladder BTØØ
Kidney and Ureter BTØ4
Bladder and Urethra BTØB
Bone
Facial BNØ5ZZZ
Nasal BNØ4ZZZ
Bones, Long, All BWØBZZZ
Breast
Bilateral BHØ2ZZZ
Left BHØ1ZZZ
Right BHØØZZZ
Calcaneus
Left BQØKZZZ
Right BQØJZZZ
Chest BWØ3ZZZ
Clavicle
Left BPØ5ZZZ
Right BPØ4ZZZ
Coccyx BRØFZZZ
Corpora Cavernosa BVØØ
Dialysis Fistula B5ØW
Dialysis Shunt B5ØW
Disc
Cervical BRØ1
Lumbar BRØ3
Thoracic BRØ2
Duct
Lacrimal
Bilateral B8Ø2
Left B8Ø1
Right B8ØØ
Mammary
Multiple
Left BHØ6
Right BHØ5
Single
Left BHØ4
Right BHØ3
Elbow
Left BPØH
Right BPØG
Epididymis
Left BVØ2
Right BVØ1
Extremity
Lower BWØCZZZ
Upper BWØJZZZ
Eye
Bilateral B8Ø7ZZZ
Left B8Ø6ZZZ
Right B8Ø5ZZZ
Facet Joint
Cervical BRØ4
Lumbar BRØ6
Thoracic BRØ5

Plain Radiography *(Continued)*
Fallopian Tube
Bilateral BUØ2
Left BUØ1
Right BUØØ
Fallopian Tube and Uterus BUØ8
Femur
Left, Densitometry BQØ4ZZ1
Right, Densitometry BQØ3ZZ1
Finger
Left BPØSZZZ
Right BPØRZZZ
Foot
Left BQØMZZZ
Right BQØLZZZ
Forearm
Left BPØKZZZ
Right BPØJZZZ
Gallbladder and Bile Duct BFØ3
Gland
Parotid
Bilateral B9Ø6
Left B9Ø5
Right B9Ø4
Salivary
Bilateral B9ØD
Left B9ØC
Right B9ØB
Submandibular
Bilateral B9Ø9
Left B9Ø8
Right B9Ø7
Hand
Left BPØPZZZ
Right BPØNZZZ
Heart
Left B2Ø5
Right B2Ø4
Right and Left B2Ø6
Hepatobiliary System, All BFØC
Hip
Left BQØ1
Densitometry BQØ1ZZ1
Right BQØØ
Densitometry BQØØZZ1
Humerus
Left BPØBZZZ
Right BPØAZZZ
Ileal Diversion Loop BTØC
Intracranial Sinus B5Ø2
Joint
Acromioclavicular, Bilateral BPØ3ZZZ
Finger
Left BPØD
Right BPØC
Foot
Left BQØY
Right BQØX
Hand
Left BPØD
Right BPØC
Lumbosacral BRØBZZZ
Sacroiliac BRØD
Sternoclavicular
Bilateral BPØ2ZZZ
Left BPØ1ZZZ
Right BPØØZZZ
Temporomandibular
Bilateral BNØ9
Left BNØ8
Right BNØ7
Thoracolumbar BRØ8ZZZ
Toe
Left BQØY
Right BQØX
Kidney
Bilateral BTØ3
Left BTØ2
Right BTØ1
Ureter and Bladder BTØ4

P

Plain Radiography *(Continued)*
Knee
Left BQØ8
Right BQØ7
Leg
Left BQØFZZZ
Right BQØDZZZ
Lymphatic
Head B7Ø4
Lower Extremity
Bilateral B7ØB
Left B7Ø9
Right B7Ø8
Neck B7Ø4
Pelvic B7ØC
Upper Extremity
Bilateral B7Ø7
Left B7Ø6
Right B7Ø5
Mandible BNØ6ZZZ
Mastoid B9ØHZZZ
Nasopharynx B9ØFZZZ
Optic Foramina
Left B8Ø4ZZZ
Right B8Ø3ZZZ
Orbit
Bilateral BNØ3ZZZ
Left BNØ2ZZZ
Right BNØ1ZZZ
Oropharynx B9ØFZZZ
Patella
Left BQØWZZZ
Right BQØVZZZ
Pelvis BRØCZZZ
Pelvis and Abdomen BWØ1ZZZ
Prostate BVØ3
Retroperitoneal Lymphatic
Bilateral B7Ø1
Unilateral B7ØØ
Ribs
Left BPØYZZZ
Right BPØXZZZ
Sacrum BRØFZZZ
Scapula
Left BPØ7ZZZ
Right BPØ6ZZZ
Shoulder
Left BPØ9
Right BPØ8
Sinus
Intracranial B5Ø2
Paranasal B9Ø2ZZZ
Skull BNØØZZZ
Spinal Cord BØØB
Spine
Cervical, Densitometry BRØØZZ1
Lumbar, Densitometry BRØ9ZZ1
Thoracic, Densitometry BRØ7ZZ1
Whole, Densitometry BRØGZZ1
Sternum BRØHZZZ
Teeth
All BNØJZZZ
Multiple BNØHZZZ
Testicle
Left BVØ6
Right BVØ5
Toe
Left BQØQZZZ
Right BQØPZZZ
Tooth, Single BNØGZZZ
Tracheobronchial Tree
Bilateral BBØ9YZZ
Left BBØ8YZZ
Right BBØ7YZZ
Ureter
Bilateral BTØ8
Kidney and Bladder BTØ4
Left BTØ7
Right BTØ6
Urethra BTØ5

Plain Radiography *(Continued)*
Urethra and Bladder BTØB
Uterus BUØ6
Uterus and Fallopian Tube BUØ8
Vagina BUØ9
Vasa Vasorum BVØ8
Vein
Cerebellar B5Ø1
Cerebral B5Ø1
Epidural B5ØØ
Jugular
Bilateral B5Ø5
Left B5Ø4
Right B5Ø3
Lower Extremity
Bilateral B5ØD
Left B5ØC
Right B5ØB
Other B5ØV
Pelvic (Iliac)
Left B5ØG
Right B5ØF
Pelvic (Iliac) Bilateral B5ØH
Portal B5ØT
Pulmonary
Bilateral B5ØS
Left B5ØR
Right B5ØQ
Renal
Bilateral B5ØL
Left B5ØK
Right B5ØJ
~~Spanchnic B5ØT~~
▶Splanchnic B5ØT
Subclavian
Left B5Ø7
Right B5Ø6
Upper Extremity
Bilateral B5ØP
Left B5ØN
Right B5ØM
Vena Cava
Inferior B5Ø9
Superior B5Ø8
Whole Body BWØKZZZ
Infant BWØMZZZ
Whole Skeleton BWØLZZZ
Wrist
Left BPØM
Right BPØL
Planar Nuclear Medicine Imaging
Abdomen CW1Ø
Abdomen and Chest CW14
Abdomen and Pelvis CW11
Anatomical Region, Other CW1ZZZZ
Anatomical Regions, Multiple CW1YYZZ
Bladder, Kidneys and Ureters CT13
Bladder and Ureters CT1H
Blood C713
Bone Marrow C71Ø
Brain CØ1Ø
Breast CH1YYZZ
Bilateral CH12
Left CH11
Right CH1Ø
Bronchi and Lungs CB12
Central Nervous System CØ1YYZZ
Cerebrospinal Fluid CØ15
Chest CW13
Chest and Abdomen CW14
Chest and Neck CW16
Digestive System CD1YYZZ
Ducts, Lacrimal, Bilateral C819
Ear, Nose, Mouth and Throat C91YYZZ
Endocrine System CG1YYZZ
Extremity
Lower CW1D
Bilateral CP1F
Left CP1D
Right CP1C

Planar Nuclear Medicine Imaging *(Continued)*
Extremity *(Continued)*
Upper CW1M
Bilateral CP1B
Left CP19
Right CP18
Eye C81YYZZ
Gallbladder CF14
Gastrointestinal Tract CD17
Upper CD15
Gland
Adrenal, Bilateral CG14
Parathyroid CG11
Thyroid CG12
Glands, Salivary, Bilateral C91B
Head and Neck CW1B
Heart C21YYZZ
Right and Left C216
Hepatobiliary System, All CF1C
Hepatobiliary System and Pancreas CF1YYZZ
Kidneys, Ureters and Bladder CT13
Liver CF15
Liver and Spleen CF16
Lungs and Bronchi CB12
Lymphatics
Head C71J
Head and Neck C715
Lower Extremity C71P
Neck C71K
Pelvic C71D
Trunk C71M
Upper Chest C71L
Upper Extremity C71N
Lymphatics and Hematologic System C71YYZZ
Musculoskeletal System
All CP1Z
Other CP1YYZZ
Myocardium C21G
Neck and Chest CW16
Neck and Head CW1B
Pancreas and Hepatobiliary System CF1YYZZ
Pelvic Region CW1J
Pelvis CP16
Pelvis and Abdomen CW11
Pelvis and Spine CP17
Reproductive System, Male CV1YYZZ
Respiratory System CB1YYZZ
Skin CH1YYZZ
Skull CP11
Spine CP15
Spine and Pelvis CP17
Spleen C712
Spleen and Liver CF16
Subcutaneous Tissue CH1YYZZ
Testicles, Bilateral CV19
Thorax CP14
Ureters, Kidneys and Bladder CT13
Ureters and Bladder CT1H
Urinary System CT1YYZZ
Veins C51YYZZ
Central C51R
Lower Extremity
Bilateral C51D
Left C51C
Right C51B
Upper Extremity
Bilateral C51Q
Left C51P
Right C51N
Whole Body CW1N
Plantar digital vein
use Foot Vein, Right
use Foot Vein, Left
Plantar fascia (aponeurosis)
use Foot Subcutaneous Tissue and Fascia, Right
use Foot Subcutaneous Tissue and Fascia, Left
Plantar metatarsal vein
use Foot Vein, Right
use Foot Vein, Left

P

Plantar venous arch
use Foot Vein, Right
use Foot Vein, Left
▶Plantaris muscle
▶use Lower Leg Muscle, Right
▶use Lower Leg Muscle, Left
Plaque Radiation
Abdomen DWY3FZZ
Adrenal Gland DGY2FZZ
Anus DDY8FZZ
Bile Ducts DFY2FZZ
Bladder DTY2FZZ
Bone, Other DPYCFZZ
Bone Marrow D7YØFZZ
Brain DØYØFZZ
Brain Stem DØY1FZZ
Breast
Left DMYØFZZ
Right DMY1FZZ
Bronchus DBY1FZZ
Cervix DUY1FZZ
Chest DWY2FZZ
Chest Wall DBY7FZZ
Colon DDY5FZZ
Diaphragm DBY8FZZ
Duodenum DDY2FZZ
Ear D9YØFZZ
Esophagus DDYØFZZ
Eye D8YØFZZ
Femur DPY9FZZ
Fibula DPYBFZZ
Gallbladder DFY1FZZ
Gland
Adrenal DGY2FZZ
Parathyroid DGY4FZZ
Pituitary DGYØFZZ
Thyroid DGY5FZZ
Glands, Salivary D9Y6FZZ
Head and Neck DWY1FZZ
Hemibody DWY4FZZ
Humerus DPY6FZZ
Ileum DDY4FZZ
Jejunum DDY3FZZ
Kidney DTYØFZZ
Larynx D9YBFZZ
Liver DFYØFZZ
Lung DBY2FZZ
Lymphatics
Abdomen D7Y6FZZ
Axillary D7Y4FZZ
Inguinal D7Y8FZZ
Neck D7Y3FZZ
Pelvis D7Y7FZZ
Thorax D7Y5FZZ
Mandible DPY3FZZ
Maxilla DPY2FZZ
Mediastinum DBY6FZZ
Mouth D9Y4FZZ
Nasopharynx D9YDFZZ
Neck and Head DWY1FZZ
Nerve, Peripheral DØY7FZZ
Nose D9Y1FZZ
Ovary DUYØFZZ
Palate
Hard D9Y8FZZ
Soft D9Y9FZZ
Pancreas DFY3FZZ
Parathyroid Gland DGY4FZZ
Pelvic Bones DPY8FZZ
Pelvic Region DWY6FZZ
Pharynx D9YCFZZ
Pineal Body DGY1FZZ
Pituitary Gland DGYØFZZ
Pleura DBY5FZZ
Prostate DVYØFZZ
Radius DPY7FZZ
Rectum DDY7FZZ
Rib DPY5FZZ
Sinuses D9Y7FZZ
Plaque Radiation (Continued)
Skin
Abdomen DHY8FZZ
Arm DHY4FZZ
Back DHY7FZZ
Buttock DHY9FZZ
Chest DHY6FZZ
Face DHY2FZZ
Foot DHYCFZZ
Hand DHY5FZZ
Leg DHYBFZZ
Neck DHY3FZZ
Skull DPYØFZZ
Spinal Cord DØY6FZZ
Spleen D7Y2FZZ
Sternum DPY4FZZ
Stomach DDY1FZZ
Testis DVY1FZZ
Thymus D7Y1FZZ
Thyroid Gland DGY5FZZ
Tibia DPYBFZZ
Tongue D9Y5FZZ
Trachea DBYØFZZ
Ulna DPY7FZZ
Ureter DTY1FZZ
Urethra DTY3FZZ
Uterus DUY2FZZ
Whole Body DWY5FZZ
Plasma, convalescent (Nonautologous) XW1
Plasmapheresis, therapeutic see Pheresis, Physiological Systems 6A5
Plateletpheresis, therapeutic see Pheresis, Physiological Systems 6A5
Platysma muscle
use Neck Muscle, Right
use Neck Muscle, Left
Plazomicin use Other Anti-infective
Pleurectomy
see Excision, Respiratory System ØBB
see Resection, Respiratory System ØBT
Pleurocentesis see Drainage, Anatomical Regions, General ØW9
Pleurodesis, pleurosclerosis
Chemical Injection see Introduction of substance in or on, Pleural Cavity 3EØL
Surgical see Destruction, Respiratory System ØB5
Pleurolysis see Release, Respiratory System ØBN
Pleuroscopy ØBJQ4ZZ
Pleurotomy see Drainage, Respiratory System ØB9
Plica semilunaris
use Conjunctiva, Right
use Conjunctiva, Left
Plication see Restriction
Pneumectomy
see Excision, Respiratory System ØBB
see Resection, Respiratory System ØBT
Pneumocentesis see Drainage, Respiratory System ØB9
Pneumogastric nerve use Vagus Nerve
Pneumolysis see Release, Respiratory System ØBN
Pneumonectomy see Resection, Respiratory System ØBT
Pneumonolysis see Release, Respiratory System ØBN
Pneumonopexy
see Repair, Respiratory System ØBQ
see Reposition, Respiratory System ØBS
Pneumonorrhaphy see Repair, Respiratory System ØBQ
Pneumonotomy see Drainage, Respiratory System ØB9
Pneumotaxic center use Pons
Pneumotomy see Drainage, Respiratory System ØB9
Pollicization see Transfer, Anatomical Regions, Upper Extremities ØXX
Polyclonal hyperimmune globulin use Globulin
Polyethylene socket use Synthetic Substitute, Polyethylene in ØSR
Polymethylmethacrylate (PMMA) use Synthetic Substitute
Polypectomy, gastrointestinal see Excision, Gastrointestinal System ØDB
Polypropylene mesh use Synthetic Substitute
Polysomnogram 4A1ZXQZ
Pontine tegmentum use Pons
▶Popliteal fossa
▶use Knee Region, Right
▶use Knee Region, Left
Popliteal ligament
use Knee Bursa and Ligament, Right
use Knee Bursa and Ligament, Left
Popliteal lymph node
use Lymphatic, Right Lower Extremity
use Lymphatic, Left Lower Extremity
Popliteal vein
use Femoral Vein, Right
use Femoral Vein, Left
Popliteus muscle
use Lower Leg Muscle, Right
use Lower Leg Muscle, Left
Porcine (bioprosthetic) valve use Zooplastic Tissue in Heart and Great Vessels
Positive Blood Culture Fluorescence Hybridization for Organism Identification, Concentration and Susceptibility XXE5XN6
▶Positive Blood Culture Small Molecule Sensor Array Technology XXE5X4A
Positive end expiratory pressure see Performance, Respiratory 5A19
Positron Emission Tomographic (PET) Imaging
Brain CØ3Ø
Bronchi and Lungs CB32
Central Nervous System CØ3YYZZ
Heart C23YYZZ
Lungs and Bronchi CB32
Myocardium C23G
Respiratory System CB3YYZZ
Whole Body CW3NYZZ
Positron emission tomography see Positron Emission Tomographic (PET) Imaging
Posoleucel XWØ
Postauricular (mastoid) lymph node
use Lymphatic, Right Neck
use Lymphatic, Left Neck
Postcava use Inferior Vena Cava
Posterior (subscapular) lymph node
use Lymphatic, Right Axillary
use Lymphatic, Left Axillary
Posterior auricular artery
use External Carotid Artery, Right
use External Carotid Artery, Left
Posterior auricular nerve use Facial Nerve
Posterior auricular vein
use External Jugular Vein, Right
use External Jugular Vein, Left
Posterior cerebral artery use Intracranial Artery
Posterior chamber
use Eye, Right
use Eye, Left
Posterior circumflex humeral artery
use Axillary Artery, Right
use Axillary Artery, Left
Posterior communicating artery use Intracranial Artery
Posterior cruciate ligament (PCL)
use Knee Bursa and Ligament, Right
use Knee Bursa and Ligament, Left
Posterior (dynamic) distraction device
Lumbar XNSØ
Thoracic XNS4
Posterior facial (retromandibular) vein
use Face Vein, Right
use Face Vein, Left
Posterior femoral cutaneous nerve use Sacral Plexus Nerve

P

▶ New ➡ Revised ~~deleted~~ Deleted

Posterior inferior cerebellar artery (PICA) *use* Intracranial Artery
Posterior interosseous nerve *use* Radial Nerve
Posterior labial nerve *use* Pudendal Nerve
Posterior scrotal nerve *use* Pudendal Nerve
Posterior spinal artery
use Vertebral Artery, Right
use Vertebral Artery, Left
Posterior tibial recurrent artery
use Anterior Tibial Artery, Right
use Anterior Tibial Artery, Left
Posterior ulnar recurrent artery
use Ulnar Artery, Right
use Ulnar Artery, Left
Posterior vagal trunk *use* Vagus Nerve
PPN (peripheral parenteral nutrition) *see* Introduction of Nutritional Substance
Prademagene Zamikeracel, Genetically Engineered Autologous Cell Therapy
▶Abdomen XHR2XGA
▶Back XHR3XGA
▶Chest XHR1XGA
▶Head and Neck XHRØXGA
▶Lower Extremity
▶Left XHR7XGA
▶Right XHR6XGA
▶Upper Extremity
▶Left XHR5XGA
▶Right XHR4XGA
Praxbind® (idarucizumab), Pradaxa® (dabigatran) reversal agent *use* Other Therapeutic Substance
Preauricular lymph node *use* Lymphatic, Head
Precava *use* Superior Vena Cava
PRECICE intramedullary limb lengthening system
use Internal Fixation Device, Intramedullary Limb Lengthening in ØPH
use Internal Fixation Device, Intramedullary Limb Lengthening in ØQH
Precision TAVI™ Coronary Obstruction Module XXE3X68
Prepatellar bursa
use Knee Bursa and Ligament, Right
use Knee Bursa and Ligament, Left
Preputiotomy *see* Drainage, Male Reproductive System ØV9
Pressure support ventilation *see* Performance, Respiratory 5A19
PRESTIGE® Cervical Disc *use* Synthetic Substitute
Pretracheal fascia
use Subcutaneous Tissue and Fascia, Right Neck
use Subcutaneous Tissue and Fascia, Left Neck
Prevertebral fascia
use Subcutaneous Tissue and Fascia, Right Neck
use Subcutaneous Tissue and Fascia, Left Neck
Prevesical space *use* Pelvic Cavity
PrimeAdvanced neurostimulator (SureScan) (MRI Safe) *use* Stimulator Generator, Multiple Array in ØJH
Princeps pollicis artery
use Hand Artery, Right
use Hand Artery, Left
Probing, duct
Diagnostic *see* Inspection
Dilation *see* Dilation
PROCEED™ Ventral Patch *use* Synthetic Substitute
Procerus muscle *use* Facial Muscle
Proctectomy
see Excision, Rectum ØDBP
see Resection, Rectum ØDTP
Proctoclysis *see* Introduction of substance in or on, Gastrointestinal Tract, Lower 3EØH
Proctocolectomy
see Excision, Gastrointestinal System ØDB
see Resection, Gastrointestinal System ØDT
Proctocolpoplasty
see Repair, Gastrointestinal System ØDQ
see Supplement, Gastrointestinal System ØDU
Proctoperineoplasty
see Repair, Gastrointestinal System ØDQ
see Supplement, Gastrointestinal System ØDU
Proctoperineorrhaphy *see* Repair, Gastrointestinal System ØDQ
Proctopexy
see Repair, Rectum ØDQP
see Reposition, Rectum ØDSP
Proctoplasty
see Repair, Rectum ØDQP
see Supplement, Rectum ØDUP
Proctorrhaphy *see* Repair, Rectum ØDQP
Proctoscopy ØDJD8ZZ
Proctosigmoidectomy
see Excision, Gastrointestinal System ØDB
see Resection, Gastrointestinal System ØDT
Proctosigmoidoscopy ØDJD8ZZ
Proctostomy *see* Drainage, Rectum ØD9P
Proctotomy *see* Drainage, Rectum ØD9P
Prodisc-C *use* Synthetic Substitute
Prodisc-L *use* Synthetic Substitute
Production, atrial septal defect *see* Excision, Septum, Atrial Ø2B5
Profunda brachii
use Brachial Artery, Right
use Brachial Artery, Left
Profunda femoris (deep femoral) vein
use Femoral Vein, Right
use Femoral Vein, Left
PROLENE Polypropylene Hernia System (PHS) *use* Synthetic Substitute
Pronator quadratus muscle
use Lower Arm and Wrist Muscle, Right
use Lower Arm and Wrist Muscle, Left
Pronator teres muscle
use Lower Arm and Wrist Muscle, Right
use Lower Arm and Wrist Muscle, Left
Prone positioning, intubated *see* Assistance, Respiratory 5AØ9
Prostatectomy
see Excision, Prostate ØVBØ
see Resection, Prostate ØVTØ
Prostatic artery
use Internal Iliac Artery, Right
use Internal Iliac Artery, Left
Prostatic urethra *use* Urethra
Prostatomy, prostatotomy *see* Drainage, Prostate ØV9Ø
Protecta XT CRT-D *use* Cardiac Resynchronization Defibrillator Pulse Generator in ØJH
Protecta XT DR (XT VR) *use* Defibrillator Generator in ØJH
Protégé® RX Carotid Stent System *use* Intraluminal Device
▶**Provizio® SEM Scanner XX2KXP9**
Proximal radioulnar joint
use Elbow Joint, Right
use Elbow Joint, Left
Psoas muscle
use Hip Muscle, Right
use Hip Muscle, Left
PSV (pressure support ventilation) *see* Performance, Respiratory 5A19
Psychoanalysis GZ54ZZZ
Psychological Tests
Cognitive Status GZ14ZZZ
Developmental GZ1ØZZZ
Intellectual and Psychoeducational GZ12ZZZ
Neurobehavioral Status GZ14ZZZ
Neuropsychological GZ13ZZZ
Personality and Behavioral GZ11ZZZ
Psychotherapy
Family, Mental Health Services GZ72ZZZ
Group
GZHZZZZ
Mental Health Services GZHZZZZ
Individual
see Psychotherapy, Individual, Mental Health Services
for substance abuse
12-Step HZ53ZZZ
Behavioral HZ51ZZZ
Cognitive HZ5ØZZZ
Cognitive-Behavioral HZ52ZZZ
Confrontational HZ58ZZZ
Interactive HZ55ZZZ
Interpersonal HZ54ZZZ
Motivational Enhancement HZ57ZZZ
Psychoanalysis HZ5BZZZ
Psychodynamic HZ5CZZZ
Psychoeducation HZ56ZZZ
Psychophysiological HZ5DZZZ
Supportive HZ59ZZZ
Mental Health Services
Behavioral GZ51ZZZ
Cognitive GZ52ZZZ
Cognitive-Behavioral GZ58ZZZ
Interactive GZ5ØZZZ
Interpersonal GZ53ZZZ
Psychoanalysis GZ54ZZZ
Psychodynamic GZ55ZZZ
Psychophysiological GZ59ZZZ
Supportive GZ56ZZZ
PTCA (percutaneous transluminal coronary angioplasty) *see* Dilation, Heart and Great Vessels Ø27
Pterygoid muscle *use* Head Muscle
Pterygoid process *use* Sphenoid Bone
Pterygopalatine (sphenopalatine) ganglion *use* Head and Neck Sympathetic Nerve
Pubis
use Pelvic Bone, Right
use Pelvic Bone, Left
Pubofemoral ligament
use Hip Bursa and Ligament, Right
use Hip Bursa and Ligament, Left
Pudendal nerve *use* Sacral Plexus
Pull-through, laparoscopic-assisted transanal
see Excision, Gastrointestinal System ØDB
see Resection, Gastrointestinal System ØDT
Pull-through, rectal *see* Resection, Rectum ØDTP
Pulmoaortic canal *use* Pulmonary Artery, Left
Pulmonary annulus *use* Pulmonary Valve
Pulmonary artery wedge monitoring *see* Monitoring, Arterial 4A13
Pulmonary plexus
use Vagus Nerve
use Thoracic Sympathetic Nerve
Pulmonic valve *use* Pulmonary Valve
Pulpectomy *see* Excision, Mouth and Throat ØCB
▶**PulseSelect™ PFA System, for cardiac IRE (Irreversible Electroporation) Ø2583ZF**
Pulverization *see* Fragmentation
Pulvinar *use* Thalamus
Pump reservoir *use* Infusion Device, Pump in Subcutaneous Tissue and Fascia
Punch biopsy *see* Excision with qualifier Diagnostic
Puncture *see* Drainage
Puncture, lumbar *see* Drainage, Spinal Canal ØØ9U
Pure-Vu® system XDPH8K7
Pyelography
see Plain Radiography, Urinary System BTØ
see Fluoroscopy, Urinary System BT1
Pyeloileostomy, urinary diversion *see* Bypass, Urinary System ØT1
Pyeloplasty
see Repair, Urinary System ØTQ
see Replacement, Urinary System ØTR
see Supplement, Urinary System ØTU

P

Pyeloplasty, dismembered
see Repair, Kidney Pelvis
Pyelorrhaphy *see* Repair, Urinary System ØTQ
Pyeloscopy ØTJ58ZZ
Pyelostomy
see Bypass, Urinary System ØT1
see Drainage, Urinary System ØT9
Pyelotomy *see* Drainage, Urinary System ØT9
Pylorectomy
see Excision, Stomach, Pylorus ØDB7
see Resection, Stomach, Pylorus ØDT7
Pyloric antrum *use* Stomach, Pylorus
Pyloric canal *use* Stomach, Pylorus
Pyloric sphincter *use* Stomach, Pylorus
Pylorodiosis *see* Dilation, Stomach, Pylorus ØD77
Pylorogastrectomy
see Excision, Gastrointestinal System ØDB
see Resection, Gastrointestinal System ØDT
Pyloroplasty
see Repair, Stomach, Pylorus ØDQ7
see Supplement, Stomach, Pylorus ØDU7
Pyloroscopy ØDJ68ZZ
Pylorotomy *see* Drainage, Stomach, Pylorus ØD97
Pyramidalis muscle
use Abdomen Muscle, Right
use Abdomen Muscle, Left
▶ **pz-cel** *use* Prademagene Zamikeracel, Genetically Engineered Autologous Cell Therapy in NewTechnology

Q

QAngio XA® 3D XXE3X58
QFR® (Quantitative Flow Ratio) analysis of coronary angiography XXE3X58
Quadrangular cartilage *use* Nasal Septum
Quadrant resection of breast *see* Excision, Skin and Breast ØHB
Quadrate lobe *use* Liver
Quadratus femoris muscle
use Hip Muscle, Right
use Hip Muscle, Left
Quadratus lumborum muscle
use Trunk Muscle, Right
use Trunk Muscle, Left
Quadratus plantae muscle
use Foot Muscle, Right
use Foot Muscle, Left
Quadriceps (femoris)
use Upper Leg Muscle, Right
use Upper Leg Muscle, Left
Quantitative Flow Ratio Analysis, Coronary Artery Flow XXE3X58
Quarantine 8EØZXY6
▶ **Quicktome** ØØKØXZ1
Quizartinib Antineoplastic XWØDXJ9

R

Radial artery arteriovenous fistula, using thermal resistance energy X2K
Radial collateral carpal ligament
use Wrist Bursa and Ligament, Right
use Wrist Bursa and Ligament, Left
Radial collateral ligament
use Elbow Bursa and Ligament, Right
use Elbow Bursa and Ligament, Left
Radial notch
use Ulna, Right
use Ulna, Left
Radial recurrent artery
use Radial Artery, Right
use Radial Artery, Left
Radial vein
use Brachial Vein, Right
use Brachial Vein, Left
Radialis indicis
use Hand Artery, Right
use Hand Artery, Left
Radiation Therapy
see Beam Radiation
see Brachytherapy
see Other Radiation
see Stereotactic Radiosurgery
Radiation treatment *see* Radiation Therapy
Radiocarpal joint
use Wrist Joint, Right
use Wrist Joint, Left
Radiocarpal ligament
use Wrist Bursa and Ligament, Right
use Wrist Bursa and Ligament, Left
Radiofrequency Ablation
▶*see* Destruction
▶Brain, Stereoelectroencephalographic (sEEG) ØØ5Ø3Z4
▶Renal Sympathetic Nerve(s) XØ5133A
Radiography *see* Plain Radiography
Radiology, analog *see* Plain Radiography
Radiology, diagnostic *see* Imaging, Diagnostic
Radioulnar ligament
use Wrist Bursa and Ligament, Right
use Wrist Bursa and Ligament, Left
Range of motion testing *see* Motor Function Assessment, Rehabilitation FØ1
Rapid ASPECTS XXEØXØ7
REALIZE® Adjustable Gastric Band *use* Extraluminal Device
Reattachment
Abdominal Wall ØWMFØZZ
Ampulla of Vater ØFMC
Ankle Region
Left ØYMLØZZ
Right ØYMKØZZ
Arm
Lower
Left ØXMFØZZ
Right ØXMDØZZ
Upper
Left ØXM9ØZZ
Right ØXM8ØZZ
Axilla
Left ØXM5ØZZ
Right ØXM4ØZZ
Back
Lower ØWMLØZZ
Upper ØWMKØZZ
Bladder ØTMB
Bladder Neck ØTMC
Breast
Bilateral ØHMVXZZ
Left ØHMUXZZ
Right ØHMTXZZ
Bronchus
Lingula ØBM9ØZZ
Lower Lobe
Left ØBMBØZZ
Right ØBM6ØZZ

Reattachment *(Continued)*
Bronchus *(Continued)*
Main
Left ØBM7ØZZ
Right ØBM3ØZZ
Middle Lobe, Right ØBM5ØZZ
Upper Lobe
Left ØBM8ØZZ
Right ØBM4ØZZ
Bursa and Ligament
Abdomen
Left ØMMJ
Right ØMMH
Ankle
Left ØMMR
Right ØMMQ
Elbow
Left ØMM4
Right ØMM3
Foot
Left ØMMT
Right ØMMS
Hand
Left ØMM8
Right ØMM7
Head and Neck ØMMØ
Hip
Left ØMMM
Right ØMML
Knee
Left ØMMP
Right ØMMN
Lower Extremity
Left ØMMW
Right ØMMV
Perineum ØMMK
Rib(s) ØMMG
Shoulder
Left ØMM2
Right ØMM1
Spine
Lower ØMMD
Upper ØMMC
Sternum ØMMF
Upper Extremity
Left ØMMB
Right ØMM9
Wrist
Left ØMM6
Right ØMM5
Buttock
Left ØYM1ØZZ
Right ØYMØØZZ
Carina ØBM2ØZZ
Cecum ØDMH
Cervix ØUMC
Chest Wall ØWM8ØZZ
Clitoris ØUMJXZZ
Colon
Ascending ØDMK
Descending ØDMM
Sigmoid ØDMN
Transverse ØDML
Cord
Bilateral ØVMH
Left ØVMG
Right ØVMF
Cul-de-sac ØUMF
Diaphragm ØBMTØZZ
Duct
Common Bile ØFM9
Cystic ØFM8
Hepatic
Common ØFM7
Left ØFM6
Right ØFM5
Pancreatic ØFMD
Accessory ØFMF
Duodenum ØDM9
Ear
Left Ø9M1XZZ
Right Ø9MØXZZ

Reattachment *(Continued)*
Elbow Region
Left ØXMCØZZ
Right ØXMBØZZ
Esophagus ØDM5
Extremity
Lower
Left ØYMBØZZ
Right ØYM9ØZZ
Upper
Left ØXM7ØZZ
Right ØXM6ØZZ
Eyelid
Lower
Left Ø8MRXZZ
Right Ø8MQXZZ
Upper
Left Ø8MPXZZ
Right Ø8MNXZZ
Face ØWM2ØZZ
Fallopian Tube
Left ØUM6
Right ØUM5
Fallopian Tubes, Bilateral ØUM7
Femoral Region
Left ØYM8ØZZ
Right ØYM7ØZZ
Finger
Index
Left ØXMPØZZ
Right ØXMNØZZ
Little
Left ØXMWØZZ
Right ØXMVØZZ
Middle
Left ØXMRØZZ
Right ØXMQØZZ
Ring
Left ØXMTØZZ
Right ØXMSØZZ
Foot
Left ØYMNØZZ
Right ØYMMØZZ
Forequarter
Left ØXM1ØZZ
Right ØXMØØZZ
Gallbladder ØFM4
Gland
Adrenal
Left ØGM2
Right ØGM3
Hand
Left ØXMKØZZ
Right ØXMJØZZ
Hindquarter
Bilateral ØYM4ØZZ
Left ØYM3ØZZ
Right ØYM2ØZZ
Hymen ØUMK
Ileum ØDMB
Inguinal Region
Left ØYM6ØZZ
Right ØYM5ØZZ
Intestine
Large ØDME
Left ØDMG
Right ØDMF
Small ØDM8
Jaw
Lower ØWM5ØZZ
Upper ØWM4ØZZ
Jejunum ØDMA
Kidney
Left ØTM1
Right ØTMØ
Kidney Pelvis
Left ØTM4
Right ØTM3
Kidneys, Bilateral ØTM2
Knee Region
Left ØYMGØZZ
Right ØYMFØZZ

R

Reattachment *(Continued)*
Leg
Lower
Left ØYMJØZZ
Right ØYMHØZZ
Upper
Left ØYMDØZZ
Right ØYMCØZZ
Lip
Lower ØCM1ØZZ
Upper ØCMØØZZ
Liver ØFMØ
Left Lobe ØFM2
Right Lobe ØFM1
Lung
Left ØBMLØZZ
Lower Lobe
Left ØBMJØZZ
Right ØBMFØZZ
Middle Lobe, Right ØBMDØZZ
Right ØBMKØZZ
Upper Lobe
Left ØBMGØZZ
Right ØBMCØZZ
Lung Lingula ØBMHØZZ
Muscle
Abdomen
Left ØKML
Right ØKMK
Facial ØKM1
Foot
Left ØKMW
Right ØKMV
Hand
Left ØKMD
Right ØKMC
Head ØKMØ
Hip
Left ØKMP
Right ØKMN
Lower Arm and Wrist
Left ØKMB
Right ØKM9
Lower Leg
Left ØKMT
Right ØKMS
Neck
Left ØKM3
Right ØKM2
Perineum ØKMM
Shoulder
Left ØKM6
Right ØKM5
Thorax
Left ØKMJ
Right ØKMH
Tongue, Palate, Pharynx ØKM4
Trunk
Left ØKMG
Right ØKMF
Upper Arm
Left ØKM8
Right ØKM7
Upper Leg
Left ØKMR
Right ØKMQ
Nasal Mucosa and Soft Tissue Ø9MKXZZ
Neck ØWM6ØZZ
Nipple
Left ØHMXXZZ
Right ØHMWXZZ
Ovary
Bilateral ØUM2
Left ØUM1
Right ØUMØ
Palate, Soft ØCM3ØZZ
Pancreas ØFMG
Parathyroid Gland ØGMR
Inferior
Left ØGMP
Right ØGMN
Multiple ØGMQ

Reattachment *(Continued)*
Parathyroid Gland *(Continued)*
Superior
Left ØGMM
Right ØGML
Penis ØVMSXZZ
Perineum
Female ØWMNØZZ
Male ØWMMØZZ
Rectum ØDMP
Scrotum ØVM5XZZ
Shoulder Region
Left ØXM3ØZZ
Right ØXM2ØZZ
Skin
Abdomen ØHM7XZZ
Back ØHM6XZZ
Buttock ØHM8XZZ
Chest ØHM5XZZ
Ear
Left ØHM3XZZ
Right ØHM2XZZ
Face ØHM1XZZ
Foot
Left ØHMNXZZ
Right ØHMMXZZ
Hand
Left ØHMGXZZ
Right ØHMFXZZ
Inguinal ØHMAXZZ
Lower Arm
Left ØHMEXZZ
Right ØHMDXZZ
Lower Leg
Left ØHMLXZZ
Right ØHMKXZZ
Neck ØHM4XZZ
Perineum ØHM9XZZ
Scalp ØHMØXZZ
Upper Arm
Left ØHMCXZZ
Right ØHMBXZZ
Upper Leg
Left ØHMJXZZ
Right ØHMHXZZ
Stomach ØDM6
Tendon
Abdomen
Left ØLMG
Right ØLMF
Ankle
Left ØLMT
Right ØLMS
Foot
Left ØLMW
Right ØLMV
Hand
Left ØLM8
Right ØLM7
Head and Neck ØLMØ
Hip
Left ØLMK
Right ØLMJ
Knee
Left ØLMR
Right ØLMQ
Lower Arm and Wrist
Left ØLM6
Right ØLM5
Lower Leg
Left ØLMP
Right ØLMN
Perineum ØLMH
Shoulder
Left ØLM2
Right ØLM1
Thorax
Left ØLMD
Right ØLMC

Reattachment *(Continued)*
Tendon *(Continued)*
Trunk
Left ØLMB
Right ØLM9
Upper Arm
Left ØLM4
Right ØLM3
Upper Leg
Left ØLMM
Right ØLML
Testis
Bilateral ØVMC
Left ØVMB
Right ØVM9
Thumb
Left ØXMMØZZ
Right ØXMLØZZ
Thyroid Gland
Left Lobe ØGMG
Right Lobe ØGMH
Toe
1st
Left ØYMQØZZ
Right ØYMPØZZ
2nd
Left ØYMSØZZ
Right ØYMRØZZ
3rd
Left ØYMUØZZ
Right ØYMTØZZ
4th
Left ØYMWØZZ
Right ØYMVØZZ
5th
Left ØYMYØZZ
Right ØYMXØZZ
Tongue ØCM7ØZZ
Tooth
Lower ØCMX
Upper ØCMW
Trachea ØBM1ØZZ
Tunica Vaginalis
Left ØVM7
Right ØVM6
Ureter
Left ØTM7
Right ØTM6
Ureters, Bilateral ØTM8
Urethra ØTMD
Uterine Supporting Structure ØUM4
Uterus ØUM9
Uvula ØCMNØZZ
Vagina ØUMG
Vulva ØUMMXZZ
Wrist Region
Left ØXMHØZZ
Right ØXMGØZZ
REBOA (resuscitative endovascular balloon occlusion of the aorta)
Ø2LW3DJ
Ø4LØ3DJ
Rebound HRD® (Hernia Repair Device) *use* Synthetic Substitute
REBYOTA® *use* Broad Consortium Microbiota-based Live Biotherapeutic Suspension
▶ **RECARBRIO™** (Imipenem-cilastatin-relebactam Anti-infective) *use* Other Anti-infective
RECELL® cell suspension autograft *see* Replacement, Skin and Breast ØHR
Recession
see Repair
see Reposition
Reclosure, disrupted abdominal wall ØWQFXZZ
Reconstruction
see Repair
see Replacement
see Supplement

Rectectomy
see Excision, Rectum ØDBP
see Resection, Rectum ØDTP
Rectocele repair
see Repair, Subcutaneous Tissue and Fascia, Pelvic Region ØJQC
Rectopexy
see Repair, Gastrointestinal System ØDQ
see Reposition, Gastrointestinal System ØDS
Rectoplasty
see Repair, Gastrointestinal System ØDQ
see Supplement, Gastrointestinal System ØDU
Rectorrhaphy see Repair, Gastrointestinal System ØDQ
Rectoscopy ØDJD8ZZ
Rectosigmoid junction use Colon, Sigmoid
Rectosigmoidectomy
see Excision, Gastrointestinal System ØDB
see Resection, Gastrointestinal System ØDT
Rectostomy see Drainage, Rectum ØD9P
Rectotomy see Drainage, Rectum ØD9P
Rectus abdominis muscle
use Abdomen Muscle, Right
use Abdomen Muscle, Left
Rectus femoris muscle
use Upper Leg Muscle, Right
use Upper Leg Muscle, Left
Recurrent laryngeal nerve use Vagus Nerve
Reducer™ system use Reduction Device in New Technology
Reduction
Dislocation see Reposition
Fracture see Reposition
Intussusception, intestinal see Reposition, Gastrointestinal System ØDS
Mammoplasty see Excision, Skin and Breast ØHB
Prolapse see Reposition
Torsion see Reposition
Volvulus, gastrointestinal see Reposition, Gastrointestinal System ØDS
Reduction device, coronary sinus X2V73Q7
Refusion see Fusion
REGN-COV2 monoclonal antibody XWØ
Rehabilitation
see Speech Assessment, Rehabilitation FØØ
see Motor Function Assessment, Rehabilitation FØ1
see Activities of Daily Living Assessment, Rehabilitation FØ2
see Speech Treatment, Rehabilitation FØ6
see Motor Treatment, Rehabilitation FØ7
see Activities of Daily Living Treatment, Rehabilitation FØ8
see Hearing Treatment, Rehabilitation FØ9
see Cochlear Implant Treatment, Rehabilitation FØB
see Vestibular Treatment, Rehabilitation FØC
see Device Fitting, Rehabilitation FØD
see Caregiver Training, Rehabilitation FØF
Reimplantation
see Reattachment
see Reposition
see Transfer
Reinforcement
see Repair
see Supplement
Relaxation, scar tissue see Release
Release
Acetabulum
Left ØQN5
Right ØQN4
Adenoids ØCNQ
Ampulla of Vater ØFNC
Anal Sphincter ØDNR
Anterior Chamber
Left Ø8N33ZZ
Right Ø8N23ZZ
Anus ØDNQ
Aorta
Abdominal Ø4NØ

Release (Continued)
Aorta (Continued)
Thoracic
Ascending/Arch Ø2NX
Descending Ø2NW
Aortic Body ØGND
Appendix ØDNJ
Artery
Anterior Tibial
Left Ø4NQ
Right Ø4NP
Axillary
Left Ø3N6
Right Ø3N5
Brachial
Left Ø3N8
Right Ø3N7
Celiac Ø4N1
Colic
Left Ø4N7
Middle Ø4N8
Right Ø4N6
Common Carotid
Left Ø3NJ
Right Ø3NH
Common Iliac
Left Ø4ND
Right Ø4NC
Coronary
Four or More Arteries Ø2N3
One Artery Ø2NØ
Three Arteries Ø2N2
Two Arteries Ø2N1
External Carotid
Left Ø3NN
Right Ø3NM
External Iliac
Left Ø4NJ
Right Ø4NH
Face Ø3NR
Femoral
Left Ø4NL
Right Ø4NK
Foot
Left Ø4NW
Right Ø4NV
Gastric Ø4N2
Hand
Left Ø3NF
Right Ø3ND
Hepatic Ø4N3
Inferior Mesenteric Ø4NB
Innominate Ø3N2
Internal Carotid
Left Ø3NL
Right Ø3NK
Internal Iliac
Left Ø4NF
Right Ø4NE
Internal Mammary
Left Ø3N1
Right Ø3NØ
Intracranial Ø3NG
Lower Ø4NY
Peroneal
Left Ø4NU
Right Ø4NT
Popliteal
Left Ø4NN
Right Ø4NM
Posterior Tibial
Left Ø4NS
Right Ø4NR
Pulmonary
Left Ø2NR
Right Ø2NQ
Pulmonary Trunk Ø2NP
Radial
Left Ø3NC
Right Ø3NB

Release (Continued)
Artery (Continued)
Renal
Left Ø4NA
Right Ø4N9
Splenic Ø4N4
Subclavian
Left Ø3N4
Right Ø3N3
Superior Mesenteric Ø4N5
Temporal
Left Ø3NT
Right Ø3NS
Thyroid
Left Ø3NV
Right Ø3NU
Ulnar
Left Ø3NA
Right Ø3N9
Upper Ø3NY
Vertebral
Left Ø3NQ
Right Ø3NP
Atrium
Left Ø2N7
Right Ø2N6
Auditory Ossicle
Left Ø9NA
Right Ø9N9
Basal Ganglia ØØN8
Bladder ØTNB
Bladder Neck ØTNC
Bone
Ethmoid
Left ØNNG
Right ØNNF
Frontal ØNN1
Hyoid ØNNX
Lacrimal
Left ØNNJ
Right ØNNH
Nasal ØNNB
Occipital ØNN7
Palatine
Left ØNNL
Right ØNNK
Parietal
Left ØNN4
Right ØNN3
Pelvic
Left ØQN3
Right ØQN2
Sphenoid ØNNC
Temporal
Left ØNN6
Right ØNN5
Zygomatic
Left ØNNN
Right ØNNM
Brain ØØNØ
Breast
Bilateral ØHNV
Left ØHNU
Right ØHNT
Bronchus
Lingula ØBN9
Lower Lobe
Left ØBNB
Right ØBN6
Main
Left ØBN7
Right ØBN3
Middle Lobe, Right ØBN5
Upper Lobe
Left ØBN8
Right ØBN4
Buccal Mucosa ØCN4

R

- **Release** *(Continued)*
  - Bursa and Ligament
    - Abdomen
      - Left ØMNJ
      - Right ØMNH
    - Ankle
      - Left ØMNR
      - Right ØMNQ
    - Elbow
      - Left ØMN4
      - Right ØMN3
    - Foot
      - Left ØMNT
      - Right ØMNS
    - Hand
      - Left ØMN8
      - Right ØMN7
    - Head and Neck ØMNØ
    - Hip
      - Left ØMNM
      - Right ØMNL
    - Knee
      - Left ØMNP
      - Right ØMNN
    - Lower Extremity
      - Left ØMNW
      - Right ØMNV
    - Perineum ØMNK
    - Rib(s) ØMNG
    - Shoulder
      - Left ØMN2
      - Right ØMN1
    - Spine
      - Lower ØMND
      - Upper ØMNC
    - Sternum ØMNF
    - Upper Extremity
      - Left ØMNB
      - Right ØMN9
    - Wrist
      - Left ØMN6
      - Right ØMN5
  - Carina ØBN2
  - Carotid Bodies, Bilateral ØGN8
  - Carotid Body
    - Left ØGN6
    - Right ØGN7
  - Carpal
    - Left ØPNN
    - Right ØPNM
  - Cecum ØDNH
  - Cerebellum ØØNC
  - Cerebral Hemisphere ØØN7
  - Cerebral Meninges ØØN1
  - Cerebral Ventricle ØØN6
  - Cervix ØUNC
  - Chordae Tendineae Ø2N9
  - Choroid
    - Left Ø8NB
    - Right Ø8NA
  - Cisterna Chyli Ø7NL
  - Clavicle
    - Left ØPNB
    - Right ØPN9
  - Clitoris ØUNJ
  - Coccygeal Glomus ØGNB
  - Coccyx ØQNS
  - Colon
    - Ascending ØDNK
    - Descending ØDNM
    - Sigmoid ØDNN
    - Transverse ØDNL
  - Conduction Mechanism Ø2N8
  - Conjunctiva
    - Left Ø8NTXZZ
    - Right Ø8NSXZZ
  - Cord
    - Bilateral ØVNH
    - Left ØVNG
    - Right ØVNF
- **Release** *(Continued)*
  - Cornea
    - Left Ø8N9XZZ
    - Right Ø8N8XZZ
  - Cul-de-sac ØUNF
  - Diaphragm ØBNT
  - Disc
    - Cervical Vertebral ØRN3
    - Cervicothoracic Vertebral ØRN5
    - Lumbar Vertebral ØSN2
    - Lumbosacral ØSN4
    - Thoracic Vertebral ØRN9
    - Thoracolumbar Vertebral ØRNB
  - Duct
    - Common Bile ØFN9
    - Cystic ØFN8
    - Hepatic
      - Common ØFN7
      - Left ØFN6
      - Right ØFN5
    - Lacrimal
      - Left Ø8NY
      - Right Ø8NX
    - Pancreatic ØFND
      - Accessory ØFNF
    - Parotid
      - Left ØCNC
      - Right ØCNB
  - Duodenum ØDN9
  - Dura Mater ØØN2
  - Ear
    - External
      - Left Ø9N1
      - Right Ø9NØ
    - External Auditory Canal
      - Left Ø9N4
      - Right Ø9N3
    - Inner
      - Left Ø9NE
      - Right Ø9ND
    - Middle
      - Left Ø9N6
      - Right Ø9N5
  - Epididymis
    - Bilateral ØVNL
    - Left ØVNK
    - Right ØVNJ
  - Epiglottis ØCNR
  - Esophagogastric Junction ØDN4
  - Esophagus ØDN5
    - Lower ØDN3
    - Middle ØDN2
    - Upper ØDN1
  - Eustachian Tube
    - Left Ø9NG
    - Right Ø9NF
  - Eye
    - Left Ø8N1XZZ
    - Right Ø8NØXZZ
  - Eyelid
    - Lower
      - Left Ø8NR
      - Right Ø8NQ
    - Upper
      - Left Ø8NP
      - Right Ø8NN
  - Fallopian Tube
    - Left ØUN6
    - Right ØUN5
  - Fallopian Tubes, Bilateral ØUN7
  - Femoral Shaft
    - Left ØQN9
    - Right ØQN8
  - Femur
    - Lower
      - Left ØQNC
      - Right ØQNB
- **Release** *(Continued)*
  - Femur *(Continued)*
    - Upper
      - Left ØQN7
      - Right ØQN6
  - Fibula
    - Left ØQNK
    - Right ØQNJ
  - Finger Nail ØHNQXZZ
  - Gallbladder ØFN4
  - Gingiva
    - Lower ØCN6
    - Upper ØCN5
  - Gland
    - Adrenal
      - Bilateral ØGN4
      - Left ØGN2
      - Right ØGN3
    - Lacrimal
      - Left Ø8NW
      - Right Ø8NV
    - Minor Salivary ØCNJ
  - Parotid
    - Left ØCN9
    - Right ØCN8
    - Pituitary ØGNØ
    - Sublingual
      - Left ØCNF
      - Right ØCND
    - Submaxillary
      - Left ØCNH
      - Right ØCNG
    - Vestibular ØUNL
  - Glenoid Cavity
    - Left ØPN8
    - Right ØPN7
  - Glomus Jugulare ØGNC
  - Humeral Head
    - Left ØPND
    - Right ØPNC
  - Humeral Shaft
    - Left ØPNG
    - Right ØPNF
  - Hymen ØUNK
  - Hypothalamus ØØNA
  - Ileocecal Valve ØDNC
  - Ileum ØDNB
  - Intestine
    - Large ØDNE
      - Left ØDNG
      - Right ØDNF
    - Small ØDN8
  - Iris
    - Left Ø8ND3ZZ
    - Right Ø8NC3ZZ
  - Jejunum ØDNA
  - Joint
    - Acromioclavicular
      - Left ØRNH
      - Right ØRNG
    - Ankle
      - Left ØSNG
      - Right ØSNF
    - Carpal
      - Left ØRNR
      - Right ØRNQ
    - Carpometacarpal
      - Left ØRNT
      - Right ØRNS
    - Cervical Vertebral ØRN1
    - Cervicothoracic Vertebral ØRN4
    - Coccygeal ØSN6
    - Elbow
      - Left ØRNM
      - Right ØRNL
    - Finger Phalangeal
      - Left ØRNX
      - Right ØRNW

R

Release (Continued)
Joint (Continued)
Hip
Left ØSNB
Right ØSN9
Knee
Left ØSND
Right ØSNC
Lumbar Vertebral ØSNØ
Lumbosacral ØSN3
Metacarpophalangeal
Left ØRNV
Right ØRNU
Metatarsal-Phalangeal
Left ØSNN
Right ØSNM
Occipital-cervical ØRNØ
Sacrococcygeal ØSN5
Sacroiliac
Left ØSN8
Right ØSN7
Shoulder
Left ØRNK
Right ØRNJ
Sternoclavicular
Left ØRNF
Right ØRNE
Tarsal
Left ØSNJ
Right ØSNH
Tarsometatarsal
Left ØSNL
Right ØSNK
Temporomandibular
Left ØRND
Right ØRNC
Thoracic Vertebral ØRN6
Thoracolumbar Vertebral ØRNA
Toe Phalangeal
Left ØSNQ
Right ØSNP
Wrist
Left ØRNP
Right ØRNN
Kidney
Left ØTN1
Right ØTNØ
Kidney Pelvis
Left ØTN4
Right ØTN3
Larynx ØCNS
Lens
Left Ø8NK3ZZ
Right Ø8NJ3ZZ
Lip
Lower ØCN1
Upper ØCNØ
Liver ØFNØ
Left Lobe ØFN2
Right Lobe ØFN1
Lung
Bilateral ØBNM
Left ØBNL
Lower Lobe
Left ØBNJ
Right ØBNF
Middle Lobe, Right ØBND
Right ØBNK
Upper Lobe
Left ØBNG
Right ØBNC
Lung Lingula ØBNH
Lymphatic
Aortic Ø7ND
Axillary
Left Ø7N6
Right Ø7N5
Head Ø7NØ

Release (Continued)
Lymphatic (Continued)
Inguinal
Left Ø7NJ
Right Ø7NH
Internal Mammary
Left Ø7N9
Right Ø7N8
Lower Extremity
Left Ø7NG
Right Ø7NF
Mesenteric Ø7NB
Neck
Left Ø7N2
Right Ø7N1
Pelvis Ø7NC
Thoracic Duct Ø7NK
Thorax Ø7N7
Upper Extremity
Left Ø7N4
Right Ø7N3
Mandible
Left ØNNV
Right ØNNT
Maxilla ØNNR
Medulla Oblongata ØØND
Mesentery ØDNV
Metacarpal
Left ØPNQ
Right ØPNP
Metatarsal
Left ØQNP
Right ØQNN
Muscle
Abdomen
Left ØKNL
Right ØKNK
Extraocular
Left Ø8NM
Right Ø8NL
Facial ØKN1
Foot
Left ØKNW
Right ØKNV
Hand
Left ØKND
Right ØKNC
Head ØKNØ
Hip
Left ØKNP
Right ØKNN
Lower Arm and Wrist
Left ØKNB
Right ØKN9
Lower Leg
Left ØKNT
Right ØKNS
Neck
Left ØKN3
Right ØKN2
Papillary Ø2ND
Perineum ØKNM
Shoulder
Left ØKN6
Right ØKN5
Thorax
Left ØKNJ
Right ØKNH
Tongue, Palate, Pharynx ØKN4
Trunk
Left ØKNG
Right ØKNF
Upper Arm
Left ØKN8
Right ØKN7
Upper Leg
Left ØKNR
Right ØKNQ

Release (Continued)
Myocardial Bridge *see* Release, Artery, Coronary
Nasal Mucosa and Soft Tissue Ø9NK
Nasopharynx Ø9NN
Nerve
Abdominal Sympathetic Ø1NM
Abducens ØØNL
Accessory ØØNR
Acoustic ØØNN
Brachial Plexus Ø1N3
Cervical Ø1N1
Cervical Plexus Ø1NØ
Facial ØØNM
Femoral Ø1ND
Glossopharyngeal ØØNP
Head and Neck Sympathetic Ø1NK
Hypoglossal ØØNS
Lumbar Ø1NB
Lumbar Plexus Ø1N9
Lumbar Sympathetic Ø1NN
Lumbosacral Plexus Ø1NA
Median Ø1N5
Oculomotor ØØNH
Olfactory ØØNF
Optic ØØNG
Peroneal Ø1NH
Phrenic Ø1N2
Pudendal Ø1NC
Radial Ø1N6
Sacral Ø1NR
Sacral Plexus Ø1NQ
Sacral Sympathetic Ø1NP
Sciatic Ø1NF
Thoracic Ø1N8
Thoracic Sympathetic Ø1NL
Tibial Ø1NG
Trigeminal ØØNK
Trochlear ØØNJ
Ulnar Ø1N4
Vagus ØØNQ
Nipple
Left ØHNX
Right ØHNW
Omentum ØDNU
Orbit
Left ØNNQ
Right ØNNP
Ovary
Bilateral ØUN2
Left ØUN1
Right ØUNØ
Palate
Hard ØCN2
Soft ØCN3
Pancreas ØFNG
Para-aortic Body ØGN9
Paraganglion Extremity ØGNF
Parathyroid Gland ØGNR
Inferior
Left ØGNP
Right ØGNN
Multiple ØGNQ
Superior
Left ØGNM
Right ØGNL
Patella
Left ØQNF
Right ØQND
Penis ØVNS
Pericardium Ø2NN
Peritoneum ØDNW
Phalanx
Finger
Left ØPNV
Right ØPNT
Thumb
Left ØPNS
Right ØPNR

Release (Continued)
Phalanx (Continued)
Toe
Left ØQNR
Right ØQNQ
Pharynx ØCNM
Pineal Body ØGN1
Pleura
Left ØBNP
Right ØBNN
Pons ØØNB
Prepuce ØVNT
Prostate ØVNØ
Radius
Left ØPNJ
Right ØPNH
Rectum ØDNP
Retina
Left Ø8NF3ZZ
Right Ø8NE3ZZ
Retinal Vessel
Left Ø8NH3ZZ
Right Ø8NG3ZZ
Ribs
1 to 2 ØPN1
3 or More ØPN2
Sacrum ØQN1
Scapula
Left ØPN6
Right ØPN5
Sclera
Left Ø8N7XZZ
Right Ø8N6XZZ
Scrotum ØVN5
Septum
Atrial Ø2N5
Nasal Ø9NM
Ventricular Ø2NM
Sinus
Accessory Ø9NP
Ethmoid
Left Ø9NV
Right Ø9NU
Frontal
Left Ø9NT
Right Ø9NS
Mastoid
Left Ø9NC
Right Ø9NB
Maxillary
Left Ø9NR
Right Ø9NQ
Sphenoid
Left Ø9NX
Right Ø9NW
Skin
Abdomen ØHN7XZZ
Back ØHN6XZZ
Buttock ØHN8XZZ
Chest ØHN5XZZ
Ear
Left ØHN3XZZ
Right ØHN2XZZ
Face ØHN1XZZ
Foot
Left ØHNNXZZ
Right ØHNMXZZ
Hand
Left ØHNGXZZ
Right ØHNFXZZ
Inguinal ØHNAXZZ
Lower Arm
Left ØHNEXZZ
Right ØHNDXZZ
Lower Leg
Left ØHNLXZZ
Right ØHNKXZZ
Neck ØHN4XZZ
Perineum ØHN9XZZ
Scalp ØHNØXZZ

Release (Continued)
Skin (Continued)
Upper Arm
Left ØHNCXZZ
Right ØHNBXZZ
Upper Leg
Left ØHNJXZZ
Right ØHNHXZZ
Spinal Cord
Cervical ØØNW
Lumbar ØØNY
Thoracic ØØNX
Spinal Meninges ØØNT
Spleen Ø7NP
Sternum ØPNØ
Stomach ØDN6
Pylorus ØDN7
Subcutaneous Tissue and Fascia
Abdomen ØJN8
Back ØJN7
Buttock ØJN9
Chest ØJN6
Face ØJN1
Foot
Left ØJNR
Right ØJNQ
Hand
Left ØJNK
Right ØJNJ
Lower Arm
Left ØJNH
Right ØJNG
Lower Leg
Left ØJNP
Right ØJNN
Neck
Left ØJN5
Right ØJN4
Pelvic Region ØJNC
Perineum ØJNB
Scalp ØJNØ
Upper Arm
Left ØJNF
Right ØJND
Upper Leg
Left ØJNM
Right ØJNL
Tarsal
Left ØQNM
Right ØQNL
Tendon
Abdomen
Left ØLNG
Right ØLNF
Ankle
Left ØLNT
Right ØLNS
Foot
Left ØLNW
Right ØLNV
Hand
Left ØLN8
Right ØLN7
Head and Neck ØLNØ
Hip
Left ØLNK
Right ØLNJ
Knee
Left ØLNR
Right ØLNQ
Lower Arm and Wrist
Left ØLN6
Right ØLN5
Lower Leg
Left ØLNP
Right ØLNN
Perineum ØLNH
Shoulder
Left ØLN2
Right ØLN1

Release (Continued)
Tendon (Continued)
Thorax
Left ØLND
Right ØLNC
Trunk
Left ØLNB
Right ØLN9
Upper Arm
Left ØLN4
Right ØLN3
Upper Leg
Left ØLNM
Right ØLNL
Testis
Bilateral ØVNC
Left ØVNB
Right ØVN9
Thalamus ØØN9
Thymus Ø7NM
Thyroid Gland ØGNK
Left Lobe ØGNG
Right Lobe ØGNH
Tibia
Left ØQNH
Right ØQNG
Toe Nail ØHNRXZZ
Tongue ØCN7
Tonsils ØCNP
Tooth
Lower ØCNX
Upper ØCNW
Trachea ØBN1
Tunica Vaginalis
Left ØVN7
Right ØVN6
Turbinate, Nasal Ø9NL
Tympanic Membrane
Left Ø9N8
Right Ø9N7
Ulna
Left ØPNL
Right ØPNK
Ureter
Left ØTN7
Right ØTN6
Urethra ØTND
Uterine Supporting Structure ØUN4
Uterus ØUN9
Uvula ØCNN
Vagina ØUNG
Valve
Aortic Ø2NF
Mitral Ø2NG
Pulmonary Ø2NH
Tricuspid Ø2NJ
Vas Deferens
Bilateral ØVNQ
Left ØVNP
Right ØVNN
Vein
Axillary
Left Ø5N8
Right Ø5N7
Azygos Ø5NØ
Basilic
Left Ø5NC
Right Ø5NB
Brachial
Left Ø5NA
Right Ø5N9
Cephalic
Left Ø5NF
Right Ø5ND
Colic Ø6N7
Common Iliac
Left Ø6ND
Right Ø6NC
Coronary Ø2N4
Esophageal Ø6N3

R

Release *(Continued)*
- Vein *(Continued)*
  - External Iliac
    - Left Ø6NG
    - Right Ø6NF
  - External Jugular
    - Left Ø5NQ
    - Right Ø5NP
  - Face
    - Left Ø5NV
    - Right Ø5NT
  - Femoral
    - Left Ø6NN
    - Right Ø6NM
  - Foot
    - Left Ø6NV
    - Right Ø6NT
  - Gastric Ø6N2
  - Hand
    - Left Ø5NH
    - Right Ø5NG
  - Hemiazygos Ø5N1
  - Hepatic Ø6N4
  - Hypogastric
    - Left Ø6NJ
    - Right Ø6NH
  - Inferior Mesenteric Ø6N6
  - Innominate
    - Left Ø5N4
    - Right Ø5N3
  - Internal Jugular
    - Left Ø5NN
    - Right Ø5NM
  - Intracranial Ø5NL
  - Lesser Saphenous
    - Left Ø6NS
    - Right Ø6NR
  - Lower Ø6NY
  - Portal Ø6N8
  - Pulmonary
    - Left Ø2NT
    - Right Ø2NS
  - Renal
    - Left Ø6NB
    - Right Ø6N9
  - Saphenous
    - Left Ø6NQ
    - Right Ø6NP
  - Splenic Ø6N1
  - Subclavian
    - Left Ø5N6
    - Right Ø5N5
  - Superior Mesenteric Ø6N5
  - Upper Ø5NY
  - Vertebral
    - Left Ø5NS
    - Right Ø5NR
- Vena Cava
  - Inferior Ø6NØ
  - Superior Ø2NV
- Ventricle
  - Left Ø2NL
  - Right Ø2NK
- Vertebra
  - Cervical ØPN3
  - Lumbar ØQNØ
  - Thoracic ØPN4
- Vesicle
  - Bilateral ØVN3
  - Left ØVN2
  - Right ØVN1
- Vitreous
  - Left Ø8N53ZZ
  - Right Ø8N43ZZ
- Vocal Cord
  - Left ØCNV
  - Right ØCNT
- Vulva ØUNM

Relocation *see* Reposition

Remdesivir anti-infection XWØ

Removal
- Abdominal Wall 2W53X
- Anorectal 2Y53X5Z
- Arm
  - Lower
    - Left 2W5DX
    - Right 2W5CX
  - Upper
    - Left 2W5BX
    - Right 2W5AX
- Back 2W55X
- Chest Wall 2W54X
- Ear 2Y52X5Z
- Extremity
  - Lower
    - Left 2W5MX
    - Right 2W5LX
  - Upper
    - Left 2W59X
    - Right 2W58X
- Face 2W51X
- Finger
  - Left 2W5KX
  - Right 2W5JX
- Foot
  - Left 2W5TX
  - Right 2W5SX
- Genital Tract, Female 2Y54X5Z
- Hand
  - Left 2W5FX
  - Right 2W5EX
- Head 2W5ØX
- Inguinal Region
  - Left 2W57X
  - Right 2W56X
- Leg
  - Lower
    - Left 2W5RX
    - Right 2W5QX
  - Upper
    - Left 2W5PX
    - Right 2W5NX
- Mouth and Pharynx 2Y5ØX5Z
- Nasal 2Y51X5Z
- Neck 2W52X
- Thumb
  - Left 2W5HX
  - Right 2W5GX
- Toe
  - Left 2W5VX
  - Right 2W5UX
- Urethra 2Y55X5Z

Removal of device from
- Abdominal Wall ØWPF
- Acetabulum
  - Left ØQP5
  - Right ØQP4
- Anal Sphincter ØDPR
- Anus ØDPQ
- Aorta, Thoracic, Descending Ø2PW3RZ
- Artery
  - Lower Ø4PY
  - Upper Ø3PY
- Back
  - Lower ØWPL
  - Upper ØWPK
- Bladder ØTPB
- Bone
  - Facial ØNPW
  - Lower ØQPY
  - Nasal ØNPB
  - Pelvic
    - Left ØQP3
    - Right ØQP2
  - Upper ØPPY
- Bone Marrow Ø7PT
- Brain ØØPØ
- Breast
  - Left ØHPU
  - Right ØHPT

Removal of device from *(Continued)*
- Bursa and Ligament
  - Lower ØMPY
  - Upper ØMPX
- Carpal
  - Left ØPPN
  - Right ØPPM
- Cavity, Cranial ØWP1
- Cerebral Ventricle ØØP6
- Chest Wall ØWP8
- Cisterna Chyli Ø7PL
- Clavicle
  - Left ØPPB
  - Right ØPP9
- Coccyx ØQPS
- Diaphragm ØBPT
- Disc
  - Cervical Vertebral ØRP3
  - Cervicothoracic Vertebral ØRP5
  - Lumbar Vertebral ØSP2
  - Lumbosacral ØSP4
  - Thoracic Vertebral ØRP9
  - Thoracolumbar Vertebral ØRPB
- Duct
  - Hepatobiliary ØFPB
  - Pancreatic ØFPD
- Ear
  - Inner
    - Left Ø9PE
    - Right Ø9PD
  - Left Ø9PJ
  - Right Ø9PH
- Epididymis and Spermatic Cord ØVPM
- Esophagus ØDP5
- Extremity
  - Lower
    - Left ØYPB
    - Right ØYP9
  - Upper
    - Left ØXP7
    - Right ØXP6
- Eye
  - Left Ø8P1
  - Right Ø8PØ
- Face ØWP2
- Fallopian Tube ØUP8
- Femoral Shaft
  - Left ØQP9
  - Right ØQP8
- Femur
  - Lower
    - Left ØQPC
    - Right ØQPB
  - Upper
    - Left ØQP7
    - Right ØQP6
- Fibula
  - Left ØQPK
  - Right ØQPJ
- Finger Nail ØHPQX
- Gallbladder ØFP4
- Gastrointestinal Tract ØWPP
- Genitourinary Tract ØWPR
- Gland
  - Adrenal ØGP5
  - Endocrine ØGPS
  - Pituitary ØGPØ
  - Salivary ØCPA
- Glenoid Cavity
  - Left ØPP8
  - Right ØPP7
- Great Vessel Ø2PY
- Hair ØHPSX
- Head ØWPØ
- Heart Ø2PA
- Humeral Head
  - Left ØPPD
  - Right ØPPC
- Humeral Shaft
  - Left ØPPG
  - Right ØPPF

Removal of device from *(Continued)*
Intestinal Tract
Lower Intestinal Tract ØDPD
Upper Intestinal Tract ØDPØ
Jaw
Lower ØWP5
Upper ØWP4
Joint
Acromioclavicular
Left ØRPH
Right ØRPG
Ankle
Left ØSPG
Right ØSPF
Carpal
Left ØRPR
Right ØRPQ
Carpometacarpal
Left ØRPT
Right ØRPS
Cervical Vertebral ØRP1
Cervicothoracic Vertebral ØRP4
Coccygeal ØSP6
Elbow
Left ØRPM
Right ØRPL
Finger Phalangeal
Left ØRPX
Right ØRPW
Hip
Left ØSPB
Acetabular Surface ØSPE
Femoral Surface ØSPS
Right ØSP9
Acetabular Surface ØSPA
Femoral Surface ØSPR
Knee
Left ØSPD
Femoral Surface ØSPU
Tibial Surface ØSPW
Right ØSPC
Femoral Surface ØSPT
Tibial Surface ØSPV
Lumbar Vertebral ØSPØ
Lumbosacral ØSP3
Metacarpophalangeal
Left ØRPV
Right ØRPU
Metatarsal-Phalangeal
Left ØSPN
Right ØSPM
Occipital-cervical ØRPØ
Sacrococcygeal ØSP5
Sacroiliac
Left ØSP8
Right ØSP7
Shoulder
Left ØRPK
Right ØRPJ
Sternoclavicular
Left ØRPF
Right ØRPE
Tarsal
Left ØSPJ
Right ØSPH
Tarsometatarsal
Left ØSPL
Right ØSPK
Temporomandibular
Left ØRPD
Right ØRPC
Thoracic Vertebral ØRP6
Thoracolumbar Vertebral ØRPA
Toe Phalangeal
Left ØSPQ
Right ØSPP
Wrist
Left ØRPP
Right ØRPN
Kidney ØTP5
Larynx ØCPS

Removal of device from *(Continued)*
Lens
Left Ø8PK3
Right Ø8PJ3
Liver ØFPØ
Lung
Left ØBPL
Right ØBPK
Lymphatic Ø7PN
Thoracic Duct Ø7PK
Mediastinum ØWPC
Mesentery ØDPV
Metacarpal
Left ØPPQ
Right ØPPP
Metatarsal
Left ØQPP
Right ØQPN
Mouth and Throat ØCPY
Muscle
Extraocular
Left Ø8PM
Right Ø8PL
Lower ØKPY
Upper ØKPX
Nasal Mucosa and Soft Tissue Ø9PK
Neck ØWP6
Nerve
Cranial ØØPE
Peripheral Ø1PY
Omentum ØDPU
Ovary ØUP3
Pancreas ØFPG
Parathyroid Gland ØGPR
Patella
Left ØQPF
Right ØQPD
Pelvic Cavity ØWPJ
Penis ØVPS
Pericardial Cavity ØWPD
Perineum
Female ØWPN
Male ØWPM
Peritoneal Cavity ØWPG
Peritoneum ØDPW
Phalanx
Finger
Left ØPPV
Right ØPPT
Thumb
Left ØPPS
Right ØPPR
Toe
Left ØQPR
Right ØQPQ
Pineal Body ØGP1
Pleura ØBPQ
Pleural Cavity
Left ØWPB
Right ØWP9
Products of Conception 1ØPØ
Prostate and Seminal Vesicles ØVP4
Radius
Left ØPPJ
Right ØPPH
Rectum ØDPP
Respiratory Tract ØWPQ
Retroperitoneum ØWPH
Ribs
1 to 2 ØPP1
3 or More ØPP2
Sacrum ØQP1
Scapula
Left ØPP6
Right ØPP5
Scrotum and Tunica Vaginalis ØVP8
Sinus Ø9PY
Skin ØHPPX
Skull ØNPØ
Spinal Canal ØØPU

Removal of device from *(Continued)*
Spinal Cord ØØPV
Spleen Ø7PP
Sternum ØPPØ
Stomach ØDP6
Subcutaneous Tissue and Fascia
Head and Neck ØJPS
Lower Extremity ØJPW
Trunk ØJPT
Upper Extremity ØJPV
Tarsal
Left ØQPM
Right ØQPL
Tendon
Lower ØLPY
Upper ØLPX
Testis ØVPD
Thymus Ø7PM
Thyroid Gland ØGPK
Tibia
Left ØQPH
Right ØQPG
Toe Nail ØHPRX
Trachea ØBP1
Tracheobronchial Tree ØBPØ
Tympanic Membrane
Left Ø9P8
Right Ø9P7
Ulna
Left ØPPL
Right ØPPK
Ureter ØTP9
Urethra ØTPD
Uterus and Cervix ØUPD
Vagina and Cul-de-sac ØUPH
Vas Deferens ØVPR
Vein
Azygos Ø5PØ
Innominate
Left Ø5P4
Right Ø5P3
Lower Ø6PY
Upper Ø5PY
Vertebra
Cervical ØPP3
Lumbar ØQPØ
Thoracic ØPP4
Vulva ØUPM
Renal calyx
use Kidney, Right
use Kidney, Left
use Kidneys, Bilateral
use Kidney
Renal capsule
use Kidney, Right
use Kidney, Left
use Kidneys, Bilateral
use Kidney
Renal cortex
use Kidney, Right
use Kidney, Left
use Kidneys, Bilateral
use Kidney
Renal dialysis *see* Performance, Urinary 5A1D
Renal nerve *use* Abdominal Sympathetic Nerve
Renal plexus *use* Abdominal Sympathetic Nerve
Renal segment
use Kidney, Right
use Kidney, Left
use Kidneys, Bilateral
use Kidney
Renal segmental artery
use Renal Artery, Right
use Renal Artery, Left
Reopening, operative site
Control of bleeding *see* Control bleeding in
Inspection only *see* Inspection

R

▶ New ➡ Revised ~~deleted~~ Deleted

- Repair
  - Abdominal Wall ØWQF
  - Acetabulum
    - Left ØQQ5
    - Right ØQQ4
  - Adenoids ØCQQ
  - Ampulla of Vater ØFQC
  - Anal Sphincter ØDQR
  - Ankle Region
    - Left ØYQL
    - Right ØYQK
  - Anterior Chamber
    - Left Ø8Q33ZZ
    - Right Ø8Q23ZZ
  - Anus ØDQQ
  - Aorta
    - Abdominal Ø4QØ
    - Thoracic
      - Ascending/Arch Ø2QX
      - Descending Ø2QW
  - Aortic Body ØGQD
  - Appendix ØDQJ
  - Arm
    - Lower
      - Left ØXQF
      - Right ØXQD
    - Upper
      - Left ØXQ9
      - Right ØXQ8
  - Artery
    - Anterior Tibial
      - Left Ø4QQ
      - Right Ø4QP
    - Axillary
      - Left Ø3Q6
      - Right Ø3Q5
    - Brachial
      - Left Ø3Q8
      - Right Ø3Q7
    - Celiac Ø4Q1
    - Colic
      - Left Ø4Q7
      - Middle Ø4Q8
      - Right Ø4Q6
    - Common Carotid
      - Left Ø3QJ
      - Right Ø3QH
    - Common Iliac
      - Left Ø4QD
      - Right Ø4QC
    - Coronary
      - Four or More Arteries Ø2Q3
      - One Artery Ø2QØ
      - Three Arteries Ø2Q2
      - Two Arteries Ø2Q1
    - External Carotid
      - Left Ø3QN
      - Right Ø3QM
    - External Iliac
      - Left Ø4QJ
      - Right Ø4QH
    - Face Ø3QR
    - Femoral
      - Left Ø4QL
      - Right Ø4QK
    - Foot
      - Left Ø4QW
      - Right Ø4QV
    - Gastric Ø4Q2
    - Hand
      - Left Ø3QF
      - Right Ø3QD
    - Hepatic Ø4Q3
    - Inferior Mesenteric Ø4QB
    - Innominate Ø3Q2
    - Internal Carotid
      - Left Ø3QL
      - Right Ø3QK
    - Internal Iliac
      - Left Ø4QF
      - Right Ø4QE

Repair *(Continued)*
  - Artery *(Continued)*
    - Internal Mammary
      - Left Ø3Q1
      - Right Ø3QØ
    - Intracranial Ø3QG
    - Lower Ø4QY
    - Peroneal
      - Left Ø4QU
      - Right Ø4QT
    - Popliteal
      - Left Ø4QN
      - Right Ø4QM
    - Posterior Tibial
      - Left Ø4QS
      - Right Ø4QR
    - Pulmonary
      - Left Ø2QR
      - Right Ø2QQ
    - Pulmonary Trunk Ø2QP
    - Radial
      - Left Ø3QC
      - Right Ø3QB
    - Renal
      - Left Ø4QA
      - Right Ø4Q9
    - Splenic Ø4Q4
    - Subclavian
      - Left Ø3Q4
      - Right Ø3Q3
    - Superior Mesenteric Ø4Q5
    - Temporal
      - Left Ø3QT
      - Right Ø3QS
    - Thyroid
      - Left Ø3QV
      - Right Ø3QU
    - Ulnar
      - Left Ø3QA
      - Right Ø3Q9
    - Upper Ø3QY
    - Vertebral
      - Left Ø3QQ
      - Right Ø3QP
  - Atrium
    - Left Ø2Q7
    - Right Ø2Q6
  - Auditory Ossicle
    - Left Ø9QA
    - Right Ø9Q9
  - Axilla
    - Left ØXQ5
    - Right ØXQ4
  - Back
    - Lower ØWQL
    - Upper ØWQK
  - Basal Ganglia ØØQ8
  - Bladder ØTQB
  - Bladder Neck ØTQC
  - Bone
    - Ethmoid
      - Left ØNQG
      - Right ØNQF
    - Frontal ØNQ1
    - Hyoid ØNQX
    - Lacrimal
      - Left ØNQJ
      - Right ØNQH
    - Nasal ØNQB
    - Occipital ØNQ7
    - Palatine
      - Left ØNQL
      - Right ØNQK
    - Parietal
      - Left ØNQ4
      - Right ØNQ3
    - Pelvic
      - Left ØQQ3
      - Right ØQQ2
    - Sphenoid ØNQC

Repair *(Continued)*
  - Bone *(Continued)*
    - Temporal
      - Left ØNQ6
      - Right ØNQ5
    - Zygomatic
      - Left ØNQN
      - Right ØNQM
  - Brain ØØQØ
  - Breast
    - Bilateral ØHQV
    - Left ØHQU
    - Right ØHQT
    - Supernumerary ØHQY
  - Bronchus
    - Lingula ØBQ9
    - Lower Lobe
      - Left ØBQB
      - Right ØBQ6
    - Main
      - Left ØBQ7
      - Right ØBQ3
    - Middle Lobe, Right ØBQ5
    - Upper Lobe
      - Left ØBQ8
      - Right ØBQ4
  - Buccal Mucosa ØCQ4
  - Bursa and Ligament
    - Abdomen
      - Left ØMQJ
      - Right ØMQH
    - Ankle
      - Left ØMQR
      - Right ØMQQ
    - Elbow
      - Left ØMQ4
      - Right ØMQ3
    - Foot
      - Left ØMQT
      - Right ØMQS
    - Hand
      - Left ØMQ8
      - Right ØMQ7
    - Head and Neck ØMQØ
    - Hip
      - Left ØMQM
      - Right ØMQL
    - Knee
      - Left ØMQP
      - Right ØMQN
    - Lower Extremity
      - Left ØMQW
      - Right ØMQV
    - Perineum ØMQK
    - Rib(s) ØMQG
    - Shoulder
      - Left ØMQ2
      - Right ØMQ1
    - Spine
      - Lower ØMQD
      - Upper ØMQC
    - Sternum ØMQF
    - Upper Extremity
      - Left ØMQB
      - Right ØMQ9
    - Wrist
      - Left ØMQ6
      - Right ØMQ5
  - Buttock
    - Left ØYQ1
    - Right ØYQØ
  - Carina ØBQ2
  - Carotid Bodies, Bilateral ØGQ8
  - Carotid Body
    - Left ØGQ6
    - Right ØGQ7
  - Carpal
    - Left ØPQN
    - Right ØPQM
  - Cecum ØDQH
  - Cerebellum ØØQC

▶ New   ➡ Revised   ~~deleted~~ Deleted

Repair *(Continued)*
Cerebral Hemisphere ØØQ7
Cerebral Meninges ØØQ1
Cerebral Ventricle ØØQ6
Cervix ØUQC
Chest Wall ØWQ8
Chordae Tendineae Ø2Q9
Choroid
Left Ø8QB
Right Ø8QA
Cisterna Chyli Ø7QL
Clavicle
Left ØPQB
Right ØPQ9
Clitoris ØUQJ
Coccygeal Glomus ØGQB
Coccyx ØQQS
Colon
Ascending ØDQK
Descending ØDQM
Sigmoid ØDQN
Transverse ØDQL
Conduction Mechanism Ø2Q8
Conjunctiva
Left Ø8QTXZZ
Right Ø8QSXZZ
Cord
Bilateral ØVQH
Left ØVQG
Right ØVQF
Cornea
Left Ø8Q9XZZ
Right Ø8Q8XZZ
Cul-de-sac ØUQF
Diaphragm ØBQT
Disc
Cervical Vertebral ØRQ3
Cervicothoracic Vertebral ØRQ5
Lumbar Vertebral ØSQ2
Lumbosacral ØSQ4
Thoracic Vertebral ØRQ9
Thoracolumbar Vertebral ØRQB
Duct
Common Bile ØFQ9
Cystic ØFQ8
Hepatic
Common ØFQ7
Left ØFQ6
Right ØFQ5
Lacrimal
Left Ø8QY
Right Ø8QX
Pancreatic ØFQD
Accessory ØFQF
Parotid
Left ØCQC
Right ØCQB
Duodenum ØDQ9
Dura Mater ØØQ2
Ear
External
Bilateral Ø9Q2
Left Ø9Q1
Right Ø9QØ
External Auditory Canal
Left Ø9Q4
Right Ø9Q3
Inner
Left Ø9QE
Right Ø9QD
Middle
Left Ø9Q6
Right Ø9Q5
Elbow Region
Left ØXQC
Right ØXQB
Epididymis
Bilateral ØVQL
Left ØVQK
Right ØVQJ
Epiglottis ØCQR

Repair *(Continued)*
Esophagogastric Junction ØDQ4
Esophagus ØDQ5
Lower ØDQ3
Middle ØDQ2
Upper ØDQ1
Eustachian Tube
Left Ø9QG
Right Ø9QF
Extremity
Lower
Left ØYQB
Right ØYQ9
Upper
Left ØXQ7
Right ØXQ6
Eye
Left Ø8Q1XZZ
Right Ø8QØXZZ
Eyelid
Lower
Left Ø8QR
Right Ø8QQ
Upper
Left Ø8QP
Right Ø8QN
Face ØWQ2
Fallopian Tube
Left ØUQ6
Right ØUQ5
Fallopian Tubes, Bilateral ØUQ7
Femoral Region
Bilateral ØYQE
Left ØYQ8
Right ØYQ7
Femoral Shaft
Left ØQQ9
Right ØQQ8
Femur
Lower
Left ØQQC
Right ØQQB
Upper
Left ØQQ7
Right ØQQ6
Fibula
Left ØQQK
Right ØQQJ
Finger
Index
Left ØXQP
Right ØXQN
Little
Left ØXQW
Right ØXQV
Middle
Left ØXQR
Right ØXQQ
Ring
Left ØXQT
Right ØXQS
Finger Nail ØHQQXZZ
Floor of mouth *see* Repair, Oral Cavity and Throat ØWQ3
Foot
Left ØYQN
Right ØYQM
Gallbladder ØFQ4
Gingiva
Lower ØCQ6
Upper ØCQ5
Gland
Adrenal
Bilateral ØGQ4
Left ØGQ2
Right ØGQ3
Lacrimal
Left Ø8QW
Right Ø8QV
Minor Salivary ØCQJ

Repair *(Continued)*
Gland *(Continued)*
Parotid
Left ØCQ9
Right ØCQ8
Pituitary ØGQØ
Sublingual
Left ØCQF
Right ØCQD
Submaxillary
Left ØCQH
Right ØCQG
Vestibular ØUQL
Glenoid Cavity
Left ØPQ8
Right ØPQ7
Glomus Jugulare ØGQC
Hand
Left ØXQK
Right ØXQJ
Head ØWQØ
Heart Ø2QA
Left Ø2QC
Right Ø2QB
Humeral Head
Left ØPQD
Right ØPQC
Humeral Shaft
Left ØPQG
Right ØPQF
Hymen ØUQK
Hypothalamus ØØQA
Ileocecal Valve ØDQC
Ileum ØDQB
Inguinal Region
Bilateral ØYQA
Left ØYQ6
Right ØYQ5
Intestine
Large ØDQE
Left ØDQG
Right ØDQF
Small ØDQ8
Iris
Left Ø8QD3ZZ
Right Ø8QC3ZZ
Jaw
Lower ØWQ5
Upper ØWQ4
Jejunum ØDQA
Joint
Acromioclavicular
Left ØRQH
Right ØRQG
Ankle
Left ØSQG
Right ØSQF
Carpal
Left ØRQR
Right ØRQQ
Carpometacarpal
Left ØRQT
Right ØRQS
Cervical Vertebral ØRQ1
Cervicothoracic Vertebral ØRQ4
Coccygeal ØSQ6
Elbow
Left ØRQM
Right ØRQL
Finger Phalangeal
Left ØRQX
Right ØRQW
Hip
Left ØSQB
Right ØSQ9
Knee
Left ØSQD
Right ØSQC
Lumbar Vertebral ØSQØ
Lumbosacral ØSQ3

R

▶ New ➠ Revised ~~deleted~~ Deleted

- Repair *(Continued)*
  - Joint *(Continued)*
    - Metacarpophalangeal
      - Left ØRQV
      - Right ØRQU
    - Metatarsal-Phalangeal
      - Left ØSQN
      - Right ØSQM
    - Occipital-cervical ØRQØ
    - Sacrococcygeal ØSQ5
    - Sacroiliac
      - Left ØSQ8
      - Right ØSQ7
    - Shoulder
      - Left ØRQK
      - Right ØRQJ
    - Sternoclavicular
      - Left ØRQF
      - Right ØRQE
    - Tarsal
      - Left ØSQJ
      - Right ØSQH
    - Tarsometatarsal
      - Left ØSQL
      - Right ØSQK
    - Temporomandibular
      - Left ØRQD
      - Right ØRQC
    - Thoracic Vertebral ØRQ6
    - Thoracolumbar Vertebral ØRQA
    - Toe Phalangeal
      - Left ØSQQ
      - Right ØSQP
    - Wrist
      - Left ØRQP
      - Right ØRQN
  - Kidney
    - Left ØTQ1
    - Right ØTQØ
  - Kidney Pelvis
    - Left ØTQ4
    - Right ØTQ3
  - Knee Region
    - Left ØYQG
    - Right ØYQF
  - Larynx ØCQS
  - Leg
    - Lower
      - Left ØYQJ
      - Right ØYQH
    - Upper
      - Left ØYQD
      - Right ØYQC
  - Lens
    - Left Ø8QK3ZZ
    - Right Ø8QJ3ZZ
  - Lip
    - Lower ØCQ1
    - Upper ØCQØ
  - Liver ØFQØ
    - Left Lobe ØFQ2
    - Right Lobe ØFQ1
  - Lung
    - Bilateral ØBQM
    - Left ØBQL
    - Lower Lobe
      - Left ØBQJ
      - Right ØBQF
    - Middle Lobe, Right ØBQD
    - Right ØBQK
    - Upper Lobe
      - Left ØBQG
      - Right ØBQC
  - Lung Lingula ØBQH
  - Lymphatic
    - Aortic Ø7QD
    - Axillary
      - Left Ø7Q6
      - Right Ø7Q5
    - Head Ø7QØ

- Repair *(Continued)*
  - Lymphatic *(Continued)*
    - Inguinal
      - Left Ø7QJ
      - Right Ø7QH
    - Internal Mammary
      - Left Ø7Q9
      - Right Ø7Q8
    - Lower Extremity
      - Left Ø7QG
      - Right Ø7QF
    - Mesenteric Ø7QB
    - Neck
      - Left Ø7Q2
      - Right Ø7Q1
    - Pelvis Ø7QC
    - Thoracic Duct Ø7QK
    - Thorax Ø7Q7
    - Upper Extremity
      - Left Ø7Q4
      - Right Ø7Q3
  - Mandible
    - Left ØNQV
    - Right ØNQT
  - Maxilla ØNQR
  - Mediastinum ØWQC
  - Medulla Oblongata ØØQD
  - Mesentery ØDQV
  - Metacarpal
    - Left ØPQQ
    - Right ØPQP
  - Metatarsal
    - Left ØQQP
    - Right ØQQN
  - Muscle
    - Abdomen
      - Left ØKQL
      - Right ØKQK
    - Extraocular
      - Left Ø8QM
      - Right Ø8QL
    - Facial ØKQ1
    - Foot
      - Left ØKQW
      - Right ØKQV
    - Hand
      - Left ØKQD
      - Right ØKQC
    - Head ØKQØ
    - Hip
      - Left ØKQP
      - Right ØKQN
    - Lower Arm and Wrist
      - Left ØKQB
      - Right ØKQ9
    - Lower Leg
      - Left ØKQT
      - Right ØKQS
    - Neck
      - Left ØKQ3
      - Right ØKQ2
    - Papillary Ø2QD
    - Perineum ØKQM
    - Shoulder
      - Left ØKQ6
      - Right ØKQ5
    - Thorax
      - Left ØKQJ
      - Right ØKQH
    - Tongue, Palate, Pharynx ØKQ4
    - Trunk
      - Left ØKQG
      - Right ØKQF
    - Upper Arm
      - Left ØKQ8
      - Right ØKQ7
    - Upper Leg
      - Left ØKQR
      - Right ØKQQ
  - Nasal Mucosa and Soft Tissue Ø9QK
  - Nasopharynx Ø9QN

- Repair *(Continued)*
  - Neck ØWQ6
  - Nerve
    - Abdominal Sympathetic Ø1QM
    - Abducens ØØQL
    - Accessory ØØQR
    - Acoustic ØØQN
    - Brachial Plexus Ø1Q3
    - Cervical Ø1Q1
    - Cervical Plexus Ø1QØ
    - Facial ØØQM
    - Femoral Ø1QD
    - Glossopharyngeal ØØQP
    - Head and Neck Sympathetic Ø1QK
    - Hypoglossal ØØQS
    - Lumbar Ø1QB
    - Lumbar Plexus Ø1Q9
    - Lumbar Sympathetic Ø1QN
    - Lumbosacral Plexus Ø1QA
    - Median Ø1Q5
    - Oculomotor ØØQH
    - Olfactory ØØQF
    - Optic ØØQG
    - Peroneal Ø1QH
    - Phrenic Ø1Q2
    - Pudendal Ø1QC
    - Radial Ø1Q6
    - Sacral Ø1QR
    - Sacral Plexus Ø1QQ
    - Sacral Sympathetic Ø1QP
    - Sciatic Ø1QF
    - Thoracic Ø1Q8
    - Thoracic Sympathetic Ø1QL
    - Tibial Ø1QG
    - Trigeminal ØØQK
    - Trochlear ØØQJ
    - Ulnar Ø1Q4
    - Vagus ØØQQ
  - Nipple
    - Left ØHQX
    - Right ØHQW
  - Omentum ØDQU
  - Orbit
    - Left ØNQQ
    - Right ØNQP
  - Ovary
    - Bilateral ØUQ2
    - Left ØUQ1
    - Right ØUQØ
  - Palate
    - Hard ØCQ2
    - Soft ØCQ3
  - Pancreas ØFQG
  - Para-aortic Body ØGQ9
  - Paraganglion Extremity ØGQF
  - Parathyroid Gland ØGQR
    - Inferior
      - Left ØGQP
      - Right ØGQN
    - Multiple ØGQQ
    - Superior
      - Left ØGQM
      - Right ØGQL
  - Patella
    - Left ØQQF
    - Right ØQQD
  - Penis ØVQS
  - Pericardium Ø2QN
  - Perineum
    - Female ØWQN
    - Male ØWQM
  - Peritoneum ØDQW
  - Phalanx
    - Finger
      - Left ØPQV
      - Right ØPQT
    - Thumb
      - Left ØPQS
      - Right ØPQR
    - Toe
      - Left ØQQR
      - Right ØQQQ

Repair (Continued)
- Pharynx ØCQM
- Pineal Body ØGQ1
- Pleura
  - Left ØBQP
  - Right ØBQN
- Pons ØØQB
- Prepuce ØVQT
- Products of Conception 1ØQØ
- Prostate ØVQØ
- Radius
  - Left ØPQJ
  - Right ØPQH
- Rectum ØDQP
- Retina
  - Left Ø8QF3ZZ
  - Right Ø8QE3ZZ
- Retinal Vessel
  - Left Ø8QH3ZZ
  - Right Ø8QG3ZZ
- Ribs
  - 1 to 2 ØPQ1
  - 3 or More ØPQ2
- Sacrum ØQQ1
- Scapula
  - Left ØPQ6
  - Right ØPQ5
- Sclera
  - Left Ø8Q7XZZ
  - Right Ø8Q6XZZ
- Scrotum ØVQ5
- Septum
  - Atrial Ø2Q5
  - Nasal Ø9QM
  - Ventricular Ø2QM
- Shoulder Region
  - Left ØXQ3
  - Right ØXQ2
- Sinus
  - Accessory Ø9QP
  - Ethmoid
    - Left Ø9QV
    - Right Ø9QU
  - Frontal
    - Left Ø9QT
    - Right Ø9QS
  - Mastoid
    - Left Ø9QC
    - Right Ø9QB
  - Maxillary
    - Left Ø9QR
    - Right Ø9QQ
  - Sphenoid
    - Left Ø9QX
    - Right Ø9QW
- Skin
  - Abdomen ØHQ7XZZ
  - Back ØHQ6XZZ
  - Buttock ØHQ8XZZ
  - Chest ØHQ5XZZ
  - Ear
    - Left ØHQ3XZZ
    - Right ØHQ2XZZ
  - Face ØHQ1XZZ
  - Foot
    - Left ØHQNXZZ
    - Right ØHQMXZZ
  - Hand
    - Left ØHQGXZZ
    - Right ØHQFXZZ
  - Inguinal ØHQAXZZ
  - Lower Arm
    - Left ØHQEXZZ
    - Right ØHQDXZZ
  - Lower Leg
    - Left ØHQLXZZ
    - Right ØHQKXZZ
  - Neck ØHQ4XZZ
  - Perineum ØHQ9XZZ
  - Scalp ØHQØXZZ

Repair (Continued)
- Skin (Continued)
  - Upper Arm
    - Left ØHQCXZZ
    - Right ØHQBXZZ
  - Upper Leg
    - Left ØHQJXZZ
    - Right ØHQHXZZ
- Skull ØNQØ
- Spinal Cord
  - Cervical ØØQW
  - Lumbar ØØQY
  - Thoracic ØØQX
- Spinal Meninges ØØQT
- Spleen Ø7QP
- Sternum ØPQØ
- Stomach ØDQ6
  - Pylorus ØDQ7
- Subcutaneous Tissue and Fascia
  - Abdomen ØJQ8
  - Back ØJQ7
  - Buttock ØJQ9
  - Chest ØJQ6
  - Face ØJQ1
  - Foot
    - Left ØJQR
    - Right ØJQQ
  - Hand
    - Left ØJQK
    - Right ØJQJ
  - Lower Arm
    - Left ØJQH
    - Right ØJQG
  - Lower Leg
    - Left ØJQP
    - Right ØJQN
  - Neck
    - Left ØJQ5
    - Right ØJQ4
  - Pelvic Region ØJQC
  - Perineum ØJQB
  - Scalp ØJQØ
  - Upper Arm
    - Left ØJQF
    - Right ØJQD
  - Upper Leg
    - Left ØJQM
    - Right ØJQL
- Tarsal
  - Left ØQQM
  - Right ØQQL
- Tendon
  - Abdomen
    - Left ØLQG
    - Right ØLQF
  - Ankle
    - Left ØLQT
    - Right ØLQS
  - Foot
    - Left ØLQW
    - Right ØLQV
  - Hand
    - Left ØLQ8
    - Right ØLQ7
  - Head and Neck ØLQØ
  - Hip
    - Left ØLQK
    - Right ØLQJ
  - Knee
    - Left ØLQR
    - Right ØLQQ
  - Lower Arm and Wrist
    - Left ØLQ6
    - Right ØLQ5
  - Lower Leg
    - Left ØLQP
    - Right ØLQN
  - Perineum ØLQH
  - Shoulder
    - Left ØLQ2
    - Right ØLQ1

Repair (Continued)
- Tendon (Continued)
  - Thorax
    - Left ØLQD
    - Right ØLQC
  - Trunk
    - Left ØLQB
    - Right ØLQ9
  - Upper Arm
    - Left ØLQ4
    - Right ØLQ3
  - Upper Leg
    - Left ØLQM
    - Right ØLQL
- Testis
  - Bilateral ØVQC
  - Left ØVQB
  - Right ØVQ9
- Thalamus ØØQ9
- Thumb
  - Left ØXQM
  - Right ØXQL
- Thymus Ø7QM
- Thyroid Gland ØGQK
  - Left Lobe ØGQG
  - Right Lobe ØGQH
- Thyroid Gland Isthmus ØGQJ
- Tibia
  - Left ØQQH
  - Right ØQQG
- Toe
  - 1st
    - Left ØYQQ
    - Right ØYQP
  - 2nd
    - Left ØYQS
    - Right ØYQR
  - 3rd
    - Left ØYQU
    - Right ØYQT
  - 4th
    - Left ØYQW
    - Right ØYQV
  - 5th
    - Left ØYQY
    - Right ØYQX
- Toe Nail ØHQRXZZ
- Tongue ØCQ7
- Tonsils ØCQP
- Tooth
  - Lower ØCQX
  - Upper ØCQW
- Trachea ØBQ1
- Tunica Vaginalis
  - Left ØVQ7
  - Right ØVQ6
- Turbinate, Nasal Ø9QL
- Tympanic Membrane
  - Left Ø9Q8
  - Right Ø9Q7
- Ulna
  - Left ØPQL
  - Right ØPQK
- Ureter
  - Left ØTQ7
  - Right ØTQ6
- Urethra ØTQD
- Uterine Supporting Structure ØUQ4
- Uterus ØUQ9
- Uvula ØCQN
- Vagina ØUQG
- Valve
  - Aortic Ø2QF
  - Mitral Ø2QG
  - Pulmonary Ø2QH
  - Tricuspid Ø2QJ
- Vas Deferens
  - Bilateral ØVQQ
  - Left ØVQP
  - Right ØVQN

Repair *(Continued)*
- Vein
  - Axillary
    - Left Ø5Q8
    - Right Ø5Q7
  - Azygos Ø5QØ
  - Basilic
    - Left Ø5QC
    - Right Ø5QB
  - Brachial
    - Left Ø5QA
    - Right Ø5Q9
  - Cephalic
    - Left Ø5QF
    - Right Ø5QD
  - Colic Ø6Q7
  - Common Iliac
    - Left Ø6QD
    - Right Ø6QC
  - Coronary Ø2Q4
  - Esophageal Ø6Q3
  - External Iliac
    - Left Ø6QG
    - Right Ø6QF
  - External Jugular
    - Left Ø5QQ
    - Right Ø5QP
  - Face
    - Left Ø5QV
    - Right Ø5QT
  - Femoral
    - Left Ø6QN
    - Right Ø6QM
  - Foot
    - Left Ø6QV
    - Right Ø6QT
  - Gastric Ø6Q2
  - Hand
    - Left Ø5QH
    - Right Ø5QG
  - Hemiazygos Ø5Q1
  - Hepatic Ø6Q4
  - Hypogastric
    - Left Ø6QJ
    - Right Ø6QH
  - Inferior Mesenteric Ø6Q6
  - Innominate
    - Left Ø5Q4
    - Right Ø5Q3
  - Internal Jugular
    - Left Ø5QN
    - Right Ø5QM
  - Intracranial Ø5QL
  - Lower Ø6QY
  - Portal Ø6Q8
  - Pulmonary
    - Left Ø2QT
    - Right Ø2QS
  - Renal
    - Left Ø6QB
    - Right Ø6Q9
  - Saphenous
    - Left Ø6QQ
    - Right Ø6QP
  - Splenic Ø6Q1
  - Subclavian
    - Left Ø5Q6
    - Right Ø5Q5
  - Superior Mesenteric Ø6Q5
  - Upper Ø5QY
  - Vertebral
    - Left Ø5QS
    - Right Ø5QR
- Vena Cava
  - Inferior Ø6QØ
  - Superior Ø2QV
- Ventricle
  - Left Ø2QL
  - Right Ø2QK

Repair *(Continued)*
- Vertebra
  - Cervical ØPQ3
  - Lumbar ØQQØ
  - Thoracic ØPQ4
- Vesicle
  - Bilateral ØVQ3
  - Left ØVQ2
  - Right ØVQ1
- Vitreous
  - Left Ø8Q53ZZ
  - Right Ø8Q43ZZ
- Vocal Cord
  - Left ØCQV
  - Right ØCQT
- Vulva ØUQM
- Wrist Region
  - Left ØXQH
  - Right ØXQG

Repair, obstetric laceration, periurethral ØUQMXZZ

Replacement
- Acetabulum
  - Left ØQR5
  - Right ØQR4
- Ampulla of Vater ØFRC
- Anal Sphincter ØDRR
- Aorta
  - Abdominal Ø4RØ
  - Thoracic
    - Ascending/Arch Ø2RX
    - Descending Ø2RW
- Artery
  - Anterior Tibial
    - Left Ø4RQ
    - Right Ø4RP
  - Axillary
    - Left Ø3R6
    - Right Ø3R5
  - Brachial
    - Left Ø3R8
    - Right Ø3R7
  - Celiac Ø4R1
  - Colic
    - Left Ø4R7
    - Middle Ø4R8
    - Right Ø4R6
  - Common Carotid
    - Left Ø3RJ
    - Right Ø3RH
  - Common Iliac
    - Left Ø4RD
    - Right Ø4RC
  - External Carotid
    - Left Ø3RN
    - Right Ø3RM
  - External Iliac
    - Left Ø4RJ
    - Right Ø4RH
  - Face Ø3RR
  - Femoral
    - Left Ø4RL
    - Right Ø4RK
  - Foot
    - Left Ø4RW
    - Right Ø4RV
  - Gastric Ø4R2
  - Hand
    - Left Ø3RF
    - Right Ø3RD
  - Hepatic Ø4R3
  - Inferior Mesenteric Ø4RB
  - Innominate Ø3R2
  - Internal Carotid
    - Left Ø3RL
    - Right Ø3RK
  - Internal Iliac
    - Left Ø4RF
    - Right Ø4RE

Replacement *(Continued)*
- Artery *(Continued)*
  - Internal Mammary
    - Left Ø3R1
    - Right Ø3RØ
  - Intracranial Ø3RG
  - Lower Ø4RY
  - Peroneal
    - Left Ø4RU
    - Right Ø4RT
  - Popliteal
    - Left Ø4RN
    - Right Ø4RM
  - Posterior Tibial
    - Left Ø4RS
    - Right Ø4RR
  - Pulmonary
    - Left Ø2RR
    - Right Ø2RQ
  - Pulmonary Trunk Ø2RP
  - Radial
    - Left Ø3RC
    - Right Ø3RB
  - Renal
    - Left Ø4RA
    - Right Ø4R9
  - Splenic Ø4R4
  - Subclavian
    - Left Ø3R4
    - Right Ø3R3
  - Superior Mesenteric Ø4R5
  - Temporal
    - Left Ø3RT
    - Right Ø3RS
  - Thyroid
    - Left Ø3RV
    - Right Ø3RU
  - Ulnar
    - Left Ø3RA
    - Right Ø3R9
  - Upper Ø3RY
  - Vertebral
    - Left Ø3RQ
    - Right Ø3RP
- Atrium
  - Left Ø2R7
  - Right Ø2R6
- Auditory Ossicle
  - Left Ø9RAØ
  - Right Ø9R9Ø
- Bladder ØTRB
- Bladder Neck ØTRC
- Bone
  - Ethmoid
    - Left ØNRG
    - Right ØNRF
  - Frontal ØNR1
  - Hyoid ØNRX
  - Lacrimal
    - Left ØNRJ
    - Right ØNRH
  - Nasal ØNRB
  - Occipital ØNR7
  - Palatine
    - Left ØNRL
    - Right ØNRK
  - Parietal
    - Left ØNR4
    - Right ØNR3
  - Pelvic
    - Left ØQR3
    - Right ØQR2
  - Sphenoid ØNRC
  - Temporal
    - Left ØNR6
    - Right ØNR5
  - Zygomatic
    - Left ØNRN
    - Right ØNRM

R

Replacement *(Continued)*
- Breast
  - Bilateral ØHRV
  - Left ØHRU
  - Right ØHRT
- Bronchus
  - Lingula ØBR9
  - Lower Lobe
    - Left ØBRB
    - Right ØBR6
  - Main
    - Left ØBR7
    - Right ØBR3
  - Middle Lobe, Right ØBR5
  - Upper Lobe
    - Left ØBR8
    - Right ØBR4
- Buccal Mucosa ØCR4
- Bursa and Ligament
  - Abdomen
    - Left ØMRJ
    - Right ØMRH
  - Ankle
    - Left ØMRR
    - Right ØMRQ
  - Elbow
    - Left ØMR4
    - Right ØMR3
  - Foot
    - Left ØMRT
    - Right ØMRS
  - Hand
    - Left ØMR8
    - Right ØMR7
  - Head and Neck ØMRØ
  - Hip
    - Left ØMRM
    - Right ØMRL
  - Knee
    - Left ØMRP
    - Right ØMRN
  - Lower Extremity
    - Left ØMRW
    - Right ØMRV
  - Perineum ØMRK
  - Rib(s) ØMRG
  - Shoulder
    - Left ØMR2
    - Right ØMR1
  - Spine
    - Lower ØMRD
    - Upper ØMRC
  - Sternum ØMRF
  - Upper Extremity
    - Left ØMRB
    - Right ØMR9
  - Wrist
    - Left ØMR6
    - Right ØMR5
  - Carina ØBR2
- Carpal
  - Left ØPRN
  - Right ØPRM
- Cerebral Meninges ØØR1
- Cerebral Ventricle ØØR6
- Chordae Tendineae Ø2R9
- Choroid
  - Left Ø8RB
  - Right Ø8RA
- Clavicle
  - Left ØPRB
  - Right ØPR9
- Coccyx ØQRS
- Conjunctiva
  - Left Ø8RTX
  - Right Ø8RSX
- Cornea
  - Left Ø8R9
  - Right Ø8R8
- Diaphragm ØBRT
- Disc

Replacement *(Continued)*
- Bursa and Ligament *(Continued)*
  - Cervical Vertebral ØRR3Ø
  - Cervicothoracic Vertebral ØRR5Ø
  - Lumbar Vertebral ØSR2Ø
  - Lumbosacral ØSR4Ø
  - Thoracic Vertebral ØRR9Ø
  - Thoracolumbar Vertebral ØRRBØ
- Duct
  - Common Bile ØFR9
  - Cystic ØFR8
  - Hepatic
    - Common ØFR7
    - Left ØFR6
    - Right ØFR5
  - Lacrimal
    - Left Ø8RY
    - Right Ø8RX
  - Pancreatic ØFRD
    - Accessory ØFRF
  - Parotid
    - Left ØCRC
    - Right ØCRB
- Dura Mater ØØR2
- Ear
  - External
    - Bilateral Ø9R2
    - Left Ø9R1
    - Right Ø9RØ
  - Inner
    - Left Ø9REØ
    - Right Ø9RDØ
  - Middle
    - Left Ø9R6Ø
    - Right Ø9R5Ø
- Epiglottis ØCRR
- Esophagus ØDR5
- Eye
  - Left Ø8R1
  - Right Ø8RØ
- Eyelid
  - Lower
    - Left Ø8RR
    - Right Ø8RQ
  - Upper
    - Left Ø8RP
    - Right Ø8RN
- Femoral Shaft
  - Left ØQR9
  - Right ØQR8
- Femur
  - Lower
    - Left ØQRC
    - Right ØQRB
  - Upper
    - Left ØQR7
    - Right ØQR6
- Fibula
  - Left ØQRK
  - Right ØQRJ
- Finger Nail ØHRQX
- Gingiva
  - Lower ØCR6
  - Upper ØCR5
- Glenoid Cavity
  - Left ØPR8
  - Right ØPR7
- Heart Ø2RAØ
- Hair ØHRSX
- Humeral Head
  - Left ØPRD
  - Right ØPRC
- Humeral Shaft
  - Left ØPRG
  - Right ØPRF
- Iris
  - Left Ø8RD3
  - Right Ø8RC3

Replacement *(Continued)*
- Joint
  - Acromioclavicular
    - Left ØRRHØ
    - Right ØRRGØ
  - Ankle
    - Left ØSRG
    - Right ØSRF
  - Carpal
    - Left ØRRRØ
    - Right ØRRQØ
  - Carpometacarpal
    - Left ØRRTØ
    - Right ØRRSØ
  - Cervical Vertebral ØRR1Ø
  - Cervicothoracic Vertebral ØRR4Ø
  - Coccygeal ØSR6Ø
  - Elbow
    - Left ØRRMØ
    - Right ØRRLØ
  - Finger Phalangeal
    - Left ØRRXØ
    - Right ØRRWØ
  - Hip
    - Left ØSRB
      - Acetabular Surface ØSRE
      - Femoral Surface ØSRS
    - Right ØSR9
      - Acetabular Surface ØSRA
      - Femoral Surface ØSRR
  - Knee
    - Left ØSRD
      - Femoral Surface ØSRU
      - Tibial Surface ØSRW
    - Right ØSRC
      - Femoral Surface ØSRT
      - Tibial Surface ØSRV
  - Lumbar Vertebral ØSRØØ
  - Lumbosacral ØSR3Ø
  - Metacarpophalangeal
    - Left ØRRVØ
    - Right ØRRUØ
  - Metatarsal-Phalangeal
    - Left ØSRNØ
    - Right ØSRMØ
  - Occipital-cervical ØRRØØ
  - Sacrococcygeal ØSR5Ø
  - Sacroiliac
    - Left ØSR8Ø
    - Right ØSR7Ø
  - Shoulder
    - Left ØRRK
    - Right ØRRJ
  - Sternoclavicular
    - Left ØRRFØ
    - Right ØRREØ
  - Tarsal
    - Left ØSRJØ
    - Right ØSRHØ
  - Tarsometatarsal
    - Left ØSRLØ
    - Right ØSRKØ
  - Temporomandibular
    - Left ØRRDØ
    - Right ØRRCØ
  - Thoracic Vertebral ØRR6Ø
  - Thoracolumbar Vertebral ØRRAØ
  - Toe Phalangeal
    - Left ØSRQØ
    - Right ØSRPØ
  - Wrist
    - Left ØRRPØ
    - Right ØRRNØ
- Kidney Pelvis
  - Left ØTR4
  - Right ØTR3
- Larynx ØCRS
- Lens
  - Left Ø8RK3ØZ
  - Right Ø8RJ3ØZ

Replacement *(Continued)*
Lip
Lower ØCR1
Upper ØCRØ
Mandible
Left ØNRV
Right ØNRT
Maxilla ØNRR
Mesentery ØDRV
Metacarpal
Left ØPRQ
Right ØPRP
Metatarsal
Left ØQRP
Right ØQRN
Muscle
Abdomen
Left ØKRL
Right ØKRK
Facial ØKR1
Foot
Left ØKRW
Right ØKRV
Hand
Left ØKRD
Right ØKRC
Head ØKRØ
Hip
Left ØKRP
Right ØKRN
Lower Arm and Wrist
Left ØKRB
Right ØKR9
Lower Leg
Left ØKRT
Right ØKRS
Neck
Left ØKR3
Right ØKR2
Papillary Ø2RD
Perineum ØKRM
Shoulder
Left ØKR6
Right ØKR5
Thorax
Left ØKRJ
Right ØKRH
Tongue, Palate, Pharynx ØKR4
Trunk
Left ØKRG
Right ØKRF
Upper Arm
Left ØKR8
Right ØKR7
Upper Leg
Left ØKRR
Right ØKRQ
Nasal Mucosa and Soft Tissue Ø9RK
Nasopharynx Ø9RN
Nerve
Abducens ØØRL
Accessory ØØRR
Acoustic ØØRN
Cervical Ø1R1
Facial ØØRM
Femoral Ø1RD
Glossopharyngeal ØØRP
Hypoglossal ØØRS
Lumbar Ø1RB
Median Ø1R5
Oculomotor ØØRH
Olfactory ØØRF
Optic ØØRG
Peroneal Ø1RH
Phrenic Ø1R2
Pudendal Ø1RC
Radial Ø1R6
Sacral Ø1RR
Sciatic Ø1RF
Thoracic Ø1R8
Tibial Ø1RG
Trigeminal ØØRK

Replacement *(Continued)*
Nerve *(Continued)*
Trochlear ØØRJ
Ulnar Ø1R4
Vagus ØØRQ
Nipple
Left ØHRX
Right ØHRW
Omentum ØDRU
Orbit
Left ØNRQ
Right ØNRP
Palate
Hard ØCR2
Soft ØCR3
Patella
Left ØQRF
Right ØQRD
Pericardium Ø2RN
Peritoneum ØDRW
Phalanx
Finger
Left ØPRV
Right ØPRT
Thumb
Left ØPRS
Right ØPRR
Toe
Left ØQRR
Right ØQRQ
Pharynx ØCRM
Radius
Left ØPRJ
Right ØPRH
Retinal Vessel
Left Ø8RH3
Right Ø8RG3
Ribs
1 to 2 ØPR1
3 or More ØPR2
Sacrum ØQR1
Scapula
Left ØPR6
Right ØPR5
Sclera
Left Ø8R7X
Right Ø8R6X
Septum
Atrial Ø2R5
Nasal Ø9RM
Ventricular Ø2RM
Skin
Abdomen ØHR7
Back ØHR6
Buttock ØHR8
Chest ØHR5
Ear
Left ØHR3
Right ØHR2
Face ØHR1
Foot
Left ØHRN
Right ØHRM
Hand
Left ØHRG
Right ØHRF
Inguinal ØHRA
Lower Arm
Left ØHRE
Right ØHRD
Lower Leg
Left ØHRL
Right ØHRK
Neck ØHR4
Perineum ØHR9
Scalp ØHRØ
Upper Arm
Left ØHRC
Right ØHRB
Upper Leg
Left ØHRJ
Right ØHRH

Replacement *(Continued)*
Skull ØNRØ
Spinal Meninges ØØRT
Sternum ØPRØ
Subcutaneous Tissue and Fascia
Abdomen ØJR8
Back ØJR7
Buttock ØJR9
Chest ØJR6
Face ØJR1
Foot
Left ØJRR
Right ØJRQ
Hand
Left ØJRK
Right ØJRJ
Lower Arm
Left ØJRH
Right ØJRG
Lower Leg
Left ØJRP
Right ØJRN
Neck
Left ØJR5
Right ØJR4
Pelvic Region ØJRC
Perineum ØJRB
Scalp ØJRØ
Upper Arm
Left ØJRF
Right ØJRD
Upper Leg
Left ØJRM
Right ØJRL
Tarsal
Left ØQRM
Right ØQRL
Tendon
Abdomen
Left ØLRG
Right ØLRF
Ankle
Left ØLRT
Right ØLRS
Foot
Left ØLRW
Right ØLRV
Hand
Left ØLR8
Right ØLR7
Head and Neck ØLRØ
Hip
Left ØLRK
Right ØLRJ
Knee
Left ØLRR
Right ØLRQ
Lower Arm and Wrist
Left ØLR6
Right ØLR5
Lower Leg
Left ØLRP
Right ØLRN
Perineum ØLRH
Shoulder
Left ØLR2
Right ØLR1
Thorax
Left ØLRD
Right ØLRC
Trunk
Left ØLRB
Right ØLR9
Upper Arm
Left ØLR4
Right ØLR3
Upper Leg
Left ØLRM
Right ØLRL

R

Replacement *(Continued)*
- Testis
  - Bilateral ØVRCØJZ
  - Left ØVRBØJZ
  - Right ØVR9ØJZ
- Thumb
  - Left ØXRM
  - Right ØXRL
- Tibia
  - Left ØQRH
  - Right ØQRG
- Toe Nail ØHRRX
- Tongue ØCR7
- Tooth
  - Lower ØCRX
  - Upper ØCRW
- Trachea ØBR1
- Turbinate, Nasal Ø9RL
- Tympanic Membrane
  - Left Ø9R8
  - Right Ø9R7
- Ulna
  - Left ØPRL
  - Right ØPRK
- Ureter
  - Left ØTR7
  - Right ØTR6
- Urethra ØTRD
- Uvula ØCRN
- Valve
  - Aortic Ø2RF
  - Mitral Ø2RG
  - Pulmonary Ø2RH
  - Tricuspid Ø2RJ
- Vein
  - Axillary
    - Left Ø5R8
    - Right Ø5R7
  - Azygos Ø5RØ
  - Basilic
    - Left Ø5RC
    - Right Ø5RB
  - Brachial
    - Left Ø5RA
    - Right Ø5R9
  - Cephalic
    - Left Ø5RF
    - Right Ø5RD
  - Colic Ø6R7
  - Common Iliac
    - Left Ø6RD
    - Right Ø6RC
  - Esophageal Ø6R3
  - External Iliac
    - Left Ø6RG
    - Right Ø6RF
  - External Jugular
    - Left Ø5RQ
    - Right Ø5RP
  - Face
    - Left Ø5RV
    - Right Ø5RT
  - Femoral
    - Left Ø6RN
    - Right Ø6RM
  - Foot
    - Left Ø6RV
    - Right Ø6RT
  - Gastric Ø6R2
  - Hand
    - Left Ø5RH
    - Right Ø5RG
  - Hemiazygos Ø5R1
  - Hepatic Ø6R4
  - Hypogastric
    - Left Ø6RJ
    - Right Ø6RH
  - Inferior Mesenteric Ø6R6
  - Innominate
    - Left Ø5R4
    - Right Ø5R3

Replacement *(Continued)*
- Vein *(Continued)*
  - Internal Jugular
    - Left Ø5RN
    - Right Ø5RM
  - Intracranial Ø5RL
  - Lower Ø6RY
  - Portal Ø6R8
  - Pulmonary
    - Left Ø2RT
    - Right Ø2RS
  - Renal
    - Left Ø6RB
    - Right Ø6R9
  - Saphenous
    - Left Ø6RQ
    - Right Ø6RP
  - Splenic Ø6R1
  - Subclavian
    - Left Ø5R6
    - Right Ø5R5
  - Superior Mesenteric Ø6R5
  - Upper Ø5RY
  - Vertebral
    - Left Ø5RS
    - Right Ø5RR
- Vena Cava
  - Inferior Ø6RØ
  - Superior Ø2RV
- Ventricle
  - Left Ø2RL
  - Right Ø2RK
- Vertebra
  - Cervical ØPR3
  - Lumbar ØQRØ
  - Thoracic ØPR4
- Vitreous
  - Left Ø8R53
  - Right Ø8R43
- Vocal Cord
  - Left ØCRV
  - Right ØCRT

Replacement, hip
- Partial or total *see* Replacement, Lower Joints ØSR
- Resurfacing only *see* Supplement, Lower Joints ØSU

Replacement, knee
- Meniscus implant only *see* New Technology, Joints XRR
- Partial or total *see* Replacement, Lower Joints ØSR

Replantation *see* Reposition

Replantation, scalp *see* Reattachment, Skin, Scalp ØHMØ

Reposition
- Acetabulum
  - Left ØQS5
  - Right ØQS4
- Ampulla of Vater ØFSC
- Anus ØDSQ
- Aorta
  - Abdominal Ø4SØ
  - Thoracic
    - Ascending/Arch Ø2SXØZZ
    - Descending Ø2SWØZZ
- Artery
  - Anterior Tibial
    - Left Ø4SQ
    - Right Ø4SP
  - Axillary
    - Left Ø3S6
    - Right Ø3S5
  - Brachial
    - Left Ø3S8
    - Right Ø3S7
  - Celiac Ø4S1
  - Colic
    - Left Ø4S7
    - Middle Ø4S8
    - Right Ø4S6

Reposition *(Continued)*
- Artery *(Continued)*
  - Common Carotid
    - Left Ø3SJ
    - Right Ø3SH
  - Common Iliac
    - Left Ø4SD
    - Right Ø4SC
  - Coronary
    - One Artery Ø2SØØZZ
    - Two Arteries Ø2S1ØZZ
  - External Carotid
    - Left Ø3SN
    - Right Ø3SM
  - External Iliac
    - Left Ø4SJ
    - Right Ø4SH
  - Face Ø3SR
  - Femoral
    - Left Ø4SL
    - Right Ø4SK
  - Foot
    - Left Ø4SW
    - Right Ø4SV
  - Gastric Ø4S2
  - Hand
    - Left Ø3SF
    - Right Ø3SD
  - Hepatic Ø4S3
  - Inferior Mesenteric Ø4SB
  - Innominate Ø3S2
  - Internal Carotid
    - Left Ø3SL
    - Right Ø3SK
  - Internal Iliac
    - Left Ø4SF
    - Right Ø4SE
  - Internal Mammary
    - Left Ø3S1
    - Right Ø3SØ
  - Intracranial Ø3SG
  - Lower Ø4SY
  - Peroneal
    - Left Ø4SU
    - Right Ø4ST
  - Popliteal
    - Left Ø4SN
    - Right Ø4SM
  - Posterior Tibial
    - Left Ø4SS
    - Right Ø4SR
  - Pulmonary
    - Left Ø2SRØZZ
    - Right Ø2SQØZZ
  - Pulmonary Trunk Ø2SPØZZ
  - Radial
    - Left Ø3SC
    - Right Ø3SB
  - Renal
    - Left Ø4SA
    - Right Ø4S9
  - Splenic Ø4S4
  - Subclavian
    - Left Ø3S4
    - Right Ø3S3
  - Superior Mesenteric Ø4S5
  - Temporal
    - Left Ø3ST
    - Right Ø3SS
  - Thyroid
    - Left Ø3SV
    - Right Ø3SU
  - Ulnar
    - Left Ø3SA
    - Right Ø3S9
  - Upper Ø3SY
  - Vertebral
    - Left Ø3SQ
    - Right Ø3SP
- Auditory Ossicle
  - Left Ø9SA
  - Right Ø9S9

- **Reposition** *(Continued)*
  - Bladder ØTSB
  - Bladder Neck ØTSC
  - Bone
    - Ethmoid
      - Left ØNSG
      - Right ØNSF
    - Frontal ØNS1
    - Hyoid ØNSX
    - Lacrimal
      - Left ØNSJ
      - Right ØNSH
    - Nasal ØNSB
    - Occipital ØNS7
    - Palatine
      - Left ØNSL
      - Right ØNSK
    - Parietal
      - Left ØNS4
      - Right ØNS3
    - Pelvic
      - Left ØQS3
      - Right ØQS2
    - Sphenoid ØNSC
    - Temporal
      - Left ØNS6
      - Right ØNS5
    - Zygomatic
      - Left ØNSN
      - Right ØNSM
  - Breast
    - Bilateral ØHSVØZZ
    - Left ØHSUØZZ
    - Right ØHSTØZZ
  - Bronchus
    - Lingula ØBS9ØZZ
    - Lower Lobe
      - Left ØBSBØZZ
      - Right ØBS6ØZZ
    - Main
      - Left ØBS7ØZZ
      - Right ØBS3ØZZ
    - Middle Lobe, Right ØBS5ØZZ
    - Upper Lobe
      - Left ØBS8ØZZ
      - Right ØBS4ØZZ
  - Bursa and Ligament
    - Abdomen
      - Left ØMSJ
      - Right ØMSH
    - Ankle
      - Left ØMSR
      - Right ØMSQ
    - Elbow
      - Left ØMS4
      - Right ØMS3
    - Foot
      - Left ØMST
      - Right ØMSS
    - Hand
      - Left ØMS8
      - Right ØMS7
    - Head and Neck ØMSØ
    - Hip
      - Left ØMSM
      - Right ØMSL
    - Knee
      - Left ØMSP
      - Right ØMSN
    - Lower Extremity
      - Left ØMSW
      - Right ØMSV
    - Perineum ØMSK
    - Rib(s) ØMSG
    - Shoulder
      - Left ØMS2
      - Right ØMS1
    - Spine
      - Lower ØMSD
      - Upper ØMSC
    - Sternum ØMSF

- **Reposition** *(Continued)*
  - Bursa and Ligament *(Continued)*
    - Upper Extremity
      - Left ØMSB
      - Right ØMS9
    - Wrist
      - Left ØMS6
      - Right ØMS5
  - Carina ØBS2ØZZ
  - Carpal
    - Left ØPSN
    - Right ØPSM
  - Cecum ØDSH
  - Cervix ØUSC
  - Clavicle
    - Left ØPSB
    - Right ØPS9
  - Coccyx ØQSS
  - Colon
    - Ascending ØDSK
    - Descending ØDSM
    - Sigmoid ØDSN
    - Transverse ØDSL
  - Cord
    - Bilateral ØVSH
    - Left ØVSG
    - Right ØVSF
  - Cul-de-sac ØUSF
  - Diaphragm ØBSTØZZ
  - Duct
    - Common Bile ØFS9
    - Cystic ØFS8
    - Hepatic
      - Common ØFS7
      - Left ØFS6
      - Right ØFS5
    - Lacrimal
      - Left Ø8SY
      - Right Ø8SX
    - Pancreatic ØFSD
      - Accessory ØFSF
    - Parotid
      - Left ØCSC
      - Right ØCSB
  - Duodenum ØDS9
  - Ear
    - Bilateral Ø9S2
      - Left Ø9S1
      - Right Ø9SØ
  - Epiglottis ØCSR
  - Esophagus ØDS5
  - Eustachian Tube
    - Left Ø9SG
    - Right Ø9SF
  - Eyelid
    - Lower
      - Left Ø8SR
      - Right Ø8SQ
    - Upper
      - Left Ø8SP
      - Right Ø8SN
  - Fallopian Tube
    - Left ØUS6
    - Right ØUS5
  - Fallopian Tubes, Bilateral ØUS7
  - Femoral Shaft
    - Left ØQS9
    - Right ØQS8
  - Femur
    - Lower
      - Left ØQSC
      - Right ØQSB
    - Upper
      - Left ØQS7
      - Right ØQS6
  - Fibula
    - Left ØQSK
    - Right ØQSJ
  - Gallbladder ØFS4

- **Reposition** *(Continued)*
  - Gland
    - Adrenal
      - Left ØGS2
      - Right ØGS3
    - Lacrimal
      - Left Ø8SW
      - Right Ø8SV
  - Glenoid Cavity
    - Left ØPS8
    - Right ØPS7
  - Hair ØHSSXZZ
  - Humeral Head
    - Left ØPSD
    - Right ØPSC
  - Humeral Shaft
    - Left ØPSG
    - Right ØPSF
  - Ileum ØDSB
  - Intestine
    - Large ØDSE
    - Small ØDS8
  - Iris
    - Left Ø8SD3ZZ
    - Right Ø8SC3ZZ
  - Jejunum ØDSA
  - Joint
    - Acromioclavicular
      - Left ØRSH
      - Right ØRSG
    - Ankle
      - Left ØSSG
      - Right ØSSF
    - Carpal
      - Left ØRSR
      - Right ØRSQ
    - Carpometacarpal
      - Left ØRST
      - Right ØRSS
    - Cervical Vertebral ØRS1
    - Cervicothoracic Vertebral ØRS4
    - Coccygeal ØSS6
    - Elbow
      - Left ØRSM
      - Right ØRSL
    - Finger Phalangeal
      - Left ØRSX
      - Right ØRSW
    - Hip
      - Left ØSSB
      - Right ØSS9
    - Knee
      - Left ØSSD
      - Right ØSSC
    - Lumbar Vertebral ØSSØ
    - Lumbosacral ØSS3
    - Metacarpophalangeal
      - Left ØRSV
      - Right ØRSU
    - Metatarsal-Phalangeal
      - Left ØSSN
      - Right ØSSM
    - Occipital-cervical ØRSØ
    - Sacrococcygeal ØSS5
    - Sacroiliac
      - Left ØSS8
      - Right ØSS7
    - Shoulder
      - Left ØRSK
      - Right ØRSJ
    - Sternoclavicular
      - Left ØRSF
      - Right ØRSE
    - Tarsal
      - Left ØSSJ
      - Right ØSSH
    - Tarsometatarsal
      - Left ØSSL
      - Right ØSSK
    - Temporomandibular
      - Left ØRSD
      - Right ØRSC

R

- **Reposition** *(Continued)*
  - Joint *(Continued)*
    - Thoracic Vertebral ØRS6
    - Thoracolumbar Vertebral ØRSA
    - Toe Phalangeal
      - Left ØSSQ
      - Right ØSSP
    - Wrist
      - Left ØRSP
      - Right ØRSN
  - Kidney
    - Left ØTS1
    - Right ØTSØ
  - Kidney Pelvis
    - Left ØTS4
    - Right ØTS3
  - Kidneys, Bilateral ØTS2
  - Larynx ØCSS
  - Lens
    - Left Ø8SK3ZZ
    - Right Ø8SJ3ZZ
  - Lip
    - Lower ØCS1
    - Upper ØCSØ
  - Liver ØFSØ
  - Lung
    - Left ØBSLØZZ
    - Lower Lobe
      - Left ØBSJØZZ
      - Right ØBSFØZZ
    - Middle Lobe, Right ØBSDØZZ
    - Right ØBSKØZZ
    - Upper Lobe
      - Left ØBSGØZZ
      - Right ØBSCØZZ
  - Lung Lingula ØBSHØZZ
  - Mandible
    - Left ØNSV
    - Right ØNST
  - Maxilla ØNSR
  - Metacarpal
    - Left ØPSQ
    - Right ØPSP
  - Metatarsal
    - Left ØQSP
    - Right ØQSN
  - Muscle
    - Abdomen
      - Left ØKSL
      - Right ØKSK
    - Extraocular
      - Left Ø8SM
      - Right Ø8SL
    - Facial ØKS1
    - Foot
      - Left ØKSW
      - Right ØKSV
    - Hand
      - Left ØKSD
      - Right ØKSC
    - Head ØKSØ
    - Hip
      - Left ØKSP
      - Right ØKSN
    - Lower Arm and Wrist
      - Left ØKSB
      - Right ØKS9
    - Lower Leg
      - Left ØKST
      - Right ØKSS
    - Neck
      - Left ØKS3
      - Right ØKS2
    - Perineum ØKSM
    - Shoulder
      - Left ØKS6
      - Right ØKS5
    - Thorax
      - Left ØKSJ
      - Right ØKSH
    - Tongue, Palate, Pharynx ØKS4

- **Reposition** *(Continued)*
  - Muscle *(Continued)*
    - Trunk
      - Left ØKSG
      - Right ØKSF
    - Upper Arm
      - Left ØKS8
      - Right ØKS7
    - Upper Leg
      - Left ØKSR
      - Right ØKSQ
  - Nasal Mucosa and Soft Tissue Ø9SK
  - Nerve
    - Abducens ØØSL
    - Accessory ØØSR
    - Acoustic ØØSN
    - Brachial Plexus Ø1S3
    - Cervical Ø1S1
    - Cervical Plexus Ø1SØ
    - Facial ØØSM
    - Femoral Ø1SD
    - Glossopharyngeal ØØSP
    - Hypoglossal ØØSS
    - Lumbar Ø1SB
    - Lumbar Plexus Ø1S9
    - Lumbosacral Plexus Ø1SA
    - Median Ø1S5
    - Oculomotor ØØSH
    - Olfactory ØØSF
    - Optic ØØSG
    - Peroneal Ø1SH
    - Phrenic Ø1S2
    - Pudendal Ø1SC
    - Radial Ø1S6
    - Sacral Ø1SR
    - Sacral Plexus Ø1SQ
    - Sciatic Ø1SF
    - Thoracic Ø1S8
    - Tibial Ø1SG
    - Trigeminal ØØSK
    - Trochlear ØØSJ
    - Ulnar Ø1S4
    - Vagus ØØSQ
  - Nipple
    - Left ØHSXXZZ
    - Right ØHSWXZZ
  - Orbit
    - Left ØNSQ
    - Right ØNSP
  - Ovary
    - Bilateral ØUS2
    - Left ØUS1
    - Right ØUSØ
  - Palate
    - Hard ØCS2
    - Soft ØCS3
  - Pancreas ØFSG
  - Parathyroid Gland ØGSR
    - Inferior
      - Left ØGSP
      - Right ØGSN
    - Multiple ØGSQ
    - Superior
      - Left ØGSM
      - Right ØGSL
  - Patella
    - Left ØQSF
    - Right ØQSD
  - Phalanx
    - Finger
      - Left ØPSV
      - Right ØPST
    - Thumb
      - Left ØPSS
      - Right ØPSR
    - Toe
      - Left ØQSR
      - Right ØQSQ
  - Products of Conception 1ØSØ
    - Ectopic 1ØS2

- **Reposition** *(Continued)*
  - Radius
    - Left ØPSJ
    - Right ØPSH
  - Rectum ØDSP
  - Retinal Vessel
    - Left Ø8SH3ZZ
    - Right Ø8SG3ZZ
  - Ribs
    - 1 to 2 ØPS1
    - 3 or More ØPS2
  - Sacrum ØQS1
  - Scapula
    - Left ØPS6
    - Right ØPS5
  - Septum, Nasal Ø9SM
  - Sesamoid Bone(s) 1st Toe
    - *see* Reposition, Metatarsal, Right ØQSN
    - *see* Reposition, Metatarsal, Left ØQSP
  - Skull ØNSØ
  - Spinal Cord
    - Cervical ØØSW
    - Lumbar ØØSY
    - Thoracic ØØSX
  - Spleen Ø7SPØZZ
  - Sternum ØPSØ
  - Stomach ØDS6
  - Tarsal
    - Left ØQSM
    - Right ØQSL
  - Tendon
    - Abdomen
      - Left ØLSG
      - Right ØLSF
    - Ankle
      - Left ØLST
      - Right ØLSS
    - Foot
      - Left ØLSW
      - Right ØLSV
    - Hand
      - Left ØLS8
      - Right ØLS7
    - Head and Neck ØLSØ
    - Hip
      - Left ØLSK
      - Right ØLSJ
    - Knee
      - Left ØLSR
      - Right ØLSQ
    - Lower Arm and Wrist
      - Left ØLS6
      - Right ØLS5
    - Lower Leg
      - Left ØLSP
      - Right ØLSN
    - Perineum ØLSH
    - Shoulder
      - Left ØLS2
      - Right ØLS1
    - Thorax
      - Left ØLSD
      - Right ØLSC
    - Trunk
      - Left ØLSB
      - Right ØLS9
    - Upper Arm
      - Left ØLS4
      - Right ØLS3
    - Upper Leg
      - Left ØLSM
      - Right ØLSL
  - Testis
    - Bilateral ØVSC
      - Left ØVSB
      - Right ØVS9
  - Thymus Ø7SMØZZ
  - Thyroid Gland
    - Left Lobe ØGSG
    - Right Lobe ØGSH

Reposition (Continued)
Tibia
Left ØQSH
Right ØQSG
Tongue ØCS7
Tooth
Lower ØCSX
Upper ØCSW
Trachea ØBS1ØZZ
Turbinate, Nasal Ø9SL
Tympanic Membrane
Left Ø9S8
Right Ø9S7
Ulna
Left ØPSL
Right ØPSK
Ureter
Left ØTS7
Right ØTS6
Ureters, Bilateral ØTS8
Urethra ØTSD
Uterine Supporting Structure ØUS4
Uterus ØUS9
Uvula ØCSN
Vagina ØUSG
Vein
Axillary
Left Ø5S8
Right Ø5S7
Azygos Ø5SØ
Basilic
Left Ø5SC
Right Ø5SB
Brachial
Left Ø5SA
Right Ø5S9
Cephalic
Left Ø5SF
Right Ø5SD
Colic Ø6S7
Common Iliac
Left Ø6SD
Right Ø6SC
Esophageal Ø6S3
External Iliac
Left Ø6SG
Right Ø6SF
External Jugular
Left Ø5SQ
Right Ø5SP
Face
Left Ø5SV
Right Ø5ST
Femoral
Left Ø6SN
Right Ø6SM
Foot
Left Ø6SV
Right Ø6ST
Gastric Ø6S2
Hand
Left Ø5SH
Right Ø5SG
Hemiazygos Ø5S1
Hepatic Ø6S4
Hypogastric
Left Ø6SJ
Right Ø6SH
Inferior Mesenteric Ø6S6
Innominate
Left Ø5S4
Right Ø5S3
Internal Jugular
Left Ø5SN
Right Ø5SM
Intracranial Ø5SL
Lower Ø6SY
Portal Ø6S8

Reposition (Continued)
Vein (Continued)
Pulmonary
Left Ø2STØZZ
Right Ø2SSØZZ
Renal
Left Ø6SB
Right Ø6S9
Saphenous
Left Ø6SQ
Right Ø6SP
Splenic Ø6S1
Subclavian
Left Ø5S6
Right Ø5S5
Superior Mesenteric Ø6S5
Upper Ø5SY
Vertebral
Left Ø5SS
Right Ø5SR
Vena Cava
Inferior Ø6SØ
Superior Ø2SVØZZ
Vertebra
Cervical ØPS3
Magnetically Controlled Growth Rod(s) XNS3
Lumbar ØQSØ
Magnetically Controlled Growth Rod(s) XNSØ
Posterior (Dynamic) Distraction Device XNSØ
Thoracic ØPS4
Magnetically Controlled Growth Rod(s) XNS4
Posterior (Dynamic) Distraction Device ØPS4
Vocal Cord
Left ØCSV
Right ØCST

Resection
Acetabulum
Left ØQT5ØZZ
Right ØQT4ØZZ
Adenoids ØCTQ
Ampulla of Vater ØFTC
Anal Sphincter ØDTR
Anus ØDTQ
Aortic Body ØGTD
Appendix ØDTJ
Auditory Ossicle
Left Ø9TA
Right Ø9T9
Bladder ØTTB
Bladder Neck ØTTC
Bone
Ethmoid
Left ØNTGØZZ
Right ØNTFØZZ
Frontal ØNT1ØZZ
Hyoid ØNTXØZZ
Lacrimal
Left ØNTJØZZ
Right ØNTHØZZ
Nasal ØNTBØZZ
Occipital ØNT7ØZZ
Palatine
Left ØNTLØZZ
Right ØNTKØZZ
Parietal
Left ØNT4ØZZ
Right ØNT3ØZZ
Pelvic
Left ØQT3ØZZ
Right ØQT2ØZZ
Sphenoid ØNTCØZZ
Temporal
Left ØNT6ØZZ
Right ØNT5ØZZ
Zygomatic
Left ØNTNØZZ
Right ØNTMØZZ

Resection (Continued)
Breast
Bilateral ØHTVØZZ
Left ØHTUØZZ
Right ØHTTØZZ
Supernumerary ØHTYØZZ
Bronchus
Lingula ØBT9
Lower Lobe
Left ØBTB
Right ØBT6
Main
Left ØBT7
Right ØBT3
Middle Lobe, Right ØBT5
Upper Lobe
Left ØBT8
Right ØBT4
Bursa and Ligament
Abdomen
Left ØMTJ
Right ØMTH
Ankle
Left ØMTR
Right ØMTQ
Elbow
Left ØMT4
Right ØMT3
Foot
Left ØMTT
Right ØMTS
Hand
Left ØMT8
Right ØMT7
Head and Neck ØMTØ
Hip
Left ØMTM
Right ØMTL
Knee
Left ØMTP
Right ØMTN
Lower Extremity
Left ØMTW
Right ØMTV
Perineum ØMTK
Rib(s) ØMTG
Shoulder
Left ØMT2
Right ØMT1
Spine
Lower ØMTD
Upper ØMTC
Sternum ØMTF
Upper Extremity
Left ØMTB
Right ØMT9
Wrist
Left ØMT6
Right ØMT5
Carina ØBT2
Carotid Bodies, Bilateral ØGT8
Carotid Body
Left ØGT6
Right ØGT7
Carpal
Left ØPTNØZZ
Right ØPTMØZZ
Cecum ØDTH
Cerebral Hemisphere ØØT7
Cervix ØUTC
Chordae Tendineae Ø2T9
Cisterna Chyli Ø7TL
Clavicle
Left ØPTBØZZ
Right ØPT9ØZZ
Clitoris ØUTJ
Coccygeal Glomus ØGTB
Coccyx ØQTSØZZ
Colon
Ascending ØDTK
Descending ØDTM

R

- Resection *(Continued)*
  - Colon *(Continued)*
    - Sigmoid ØDTN
    - Transverse ØDTL
  - Conduction Mechanism Ø2T8
  - Cord
    - Bilateral ØVTH
    - Left ØVTG
    - Right ØVTF
  - Cornea
    - Left Ø8T9XZZ
    - Right Ø8T8XZZ
  - Cul-de-sac ØUTF
  - Diaphragm ØBTT
  - Disc
    - Cervical Vertebral ØRT3ØZZ
    - Cervicothoracic Vertebral ØRT5ØZZ
    - Lumbar Vertebral ØST2ØZZ
    - Lumbosacral ØST4ØZZ
    - Thoracic Vertebral ØRT9ØZZ
    - Thoracolumbar Vertebral ØRTBØZZ
  - Duct
    - Common Bile ØFT9
    - Cystic ØFT8
    - Hepatic
      - Common ØFT7
      - Left ØFT6
      - Right ØFT5
    - Lacrimal
      - Left Ø8TY
      - Right Ø8TX
    - Pancreatic ØFTD
      - Accessory ØFTF
    - Parotid
      - Left ØCTCØZZ
      - Right ØCTBØZZ
  - Duodenum ØDT9
  - Ear
    - External
      - Left Ø9T1
      - Right Ø9TØ
    - Inner
      - Left Ø9TE
      - Right Ø9TD
    - Middle
      - Left Ø9T6
      - Right Ø9T5
  - Epididymis
    - Bilateral ØVTL
    - Left ØVTK
    - Right ØVTJ
  - Epiglottis ØCTR
  - Esophagogastric Junction ØDT4
  - Esophagus ØDT5
    - Lower ØDT3
    - Middle ØDT2
    - Upper ØDT1
  - Eustachian Tube
    - Left Ø9TG
    - Right Ø9TF
  - Eye
    - Left Ø8T1XZZ
    - Right Ø8TØXZZ
  - Eyelid
    - Lower
      - Left Ø8TR
      - Right Ø8TQ
    - Upper
      - Left Ø8TP
      - Right Ø8TN
  - Fallopian Tube
    - Left ØUT6
    - Right ØUT5
  - Fallopian Tubes, Bilateral ØUT7
  - Femoral Shaft
    - Left ØQT9ØZZ
    - Right ØQT8ØZZ

- Resection *(Continued)*
  - Femur
    - Lower
      - Left ØQTCØZZ
      - Right ØQTBØZZ
    - Upper
      - Left ØQT7ØZZ
      - Right ØQT6ØZZ
  - Fibula
    - Left ØQTKØZZ
    - Right ØQTJØZZ
  - Finger Nail ØHTQXZZ
  - Gallbladder ØFT4
  - Gland
    - Adrenal
      - Bilateral ØGT4
      - Left ØGT2
      - Right ØGT3
    - Lacrimal
      - Left Ø8TW
      - Right Ø8TV
    - Minor Salivary ØCTJØZZ
    - Parotid
      - Left ØCT9ØZZ
      - Right ØCT8ØZZ
    - Pituitary ØGTØ
    - Sublingual
      - Left ØCTFØZZ
      - Right ØCTDØZZ
    - Submaxillary
      - Left ØCTHØZZ
      - Right ØCTGØZZ
    - Vestibular ØUTL
  - Glenoid Cavity
    - Left ØPT8ØZZ
    - Right ØPT7ØZZ
  - Glomus Jugulare ØGTC
  - Humeral Head
    - Left ØPTDØZZ
    - Right ØPTCØZZ
  - Humeral Shaft
    - Left ØPTGØZZ
    - Right ØPTFØZZ
  - Hymen ØUTK
  - Ileocecal Valve ØDTC
  - Ileum ØDTB
  - Intestine
    - Large ØDTE
      - Left ØDTG
      - Right ØDTF
    - Small ØDT8
  - Iris
    - Left Ø8TD3ZZ
    - Right Ø8TC3ZZ
  - Jejunum ØDTA
  - Joint
    - Acromioclavicular
      - Left ØRTHØZZ
      - Right ØRTGØZZ
    - Ankle
      - Left ØSTGØZZ
      - Right ØSTFØZZ
    - Carpal
      - Left ØRTRØZZ
      - Right ØRTQØZZ
    - Carpometacarpal
      - Left ØRTTØZZ
      - Right ØRTSØZZ
    - Cervicothoracic Vertebral ØRT4ØZZ
    - Coccygeal ØST6ØZZ
    - Elbow
      - Left ØRTMØZZ
      - Right ØRTLØZZ
    - Finger Phalangeal
      - Left ØRTXØZZ
      - Right ØRTWØZZ
    - Hip
      - Left ØSTBØZZ
      - Right ØST9ØZZ

- Resection *(Continued)*
  - Joint *(Continued)*
    - Knee
      - Left ØSTDØZZ
      - Right ØSTCØZZ
    - Metacarpophalangeal
      - Left ØRTVØZZ
      - Right ØRTUØZZ
    - Metatarsal-Phalangeal
      - Left ØSTNØZZ
      - Right ØSTMØZZ
    - Sacrococcygeal ØST5ØZZ
    - Sacroiliac
      - Left ØST8ØZZ
      - Right ØST7ØZZ
    - Shoulder
      - Left ØRTKØZZ
      - Right ØRTJØZZ
    - Sternoclavicular
      - Left ØRTFØZZ
      - Right ØRTEØZZ
    - Tarsal
      - Left ØSTJØZZ
      - Right ØSTHØZZ
    - Tarsometatarsal
      - Left ØSTLØZZ
      - Right ØSTKØZZ
    - Temporomandibular
      - Left ØRTDØZZ
      - Right ØRTCØZZ
    - Toe Phalangeal
      - Left ØSTQØZZ
      - Right ØSTPØZZ
    - Wrist
      - Left ØRTPØZZ
      - Right ØRTNØZZ
  - Kidney
    - Left ØTT1
    - Right ØTTØ
  - Kidney Pelvis
    - Left ØTT4
    - Right ØTT3
  - Kidneys, Bilateral ØTT2
  - Larynx ØCTS
  - Lens
    - Left Ø8TK3ZZ
    - Right Ø8TJ3ZZ
  - Lip
    - Lower ØCT1
    - Upper ØCTØ
  - Liver ØFTØ
    - Left Lobe ØFT2
    - Right Lobe ØFT1
  - Lung
    - Bilateral ØBTM
    - Left ØBTL
    - Lower Lobe
      - Left ØBTJ
      - Right ØBTF
    - Middle Lobe, Right ØBTD
    - Right ØBTK
    - Upper Lobe
      - Left ØBTG
      - Right ØBTC
  - Lung Lingula ØBTH
  - Lymphatic
    - Aortic Ø7TD
    - Axillary
      - Left Ø7T6
      - Right Ø7T5
    - Head Ø7TØ
    - Inguinal
      - Left Ø7TJ
      - Right Ø7TH
    - Internal Mammary
      - Left Ø7T9
      - Right Ø7T8

R

New Revised ~~deleted~~ Deleted

Resection *(Continued)*
Lymphatic *(Continued)*
Lower Extremity
Left Ø7TG
Right Ø7TF
Mesenteric Ø7TB
Neck
Left Ø7T2
Right Ø7T1
Pelvis Ø7TC
Thoracic Duct Ø7TK
Thorax Ø7T7
Upper Extremity
Left Ø7T4
Right Ø7T3
Mandible
Left ØNTVØZZ
Right ØNTTØZZ
Maxilla ØNTRØZZ
Metacarpal
Left ØPTQØZZ
Right ØPTPØZZ
Metatarsal
Left ØQTPØZZ
Right ØQTNØZZ
Muscle
Abdomen
Left ØKTL
Right ØKTK
Extraocular
Left Ø8TM
Right Ø8TL
Facial ØKT1
Foot
Left ØKTW
Right ØKTV
Hand
Left ØKTD
Right ØKTC
Head ØKTØ
Hip
Left ØKTP
Right ØKTN
Lower Arm and Wrist
Left ØKTB
Right ØKT9
Lower Leg
Left ØKTT
Right ØKTS
Neck
Left ØKT3
Right ØKT2
Papillary Ø2TD
Perineum ØKTM
Shoulder
Left ØKT6
Right ØKT5
Thorax
Left ØKTJ
Right ØKTH
Tongue, Palate, Pharynx ØKT4
Trunk
Left ØKTG
Right ØKTF
Upper Arm
Left ØKT8
Right ØKT7
Upper Leg
Left ØKTR
Right ØKTQ
Nasal Mucosa and Soft Tissue Ø9TK
Nasopharynx Ø9TN
Nipple
Left ØHTXXZZ
Right ØHTWXZZ
Omentum ØDTU
Orbit
Left ØNTQØZZ
Right ØNTPØZZ

Resection *(Continued)*
Ovary
Bilateral ØUT2
Left ØUT1
Right ØUTØ
Palate
Hard ØCT2
Soft ØCT3
Pancreas ØFTG
Para-aortic Body ØGT9
Paraganglion Extremity ØGTF
Parathyroid Gland ØGTR
Inferior
Left ØGTP
Right ØGTN
Multiple ØGTQ
Superior
Left ØGTM
Right ØGTL
Patella
Left ØQTFØZZ
Right ØQTDØZZ
Penis ØVTS
Pericardium Ø2TN
Phalanx
Finger
Left ØPTVØZZ
Right ØPTTØZZ
Thumb
Left ØPTSØZZ
Right ØPTRØZZ
Toe
Left ØQTRØZZ
Right ØQTQØZZ
Pharynx ØCTM
Pineal Body ØGT1
Prepuce ØVTT
Products of Conception, Ectopic 1ØT2
Prostate ØVTØ
Radius
Left ØPTJØZZ
Right ØPTHØZZ
Rectum ØDTP
Ribs
1 to 2 ØPT1ØZZ
3 or More ØPT2ØZZ
Scapula
Left ØPT6ØZZ
Right ØPT5ØZZ
Scrotum ØVT5
Septum
Atrial Ø2T5
Nasal Ø9TM
Ventricular Ø2TM
Sinus
Accessory Ø9TP
Ethmoid
Left Ø9TV
Right Ø9TU
Frontal
Left Ø9TT
Right Ø9TS
Mastoid
Left Ø9TC
Right Ø9TB
Maxillary
Left Ø9TR
Right Ø9TQ
Sphenoid
Left Ø9TX
Right Ø9TW
Spleen Ø7TP
Sternum ØPTØØZZ
Stomach ØDT6
Pylorus ØDT7
Tarsal
Left ØQTMØZZ
Right ØQTLØZZ

Resection *(Continued)*
Tendon
Abdomen
Left ØLTG
Right ØLTF
Ankle
Left ØLTT
Right ØLTS
Foot
Left ØLTW
Right ØLTV
Hand
Left ØLT8
Right ØLT7
Head and Neck ØLTØ
Hip
Left ØLTK
Right ØLTJ
Knee
Left ØLTR
Right ØLTQ
Lower Arm and Wrist
Left ØLT6
Right ØLT5
Lower Leg
Left ØLTP
Right ØLTN
Perineum ØLTH
Shoulder
Left ØLT2
Right ØLT1
Thorax
Left ØLTD
Right ØLTC
Trunk
Left ØLTB
Right ØLT9
Upper Arm
Left ØLT4
Right ØLT3
Upper Leg
Left ØLTM
Right ØLTL
Testis
Bilateral ØVTC
Left ØVTB
Right ØVT9
Thymus Ø7TM
Thyroid Gland ØGTK
Left Lobe ØGTG
Right Lobe ØGTH
Thyroid Gland Isthmus ØGTJ
Tibia
Left ØQTHØZZ
Right ØQTGØZZ
Toe Nail ØHTRXZZ
Tongue ØCT7
Tonsils ØCTP
Tooth
Lower ØCTXØZ
Upper ØCTWØZ
Trachea ØBT1
Tunica Vaginalis
Left ØVT7
Right ØVT6
Turbinate, Nasal Ø9TL
Tympanic Membrane
Left Ø9T8
Right Ø9T7
Ulna
Left ØPTLØZZ
Right ØPTKØZZ
Ureter
Left ØTT7
Right ØTT6
Urethra ØTTD
Uterine Supporting Structure ØUT4
Uterus ØUT9

R

Resection *(Continued)*
Uvula ØCTN
Vagina ØUTG
Valve, Pulmonary Ø2TH
Vas Deferens
Bilateral ØVTQ
Left ØVTP
Right ØVTN
Vesicle
Bilateral ØVT3
Left ØVT2
Right ØVT1
Vitreous
Left Ø8T53ZZ
Right Ø8T43ZZ
Vocal Cord
Left ØCTV
Right ØCTT
Vulva ØUTM
Resection, Left ventricular outflow tract obstruction (LVOT) *see* Dilation, Ventricle, Left Ø27L
Resection, Subaortic membrane (Left ventricular outflow tract obstruction) *see* Dilation, Ventricle, Left Ø27L
Restoration, Cardiac, Single, Rhythm 5A22Ø4Z
▶ **restor3d TIDAL™ Fusion Cage** *use* Internal Fixation Device, Gyroid-Sheet Lattice Design in New Technology
RestoreAdvanced neurostimulator (SureScan) (MRI Safe) *use* Stimulator Generator, Multiple Array Rechargeable in ØJH
RestoreSensor neurostimulator (SureScan) (MRI Safe) *use* Stimulator Generator, Multiple Array Rechargeable in ØJH
RestoreUltra neurostimulator (SureScan) (MRI Safe) *use* Stimulator Generator, Multiple Array Rechargeable in ØJH
Restriction
Ampulla of Vater ØFVC
Anus ØDVQ
Aorta
Abdominal Ø4VØ
Ascending/Arch, Intraluminal Device, Branched or Fenestrated Ø2VX
Descending, Intraluminal Device, Branched or Fenestrated Ø2VW
Thoracic
Intraluminal Device, Branched or Fenestrated Ø4VØ
Artery
Anterior Tibial
Left Ø4VQ
Right Ø4VP
Axillary
Left Ø3V6
Right Ø3V5
Brachial
Left Ø3V8
Right Ø3V7
Celiac Ø4V1
Colic
Left Ø4V7
Middle Ø4V8
Right Ø4V6
Common Carotid
Left Ø3VJ
Right Ø3VH
Common Iliac
Left Ø4VD
Right Ø4VC
External Carotid
Left Ø3VN
Right Ø3VM
External Iliac
Left Ø4VJ
Right Ø4VH
Face Ø3VR

Restriction *(Continued)*
Artery *(Continued)*
Femoral
Left Ø4VL
Right Ø4VK
Foot
Left Ø4VW
Right Ø4VV
Gastric Ø4V2
Hand
Left Ø3VF
Right Ø3VD
Hepatic Ø4V3
Inferior Mesenteric Ø4VB
Innominate Ø3V2
Internal Carotid
Left Ø3VL
Right Ø3VK
Internal Iliac
Left Ø4VF
Right Ø4VE
Internal Mammary
Left Ø3V1
Right Ø3VØ
Intracranial Ø3VG
Lower Ø4VY
Peroneal
Left Ø4VU
Right Ø4VT
Popliteal
Left Ø4VN
Right Ø4VM
Posterior Tibial
Left Ø4VS
Right Ø4VR
Pulmonary
Left Ø2VR
Right Ø2VQ
Pulmonary Trunk Ø2VP
Radial
Left Ø3VC
Right Ø3VB
Renal
Left Ø4VA
Right Ø4V9
Splenic Ø4V4
Subclavian
Left Ø3V4
Right Ø3V3
Superior Mesenteric Ø4V5
Temporal
Left Ø3VT
Right Ø3VS
Thyroid
Left Ø3VV
Right Ø3VU
Ulnar
Left Ø3VA
Right Ø3V9
Upper Ø3VY
Vertebral
Left Ø3VQ
Right Ø3VP
Bladder ØTVB
Bladder Neck ØTVC
Bronchus
Lingula ØBV9
Lower Lobe
Left ØBVB
Right ØBV6
Main
Left ØBV7
Right ØBV3
Middle Lobe, Right ØBV5
Upper Lobe
Left ØBV8
Right ØBV4
Carina ØBV2

Restriction *(Continued)*
Cecum ØDVH
Cervix ØUVC
Cisterna Chyli Ø7VL
Colon
Ascending ØDVK
Descending ØDVM
Sigmoid ØDVN
Transverse ØDVL
Duct
Common Bile ØFV9
Cystic ØFV8
Hepatic
Common ØFV7
Left ØFV6
Right ØFV5
Lacrimal
Left Ø8VY
Right Ø8VX
Pancreatic ØFVD
Accessory ØFVF
Parotid
Left ØCVC
Right ØCVB
Duodenum ØDV9
Esophagogastric Junction ØDV4
Esophagus ØDV5
Lower ØDV3
Middle ØDV2
Upper ØDV1
Heart Ø2VA
Ileocecal Valve ØDVC
Ileum ØDVB
Intestine
Large ØDVE
Left ØDVG
Right ØDVF
Small ØDV8
Jejunum ØDVA
Kidney Pelvis
Left ØTV4
Right ØTV3
Lymphatic
Aortic Ø7VD
Axillary
Left Ø7V6
Right Ø7V5
Head Ø7VØ
Inguinal
Left Ø7VJ
Right Ø7VH
Internal Mammary
Left Ø7V9
Right Ø7V8
Lower Extremity
Left Ø7VG
Right Ø7VF
Mesenteric Ø7VB
Neck
Left Ø7V2
Right Ø7V1
Pelvis Ø7VC
Thoracic Duct Ø7VK
Thorax Ø7V7
Upper Extremity
Left Ø7V4
Right Ø7V3
Rectum ØDVP
Stomach ØDV6
Pylorus ØDV7
Trachea ØBV1
Ureter
Left ØTV7
Right ØTV6
Urethra ØTVD
Valve, Mitral Ø2VG

R

Restriction *(Continued)*
Vein
Axillary
Left Ø5V8
Right Ø5V7
Azygos Ø5VØ
Basilic
Left Ø5VC
Right Ø5VB
Brachial
Left Ø5VA
Right Ø5V9
Cephalic
Left Ø5VF
Right Ø5VD
Colic Ø6V7
Common Iliac
Left Ø6VD
Right Ø6VC
Esophageal Ø6V3
External Iliac
Left Ø6VG
Right Ø6VF
External Jugular
Left Ø5VQ
Right Ø5VP
Face
Left Ø5VV
Right Ø5VT
Femoral
Left Ø6VN
Right Ø6VM
Foot
Left Ø6VV
Right Ø6VT
Gastric Ø6V2
Hand
Left Ø5VH
Right Ø5VG
Hemiazygos Ø5V1
Hepatic Ø6V4
Hypogastric
Left Ø6VJ
Right Ø6VH
Inferior Mesenteric Ø6V6
Innominate
Left Ø5V4
Right Ø5V3
Internal Jugular
Left Ø5VN
Right Ø5VM
Intracranial Ø5VL
Lower Ø6VY
Portal Ø6V8
Pulmonary
Left Ø2VT
Right Ø2VS
Renal
Left Ø6VB
Right Ø6V9
Saphenous
Left Ø6VQ
Right Ø6VP
Splenic Ø6V1
Subclavian
Left Ø5V6
Right Ø5V5
Superior Mesenteric Ø6V5
Upper Ø5VY
Vertebral
Left Ø5VS
Right Ø5VR
Vena Cava
Inferior Ø6VØ
Superior Ø2VV
Ventricle, Left Ø2VL

Resurfacing Device
Removal of device from
Left ØSPBØBZ
Right ØSP9ØBZ
Revision of device in
Left ØSWBØBZ
Right ØSW9ØBZ
Supplement
Left ØSUBØBZ
Acetabular Surface ØSUEØBZ
Femoral Surface ØSUSØBZ
Right ØSU9ØBZ
Acetabular Surface ØSUAØBZ
Femoral Surface ØSURØBZ
Resuscitation
Cardiopulmonary *see* Assistance, Cardiac 5AØ2
Cardioversion 5A22Ø4Z
Defibrillation 5A22Ø4Z
Endotracheal intubation *see* Insertion of device in, Trachea ØBH1
External chest compression, manual 5A12Ø12
External chest compression, mechanical 5A1221J
Pulmonary 5A19Ø54
Resuscitative endovascular balloon occlusion of the aorta (REBOA)
Ø2LW3DJ
Ø4LØ3DJ
▶ **Resuscitative thoracotomy**
▶ *see* Control bleeding in, Mediastinum ØW3C
▶ *see* Control bleeding in, Pericardial Cavity ØW3D
Resuture, Heart valve prosthesis *see* Revision of device in, Heart and Great Vessels Ø2W
Retained placenta, manual removal *see* Extraction, Products of Conception, Retained 1ØD1
RETHYMIC® *use* Engineered Allogeneic Thymus Tissue
Retraining
Cardiac *see* Motor Treatment, Rehabilitation FØ7
Vocational *see* Activities of Daily Living Treatment, Rehabilitation FØ8
Retrogasserian rhizotomy *see* Division, Nerve, Trigeminal ØØ8K
Retroperitoneal cavity *use* Retroperitoneum
Retroperitoneal lymph node *use* Lymphatic, Aortic
Retroperitoneal space *use* Retroperitoneum
Retropharyngeal lymph node
use Lymphatic, Right Neck
use Lymphatic, Left Neck
Retropharyngeal space *use* Neck
Retropubic space *use* Pelvic Cavity
Reveal (LINQ) (DX) (XT) *use* Monitoring Device
Reverse total shoulder replacement *see* Replacement, Upper Joints ØRR
Reverse® Shoulder Prosthesis *use* Synthetic Substitute, Reverse Ball and Socket in ØRR
Revision
Correcting a portion of existing device *see* Revision of device in
Removal of device without replacement *see* Removal of device from
Replacement of existing device
see Removal of device from
see Root operation to place new device, e.g., Insertion, Replacement, Supplement
Revision of device in
Abdominal Wall ØWWF
Acetabulum
Left ØQW5
Right ØQW4

Revision of device in *(Continued)*
Anal Sphincter ØDWR
Anus ØDWQ
Aorta, Thoracic, Descending Ø2WW3RZ
Artery
Lower Ø4WY
Upper Ø3WY
Auditory Ossicle
Left Ø9WA
Right Ø9W9
Back
Lower ØWWL
Upper ØWWK
Bladder ØTWB
Bone
Facial ØNWW
Lower ØQWY
Nasal ØNWB
Pelvic
Left ØQW3
Right ØQW2
Upper ØPWY
Bone Marrow Ø7WT
Brain ØØWØ
Breast
Left ØHWU
Right ØHWT
Bursa and Ligament
Lower ØMWY
Upper ØMWX
Carpal
Left ØPWN
Right ØPWM
Cavity, Cranial ØWW1
Cerebral Ventricle ØØW6
Chest Wall ØWW8
Cisterna Chyli Ø7WL
Clavicle
Left ØPWB
Right ØPW9
Coccyx ØQWS
Diaphragm ØBWT
Disc
Cervical Vertebral ØRW3
Cervicothoracic Vertebral ØRW5
Lumbar Vertebral ØSW2
Lumbosacral ØSW4
Thoracic Vertebral ØRW9
Thoracolumbar Vertebral ØRWB
Duct
Hepatobiliary ØFWB
Pancreatic ØFWD
Thoracic Ø7WK
Ear
Inner
Left Ø9WE
Right Ø9WD
Left Ø9WJ
Right Ø9WH
Epididymis and Spermatic Cord ØVWM
Esophagus ØDW5
Extremity
Lower
Left ØYWB
Right ØYW9
Upper
Left ØXW7
Right ØXW6
Eye
Left Ø8W1
Right Ø8WØ
Face ØWW2
Fallopian Tube ØUW8
Femoral Shaft
Left ØQW9
Right ØQW8
Femur
Lower
Left ØQWC
Right ØQWB

R

Revision of device in (Continued)
Femur (Continued)
Upper
Left ØQW7
Right ØQW6
Fibula
Left ØQWK
Right ØQWJ
Finger Nail ØHWQX
Gallbladder ØFW4
Gastrointestinal Tract ØWWP
Genitourinary Tract ØWWR
Gland
Adrenal ØGW5
Endocrine ØGWS
Pituitary ØGWØ
Salivary ØCWA
Glenoid Cavity
Left ØPW8
Right ØPW7
Great Vessel Ø2WY
Hair ØHWSX
Head ØWWØ
Heart Ø2WA
Humeral Head
Left ØPWD
Right ØPWC
Humeral Shaft
Left ØPWG
Right ØPWF
Intestinal Tract
Lower Intestinal Tract ØDWD
Upper Intestinal Tract ØDWØ
Intestine
Large ØDWE
Small ØDW8
Jaw
Lower ØWW5
Upper ØWW4
Joint
Acromioclavicular
Left ØRWH
Right ØRWG
Ankle
Left ØSWG
Right ØSWF
Carpal
Left ØRWR
Right ØRWQ
Carpometacarpal
Left ØRWT
Right ØRWS
Cervical Vertebral ØRW1
Cervicothoracic Vertebral ØRW4
Coccygeal ØSW6
Elbow
Left ØRWM
Right ØRWL
Finger Phalangeal
Left ØRWX
Right ØRWW
Hip
Left ØSWB
Acetabular Surface ØSWE
Femoral Surface ØSWS
Right ØSW9
Acetabular Surface ØSWA
Femoral Surface ØSWR
Knee
Left ØSWD
Femoral Surface ØSWU
Tibial Surface ØSWW
Right ØSWC
Femoral Surface ØSWT
Tibial Surface ØSWV
Lumbar Vertebral ØSWØ
Lumbosacral ØSW3
Metacarpophalangeal
Left ØRWV
Right ØRWU

Revision of device in (Continued)
Knee (Continued)
Metatarsal-Phalangeal
Left ØSWN
Right ØSWM
Occipital-cervical ØRWØ
Sacrococcygeal ØSW5
Sacroiliac
Left ØSW8
Right ØSW7
Shoulder
Left ØRWK
Right ØRWJ
Sternoclavicular
Left ØRWF
Right ØRWE
Tarsal
Left ØSWJ
Right ØSWH
Tarsometatarsal
Left ØSWL
Right ØSWK
Temporomandibular
Left ØRWD
Right ØRWC
Thoracic Vertebral ØRW6
Thoracolumbar Vertebral ØRWA
Toe Phalangeal
Left ØSWQ
Right ØSWP
Wrist
Left ØRWP
Right ØRWN
Kidney ØTW5
Larynx ØCWS
Lens
Left Ø8WK
Right Ø8WJ
Liver ØFWØ
Lung
Left ØBWL
Right ØBWK
Lymphatic Ø7WN
Thoracic Duct Ø7WK
Mediastinum ØWWC
Mesentery ØDWV
Metacarpal
Left ØPWQ
Right ØPWP
Metatarsal
Left ØQWP
Right ØQWN
Mouth and Throat ØCWY
Muscle
Extraocular
Left Ø8WM
Right Ø8WL
Lower ØKWY
Upper ØKWX
Nasal Mucosa and Soft Tissue Ø9WK
Neck ØWW6
Nerve
Cranial ØØWE
Peripheral Ø1WY
Omentum ØDWU
Ovary ØUW3
Pancreas ØFWG
Parathyroid Gland ØGWR
Patella
Left ØQWF
Right ØQWD
Pelvic Cavity ØWWJ
Penis ØVWS
Pericardial Cavity ØWWD
Perineum
Female ØWWN
Male ØWWM
Peritoneal Cavity ØWWG
Peritoneum ØDWW

Revision of device in (Continued)
Phalanx
Finger
Left ØPWV
Right ØPWT
Thumb
Left ØPWS
Right ØPWR
Toe
Left ØQWR
Right ØQWQ
Pineal Body ØGW1
Pleura ØBWQ
Pleural Cavity
Left ØWWB
Right ØWW9
Prostate and Seminal Vesicles ØVW4
Radius
Left ØPWJ
Right ØPWH
Respiratory Tract ØWWQ
Retroperitoneum ØWWH
Ribs
1 to 2 ØPW1
3 or More ØPW2
Sacrum ØQW1
Scapula
Left ØPW6
Right ØPW5
Scrotum and Tunica Vaginalis ØVW8
Septum
Atrial Ø2W5
Ventricular Ø2WM
Sinus Ø9WY
Skin ØHWPX
Skull ØNWØ
Spinal Canal ØØWU
Spinal Cord ØØWV
Spleen Ø7WP
Sternum ØPWØ
Stomach ØDW6
Subcutaneous Tissue and Fascia
Head and Neck ØJWS
Lower Extremity ØJWW
Trunk ØJWT
Upper Extremity ØJWV
Tarsal
Left ØQWM
Right ØQWL
Tendon
Lower ØLWY
Upper ØLWX
Testis ØVWD
Thymus Ø7WM
Thyroid Gland ØGWK
Tibia
Left ØQWH
Right ØQWG
Toe Nail ØHWRX
Trachea ØBW1
Tracheobronchial Tree ØBWØ
Tympanic Membrane
Left Ø9W8
Right Ø9W7
Ulna
Left ØPWL
Right ØPWK
Ureter ØTW9
Urethra ØTWD
Uterus and Cervix ØUWD
Vagina and Cul-de-sac ØUWH
Valve
Aortic Ø2WF
Mitral Ø2WG
Pulmonary Ø2WH
Tricuspid Ø2WJ
Vas Deferens ØVWR
Vein
Azygos Ø5WØ

R

- **Revision of device in** *(Continued)*
  - Vein *(Continued)*
    - Innominate
      - Left Ø5W4
      - Right Ø5W3
    - Lower Ø6WY
    - Upper Ø5WY
  - Vertebra
    - Cervical ØPW3
    - Lumbar ØQWØ
    - Thoracic ØPW4
  - Vulva ØUWM
- **Revo MRI™ SureScan® pacemaker** *use* Pacemaker, Dual Chamber in ØJH
- **Rezafungin** XWØ
- **rhBMP-2** *use* Recombinant Bone Morphogenetic Protein
- **Rheos® System device** *use* Stimulator Generator in Subcutaneous Tissue and Fascia
- **Rheos® System lead** *use* Stimulator Lead in Upper Arteries
- **Rhinopharynx** *use* Nasopharynx
- **Rhinoplasty**
  - *see* Alteration, Nasal Mucosa and Soft Tissue Ø9ØK
  - *see* Repair, Nasal Mucosa and Soft Tissue Ø9QK
  - *see* Replacement, Nasal Mucosa and Soft Tissue Ø9RK
  - *see* Supplement, Nasal Mucosa and Soft Tissue Ø9UK
- **Rhinorrhaphy** *see* Repair, Nasal Mucosa and Soft Tissue Ø9QK
- **Rhinoscopy** Ø9JKXZZ
- **Rhizotomy**
  - *see* Division, Central Nervous System and Cranial Nerves ØØ8
  - *see* Division, Peripheral Nervous System Ø18
- **Rhomboid major muscle**
  - *use* Trunk Muscle, Right
  - *use* Trunk Muscle, Left
- **Rhomboid minor muscle**
  - *use* Trunk Muscle, Right
  - *use* Trunk Muscle, Left
- **Rhythm electrocardiogram** *see* Measurement, Cardiac 4AØ2
- **Rhytidectomy** *see* Alteration, Face ØwØ2
- **Right ascending lumbar vein** *use* Azygos Vein
- **Right atrioventricular valve** *use* Tricuspid Valve
- **Right auricular appendix** *use* Atrium, Right
- **Right colic vein** *use* Colic Vein
- **Right coronary sulcus** *use* Heart, Right
- **Right gastric artery** *use* Gastric Artery
- **Right gastroepiploic vein** *use* Superior Mesenteric Vein
- **Right inferior phrenic vein** *use* Inferior Vena Cava
- **Right inferior pulmonary vein** *use* Pulmonary Vein, Right
- **Right jugular trunk** *use* Lymphatic, Right Neck
- **Right lateral ventricle** *use* Cerebral Ventricle
- **Right lymphatic duct** *use* Lymphatic, Right Neck
- **Right ovarian vein** *use* Inferior Vena Cava
- **Right second lumbar vein** *use* Inferior Vena Cava
- **Right subclavian trunk** *use* Lymphatic, Right Neck
- **Right subcostal vein** *use* Azygos Vein
- **Right superior pulmonary vein** *use* Pulmonary Vein, Right
- **Right suprarenal vein** *use* Inferior Vena Cava
- **Right testicular vein** *use* Inferior Vena Cava
- **Rima glottidis** *use* Larynx
- **Risorius muscle** *use* Facial Muscle
- **RNS System lead** *use* Neurostimulator Lead in Central Nervous System and Cranial Nerves
- **RNS system neurostimulator generator** *use* Neurostimulator Generator in Head and Facial Bones
- **Robotic Assisted Procedure**
  - Extremity
    - Lower 8EØY
    - Upper 8EØX
  - Head and Neck Region 8EØ9
  - Trunk Region 8EØW
- **Rotation of fetal head**
  - Forceps 1ØSØ7ZZ
  - Manual 1ØSØXZZ
- **Round ligament of uterus** *use* Uterine Supporting Structure
- **Round window**
  - *use* Inner Ear, Right
  - *use* Inner Ear, Left
- **Roux-en-Y operation**
  - *see* Bypass, Gastrointestinal System ØD1
  - *see* Bypass, Hepatobiliary System and Pancreas ØF1
- ▶**RP-L2Ø1** *use* Marnetegragene Autotemcel
- **Rupture**
  - Adhesions *see* Release
  - Fluid collection *see* Drainage
- ➠**Ruxolitinib** *use* Other Substance ~~XWØDWT5~~

R

S

S-ICD™ lead *use* Subcutaneous Defibrillator Lead in Subcutaneous Tissue and Fascia
Sabizabulin XWØ
Sacral ganglion *use* Sacral Sympathetic Nerve
Sacral lymph node *use* Lymphatic, Pelvis
Sacral nerve modulation (SNM) lead *use* Stimulator Lead in Urinary System
Sacral neuromodulation lead *use* Stimulator Lead in Urinary System
Sacral splanchnic nerve *use* Sacral Sympathetic Nerve
Sacrectomy *see* Excision, Lower Bones ØQB
Sacrococcygeal ligament *use* Lower Spine Bursa and Ligament
Sacrococcygeal symphysis *use* Sacrococcygeal Joint
Sacroiliac ligament *use* Lower Spine Bursa and Ligament
Sacrospinous ligament *use* Lower Spine Bursa and Ligament
Sacrotuberous ligament *use* Lower Spine Bursa and Ligament
Salpingectomy
- *see* Excision, Female Reproductive System ØUB
- *see* Resection, Female Reproductive System ØUT

Salpingolysis *see* Release, Female Reproductive System ØUN
Salpingopexy
- *see* Repair, Female Reproductive System ØUQ
- *see* Reposition, Female Reproductive System ØUS

Salpingopharyngeus muscle *use* Tongue, Palate, Pharynx Muscle
Salpingoplasty
- *see* Repair, Female Reproductive System ØUQ
- *see* Supplement, Female Reproductive System ØUU

Salpingorrhaphy *see* Repair, Female Reproductive System ØUQ
Salpingoscopy ØUJ88ZZ
Salpingostomy *see* Drainage, Female Reproductive System ØU9
Salpingotomy *see* Drainage, Female Reproductive System ØU9
Salpinx
- *use* Fallopian Tube, Right
- *use* Fallopian Tube, Left

Saphenous nerve *use* Femoral Nerve
SAPIEN transcatheter aortic valve *use* Zooplastic Tissue in Heart and Great Vessels
Sarilumab XWØ
SARS-CoV-2 antibody detection, serum/plasma nanoparticle fluorescence XXE5XV7
SARS-CoV-2 polymerase chain reaction, nasopharyngeal fluid XXE97U7
Sartorius muscle
- *use* Upper Leg Muscle, Right
- *use* Upper Leg Muscle, Left

Satralizumab-mwge XWØ1397
SAVAL below-the-knee (BTK) drug-eluting stent system
- ~~use Intraluminal Device, Sustained Release Drug-eluting in New Technology~~
- ~~use Intraluminal Device, Sustained Release Drug-eluting, Two in New Technology~~
- ~~use Intraluminal Device, Sustained Release Drug-eluting, Three in New Technology~~
- ~~use Intraluminal Device, Sustained Release Drug-eluting, Four or More in New Technology~~
- ▶ *use* Intraluminal Device, Drug-eluting in Lower Arteries
- ▶ *use* Intraluminal Device, Drug-eluting, Two in Lower Arteries
- ▶ *use* Intraluminal Device, Drug-eluting, Three in Lower Arteries
- ▶ *use* Intraluminal Device, Drug-eluting, Four or More in Lower Arteries

Scalene muscle
- *use* Neck Muscle, Right
- *use* Neck Muscle, Left

Scan
- Computerized Tomography (CT) *see* Computerized Tomography (CT Scan)
- Radioisotope *see* Planar Nuclear Medicine Imaging

Scaphoid bone
- *use* Carpal, Right
- *use* Carpal, Left

Scapholunate ligament
- *use* Wrist Bursa and Ligament, Right
- *use* Wrist Bursa and Ligament, Left

Scaphotrapezium ligament
- *use* Hand Bursa and Ligament, Right
- *use* Hand Bursa and Ligament, Left

Scapulectomy
- *see* Excision, Upper Bones ØPB
- *see* Resection, Upper Bones ØPT

Scapulopexy
- *see* Repair, Upper Bones ØPQ
- *see* Reposition, Upper Bones ØPS

Scarpa's (vestibular) ganglion *use* Acoustic Nerve
Sclerectomy *see* Excision, Eye Ø8B
Sclerotherapy, mechanical *see* Destruction
Sclerotherapy, via injection of sclerosing agent *see* Introduction, Destructive Agent
Sclerotomy *see* Drainage, Eye Ø89
Scrotectomy
- *see* Excision, Male Reproductive System ØVB
- *see* Resection, Male Reproductive System ØVT

Scrotoplasty
- *see* Repair, Male Reproductive System ØVQ
- *see* Supplement, Male Reproductive System ØVU

Scrotorrhaphy *see* Repair, Male Reproductive System ØVQ
Scrototomy *see* Drainage, Male Reproductive System ØV9
Sebaceous gland *use* Skin
Second cranial nerve *use* Optic Nerve
Section, cesarean *see* Extraction, Pregnancy 1ØD
Secura (DR) (VR) *use* Defibrillator Generator in ØJH
▶ **sEEG radiofrequency ablation (RFA)** ØØ5Ø3Z4
Sella turcica *use* Sphenoid Bone
Selux Rapid AST Platform XXE5XY9
Semicircular canal
- *use* Inner Ear, Right
- *use* Inner Ear, Left

Semimembranosus muscle
- *use* Upper Leg Muscle, Right
- *use* Upper Leg Muscle, Left

Semitendinosus muscle
- *use* Upper Leg Muscle, Right
- *use* Upper Leg Muscle, Left

Sentinel™ Cerebral Protection System (CPS) X2A5312
Seprafilm *use* Adhesion Barrier
Septal cartilage *use* Nasal Septum
Septectomy
- *see* Excision, Heart and Great Vessels Ø2B
- *see* Resection, Heart and Great Vessels Ø2T
- *see* Excision, Ear, Nose, Sinus Ø9B
- *see* Resection, Ear, Nose, Sinus Ø9T

SeptiCyte® RAPID XXE5X38
Septoplasty
- *see* Repair, Heart and Great Vessels Ø2Q
- *see* Replacement, Heart and Great Vessels Ø2R
- *see* Supplement, Heart and Great Vessels Ø2U
- *see* Repair, Ear, Nose, Sinus Ø9Q
- *see* Replacement, Ear, Nose, Sinus Ø9R
- *see* Reposition, Ear, Nose, Sinus Ø9S
- *see* Supplement, Ear, Nose, Sinus Ø9U

Septostomy, balloon atrial Ø2163Z7
Septotomy *see* Drainage, Ear, Nose, Sinus Ø99
Sequestrectomy, bone *see* Extirpation
SER-109 XWØDXN9
▶ **Seraph® 1ØØ Microbind® Affinity Blood Filter** XXA536A
Serratus anterior muscle
- *use* Thorax Muscle, Right
- *use* Thorax Muscle, Left

Serratus posterior muscle
- *use* Trunk Muscle, Right
- *use* Trunk Muscle, Left

Seventh cranial nerve *use* Facial Nerve
Sheffield hybrid external fixator
- *use* External Fixation Device, Hybrid in ØPH
- *use* External Fixation Device, Hybrid in ØPS
- *use* External Fixation Device, Hybrid in ØQH
- *use* External Fixation Device, Hybrid in ØQS

Sheffield ring external fixator
- *use* External Fixation Device, Ring in ØPH
- *use* External Fixation Device, Ring in ØPS
- *use* External Fixation Device, Ring in ØQH
- *use* External Fixation Device, Ring in ØQS

Shirodkar cervical cerclage ØUVC7ZZ
Shockwave Intravascular Lithotripsy (Shockwave IVL) *see* Fragmentation
Shock Wave Therapy, Musculoskeletal 6A93
▶ **ShortCut™, used during transcatheter aortic valve replacement (TAVR) procedure** X28F3VA
Short gastric artery *use* Splenic Artery
Shortening
- *see* Excision
- *see* Repair
- *see* Reposition

Shunt creation *see* Bypass
Sialoadenectomy
- Complete *see* Resection, Mouth and Throat ØCT
- Partial *see* Excision, Mouth and Throat ØCB

Sialodochoplasty
- *see* Repair, Mouth and Throat ØCQ
- *see* Replacement, Mouth and Throat ØCR
- *see* Supplement, Mouth and Throat ØCU

Sialoectomy
- *see* Excision, Mouth and Throat ØCB
- *see* Resection, Mouth and Throat ØCT

Sialography *see* Plain Radiography, Ear, Nose, Mouth and Throat B9Ø
Sialolithotomy *see* Extirpation, Mouth and Throat ØCC
Sigmoid artery *use* Inferior Mesenteric Artery
Sigmoid flexure *use* Sigmoid Colon
Sigmoid vein *use* Inferior Mesenteric Vein
Sigmoidectomy
- *see* Excision, Gastrointestinal System ØDB
- *see* Resection, Gastrointestinal System ØDT

Sigmoidorrhaphy *see* Repair, Gastrointestinal System ØDQ
Sigmoidoscopy ØDJD8ZZ
Sigmoidotomy *see* Drainage, Gastrointestinal System ØD9
Single lead pacemaker (atrium) (ventricle) *use* Pacemaker, Single Chamber in ØJH
Single lead rate responsive pacemaker (atrium) (ventricle) *use* Pacemaker, Single Chamber Rate Responsive in ØJH
Single-use duodenoscope XFJ
Single-use oversleeve with intraoperative colonic irrigation XDPH8K7
Sinoatrial node *use* Conduction Mechanism
Sinogram
- Abdominal Wall *see* Fluoroscopy, Abdomen and Pelvis BW11
- Chest Wall *see* Plain Radiography, Chest BWØ3
- Retroperitoneum *see* Fluoroscopy, Abdomen and Pelvis BW11

Sinus venosus *use* Atrium, Right
Sinusectomy
- *see* Excision, Ear, Nose, Sinus Ø9B
- *see* Resection, Ear, Nose, Sinus Ø9T

Sinusoscopy Ø9JY4ZZ
Sinusotomy *see* Drainage, Ear, Nose, Sinus Ø99
Sirolimus-eluting coronary stent *use* Intraluminal Device, Drug-eluting in Heart and Great Vessels

Sixth cranial nerve *use* Abducens Nerve
Size reduction, breast *see* Excision, Skin and Breast ØHB
SJM Biocor® Stented Valve System *use* Zooplastic Tissue in Heart and Great Vessels
Skene's (paraurethral) gland *use* Vestibular Gland
Sling
- Fascial, orbicularis muscle (mouth) *see* Supplement, Muscle, Facial ØKU1
- Levator muscle, for urethral suspension *see* Reposition, Bladder Neck ØTSC
- Pubococcygeal, for urethral suspension *see* Reposition, Bladder Neck ØTSC
- Rectum *see* Reposition, Rectum ØDSP

Small bowel series *see* Fluoroscopy, Bowel, Small BD13
Small saphenous vein
- *use* Saphenous Vein, Right
- *use* Saphenous Vein, Left

Snapshot_NIR 8EØ2XDZ
Snaring, polyp, colon *see* Excision, Gastrointestinal System ØDB
Solar (celiac) plexus *use* Abdominal Sympathetic Nerve
Soleus muscle
- *use* Lower Leg Muscle, Right
- *use* Lower Leg Muscle, Left

Soliris® *use* Eculizumab
Space of Retzius *use* Pelvic Cavity
Spacer
- Insertion of device in
  - Disc
    - Lumbar Vertebral ØSH2
    - Lumbosacral ØSH4
  - Joint
    - Acromioclavicular
      - Left ØRHH
      - Right ØRHG
    - Ankle
      - Left ØSHG
      - Right ØSHF
    - Carpal
      - Left ØRHR
      - Right ØRHQ
    - Carpometacarpal
      - Left ØRHT
      - Right ØRHS
    - Cervical Vertebral ØRH1
    - Cervicothoracic Vertebral ØRH4
    - Coccygeal ØSH6
    - Elbow
      - Left ØRHM
      - Right ØRHL
    - Finger Phalangeal
      - Left ØRHX
      - Right ØRHW
    - Hip
      - Left ØSHB
      - Right ØSH9
    - Knee
      - Left ØSHD
      - Right ØSHC
    - Lumbar Vertebral ØSHØ
    - Lumbosacral ØSH3
    - Metacarpophalangeal
      - Left ØRHV
      - Right ØRHU
    - Metatarsal-Phalangeal
      - Left ØSHN
      - Right ØSHM
    - Occipital-cervical ØRHØ
    - Sacrococcygeal ØSH5
    - Sacroiliac
      - Left ØSH8
      - Right ØSH7
    - Shoulder
      - Left ØRHK
      - Right ØRHJ
    - Sternoclavicular
      - Left ØRHF
      - Right ØRHE

Spacer *(Continued)*
- Insertion of device in *(Continued)*
  - Joint *(Continued)*
    - Tarsal
      - Left ØSHJ
      - Right ØSHH
    - Tarsometatarsal
      - Left ØSHL
      - Right ØSHK
    - Temporomandibular
      - Left ØRHD
      - Right ØRHC
    - Thoracic Vertebral ØRH6
    - Thoracolumbar Vertebral ØRHA
    - Toe Phalangeal
      - Left ØSHQ
      - Right ØSHP
    - Wrist
      - Left ØRHP
      - Right ØRHN
- Removal of device from
  - Acromioclavicular
    - Left ØRPH
    - Right ØRPG
  - Ankle
    - Left ØSPG
    - Right ØSPF
  - Carpal
    - Left ØRPR
    - Right ØRPQ
  - Carpometacarpal
    - Left ØRPT
    - Right ØRPS
  - Cervical Vertebral ØRP1
  - Cervicothoracic Vertebral ØRP4
  - Coccygeal ØSP6
  - Elbow
    - Left ØRPM
    - Right ØRPL
  - Finger Phalangeal
    - Left ØRPX
    - Right ØRPW
  - Hip
    - Left ØSPB
    - Right ØSP9
  - Knee
    - Left ØSPD
    - Right ØSPC
  - Lumbar Vertebral ØSPØ
  - Lumbosacral ØSP3
  - Metacarpophalangeal
    - Left ØRPV
    - Right ØRPU
  - Metatarsal-Phalangeal
    - Left ØSPN
    - Right ØSPM
  - Occipital-cervical ØRPØ
  - Sacrococcygeal ØSP5
  - Sacroiliac
    - Left ØSP8
    - Right ØSP7
  - Shoulder
    - Left ØRPK
    - Right ØRPJ
  - Sternoclavicular
    - Left ØRPF
    - Right ØRPE
  - Tarsal
    - Left ØSPJ
    - Right ØSPH
  - Tarsometatarsal
    - Left ØSPL
    - Right ØSPK
  - Temporomandibular
    - Left ØRPD
    - Right ØRPC
  - Thoracic Vertebral ØRP6
  - Thoracolumbar Vertebral ØRPA
  - Toe Phalangeal
    - Left ØSPQ
    - Right ØSPP

Spacer *(Continued)*
- Removal of device from *(Continued)*
  - Wrist
    - Left ØRPP
    - Right ØRPN
- Revision of device in
  - Acromioclavicular
    - Left ØRWH
    - Right ØRWG
  - Ankle
    - Left ØSWG
    - Right ØSWF
  - Carpal
    - Left ØRWR
    - Right ØRWQ
  - Carpometacarpal
    - Left ØRWT
    - Right ØRWS
  - Cervical Vertebral ØRW1
  - Cervicothoracic Vertebral ØRW4
  - Coccygeal ØSW6
  - Elbow
    - Left ØRWM
    - Right ØRWL
  - Finger Phalangeal
    - Left ØRWX
    - Right ØRWW
  - Hip
    - Left ØSWB
    - Right ØSW9
  - Knee
    - Left ØSWD
    - Right ØSWC
  - Lumbar Vertebral ØSWØ
  - Lumbosacral ØSW3
  - Metacarpophalangeal
    - Left ØRWV
    - Right ØRWU
  - Metatarsal-Phalangeal
    - Left ØSWN
    - Right ØSWM
  - Occipital-cervical ØRWØ
  - Sacrococcygeal ØSW5
  - Sacroiliac
    - Left ØSW8
    - Right ØSW7
  - Shoulder
    - Left ØRWK
    - Right ØRWJ
  - Sternoclavicular
    - Left ØRWF
    - Right ØRWE
  - Tarsal
    - Left ØSWJ
    - Right ØSWH
  - Tarsometatarsal
    - Left ØSWL
    - Right ØSWK
  - Temporomandibular
    - Left ØRWD
    - Right ØRWC
  - Thoracic Vertebral ØRW6
  - Thoracolumbar Vertebral ØRWA
  - Toe Phalangeal
    - Left ØSWQ
    - Right ØSWP
  - Wrist
    - Left ØRWP
    - Right ØRWN

Spacer, Articulating (Antibiotic) *use* Articulating Spacer in Lower Joints
Spacer, Static (Antibiotic) *use* Spacer in Lower Joints
Spectroscopy
- Intravascular Near Infrared 8EØ23DZ
- Near Infrared *see* Physiological Systems and Anatomical Regions 8EØ

Speech Assessment FØØ

Speech therapy *see* Speech Treatment, Rehabilitation F06
Speech Treatment F06
Spesolimab Monoclonal Antibody XW0
▶**SPEVIGO®** *use* Spesolimab Monoclonal Antibody
Sphenoidectomy
- *see* Excision, Ear, Nose, Sinus 09B
- *see* Resection, Ear, Nose, Sinus 09T
- *see* Excision, Head and Facial Bones 0NB
- *see* Resection, Head and Facial Bones 0NT

Sphenoidotomy *see* Drainage, Ear, Nose, Sinus 099
Sphenomandibular ligament *use* Head and Neck Bursa and Ligament
Sphenopalatine (pterygopalatine) ganglion *use* Head and Neck Sympathetic Nerve
Sphincterorrhaphy, anal *see* Repair, Sphincter, Anal 0DQR
Sphincterotomy, anal
- *see* Division, Sphincter, Anal 0D8R
- *see* Drainage, Sphincter, Anal 0D9R

SPIKEVAX™
- *use* COVID-19 Vaccine Dose 1
- *use* COVID-19 Vaccine Dose 2
- *use* COVID-19 Vaccine
- *use* COVID-19 Vaccine Dose 3
- *use* COVID-19 Vaccine Booster

Spinal cord neurostimulator lead *use* Neurostimulator Lead in Central Nervous System and Cranial Nerves
Spinal growth rods, magnetically controlled *use* Magnetically Controlled Growth Rod(s) in New Technology
Spinal nerve, cervical *use* Cervical Nerve
Spinal nerve, lumbar *use* Lumbar Nerve
Spinal nerve, sacral *use* Sacral Nerve
Spinal nerve, thoracic *use* Thoracic Nerve
Spinal Stabilization Device
- Facet Replacement
  - Cervical Vertebral 0RH1
  - Cervicothoracic Vertebral 0RH4
  - Lumbar Vertebral 0SH0
  - Lumbosacral 0SH3
  - Occipital-cervical 0RH0
  - Thoracic Vertebral 0RH6
  - Thoracolumbar Vertebral 0RHA
- Interspinous Process
  - Cervical Vertebral 0RH1
  - Cervicothoracic Vertebral 0RH4
  - Lumbar Vertebral 0SH0
  - Lumbosacral 0SH3
  - Occipital-cervical 0RH0
  - Thoracic Vertebral 0RH6
  - Thoracolumbar Vertebral 0RHA
- Pedicle-Based
  - Cervical Vertebral 0RH1
  - Cervicothoracic Vertebral 0RH4
  - Lumbar Vertebral 0SH0
  - Lumbosacral 0SH3
  - Occipital-cervical 0RH0
  - Thoracic Vertebral 0RH6
  - Thoracolumbar Vertebral 0RHA

SpineJack® system *use* Synthetic Substitute, Mechanically Expandable (Paired) in New Technology
Spinous process
- *use* Cervical Vertebra
- *use* Thoracic Vertebra
- *use* Lumbar Vertebra

Spiral ganglion *use* Acoustic Nerve
Spiration IBV™ Valve System *use* Intraluminal Device, Endobronchial Valve in Respiratory System
Splenectomy
- *see* Excision, Lymphatic and Hemic Systems 07B
- *see* Resection, Lymphatic and Hemic Systems 07T

Splenic flexure *use* Transverse Colon
Splenic plexus *use* Abdominal Sympathetic Nerve
Splenius capitis muscle *use* Head Muscle
Splenius cervicis muscle
- *use* Neck Muscle, Right
- *use* Neck Muscle, Left

Splenolysis *see* Release, Lymphatic and Hemic Systems 07N
Splenopexy
- *see* Repair, Lymphatic and Hemic Systems 07Q
- *see* Reposition, Lymphatic and Hemic Systems 07S

Splenoplasty *see* Repair, Lymphatic and Hemic Systems 07Q
Splenorrhaphy *see* Repair, Lymphatic and Hemic Systems 07Q
Splenotomy *see* Drainage, Lymphatic and Hemic Systems 079
Splinting, musculoskeletal *see* Immobilization, Anatomical Regions 2W3
~~SPRAVATO™ use Esketamine Hydrochloride~~
▶**SPRAVATO™** (Esketamine Hydrochloride) *use* Other Substance
SPY PINPOINT fluorescence imaging system
- *see* Monitoring, Physiological Systems 4A1
- *see* Other Imaging, Hepatobiliary System and Pancreas BF5

SPY system intraoperative fluorescence cholangiography *see* Other Imaging, Hepatobiliary System and Pancreas BF5
SPY system intravascular fluorescence angiography *see* Monitoring, Physiological Systems 4A1
SSO2 (Supersaturated Oxygen) therapy, cardiac intra-arterial 5A0222C
Staged hepatectomy
- *see* Division, Hepatobiliary System and Pancreas 0F8
- *see* Resection, Hepatobiliary System and Pancreas 0FT

Stapedectomy
- *see* Excision, Ear, Nose, Sinus 09B
- *see* Resection, Ear, Nose, Sinus 09T

Stapediolysis *see* Release, Ear, Nose, Sinus 09N
Stapedioplasty
- *see* Repair, Ear, Nose, Sinus 09Q
- *see* Replacement, Ear, Nose, Sinus 09R
- *see* Supplement, Ear, Nose, Sinus 09U

Stapedotomy *see* Drainage, Ear, Nose, Sinus 099
Stapes
- *use* Auditory Ossicle, Right
- *use* Auditory Ossicle, Left

Static Spacer (Antibiotic) *use* Spacer in Lower Joints
STELARA® *use* Other New Technology Therapeutic Substance
Stellate ganglion *use* Head and Neck Sympathetic Nerve
Stem cell transplant *see* Transfusion, Circulatory 302
Stensen's duct
- *use* Parotid Duct, Right
- *use* Parotid Duct, Left

Stent, intraluminal (cardiovascular)(gastrointestinal)(hepatobiliary)(urinary) *use* Intraluminal Device
Stent retriever thrombectomy *see* Extirpation, Upper Arteries 03C
Stented tissue valve *use* Zooplastic Tissue in Heart and Great Vessels
▶**Stereoelectroencephalographic Radiofrequency (sEEG) Ablation** 00503Z4
Stereotactic Radiosurgery
- Abdomen DW23
- Adrenal Gland DG22
- Bile Ducts DF22
- Bladder DT22
- Bone Marrow D720
- Brain D020
- Brain Stem D021
- Breast
  - Left DM20
  - Right DM21
- Bronchus DB21
- Cervix DU21
- Chest DW22
- Chest Wall DB27
- Colon DD25
- Diaphragm DB28
- Duodenum DD22
- Ear D920
- Esophagus DD20
- Eye D820
- Gallbladder DF21
- Gamma Beam
  - Abdomen DW23JZZ
  - Adrenal Gland DG22JZZ
  - Bile Ducts DF22JZZ
  - Bladder DT22JZZ
  - Bone Marrow D720JZZ
  - Brain D020JZZ
  - Brain Stem D021JZZ
  - Breast
    - Left DM20JZZ
    - Right DM21JZZ
  - Bronchus DB21JZZ
  - Cervix DU21JZZ
  - Chest DW22JZZ
  - Chest Wall DB27JZZ
  - Colon DD25JZZ
  - Diaphragm DB28JZZ
  - Duodenum DD22JZZ
  - Ear D920JZZ
  - Esophagus DD20JZZ
  - Eye D820JZZ
  - Gallbladder DF21JZZ
  - Gland
    - Adrenal DG22JZZ
    - Parathyroid DG24JZZ
    - Pituitary DG20JZZ
    - Thyroid DG25JZZ
  - Glands, Salivary D926JZZ
  - Head and Neck DW21JZZ
  - Ileum DD24JZZ
  - Jejunum DD23JZZ
  - Kidney DT20JZZ
  - Larynx D92BJZZ
  - Liver DF20JZZ
  - Lung DB22JZZ
  - Lymphatics
    - Abdomen D726JZZ
    - Axillary D724JZZ
    - Inguinal D728JZZ
    - Neck D723JZZ
    - Pelvis D727JZZ
    - Thorax D725JZZ
  - Mediastinum DB26JZZ
  - Mouth D924JZZ
  - Nasopharynx D92DJZZ
  - Neck and Head DW21JZZ
  - Nerve, Peripheral D027JZZ
  - Nose D921JZZ
  - Ovary DU20JZZ
  - Palate
    - Hard D928JZZ
    - Soft D929JZZ
  - Pancreas DF23JZZ
  - Parathyroid Gland DG24JZZ
  - Pelvic Region DW26JZZ
  - Pharynx D92CJZZ
  - Pineal Body DG21JZZ
  - Pituitary Gland DG20JZZ
  - Pleura DB25JZZ
  - Prostate DV20JZZ
  - Rectum DD27JZZ
  - Sinuses D927JZZ
  - Spinal Cord D026JZZ
  - Spleen D722JZZ
  - Stomach DD21JZZ
  - Testis DV21JZZ

▶ New ➡ Revised ~~deleted~~ Deleted

Stereotactic Radiosurgery *(Continued)*
Gamma Beam *(Continued)*
Thymus D721JZZ
Thyroid Gland DG25JZZ
Tongue D925JZZ
Trachea DB20JZZ
Ureter DT21JZZ
Urethra DT23JZZ
Uterus DU22JZZ
Gland
Adrenal DG22
Parathyroid DG24
Pituitary DG20
Thyroid DG25
Glands, Salivary D926
Head and Neck DW21
Ileum DD24
Jejunum DD23
Kidney DT20
Larynx D92B
Liver DF20
Lung DB22
Lymphatics
Abdomen D726
Axillary D724
Inguinal D728
Neck D723
Pelvis D727
Thorax D725
Mediastinum DB26
Mouth D924
Nasopharynx D92D
Neck and Head DW21
Nerve, Peripheral D027
Nose D921
Other Photon
Abdomen DW23DZZ
Adrenal Gland DG22DZZ
Bile Ducts DF22DZZ
Bladder DT22DZZ
Bone Marrow D720DZZ
Brain D020DZZ
Brain Stem D021DZZ
Breast
Left DM20DZZ
Right DM21DZZ
Bronchus DB21DZZ
Cervix DU21DZZ
Chest DW22DZZ
Chest Wall DB27DZZ
Colon DD25DZZ
Diaphragm DB28DZZ
Duodenum DD22DZZ
Ear D920DZZ
Esophagus DD20DZZ
Eye D820DZZ
Gallbladder DF21DZZ
Gland
Adrenal DG22DZZ
Parathyroid DG24DZZ
Pituitary DG20DZZ
Thyroid DG25DZZ
Glands, Salivary D926DZZ
Head and Neck DW21DZZ
Ileum DD24DZZ
Jejunum DD23DZZ
Kidney DT20DZZ
Larynx D92BDZZ
Liver DF20DZZ
Lung DB22DZZ
Lymphatics
Abdomen D726DZZ
Axillary D724DZZ
Inguinal D728DZZ
Neck D723DZZ
Pelvis D727DZZ
Thorax D725DZZ
Mediastinum DB26DZZ
Mouth D924DZZ
Nasopharynx D92DDZZ

Stereotactic Radiosurgery *(Continued)*
Other Photon *(Continued)*
Neck and Head DW21DZZ
Nerve, Peripheral D027DZZ
Nose D921DZZ
Ovary DU20DZZ
Palate
Hard D928DZZ
Soft D929DZZ
Pancreas DF23DZZ
Parathyroid Gland DG24DZZ
Pelvic Region DW26DZZ
Pharynx D92CDZZ
Pineal Body DG21DZZ
Pituitary Gland DG20DZZ
Pleura DB25DZZ
Prostate DV20DZZ
Rectum DD27DZZ
Sinuses D927DZZ
Spinal Cord D026DZZ
Spleen D722DZZ
Stomach DD21DZZ
Testis DV21DZZ
Thymus D721DZZ
Thyroid Gland DG25DZZ
Tongue D925DZZ
Trachea DB20DZZ
Ureter DT21DZZ
Urethra DT23DZZ
Uterus DU22DZZ
Ovary DU20
Palate
Hard D928
Soft D929
Pancreas DF23
Parathyroid Gland DG24
Particulate
Abdomen DW23HZZ
Adrenal Gland DG22HZZ
Bile Ducts DF22HZZ
Bladder DT22HZZ
Bone Marrow D720HZZ
Brain D020HZZ
Brain Stem D021HZZ
Breast
Left DM20HZZ
Right DM21HZZ
Bronchus DB21HZZ
Cervix DU21HZZ
Chest DW22HZZ
Chest Wall DB27HZZ
Colon DD25HZZ
Diaphragm DB28HZZ
Duodenum DD22HZZ
Ear D920HZZ
Esophagus DD20HZZ
Eye D820HZZ
Gallbladder DF21HZZ
Gland
Adrenal DG22HZZ
Parathyroid DG24HZZ
Pituitary DG20HZZ
Thyroid DG25HZZ
Glands, Salivary D926HZZ
Head and Neck DW21HZZ
Ileum DD24HZZ
Jejunum DD23HZZ
Kidney DT20HZZ
Larynx D92BHZZ
Liver DF20HZZ
Lung DB22HZZ
Lymphatics
Abdomen D726HZZ
Axillary D724HZZ
Inguinal D728HZZ
Neck D723HZZ
Pelvis D727HZZ
Thorax D725HZZ
Mediastinum DB26HZZ
Mouth D924HZZ

Stereotactic Radiosurgery *(Continued)*
Particulate *(Continued)*
Nasopharynx D92DHZZ
Neck and Head DW21HZZ
Nerve, Peripheral D027HZZ
Nose D921HZZ
Ovary DU20HZZ
Palate
Hard D928HZZ
Soft D929HZZ
Pancreas DF23HZZ
Parathyroid Gland DG24HZZ
Pelvic Region DW26HZZ
Pharynx D92CHZZ
Pineal Body DG21HZZ
Pituitary Gland DG20HZZ
Pleura DB25HZZ
Prostate DV20HZZ
Rectum DD27HZZ
Sinuses D927HZZ
Spinal Cord D026HZZ
Spleen D722HZZ
Stomach DD21HZZ
Testis DV21HZZ
Thymus D721HZZ
Thyroid Gland DG25HZZ
Tongue D925HZZ
Trachea DB20HZZ
Ureter DT21HZZ
Urethra DT23HZZ
Uterus DU22HZZ
Pelvic Region DW26
Pharynx D92C
Pineal Body DG21
Pituitary Gland DG20
Pleura DB25
Prostate DV20
Rectum DD27
Sinuses D927
Spinal Cord D026
Spleen D722
Stomach DD21
Testis DV21
Thymus D721
Thyroid Gland DG25
Tongue D925
Trachea DB20
Ureter DT21
Urethra DT23
Uterus DU22
Steripath® Micro™ Blood Collection System XXE5XR7
Sternoclavicular ligament
use Shoulder Bursa and Ligament, Right
use Shoulder Bursa and Ligament, Left
Sternocleidomastoid artery
use Thyroid Artery, Right
use Thyroid Artery, Left
Sternocleidomastoid muscle
use Neck Muscle, Right
use Neck Muscle, Left
Sternocostal ligament *use* Sternum Bursa and Ligament
Sternotomy
see Division, Sternum 0P80
see Drainage, Sternum 0P90
Stimulation, cardiac
Cardioversion 5A2204Z
Electrophysiologic testing *see* Measurement, Cardiac 4A02
Stimulator Generator
Insertion of device in
Abdomen 0JH8
Back 0JH7
Chest 0JH6
Multiple Array
Abdomen 0JH8
Back 0JH7
Chest 0JH6

S

Stimulator Generator *(Continued)*
Multiple Array Rechargeable
Abdomen ØJH8
Back ØJH7
Chest ØJH6
Removal of device from, Subcutaneous Tissue and Fascia, Trunk ØJPT
Revision of device in, Subcutaneous Tissue and Fascia, Trunk ØJWT
Single Array
Abdomen ØJH8
Back ØJH7
Chest ØJH6
Single Array Rechargeable
Abdomen ØJH8
Back ØJH7
Chest ØJH6
Stimulator Lead
Insertion of device in
Anal Sphincter ØDHR
Artery
Left Ø3HL
Right Ø3HK
Bladder ØTHB
Muscle
Lower ØKHY
Upper ØKHX
Stomach ØDH6
Ureter ØTH9
Removal of device from
Anal Sphincter ØDPR
Artery, Upper Ø3PY
Bladder ØTPB
Muscle
Lower ØKPY
Upper ØKPX
Stomach ØDP6
Ureter ØTP9
Revision of device in
Anal Sphincter ØDWR
Artery, Upper Ø3WY
Bladder ØTWB
Muscle
Lower ØKWY
Upper ØKWX
Stomach ØDW6
Ureter ØTW9
Stoma
Excision
Abdominal Wall ØWBFXZ2
Neck ØWB6XZ2
Repair
Abdominal Wall ØWQFXZ2
Neck ØWQ6XZ2
Stomatoplasty
see Repair, Mouth and Throat ØCQ
see Replacement, Mouth and Throat ØCR
see Supplement, Mouth and Throat ØCU
Stomatorrhaphy *see* Repair, Mouth and Throat ØCQ
StrataGraft® *use* Bioengineered Allogeneic Construct
Stratos LV *use* Cardiac Resynchronization Pacemaker Pulse Generator in ØJH
Stress test
4AØ2XM4
4A12XM4
Stripping *see* Extraction
Study
Electrophysiologic stimulation, cardiac *see* Measurement, Cardiac 4AØ2
Ocular motility 4AØ7X7Z
Pulmonary airway flow measurement *see* Measurement, Respiratory 4AØ9
Visual acuity 4AØ7XØZ
Styloglossus muscle *use* Tongue, Palate, Pharynx Muscle
Stylomandibular ligament *use* Head and Neck Bursa and Ligament
Stylopharyngeus muscle *use* Tongue, Palate, Pharynx Muscle
Subacromial bursa
use Shoulder Bursa and Ligament, Right
use Shoulder Bursa and Ligament, Left
Subaortic (common iliac) lymph node *use* Lymphatic, Pelvis
Subarachnoid space, spinal *use* Spinal Canal
Subclavicular (apical) lymph node
use Lymphatic, Right Axillary
use Lymphatic, Left Axillary
Subclavius muscle
use Thorax Muscle, Right
use Thorax Muscle, Left
Subclavius nerve *use* Brachial Plexus Nerve
Subcostal artery *use* Upper Artery
Subcostal muscle
use Thorax Muscle, Right
use Thorax Muscle, Left
Subcostal nerve *use* Thoracic Nerve
Subcutaneous Defibrillator Lead
Insertion of device in, Subcutaneous Tissue and Fascia, Chest ØJH6
Removal of device from, Subcutaneous Tissue and Fascia, Trunk ØJPT
Revision of device in, Subcutaneous Tissue and Fascia, Trunk ØJWT
Subcutaneous injection reservoir, port *use* Vascular Access Device, Totally Implantable in Subcutaneous Tissue and Fascia
Subcutaneous injection reservoir, pump *use* Infusion Device, Pump in Subcutaneous Tissue and Fascia
Subdermal progesterone implant *use* Contraceptive Device in Subcutaneous Tissue and Fascia
Subdural space, spinal *use* Spinal Canal
Submandibular ganglion
use Head and Neck Sympathetic Nerve
use Facial Nerve
Submandibular gland
use Submaxillary Gland, Right
use Submaxillary Gland, Left
Submandibular lymph node *use* Lymphatic, Head
Submandibular space *use* Subcutaneous Tissue and Fascia, Face
Submaxillary ganglion *use* Head and Neck Sympathetic Nerve
Submaxillary lymph node *use* Lymphatic, Head
Submental artery *use* Face Artery
Submental lymph node *use* Lymphatic, Head
Submucous (Meissner's) plexus *use* Abdominal Sympathetic Nerve
Suboccipital nerve *use* Cervical Nerve
Suboccipital venous plexus
use Vertebral Vein, Right
use Vertebral Vein, Left
Subparotid lymph node *use* Lymphatic, Head
Subscapular (posterior) lymph node
use Lymphatic, Right Axillary
use Lymphatic, Left Axillary
Subscapular aponeurosis
use Subcutaneous Tissue and Fascia, Right Upper Arm
use Subcutaneous Tissue and Fascia, Left Upper Arm
Subscapular artery
use Axillary Artery, Right
use Axillary Artery, Left
Subscapularis muscle
use Shoulder Muscle, Right
use Shoulder Muscle, Left
Substance Abuse Treatment
Counseling
Family, for substance abuse, Other Family Counseling HZ63ZZZ
Substance Abuse Treatment *(Continued)*
Counseling *(Continued)*
Group
12-Step HZ43ZZZ
Behavioral HZ41ZZZ
Cognitive HZ4ØZZZ
Cognitive-Behavioral HZ42ZZZ
Confrontational HZ48ZZZ
Continuing Care HZ49ZZZ
Infectious Disease
Post-Test HZ4CZZZ
Pre-Test HZ4CZZZ
Interpersonal HZ44ZZZ
Motivational Enhancement HZ47ZZZ
Psychoeducation HZ46ZZZ
Spiritual HZ4BZZZ
Vocational HZ45ZZZ
Individual
12-Step HZ33ZZZ
Behavioral HZ31ZZZ
Cognitive HZ3ØZZZ
Cognitive-Behavioral HZ32ZZZ
Confrontational HZ38ZZZ
Continuing Care HZ39ZZZ
Infectious Disease
Post-Test HZ3CZZZ
Pre-Test HZ3CZZZ
Interpersonal HZ34ZZZ
Motivational Enhancement HZ37ZZZ
Psychoeducation HZ36ZZZ
Spiritual HZ3BZZZ
Vocational HZ35ZZZ
Detoxification Services, for substance abuse HZ2ZZZZ
Medication Management
Antabuse HZ83ZZZ
Bupropion HZ87ZZZ
Clonidine HZ86ZZZ
Levo-alpha-acetyl-methadol (LAAM) HZ82ZZZ
Methadone Maintenance HZ81ZZZ
Naloxone HZ85ZZZ
Naltrexone HZ84ZZZ
Nicotine Replacement HZ8ØZZZ
Other Replacement Medication HZ89ZZZ
Psychiatric Medication HZ88ZZZ
Pharmacotherapy
Antabuse HZ93ZZZ
Bupropion HZ97ZZZ
Clonidine HZ96ZZZ
Levo-alpha-acetyl-methadol (LAAM) HZ92ZZZ
Methadone Maintenance HZ91ZZZ
Naloxone HZ95ZZZ
Naltrexone HZ94ZZZ
Nicotine Replacement HZ9ØZZZ
Psychiatric Medication HZ98ZZZ
Replacement Medication, Other HZ99ZZZ
Psychotherapy
12-Step HZ53ZZZ
Behavioral HZ51ZZZ
Cognitive HZ5ØZZZ
Cognitive-Behavioral HZ52ZZZ
Confrontational HZ58ZZZ
Interactive HZ55ZZZ
Interpersonal HZ54ZZZ
Motivational Enhancement HZ57ZZZ
Psychoanalysis HZ5BZZZ
Psychodynamic HZ5CZZZ
Psychoeducation HZ56ZZZ
Psychophysiological HZ5DZZZ
Supportive HZ59ZZZ
Substantia nigra *use* Basal Ganglia
Subtalar (talocalcaneal) joint
use Tarsal Joint, Right
use Tarsal Joint, Left
Subtalar ligament
use Foot Bursa and Ligament, Right
use Foot Bursa and Ligament, Left

Subthalamic nucleus *use* Basal Ganglia
Suction curettage (D&C), nonobstetric *see* Extraction, Endometrium ØUDB
Suction curettage, obstetric post-delivery *see* Extraction, Products of Conception, Retained 1ØD1
SUL-DUR *use* Sulbactam-Durlobactam
Sulbactam-Durlobactam XWØ
Superficial circumflex iliac vein
use Saphenous Vein, Right
use Saphenous Vein, Left
Superficial epigastric artery
use Femoral Artery, Right
use Femoral Artery, Left
Superficial epigastric vein
use Saphenous Vein, Right
use Saphenous Vein, Left
Superficial Inferior Epigastric Artery Flap
Replacement
Bilateral ØHRVØ78
Left ØHRUØ78
Right ØHRTØ78
Transfer
Left ØKXG
Right ØKXF
Superficial palmar arch
use Hand Artery, Right
use Hand Artery, Left
Superficial palmar venous arch
use Hand Vein, Right
use Hand Vein, Left
Superficial temporal artery
use Temporal Artery, Right
use Temporal Artery, Left
Superficial transverse perineal muscle *use* Perineum Muscle
Superior cardiac nerve *use* Thoracic Sympathetic Nerve
Superior cerebellar vein *use* Intracranial Vein
Superior cerebral vein *use* Intracranial Vein
Superior clunic (cluneal) nerve *use* Lumbar Nerve
Superior epigastric artery
use Internal Mammary Artery, Right
use Internal Mammary Artery, Left
Superior genicular artery
use Popliteal Artery, Right
use Popliteal Artery, Left
Superior gluteal artery
use Internal Iliac Artery, Right
use Internal Iliac Artery, Left
Superior gluteal nerve *use* Lumbar Plexus Nerve
Superior hypogastric plexus *use* Abdominal Sympathetic Nerve
Superior labial artery *use* Face Artery
Superior laryngeal artery
use Thyroid Artery, Right
use Thyroid Artery, Left
Superior laryngeal nerve *use* Vagus Nerve
Superior longitudinal muscle *use* Tongue, Palate, Pharynx Muscle
Superior mesenteric ganglion *use* Abdominal Sympathetic Nerve
Superior mesenteric lymph node *use* Lymphatic, Mesenteric
Superior mesenteric plexus *use* Abdominal Sympathetic Nerve
Superior oblique muscle
use Extraocular Muscle, Right
use Extraocular Muscle, Left
Superior olivary nucleus *use* Pons
Superior rectal artery *use* Inferior Mesenteric Artery
Superior rectal vein *use* Inferior Mesenteric Vein
Superior rectus muscle
use Extraocular Muscle, Right
use Extraocular Muscle, Left
Superior tarsal plate
use Upper Eyelid, Right
use Upper Eyelid, Left
Superior thoracic artery
use Axillary Artery, Right
use Axillary Artery, Left
Superior thyroid artery
use External Carotid Artery, Right
use External Carotid Artery, Left
use Thyroid Artery, Right
use Thyroid Artery, Left
Superior turbinate *use* Nasal Turbinate
Superior ulnar collateral artery
use Brachial Artery, Right
use Brachial Artery, Left
Superior vesical artery
use Internal Iliac Artery, Right
use Internal Iliac Artery, Left
Supersaturated Oxygen (SSO2) therapy, cardiac intra-arterial 5AØ222C
Supplement
Abdominal Wall ØWUF
Acetabulum
Left ØQU5
Right ØQU4
Ampulla of Vater ØFUC
Anal Sphincter ØDUR
Ankle Region
Left ØYUL
Right ØYUK
Anus ØDUQ
Aorta
Abdominal Ø4UØ
Thoracic
Ascending/Arch Ø2UX
Descending Ø2UW
Arm
Lower
Left ØXUF
Right ØXUD
Upper
Left ØXU9
Right ØXU8
Arteriovenous Fistula, Extraluminal Support Device X2U
Artery
Anterior Tibial
Left Ø4UQ
Right Ø4UP
Axillary
Left Ø3U6
Right Ø3U5
Brachial
Left Ø3U8
Right Ø3U7
Celiac Ø4U1
Colic
Left Ø4U7
Middle Ø4U8
Right Ø4U6
Common Carotid
Left Ø3UJ
Right Ø3UH
Common Iliac
Left Ø4UD
Right Ø4UC
Coronary
Four or More Arteries Ø2U3
One Artery Ø2UØ
Three Arteries Ø2U2
Two Arteries Ø2U1
External Carotid
Left Ø3UN
Right Ø3UM
External Iliac
Left Ø4UJ
Right Ø4UH
Face Ø3UR
Supplement *(Continued)*
Artery *(Continued)*
Femoral
Left Ø4UL
Right Ø4UK
Foot
Left Ø4UW
Right Ø4UV
Gastric Ø4U2
Hand
Left Ø3UF
Right Ø3UD
Hepatic Ø4U3
Inferior Mesenteric Ø4UB
Innominate Ø3U2
Internal Carotid
Left Ø3UL
Right Ø3UK
Internal Iliac
Left Ø4UF
Right Ø4UE
Internal Mammary
Left Ø3U1
Right Ø3UØ
Intracranial Ø3UG
Lower Ø4UY
Peroneal
Left Ø4UU
Right Ø4UT
Popliteal
Left Ø4UN
Right Ø4UM
Posterior Tibial
Left Ø4US
Right Ø4UR
Pulmonary
Left Ø2UR
Right Ø2UQ
Pulmonary Trunk Ø2UP
Radial
Left Ø3UC
Right Ø3UB
Renal
Left Ø4UA
Right Ø4U9
Splenic Ø4U4
Subclavian
Left Ø3U4
Right Ø3U3
Superior Mesenteric Ø4U5
Temporal
Left Ø3UT
Right Ø3US
Thyroid
Left Ø3UV
Right Ø3UU
Ulnar
Left Ø3UA
Right Ø3U9
Upper Ø3UY
Vertebral
Left Ø3UQ
Right Ø3UP
Atrium
Left Ø2U7
Right Ø2U6
Auditory Ossicle
Left Ø9UA
Right Ø9U9
Axilla
Left ØXU5
Right ØXU4
Back
Lower ØWUL
Upper ØWUK
Bladder ØTUB
Bladder Neck ØTUC
Bone
Ethmoid
Left ØNUG
Right ØNUF

S

Supplement *(Continued)*
Bone *(Continued)*
Frontal ØNU1
Hyoid ØNUX
Lacrimal
Left ØNUJ
Right ØNUH
Nasal ØNUB
Occipital ØNU7
Palatine
Left ØNUL
Right ØNUK
Parietal
Left ØNU4
Right ØNU3
Pelvic
Left ØQU3
Right ØQU2
Sphenoid ØNUC
Temporal
Left ØNU6
Right ØNU5
Zygomatic
Left ØNUN
Right ØNUM
Breast
Bilateral ØHUV
Left ØHUU
Right ØHUT
Bronchus
Lingula ØBU9
Lower Lobe
Left ØBUB
Right ØBU6
Main
Left ØBU7
Right ØBU3
Middle Lobe, Right ØBU5
Upper Lobe
Left ØBU8
Right ØBU4
Buccal Mucosa ØCU4
Bursa and Ligament
Abdomen
Left ØMUJ
Right ØMUH
Ankle
Left ØMUR
Right ØMUQ
Elbow
Left ØMU4
Right ØMU3
Foot
Left ØMUT
Right ØMUS
Hand
Left ØMU8
Right ØMU7
Head and Neck ØMUØ
Hip
Left ØMUM
Right ØMUL
Knee
Left ØMUP
Right ØMUN
Lower Extremity
Left ØMUW
Right ØMUV
Perineum ØMUK
Rib(s) ØMUG
Shoulder
Left ØMU2
Right ØMU1
Spine
Lower ØMUD
Posterior Vertebral Tether XKU
Upper ØMUC
Sternum ØMUF
Upper Extremity
Left ØMUB
Right ØMU9

Supplement *(Continued)*
Bursa and Ligament *(Continued)*
Wrist
Left ØMU6
Right ØMU5
Buttock
Left ØYU1
Right ØYUØ
Carina ØBU2
Carpal
Left ØPUN
Right ØPUM
Cecum ØDUH
Cerebral Meninges ØØU1
Cerebral Ventricle ØØU6
Chest Wall ØWU8
Chordae Tendineae Ø2U9
Cisterna Chyli Ø7UL
Clavicle
Left ØPUB
Right ØPU9
Clitoris ØUUJ
Coccyx ØQUS
Colon
Ascending ØDUK
Descending ØDUM
Sigmoid ØDUN
Transverse ØDUL
Cord
Bilateral ØVUH
Left ØVUG
Right ØVUF
Cornea
Left Ø8U9
Right Ø8U8
Coronary Artery/Arteries, Vein Graft
Extraluminal Support Device(s) X2U4Ø79
Cul-de-sac ØUUF
Diaphragm ØBUT
Disc
Cervical Vertebral ØRU3
Cervicothoracic Vertebral ØRU5
Lumbar Vertebral ØSU2
Lumbosacral ØSU4
Thoracic Vertebral ØRU9
Thoracolumbar Vertebral ØRUB
Duct
Common Bile ØFU9
Cystic ØFU8
Hepatic
Common ØFU7
Left ØFU6
Right ØFU5
Lacrimal
Left Ø8UY
Right Ø8UX
Pancreatic ØFUD
Accessory ØFUF
Duodenum ØDU9
Dura Mater ØØU2
Ear
External
Bilateral Ø9U2
Left Ø9U1
Right Ø9UØ
Inner
Left Ø9UE
Right Ø9UD
Middle
Left Ø9U6
Right Ø9U5
Elbow Region
Left ØXUC
Right ØXUB
Epididymis
Bilateral ØVUL
Left ØVUK
Right ØVUJ
Epiglottis ØCUR
Esophagogastric Junction ØDU4

Supplement *(Continued)*
Esophagus ØDU5
Lower ØDU3
Middle ØDU2
Upper ØDU1
Extremity
Lower
Left ØYUB
Right ØYU9
Upper
Left ØXU7
Right ØXU6
Eye
Left Ø8U1
Right Ø8UØ
Eyelid
Lower
Left Ø8UR
Right Ø8UQ
Upper
Left Ø8UP
Right Ø8UN
Face ØWU2
Fallopian Tube
Left ØUU6
Right ØUU5
Fallopian Tubes, Bilateral ØUU7
Femoral Region
Bilateral ØYUE
Left ØYU8
Right ØYU7
Femoral Shaft
Left ØQU9
Right ØQU8
Femur
Lower
Left ØQUC
Right ØQUB
Upper
Left ØQU7
Right ØQU6
Fibula
Left ØQUK
Right ØQUJ
Finger
Index
Left ØXUP
Right ØXUN
Little
Left ØXUW
Right ØXUV
Middle
Left ØXUR
Right ØXUQ
Ring
Left ØXUT
Right ØXUS
Foot
Left ØYUN
Right ØYUM
Gingiva
Lower ØCU6
Upper ØCU5
Glenoid Cavity
Left ØPU8
Right ØPU7
Hand
Left ØXUK
Right ØXUJ
Head ØWUØ
Heart Ø2UA
Humeral Head
Left ØPUD
Right ØPUC
Humeral Shaft
Left ØPUG
Right ØPUF
Hymen ØUUK
Ileocecal Valve ØDUC
Ileum ØDUB

S

Supplement *(Continued)*
- Inguinal Region
  - Bilateral 0YUA
  - Left 0YU6
  - Right 0YU5
- Intestine
  - Large 0DUE
    - Left 0DUG
    - Right 0DUF
  - Small 0DU8
- Iris
  - Left 08UD
  - Right 08UC
- Jaw
  - Lower 0WU5
  - Upper 0WU4
- Jejunum 0DUA
- Joint
  - Acromioclavicular
    - Left 0RUH
    - Right 0RUG
  - Ankle
    - Left 0SUG
    - Right 0SUF
  - Carpal
    - Left 0RUR
    - Right 0RUQ
  - Carpometacarpal
    - Left 0RUT
    - Right 0RUS
  - Cervical Vertebral 0RU1
  - Cervicothoracic Vertebral 0RU4
  - Coccygeal 0SU6
  - Elbow
    - Left 0RUM
    - Right 0RUL
  - Finger Phalangeal
    - Left 0RUX
    - Right 0RUW
  - Hip
    - Left 0SUB
      - Acetabular Surface 0SUE
      - Femoral Surface 0SUS
    - Right 0SU9
      - Acetabular Surface 0SUA
      - Femoral Surface 0SUR
  - Knee
    - Left 0SUD
      - Femoral Surface 0SUU09Z
      - Tibial Surface 0SUW09Z
    - Right 0SUC
      - Femoral Surface 0SUT09Z
      - Tibial Surface 0SUV09Z
  - Lumbar Vertebral 0SU0
  - Lumbosacral 0SU3
  - Metacarpophalangeal
    - Left 0RUV
    - Right 0RUU
  - Metatarsal-Phalangeal
    - Left 0SUN
    - Right 0SUM
  - Occipital-cervical 0RU0
  - Sacrococcygeal 0SU5
  - Sacroiliac
    - Left 0SU8
    - Right 0SU7
  - Shoulder
    - Left 0RUK
    - Right 0RUJ
  - Sternoclavicular
    - Left 0RUF
    - Right 0RUE
  - Tarsal
    - Left 0SUJ
    - Right 0SUH
  - Tarsometatarsal
    - Left 0SUL
    - Right 0SUK
  - Temporomandibular
    - Left 0RUD
    - Right 0RUC

Supplement *(Continued)*
- Joint *(Continued)*
  - Thoracic Vertebral 0RU6
  - Thoracolumbar Vertebral 0RUA
  - Toe Phalangeal
    - Left 0SUQ
    - Right 0SUP
  - Wrist
    - Left 0RUP
    - Right 0RUN
- Kidney Pelvis
  - Left 0TU4
  - Right 0TU3
- Knee Region
  - Left 0YUG
  - Right 0YUF
- Larynx 0CUS
- Leg
  - Lower
    - Left 0YUJ
    - Right 0YUH
  - Upper
    - Left 0YUD
    - Right 0YUC
- Lip
  - Lower 0CU1
  - Upper 0CU0
- Lymphatic
  - Aortic 07UD
  - Axillary
    - Left 07U6
    - Right 07U5
  - Head 07U0
  - Inguinal
    - Left 07UJ
    - Right 07UH
  - Internal Mammary
    - Left 07U9
    - Right 07U8
  - Lower Extremity
    - Left 07UG
    - Right 07UF
  - Mesenteric 07UB
  - Neck
    - Left 07U2
    - Right 07U1
  - Pelvis 07UC
  - Thoracic Duct 07UK
  - Thorax 07U7
  - Upper Extremity
    - Left 07U4
    - Right 07U3
- Mandible
  - Left 0NUV
  - Right 0NUT
- Maxilla 0NUR
- Mediastinum 0WUC
- Mesentery 0DUV
- Metacarpal
  - Left 0PUQ
  - Right 0PUP
- Metatarsal
  - Left 0QUP
  - Right 0QUN
- Muscle
  - Abdomen
    - Left 0KUL
    - Right 0KUK
  - Extraocular
    - Left 08UM
    - Right 08UL
  - Facial 0KU1
  - Foot
    - Left 0KUW
    - Right 0KUV
  - Hand
    - Left 0KUD
    - Right 0KUC
  - Head 0KU0

Supplement *(Continued)*
- Muscle *(Continued)*
  - Hip
    - Left 0KUP
    - Right 0KUN
  - Lower Arm and Wrist
    - Left 0KUB
    - Right 0KU9
  - Lower Leg
    - Left 0KUT
    - Right 0KUS
  - Neck
    - Left 0KU3
    - Right 0KU2
  - Papillary 02UD
  - Perineum 0KUM
  - Shoulder
    - Left 0KU6
    - Right 0KU5
  - Thorax
    - Left 0KUJ
    - Right 0KUH
  - Tongue, Palate, Pharynx 0KU4
  - Trunk
    - Left 0KUG
    - Right 0KUF
  - Upper Arm
    - Left 0KU8
    - Right 0KU7
  - Upper Leg
    - Left 0KUR
    - Right 0KUQ
- Nasal Mucosa and Soft Tissue 09UK
- Nasopharynx 09UN
- Neck 0WU6
- Nerve
  - Abducens 00UL
  - Accessory 00UR
  - Acoustic 00UN
  - Cervical 01U1
  - Facial 00UM
  - Femoral 01UD
  - Glossopharyngeal 00UP
  - Hypoglossal 00US
  - Lumbar 01UB
  - Median 01U5
  - Oculomotor 00UH
  - Olfactory 00UF
  - Optic 00UG
  - Peroneal 01UH
  - Phrenic 01U2
  - Pudendal 01UC
  - Radial 01U6
  - Sacral 01UR
  - Sciatic 01UF
  - Thoracic 01U8
  - Tibial 01UG
  - Trigeminal 00UK
  - Trochlear 00UJ
  - Ulnar 01U4
  - Vagus 00UQ
- Nipple
  - Left 0HUX
  - Right 0HUW
- Omentum 0DUU
- Orbit
  - Left 0NUQ
  - Right 0NUP
- Palate
  - Hard 0CU2
  - Soft 0CU3
- Patella
  - Left 0QUF
  - Right 0QUD
- Penis 0VUS
- Pericardium 02UN
- Perineum
  - Female 0WUN
  - Male 0WUM
- Peritoneum 0DUW

Supplement (Continued)
Phalanx
Finger
Left ØPUV
Right ØPUT
Thumb
Left ØPUS
Right ØPUR
Toe
Left ØQUR
Right ØQUQ
Pharynx ØCUM
Prepuce ØVUT
Radius
Left ØPUJ
Right ØPUH
Rectum ØDUP
Retina
Left Ø8UF
Right Ø8UE
Retinal Vessel
Left Ø8UH
Right Ø8UG
Ribs
1 to 2 ØPU1
3 or More ØPU2
Sacrum ØQU1
Scapula
Left ØPU6
Right ØPU5
Scrotum ØVU5
Septum
Atrial Ø2U5
Nasal Ø9UM
Ventricular Ø2UM
Shoulder Region
Left ØXU3
Right ØXU2
Sinus
Accessory Ø9UP
Ethmoid
Left Ø9UV
Right Ø9UU
Frontal
Left Ø9UT
Right Ø9US
Mastoid
Left Ø9UC
Right Ø9UB
Maxillary
Left Ø9UR
Right Ø9UQ
Sphenoid
Left Ø9UX
Right Ø9UW
Skull ØNUØ
Spinal Meninges ØØUT
Sternum ØPUØ
Stomach ØDU6
Pylorus ØDU7
Subcutaneous Tissue and Fascia
Abdomen ØJU8
Back ØJU7
Buttock ØJU9
Chest ØJU6
Face ØJU1
Foot
Left ØJUR
Right ØJUQ
Hand
Left ØJUK
Right ØJUJ
Lower Arm
Left ØJUH
Right ØJUG
Lower Leg
Left ØJUP
Right ØJUN
Neck
Left ØJU5
Right ØJU4

Supplement (Continued)
Subcutaneous Tissue and Fascia (Continued)
Pelvic Region ØJUC
Perineum ØJUB
Scalp ØJUØ
Upper Arm
Left ØJUF
Right ØJUD
Upper Leg
Left ØJUM
Right ØJUL
Tarsal
Left ØQUM
Right ØQUL
Tendon
Abdomen
Left ØLUG
Right ØLUF
Ankle
Left ØLUT
Right ØLUS
Foot
Left ØLUW
Right ØLUV
Hand
Left ØLU8
Right ØLU7
Head and Neck ØLUØ
Hip
Left ØLUK
Right ØLUJ
Knee
Left ØLUR
Right ØLUQ
Lower Arm and Wrist
Left ØLU6
Right ØLU5
Lower Leg
Left ØLUP
Right ØLUN
Perineum ØLUH
Shoulder
Left ØLU2
Right ØLU1
Thorax
Left ØLUD
Right ØLUC
Trunk
Left ØLUB
Right ØLU9
Upper Arm
Left ØLU4
Right ØLU3
Upper Leg
Left ØLUM
Right ØLUL
Testis
Bilateral ØVUCØ
Left ØVUBØ
Right ØVU9Ø
Thumb
Left ØXUM
Right ØXUL
Tibia
Left ØQUH
Right ØQUG
Toe
1st
Left ØYUQ
Right ØYUP
2nd
Left ØYUS
Right ØYUR
3rd
Left ØYUU
Right ØYUT

Supplement (Continued)
Toe (Continued)
4th
Left ØYUW
Right ØYUV
5th
Left ØYUY
Right ØYUX
Tongue ØCU7
Trachea ØBU1
Tunica Vaginalis
Left ØVU7
Right ØVU6
Turbinate, Nasal Ø9UL
Tympanic Membrane
Left Ø9U8
Right Ø9U7
Ulna
Left ØPUL
Right ØPUK
Ureter
Left ØTU7
Right ØTU6
Urethra ØTUD
Uterine Supporting Structure ØUU4
Uvula ØCUN
Vagina ØUUG
Valve
Aortic Ø2UF
Mitral Ø2UG
Pulmonary Ø2UH
Tricuspid Ø2UJ
Vas Deferens
Bilateral ØVUQ
Left ØVUP
Right ØVUN
Vein
Axillary
Left Ø5U8
Right Ø5U7
Azygos Ø5UØ
Basilic
Left Ø5UC
Right Ø5UB
Brachial
Left Ø5UA
Right Ø5U9
Cephalic
Left Ø5UF
Right Ø5UD
Colic Ø6U7
Common Iliac
Left Ø6UD
Right Ø6UC
Esophageal Ø6U3
External Iliac
Left Ø6UG
Right Ø6UF
External Jugular
Left Ø5UQ
Right Ø5UP
Face
Left Ø5UV
Right Ø5UT
Femoral
Left Ø6UN
Right Ø6UM
Foot
Left Ø6UV
Right Ø6UT
Gastric Ø6U2
Hand
Left Ø5UH
Right Ø5UG
Hemiazygos Ø5U1
Hepatic Ø6U4
Hypogastric
Left Ø6UJ
Right Ø6UH

Supplement *(Continued)*
Vein *(Continued)*
Inferior Mesenteric Ø6U6
Innominate
Left Ø5U4
Right Ø5U3
Internal Jugular
Left Ø5UN
Right Ø5UM
Intracranial Ø5UL
Lower Ø6UY
Portal Ø6U8
Pulmonary
Left Ø2UT
Right Ø2US
Renal
Left Ø6UB
Right Ø6U9
Saphenous
Left Ø6UQ
Right Ø6UP
Splenic Ø6U1
Subclavian
Left Ø5U6
Right Ø5U5
Superior Mesenteric Ø6U5
Upper Ø5UY
Vertebral
Left Ø5US
Right Ø5UR
Vena Cava
Inferior Ø6UØ
Superior Ø2UV
Ventricle
Left Ø2UL
Right Ø2UK
Vertebra
Cervical ØPU3
Lumbar ØQUØ
Mechanically Expandable (Paired) Synthetic Substitute XNUØ356
Thoracic ØPU4
Mechanically Expandable (Paired) Synthetic Substitute XNUØ356
Vesicle
Bilateral ØVU3
Left ØVU2
Right ØVU1
Vocal Cord
Left ØCUV
Right ØCUT
Vulva ØUUM
Wrist Region
Left ØXUH
Right ØXUG
Supraclavicular (Virchow's) lymph node
use Lymphatic, Right Neck
use Lymphatic, Left Neck
Supraclavicular nerve *use* Cervical Plexus
Suprahyoid lymph node *use* Lymphatic, Head
Suprahyoid muscle
use Neck Muscle, Right
use Neck Muscle, Left
Suprainguinal lymph node *use* Lymphatic, Pelvis
Supraorbital vein
use Face Vein, Right
use Face Vein, Left
Suprarenal gland
use Adrenal Gland, Left
use Adrenal Gland, Right
use Adrenal Gland, Bilateral
use Adrenal Gland
Suprarenal plexus *use* Abdominal Sympathetic Nerve
Suprascapular nerve *use* Brachial Plexus Nerve
Supraspinatus fascia
use Subcutaneous Tissue and Fascia, Right Upper Arm
use Subcutaneous Tissue and Fascia, Left Upper Arm
Supraspinatus muscle
use Shoulder Muscle, Right
use Shoulder Muscle, Left
Supraspinous ligament
use Upper Spine Bursa and Ligament
use Lower Spine Bursa and Ligament
Suprasternal notch *use* Sternum
Supratrochlear lymph node
use Lymphatic, Right Upper Extremity
use Lymphatic, Left Upper Extremity
Sural artery
use Popliteal Artery, Right
use Popliteal Artery, Left
Surpass Streamline™ Flow Diverter *use* Intraluminal Device, Flow Diverter in Ø3V
Suspension
Bladder Neck *see* Reposition, Bladder Neck ØTSC
Kidney *see* Reposition, Urinary System ØTS
Urethra *see* Reposition, Urinary System ØTS
Urethrovesical *see* Reposition, Bladder Neck ØTSC
Uterus *see* Reposition, Uterus ØUS9
Vagina *see* Reposition, Vagina ØUSG
~~Sustained Release Drug-eluting Intraluminal Device~~
~~Dilation~~
~~Anterior Tibial~~
~~Left X27Q385~~
~~Right X27P385~~
~~Femoral~~
~~Left X27J385~~
~~Right X27H385~~
~~Peroneal~~
~~Left X27U385~~
~~Right X27T385~~
~~Popliteal~~
~~Left Distal X27N385~~
~~Left Proximal X27L385~~
~~Right Distal X27M385~~
~~Right Proximal X27K385~~
~~Posterior Tibial~~
~~Left X27S385~~
~~Right X27R385~~
~~Four or More~~
~~Anterior Tibial~~
~~Left X27Q3C5~~
~~Right X27P3C5~~
~~Femoral~~
~~Left X27J3C5~~
~~Right X27H3C5~~
~~Peroneal~~
~~Left X27U3C5~~
~~Right X27T3C5~~
~~Popliteal~~
~~Left Distal X27N3C5~~
~~Left Proximal X27L3C5~~
~~Right Distal X27M3C5~~
~~Right Proximal X27K3C5~~
~~Posterior Tibial~~
~~Left X27S3C5~~
~~Right X27R3C5~~
~~Three~~
~~Anterior Tibial~~
~~Left X27Q3B5~~
~~Right X27P3B5~~
~~Femoral~~
~~Left X27J3B5~~
~~Right X27H3B5~~
~~Peroneal~~
~~Left X27U3B5~~
~~Right X27T3B5~~
~~Popliteal~~
~~Left Distal X27N3B5~~
~~Left Proximal X27L3B5~~
~~Right Distal X27M3B5~~
~~Right Proximal X27K3B5~~
~~Posterior Tibial~~
~~Left X27S3B5~~
~~Right X27R3B5~~
~~Two~~
~~Anterior Tibial~~
~~Left X27Q395~~
~~Right X27P395~~
~~Femoral~~
~~Left X27J395~~
~~Right X27H395~~
~~Peroneal~~
~~Left X27U395~~
~~Right X27T395~~
~~Popliteal~~
~~Left Distal X27N395~~
~~Left Proximal X27L395~~
~~Right Distal X27M395~~
~~Right Proximal X27K395~~
~~Posterior Tibial~~
~~Left X27S395~~
~~Right X27R395~~
Suture
Laceration repair *see* Repair
Ligation *see* Occlusion
Suture Removal
Extremity
Lower 8EØYXY8
Upper 8EØXXY8
Head and Neck Region 8EØ9XY8
Trunk Region 8EØWXY8
Sutureless valve, Perceval (rapid deployment technique) *see* Replacement, Valve, Aortic Ø2RF
Sweat gland *use* Skin
Sympathectomy
see Excision, Peripheral Nervous System Ø1B
▶ **Symplicity Spyral™ Renal Denervation System** XØ5133A
SynCardia Total Artificial Heart *use* Synthetic Substitute
SynCardia (temporary) total artificial heart (TAH) *use* Synthetic Substitute, Pneumatic in Ø2R
~~Synchra CRT-P use Cardiac Resynchronization Pacemaker Pulse Generator in ØJH~~
SynchroMed pump *use* Infusion Device, Pump in Subcutaneous Tissue and Fascia
▶ **Syncra CRT-P** *use* Cardiac Resynchronization Pacemaker Pulse Generator in ØJH
Synechiotomy, iris *see* Release, Eye Ø8N
Synovectomy
Lower joint *see* Excision, Lower Joints ØSB
Upper joint *see* Excision, Upper Joints ØRB
Systemic Nuclear Medicine Therapy
Abdomen CW7Ø
Anatomical Regions, Multiple CW7YYZZ
Chest CW73
Thyroid CW7G
Whole Body CW7N

S

T

tab-cel® *use* Tabelecleucel Immunotherapy
Tabelecleucel Immunotherapy XWØ
Tagraxofusp-erzs Antineoplastic XWØ
Takedown
Arteriovenous shunt *see* Removal of device from, Upper Arteries Ø3P
Arteriovenous shunt, with creation of new shunt *see* Bypass, Upper Arteries Ø31
Stoma
see Excision
see Reposition
Talent® Converter *use* Intraluminal Device
Talent® Occluder *use* Intraluminal Device
Talent® Stent Graft (abdominal) (thoracic) *use* Intraluminal Device
Talocalcaneal (subtalar) joint
use Tarsal Joint, Right
use Tarsal Joint, Left
Talocalcaneal ligament
use Foot Bursa and Ligament, Right
use Foot Bursa and Ligament, Left
Talocalcaneonavicular joint
use Tarsal Joint, Right
use Tarsal Joint, Left
Talocalcaneonavicular ligament
use Foot Bursa and Ligament, Right
use Foot Bursa and Ligament, Left
Talocrural joint
use Ankle Joint, Right
use Ankle Joint, Left
Talofibular ligament
use Ankle Bursa and Ligament, Right
use Ankle Bursa and Ligament, Left
▶**Talquetamab Antineoplastic XWØ1329]**
Talus bone
use Tarsal, Right
use Tarsal, Left
▶**TALVEY™** *use* Talquetamab Antineoplastic
▶**TAMBE Device** (Thoracoabdominal Branch Endoprosthesis), GORE® EXCLUDER® *use* Branched Intraluminal Device, Manufactured Integrated System, Four or More Arteries in New Technology
TandemHeart® System *use* Short-term External Heart Assist System in Heart and Great Vessels
Tarsectomy
see Excision, Lower Bones ØQB
see Resection, Lower Bones ØQT
Tarsometatarsal ligament
use Foot Bursa and Ligament, Right
use Foot Bursa and Ligament, Left
Tarsorrhaphy *see* Repair, Eye Ø8Q
Tattooing
Cornea 3EØCXMZ
Skin *see* Introduction of substance in or on Skin 3EØØ
Taurolidine Anti-infective and Heparin Anticoagulant XYØYX28
TAXUS® Liberté® Paclitaxel-eluting Coronary Stent System *use* Intraluminal Device, Drug-eluting in Heart and Great Vessels
TBNA (transbronchial needle aspiration)
Fluid or gas *see* Drainage, Respiratory System ØB9
Tissue biopsy *see* Extraction, Respiratory System ØBD
▶**T-cell Antigen Coupler T-cell (TAC-T) Therapy** *use* Non-Chimeric Antigen Receptor T-cell Immune Effector Cell Therapy
▶**T-cell Receptor-Engineered T-cell (TCR-T) Therapy** *use* Non-Chimeric Antigen Receptor T-cell Immune Effector Cell Therapy
Tecartus™ *use* Brexucabtagene Autoleucel Immunotherapy
TECENTRIQ® *use* Atezolizumab Antineoplastic
Teclistamab Antineoplastic XWØ1348
▶**TECVAYLI™** *use* Teclistamab Antineoplastic
Telemetry
4A12X4Z
Ambulatory 4A12X45
▶**Temperature-controlled sEEG radiofrequency ablation** ØØ5Ø3Z4
Temperature gradient study 4AØZXKZ
Temporal lobe *use* Cerebral Hemisphere
Temporalis muscle *use* Head Muscle
Temporoparietalis muscle *use* Head Muscle
Tendolysis *see* Release, Tendons ØLN
Tendonectomy
see Excision, Tendons ØLB
see Resection, Tendons ØLT
Tendonoplasty, tenoplasty
see Repair, Tendons ØLQ
see Replacement, Tendons ØLR
see Supplement, Tendons ØLU
Tendorrhaphy *see* Repair, Tendons ØLQ
Tendototomy
see Division, Tendons ØL8
see Drainage, Tendons ØL9
Tenectomy, tenonectomy
see Excision, Tendons ØLB
see Resection, Tendons ØLT
Tenolysis *see* Release, Tendons ØLN
Tenontorrhaphy *see* Repair, Tendons ØLQ
Tenontotomy
see Division, Tendons ØL8
see Drainage, Tendons ØL9
Tenorrhaphy *see* Repair, Tendons ØLQ
Tenosynovectomy
see Excision, Tendons ØLB
see Resection, Tendons ØLT
Tenotomy
see Division, Tendons ØL8
see Drainage, Tendons ØL9
Tensor fasciae latae muscle
use Hip Muscle, Right
use Hip Muscle, Left
Tensor veli palatini muscle *use* Tongue, Palate, Pharynx Muscle
Tenth cranial nerve *use* Vagus Nerve
Tentorium cerebelli *use* Dura Mater
Teres major muscle
use Shoulder Muscle, Right
use Shoulder Muscle, Left
Teres minor muscle
use Shoulder Muscle, Right
use Shoulder Muscle, Left
Terlipressin XWØ
TERLIVAZ® *use* Terlipressin
Termination of pregnancy
Aspiration curettage 1ØAØ7ZZ
Dilation and curettage 1ØAØ7ZZ
Hysterotomy 1ØAØØZZ
Intra-amniotic injection 1ØAØ3ZZ
Laminaria 1ØAØ7ZW
Vacuum 1ØAØ7Z6
Testectomy
see Excision, Male Reproductive System ØVB
see Resection, Male Reproductive System ØVT
Testicular artery *use* Abdominal Aorta
Testing
Glaucoma 4AØ7XBZ
Hearing *see* Hearing Assessment, Diagnostic Audiology F13
Mental health *see* Psychological Tests
Muscle function, electromyography (EMG) *see* Measurement, Musculoskeletal 4AØF
Muscle function, manual *see* Motor Function Assessment, Rehabilitation FØ1
Neurophysiologic monitoring, intra-operative *see* Monitoring, Physiological Systems 4A1
Testing *(Continued)*
Range of motion *see* Motor Function Assessment, Rehabilitation FØ1
Vestibular function *see* Vestibular Assessment, Diagnostic Audiology F15
Thalamectomy *see* Excision, Thalamus ØØB9
Thalamotomy
see Drainage, Thalamus ØØ99
Thenar muscle
use Hand Muscle, Right
use Hand Muscle, Left
Therapeutic Massage
Musculoskeletal System 8EØKX1Z
Reproductive System
Prostate 8EØVX1C
Rectum 8EØVX1D
Therapeutic occlusion coil(s) *use* Intraluminal Device
Thermography 4AØZXKZ
Thermotherapy, prostate *see* Destruction, Prostate ØV5Ø
Third cranial nerve *use* Oculomotor Nerve
Third occipital nerve *use* Cervical Nerve
Third ventricle *use* Cerebral Ventricle
Thoracectomy *see* Excision, Anatomical Regions, General ØWB
Thoracentesis *see* Drainage, Anatomical Regions, General ØW9
Thoracic aortic plexus *use* Thoracic Sympathetic Nerve
Thoracic esophagus *use* Esophagus, Middle
Thoracic facet joint *use* Thoracic Vertebral Joint
Thoracic ganglion *use* Thoracic Sympathetic Nerve
Thoracoacromial artery
use Axillary Artery, Right
use Axillary Artery, Left
Thoracocentesis *see* Drainage, Anatomical Regions, General ØW9
Thoracolumbar facet joint *use* Thoracolumbar Vertebral Joint
Thoracoplasty
see Repair, Anatomical Regions, General ØWQ
see Supplement, Anatomical Regions, General ØWU
Thoracostomy tube *use* Drainage Device
Thoracostomy, for lung collapse *see* Drainage, Respiratory System ØB9
➠**Thoracotomy** ~~see Drainage, Anatomical Regions, General ØW9~~
▶*see* Control bleeding in, Mediastinum ØW3C
▶*see* Control bleeding in, Pericardial Cavity ØW3D
▶*see* Drainage, Anatomical Regions, General ØW9
▶Exploratory *see* Inspection, Anatomical Regions, General ØWJ
Thoraflex™ hybrid device *use* Branched Synthetic Substitute with Intraluminal Device in New Technology
Thoratec IVAD (Implantable Ventricular Assist Device) *use* Implantable Heart Assist System in Heart and Great Vessels
Thoratec Paracorporeal Ventricular Assist Device *use* Short-term External Heart Assist System in Heart and Great Vessels
Thrombectomy *see* Extirpation
~~Thrombolysis, Ultrasound assisted see Fragmentation, Artery~~
▶**Thrombolysis**
▶Catheter-directed *see* Fragmentation
▶Systemic *see* Introduction of substance in or on, Physiological Systems and Anatomical Regions 3EØ
▶Ultrasound assisted
▶*see* Fragmentation, Artery
▶*see* Fragmentation, Vein

▶ New ➠ Revised ~~deleted~~ Deleted

Thymectomy
see Excision, Lymphatic and Hemic Systems Ø7B
see Resection, Lymphatic and Hemic Systems Ø7T
Thymopexy
see Repair, Lymphatic and Hemic Systems Ø7Q
see Reposition, Lymphatic and Hemic Systems Ø7S
Thymus gland *use* Thymus
Thyroarytenoid muscle
use Neck Muscle, Right
use Neck Muscle, Left
Thyrocervical trunk
use Thyroid Artery, Right
use Thyroid Artery, Left
Thyroid cartilage *use* Larynx
Thyroidectomy
see Excision, Endocrine System ØGB
see Resection, Endocrine System ØGT
Thyroidorrhaphy *see* Repair, Endocrine System ØGQ
Thyroidoscopy ØGJK4ZZ
Thyroidotomy *see* Drainage, Endocrine System ØG9
Tibial Extension with Motion Sensors, Insertion XNH
Tibial insert *use* Liner in Lower Joints
Tibial sesamoid
use Metatarsal, Right
use Metatarsal, Left
Tibialis anterior muscle
use Lower Leg Muscle, Right
use Lower Leg Muscle, Left
Tibialis posterior muscle
use Lower Leg Muscle, Right
use Lower Leg Muscle, Left
Tibiofemoral joint
use Knee Joint, Right
use Knee Joint, Left
use Knee Joint, Tibial Surface, Right
use Knee Joint, Tibial Surface, Left
Tibioperoneal trunk
use Popliteal Artery, Right
use Popliteal Artery, Left
Tisagenlecleucel *use* Tisagenlecleucel Immunotherapy
Tisagenlecleucel immunotherapy XWØ
Tissue bank graft *use* Nonautologous Tissue Substitute
Tissue Expander
Insertion of device in
Breast
Bilateral ØHHV
Left ØHHU
Right ØHHT
Nipple
Left ØHHX
Right ØHHW
Subcutaneous Tissue and Fascia
Abdomen ØJH8
Back ØJH7
Buttock ØJH9
Chest ØJH6
Face ØJH1
Foot
Left ØJHR
Right ØJHQ
Hand
Left ØJHK
Right ØJHJ
Lower Arm
Left ØJHH
Right ØJHG
Lower Leg
Left ØJHP
Right ØJHN
Tissue Expander *(Continued)*
Insertion of device in *(Continued)*
Subcutaneous Tissue and Fascia *(Continued)*
Neck
Left ØJH5
Right ØJH4
Pelvic Region ØJHC
Perineum ØJHB
Scalp ØJHØ
Upper Arm
Left ØJHF
Right ØJHD
Upper Leg
Left ØJHM
Right ØJHL
Removal of device from
Breast
Left ØHPU
Right ØHPT
Subcutaneous Tissue and Fascia
Head and Neck ØJPS
Lower Extremity ØJPW
Trunk ØJPT
Upper Extremity ØJPV
Revision of device in
Breast
Left ØHWU
Right ØHWT
Subcutaneous Tissue and Fascia
Head and Neck ØJWS
Lower Extremity ØJWW
Trunk ØJWT
Upper Extremity ØJWV
Tissue expander (inflatable) (injectable)
use Tissue Expander in Skin and Breast
use Tissue Expander in Subcutaneous Tissue and Fascia
Tissue Plasminogen Activator (tPA)(r-tPA) *use* Thrombolytic, Other
Titan Endoskeleton™
use Interbody Fusion Device in Upper Joints
use Interbody Fusion Device in Lower Joints
Titanium Sternal Fixation System (TSFS)
use Internal Fixation Device, Rigid Plate in ØPS
use Internal Fixation Device, Rigid Plate in ØPH
Tocilizumab XWØ
Tomographic (Tomo) Nuclear Medicine Imaging
Abdomen CW2Ø
Abdomen and Chest CW24
Abdomen and Pelvis CW21
Anatomical Regions, Multiple CW2YYZZ
Bladder, Kidneys and Ureters CT23
Brain CØ2Ø
Breast CH2YYZZ
Bilateral CH22
Left CH21
Right CH2Ø
Bronchi and Lungs CB22
Central Nervous System CØ2YYZZ
Cerebrospinal Fluid CØ25
Chest CW23
Chest and Abdomen CW24
Chest and Neck CW26
Digestive System CD2YYZZ
Endocrine System CG2YYZZ
Extremity
Lower CW2D
Bilateral CP2F
Left CP2D
Right CP2C
Upper CW2M
Bilateral CP2B
Left CP29
Right CP28
Gallbladder CF24
Gastrointestinal Tract CD27
Gland, Parathyroid CG21
Tomographic (Tomo) Nuclear Medicine Imaging *(Continued)*
Head and Neck CW2B
Heart C22YYZZ
Right and Left C226
Hepatobiliary System and Pancreas CF2YYZZ
Kidneys, Ureters and Bladder CT23
Liver CF25
Liver and Spleen CF26
Lungs and Bronchi CB22
Lymphatics and Hematologic System C72YYZZ
Musculoskeletal System, Other CP2YYZZ
Myocardium C22G
Neck and Chest CW26
Neck and Head CW2B
Pancreas and Hepatobiliary System CF2YYZZ
Pelvic Region CW2J
Pelvis CP26
Pelvis and Abdomen CW21
Pelvis and Spine CP27
Respiratory System CB2YYZZ
Skin CH2YYZZ
Skull CP21
Skull and Cervical Spine CP23
Spine
Cervical CP22
Cervical and Skull CP23
Lumbar CP2H
Thoracic CP2G
Thoracolumbar CP2J
Spine and Pelvis CP27
Spleen C722
Spleen and Liver CF26
Subcutaneous Tissue CH2YYZZ
Thorax CP24
Ureters, Kidneys and Bladder CT23
Urinary System CT2YYZZ
Tomography, computerized *see* Computerized Tomography (CT Scan)
Tongue, base of *use* Pharynx
Tonometry 4AØ7XBZ
Tonsillectomy
see Excision, Mouth and Throat ØCB
see Resection, Mouth and Throat ØCT
Tonsillotomy *see* Drainage, Mouth and Throat ØC9
TOPS™ System *use* Posterior Spinal Motion Preservation Device in New Technology
Total Ankle Talar Replacement™ (TATR) *use* Synthetic Substitute, Talar Prosthesis in New Technology
Total Anomalous Pulmonary Venous Return (TAPVR) repair
see Bypass, Atrium, Left Ø217
see Bypass, Vena Cava, Superior Ø21V
Total artificial (replacement) heart *use* Synthetic Substitute
Total parenteral nutrition (TPN) *see* Introduction of Nutritional Substance
Tourniquet, external *see* Compression, Anatomical Regions 2W1
Trachectomy
see Excision, Trachea ØBB1
see Resection, Trachea ØBT1
Trachelectomy
see Excision, Cervix ØUBC
see Resection, Cervix ØUTC
Trachelopexy
see Repair, Cervix ØUQC
see Reposition, Cervix ØUSC
Tracheloplasty
see Repair, Cervix ØUQC
Trachelorrhaphy *see* Repair, Cervix ØUQC
Trachelotomy *see* Drainage, Cervix ØU9C
Tracheobronchial lymph node *see* Lymphatic, Thorax
Tracheoesophageal fistulization ØB11ØD6
▶**Tracheoesophageal Puncture (TEP)** ØB11ØD6

▶ New ▶ Revised ~~deleted~~ Deleted

Tracheolysis *see* Release, Respiratory System ØBN
Tracheoplasty
  see Repair, Respiratory System ØBQ
  see Supplement, Respiratory System ØBU
Tracheorrhaphy *see* Repair, Respiratory System ØBQ
Tracheoscopy ØBJ18ZZ
Tracheostomy *see* Bypass, Respiratory System ØB1
Tracheostomy Device
  Bypass, Trachea ØB11
  Change device in, Trachea ØB21XFZ
  Removal of device from, Trachea ØBP1
  Revision of device in, Trachea ØBW1
Tracheostomy tube *use* Tracheostomy Device in Respiratory System
Tracheotomy *see* Drainage, Respiratory System ØB9
Traction
  Abdominal Wall 2W63X
  Arm
    Lower
      Left 2W6DX
      Right 2W6CX
    Upper
      Left 2W6BX
      Right 2W6AX
  Back 2W65X
  Chest Wall 2W64X
  Extremity
    Lower
      Left 2W6MX
      Right 2W6LX
    Upper
      Left 2W69X
      Right 2W68X
  Face 2W61X
  Finger
    Left 2W6KX
    Right 2W6JX
  Foot
    Left 2W6TX
    Right 2W6SX
  Hand
    Left 2W6FX
    Right 2W6EX
  Head 2W60X
  Inguinal Region
    Left 2W67X
    Right 2W66X
  Leg
    Lower
      Left 2W6RX
      Right 2W6QX
    Upper
      Left 2W6PX
      Right 2W6NX
  Neck 2W62X
  Thumb
    Left 2W6HX
    Right 2W6GX
  Toe
    Left 2W6VX
    Right 2W6UX
Tractotomy *see* Division, Central Nervous System and Cranial Nerves ØØ8
Tragus
  use External Ear, Right
  use External Ear, Left
  use External Ear, Bilateral
Training, caregiver *see* Caregiver Training
TRAM (transverse rectus abdominis myocutaneous) flap reconstruction
  Free *see* Replacement, Skin and Breast ØHR
  Pedicled *see* Transfer, Muscles ØKX
Transcatheter pulmonary valve (TPV) placement
  In Conduit Ø2RH38L
  Native Site Ø2RH38M
▶Transcatheter tricuspid valve replacement
  ▶EVOQUE valve/system (Edwards) X2RJ3RA
  ▶Other valve/system Ø2RJ38Z
Transection *see* Division
Transdermal Glomerular Filtration Rate (GFR) Measurement System XT25XE5
Transfer
  Buccal Mucosa ØCX4
  Bursa and Ligament
    Abdomen
      Left ØMXJ
      Right ØMXH
    Ankle
      Left ØMXR
      Right ØMXQ
    Elbow
      Left ØMX4
      Right ØMX3
    Foot
      Left ØMXT
      Right ØMXS
    Hand
      Left ØMX8
      Right ØMX7
    Head and Neck ØMXØ
    Hip
      Left ØMXM
      Right ØMXL
    Knee
      Left ØMXP
      Right ØMXN
    Lower Extremity
      Left ØMXW
      Right ØMXV
    Perineum ØMXK
    Rib(s) ØMXG
    Shoulder
      Left ØMX2
      Right ØMX1
    Spine
      Lower ØMXD
      Upper ØMXC
    Sternum ØMXF
    Upper Extremity
      Left ØMXB
      Right ØMX9
    Wrist
      Left ØMX6
      Right ØMX5
  Finger
    Left ØXXPØZM
    Right ØXXNØZL
  Gingiva
    Lower ØCX6
    Upper ØCX5
  Intestine
    Large ØDXE
    Small ØDX8
  Lip
    Lower ØCX1
    Upper ØCXØ
  Muscle
    Abdomen
      Left ØKXL
      Right ØKXK
    Extraocular
      Left Ø8XM
      Right Ø8XL
    Facial ØKX1
    Foot
      Left ØKXW
      Right ØKXV
    Hand
      Left ØKXD
      Right ØKXC
    Head ØKXØ
    Hip
      Left ØKXP
      Right ØKXN
Transfer *(Continued)*
  Muscle *(Continued)*
    Lower Arm and Wrist
      Left ØKXB
      Right ØKX9
    Lower Leg
      Left ØKXT
      Right ØKXS
    Neck
      Left ØKX3
      Right ØKX2
    Perineum ØKXM
    Shoulder
      Left ØKX6
      Right ØKX5
    Thorax
      Left ØKXJ
      Right ØKXH
    Tongue, Palate, Pharynx ØKX4
    Trunk
      Left ØKXG
      Right ØKXF
    Upper Arm
      Left ØKX8
      Right ØKX7
    Upper Leg
      Left ØKXR
      Right ØKXQ
  Nerve
    Abducens ØØXL
    Accessory ØØXR
    Acoustic ØØXN
    Cervical Ø1X1
    Facial ØØXM
    Femoral Ø1XD
    Glossopharyngeal ØØXP
    Hypoglossal ØØXS
    Lumbar Ø1XB
    Median Ø1X5
    Oculomotor ØØXH
    Olfactory ØØXF
    Optic ØØXG
    Peroneal Ø1XH
    Phrenic Ø1X2
    Pudendal Ø1XC
    Radial Ø1X6
    Sciatic Ø1XF
    Thoracic Ø1X8
    Tibial Ø1XG
    Trigeminal ØØXK
    Trochlear ØØXJ
    Ulnar Ø1X4
    Vagus ØØXQ
  ▶Omentum ØDXU
  Palate, Soft ØCX3
  Prepuce ØVXT
  Skin
    Abdomen ØHX7XZZ
    Back ØHX6XZZ
    Buttock ØHX8XZZ
    Chest ØHX5XZZ
    Ear
      Left ØHX3XZZ
      Right ØHX2XZZ
    Face ØHX1XZZ
    Foot
      Left ØHXNXZZ
      Right ØHXMXZZ
    Hand
      Left ØHXGXZZ
      Right ØHXFXZZ
    Inguinal ØHXAXZZ
    Lower Arm
      Left ØHXEXZZ
      Right ØHXDXZZ
    Lower Leg
      Left ØHXLXZZ
      Right ØHXKXZZ

Transfer *(Continued)*
Subcutaneous Tissue and Fascia
Neck ØHX4XZZ
Perineum ØHX9XZZ
Scalp ØHXØXZZ
Upper Arm
Left ØHXCXZZ
Right ØHXBXZZ
Upper Leg
Left ØHXJXZZ
Right ØHXHXZZ
Stomach ØDX6
Abdomen ØJX8
Back ØJX7
Buttock ØJX9
Chest ØJX6
Face ØJX1
Foot
Left ØJXR
Right ØJXQ
Hand
Left ØJXK
Right ØJXJ
Lower Arm
Left ØJXH
Right ØJXG
Lower Leg
Left ØJXP
Right ØJXN
Neck
Left ØJX5
Right ØJX4
Pelvic Region ØJXC
Perineum ØJXB
Scalp ØJXØ
Upper Arm
Left ØJXF
Right ØJXD
Upper Leg
Left ØJXM
Right ØJXL
Tendon
Abdomen
Left ØLXG
Right ØLXF
Ankle
Left ØLXT
Right ØLXS
Foot
Left ØLXW
Right ØLXV
Hand
Left ØLX8
Right ØLX7
Head and Neck ØLXØ
Hip
Left ØLXK
Right ØLXJ
Knee
Left ØLXR
Right ØLXQ
Lower Arm and Wrist
Left ØLX6
Right ØLX5
Lower Leg
Left ØLXP
Right ØLXN
Perineum ØLXH
Shoulder
Left ØLX2
Right ØLX1
Thorax
Left ØLXD
Right ØLXC
Trunk
Left ØLXB
Right ØLX9
Upper Arm
Left ØLX4
Right ØLX3

Transfer *(Continued)*
Tendon *(Continued)*
Upper Leg
Left ØLXM
Right ØLXL
Tongue ØCX7
Transfusion
Bone Marrow
Blood
Platelets 3Ø2A3R
Red Cells 3Ø2A3N
Frozen 3Ø2A3P
Whole 3Ø2A3H
Plasma
Fresh 3Ø2A3L
Frozen 3Ø2A3K
Serum Albumin 3Ø2A3J
New Technology *see* New Technology, Anatomical Regions XW1
Products of Conception
Antihemophilic Factors 3Ø27
Blood
Platelets 3Ø27
Red Cells 3Ø27
Frozen 3Ø27
White Cells 3Ø27
Whole 3Ø27
Factor IX 3Ø27
Fibrinogen 3Ø27
Globulin 3Ø27
Plasma
Fresh 3Ø27
Frozen 3Ø27
Plasma Cryoprecipitate 3Ø27
Serum Albumin 3Ø27
Vein
4-Factor Prothrombin Complex Concentrate 3Ø283B1
Central
Antihemophilic Factors 3Ø243V
Blood
Platelets 3Ø243R
Red Cells 3Ø243N
Frozen 3Ø243P
White Cells 3Ø243Q
Whole 3Ø243H
Bone Marrow 3Ø243G
Factor IX 3Ø243W
Fibrinogen 3Ø243T
Globulin 3Ø243S
Hematopoietic Stem/Progenitor Cells (HSPC), Genetically Modified 3Ø243CØ
Pathogen Reduced Cryoprecipitated Fibrinogen Complex 3Ø243D1
Plasma
Fresh 3Ø243L
Frozen 3Ø243K
Plasma Cryoprecipitate 3Ø243M
Serum Albumin 3Ø243J
Stem Cells
Cord Blood 3Ø243X
Embryonic 3Ø243AZ
Hematopoietic 3Ø243Y
T-cell Depleted Hematopoietic 3Ø243U
Peripheral
Antihemophilic Factors 3Ø233V
Blood
Platelets 3Ø233R
Red Cells 3Ø233N
Frozen 3Ø233P
White Cells 3Ø233Q
Whole 3Ø233H
Bone Marrow 3Ø233G
Factor IX 3Ø233W
Fibrinogen 3Ø233T
Globulin 3Ø233S
Hematopoietic Stem/Progenitor Cells (HSPC), Genetically Modified 3Ø233CØ

Transfusion *(Continued)*
Vein *(Continued)*
Peripheral *(Continued)*
Pathogen Reduced Cryoprecipitated Fibrinogen Complex 3Ø243D1
Plasma
Fresh 3Ø233L
Frozen 3Ø233K
Plasma Cryoprecipitate 3Ø233M
Serum Albumin 3Ø233J
Stem Cells
Cord Blood 3Ø233X
Embryonic 3Ø233Z
Hematopoietic 3Ø233Y
T-cell Depleted Hematopoietic 3Ø233U
Transplant *see* Transplantation
Transplantation
Bone marrow ~~see Transfusion, Circulatory 302~~
see Transfusion, Vein, Peripheral 3Ø233G
see Transfusion, Vein, Central 3Ø243G
Esophagus ØDY5ØZ
Face ØWY2ØZ
Hand
Left ØXYKØZ
Right ØXYJØZ
Heart Ø2YAØZ
Hematopoietic cell *see* Transfusion, Circulatory 3Ø2
Intestine
Large ØDYEØZ
Small ØDY8ØZ
Kidney
Left ØTY1ØZ
Right ØTYØØZ
Liver ØFYØØZ
Lung
Bilateral ØBYMØZ
Left ØBYLØZ
Lower Lobe
Left ØBYJØZ
Right ØBYFØZ
Middle Lobe, Right ØBYDØZ
Right ØBYKØZ
Upper Lobe
Left ØBYGØZ
Right ØBYCØZ
Lung Lingula ØBYHØZ
Ovary
Left ØUY1ØZ
Right ØUYØØZ
Pancreas ØFYGØZ
Penis ØVYSØZ
Products of Conception 1ØYØ
Scrotum ØVY5ØZ
Spleen Ø7YPØZ
Stem cell *see* Transfusion, Circulatory 3Ø2
Stomach ØDY6ØZ
Thymus Ø7YMØZ
Uterus ØUY9ØZ
Transposition
see Bypass
see Reposition
see Transfer
Transversalis fascia *use* Subcutaneous Tissue and Fascia, Trunk
Transverse (cutaneous) cervical nerve *use* Cervical Plexus
Transverse acetabular ligament
use Hip Bursa and Ligament, Right
use Hip Bursa and Ligament, Left
Transverse facial artery
use Temporal Artery, Right
use Temporal Artery, Left
Transverse foramen *use* Cervical Vertebra
Transverse humeral ligament
use Shoulder Bursa and Ligament, Right
use Shoulder Bursa and Ligament, Left
Transverse ligament of atlas *use* Head and Neck Bursa and Ligament

Transverse process
use Cervical Vertebra
use Thoracic Vertebra
use Lumbar Vertebra
Transverse Rectus Abdominis Myocutaneous Flap
Replacement
Bilateral ØHRVØ76
Left ØHRUØ76
Right ØHRTØ76
Transfer
Left ØKXL
Right ØKXK
Transverse scapular ligament
use Shoulder Bursa and Ligament, Right
use Shoulder Bursa and Ligament, Left
Transverse thoracis muscle
use Thorax Muscle, Right
use Thorax Muscle, Left
Transversospinalis muscle
use Trunk Muscle, Right
use Trunk Muscle, Left
Transversus abdominis muscle
use Abdomen Muscle, Right
use Abdomen Muscle, Left
Trapezium bone
use Carpal, Right
use Carpal, Left
Trapezius muscle
use Trunk Muscle, Right
use Trunk Muscle, Left
Trapezoid bone
use Carpal, Right
use Carpal, Left
Treosulfan XWØ
Triceps brachii muscle
use Upper Arm Muscle, Right
use Upper Arm Muscle, Left
Tricuspid annulus *use* Tricuspid Valve
TricValve® Transcatheter Bicaval Valve System *use* Intraluminal Device, Bioprosthetic Valve in New Technology
Trifacial nerve *use* Trigeminal Nerve
Trifecta™ Valve (aortic) *use* Zooplastic Tissue in Heart and Great Vessels
Trigone of bladder *use* Bladder
TriGuard 3™ CEPD (cerebral embolic protection device) X2A6325
Trilaciclib XWØ
Trimming, excisional *see* Excision
Triquetral bone
use Carpal, Right
use Carpal, Left
Trochanteric bursa
use Hip Bursa and Ligament, Right
use Hip Bursa and Ligament, Left
▶**TTVR** *see* Transcatheter tricuspid valve replacement
▶**Tumor-Infiltrating Lymphocyte (TIL) Therapy** *use* Non-Chimeric Antigen Receptor T-cell Immune Effector Cell Therapy
TUMT (Transurethral microwave thermotherapy of prostate) ØV5Ø7ZZ
TUNA (transurethral needle ablation of prostate) ØV5Ø7ZZ
Tunneled central venous catheter *use* Vascular Access Device, Tunneled in Subcutaneous Tissue and Fascia
Tunneled spinal (intrathecal) catheter *use* Infusion Device
Turbinectomy
see Excision, Ear, Nose, Sinus Ø9B
see Resection, Ear, Nose, Sinus Ø9T
Turbinoplasty
see Repair, Ear, Nose, Sinus Ø9Q
see Replacement, Ear, Nose, Sinus Ø9R
see Supplement, Ear, Nose, Sinus Ø9U
Turbinotomy
see Division, Ear, Nose, Sinus Ø98
see Drainage, Ear, Nose, Sinus Ø99
TURP (transurethral resection of prostate)
see Excision, Prostate ØVBØ
see Resection, Prostate ØVTØ
Twelfth cranial nerve *use* Hypoglossal Nerve
Two lead pacemaker *use* Pacemaker, Dual Chamber in ØJH
Tympanic cavity
use Middle Ear, Right
use Middle Ear, Left
Tympanic nerve *use* Glossopharyngeal Nerve
Tympanic part of temoporal bone
use Temporal Bone, Right
use Temporal Bone, Left
Tympanogram *see* Hearing Assessment, Diagnostic Audiology F13
Tympanoplasty
see Repair, Ear, Nose, Sinus Ø9Q
see Replacement, Ear, Nose, Sinus Ø9R
see Supplement, Ear, Nose, Sinus Ø9U
Tympanosympathectomy *see* Excision, Nerve, Head and Neck Sympathetic Ø1BK
Tympanotomy *see* Drainage, Ear, Nose, Sinus Ø99
TYRX Antibacterial Envelope *use* Anti-Infective Envelope

T

▶ New ➠ Revised ~~deleted~~ Deleted

U

Ulnar collateral carpal ligament
use Wrist Bursa and Ligament, Right
use Wrist Bursa and Ligament, Left
Ulnar collateral ligament
use Elbow Bursa and Ligament, Right
use Elbow Bursa and Ligament, Left
Ulnar notch
use Radius, Right
use Radius, Left
Ulnar vein
use Brachial Vein, Right
use Brachial Vein, Left
Ultrafiltration
Hemodialysis *see* Performance, Urinary 5A1D
Therapeutic plasmapheresis *see* Pheresis, Circulatory 6A55
Ultraflex™ Precision Colonic Stent System *use* Intraluminal Device
ULTRAPRO Hernia System (UHS) *use* Synthetic Substitute
ULTRAPRO Partially Absorbable Lightweight Mesh *use* Synthetic Substitute
ULTRAPRO Plug *use* Synthetic Substitute
Ultrasonic osteogenic stimulator
use Bone Growth Stimulator in Head and Facial Bones
use Bone Growth Stimulator in Upper Bones
use Bone Growth Stimulator in Lower Bones
Ultrasonography
Abdomen BW40ZZZ
Abdomen and Pelvis BW41ZZZ
Abdominal Wall BH49ZZZ
Aorta
Abdominal, Intravascular B440ZZ3
Thoracic, Intravascular B340ZZ3
Appendix BD48ZZZ
Artery
Brachiocephalic-Subclavian, Right, Intravascular B341ZZ3
Celiac and Mesenteric, Intravascular B44KZZ3
Common Carotid
Bilateral, Intravascular B345ZZ3
Left, Intravascular B344ZZ3
Right, Intravascular B343ZZ3
Coronary
Multiple B241YZZ
Intravascular B241ZZ3
Transesophageal B241ZZ4
Single B240YZZ
Intravascular B240ZZ3
Transesophageal B240ZZ4
Femoral, Intravascular B44LZZ3
Inferior Mesenteric, Intravascular B445ZZ3
Internal Carotid
Bilateral, Intravascular B348ZZ3
Left, Intravascular B347ZZ3
Right, Intravascular B346ZZ3
Intra-Abdominal, Other, Intravascular B44BZZ3
Intracranial, Intravascular B34RZZ3
Lower Extremity
Bilateral, Intravascular B44HZZ3
Left, Intravascular B44GZZ3
Right, Intravascular B44FZZ3
Mesenteric and Celiac, Intravascular B44KZZ3
Ophthalmic, Intravascular B34VZZ3
Penile, Intravascular B44NZZ3
Pulmonary
Left, Intravascular B34TZZ3
Right, Intravascular B34SZZ3
Renal
Bilateral, Intravascular B448ZZ3
Left, Intravascular B447ZZ3
Right, Intravascular B446ZZ3
Subclavian, Left, Intravascular B342ZZ3

Ultrasonography *(Continued)*
Artery *(Continued)*
Superior Mesenteric, Intravascular B444ZZ3
Upper Extremity
Bilateral, Intravascular B34KZZ3
Left, Intravascular B34JZZ3
Right, Intravascular B34HZZ3
Bile Duct BF40ZZZ
Bile Duct and Gallbladder BF43ZZZ
Bladder BT40ZZZ
and Kidney BT4JZZZ
Brain B040ZZZ
Breast
Bilateral BH42ZZZ
Left BH41ZZZ
Right BH40ZZZ
Chest Wall BH4BZZZ
Coccyx BR4FZZZ
Connective Tissue
Lower Extremity BL41ZZZ
Upper Extremity BL40ZZZ
Duodenum BD49ZZZ
Elbow
Left, Densitometry BP4HZZ1
Right, Densitometry BP4GZZ1
Esophagus BD41ZZZ
Extremity
Lower BH48ZZZ
Upper BH47ZZZ
Eye
Bilateral B847ZZZ
Left B846ZZZ
Right B845ZZZ
Fallopian Tube
Bilateral BU42
Left BU41
Right BU40
Fetal Umbilical Cord BY47ZZZ
Fetus
First Trimester, Multiple Gestation BY4BZZZ
Second Trimester, Multiple Gestation BY4DZZZ
Single
First Trimester BY49ZZZ
Second Trimester BY4CZZZ
Third Trimester BY4FZZZ
Third Trimester, Multiple Gestation BY4GZZZ
Gallbladder BF42ZZZ
Gallbladder and Bile Duct BF43ZZZ
Gastrointestinal Tract BD47ZZZ
Gland
Adrenal
Bilateral BG42ZZZ
Left BG41ZZZ
Right BG40ZZZ
Parathyroid BG43ZZZ
Thyroid BG44ZZZ
Hand
Left, Densitometry BP4PZZ1
Right, Densitometry BP4NZZ1
Head and Neck BH4CZZZ
Heart
Left B245YZZ
Intravascular B245ZZ3
Transesophageal B245ZZ4
Pediatric B24DYZZ
Intravascular B24DZZ3
Transesophageal B24DZZ4
Right B244YZZ
Intravascular B244ZZ3
Transesophageal B244ZZ4
Right and Left B246YZZ
Intravascular B246ZZ3
Transesophageal B246ZZ4
Heart with Aorta B24BYZZ
Intravascular B24BZZ3
Transesophageal B24BZZ4
Hepatobiliary System, All BF4CZZZ

Ultrasonography *(Continued)*
Hip
Bilateral BQ42ZZZ
Left BQ41ZZZ
Right BQ40ZZZ
Kidney
and Bladder BT4JZZZ
Bilateral BT43ZZZ
Left BT42ZZZ
Right BT41ZZZ
Transplant BT49ZZZ
Knee
Bilateral BQ49ZZZ
Left BQ48ZZZ
Right BQ47ZZZ
Liver BF45ZZZ
Liver and Spleen BF46ZZZ
Mediastinum BB4CZZZ
Neck BW4FZZZ
Ovary
Bilateral BU45
Left BU44
Right BU43
Ovary and Uterus BU4C
Pancreas BF47ZZZ
Pelvic Region BW4GZZZ
Pelvis and Abdomen BW41ZZZ
Penis BV4BZZZ
Pericardium B24CYZZ
Intravascular B24CZZ3
Transesophageal B24CZZ4
Placenta BY48ZZZ
Pleura BB4BZZZ
Prostate and Seminal Vesicle BV49ZZZ
Rectum BD4CZZZ
Sacrum BR4FZZZ
Scrotum BV44ZZZ
Seminal Vesicle and Prostate BV49ZZZ
Shoulder
Left, Densitometry BP49ZZ1
Right, Densitometry BP48ZZ1
Spinal Cord B04BZZZ
Spine
Cervical BR40ZZZ
Lumbar BR49ZZZ
Thoracic BR47ZZZ
Spleen and Liver BF46ZZZ
Stomach BD42ZZZ
Tendon
Lower Extremity BL43ZZZ
Upper Extremity BL42ZZZ
Ureter
Bilateral BT48ZZZ
Left BT47ZZZ
Right BT46ZZZ
Urethra BT45ZZZ
Uterus BU46
Uterus and Ovary BU4C
Vein
Jugular
Left, Intravascular B544ZZ3
Right, Intravascular B543ZZ3
Lower Extremity
Bilateral, Intravascular B54DZZ3
Left, Intravascular B54CZZ3
Right, Intravascular B54BZZ3
Portal, Intravascular B54TZZ3
Renal
Bilateral, Intravascular B54LZZ3
Left, Intravascular B54KZZ3
Right, Intravascular B54JZZ3
~~Spanchnic, Intravascular B54TZZ3~~
▶ Splanchnic, Intravascular B54TZZ3
Subclavian
Left, Intravascular B547ZZ3
Right, Intravascular B546ZZ3

Ultrasonography *(Continued)*
Vein *(Continued)*
Upper Extremity
Bilateral, Intravascular B54PZZ3
Left, Intravascular B54NZZ3
Right, Intravascular B54MZZ3
Vena Cava
Inferior, Intravascular B549ZZ3
Superior, Intravascular B548ZZ3
Wrist
Left, Densitometry BP4MZZ1
Right, Densitometry BP4LZZ1
Ultrasound Ablation, Destruction, Renal Sympathetic Nerve(s) XØ51329
Ultrasound bone healing system
use Bone Growth Stimulator in Head and Facial Bones
use Bone Growth Stimulator in Upper Bones
use Bone Growth Stimulator in Lower Bones
Ultrasound Penetrable Synthetic Substitute, Skull XNR8ØD9
Ultrasound Therapy
Heart 6A75
No Qualifier 6A75
Vessels
Head and Neck 6A75
Other 6A75
Peripheral 6A75
Ultraviolet Light Therapy, Skin 6A8Ø
Umbilical artery
use Internal Iliac Artery, Right
use Internal Iliac Artery, Left
use Lower Artery
Uniplanar external fixator
use External Fixation Device, Monoplanar in ØPH
use External Fixation Device, Monoplanar in ØPS
use External Fixation Device, Monoplanar in ØQH
use External Fixation Device, Monoplanar in ØQS
UPLIZNA® *use* Inebilizumab-cdon
Upper GI series *see* Fluoroscopy, Gastrointestinal, Upper BD15
Ureteral orifice
use Ureter, Left
use Ureter
use Ureter, Right
use Ureters, Bilateral
Ureterectomy
see Excision, Urinary System ØTB
see Resection, Urinary System ØTT
Ureterocolostomy *see* Bypass, Urinary System ØT1
Ureterocystostomy *see* Bypass, Urinary System ØT1
Ureteroenterostomy *see* Bypass, Urinary System ØT1
Ureteroileostomy *see* Bypass, Urinary System ØT1
Ureterolithotomy *see* Extirpation, Urinary System ØTC
Ureterolysis *see* Release, Urinary System ØTN
Ureteroneocystostomy
see Bypass, Urinary System ØT1
see Reposition, Urinary System ØTS
Ureteropelvic junction (UPJ)
use Kidney Pelvis, Right
use Kidney Pelvis, Left
Ureteropexy
see Repair, Urinary System ØTQ
see Reposition, Urinary System ØTS
Ureteroplasty
see Repair, Urinary System ØTQ
see Replacement, Urinary System ØTR
see Supplement, Urinary System ØTU
Ureteroplication *see* Restriction, Urinary System ØTV
Ureteropyelography *see* Fluoroscopy, Urinary System BT1
Ureterorrhaphy *see* Repair, Urinary System ØTQ
Ureteroscopy ØTJ98ZZ
Ureterostomy
see Bypass, Urinary System ØT1
see Drainage, Urinary System ØT9
Ureterotomy *see* Drainage, Urinary System ØT9
Ureteroureterostomy *see* Bypass, Urinary System ØT1
Ureterovesical orifice
use Ureter, Right
use Ureter, Left
use Ureters, Bilateral
use Ureter
Urethral catheterization, indwelling ØT9B7ØZ
Urethrectomy
see Excision, Urethra ØTBD
see Resection, Urethra ØTTD
Urethrolithotomy *see* Extirpation, Urethra ØTCD
Urethrolysis *see* Release, Urethra ØTND
Urethropexy
see Repair, Urethra ØTQD
see Reposition, Urethra ØTSD
Urethroplasty
see Repair, Urethra ØTQD
see Replacement, Urethra ØTRD
see Supplement, Urethra ØTUD
Urethrorrhaphy *see* Repair, Urethra ØTQD
Urethroscopy ØTJD8ZZ
Urethrotomy *see* Drainage, Urethra ØT9D
Uridine Triacetate XWØDX82
Urinary incontinence stimulator lead *use* Stimulator Lead in Urinary System
Urography *see* Fluoroscopy, Urinary System BT1
Ustekinumab *use* Other New Technology Therapeutic Substance
Uterine Artery
use Internal Iliac Artery, Right
use Internal Iliac Artery, Left
Uterine artery embolization (UAE) *see* Occlusion, Lower Arteries Ø4L
Uterine cornu *use* Uterus
Uterine tube
use Fallopian Tube, Right
use Fallopian Tube, Left
Uterine vein
use Hypogastric Vein, Right
use Hypogastric Vein, Left
Uvulectomy
see Excision, Uvula ØCBN
see Resection, Uvula ØCTN
Uvulorrhaphy *see* Repair, Uvula ØCQN
Uvulotomy *see* Drainage, Uvula ØC9N

V

- **V-Wave Interatrial Shunt System** *use* Synthetic Substitute
- ~~Vabomere™ use Meropenem-vaborbactam Anti-infective~~
- ▶ **VABOMERE™** (Meropenem-vaborbactam Anti-infective) *use* Other Anti-infective
- **Vaccination** *see* Introduction of Serum, Toxoid, and Vaccine
- **Vacuum extraction, obstetric** 10D07Z6
- ▶ **VADER® Pedicle System** *use* Carbon/PEEK Spinal Stabilization Device, Pedicle Based in New Technology
- **Vaginal artery**
  - *use* Internal Iliac Artery, Right
  - *use* Internal Iliac Artery, Left
- **Vaginal pessary** *use* Intraluminal Device, Pessary in Female Reproductive System
- **Vaginal vein**
  - *use* Hypogastric Vein, Right
  - *use* Hypogastric Vein, Left
- **Vaginectomy**
  - *see* Excision, Vagina 0UBG
  - *see* Resection, Vagina 0UTG
- **Vaginofixation**
  - *see* Repair, Vagina 0UQG
  - *see* Reposition, Vagina 0USG
- **Vaginoplasty**
  - *see* Repair, Vagina 0UQG
  - *see* Supplement, Vagina 0UUG
- **Vaginorrhaphy** *see* Repair, Vagina 0UQG
- **Vaginoscopy** 0UJH8ZZ
- **Vaginotomy** *see* Drainage, Female Reproductive System 0U9
- **Vagotomy** *see* Division, Nerve, Vagus 008Q
- **Valiant Thoracic Stent Graft** *use* Intraluminal Device
- **Valvotomy, valvulotomy**
  - *see* Division, Heart and Great Vessels 028
  - *see* Release, Heart and Great Vessels 02N
- **Valvuloplasty**
  - *see* Repair, Heart and Great Vessels 02Q
  - *see* Replacement, Heart and Great Vessels 02R
  - *see* Supplement, Heart and Great Vessels 02U
- **Valvuloplasty, Alfieri Stitch** *see* Restriction, Valve, Mitral 02VG
- ▶ **Vancomycin Hydrochloride and Tobramycin Sulfate Anti-Infective, Temporary Irrigation Spacer System** XW0U0GA
- **Vanta™ PC neurostimulator** *use* Stimulator Generator, Multiple Array in 0JH
- **Vascular Access Device**
  - Totally Implantable
    - Insertion of device in
      - Abdomen 0JH8
      - Chest 0JH6
      - Lower Arm
        - Left 0JHH
        - Right 0JHG
      - Lower Leg
        - Left 0JHP
        - Right 0JHN
      - Upper Arm
        - Left 0JHF
        - Right 0JHD
      - Upper Leg
        - Left 0JHM
        - Right 0JHL
    - Removal of device from
      - Lower Extremity 0JPW
      - Trunk 0JPT
      - Upper Extremity 0JPV
    - Revision of device in
      - Lower Extremity 0JWW
      - Trunk 0JWT
      - Upper Extremity 0JWV
  - Tunneled
    - Insertion of device in
      - Abdomen 0JH8
      - Chest 0JH6

- **Vascular Access Device** *(Continued)*
  - Tunneled *(Continued)*
    - Insertion of device in *(Continued)*
      - Lower Arm
        - Left 0JHH
        - Right 0JHG
      - Lower Leg
        - Left 0JHP
        - Right 0JHN
      - Upper Arm
        - Left 0JHF
        - Right 0JHD
      - Upper Leg
        - Left 0JHM
        - Right 0JHL
    - Removal of device from
      - Lower Extremity 0JPW
      - Trunk 0JPT
      - Upper Extremity 0JPV
    - Revision of device in
      - Lower Extremity 0JWW
      - Trunk 0JWT
      - Upper Extremity 0JWV
- **Vasectomy** *see* Excision, Male Reproductive System 0VB
- **Vasography**
  - *see* Plain Radiography, Male Reproductive System BV0
  - *see* Fluoroscopy, Male Reproductive System BV1
- **Vasoligation** *see* Occlusion, Male Reproductive System 0VL
- **Vasorrhaphy** *see* Repair, Male Reproductive System 0VQ
- **Vasostomy** *see* Bypass, Male Reproductive System 0V1
- **Vasotomy**
  - Drainage *see* Drainage, Male Reproductive System 0V9
  - With ligation *see* Occlusion, Male Reproductive System 0VL
- **Vasovasostomy** *see* Repair, Male Reproductive System 0VQ
- **VasQ™ External Support device** *use* Synthetic Substitute, Extraluminal Support Device in New Technology
- **Vastus intermedius muscle**
  - *use* Upper Leg Muscle, Right
  - *use* Upper Leg Muscle, Left
- **Vastus lateralis muscle**
  - *use* Upper Leg Muscle, Right
  - *use* Upper Leg Muscle, Left
- **Vastus medialis muscle**
  - *use* Upper Leg Muscle, Right
  - *use* Upper Leg Muscle, Left
- **VCG (vectorcardiogram)** *see* Measurement, Cardiac 4A02
- **Vectra® Vascular Access Graft** *use* Vascular Access Device, Tunneled in Subcutaneous Tissue and Fascia
- **Vein Graft Extraluminal Support Device(s), Supplement, Coronary Artery/Arteries** X2U4079
- **Veklury** *use* Remdesivir Anti-infective
- ~~Venclexta® use Venetoclax Antineoplastic~~
- ▶ **Venclexta®** (Venetoclax Antineoplastic tablets) *use* Other Antineoplastic
- **Venectomy**
  - *see* Excision, Upper Veins 05B
  - *see* Excision, Lower Veins 06B
- ~~Venetoclax Antineoplastic XW0DXR5~~
- ▶ **Venetoclax Antineoplastic** (tablets) *use* Other Antineoplastic
- **Venography**
  - *see* Plain Radiography, Veins B50
  - *see* Fluoroscopy, Veins B51
- **Venorrhaphy**
  - *see* Repair, Upper Veins 05Q
  - *see* Repair, Lower Veins 06Q
- **Venotripsy**
  - *see* Occlusion, Upper Veins 05L
  - *see* Occlusion, Lower Veins 06L
- **VenoValve®** *use* Intraluminal Device, Bioprosthetic Valve in New Technology
- ▶ **Veno-venous bypass, during percutaneous thrombectomy** 5A05A0L
- ▶ **Veno-venous circuit, during percutaneous thrombectomy** 5A05A0L
- **Ventricular fold** *use* Larynx
- **Ventriculoatriostomy** *see* Bypass, Central Nervous System and Cranial Nerves 001
- **Ventriculocisternostomy** *see* Bypass, Central Nervous System and Cranial Nerves 001
- **Ventriculogram, cardiac**
  - Combined left and right heart *see* Fluoroscopy, Heart, Right and Left B216
  - Left ventricle *see* Fluoroscopy, Heart, Left B215
  - Right ventricle *see* Fluoroscopy, Heart, Right B214
- **Ventriculopuncture, through previously implanted catheter** 8C01X6J
- **Ventriculoscopy** 00J04ZZ
- **Ventriculostomy**
  - External drainage *see* Drainage, Cerebral Ventricle 0096
  - Internal shunt *see* Bypass, Cerebral Ventricle 0016
- **Ventriculovenostomy** *see* Bypass, Cerebral Ventricle 0016
- **Ventrio™ Hernia Patch** *use* Synthetic Substitute
- **VEP (visual evoked potential)** 4A07X0Z
- **Vermiform appendix** *use* Appendix
- **Vermilion border**
  - *use* Upper Lip
  - *use* Lower Lip
- **Versa** *use* Pacemaker, Dual Chamber in 0JH
- **Version, obstetric**
  - External 10S0XZZ
  - Internal 10S07ZZ
- **Vertebral arch**
  - *use* Cervical Vertebra
  - *use* Thoracic Vertebra
  - *use* Lumbar Vertebra
- **Vertebral artery, intracranial portion** *use* Intracranial Artery
- **Vertebral body**
  - *use* Cervical Vertebra
  - *use* Thoracic Vertebra
  - *use* Lumbar Vertebra
- **Vertebral canal** *use* Spinal Canal
- **Vertebral foramen**
  - *use* Cervical Vertebra
  - *use* Thoracic Vertebra
  - *use* Lumbar Vertebra
- **Vertebral lamina**
  - *use* Cervical Vertebra
  - *use* Thoracic Vertebra
  - *use* Lumbar Vertebra
- **Vertebral pedicle**
  - *use* Cervical Vertebra
  - *use* Thoracic Vertebra
  - *use* Lumbar Vertebra
- **Vesical vein**
  - *use* Hypogastric Vein, Right
  - *use* Hypogastric Vein, Left
- **Vesicotomy** *see* Drainage, Urinary System 0T9
- **Vesiculectomy**
  - *see* Excision, Male Reproductive System 0VB
  - *see* Resection, Male Reproductive System 0VT
- **Vesiculogram, seminal** *see* Plain Radiography, Male Reproductive System BV0
- **Vesiculotomy** *see* Drainage, Male Reproductive System 0V9
- **VEST™ Venous External Support device** *use* Vein Graft Extraluminal Support Device(s) in New Technology

Vestibular (Scarpa's) ganglion *use* Acoustic Nerve
Vestibular Assessment F15Z
Vestibular nerve *use* Acoustic Nerve
Vestibular Treatment FØC
Vestibulocochlear nerve *use* Acoustic Nerve
VH-IVUS (virtual histology intravascular ultrasound) *see* Ultrasonography, Heart B24
Virchow's (supraclavicular) lymph node
use Lymphatic, Right Neck
use Lymphatic, Left Neck
Virtuoso (II) (DR) (VR) *use* Defibrillator Generator in ØJH
Vistogard® *use* Uridine Triacetate
Visualase™ MRI-Guided Laser Ablation System *see* Destruction
▶**VITEK® REVEAL™ Rapid AST System** XXE5X4A
Vitrectomy
see Excision, Eye Ø8B
see Resection, Eye Ø8T
Vitreous body
use Vitreous, Right
use Vitreous, Left
Viva (XT)(S) *use* Cardiac Resynchronization Defibrillator Pulse Generator in ØJH
Vivistim® Paired VNS System Lead *use* Neurostimulator Lead with Paired Stimulation System in New Technology
Vocal fold
use Vocal Cord, Right
use Vocal Cord, Left
Vocational
Assessment *see* Activities of Daily Living Assessment, Rehabilitation FØ2
Retraining *see* Activities of Daily Living Treatment, Rehabilitation FØ8
Volar (palmar) digital vein
use Hand Vein, Right
use Hand Vein, Left
Volar (palmar) metacarpal vein
use Hand Vein, Right
use Hand Vein, Left
Vomer bone *use* Nasal Septum
Vomer of nasal septum *use* Nasal Bone
Voraxaze *use* Glucarpidase
▶**VOWST™** use SER-1Ø9
▶**VT-X7** (Irrigation System) (Spacer) *use* Vancomycin Hydrochloride and Tobramycin Sulfate Anti-Infective, Temporary Irrigation Spacer System
Vulvectomy
see Excision, Female Reproductive System ØUB
see Resection, Female Reproductive System ØUT
VYXEOS™ *use* Cytarabine and Daunorubicin Liposome Antineoplastic

W

WALLSTENT® Endoprosthesis *use* Intraluminal Device
Washing *see* Irrigation
WavelinQ EndoAVF system
Radial Artery, Left Ø31C3ZF
Radial Artery, Right Ø31B3ZF
Ulnar Artery, Left Ø31A3ZF
Ulnar Artery, Right Ø3193ZF
Wedge resection, pulmonary *see* Excision, Respiratory System ØBB
~~Whole Blood Nucleic Acid-base Microbial Detection XXE5XM5~~
Whole Blood Reverse Transcription and Quantitative Real-time Polymerase Chain Reaction XXE5X38
Window *see* Drainage
Wiring, dental 2W31X9Z

X

▶**Xacduro®** *use* Sulbactam-Durlobactam
Xact Carotid Stent System *use* Intraluminal Device
XENLETA™ *use* Lefamulin Anti-infective
X-ray *see* Plain Radiography
X-Spine Axle Cage
use Spinal Stabilization Device, Interspinous Process in ØRH
use Spinal Stabilization Device, Interspinous Process in ØSH
X-STOP® Spacer
use Spinal Stabilization Device, Interspinous Process in ØRH
use Spinal Stabilization Device, Interspinous Process in ØSH
Xenograft *use* Zooplastic Tissue in Heart and Great Vessels
XENOVIEW™ BB34Z3Z
XIENCE Everolimus Eluting Coronary Stent System *use* Intraluminal Device, Drug-eluting in Heart and Great Vessels
Xiphoid process *use* Sternum
XLIF® System *use* Interbody Fusion Device in Lower Joints
~~XOSPATA® use Gilteritinib Antineoplastic~~
▶**XOSPATA®** (Gilteritinib) *use* Other Antineoplastic

Y

Yescarta® *use* Axicabtagene Ciloleucel Immunotherapy
Yoga Therapy 8EØZXY4

Z

Z-plasty, skin for scar contracture *see* Release, Skin and Breast ØHN
▶**Zanidatamab Antineoplastic** XWØ
Zenith AAA Endovascular Graft
use Intraluminal Device
Zenith® Fenestrated AAA Endovascular Graft
use Intraluminal Device, Branched or Fenestrated, One or Two Arteries in Ø4V
use Intraluminal Device, Branched or Fenestrated, Three or More Arteries in Ø4V
Zenith Flex® AAA Endovascular Graft *use* Intraluminal Device
Zenith® Renu™ AAA Ancillary Graft *use* Intraluminal Device
Zenith TX2® TAA Endovascular Graft *use* Intraluminal Device
ZEPZELCA™ *use* Lurbinectedin
ZERBAXA® *use* Ceftolozane/Tazobactam Anti-infective
Zilver® PTX® (paclitaxel) Drug-Eluting Peripheral Stent
use Intraluminal Device, Drug-eluting in Upper Arteries
use Intraluminal Device, Drug-eluting in Lower Arteries
Zimmer® NexGen® LPS Mobile Bearing Knee *use* Synthetic Substitute
Zimmer® NexGen® LPS-Flex Mobile Knee *use* Synthetic Substitute
ZINPLAVA™ infusion *see* Introduction with qualifier Other Therapeutic Monoclonal Antibody
Zonule of Zinn
use Lens, Right
use Lens, Left
Zotarolimus-eluting coronary stent *use* Intraluminal Device, Drug-eluting in Heart and Great Vessels
ZULRESSO™ *use* Brexanolone
Zygomatic process of frontal bone *use* Frontal Bone
Zygomatic process of temporal bone
use Temporal Bone, Right
use Temporal Bone, Left
Zygomaticus muscle *use* Facial Muscle
ZYNTEGLO® *use* Betibeglogene Autotemcel
Zyvox *use* Oxazolidinones

KEYS

Appendices

DEFINITIONS

SECTION-CHARACTER

Ø 3 Medical and Surgical - Operation 865
Ø 4 Medical and Surgical - Body Part 867
Ø 5 Medical and Surgical - Approach 883
Ø 6 Medical and Surgical - Device 884
1 3 Obstetrics - Operation 891
1 5 Obstetrics - Approach 891
2 3 Placement - Operation 892
2 5 Placement - Approach 892
3 3 Administration - Operation 892
3 5 Administration - Approach 892
3 6 Administration - Substance 893
4 3 Measurement and Monitoring - Operation 893
4 5 Measurement and Monitoring - Approach 894
5 3 Extracorporeal or Systemic Assistance and Performance - Operation 894
6 3 Extracorporeal or Systemic Therapies - Operation 894
7 3 Osteopathic - Operation 894
7 5 Osteopathic - Approach 895
8 3 Other Procedures - Operation 895
8 5 Other Procedures - Approach 895
9 3 Chiropractic - Operation 895
9 5 Chiropractic - Approach 895
B 3 Imaging - Type 896
C 3 Nuclear Medicine - Type 896
F 3 Physical Rehabilitation and Diagnostic Audiology - Type 897
F 5 Physical Rehabilitation and Diagnostic Audiology - Type Qualifier 897
G 3 Mental Health - Type 9Ø4
G 4 Mental Health - Qualifier 9Ø5
H 3 Substance Abuse Treatment - Type 9Ø6
X 3 New Technology - Operation 9Ø6
X 5 New Technology - Approach 9Ø7
X 6 New Technology - Device/Substance/Technology 9Ø8

SECTION Ø - MEDICAL AND SURGICAL

CHARACTER 3 - OPERATION

Alteration	**Definition:** Modifying the anatomic structure of a body part without affecting the function of the body part **Explanation:** Principal purpose is to improve appearance **Includes/Examples:** Face lift, breast augmentation
Bypass	**Definition:** Altering the route of passage of the contents of a tubular body part **Explanation:** Rerouting contents of a body part to a downstream area of the normal route, to a similar route and body part, or to an abnormal route and dissimilar body part. Includes one or more anastomoses, with or without the use of a device **Includes/Examples:** Coronary artery bypass, colostomy formation
Change	**Definition:** Taking out or off a device from a body part and putting back an identical or similar device in or on the same body part without cutting or puncturing the skin or a mucous membrane **Explanation:** All CHANGE procedures are coded using the approach EXTERNAL **Includes/Examples:** Urinary catheter change, gastrostomy tube change
Control	**Definition:** Stopping, or attempting to stop, postprocedural or other acute bleeding **Includes/Examples:** Control of post-prostatectomy hemorrhage, control of intracranial subdural hemorrhage, control of bleeding duodenal ulcer, control of retroperitoneal hemorrhage
Creation	**Definition:** Putting in or on biological or synthetic material to form a new body part that to the extent possible replicates the anatomic structure or function of an absent body part **Explanation:** Used for gender reassignment surgery and corrective procedures in individuals with congenital anomalies **Includes/Examples:** Creation of vagina in a male, creation of right and left atrioventricular valve from common atrioventricular valve
Destruction	**Definition:** Physical eradication of all or a portion of a body part by the direct use of energy, force, or a destructive agent **Explanation:** None of the body part is physically taken out **Includes/Examples:** Fulguration of rectal polyp, cautery of skin lesion

Detachment	**Definition:** Cutting off all or a portion of the upper or lower extremities **Explanation:** The body part value is the site of the detachment, with a qualifier if applicable to further specify the level where the extremity was detached **Includes/Examples:** Below knee amputation, disarticulation of shoulder
Dilation	**Definition:** Expanding an orifice or the lumen of a tubular body part **Explanation:** The orifice can be a natural orifice or an artificially created orifice. Accomplished by stretching a tubular body part using intraluminal pressure or by cutting part of the orifice or wall of the tubular body part **Includes/Examples:** Percutaneous transluminal angioplasty, internal urethrotomy
Division	**Definition:** Cutting into a body part, without draining fluids and/or gases from the body part, in order to separate or transect a body part **Explanation:** All or a portion of the body part is separated into two or more portions **Includes/Examples:** Spinal cordotomy, osteotomy
Drainage	**Definition:** Taking or letting out fluids and/or gases from a body part **Explanation:** The qualifier DIAGNOSTIC is used to identify drainage procedures that are biopsies **Includes/Examples:** Thoracentesis, incision and drainage
Excision	**Definition:** Cutting out or off, without replacement, a portion of a body part **Explanation:** The qualifier DIAGNOSTIC is used to identify excision procedures that are biopsies **Includes/Examples:** Partial nephrectomy, liver biopsy
Extirpation	**Definition:** Taking or cutting out solid matter from a body part **Explanation:** The solid matter may be an abnormal byproduct of a biological function or a foreign body; it may be imbedded in a body part or in the lumen of a tubular body part. The solid matter may or may not have been previously broken into pieces **Includes/Examples:** Thrombectomy, choledocholithotomy
Extraction	**Definition:** Pulling or stripping out or off all or a portion of a body part by the use of force **Explanation:** The qualifier DIAGNOSTIC is used to identify extraction procedures that are biopsies **Includes/Examples:** Dilation and curettage, vein stripping

SECTION Ø - MEDICAL AND SURGICAL
CHARACTER 3 - OPERATION

Fragmentation	**Definition:** Breaking solid matter in a body part into pieces **Explanation:** Physical force (e.g., manual, ultrasonic) applied directly or indirectly is used to break the solid matter into pieces. The solid matter may be an abnormal byproduct of a biological function or a foreign body. The pieces of solid matter are not taken out **Includes/Examples:** Extracorporeal shockwave lithotripsy, transurethral lithotripsy
Fusion	**Definition:** Joining together portions of an articular body part rendering the articular body part immobile **Explanation:** The body part is joined together by fixation device, bone graft, or other means **Includes/Examples:** Spinal fusion, ankle arthrodesis
Insertion	**Definition:** Putting in a nonbiological appliance that monitors, assists, performs, or prevents a physiological function but does not physically take the place of a body part **Includes/Examples:** Insertion of radioactive implant, insertion of central venous catheter
Inspection	**Definition:** Visually and/or manually exploring a body part **Explanation:** Visual exploration may be performed with or without optical instrumentation. Manual exploration may be performed directly or through intervening body layers **Includes/Examples:** Diagnostic arthroscopy, exploratory laparotomy
Map	**Definition:** Locating the route of passage of electrical impulses and/or locating functional areas in a body part **Explanation:** Applicable only to the cardiac conduction mechanism and the central nervous system **Includes/Examples:** Cardiac mapping, cortical mapping
Occlusion	**Definition:** Completely closing an orifice or the lumen of a tubular body part **Explanation:** The orifice can be a natural orifice or an artificially created orifice **Includes/Examples:** Fallopian tube ligation, ligation of inferior vena cava
Reattachment	**Definition:** Putting back in or on all or a portion of a separated body part to its normal location or other suitable location **Explanation:** Vascular circulation and nervous pathways may or may not be reestablished **Includes/Examples:** Reattachment of hand, reattachment of avulsed kidney

Release	**Definition:** Freeing a body part from an abnormal physical constraint by cutting or by the use of force **Explanation:** Some of the restraining tissue may be taken out but none of the body part is taken out **Includes/Examples:** Adhesiolysis, carpal tunnel release
Removal	**Definition:** Taking out or off a device from a body part **Explanation:** If a device is taken out and a similar device put in without cutting or puncturing the skin or mucous membrane, the procedure is coded to the root operation CHANGE. Otherwise, the procedure for taking out a device is coded to the root operation REMOVAL **Includes/Examples:** Drainage tube removal, cardiac pacemaker removal
Repair	**Definition:** Restoring, to the extent possible, a body part to its normal anatomic structure and function **Explanation:** Used only when the method to accomplish the repair is not one of the other root operations **Includes/Examples:** Colostomy takedown, suture of laceration
Replacement	**Definition:** Putting in or on biological or synthetic material that physically takes the place and/or function of all or a portion of a body part **Explanation:** The body part may have been taken out or replaced, or may be taken out, physically eradicated, or rendered nonfunctional during the Replacement procedure. A Removal procedure is coded for taking out the device used in a previous replacement procedure **Includes/Examples:** Total hip replacement, bone graft, free skin graft
Reposition	**Definition:** Moving to its normal location, or other suitable location, all or a portion of a body part **Explanation:** The body part is moved to a new location from an abnormal location, or from a normal location where it is not functioning correctly. The body part may or may not be cut out or off to be moved to the new location **Includes/Examples:** Reposition of undescended testicle, fracture reduction
Resection	**Definition:** Cutting out or off, without replacement, all of a body part **Includes/Examples:** Total nephrectomy, total lobectomy of lung

SECTION Ø - MEDICAL AND SURGICAL
CHARACTER 3 - OPERATION

Restriction	**Definition:** Partially closing an orifice or the lumen of a tubular body part **Explanation:** The orifice can be a natural orifice or an artificially created orifice **Includes/Examples:** Esophagogastric fundoplication, cervical cerclage
Revision	**Definition:** Correcting, to the extent possible, a portion of a malfunctioning device or the position of a displaced device **Explanation:** Revision can include correcting a malfunctioning or displaced device by taking out or putting in components of the device such as a screw or pin **Includes/Examples:** Adjustment of position of pacemaker lead, recementing of hip prosthesis
Supplement	**Definition:** Putting in or on biological or synthetic material that physically reinforces and/or augments the function of a portion of a body part **Explanation:** The biological material is non-living, or is living and from the same individual. The body part may have been previously replaced, and the Supplement procedure is performed to physically reinforce and/or augment the function of the replaced body part **Includes/Examples:** Herniorrhaphy using mesh, mitral valve ring annuloplasty, put a new acetabular liner in a previous hip replacement
Transfer	**Definition:** Moving, without taking out, all or a portion of a body part to another location to take over the function of all or a portion of a body part **Explanation:** The body part transferred remains connected to its vascular and nervous supply **Includes/Examples:** Tendon transfer, skin pedicle flap transfer
Transplantation	**Definition:** Putting in or on all or a portion of a living body part taken from another individual or animal to physically take the place and/or function of all or a portion of a similar body part **Explanation:** The native body part may or may not be taken out, and the transplanted body part may take over all or a portion of its function **Includes/Examples:** Kidney transplant, heart transplant

SECTION Ø - MEDICAL AND SURGICAL
CHARACTER 4 - BODY PART

1st Toe, Left 1st Toe, Right	**Includes:** Hallux
Abdomen Muscle, Left Abdomen Muscle, Right	**Includes:** External oblique muscle Internal oblique muscle Pyramidalis muscle Rectus abdominis muscle Transversus abdominis muscle
Abdominal Aorta	**Includes:** Inferior phrenic artery Lumbar artery Median sacral artery Middle suprarenal artery Ovarian artery Testicular artery
Abdominal Sympathetic Nerve	**Includes:** Abdominal aortic plexus Auerbach's (myenteric) plexus Celiac (solar) plexus Celiac ganglion Gastric plexus Hepatic plexus Inferior hypogastric plexus Inferior mesenteric ganglion Inferior mesenteric plexus Meissner's (submucous) plexus Myenteric (Auerbach's) plexus Pancreatic plexus Pelvic splanchnic nerve Renal nerve Renal plexus Solar (celiac) plexus Splenic plexus Submucous (Meissner's) plexus Superior hypogastric plexus Superior mesenteric ganglion Superior mesenteric plexus Suprarenal plexus

SECTION Ø - MEDICAL AND SURGICAL
CHARACTER 4 - BODY PART

Body Part	Includes
Abducens Nerve	**Includes:** Sixth cranial nerve
Accessory Nerve	**Includes:** Eleventh cranial nerve
Acoustic Nerve	**Includes:** Cochlear nerve Eighth cranial nerve Scarpa's (vestibular) ganglion Spiral ganglion Vestibular (Scarpa's) ganglion Vestibular nerve Vestibulocochlear nerve
Adenoids	**Includes:** Pharyngeal tonsil
Adrenal Gland Adrenal Gland, Left Adrenal Gland, Right Adrenal Glands, Bilateral	**Includes:** Suprarenal gland
Ampulla of Vater	**Includes:** Duodenal ampulla Hepatopancreatic ampulla
Anal Sphincter	**Includes:** External anal sphincter Internal anal sphincter
Ankle Bursa and Ligament, Left Ankle Bursa and Ligament, Right	**Includes:** Calcaneofibular ligament Deltoid ligament Ligament of the lateral malleolus Talofibular ligament
Ankle Joint, Left Ankle Joint, Right	**Includes:** Inferior tibiofibular joint Talocrural joint
Anterior Chamber, Left Anterior Chamber, Right	**Includes:** Aqueous humour
Anterior Tibial Artery, Left Anterior Tibial Artery, Right	**Includes:** Anterior lateral malleolar artery Anterior medial malleolar artery Anterior tibial recurrent artery Dorsalis pedis artery Posterior tibial recurrent artery
Anus	**Includes:** Anal orifice
Aortic Valve	**Includes:** Aortic annulus
Appendix	**Includes:** Vermiform appendix
Atrial Septum	**Includes:** Interatrial septum
Atrium, Left	**Includes:** Atrium pulmonale Left auricular appendix
Atrium, Right	**Includes:** Atrium dextrum cordis Right auricular appendix Sinus venosus
Auditory Ossicle, Left Auditory Ossicle, Right	**Includes:** Incus Malleus Stapes
Axillary Artery, Left Axillary Artery, Right	**Includes:** Anterior circumflex humeral artery Lateral thoracic artery Posterior circumflex humeral artery Subscapular artery Superior thoracic artery Thoracoacromial artery
Azygos Vein	**Includes:** Right ascending lumbar vein Right subcostal vein
Basal Ganglia	**Includes:** Basal nuclei Claustrum Corpus striatum Globus pallidus Substantia nigra Subthalamic nucleus
Basilic Vein, Left Basilic Vein, Right	**Includes:** Median antebrachial vein Median cubital vein
Bladder	**Includes:** Trigone of bladder
Brachial Artery, Left Brachial Artery, Right	**Includes:** Inferior ulnar collateral artery Profunda brachii Superior ulnar collateral artery
Brachial Plexus	**Includes:** Axillary nerve Dorsal scapular nerve First intercostal nerve Long thoracic nerve Musculocutaneous nerve Subclavius nerve Suprascapular nerve

SECTION Ø - MEDICAL AND SURGICAL

CHARACTER 4 - BODY PART

Body Part	Includes
Brachial Vein, Left Brachial Vein, Right	**Includes:** Radial vein Ulnar vein
Brain	**Includes:** Cerebrum Corpus callosum Encephalon
Breast, Bilateral Breast, Left Breast, Right	**Includes:** Mammary duct Mammary gland
Buccal Mucosa	**Includes:** Buccal gland Molar gland Palatine gland
Carotid Bodies, Bilateral Carotid Body, Left Carotid Body, Right	**Includes:** Carotid glomus
Carpal Joint, Left Carpal Joint, Right	**Includes:** Intercarpal joint Midcarpal joint
Carpal, Left Carpal, Right	**Includes:** Capitate bone Hamate bone Lunate bone Pisiform bone Scaphoid bone Trapezium bone Trapezoid bone Triquetral bone
Celiac Artery	**Includes:** Celiac trunk
Cephalic Vein, Left Cephalic Vein, Right	**Includes:** Accessory cephalic vein
Cerebellum	**Includes:** Culmen
Cerebral Hemisphere	**Includes:** Frontal lobe Occipital lobe Parietal lobe Temporal lobe
Cerebral Meninges	**Includes:** Arachnoid mater, intracranial Leptomeninges, intracranial Pia mater, intracranial
Cerebral Ventricle	**Includes:** Aqueduct of Sylvius Cerebral aqueduct (Sylvius) Choroid plexus Ependyma Foramen of Monro (intraventricular) Fourth ventricle Interventricular foramen (Monro) Left lateral ventricle Right lateral ventricle Third ventricle
Cervical Nerve	**Includes:** Greater occipital nerve Spinal nerve, cervical Suboccipital nerve Third occipital nerve
Cervical Plexus	**Includes:** Ansa cervicalis Cutaneous (transverse) cervical nerve Great auricular nerve Lesser occipital nerve Supraclavicular nerve Transverse (cutaneous) cervical nerve
Cervical Spinal Cord	**Includes:** Dorsal root ganglion
Cervical Vertebra	**Includes:** Dens Odontoid process Spinous process Transverse foramen Transverse process Vertebral body Vertebral arch Vertebral foramen Vertebral lamina Vertebral pedicle
Cervical Vertebral Joint	**Includes:** Atlantoaxial joint Cervical facet joint
Cervical Vertebral Joints, 2 or more	**Includes:** Cervical facet joint
Cervicothoracic Vertebral Joint	**Includes:** Cervicothoracic facet joint
Cisterna Chyli	**Includes:** Intestinal lymphatic trunk Lumbar lymphatic trunk
Coccygeal Glomus	**Includes:** Coccygeal body

APPENDIX A

SECTION Ø - MEDICAL AND SURGICAL
CHARACTER 4 - BODY PART

Body Part	Includes
Colic Vein	**Includes:** Ileocolic vein Left colic vein Middle colic vein Right colic vein
Conduction Mechanism	**Includes:** Atrioventricular node Bundle of His Bundle of Kent Sinoatrial node
Conjunctiva, Left Conjunctiva, Right	**Includes:** Plica semilunaris
Dura Mater	**Includes:** Diaphragma sellae Dura mater, intracranial Falx cerebri Tentorium cerebelli
Elbow Bursa and Ligament, Left Elbow Bursa and Ligament, Right	**Includes:** Annular ligament Olecranon bursa Radial collateral ligament Ulnar collateral ligament
Elbow Joint, Left Elbow Joint, Right	**Includes:** Distal humerus, involving joint Humeroradial joint Humeroulnar joint Proximal radioulnar joint
Epidural Space, Intracranial	**Includes:** Extradural space, intracranial
Epiglottis	**Includes:** Glossoepiglottic fold
Esophagogastric Junction	**Includes:** Cardia Cardioesophageal junction Gastroesophageal (GE) junction
Esophagus, Lower	**Includes:** Abdominal esophagus
Esophagus, Middle	**Includes:** Thoracic esophagus
Esophagus, Upper	**Includes:** Cervical esophagus
Ethmoid Bone, Left Ethmoid Bone, Right	**Includes:** Cribriform plate
Ethmoid Sinus, Left Ethmoid Sinus, Right	**Includes:** Ethmoidal air cell
Eustachian Tube, Left Eustachian Tube, Right	**Includes:** Auditory tube Pharyngotympanic tube
External Auditory Canal, Left External Auditory Canal, Right	**Includes:** External auditory meatus
External Carotid Artery, Left External Carotid Artery, Right	**Includes:** Ascending pharyngeal artery Internal maxillary artery Lingual artery Maxillary artery Occipital artery Posterior auricular artery Superior thyroid artery
External Ear, Bilateral External Ear, Left External Ear, Right	**Includes:** Antihelix Antitragus Auricle Earlobe Helix Pinna Tragus
External Iliac Artery, Left External Iliac Artery, Right	**Includes:** Deep circumflex iliac artery Inferior epigastric artery
External Jugular Vein, Left External Jugular Vein, Right	**Includes:** Posterior auricular vein
Extraocular Muscle, Left Extraocular Muscle, Right	**Includes:** Inferior oblique muscle Inferior rectus muscle Lateral rectus muscle Medial rectus muscle Superior oblique muscle Superior rectus muscle
Eye, Left Eye, Right	**Includes:** Ciliary body Posterior chamber
Face Artery	**Includes:** Angular artery Ascending palatine artery External maxillary artery Facial artery Inferior labial artery Submental artery Superior labial artery

SECTION Ø - MEDICAL AND SURGICAL

CHARACTER 4 - BODY PART

Body Part	Includes
Face Vein, Left Face Vein, Right	**Includes:** Angular vein Anterior facial vein Common facial vein Deep facial vein Frontal vein Posterior facial (retromandibular) vein Supraorbital vein
Facial Muscle	**Includes:** Buccinator muscle Corrugator supercilii muscle Depressor anguli oris muscle Depressor labii inferioris muscle Depressor septi nasi muscle Depressor supercilii muscle Levator anguli oris muscle Levator labii superioris alaeque nasi muscle Levator labii superioris muscle Mentalis muscle Nasalis muscle Occipitofrontalis muscle Orbicularis oris muscle Procerus muscle Risorius muscle Zygomaticus muscle
Facial Nerve	**Includes:** Chorda tympani Geniculate ganglion Greater superficial petrosal nerve Nerve to the stapedius Parotid plexus Posterior auricular nerve Seventh cranial nerve Submandibular ganglion
Fallopian Tube, Left Fallopian Tube, Right	**Includes:** Oviduct Salpinx Uterine tube
Femoral Artery, Left Femoral Artery, Right	**Includes:** Circumflex iliac artery Deep femoral artery Descending genicular artery External pudendal artery Superficial epigastric artery
Femoral Nerve	**Includes:** Anterior crural nerve Saphenous nerve
Femoral Shaft, Left Femoral Shaft, Right	**Includes:** Body of femur
Femoral Vein, Left Femoral Vein, Right	**Includes:** Deep femoral (profunda femoris) vein Popliteal vein Profunda femoris (deep femoral) vein
Fibula, Left Fibula, Right	**Includes:** Body of fibula Head of fibula Lateral malleolus
Finger Nail	**Includes:** Nail bed Nail plate
Finger Phalangeal Joint, Left Finger Phalangeal Joint, Right	**Includes:** Interphalangeal (IP) joint
Foot Artery, Left Foot Artery, Right	**Includes:** Arcuate artery Dorsal metatarsal artery Lateral plantar artery Lateral tarsal artery Medial plantar artery
Foot Bursa and Ligament, Left Foot Bursa and Ligament, Right	**Includes:** Calcaneocuboid ligament Cuneonavicular ligament Intercuneiform ligament Interphalangeal ligament Metatarsal ligament Metatarsophalangeal ligament Subtalar ligament Talocalcaneal ligament Talocalcaneonavicular ligament Tarsometatarsal ligament
Foot Muscle, Left Foot Muscle, Right	**Includes:** Abductor hallucis muscle Adductor hallucis muscle Extensor digitorum brevis muscle Extensor hallucis brevis muscle Flexor digitorum brevis muscle Flexor hallucis brevis muscle Quadratus plantae muscle
Foot Vein, Left Foot Vein, Right	**Includes:** Common digital vein Dorsal metatarsal vein Dorsal venous arch Plantar digital vein Plantar metatarsal vein Plantar venous arch
Frontal Bone	**Includes:** Zygomatic process of frontal bone

APPENDIX A

SECTION Ø - MEDICAL AND SURGICAL
CHARACTER 4 - BODY PART

Body Part	Includes
Gastric Artery	**Includes:** Left gastric artery Right gastric artery
Glenoid Cavity, Left Glenoid Cavity, Right	**Includes:** Glenoid fossa (of scapula)
Glomus Jugulare	**Includes:** Jugular body
Glossopharyngeal Nerve	**Includes:** Carotid sinus nerve Ninth cranial nerve Tympanic nerve
Hand Artery, Left Hand Artery, Right	**Includes:** Deep palmar arch Princeps pollicis artery Radialis indicis Superficial palmar arch
Hand Bursa and Ligament, Left Hand Bursa and Ligament, Right	**Includes:** Carpometacarpal ligament Intercarpal ligament Interphalangeal ligament Lunotriquetral ligament Metacarpal ligament Metacarpophalangeal ligament Pisohamate ligament Pisometacarpal ligament Scaphotrapezium ligament
Hand Muscle, Left Hand Muscle, Right	**Includes:** Adductor pollicis muscle Hypothenar muscle Palmar interosseous muscle Thenar muscle
Hand Vein, Left Hand Vein, Right	**Includes:** Dorsal metacarpal vein Palmar (volar) digital vein Palmar (volar) metacarpal vein Superficial palmar venous arch Volar (palmar) digital vein Volar (palmar) metacarpal vein
Head and Neck Bursa and Ligament	**Includes:** Alar ligament of axis Cervical interspinous ligament Cervical intertransverse ligament Cervical ligamentum flavum Interspinous ligament, cervical Intertransverse ligament, cervical Lateral temporomandibular ligament Ligamentum flavum, cervical Sphenomandibular ligament Stylomandibular ligament Transverse ligament of atlas
Head and Neck Sympathetic Nerve	**Includes:** Cavernous plexus Cervical ganglion Ciliary ganglion Internal carotid plexus Otic ganglion Pterygopalatine (sphenopalatine) ganglion Sphenopalatine (pterygopalatine) ganglion Stellate ganglion Submandibular ganglion Submaxillary ganglion
Head Muscle	**Includes:** Auricularis muscle Masseter muscle Pterygoid muscle Splenius capitis muscle Temporalis muscle Temporoparietalis muscle
Heart, Left	**Includes:** Left coronary sulcus Obtuse margin
Heart, Right	**Includes:** Right coronary sulcus
Hemiazygos Vein	**Includes** Left ascending lumbar vein Left subcostal vein
Hepatic Artery	**Includes:** Common hepatic artery Gastroduodenal artery Hepatic artery proper
Hip Bursa and Ligament, Left Hip Bursa and Ligament, Right	**Includes:** Iliofemoral ligament Ischiofemoral ligament Pubofemoral ligament Transverse acetabular ligament Trochanteric bursa
Hip Joint, Left Hip Joint, Right	**Includes:** Acetabulofemoral joint
Hip Muscle, Left Hip Muscle, Right	**Includes:** Gemellus muscle Gluteus maximus muscle Gluteus medius muscle Gluteus minimus muscle Iliacus muscle Iliopsoas muscle Obturator muscle Piriformis muscle Psoas muscle Quadratus femoris muscle Tensor fasciae latae muscle

SECTION Ø - MEDICAL AND SURGICAL
CHARACTER 4 - BODY PART

Body Part	Includes
Humeral Head, Left Humeral Head, Right	**Includes:** Greater tuberosity Lesser tuberosity Neck of humerus (anatomical) (surgical)
Humeral Shaft, Left Humeral Shaft, Right	**Includes:** Distal humerus Humerus, distal Lateral epicondyle of humerus Medial epicondyle of humerus
Hypogastric Vein, Left Hypogastric Vein, Right	**Includes:** Gluteal vein Internal iliac vein Internal pudendal vein Lateral sacral vein Middle hemorrhoidal vein Obturator vein Uterine vein Vaginal vein Vesical vein
Hypoglossal Nerve	**Includes:** Twelfth cranial nerve
Hypothalamus	**Includes:** Mammillary body
Inferior Mesenteric Artery	**Includes:** Sigmoid artery Superior rectal artery
Inferior Mesenteric Vein	**Includes:** Sigmoid vein Superior rectal vein
Inferior Vena Cava	**Includes:** Postcava Right inferior phrenic vein Right ovarian vein Right second lumbar vein Right suprarenal vein Right testicular vein
Inguinal Region, Bilateral Inguinal Region, Left Inguinal Region, Right	**Includes:** Inguinal canal Inguinal triangle
Inner Ear, Left Inner Ear, Right	**Includes:** Bony labyrinth Bony vestibule Cochlea Round window Semicircular canal
Innominate Artery	**Includes:** Brachiocephalic artery Brachiocephalic trunk
Innominate Vein, Left Innominate Vein, Right	**Includes:** Brachiocephalic vein Inferior thyroid vein
Internal Carotid Artery, Left Internal Carotid Artery, Right	**Includes:** Caroticotympanic artery Carotid sinus
Internal Iliac Artery, Left Internal Iliac Artery, Right	**Includes:** Deferential artery Hypogastric artery Iliolumbar artery Inferior gluteal artery Inferior vesical artery Internal pudendal artery Lateral sacral artery Middle rectal artery Obturator artery Superior gluteal artery Umbilical artery Uterine Artery Vaginal artery
Internal Mammary Artery, Left Internal Mammary Artery, Right	**Includes:** Anterior intercostal artery Internal thoracic artery Musculophrenic artery Pericardiophrenic artery Superior epigastric artery
Intracranial Artery	**Includes:** Anterior cerebral artery Anterior choroidal artery Anterior communicating artery Basilar artery Circle of Willis Internal carotid artery, intracranial portion Middle cerebral artery Middle meningeal artery, intracranial portion Ophthalmic artery Posterior cerebral artery Posterior communicating artery Posterior inferior cerebellar artery (PICA) Vertebral artery, intracranial portion

APPENDIX A

SECTION Ø - MEDICAL AND SURGICAL
CHARACTER 4 - BODY PART

Body Part	Includes
Intracranial Vein	**Includes:** Anterior cerebral vein Basal (internal) cerebral vein Dural venous sinus Great cerebral vein Inferior cerebellar vein Inferior cerebral vein Internal (basal) cerebral vein Middle cerebral vein Ophthalmic vein Superior cerebellar vein Superior cerebral vein
Jejunum	**Includes:** Duodenojejunal flexure
Kidney	**Includes:** Renal calyx Renal capsule Renal cortex Renal segment
Kidney Pelvis, Left Kidney Pelvis, Right	**Includes:** Ureteropelvic junction (UPJ)
Kidney, Left Kidney, Right Kidneys, Bilateral	**Includes:** Renal calyx Renal capsule Renal cortex Renal segment
Knee Bursa and Ligament, Left Knee Bursa and Ligament, Right	**Includes:** Anterior cruciate ligament (ACL) Lateral collateral ligament (LCL) Ligament of head of fibula Medial collateral ligament (MCL) Patellar ligament Popliteal ligament Posterior cruciate ligament (PCL) Prepatellar bursa
Knee Joint, Femoral Surface, Left Knee Joint, Femoral Surface, Right	**Includes:** Femoropatellar joint Patellofemoral joint
Knee Joint, Left Knee Joint, Right	**Includes:** Femoropatellar joint Femorotibial joint Lateral meniscus Medial meniscus Patellofemoral joint Popliteal fossa Tibiofemoral joint
Knee Joint, Tibial Surface, Left Knee Joint, Tibial Surface, Right	**Includes:** Femorotibial joint Tibiofemoral joint
Knee Tendon, Left Knee Tendon, Right	**Includes:** Patellar tendon
Lacrimal Duct, Left Lacrimal Duct, Right	**Includes:** Lacrimal canaliculus Lacrimal punctum Lacrimal sac Nasolacrimal duct
Larynx	**Includes:** Aryepiglottic fold Arytenoid cartilage Corniculate cartilage Cuneiform cartilage False vocal cord Glottis Rima glottidis Thyroid cartilage Ventricular fold
Lens, Left Lens, Right	**Includes:** Zonule of Zinn
Liver	**Includes:** Quadrate lobe
Lower Arm and Wrist Muscle, Left Lower Arm and Wrist Muscle, Right	**Includes:** Anatomical snuffbox Anconeus muscle Brachioradialis muscle Extensor carpi radialis muscle Extensor carpi ulnaris muscle Flexor carpi radialis muscle Flexor carpi ulnaris muscle Flexor pollicis longus muscle Palmaris longus muscle Pronator quadratus muscle Pronator teres muscle
Lower Artery	**Includes:** Umbilical artery
Lower Eyelid, Left Lower Eyelid, Right	**Includes:** Inferior tarsal plate Medial canthus
Lower Femur, Left Lower Femur, Right	**Includes:** Lateral condyle of femur Lateral epicondyle of femur Medial condyle of femur Medial epicondyle of femur

SECTION Ø, CHARACTER 4

SECTION Ø - MEDICAL AND SURGICAL

CHARACTER 4 - BODY PART

Lower Leg Muscle, Left Lower Leg Muscle, Right	**Includes:** Extensor digitorum longus muscle Extensor hallucis longus muscle Fibularis brevis muscle Fibularis longus muscle Flexor digitorum longus muscle Flexor hallucis longus muscle Gastrocnemius muscle Peroneus brevis muscle Peroneus longus muscle Plantaris muscle Popliteus muscle Soleus muscle Tibialis anterior muscle Tibialis posterior muscle
Lower Leg Tendon, Left Lower Leg Tendon, Right	**Includes:** Achilles tendon
Lower Lip	**Includes:** Frenulum labii inferioris Labial gland Vermilion border
Lower Spine Bursa and Ligament	**Includes:** Iliolumbar ligament Interspinous ligament, lumbar Intertransverse ligament, lumbar Ligamentum flavum, lumbar Sacrococcygeal ligament Sacroiliac ligament Sacrospinous ligament Sacrotuberous ligament Supraspinous ligament
Lumbar Nerve	**Includes:** Lumbosacral trunk Spinal nerve, lumbar Superior clunic (cluneal) nerve
Lumbar Plexus	**Includes:** Accessory obturator nerve Genitofemoral nerve Iliohypogastric nerve Ilioinguinal nerve Lateral femoral cutaneous nerve Obturator nerve Superior gluteal nerve
Lumbar Spinal Cord	**Includes:** Cauda equina Conus medullaris Dorsal root ganglion
Lumbar Sympathetic Nerve	**Includes:** Lumbar ganglion Lumbar splanchnic nerve

Lumbar Vertebra	**Includes:** Spinous process Transverse process Vertebral arch Vertebral body Vertebral foramen Vertebral lamina Vertebral pedicle
Lumbar Vertebral Joint	**Includes:** Lumbar facet joint
Lumbosacral Joint	**Includes:** Lumbosacral facet joint
Lymphatic, Aortic	**Includes:** Celiac lymph node Gastric lymph node Hepatic lymph node Lumbar lymph node Pancreaticosplenic lymph node Paraaortic lymph node Retroperitoneal lymph node
Lymphatic, Head	**Includes:** Buccinator lymph node Infraauricular lymph node Infraparotid lymph node Parotid lymph node Preauricular lymph node Submandibular lymph node Submaxillary lymph node Submental lymph node Subparotid lymph node Suprahyoid lymph node
Lymphatic, Left Axillary	**Includes:** Anterior (pectoral) lymph node Apical (subclavicular) lymph node Brachial (lateral) lymph node Central axillary lymph node Lateral (brachial) lymph node Pectoral (anterior) lymph node Posterior (subscapular) lymph node Subclavicular (apical) lymph node Subscapular (posterior) lymph node
Lymphatic, Left Lower Extremity	**Includes:** Femoral lymph node Popliteal lymph node
Lymphatic, Left Neck	**Includes:** Cervical lymph node Jugular lymph node Mastoid (postauricular) lymph node Occipital lymph node Postauricular (mastoid) lymph node Retropharyngeal lymph node Supraclavicular (Virchow's) lymph node Virchow's (supraclavicular) lymph node

APPENDIX A

SECTION Ø - MEDICAL AND SURGICAL
CHARACTER 4 - BODY PART

Body Part	Includes
Lymphatic, Left Upper Extremity	**Includes:** Cubital lymph node Deltopectoral (infraclavicular) lymph node Epitrochlear lymph node Infraclavicular (deltopectoral) lymph node Supratrochlear lymph node
Lymphatic, Mesenteric	**Includes:** Inferior mesenteric lymph node Pararectal lymph node Superior mesenteric lymph node
Lymphatic, Pelvis	**Includes:** Common iliac (subaortic) lymph node Gluteal lymph node Iliac lymph node Inferior epigastric lymph node Obturator lymph node Sacral lymph node Subaortic (common iliac) lymph node Suprainguinal lymph node
Lymphatic, Right Axillary	**Includes:** Anterior (pectoral) lymph node Apical (subclavicular) lymph node Brachial (lateral) lymph node Central axillary lymph node Lateral (brachial) lymph node Pectoral (anterior) lymph node Posterior (subscapular) lymph node Subclavicular (apical) lymph node Subscapular (posterior) lymph node
Lymphatic, Right Lower Extremity	**Includes:** Femoral lymph node Popliteal lymph node
Lymphatic, Right Neck	**Includes:** Cervical lymph node Jugular lymph node Mastoid (postauricular) lymph node Occipital lymph node Postauricular (mastoid) lymph node Retropharyngeal lymph node Right jugular trunk Right lymphatic duct Right subclavian trunk Supraclavicular (Virchow's) lymph node Virchow's (supraclavicular) lymph node
Lymphatic, Right Upper Extremity	**Includes:** Cubital lymph node Deltopectoral (infraclavicular) lymph node Epitrochlear lymph node Infraclavicular (deltopectoral) lymph node Supratrochlear lymph node
Lymphatic, Thorax	**Includes:** Intercostal lymph node Mediastinal lymph node Parasternal lymph node Paratracheal lymph node Tracheobronchial lymph node
Main Bronchus, Right	**Includes:** Bronchus Intermedius Intermediate bronchus
Mandible, Left Mandible, Right	**Includes:** Alveolar process of mandible Condyloid process Mandibular notch Mental foramen
Mastoid Sinus, Left Mastoid Sinus, Right	**Includes:** Mastoid air cells
Maxilla	**Includes:** Alveolar process of maxilla
Maxillary Sinus, Left Maxillary Sinus, Right	**Includes:** Antrum of Highmore
Median Nerve	**Includes:** Anterior interosseous nerve Palmar cutaneous nerve
Mediastinum	**Includes:** Mediastinal cavity Mediastinal space
Medulla Oblongata	**Includes:** Myelencephalon
Mesentery	**Includes:** Mesoappendix Mesocolon
Metatarsal, Left Metatarsal, Right	**Includes:** Fibular sesamoid Tibial sesamoid
Metatarsal-Phalangeal Joint, Left Metatarsal-Phalangeal Joint, Right	**Includes:** Metatarsophalangeal (MTP) joint
Middle Ear, Left Middle Ear, Right	**Includes:** Oval window Tympanic cavity
Minor Salivary Gland	**Includes:** Anterior lingual gland

SECTION Ø - MEDICAL AND SURGICAL

CHARACTER 4 - BODY PART

Body Part	Includes
Mitral Valve	**Includes:** Bicuspid valve Left atrioventricular valve Mitral annulus
Nasal Bone	**Includes:** Vomer of nasal septum
Nasal Mucosa and Soft Tissue	**Includes:** Columella External naris Greater alar cartilage Internal naris Lateral nasal cartilage Lesser alar cartilage Nasal cavity Nostril
Nasal Septum	**Includes:** Quadrangular cartilage Septal cartilage Vomer bone
Nasal Turbinate	**Includes:** Inferior turbinate Middle turbinate Nasal concha Superior turbinate
Nasopharynx	**Includes:** Choana Fossa of Rosenmuller Pharyngeal recess Rhinopharynx
Neck	**Includes:** Parapharyngeal space Retropharyngeal
Neck Muscle, Left Neck Muscle, Right	**Includes:** Anterior vertebral muscle Arytenoid muscle Cricothyroid muscle Infrahyoid muscle Levator scapulae muscle Platysma muscle Scalene muscle Splenius cervicis muscle Sternocleidomastoid muscle Suprahyoid muscle Thyroarytenoid muscle
Nipple, Left Nipple, Right	**Includes:** Areola
Occipital Bone	**Includes:** Foramen magnum
Oculomotor Nerve	**Includes:** Third cranial nerve
Olfactory Nerve	**Includes:** First cranial nerve Olfactory bulb
Omentum	**Includes:** Gastrocolic ligament Gastrocolic omentum Gastrohepatic omentum Gastrophrenic ligament Gastrosplenic ligament Greater omentum Hepatogastric ligament Lesser omentum
Optic Nerve	**Includes:** Optic chiasma Second cranial nerve
Orbit, Left Orbit, Right	**Includes:** Bony orbit Orbital portion of ethmoid bone Orbital portion of frontal bone Orbital portion of lacrimal bone Orbital portion of maxilla Orbital portion of palatine bone Orbital portion of sphenoid bone Orbital portion of zygomatic bone
Pancreatic Duct	**Includes:** Duct of Wirsung
Pancreatic Duct, Accessory	**Includes:** Duct of Santorini
Parotid Duct, Left Parotid Duct, Right	**Includes:** Stensen's duct
Pelvic Bone, Left Pelvic Bone, Right	**Includes:** Iliac crest Ilium Ischium Pubis
Pelvic Cavity	**Includes:** Prevesical space Retropubic space Space of Retzius
Penis	**Includes:** Corpus cavernosum Corpus spongiosum
Perineum Muscle	**Includes:** Bulbospongiosus muscle Cremaster muscle Deep transverse perineal muscle Ischiocavernosus muscle Levator ani muscle Superficial transverse perineal muscle
Peritoneum	**Includes:** Epiploic foramen
Peroneal Artery, Left Peroneal Artery, Right	**Includes:** Fibular artery

APPENDIX A

SECTION Ø - MEDICAL AND SURGICAL
CHARACTER 4 - BODY PART

Peroneal Nerve	**Includes:** Common fibular nerve Common peroneal nerve External popliteal nerve Lateral sural cutaneous nerve
Pharynx	**Includes:** Base of tongue Hypopharynx Laryngopharynx Lingual tonsil Oropharynx Piriform recess (sinus) Tongue, base of
Phrenic Nerve	**Includes:** Accessory phrenic nerve
Pituitary Gland	**Includes:** Adenohypophysis Hypophysis Neurohypophysis
Pons	**Includes:** Apneustic center Basis pontis Locus ceruleus Pneumotaxic center Pontine tegmentum Superior olivary nucleus
Popliteal Artery, Left Popliteal Artery, Right	**Includes:** Inferior genicular artery Middle genicular artery Superior genicular artery Sural artery Tibioperoneal trunk
Portal Vein	**Includes:** Hepatic portal vein
Prepuce	**Includes:** Foreskin Glans penis
Pudendal Nerve	**Includes:** Posterior labial nerve Posterior scrotal nerve
Pulmonary Artery, Left	**Includes:** Arterial canal (duct) Botallo's duct Pulmoaortic canal
Pulmonary Valve	**Includes:** Pulmonary annulus Pulmonic valve
Pulmonary Vein, Left	**Includes:** Left inferior pulmonary vein Left superior pulmonary vein
Pulmonary Vein, Right	**Includes:** Right inferior pulmonary vein Right superior pulmonary vein
Radial Artery, Left Radial Artery, Right	**Includes:** Radial recurrent artery
Radial Nerve	**Includes:** Dorsal digital nerve Musculospiral nerve Palmar cutaneous nerve Posterior interosseous nerve
Radius, Left Radius, Right	**Includes:** Ulnar notch
Rectum	**Includes:** Anorectal junction
Renal Artery, Left Renal Artery, Right	**Includes:** Inferior suprarenal artery Renal segmental artery
Renal Vein, Left	**Includes:** Left inferior phrenic vein Left ovarian vein Left second lumbar vein Left suprarenal vein Left testicular vein
Retina, Left Retina, Right	**Includes:** Fovea Macula Optic disc
Retroperitoneum	**Includes:** Retroperitoneal cavity Retroperitoneal space
Rib(s) Bursa and Ligament	**Includes:** Costoxiphoid ligament
Sacral Nerve	**Includes:** Spinal nerve, sacral
Sacral Plexus	**Includes:** Inferior gluteal nerve Posterior femoral cutaneous nerve Pudendal nerve
Sacral Sympathetic Nerve	**Includes:** Ganglion impar (ganglion of Walther) Pelvic splanchnic nerve Sacral ganglion Sacral splanchnic nerve
Sacrococcygeal Joint	**Includes:** Sacrococcygeal symphysis

SECTION Ø, CHARACTER 4

SECTION Ø - MEDICAL AND SURGICAL
CHARACTER 4 - BODY PART

Body Part	Includes
Saphenous Vein, Left Saphenous Vein, Right	**Includes:** External pudendal vein Great(er) saphenous vein Lesser saphenous vein Small saphenous vein Superficial circumflex iliac vein Superficial epigastric vein
Scapula, Left Scapula, Right	**Includes:** Acromion (process) Coracoid process
Sciatic Nerve	**Includes:** Ischiatic nerve
Shoulder Bursa and Ligament, Left Shoulder Bursa and Ligament, Right	**Includes:** Acromioclavicular ligament Coracoacromial ligament Coracoclavicular ligament Coracohumeral ligament Costoclavicular ligament Glenohumeral ligament Interclavicular ligament Sternoclavicular ligament Subacromial bursa Transverse humeral ligament Transverse scapular ligament
Shoulder Joint, Left Shoulder Joint, Right	**Includes:** Glenohumeral joint Glenoid ligament (labrum)
Shoulder Muscle, Left Shoulder Muscle, Right	**Includes:** Deltoid muscle Infraspinatus muscle Subscapularis muscle Supraspinatus muscle Teres major muscle Teres minor muscle
Sigmoid Colon	**Includes:** Rectosigmoid junction Sigmoid flexure
Skin	**Includes:** Dermis Epidermis Sebaceous gland Sweat gland
Skin, Chest	**Includes:** Breast procedures, skin only
Sphenoid Bone	**Includes:** Greater wing Lesser wing Optic foramen Pterygoid process Sella turcica

Body Part	Includes
Spinal Canal	**Includes:** Epidural space, spinal Extradural space, spinal Subarachnoid space, spinal Subdural space, spinal Vertebral canal
Spinal Cord	**Includes:** Dorsal root ganglion
Spinal Meninges	**Includes:** Arachnoid mater, spinal Denticulate (dentate) ligament Dura mater, spinal Filum terminale Leptomeninges, spinal Pia mater, spinal
Spleen	**Includes:** Accessory spleen
Splenic Artery	**Includes:** Left gastroepiploic artery Pancreatic artery Short gastric artery
Splenic Vein	**Includes:** Left gastroepiploic vein Pancreatic vein
Sternum	**Includes:** Manubrium Suprasternal notch Xiphoid process
Sternum Bursa and Ligament	**Includes:** Costoxiphoid ligament Sternocostal ligament
Stomach, Pylorus	**Includes:** Pyloric antrum Pyloric canal Pyloric sphincter
Subclavian Artery, Left Subclavian Artery, Right	**Includes:** Costocervical trunk Dorsal scapular artery Internal thoracic artery
Subcutaneous Tissue and Fascia, Chest	**Includes:** Pectoral fascia
Subcutaneous Tissue and Fascia, Face	**Includes:** Chin Masseteric fascia Orbital fascia Submandibular space
Subcutaneous Tissue and Fascia, Left Foot	**Includes:** Plantar fascia (aponeurosis)

APPENDIX A

SECTION Ø - MEDICAL AND SURGICAL
CHARACTER 4 - BODY PART

Body Part	Includes
Subcutaneous Tissue and Fascia, Left Hand	**Includes:** Palmar fascia (aponeurosis)
Subcutaneous Tissue and Fascia, Left Lower Arm	**Includes:** Antebrachial fascia Bicipital aponeurosis
Subcutaneous Tissue and Fascia, Left Neck	**Includes:** Deep cervical fascia Pretracheal fascia Prevertebral fascia
Subcutaneous Tissue and Fascia, Left Upper Arm	**Includes:** Axillary fascia Deltoid fascia Infraspinatus fascia Subscapular aponeurosis Supraspinatus fascia
Subcutaneous Tissue and Fascia, Left Upper Leg	**Includes:** Crural fascia Fascia lata Iliac fascia Iliotibial tract (band)
Subcutaneous Tissue and Fascia, Right Foot	**Includes:** Plantar fascia (aponeurosis)
Subcutaneous Tissue and Fascia, Right Hand	**Includes:** Palmar fascia (aponeurosis)
Subcutaneous Tissue and Fascia, Right Lower Arm	**Includes:** Antebrachial fascia Bicipital aponeurosis
Subcutaneous Tissue and Fascia, Right Neck	**Includes:** Deep cervical fascia Pretracheal fascia Prevertebral fascia
Subcutaneous Tissue and Fascia, Right Upper Arm	**Includes:** Axillary fascia Deltoid fascia Infraspinatus fascia Subscapular aponeurosis Supraspinatus fascia
Subcutaneous Tissue and Fascia, Right Upper Leg	**Includes:** Crural fascia Fascia lata Iliac fascia Iliotibial tract (band)
Subcutaneous Tissue and Fascia, Scalp	**Includes:** Galea aponeurotica
Subcutaneous Tissue and Fascia, Trunk	**Includes:** External oblique aponeurosis Transversalis fascia
Submaxillary Gland, Left Submaxillary Gland, Right	**Includes:** Submandibular gland
Superior Mesenteric Artery	**Includes:** Ileal artery Ileocolic artery Inferior pancreaticoduodenal artery Jejunal artery
Superior Mesenteric Vein	**Includes:** Right gastroepiploic vein
Superior Vena Cava	**Includes:** Precava
Tarsal Joint, Left Tarsal Joint, Right	**Includes:** Calcaneocuboid joint Cuboideonavicular joint Cuneonavicular joint Intercuneiform joint Subtalar (talocalcaneal) joint Talocalcaneal (subtalar) joint Talocalcaneonavicular joint
Tarsal, Left Tarsal, Right	**Includes:** Calcaneus Cuboid bone Intermediate cuneiform bone Lateral cuneiform bone Medial cuneiform bone Navicular bone Talus bone
Temporal Artery, Left Temporal Artery, Right	**Includes:** Middle temporal artery Superficial temporal artery Transverse facial artery
Temporal Bone, Left Temporal Bone, Right	**Includes:** Mastoid process Petrous part of temporal bone Tympanic part of temporal bone Zygomatic process of temporal bone
Thalamus	**Includes:** Epithalamus Geniculate nucleus Metathalamus Pulvinar
Thoracic Aorta, Ascending/Arch	**Includes:** Aortic arch Aortic isthmus Ascending aorta Juxtaductal aorta
Thoracic Duct	**Includes:** Left jugular trunk Left subclavian trunk

SECTION Ø - MEDICAL AND SURGICAL
CHARACTER 4 - BODY PART

Body Part	Includes
Thoracic Nerve	**Includes:** Intercostal nerve Intercostobrachial nerve Spinal nerve, thoracic Subcostal nerve
Thoracic Spinal Cord	**Includes:** Dorsal root ganglion
Thoracic Sympathetic Nerve	**Includes:** Cardiac plexus Esophageal plexus Greater splanchnic nerve Inferior cardiac nerve Least splanchnic nerve Lesser splanchnic nerve Middle cardiac nerve Pulmonary plexus Superior cardiac nerve Thoracic aortic plexus Thoracic ganglion
Thoracic Vertebra	**Includes:** Spinous process Transverse process Vertebral arch Vertebral body Vertebral foramen Vertebral lamina Vertebral pedicle
Thoracic Vertebral Joint	**Includes:** Costotransverse joint Costovertebral joint Thoracic facet joint
Thoracolumbar Vertebral Joint	**Includes:** Thoracolumbar facet joint
Thorax Muscle, Left Thorax Muscle, Right	**Includes:** Intercostal muscle Levatores costarum muscle Pectoralis major muscle Pectoralis minor muscle Serratus anterior muscle Subclavius muscle Subcostal muscle Transverse thoracis muscle
Thymus	**Includes:** Thymus gland
Thyroid Artery, Left Thyroid Artery, Right	**Includes:** Cricothyroid artery Hyoid artery Sternocleidomastoid artery Superior laryngeal artery Superior thyroid artery Thyrocervical trunk
Tibia, Left Tibia, Right	**Includes:** Lateral condyle of tibia Medial condyle of tibia Medial malleolus
Tibial Nerve	**Includes:** Lateral plantar nerve Medial plantar nerve Medial popliteal nerve Medial sural cutaneous nerve
Toe Nail	**Includes:** Nail bed Nail plate
Toe Phalangeal Joint, Left Toe Phalangeal Joint, Right	**Includes:** Interphalangeal (IP) joint
Tongue	**Includes:** Frenulum linguae
Tongue, Palate, Pharynx Muscle	**Includes:** Chrondroglossus muscle Genioglossus muscle Hyoglossus muscle Inferior longitudinal muscle Levator veli palatini muscle Palatoglossal muscle Palatopharyngeal muscle Pharyngeal constrictor muscle Salpingopharyngeus muscle Styloglossus muscle Stylopharyngeus muscle Superior longitudinal muscle Tensor veli palatini muscle
Tonsils	**Includes:** Palatine tonsil
Trachea	**Includes:** Cricoid cartilage
Transverse Colon	**Includes:** Hepatic flexure Splenic flexure
Tricuspid Valve	**Includes:** Right atrioventricular valve Tricuspid annulus
Trigeminal Nerve	**Includes:** Fifth cranial nerve Gasserian ganglion Mandibular nerve Maxillary nerve Ophthalmic nerve Trifacial nerve
Trochlear Nerve	**Includes:** Fourth cranial nerve

SECTION Ø - MEDICAL AND SURGICAL
CHARACTER 4 - BODY PART

Trunk Muscle, Left Trunk Muscle, Right	**Includes:** Coccygeus muscle Erector spinae muscle Interspinalis muscle Intertransversarius muscle Latissimus dorsi muscle Quadratus lumborum muscle Rhomboid major muscle Rhomboid minor muscle Serratus posterior muscle Transversospinalis muscle Trapezius muscle
Tympanic Membrane, Left Tympanic Membrane, Right	**Includes:** Pars flaccida
Ulna, Left Ulna, Right	**Includes:** Olecranon process Radial notch
Ulnar Artery, Left Ulnar Artery, Right	**Includes:** Anterior ulnar recurrent artery Common interosseous artery Posterior ulnar recurrent artery
Ulnar Nerve	**Includes:** Cubital nerve
Upper Arm Muscle, Left Upper Arm Muscle, Right	**Includes:** Biceps brachii muscle Brachialis muscle Coracobrachialis muscle Triceps brachii muscle
Upper Artery	**Includes:** Aortic intercostal artery Bronchial artery Esophageal artery Subcostal artery
Upper Eyelid, Left Upper Eyelid, Right	**Includes:** Lateral canthus Levator palpebrae superioris muscle Orbicularis oculi muscle Superior tarsal plate
Upper Femur, Left Upper Femur, Right	**Includes:** Femoral head Greater trochanter Lesser trochanter Neck of femur

Upper Leg Muscle, Left Upper Leg Muscle, Right	**Includes:** Adductor brevis muscle Adductor longus muscle Adductor magnus muscle Biceps femoris muscle Gracilis muscle Hamstring muscle Pectineus muscle Quadriceps (femoris) Rectus femoris muscle Sartorius muscle Semimembranosus muscle Semitendinosus muscle Vastus intermedius muscle Vastus lateralis muscle Vastus medialis muscle
Upper Lip	**Includes:** Frenulum labii superioris Labial gland Vermilion border
Upper Spine Bursa and Ligament	**Includes:** Interspinous ligament, thoracic Intertransverse ligament, thoracic Ligamentum flavum, thoracic Supraspinous ligament
Ureter Ureter, Left Ureter, Right Ureters, Bilateral	**Includes:** Ureteral orifice Ureterovesical orifice
Urethra	**Includes:** Bulbourethral (Cowper's) gland Cowper's (bulbourethral) gland External urethral sphincter Internal urethral sphincter Membranous urethra Penile urethra Prostatic urethra
Uterine Supporting Structure	**Includes:** Broad ligament Infundibulopelvic ligament Ovarian ligament Round ligament of uterus
Uterus	**Includes:** Fundus uteri Myometrium Perimetrium Uterine cornu
Uvula	**Includes:** Palatine uvula

SECTION Ø - MEDICAL AND SURGICAL
CHARACTER 4 - BODY PART

Vagus Nerve	**Includes:** Anterior vagal trunk Pharyngeal plexus Pneumogastric nerve Posterior vagal trunk Pulmonary plexus Recurrent laryngeal nerve Superior laryngeal nerve Tenth cranial nerve
Vas Deferens Vas Deferens, Bilateral Vas Deferens, Left Vas Deferens, Right	**Includes:** Ductus deferens Ejaculatory duct
Ventricle, Right	**Includes:** Conus arteriosus
Ventricular Septum	**Includes:** Interventricular septum
Vertebral Artery, Left Vertebral Artery, Right	**Includes:** Anterior spinal artery Posterior spinal artery
Vertebral Vein, Left Vertebral Vein, Right	**Includes:** Deep cervical vein Suboccipital venous plexus
Vestibular Gland	**Includes:** Bartholin's (greater vestibular) gland Greater vestibular (Bartholin's) gland Paraurethral (Skene's) gland Skene's (paraurethral) gland
Vitreous, Left Vitreous, Right	**Includes:** Vitreous body
Vocal Cord, Left Vocal Cord, Right	**Includes:** Vocal fold
Vulva	**Includes:** Labia majora Labia minora
Wrist Bursa and Ligament, Left Wrist Bursa and Ligament, Right	**Includes:** Palmar ulnocarpal ligament Radial collateral carpal ligament Radiocarpal ligament Radioulnar ligament Scapholunate ligament Ulnar collateral carpal ligament
Wrist Joint, Left Wrist Joint, Right	**Includes:** Distal radioulnar joint Radiocarpal joint

SECTION Ø - MEDICAL AND SURGICAL
CHARACTER 5 - APPROACH

External	**Definition:** Procedures performed directly on the skin or mucous membrane and procedures performed indirectly by the application of external force through the skin or mucous membrane
Open	**Definition:** Cutting through the skin or mucous membrane and any other body layers necessary to expose the site of the procedure
Percutaneous	**Definition:** Entry, by puncture or minor incision, of instrumentation through the skin or mucous membrane and any other body layers necessary to reach the site of the procedure
Percutaneous Endoscopic	**Definition:** Entry, by puncture or minor incision, of instrumentation through the skin or mucous membrane and any other body layers necessary to reach and visualize the site of the procedure
Via Natural or Artificial Opening	**Definition:** Entry of instrumentation through a natural or artificial external opening to reach the site of the procedure
Via Natural or Artificial Opening Endoscopic	**Definition:** Entry of instrumentation through a natural or artificial external opening to reach and visualize the site of the procedure
Via Natural or Artificial Opening With Percutaneous Endoscopic Assistance	**Definition:** Entry of instrumentation through a natural or artificial external opening and entry, by puncture or minor incision, of instrumentation through the skin or mucous membrane and any other body layers necessary to aid in the performance of the procedure

APPENDIX A

SECTION Ø - MEDICAL AND SURGICAL
CHARACTER 6 - DEVICE

Device	Includes
Articulating Spacer in Lower Joints	**Includes:** Articulating Spacer (Antibiotic) Spacer, Articulating (Antibiotic)
Artificial Sphincter in Gastrointestinal System	**Includes:** Artificial anal sphincter (AAS) Artificial bowel sphincter (neosphincter)
Artificial Sphincter in Urinary System	**Includes:** AMS 8ØØ® Urinary Control System Artificial urinary sphincter (AUS)
Autologous Arterial Tissue in Heart and Great Vessels	**Includes:** Autologous artery graft
Autologous Arterial Tissue in Lower Arteries	**Includes:** Autologous artery graft
Autologous Arterial Tissue in Lower Veins	**Includes:** Autologous artery graft
Autologous Arterial Tissue in Upper Arteries	**Includes:** Autologous artery graft
Autologous Arterial Tissue in Upper Veins	**Includes:** Autologous artery graft
Autologous Tissue Substitute	**Includes:** Autograft Cultured epidermal cell autograft Epicel® cultured epidermal autograft
Autologous Venous Tissue in Heart and Great Vessels	**Includes:** Autologous vein graft
Autologous Venous Tissue in Lower Arteries	**Includes:** Autologous vein graft
Autologous Venous Tissue in Lower Veins	**Includes:** Autologous vein graft
Autologous Venous Tissue in Upper Arteries	**Includes:** Autologous vein graft
Autologous Venous Tissue in Upper Veins	**Includes:** Autologous vein graft
Biologic with Synthetic Substitute, Autoregulated Electrohydraulic for Replacement in Heart and Great Vessels	**Includes:** Carmat total artificial heart (TAH)
Bone Growth Stimulator in Head and Facial Bones	**Includes:** Electrical bone growth stimulator (EBGS) Ultrasonic osteogenic stimulator Ultrasound bone healing system
Bone Growth Stimulator in Lower Bones	**Includes:** Electrical bone growth stimulator (EBGS) Ultrasonic osteogenic stimulator Ultrasound bone healing system
Bone Growth Stimulator in Upper Bones	**Includes:** Electrical bone growth stimulator (EBGS) Ultrasonic osteogenic stimulator Ultrasound bone healing system
Cardiac Lead in Heart and Great Vessels	**Includes:** Cardiac contractility modulation lead
Cardiac Lead, Defibrillator for Insertion in Heart and Great Vessels	**Includes:** ACUITY™ Steerable Lead Attain Ability® lead Attain StarFix® (OTW) lead Cardiac resynchronization therapy (CRT) lead Corox (OTW) Bipolar Lead Durata® Defibrillation Lead ENDOTAK RELIANCE® (G) Defibrillation Lead
Cardiac Lead, Pacemaker for Insertion in Heart and Great Vessels	**Includes:** ACUITY™ Steerable Lead Attain Ability® Lead Attain StarFix® (OTW) lead Cardiac resynchronization therapy (CRT) lead Corox (OTW) Bipolar Lead
Cardiac Resynchronization Defibrillator Pulse Generator for Insertion in Subcutaneous Tissue and Fascia	**Includes:** COGNIS® CRT-D Concerto II CRT-D Consulta CRT-D CONTAK RENEWAL® 3 RF (HE) CRT-D LIVIAN™ CRT-D Maximo II DR CRT-D Ovatio™ CRT-D Protecta XT CRT-D Viva (XT)(S)
Cardiac Resynchronization Pacemaker Pulse Generator for Insertion in Subcutaneous Tissue and Fascia	**Includes:** Consulta CRT-P Stratos LV ~~Synchra CRT-P~~ Syncra CRT-P
Contraceptive Device in Female Reproductive System	**Includes:** Intrauterine device (IUD)
Contraceptive Device in Subcutaneous Tissue and Fascia	**Includes:** Subdermal progesterone implant
Contractility Modulation Device for Insertion in Subcutaneous Tissue and Fascia	**Includes:** Optimizer™ III implantable pulse generator

SECTION Ø - MEDICAL AND SURGICAL

CHARACTER 6 - DEVICE

Device	Includes
Defibrillator Generator for Insertion in Subcutaneous Tissue and Fascia	**Includes:** Implantable cardioverter-defibrillator (ICD) Maximo II DR (VR) Protecta XT DR (XT VR) Secura (DR) (VR) Evera (XT)(S)(DR/VR) Virtuoso (II) (DR) (VR)
Defibrillator Lead in Anatomical Regions, General	**Includes:** EV ICD System (Extravascular implantable defibrillator lead)
Diaphragmatic Pacemaker Lead in Respiratory System	**Includes:** Phrenic nerve stimulator lead
Drainage Device	**Includes:** Cystostomy tube Foley catheter Percutaneous nephrostomy catheter Thoracostomy tube
External Fixation Device in Head and Facial Bones	**Includes:** External fixator
External Fixation Device in Lower Bones	**Includes:** External fixator
External Fixation Device in Lower Joints	**Includes:** External fixator
External Fixation Device in Upper Bones	**Includes:** External fixator
External Fixation Device in Upper Joints	**Includes:** External fixator
External Fixation Device, Hybrid for Insertion in Upper Bones	**Includes:** Delta frame external fixator Sheffield hybrid external fixator
External Fixation Device, Hybrid for Insertion in Lower Bones	**Includes:** Delta frame external fixator Sheffield hybrid external fixator
External Fixation Device, Hybrid for Reposition in Upper Bones	**Includes:** Delta frame external fixator Sheffield hybrid external fixator
External Fixation Device, Hybrid for Reposition in Lower Bones	**Includes:** Delta frame external fixator Sheffield hybrid external fixator
External Fixation Device, Limb Lengthening for Insertion in Upper Bones	**Includes:** Ilizarov-Vecklich device
External Fixation Device, Limb Lengthening for Insertion in Lower Bones	**Includes:** Ilizarov-Vecklich device
External Fixation Device, Monoplanar for Insertion in Upper Bones	**Includes:** Uniplanar external fixator
External Fixation Device, Monoplanar for Insertion in Lower Bones	**Includes:** Uniplanar external fixator
External Fixation Device, Monoplanar for Reposition in Upper Bones	**Includes:** Uniplanar external fixator
External Fixation Device, Monoplanar for Reposition in Lower Bones	**Includes:** Uniplanar external fixator
External Fixation Device, Ring for Insertion in Upper Bones	**Includes:** Ilizarov external fixator Sheffield ring external fixator
External Fixation Device, Ring for Insertion in Lower Bones	**Includes:** Ilizarov external fixator Sheffield ring external fixator
External Fixation Device, Ring for Reposition in Upper Bones	**Includes:** Ilizarov external fixator Sheffield ring external fixator
External Fixation Device, Ring for Reposition in Lower Bones	**Includes:** Ilizarov external fixator Sheffield ring external fixator
Extraluminal Device	**Includes:** AtriClip LAA Exclusion System LAP-BAND® adjustable gastric banding system REALIZE® Adjustable Gastric Band
Feeding Device in Gastrointestinal System	**Includes:** Percutaneous endoscopic gastrojejunostomy (PEG/J) tube Percutaneous endoscopic gastrostomy (PEG) tube
Hearing Device in Ear, Nose, Sinus	**Includes:** Esteem® implantable hearing system
Hearing Device in Head and Facial Bones	**Includes:** Bone anchored hearing device

APPENDIX A

SECTION Ø - MEDICAL AND SURGICAL
CHARACTER 6 - DEVICE

Device	Includes
Hearing Device, Bone Conduction for Insertion in Ear, Nose, Sinus	**Includes:** Bone anchored hearing device
Hearing Device, Multiple Channel Cochlear Prosthesis for Insertion in Ear, Nose, Sinus	**Includes:** Cochlear implant (CI), multiple channel (electrode)
Hearing Device, Single Channel Cochlear Prosthesis for Insertion in Ear, Nose, Sinus	**Includes:** Cochlear implant (CI), single channel (electrode)
Implantable Heart Assist System in Heart and Great Vessels	**Includes:** Berlin Heart Ventricular Assist Device DeBakey Left Ventricular Assist Device DuraHeart Left Ventricular Assist System HeartMate 3™ LVAS HeartMate II® Left Ventricular Assist Device (LVAD) HeartMate XVE® Left Ventricular Assist Device (LVAD) MicroMed HeartAssist Novacor Left Ventricular Assist Device Thoratec IVAD (Implantable Ventricular Assist Device)
Infusion Device	**Includes:** Ascenda Intrathecal Catheter InDura, intrathecal catheter (1P) (spinal) Non-tunneled central venous catheter Peripherally inserted central catheter (PICC) Tunneled spinal (intrathecal) catheter
Infusion Device, Pump in Subcutaneous Tissue and Fascia	**Includes:** Implantable drug infusion pump (anti-spasmodic) (chemotherapy) (pain) Injection reservoir, pump Pump reservoir Subcutaneous injection reservoir, pump SynchroMed pump
Interbody Fusion Device in Lower Joints	**Includes:** Axial Lumbar Interbody Fusion System AxiaLIF® System CoRoent® XL Direct Lateral Interbody Fusion (DLIF) device EXtreme Lateral Interbody Fusion (XLIF) device Interbody fusion (spine) cage XLIF® System
Interbody Fusion Device in Upper Joints	**Includes:** BAK/C® Interbody Cervical Fusion System Interbody fusion (spine) cage
Internal Fixation Device in Head and Facial Bones	**Includes:** Bone screw (interlocking) (lag) (pedicle) (recessed) Kirschner wire (K-wire) Neutralization plate
Internal Fixation Device in Lower Bones	**Includes:** Bone screw (interlocking) (lag) (pedicle) (recessed) Clamp and rod internal fixation system (CRIF) Kirschner wire (K-wire) Neutralization plate
Internal Fixation Device in Lower Joints	**Includes:** Fusion screw (compression) (lag) (locking) Joint fixation plate Kirschner wire (K-wire)
Internal Fixation Device in Upper Bones	**Includes:** Bone screw (interlocking) (lag) (pedicle) (recessed) Clamp and rod internal fixation system (CRIF) Kirschner wire (K-wire) Neutralization plate
Internal Fixation Device in Upper Joints	**Includes:** Fusion screw (compression) (lag) (locking) Joint fixation plate Kirschner wire (K-wire)
Internal Fixation Device, Intramedullary in Lower Bones	**Includes:** Intramedullary (IM) rod (nail) Intramedullary skeletal kinetic distractor (ISKD) Kuntscher nail
Internal Fixation Device, Intramedullary in Upper Bones	**Includes:** Intramedullary (IM) rod (nail) Intramedullary skeletal kinetic distractor (ISKD) Kuntscher nail
Internal Fixation Device, Intramedullary Limb Lengthening for Insertion in Lower Bones	**Includes:** PRECICE intramedullary limb lengthening system
Internal Fixation Device, Intramedullary Limb Lengthening for Insertion in Upper Bones	**Includes:** PRECICE intramedullary limb lengthening system
Internal Fixation Device, Rigid Plate for Insertion in Upper Bones	**Includes:** Titanium Sternal Fixation System (TSFS)
Internal Fixation Device, Rigid Plate for Reposition in Upper Bones	**Includes:** Titanium Sternal Fixation System (TSFS)

SECTION Ø - MEDICAL AND SURGICAL
CHARACTER 6 - DEVICE

Internal Fixation Device, Sustained Compression for Fusion in Lower Joints	**Includes:** DynaClip® (Delta)(Forte)(Quattro) DynaNail® (Helix)(Hybrid)(Mini)
Internal Fixation Device, Sustained Compression for Fusion in Upper Joints	**Includes:** DynaClip® (Delta)(Forte)(Quattro) DynaNail® (Helix)(Hybrid)(Mini)
Intracardiac Pacemaker in Heart and Great Vessels	**Includes:** Aveir™ VR, as single chamber
Intraluminal Device	**Includes:** Absolute Pro Vascular (OTW) Self-Expanding Stent System Acculink (RX) Carotid Stent System AFX® Endovascular AAA System AneuRx® AAA Advantage® Assurant (Cobalt) stent Carotid WALLSTENT® Monorail® Endoprosthesis CoAxia NeuroFlo catheter Colonic Z-Stent® Complete (SE) stent Cook Zenith AAA Endovascular Graft Driver stent (RX) (OTW) E-Luminexx™ (Biliary) (Vascular) Stent Embolization coil(s) Endologix AFX® Endovascular AAA System Endurant® Endovascular Stent Graft Endurant® II AAA stent graft system EXCLUDER® AAA Endoprosthesis Express® (LD) Premounted Stent System Express® Biliary SD Monorail® Premounted Stent System Express® SD Renal Monorail® Premounted Stent System FLAIR® Endovascular Stent Graft Formula™ Balloon-Expandable Renal Stent System GORE EXCLUDER® AAA Endoprosthesis GORE TAG® Thoracic Endoprosthesis Herculink (RX) Elite Renal Stent System Innova™ stent LifeStent® (Flexstar) (XL) Vascular Stent System Medtronic Endurant® II AAA stent graft system Micro-Driver stent (RX) (OTW) MULTI-LINK (VISION)(MINI-VISION)(ULTRA) Coronary Stent System Omnilink Elite Vascular Balloon Expandable Stent System Protégé® RX Carotid Stent System Stent, intraluminal (cardiovascular) (gastrointestinal)(hepatobiliary)(urinary) Talent® Converter Talent® Occluder Talent® Stent Graft (abdominal) (thoracic) Therapeutic occlusion coil(s) Ultraflex™ Precision Colonic Stent System Valiant Thoracic Stent Graft WALLSTENT® Endoprosthesis Xact Carotid Stent System Zenith AAA Endovascular Graft Zenith Flex® AAA Endovascular Graft Zenith® Renu™ AAA Ancillary Graft Zenith TX2® TAA Endovascular Graft

Intraluminal Device, Airway in Ear, Nose, Sinus	**Includes:** Nasopharyngeal airway (NPA)
Intraluminal Device, Airway in Gastrointestinal System	**Includes:** Esophageal obturator airway (EOA)
Intraluminal Device, Airway in Mouth and Throat	**Includes:** Guedel airway Oropharyngeal airway (OPA)
Intraluminal Device, Bioactive in Upper Arteries	**Includes:** Bioactive embolization coil(s) Micrus CERECYTE microcoil
Intraluminal Device, Branched or Fenestrated, One or Two Arteries for Restriction in Lower Arteries	**Includes:** Cook Zenith® Fenestrated AAA Endovascular Graft EXCLUDER® AAA Endoprosthesis EXCLUDER® IBE Endoprosthesis GORE EXCLUDER® AAA Endoprosthesis GORE EXCLUDER® IBE Endoprosthesis Zenith® Fenestrated AAA Endovascular Graft
Intraluminal Device, Branched or Fenestrated, Three or More Arteries for Restriction in Lower Arteries	**Includes:** Cook Zenith® Fenestrated AAA Endovascular Graft EXCLUDER® AAA Endoprosthesis GORE EXCLUDER® AAA Endoprosthesis Zenith® Fenestrated AAA Endovascular Graft
Intraluminal Device, Drug-eluting in Heart and Great Vessels	**Includes:** CYPHER® Stent Endeavor® (III) (IV) (Sprint) Zotarolimus-eluting Coronary Stent System Everolimus-eluting coronary stent Paclitaxel-eluting coronary stent Sirolimus-eluting coronary stent TAXUS® Liberté® Paclitaxel-eluting Coronary Stent System XIENCE Everolimus Eluting Coronary Stent System Zotarolimus-eluting coronary stent
Intraluminal Device, Drug-eluting in Lower Arteries	**Includes:** Eluvia™ Drug-Eluting Vascular Stent System Paclitaxel-eluting peripheral stent SAVAL below-the-knee (BTK) drug-eluting stent system Zilver® PTX® (paclitaxel) Drug-Eluting Peripheral Stent
Intraluminal Device, Drug-eluting, Four or More in Lower Arteries	**Includes:** Eluvia™ Drug-Eluting Vascular Stent System SAVAL below-the-knee (BTK) drug-eluting stent system
Intraluminal Device, Drug-eluting, Three in Lower Arteries	**Includes:** Eluvia™ Drug-Eluting Vascular Stent System SAVAL below-the-knee (BTK) drug-eluting stent system

APPENDIX A

SECTION Ø - MEDICAL AND SURGICAL
CHARACTER 6 - DEVICE

Intraluminal Device, Drug-eluting, Two in Lower Arteries	**Includes:** Eluvia™ Drug-Eluting Vascular Stent System SAVAL below-the-knee (BTK) drug-eluting stent system
Intraluminal Device, Drug-eluting in Upper Arteries	**Includes:** Paclitaxel-eluting peripheral stent Zilver® PTX® (paclitaxel) Drug-Eluting Peripheral Stent
Intraluminal Device, Endobronchial Valve in Respiratory System	**Includes:** Spiration IBV™ Valve System
Intraluminal Device, Endotracheal Airway in Respiratory System	**Includes:** Endotracheal tube (cuffed) (double-lumen)
Intraluminal Device, Flow Diverter for Restriction in Upper Arteries	**Includes:** Flow Diverter embolization device Pipeline™ (Flex) embolization device Surpass Streamline™ Flow Diverter
Intraluminal Device, Pessary in Female Reproductive System	**Includes:** Pessary ring Vaginal pessary
Liner in Lower Joints	**Includes:** Acetabular cup Hip (joint) liner Joint liner (insert) Knee (implant) insert Tibial insert
Magnetic Lengthening Device in Gastrointestinal System	**Includes:** Flourish® Pediatric Esophageal Atresia Device
Monitoring Device	**Includes:** Blood glucose monitoring system Cardiac event recorder Continuous Glucose Monitoring (CGM) device Implantable glucose monitoring device Loop recorder, implantable Reveal (LINQ) (DX) (XT)
Monitoring Device, Hemodynamic for Insertion in Subcutaneous Tissue and Fascia	**Includes:** Implantable hemodynamic monitor (IHM) Implantable hemodynamic monitoring system (IHMS)
Monitoring Device, Pressure Sensor for Insertion in Heart and Great Vessels	**Includes:** CardioMEMS® pressure sensor EndoSure® sensor
Neurostimulator Lead in Central Nervous System and Cranial Nerves	**Includes:** Cortical strip neurostimulator lead DBS lead Deep brain neurostimulator lead RNS System lead Spinal cord neurostimulator lead
Neurostimulator Lead in Peripheral Nervous System	**Includes:** InterStim® Therapy lead
Neurostimulator Generator in Head and Facial Bones	**Includes:** RNS system neurostimulator generator
Nonautologous Tissue Substitute	**Includes:** Acellular Hydrated Dermis Bone bank bone graft Cook Biodesign® Fistula Plug(s) Cook Biodesign® Hernia Graft(s) Cook Biodesign® Layered Graft(s) Cook Zenapro™ Layered Graft(s) Fish skin Kerecis® (GraftGuide) (MariGen) (SurgiBind) (SurgiClose) Piscine skin Tissue bank graft
Other Device	**Includes:** Alfapump® system
Pacemaker, Dual Chamber for Insertion in Subcutaneous Tissue and Fascia	**Includes:** Advisa (MRI) EnRhythm Kappa Revo MRI™ SureScan® pacemaker Two lead pacemaker Versa
Pacemaker, Single Chamber for Insertion in Subcutaneous Tissue and Fascia	**Includes:** Single lead pacemaker (atrium) (ventricle)
Pacemaker, Single Chamber Rate Responsive for Insertion in Subcutaneous Tissue and Fascia	**Includes:** Single lead rate responsive pacemaker (atrium) (ventricle)
Radioactive Element	**Includes:** Brachytherapy seeds CivaSheet®
Radioactive Element, Palladium-1Ø3 Collagen Implant for Insertion in Central Nervous System and Cranial Nerves	GammaTile™ Palladium-1Ø3 Collagen Implant
Radioactive Element, Cesium-131 Collagen Implant for Insertion in Central Nervous System and Cranial Nerves	Cesium-131 Collagen Implant GammaTile™
Resurfacing Device in Lower Joints	**Includes:** CONSERVE® PLUS Total Resurfacing Hip System Cormet Hip Resurfacing System

New/Revised Text in Green ~~deleted~~ Deleted

SECTION Ø - MEDICAL AND SURGICAL
CHARACTER 6 - DEVICE

Short-term External Heart Assist System in Heart and Great Vessels	Aortix™ System Biventricular external heart assist system BVS 5ØØØ Ventricular Assist Device Centrimag® Blood Pump Impella® heart pump TandemHeart® System Thoratec Paracorporeal Ventricular Assist Device
Spacer in Lower Joints	**Includes:** Joint spacer (antibiotic)
Spacer in Upper Joints	**Includes:** Joint spacer (antibiotic) Spacer, static (antibiotic) Static spacer (antibiotic)
Spinal Stabilization Device, Facet Replacement for Insertion in Upper Joints	**Includes:** Facet replacement spinal stabilization device
Spinal Stabilization Device, Facet Replacement for Insertion in Lower Joints	**Includes:** Facet replacement spinal stabilization device
Spinal Stabilization Device, Interspinous Process for Insertion in Upper Joints	**Includes:** Interspinous process spinal stabilization device X-STOP® Spacer
Spinal Stabilization Device, Interspinous Process for Insertion in Lower Joints	**Includes:** Interspinous process spinal stabilization device X-STOP® Spacer
Spinal Stabilization Device, Pedicle-Based for Insertion in Upper Joints	**Includes:** Dynesys® Dynamic Stabilization System Pedicle-based dynamic stabilization device
Spinal Stabilization Device, Pedicle-Based for Insertion in Lower Joints	**Includes:** Dynesys® Dynamic Stabilization System Pedicle-based dynamic stabilization device
Stimulator Generator in Subcutaneous Tissue and Fascia	**Includes:** Baroreflex Activation Therapy® (BAT®) Diaphragmatic pacemaker generator Mark IV Breathing Pacemaker System Phrenic nerve stimulator generator Rheos® System device
Stimulator Generator, Multiple Array for Insertion in Subcutaneous Tissue and Fascia	**Includes:** Activa PC neurostimulator Enterra gastric neurostimulator Neurostimulator generator, multiple channel PERCEPT™ PC neurostimulator PrimeAdvanced neurostimulator (SureScan) (MRI Safe) Vanta™ PC neurostimulator
Stimulator Generator, Multiple Array Rechargeable for Insertion in Subcutaneous Tissue and Fascia	**Includes:** Activa RC neurostimulator Intellis™ neurostimulator Neurostimulator generator, multiple channel rechargeable RestoreAdvanced neurostimulator (SureScan) (MRI Safe) RestoreSensor neurostimulator (SureScan) (MRI Safe) RestoreUltra neurostimulator (SureScan) (MRI Safe)
Stimulator Generator, Single Array for Insertion in Subcutaneous Tissue and Fascia	**Includes:** Activa SC neurostimulator InterSlim™ II Therapy neurostimulator Itrel (3) (4) neurostimulator Neurostimulator generator, single channel
Stimulator Generator, Single Array Rechargeable for Insertion in Subcutaneous Tissue and Fascia	**Includes:** InterSlim™ II Micro Therapy neurostimulator Neurostimulator generator, single channel rechargeable
Stimulator Lead in Gastrointestinal System	**Includes:** Gastric electrical stimulation (GES) lead Gastric pacemaker lead
Stimulator Lead in Muscles	**Includes:** Electrical muscle stimulation (EMS) lead Electronic muscle stimulator lead Neuromuscular electrical stimulation (NEMS) lead
Stimulator Lead in Upper Arteries	**Includes:** Baroreflex Activation Therapy® (BAT®) Carotid (artery) sinus (baroreceptor) lead Rheos® System lead
Stimulator Lead in Urinary System	**Includes:** Sacral nerve modulation (SNM) lead Sacral neuromodulation lead Urinary incontinence stimulator lead
Subcutaneous Defibrillator Lead in Subcutaneous Tissue and Fascia	**Includes:** S-ICD™ lead

APPENDIX A

SECTION Ø - MEDICAL AND SURGICAL
CHARACTER 6 - DEVICE

Device	Includes
Synthetic Substitute	**Includes:** AbioCor® Total Replacement Heart AMPLATZER® Muscular VSD Occluder Annuloplasty ring Bard® Composix® (E/X) (LP) mesh Bard® Composix® Kugel® patch Bard® Dulex™ mesh Bard® Ventralex™ hernia patch Barricaid® Annular Closure Device (ACD) BRYAN® Cervical Disc System Corvia IASD® Ex-PRESS™ mini glaucoma shunt Flexible Composite Mesh GORE® DUALMESH® Holter valve ventricular shunt IASD® (InterAtrial Shunt Device), Corvia InterAtrial Shunt Device IASD®, Corvia LimFlow™ Transcatheter Arterialization of the Deep Veins (TADV) System MitraClip valve repair system Nitinol framed polymer mesh Open Pivot (mechanical) valve Open Pivot Aortic Valve Graft (AVG) Partially absorbable mesh PHYSIOMESH™ Flexible Composite Mesh Polymethylmethacrylate (PMMA) Polypropylene mesh PRESTIGE® Cervical Disc PROCEED™ Ventral Patch Prodisc-C Prodisc-L PROLENE Polypropylene Hernia System (PHS) Rebound HRD® (Hernia Repair Device) SynCardia Total Artificial Heart Total artificial (replacement) heart ULTRAPRO Hernia System (UHS) ULTRAPRO Partially Absorbable Lightweight Mesh ULTRAPRO Plug V-Wave Interatrial Shunt System Ventrio™ Hernia Patch Zimmer® NexGen® LPS Mobile Bearing Knee Zimmer® NexGen® LPS-Flex Mobile Knee
Synthetic Substitute, Ceramic for Replacement in Lower Joints	**Includes:** Ceramic on ceramic bearing surface Novation® Ceramic AHS® (Articulation Hip System)
Synthetic Substitute, Intraocular Telescope for Replacement in Eye	**Includes:** Implantable Miniature Telescope™ (IMT)
Synthetic Substitute, Metal for Replacement in Lower Joints	**Includes:** Cobalt/chromium head and socket Metal on metal bearing surface
Synthetic Substitute, Metal on Polyethylene for Replacement in Lower Joints	**Includes:** Cobalt/chromium head and polyethylene socket
Synthetic Substitute, Oxidized Zirconium on Polyethylene for Replacement in Lower Joints	OXINIUM
Synthetic Substitute, Pneumatic for Replacement in Heart and Great Vessels	**Includes:** SynCardia (temporary) total artificial heart (TAH)
Synthetic Substitute, Polyethylene for Replacement in Lower Joints	**Includes:** Polyethylene socket
Synthetic Substitute, Reverse Ball and Socket for Replacement in Upper Joints	**Includes:** Delta III Reverse shoulder prosthesis Reverse® Shoulder Prosthesis
Tissue Expander in Skin and Breast	**Includes:** Tissue expander (inflatable) (injectable)
Tissue Expander in Subcutaneous Tissue and Fascia	**Includes:** Tissue expander (inflatable) (injectable)
Tracheostomy Device in Respiratory System	**Includes:** Tracheostomy tube
Vascular Access Device, Totally Implantable in Subcutaneous Tissue and Fascia	**Includes:** Implanted (venous) (access) port Injection reservoir, port Subcutaneous injection reservoir, port
Vascular Access Device, Tunneled in Subcutaneous Tissue and Fascia	**Includes:** Tunneled central venous catheter Vectra® Vascular Access Graft
Zooplastic Tissue in Heart and Great Vessels	**Includes:** 3f (Aortic) Bioprosthesis valve Bovine pericardial valve Bovine pericardium graft Contegra Pulmonary Valved Conduit CoreValve transcatheter aortic valve Epic™ Stented Tissue Valve (aortic) Freestyle (Stentless) Aortic Root Bioprosthesis Hancock Bioprosthesis (aortic) (mitral) valve Hancock Bioprosthetic Valved Conduit Inspiris Resilia valve Melody® transcatheter pulmonary valve Mitroflow® Aortic Pericardial Heart Valve Mosaic Bioprosthesis (aortic) (mitral) valve Porcine (bioprosthetic) valve SAPIEN transcatheter aortic valve SJM Biocor® Stented Valve System Stented tissue valve Trifecta™ Valve (aortic) Xenograft

SECTION Ø CHARACTER 6

SECTION 1 - OBSTETRICS
CHARACTER 3 - OPERATION

Abortion	**Definition:** Artificially terminating a pregnancy
Change	**Definition:** Taking out or off a device from a body part and putting back an identical or similar device in or on the same body part without cutting or puncturing the skin or a mucous membrane
Delivery	**Definition:** Assisting the passage of the products of conception from the genital canal
Drainage	**Definition:** Taking or letting out fluids and/or gases from a body part by the use of force
Extraction	**Definition:** Pulling or stripping out or off all or a portion of a body part
Insertion	**Definition:** Putting in a nonbiological appliance that monitors, assists, performs, or prevents a physiological function but does not physically take the place of a body part
Inspection	**Definition:** Visually and/or manually exploring a body part **Explanation:** Visual exploration may be performed with or without optical instrumentation. Manual exploration may be performed directly or through intervening body layers
Removal	**Definition:** Taking out or off a device from a body part, region or orifice **Explanation:** If a device is taken out and a similar device put in without cutting or puncturing the skin or mucous membrane, the procedure is coded to the root operation CHANGE. Otherwise, the procedure for taking out a device is coded to the root operation REMOVAL
Repair	**Definition:** Restoring, to the extent possible, a body part to its normal anatomic structure and function **Explanation:** Used only when the method to accomplish the repair is not one of the other root operations
Reposition	**Definition:** Moving to its normal location or other suitable location all or a portion of a body part **Explanation:** The body part is moved to a new location from an abnormal location, or from a normal location where it is not functioning correctly. The body part may or may not be cut out or off to be moved to the new location
Resection	**Definition:** Cutting out or off, without replacement, all of a body part
Transplantation	**Definition:** Putting in or on all or a portion of a living body part taken from another individual or animal to physically take the place and/or function of all or a portion of a similar body part **Explanation:** The native body part may or may not be taken out, and the transplanted body part may take over all or a portion of its function

SECTION 1 - OBSTETRICS
CHARACTER 5 - APPROACH

External	**Definition:** Procedures performed directly on the skin or mucous membrane and procedures performed indirectly by the application of external force through the skin or mucous membrane
Open	**Definition:** Cutting through the skin or mucous membrane and any other body layers necessary to expose the site of the procedure
Percutaneous	**Definition:** Entry, by puncture or minor incision, of instrumentation through the skin or mucous membrane and any other body layers necessary to reach the site of the procedure
Percutaneous Endoscopic	**Definition:** Entry, by puncture or minor incision, of instrumentation through the skin or mucous membrane and any other body layers necessary to reach and visualize the site of the procedure
Via Natural or Artificial Opening	**Definition:** Entry of instrumentation through a natural or artificial external opening to reach the site of the procedure
Via Natural or Artificial Opening Endoscopic	**Definition:** Entry of instrumentation through a natural or artificial external opening to reach and visualize the site of the procedure

APPENDIX A

SECTION 2 - PLACEMENT
CHARACTER 3 - OPERATION

Change	**Definition:** Taking out or off a device from a body part and putting back an identical or similar device in or on the same body part without cutting or puncturing the skin or a mucous membrane
Compression	**Definition:** Putting pressure on a body region
Dressing	**Definition:** Putting material on a body region for protection
Immobilization	**Definition:** Limiting or preventing motion of a body region
Packing	**Definition:** Putting material in a body region or orifice
Removal	**Definition:** Taking out or off a device from a body part
Traction	**Definition:** Exerting a pulling force on a body region in a distal direction

SECTION 2 - PLACEMENT
CHARACTER 5 - APPROACH

External	**Definition:** Procedures performed directly on the skin or mucous membrane and procedures performed indirectly by the application of external force through the skin or mucous membrane

SECTION 3 - ADMINISTRATION
CHARACTER 3 - OPERATION

Introduction	**Definition:** Putting in or on a therapeutic, diagnostic, nutritional, physiological, or prophylactic substance except blood or blood products
Irrigation	**Definition:** Putting in or on a cleansing substance
Transfusion	**Definition:** Putting in blood or blood products

SECTION 3 - ADMINISTRATION
CHARACTER 5 - APPROACH

External	**Definition:** Procedures performed directly on the skin or mucous membrane and procedures performed indirectly by the application of external force through the skin or mucous membrane
Open	**Definition:** Cutting through the skin or mucous membrane and any other body layers necessary to expose the site of the procedure
Percutaneous	**Definition:** Entry, by puncture or minor incision, of instrumentation through the skin or mucous membrane and any other body layers necessary to reach the site of the procedure
Percutaneous Endoscopic	**Definition:** Entry, by puncture or minor incision, of instrumentation through the skin or mucous membrane and any other body layers necessary to reach and visualize the site of the procedure
Via Natural or Artificial Opening	**Definition:** Entry of instrumentation through a natural or artificial external opening to reach the site of the procedure
Via Natural or Artificial Opening Endoscopic	**Definition:** Entry of instrumentation through a natural or artificial external opening to reach and visualize the site of the procedure

SECTION 3 - ADMINISTRATION
CHARACTER 6 - SUBSTANCE

4-Factor Prothrombin Complex Concentrate	**Includes:** Kcentra
Adhesion Barrier	**Includes:** Seprafilm
Anti-Infective Envelope	**Includes:** AIGISRx Antibacterial Envelope Antibacterial Envelope (TYRX) (AIGISRx) Antimicrobial envelope TYRX Antibacterial Envelope
Clofarabine	**Includes:** Clolar
Globulin	**Includes:** Gammaglobulin Hyperimmune globulin Immunoglobulin Polyclonal hyperimmune globulin
Glucarpidase	**Includes:** Voraxaze
Hematopoietic Stem/ ProgenitorCells, Genetically Modified	**Includes:** OTL-101 OTL-103
Human B-type Natriuretic Peptide	**Includes:** Nesiritide
Other Anti-infective	**Includes:** AVYCAZ® (ceftazidime-avibactam) Ceftazidime-avibactam CONTEPO™ (Fosfomycin Anti-infective) CRESEMBA® (isavuconazonium sulfate) Fosfomycin Anti-infective MI/REL mipenem-cilastatin-relebactam Anti-infective Isavuconazole (isavuconazonium sulfate) Meropenem-vaborbactam Anti-infective Plazomicin RECARBRIO™ (Imipenem-cilastatin-relebactam Anti-infective) ABOMERE™ (Meropenem-vaborbactam Anti-infective)
Other Antineoplastic	**Includes:** Apalutamide Antineoplastic Balversa™ (Erdafitinib Antineoplastic) Blinatumomab BLINCYTO® (blinatumomab) Erdafitinib Antineoplastic ERLEADA™ (Apalutamide Antineoplastic) Gilteritinib Venclexta® (Venetoclax Antineoplastic tablets) Venetoclax Antineoplastic (tablets) XOSPATA® (Gilteritinib)
Other Substance	~~Dnase (Deoxyribonuclease)~~ Dnase (Deoxyribonuclease) Esketamine Hydrochloride JAKAFI® (Ruxolitinib) Ruxolitinib SPRAVATO™ (Esketamine Hydrochloride)
Other Therapeutic Substance	**Includes:** Idarucizumab, Pradaxa® (dabigatran) reversal agent Praxbind® (idarucizumab), Pradaxa® (dabigatran) reversal agent
Other Thrombolytic	**Includes:** Tissue Plasminogen Activator (tPA)(r-tPA)
Oxazolidinones	**Includes:** Zyvox
Pathogen Reduced Cryoprecipitated Fibrinogen Complex	**Includes:** INTERCEPT Blood System for Plasma Pathogen Reduced Cryoprecipitated Fibrinogen Complex INTERCEPT Fibrinogen Complex
Recombinant Bone Morphogenetic Protein	**Includes:** Bone morphogenetic protein 2 (BMP 2) rhBMP-2
Vasopressor	**Includes:** Angiotensin II GIAPREZA™ Human angiotensin II, synthetic

SECTION 4 - MEASUREMENT AND MONITORING
CHARACTER 3 - OPERATION

Measurement	**Definition:** Determining the level of a physiological or physical function at a point in time
Monitoring	**Definition:** Determining the level of a physiological or physical function repetitively over a period of time

New/Revised Text in Green ~~deleted~~ Deleted

APPENDIX A

SECTION 4 - MEASUREMENT AND MONITORING
CHARACTER 5 - APPROACH

External	**Definition:** Procedures performed directly on the skin or mucous membrane and procedures performed indirectly by the application of external force through the skin or mucous membrane
Open	**Definition:** Cutting through the skin or mucous membrane and any other body layers necessary to expose the site of the procedure
Percutaneous	**Definition:** Entry, by puncture or minor incision, of instrumentation through the skin or mucous membrane and any other body layers necessary to reach the site of the procedure
Percutaneous Endoscopic	**Definition:** Entry, by puncture or minor incision, of instrumentation through the skin or mucous membrane and any other body layers necessary to reach and visualize the site of the procedure
Via Natural or Artificial Opening	**Definition:** Entry of instrumentation through a natural or artificial external opening to reach the site of the procedure
Via Natural or Artificial Opening Endoscopic	**Definition:** Entry of instrumentation through a natural or artificial external opening to reach and visualize the site of the procedure

SECTION 5 - EXTRACORPOREAL OR SYSTEMIC ASSISTANCE AND PERFORMANCE
CHARACTER 3 - OPERATION

Assistance	**Definition:** Taking over a portion of a physiological function by extracorporeal means
Performance	**Definition:** Completely taking over a physiological function by extracorporeal means
Restoration	**Definition:** Returning, or attempting to return, a physiological function to its original state by extracorporeal means.

SECTION 6 - EXTRACORPOREAL OR SYSTEMIC THERAPIES
CHARACTER 3 - OPERATION

Atmospheric Control	**Definition:** Extracorporeal control of atmospheric pressure and composition
Decompression	**Definition:** Extracorporeal elimination of undissolved gas from body fluids
Electromagnetic Therapy	**Definition:** Extracorporeal treatment by electromagnetic rays
Hyperthermia	**Definition:** Extracorporeal raising of body temperature
Hypothermia	**Definition:** Extracorporeal lowering of body temperature
Perfusion	**Definition:** Extracorporeal treatment by diffusion of therapeutic fluid
Pheresis	**Definition:** Extracorporeal separation of blood products
Phototherapy	**Definition:** Extracorporeal treatment by light rays
Shock Wave Therapy	**Definition:** Extracorporeal treatment by shock waves
Ultrasound Therapy	**Definition:** Extracorporeal treatment by ultrasound
Ultraviolet Light Therapy	**Definition:** Extracorporeal treatment by ultraviolet light

SECTION 7 - OSTEOPATHIC
CHARACTER 3 - OPERATION

Treatment	**Definition:** Manual treatment to eliminate or alleviate somatic dysfunction and related disorders

SECTION 7 - OSTEOPATHIC
CHARACTER 5 - APPROACH

External	**Definition:** Procedures performed directly on the skin or mucous membrane and procedures performed indirectly by the application of external force through the skin or mucous membrane

SECTION 8 - OTHER PROCEDURES
CHARACTER 3 - OPERATION

Other Procedures	**Definition:** Methodologies which attempt to remediate or cure a disorder or disease

SECTION 8 - OTHER PROCEDURES
CHARACTER 5 - APPROACH

External	**Definition:** Procedures performed directly on the skin or mucous membrane and procedures performed indirectly by the application of external force through the skin or mucous membrane
Percutaneous	**Definition:** Entry, by puncture or minor incision, of instrumentation through the skin or mucous membrane and any other body layers necessary to reach the site of the procedure
Percutaneous Endoscopic	**Definition:** Entry, by puncture or minor incision, of instrumentation through the skin or mucous membrane and any other body layers necessary to reach and visualize the site of the procedure
Via Natural or Artificial Opening	**Definition:** Entry of instrumentation through a natural or artificial external opening to reach the site of the procedure
Via Natural or Artificial Opening Endoscopic	**Definition:** Entry of instrumentation through a natural or artificial external opening to reach and visualize the site of the procedure

SECTION 9 - CHIROPRACTIC
CHARACTER 3 - OPERATION

Manipulation	**Definition:** Manual procedure that involves a directed thrust to move a joint past the physiological range of motion, without exceeding the anatomical limit

SECTION 9 - CHIROPRACTIC
CHARACTER 5 - APPROACH

External	**Definition:** Procedures performed directly on the skin or mucous membrane and procedures performed indirectly by the application of external force through the skin or mucous membrane

SECTION B - IMAGING
CHARACTER 3 - TYPE

Computerized Tomography (CT Scan)	**Definition:** Computer-reformatted digital display of multiplanar images developed from the capture of multiple exposures of external ionizing radiation
Fluoroscopy	**Definition:** Single plane or bi-plane real-time display of an image developed from the capture of external ionizing radiation on a fluorescent screen. The image may also be stored by either digital or analog means
Magnetic Resonance Imaging (MRI)	**Definition:** Computer reformatted digital display of multiplanar images developed from the capture of radiofrequency signals emitted by nuclei in a body site excited within a magnetic field
Other Imaging	**Definition:** Other specified modality for visualizing a body part
Plain Radiography	**Definition:** Planar display of an image developed from the capture of external ionizing radiation on photographic or photoconductive plate
Ultrasonography	**Definition:** Real-time display of images of anatomy or flow information developed from the capture of reflected and attenuated high-frequency sound waves

SECTION C - NUCLEAR MEDICINE
CHARACTER 3 - TYPE

Nonimaging Nuclear Medicine Assay	**Definition:** Introduction of radioactive materials into the body for the study of body fluids and blood elements, by the detection of radioactive emissions
Nonimaging Nuclear Medicine Probe	**Definition:** Introduction of radioactive materials into the body for the study of distribution and fate of certain substances by the detection of radioactive emissions; or, alternatively, measurement of absorption of radioactive emissions from an external source
Nonimaging Nuclear Medicine Uptake	**Definition:** Introduction of radioactive materials into the body for measurements of organ function, from the detection of radioactive emissions
Planar Nuclear Medicine Imaging	**Definition:** Introduction of radioactive materials into the body for single plane display of images developed from the capture of radioactive emissions
Positron Emission Tomographic (PET) Imaging	**Definition:** Introduction of radioactive materials into the body for three-dimensional display of images developed from the simultaneous capture, 180 degrees apart, of radioactive emissions
Systemic Nuclear Medicine Therapy	**Definition:** Introduction of unsealed radioactive materials into the body for treatment
Tomographic (Tomo) Nuclear Medicine Imaging	**Definition:** Introduction of radioactive materials into the body for three-dimensional display of images developed from the capture of radioactive emissions

SECTION F - PHYSICAL REHABILITATION AND DIAGNOSTIC AUDIOLOGY

CHARACTER 3 - TYPE

Activities of Daily Living Assessment	**Definition:** Measurement of functional level for activities of daily living
Activities of Daily Living Treatment	**Definition:** Exercise or activities to facilitate functional competence for activities of daily living
Caregiver Training	**Definition:** Training in activities to support patient's optimal level of function
Cochlear Implant Treatment	**Definition:** Application of techniques to improve the communication abilities of individuals with cochlear implant
Device Fitting	**Definition:** Fitting of a device designed to facilitate or support achievement of a higher level of function
Hearing Aid Assessment	**Definition:** Measurement of the appropriateness and/or effectiveness of a hearing device
Hearing Assessment	**Definition:** Measurement of hearing and related functions
Hearing Treatment	**Definition:** Application of techniques to improve, augment, or compensate for hearing and related functional impairment
Motor and/or Nerve Function Assessment	**Definition:** Measurement of motor, nerve, and related functions
Motor Treatment	**Definition:** Exercise or activities to increase or facilitate motor function
Speech Assessment	**Definition:** Measurement of speech and related functions
Speech Treatment	**Definition:** Application of techniques to improve, augment, or compensate for speech and related functional impairment
Vestibular Assessment	**Definition:** Measurement of the vestibular system and related functions
Vestibular Treatment	**Definition:** Application of techniques to improve, augment, or compensate for vestibular and related functional impairment

SECTION F - PHYSICAL REHABILITATION AND DIAGNOSTIC AUDIOLOGY

CHARACTER 5 - TYPE QUALIFIER

Acoustic Reflex Decay	**Definition:** Measures reduction in size/ strength of acoustic reflex over time **Includes/Examples:** Includes site of lesion test
Acoustic Reflex Patterns	**Definition:** Defines site of lesion based upon presence/absence of acoustic reflexes with ipsilateral vs. contralateral stimulation
Acoustic Reflex Threshold	**Definition:** Determines minimal intensity that acoustic reflex occurs with ipsilateral and/ or contralateral stimulation
Aerobic Capacity and Endurance	**Definition:** Measures autonomic responses to positional changes; perceived exertion, dyspnea or angina during activity, performance during exercise protocols; standard vital signs; and blood gas analysis or oxygen consumption
Alternate Binaural or Monaural Loudness Balance	**Definition:** Determines auditory stimulus parameter that yields the same objective sensation **Includes/Examples:** Sound intensities that yield same loudness perception
Anthropometric Characteristics	**Definition:** Measures edema, body fat composition, height, weight, length and girth
Aphasia (Assessment)	**Definition:** Measures expressive and receptive speech and language function including reading and writing
Aphasia (Treatment)	**Definition:** Applying techniques to improve, augment, or compensate for receptive/ expressive language impairments
Articulation/Phonology (Assessment)	**Definition:** Measures speech production
Articulation/Phonology (Treatment)	**Definition:** Applying techniques to correct, improve, or compensate for speech productive impairment
Assistive Listening Device	**Definition:** Assists in use of effective and appropriate assistive listening device/ system
Assistive Listening System/Device Selection	**Definition:** Measures the effectiveness and appropriateness of assistive listening systems/devices
Assistive, Adaptive,Supportive or Protective Devices	**Explanation:** Devices to facilitate or support achievement of a higher level of function in wheelchair mobility; bed mobility; transfer or ambulation ability; bath and showering ability; dressing; grooming; personal hygiene; play or leisure

SECTION F - PHYSICAL REHABILITATION AND DIAGNOSTIC AUDIOLOGY

CHARACTER 5 - TYPE QUALIFIER

Auditory Evoked Potentials	**Definition:** Measures electric responses produced by the VIIIth cranial nerve and brainstem following auditory stimulation
Auditory Processing (Assessment)	**Definition:** Evaluates ability to receive and process auditory information and comprehension of spoken language
Auditory Processing (Treatment)	**Definition:** Applying techniques to improve the receiving and processing of auditory information and comprehension of spoken language
Augmentative/ Alternative Communication System (Assessment)	**Definition:** Determines the appropriateness of aids, techniques, symbols, and/or strategies to augment or replace speech and enhance communication **Includes/Examples:** Includes the use of telephones, writing equipment, emergency equipment, and TDD
Augmentative/ Alternative Communication System (Treatment)	**Includes/Examples:** Includes augmentative communication devices and aids
Aural Rehabilitation	**Definition:** Applying techniques to improve the communication abilities associated with hearing loss
Aural Rehabilitation Status	**Definition:** Measures impact of a hearing loss including evaluation of receptive and expressive communication skills
Bathing/Showering	**Includes/Examples:** Includes obtaining and using supplies; soaping, rinsing, and drying body parts; maintaining bathing position; and transferring to and from bathing positions
Bathing/Showering Techniques	**Definition:** Activities to facilitate obtaining and using supplies, soaping, rinsing and drying body parts, maintaining bathing position, and transferring to and from bathing positions
Bed Mobility (Assessment)	**Definition:** Transitional movement within bed
Bed Mobility (Treatment)	**Definition:** Exercise or activities to facilitate transitional movements within bed
Bedside Swallowing and Oral Function	**Includes/Examples:** Bedside swallowing includes assessment of sucking, masticating, coughing, and swallowing. Oral function includes assessment of musculature for controlled movements, structures and functions to determine coordination and phonation
Bekesy Audiometry	**Definition:** Uses an instrument that provides a choice of discrete or continuously varying pure tones; choice of pulsed or continuous signal
Binaural Electroacoustic Hearing Aid Check	**Definition:** Determines mechanical and electroacoustic function of bilateral hearing aids using hearing aid test box
Binaural Hearing Aid (Assessment)	**Definition:** Measures the candidacy, effectiveness, and appropriateness of hearing aids **Explanation:** Measures bilateral fit
Binaural Hearing Aid (Treatment)	**Explanation:** Assists in achieving maximum understanding and performance
Bithermal, Binaural Caloric Irrigation	**Definition:** Measures the rhythmic eye movements stimulated by changing the temperature of the vestibular system
Bithermal, Monaural Caloric Irrigation	**Definition:** Measures the rhythmic eye movements stimulated by changing the temperature of the vestibular system in one ear
Brief Tone Stimuli	**Definition:** Measures specific central auditory process
Cerumen Management	**Definition:** Includes examination of external auditory canal and tympanic membrane and removal of cerumen from external ear canal
Cochlear Implant	**Definition:** Measures candidacy for cochlear implant
Cochlear Implant Rehabilitation	**Definition:** Applying techniques to improve the communication abilities of individuals with cochlear implant; includes programming the device, providing patients/families with information
Communicative/ Cognitive Integration Skills (Assessment)	**Definition:** Measures ability to use higher cortical functions **Includes/Examples:** Includes orientation, recognition, attention span, initiation and termination of activity, memory, sequencing, categorizing, concept formation, spatial operations, judgment, problem solving, generalization and pragmatic communication
Communicative/ Cognitive Integration Skills (Treatment)	**Definition:** Activities to facilitate the use of higher cortical functions **Includes/Examples:** Includes level of arousal, orientation, recognition, attention span, initiation and termination of activity, memory sequencing, judgment and problem solving, learning and generalization, and pragmatic communication

SECTION F - PHYSICAL REHABILITATION AND DIAGNOSTIC AUDIOLOGY
CHARACTER 5 - TYPE QUALIFIER

Computerized Dynamic Posturography	**Definition:** Measures the status of the peripheral and central vestibular system and the sensory/motor component of balance; evaluates the efficacy of vestibular rehabilitation
Conditioned Play Audiometry	**Definition:** Behavioral measures using nonspeech and speech stimuli to obtain frequency-specific and ear-specific information on auditory status from the patient **Explanation:** Obtains speech reception threshold by having patient point to pictures of spondaic words
Coordination/Dexterity (Assessment)	**Definition:** Measures large and small muscle groups for controlled goal-directed movements **Explanation:** Dexterity includes object manipulation
Coordination/Dexterity (Treatment)	**Definition:** Exercise or activities to facilitate gross coordination and fine coordination
Cranial Nerve Integrity	**Definition:** Measures cranial nerve sensory and motor functions, including tastes, smell and facial expression
Dichotic Stimuli	**Definition:** Measures specific central auditory process
Distorted Speech	**Definition:** Measures specific central auditory process
Dix-Hallpike Dynamic	**Definition:** Measures nystagmus following Dix-Hallpike maneuver
Dressing	**Includes/Examples:** Includes selecting clothing and accessories, obtaining clothing from storage, dressing and, fastening and adjusting clothing and shoes, and applying and removing personal devices, prosthesis or orthosis
Dressing Techniques	**Definition:** Activities to facilitate selecting clothing and accessories, dressing and undressing, adjusting clothing and shoes, applying and removing devices, prostheses or orthoses
Dynamic Orthosis	**Includes/Examples:** Includes customized and prefabricated splints, inhibitory casts, spinal and other braces, and protective devices; allows motion through transfer of movement from other body parts or by use of outside forces
Ear Canal Probe Microphone	**Definition:** Real ear measures
Ear Protector Attentuation	**Definition:** Measures ear protector fit and effectiveness
Electrocochleography	**Definition:** Measures the VIIIth cranial nerve action potential
Environmental, Home and Work Barriers	**Definition:** Measures current and potential barriers to optimal function, including safety hazards, access problems and home or office design
Ergonomics and Body Mechanics	**Definition:** Ergonomic measurement of job tasks, work hardening or work conditioning needs; functional capacity; and body mechanics
Eustachian Tube Function	**Definition:** Measures eustachian tube function and patency of eustachian tube
Evoked Otoacoustic Emissions, Diagnostic	**Definition:** Measures auditory evoked potentials in a diagnostic format
Evoked Otoacoustic Emissions, Screening	**Definition:** Measures auditory evoked potentials in a screening format
Facial Nerve Function	**Definition:** Measures electrical activity of the VIIth cranial nerve (facial nerve)
Feeding/Eating (Assessment)	**Includes/Examples:** Includes setting up food, selecting and using utensils and tableware, bringing food or drink to mouth, cleaning face, hands, and clothing, and management of alternative methods of nourishment
Feeding/Eating (Treatment)	**Definition:** Exercise or activities to facilitate setting up food, selecting and using utensils and tableware, bringing food or drink to mouth, cleaning face, hands, and clothing, and management of alternative methods of nourishment
Filtered Speech	**Definition:** Uses high or low pass filtered speech stimuli to assess central auditory processing disorders, site of lesion testing
Fluency (Assessment)	**Definition:** Measures speech fluency or stuttering
Fluency (Treatment)	**Definition:** Applying techniques to improve and augment fluent speech
Gait and/or Balance	**Definition:** Measures biomechanical, arthrokinematic and other spatial and temporal characteristics of gait and balance
Gait Training/ Functional Ambulation	**Definition:** Exercise or activities to facilitate ambulation on a variety of surfaces and in a variety of environments

APPENDIX A

SECTION F - PHYSICAL REHABILITATION AND DIAGNOSTIC AUDIOLOGY

CHARACTER 5 - TYPE QUALIFIER

Grooming/Personal Hygiene (Assessment)	**Includes/Examples:** Includes ability to obtain and use supplies in a sequential fashion, general grooming, oral hygiene, toilet hygiene, personal care devices, including care for artificial airways
Grooming/Personal Hygiene (Treatment)	**Definition:** Activities to facilitate obtaining and using supplies in a sequential fashion: general grooming, oral hygiene, toilet hygiene, cleaning body, and personal care devices, including artificial airways
Hearing and Related Disorders Counseling	**Definition:** Provides patients/families/caregivers with information, support, referrals to facilitate recovery from a communication disorder **Includes/Examples:** Includes strategies for psychosocial adjustment to hearing loss for clients and families/caregivers
Hearing and Related Disorders Prevention	**Definition:** Provides patients/families/caregivers with information and support to prevent communication disorders
Hearing Screening	**Definition:** Pass/refer measures designed to identify need for further audiologic assessment
Home Management (Assessment)	**Definition:** Obtaining and maintaining personal and household possessions and environment **Includes/Examples:** Includes clothing care, cleaning, meal preparation and cleanup, shopping, money management, household maintenance, safety procedures, and childcare/parenting
Home Management (Treatment)	**Definition:** Activities to facilitate obtaining and maintaining personal household possessions and environment **Includes/Examples:** Includes clothing care, cleaning, meal preparation and clean-up, shopping, money management, household maintenance, safety procedures, childcare/parenting
Instrumental Swallowing and Oral Function	**Definition:** Measures swallowing function using instrumental diagnostic procedures **Explanation:** Methods include videofluoroscopy, ultrasound, manometry, endoscopy
Integumentary Integrity	**Includes/Examples:** Includes burns, skin conditions, ecchymosis, bleeding, blisters, scar tissue, wounds and other traumas, tissue mobility, turgor and texture
Manual Therapy Techniques	**Definition:** Techniques in which the therapist uses his/her hands to administer skilled movements **Includes/Examples:** Includes connective tissue massage, joint mobilization and manipulation, manual lymph drainage, manual traction, soft tissue mobilization and manipulation
Masking Patterns	**Definition:** Measures central auditory processing status
Monaural Electroacoustic Hearing Aid Check	**Definition:** Determines mechanical and electroacoustic function of one hearing aid using hearing aid test box
Monaural Hearing Aid (Assessment)	**Definition:** Measures the candidacy, effectiveness, and appropriateness of a hearing aid **Explanation:** Measures unilateral fit
Monaural Hearing Aid (Treatment)	**Explanation:** Assists in achieving maximum understanding and performance
Motor Function (Assessment)	**Definition:** Measures the body's functional and versatile movement patterns **Includes/Examples:** Includes motor assessment scales, analysis of head, trunk and limb movement, and assessment of motor learning
Motor Function (Treatment)	**Definition:** Exercise or activities to facilitate crossing midline, laterality, bilateral integration, praxis, neuromuscular relaxation, inhibition, facilitation, motor function and motor learning
Motor Speech (Assessment)	**Definition:** Measures neurological motor aspects of speech production
Motor Speech (Treatment)	**Definition:** Applying techniques to improve and augment the impaired neurological motor aspects of speech production
Muscle Performance (Assessment)	**Definition:** Measures muscle strength, power and endurance using manual testing, dynamometry or computer-assisted electromechanical muscle test; functional muscle strength, power and endurance; muscle pain, tone, or soreness; or pelvic-floor musculature **Explanation:** Muscle endurance refers to the ability to contract a muscle repeatedly over time

SECTION F - PHYSICAL REHABILITATION AND DIAGNOSTIC AUDIOLOGY

CHARACTER 5 - TYPE QUALIFIER

Muscle Performance (Treatment)	**Definition:** Exercise or activities to increase the capacity of a muscle to do work in terms of strength, power, and/or endurance **Explanation:** Muscle strength is the force exerted to overcome resistance in one maximal effort. Muscle power is work produced per unit of time, or the product of strength and speed. Muscle endurance is the ability to contract a muscle repeatedly over time
Neuromotor Development	**Definition:** Measures motor development, righting and equilibrium reactions, and reflex and equilibrium reactions
Non-invasive Instrumental Status	**Definition:** Instrumental measures of oral, nasal, vocal, and velopharyngeal functions as they pertain to speech production
Nonspoken Language (Assessment)	**Definition:** Measures nonspoken language (print, sign, symbols) for communication
Nonspoken Language (Treatment)	**Definition:** Applying techniques that improve, augment, or compensate spoken communication
Oral Peripheral Mechanism	**Definition:** Structural measures of face, jaw, lips, tongue, teeth, hard and soft palate, pharynx as related to speech production
Orofacial Myofunctional (Assessment)	**Definition:** Measures orofacial myofunctional patterns for speech and related functions
Orofacial Myofunctional (Treatment)	**Definition:** Applying techniques to improve, alter, or augment impaired orofacial myofunctional patterns and related speech production errors
Oscillating Tracking	**Definition:** Measures ability to visually track
Pain	**Definition:** Measures muscle soreness, pain and soreness with joint movement, and pain perception **Includes/Examples:** Includes questionnaires, graphs, symptom magnification scales or visual analog scales
Perceptual Processing (Assessment)	**Definition:** Measures stereognosis, kinesthesia, body schema, right-left discrimination, form constancy, position in space, visual closure, figure-ground, depth perception, spatial relations and topographical orientation
Perceptual Processing (Treatment)	**Definition:** Exercise and activities to facilitate perceptual processing **Explanation:** Includes stereognosis, kinesthesia, body schema, right-left discrimination, form constancy, position in space, visual closure, figure-ground, depth perception, spatial relations, and topographical orientation **Includes/Examples:** Includes stereognosis, kinesthesia, body schema, right-left discrimination, form constancy, position in space, visual closure, figure-ground, depth perception, spatial relations, and topographical orientation
Performance Intensity Phonetically Balanced Speech Discrimination	**Definition:** Measures word recognition over varying intensity levels
Postural Control	**Definition:** Exercise or activities to increase postural alignment and control
Prosthesis	**Definition:** Artificial substitutes for missing body parts that augment performance or function **Includes/Examples:** Limb prosthesis, ocular prosthesis
Psychosocial Skills (Assessment)	**Definition:** The ability to interact in society and to process emotions **Includes/Examples:** Includes psychological (values, interests, self-concept); social (role performance, social conduct, interpersonal skills, self expression); self-management (coping skills, time management, self-control)
Psychosocial Skills (Treatment)	**Definition:** The ability to interact in society and to process emotions **Includes/Examples:** Includes psychological (values, interests, self-concept); social (role performance, social conduct, interpersonal skills, self expression); self-management (coping skills, time management, self-control)
Pure Tone Audiometry, Air	**Definition:** Air-conduction pure tone threshold measures with appropriate masking
Pure Tone Audiometry, Air and Bone	**Definition:** Air-conduction and bone-conduction pure tone threshold measures with appropriate masking
Pure Tone Stenger	**Definition:** Measures unilateral nonorganic hearing loss based on simultaneous presentation of pure tones of differing volume

APPENDIX A

SECTION F - PHYSICAL REHABILITATION AND DIAGNOSTIC AUDIOLOGY

CHARACTER 5 - TYPE QUALIFIER

Range of Motion and Joint Integrity	**Definition:** Measures quantity, quality, grade, and classification of joint movement and/or mobility **Explanation:** Range of Motion is the space, distance or angle through which movement occurs at a joint or series of joints. Joint integrity is the conformance of joints to expected anatomic, biomechanical and kinematic norms
Range of Motion and Joint Mobility	**Definition:** Exercise or activities to increase muscle length and joint mobility
Receptive/Expressive Language (Assessment)	**Definition:** Measures receptive and expressive language
Receptive/Expressive Language (Treatment)	**Definition:** Applying techniques tot improve and augment receptive/expressive language
Reflex Integrity	**Definition:** Measures the presence, absence, or exaggeration of developmentally appropriate, pathologic or normal reflexes
Select Picture Audiometry	**Definition:** Establishes hearing threshold levels for speech using pictures
Sensorineural Acuity Level	**Definition:** Measures sensorineural acuity masking presented via bone conduction
Sensory Aids	**Definition:** Determines the appropriateness of a sensory prosthetic device, other than a hearing aid or assistive listening system/device
Sensory Awareness/Processing/Integrity	**Includes/Examples:** Includes light touch, pressure, temperature, pain, sharp/dull, proprioception, vestibular, visual, auditory, gustatory, and olfactory
Short Increment Sensitivity Index	**Definition:** Measures the ear's ability to detect small intensity changes; site of lesion test requiring a behavioral response
Sinusoidal Vertical Axis Rotational	**Definition:** Measures nystagmus following rotation
Somatosensory Evoked Potentials	**Definition:** Measures neural activity from sites throughout the body
Speech and/or Language Screening	**Definition:** Identifies need for further speech and/or language evaluation
Speech Threshold	**Definition:** Measures minimal intensity needed to repeat spondaic words
Speech-Language Pathology and Related Disorders Counseling	**Definition:** Provides patients/families with information, support, referrals to facilitate recovery from a communication disorder
Speech-Language Pathology and Related Disorders Prevention	**Definition:** Applying techniques to avoid or minimize onset and/or development of a communication disorder
Speech/Word Recognition	**Definition:** Measures ability to repeat/identify single syllable words; scores given as a percentage; includes word recognition/speech discrimination
Staggered Spondaic Word	**Definition:** Measures central auditory processing site of lesion based upon dichotic presentation of spondaic words
Static Orthosis	**Includes/Examples:** Includes customized and prefabricated splints, inhibitory casts, spinal and other braces, and protective devices; has no moving parts, maintains joint(s) in desired position
Stenger	**Definition:** Measures unilateral nonorganic hearing loss based on simultaneous presentation of signals of differing volume
Swallowing Dysfunction	**Definition:** Activities to improve swallowing function in coordination with respiratory function **Includes/Examples:** Includes function and coordination of sucking, mastication, coughing, swallowing
Synthetic Sentence Identification	**Definition:** Measures central auditory dysfunction using identification of third order approximations of sentences and competing messages
Temporal Ordering of Stimuli	**Definition:** Measures specific central auditory process
Therapeutic Exercise	**Definition:** Exercise or activities to facilitate sensory awareness, sensory processing, sensory integration, balance training, conditioning, reconditioning **Includes/Examples:** Includes developmental activities, breathing exercises, aerobic endurance activities, aquatic exercises, stretching and ventilatory muscle training
Tinnitus Masker (Assessment)	**Definition:** Determines candidacy for tinnitus masker
Tinnitus Masker (Treatment)	**Explanation:** Used to verify physical fit, acoustic appropriateness, and benefit; assists in achieving maximum benefit

SECTION F, CHARACTER 5

SECTION F - PHYSICAL REHABILITATION AND DIAGNOSTIC AUDIOLOGY

CHARACTER 5 - TYPE QUALIFIER

Tone Decay	**Definition:** Measures decrease in hearing sensitivity to a tone; site of lesion test requiring a behavioral response
Transfer	**Definition:** Transitional movement from one surface to another
Transfer Training	**Definition:** Exercise or activities to facilitate movement from one surface to another
Tympanometry	**Definition:** Measures the integrity of the middle ear; measures ease at which sound flows through the tympanic membrane while air pressure against the membrane is varied
Unithermal Binaural Screen	**Definition:** Measures the rhythmic eye movements stimulated by changing the temperature of the vestibular system in both ears using warm water, screening format
Ventilation, Respiration and Circulation	**Definition:** Measures ventilatory muscle strength, power and endurance, pulmonary function and ventilatory mechanics **Includes/Examples:** Includes ability to clear airway, activities that aggravate or relieve edema, pain, dyspnea or other symptoms, chest wall mobility, cardiopulmonary response to performance of ADL and IAD, cough and sputum, standard vital signs
Vestibular	**Definition:** Applying techniques to compensate for balance disorders; includes habituation, exercise therapy, and balance retraining
Visual Motor Integration (Assessment)	**Definition:** Coordinating the interaction of information from the eyes with body movement during activity
Visual Motor Integration (Treatment)	**Definition:** Exercise or activities to facilitate coordinating the interaction of information from eyes with body movement during activity
Visual Reinforcement Audiometry	**Definition:** Behavioral measures using nonspeech and speech stimuli to obtain frequency/ear-specific information on auditory status **Includes/Examples:** Includes a conditioned response of looking toward a visual reinforcer (e.g., lights, animated toy) every time auditory stimuli are heard
Vocational Activities and Functional Community or Work Reintegration Skills (Assessment)	**Definition:** Measures environmental, home, work (job/school/play) barriers that keep patients from functioning optimally in their environment **Includes/Examples:** Includes assessment of vocational skill and interests, environment of work (job/school/play), injury potential and injury prevention or reduction, ergonomic stressors, transportation skills, and ability to access and use community resources
Vocational Activities and Functional Community or Work Reintegration Skills (Treatment)	**Definition:** Activities to facilitate vocational exploration, body mechanics training, job acquisition, and environmental or work (job/school/play) task adaptation **Includes/Examples:** Includes injury prevention and reduction, ergonomic stressor reduction, job coaching and simulation, work hardening and conditioning, driving training, transportation skills, and use of community resources
Voice (Assessment)	**Definition:** Measures vocal structure, function and production
Voice (Treatment)	**Definition:** Applying techniques to improve voice and vocal function
Voice Prosthetic (Assessment)	**Definition:** Determines the appropriateness of voice prosthetic/adaptive device to enhance or facilitate communication
Voice Prosthetic (Treatment)	**Includes/Examples:** Includes electrolarynx, and other assistive, adaptive, supportive devices
Wheelchair Mobility (Assessment)	**Definition:** Measures fit and functional abilities within wheelchair in a variety of environments
Wheelchair Mobility (Treatment)	**Definition:** Management, maintenance and controlled operation of a wheelchair, scooter or other device, in and on a variety of surfaces and environments
Wound Management	**Includes/Examples:** Includes non-selective and selective debridement (enzymes, autolysis, sharp debridement), dressings (wound coverings, hydrogel, vacuum-assisted closure), topical agents, etc.

APPENDIX A

SECTION G - MENTAL HEALTH
CHARACTER 3 - TYPE

Biofeedback	**Definition:** Provision of information from the monitoring and regulating of physiological processes in conjunction with cognitive-behavioral techniques to improve patient functioning or well-being **Includes/Examples:** Includes EEG, blood pressure, skin temperature or peripheral blood flow, ECG, electrooculogram, EMG, respirometry or capnometry, GSR/EDR, perineometry to monitor/regulate bowel/bladder activity, electrogastrogram to monitor/regulate gastric motility
Counseling	**Definition:** The application of psychological methods to treat an individual with normal developmental issues and psychological problems in order to increase function, improve well-being, alleviate distress, maladjustment or resolve crises
Crisis Intervention	**Definition:** Treatment of a traumatized, acutely disturbed or distressed individual for the purpose of short-term stabilization **Includes/Examples:** Includes defusing, debriefing, counseling, psychotherapy and/or coordination of care with other providers or agencies
Electroconvulsive Therapy	**Definition:** The application of controlled electrical voltages to treat a mental health disorder **Includes/Examples:** Includes appropriate sedation and other preparation of the individual
Family Psychotherapy	**Definition:** Treatment that includes one or more family members of an individual with a mental health disorder by behavioral, cognitive, psychoanalytic, psychodynamic or psychophysiological means to improve functioning or well-being **Explanation:** Remediation of emotional or behavioral problems presented by one or more family members in cases where psychotherapy with more than one family member is indicated
Group Psychotherapy	**Definition:** Treatment of two or more individuals with a mental health disorder by behavioral, cognitive, psychoanalytic, psychodynamic or psychophysiological means to improve functioning or well-being
Hypnosis	**Definition:** Induction of a state of heightened suggestibility by auditory, visual and tactile techniques to elicit an emotional or behavioral response
Individual Psychotherapy	**Definition:** Treatment of an individual with a mental health disorder by behavioral, cognitive, psychoanalytic, psychodynamic or psychophysiological means to improve functioning or well-being
Light Therapy	**Definition:** Application of specialized light treatments to improve functioning or well-being
Medication Management	**Definition:** Monitoring and adjusting the use of medications for the treatment of a mental health disorder
Narcosynthesis	**Definition:** Administration of intravenous barbiturates in order to release suppressed or repressed thoughts
Psychological Tests	**Definition:** The administration and interpretation of standardized psychological tests and measurement instruments for the assessment of psychological function

SECTION G - MENTAL HEALTH
CHARACTER 4 - QUALIFIER

Behavioral	**Definition:** Primarily to modify behavior **Includes/Examples:** Includes modeling and role playing, positive reinforcement of target behaviors, response cost, and training of self-management skills
Cognitive	**Definition:** Primarily to correct cognitive distortions and errors
Cognitive-Behavioral	**Definition:** Combining cognitive and behavioral treatment strategies to improve functioning **Explanation:** Maladaptive responses are examined to determine how cognitions relate to behavior patterns in response to an event. Uses learning principles and information-processing models
Developmental	**Definition:** Age-normed developmental status of cognitive, social and adaptive behavior skills
Intellectual and Psychoeducational	**Definition:** Intellectual abilities, academic achievement and learning capabilities (including behaviors and emotional factors affecting learning)
Interactive	**Definition:** Uses primarily physical aids and other forms of non-oral interaction with a patient who is physically, psychologically or developmentally unable to use ordinary language for communication **Includes/Examples:** Includes the use of toys in symbolic play
Interpersonal	**Definition:** Helps an individual make changes in interpersonal behaviors to reduce psychological dysfunction **Includes/Examples:** Includes exploratory techniques, encouragement of affective expression, clarification of patient statements, analysis of communication patterns, use of therapy relationship and behavior change techniques
Neurobehavioral and Cognitive Status	**Definition:** Includes neurobehavioral status exam, interview(s), and observation for the clinical assessment of thinking, reasoning and judgment, acquired knowledge, attention, memory, visual spatial abilities, language functions, and planning
Neuropsychological	**Definition:** Thinking, reasoning and judgment, acquired knowledge, attention, memory, visual spatial abilities, language functions, planning
Personality and Behavioral	**Definition:** Mood, emotion, behavior, social functioning, psychopathological conditions, personality traits and characteristics
Psychoanalysis	**Definition:** Methods of obtaining a detailed account of past and present mental and emotional experiences to determine the source and eliminate or diminish the undesirable effects of unconscious conflicts **Explanation:** Accomplished by making the individual aware of their existence, origin, and inappropriate expression in emotions and behavior
Psychodynamic	**Definition:** Exploration of past and present emotional experiences to understand motives and drives using insight-oriented techniques to reduce the undesirable effects of internal conflicts on emotions and behavior **Explanation:** Techniques include empathetic listening, clarifying self-defeating behavior patterns, and exploring adaptive alternatives
Psychophysiological	**Definition:** Monitoring and alteration of physiological processes to help the individual associate physiological reactions combined with cognitive and behavioral strategies to gain improved control of these processes to help the individual cope more effectively
Supportive	**Definition:** Formation of therapeutic relationship primarily for providing emotional support to prevent further deterioration in functioning during periods of particular stress **Explanation:** Often used in conjunction with other therapeutic approaches
Vocational	**Definition:** Exploration of vocational interests, aptitudes and required adaptive behavior skills to develop and carry out a plan for achieving a successful vocational placement **Includes/Examples:** Includes enhancing work related adjustment and/or pursuing viable options in training education or preparation

APPENDIX A

SECTION H - SUBSTANCE ABUSE TREATMENT

CHARACTER 3 - TYPE

Detoxification Services	**Definition:** Detoxification from alcohol and/or drugs **Explanation:** Not a treatment modality, but helps the patient stabilize physically and psychologically until the body becomes free of drugs and the effects of alcohol
Family Counseling	**Definition:** The application of psychological methods that includes one or more family members to treat an individual with addictive behavior **Explanation:** Provides support and education for family members of addicted individuals. Family member participation is seen as a critical area of substance abuse treatment
Group Counseling	**Definition:** The application of psychological methods to treat two or more individuals with addictive behavior **Explanation:** Provides structured group counseling sessions and healing power through the connection with others
Individual Counseling	**Definition:** The application of psychological methods to treat an individual with addictive behavior **Explanation:** Comprised of several different techniques, which apply various strategies to address drug addiction
Individual Psychotherapy	**Definition:** Treatment of an individual with addictive behavior by behavioral, cognitive, psychoanalytic, psychodynamic or psychophysiological means
Medication Management	**Definition:** Monitoring and adjusting the use of replacement medications for the treatment of addiction
Pharmacotherapy	**Definition:** The use of replacement medications for the treatment of addiction

SECTION X - NEW TECHNOLOGY

CHARACTER 3 - OPERATION

Assistance	**Definition:** Taking over a portion of a physiological function by extracorporeal means
Bypass	**Definition:** Altering the route of passage of the contents of a tubular body part
Destruction	**Definition:** Physical eradication of all or a portion of a body part by the direct use of energy, force, or a destructive agent **Explanation:** None of the body part is physically taken out **Includes/Examples:** Fulguration of rectal polyp, cautery of skin lesion
Dilation	**Definition:** Expanding an orifice or the lumen of a tubular body part **Explanation:** The orifice can be a natural orifice or an artificially created orifice. Accomplished by stretching a tubular body part using intraluminal pressure or by cutting part of the orifice or wall of the tubular body part
Extirpation	**Definition:** Taking or cutting out solid matter from a body part **Explanation:** The solid matter may be an abnormal byproduct of a biological function or foreign body; it may be imbedded in a body part or in the lumen of a tubular body part. The solid matter may or may not have been previously broken into pieces **Includes/Examples:** Thrombectomy, choledocholithotomy
Fusion	**Definition:** Joining together portions of an articular body part rendering the articular body part immobile **Explanation:** The body part is joined together by fixation device, bone graft, or other means **Includes/Examples:** Spinal fusion, ankle arthrodesis
Insertion	**Definition:** Putting in a nonbiological appliance that monitors, assists,performs, or prevents a physiological function but does not physically take the place of a body part
Inspection	**Definition:** Visually and/or manually exploring a body part
Introduction	**Definition:** Putting in or on a therapeutic, diagnostic, nutritional, physiological, or prophylactic substance except blood or blood products
Irrigation	**Definition:** Putting in or on a cleansing substance
Measurement	**Definition:** Determining the level of a physiological or physical function repetitively at a point in time
Monitoring	**Definition:** Determining the level of a physiological or physical function repetitively over a period of time

SECTION X - NEW TECHNOLOGY
CHARACTER 3 - OPERATION

Division	**Definition:** Cutting into a body part, without draining fluids and/or gasesfrom the body part, in order to separate or transect a body part **Explanation:** All or a portion of the body part is separated into two or more portions
Replacement	**Definition:** Putting in or on biological or synthetic material that physically takes the place and/or function of all or a portion of a body part **Explanation:** The body part may have been taken out or replaced, or may be taken out, physically eradicated, or rendered nonfunctional during the Replacement procedure. A Removal procedure is coded for taking out the device used in a previous replacement procedure **Includes/Examples:** Total hip replacement, bone graft, free skin graft
Reposition	**Definition:** Moving to its normal location, or other suitable location, all or a portion of a body part **Explanation:** The body part is moved to a new location from an abnormal location, or from a normal location where it is not functioning correctly. The body part may or may not be cut out or off to be moved to the new location **Includes/Examples:** Reposition of undescended testicle, fracture reduction
Restriction	Definition: Partially closing an orifice or the lumen of a tubular body part
Supplement	**Definition:** Putting in or on biological or synthetic material that physically reinforces and/or augments the function of a portion of a body part

SECTION X - NEW TECHNOLOGY
CHARACTER 5 - APPROACH

External	**Definition:** Procedures performed directly on the skin or mucous membrane and procedures performed indirectly by the application of external force through the skin or mucous membrane
Open	**Definition:** Cutting through the skin or mucous membrane and any other body layers necessary to expose the site of the procedure
Percutaneous	**Definition:** Entry, by puncture or minor incision, of instrumentation through the skin or mucous membrane and any other body layers necessary to reach the site of the procedure
Percutaneous Endoscopic	**Definition:** Entry, by puncture or minor incision, of instrumentation through the skin or mucous membrane and any other body layers necessary to reach and visualize the site of the procedure
Via Natural or Artificial Opening Endoscopic	**Definition:** Entry of instrumentation through a natural or artificial external opening to reach and visualize the site of the procedure
Via Natural or Artificial Opening	**Definition:** Entry of instrumentation through a natural or artificial external opening to reach the site of the procedure

SECTION X - NEW TECHNOLOGY

CHARACTER 6 - DEVICE / SUBSTANCE / TECHNOLOGY

AGN1 Bone Void Filler	OSSURE™ implant material
Anacaulase-bcdb	Bromelain-enriched Proteolytic Enzyme NexoBrid™
Antibiotic-eluting Bone Void Filler	CERAMENT® G
~~Apalutamide Antineoplastic~~	~~ERLEADA™~~
Atezolizumab Antineoplastic	TECENTRIQ®
Axicabtagene Ciloleucel Immunotherapy	Axicabtagene Ciloleucel Yescarta®
Betibeglogene Autotemcel	ZYNTEGLO®
Bezlotoxumab Monoclonal Antibody	ZINPLAVA™
Bioengineered Allogeneic Construct	StrataGraft®
Bioengineered Human Acellular Vessel in New Technology	HAV™ (Human Acellular Vessel) Human Acellular Vessel™ (HAV)
Branched Intraluminal Device, Manufactured Integrated System, Four or More Arteries in New Technology	GORE® EXCLUDER® TAMBE Device (Thoracoabdominal Branch Endoprosthesis) TAMBE Device (Thoracoabdominal Branch Endoprosthesis), GORE® EXCLUDER®
Branched Synthetic Substitute with Intraluminal Device in Technology	Thoraflex™ Hybrid device
Brexanolone	ZULRESSO™
Brexucabtagene Autoleucel Immunotherapy	Brexucabtagene Autoleucel Tecartus™
Carbon/PEEK Spinal Stabilization Device, Pedicle Based in New Technology	BlackArmor® Carbon/PEEK fixation system VADER® Pedicle System
Cefiderocol Anti-infective	FETROJA®
Ceftolozane/Tazobactam Anti-infective	ZEBAXA®
Ciltacabtagene Autoleucel	cilta-cel
Coagulation Factor Xa, Inactivated	Andexanet Alfa, Factor Xa Inhibitor Reversal Agent Andexxa Coagulation Factor Xa, (Recombinant) Factor Xa Inhibitor Reversal Agent, Andexanet Alfa
Concentrated Bone Marrow Aspirate	CBMA (Concentrated Bone Marrow Aspirate)
Conduit through Femoral Vein to Popliteal Artery in New Technology	DETOUR® System
Conduit through Femoral Vein to Superficial Femoral Artery in New Technology	DETOUR® System
Conduit to Short-term External Heart Assist System in New Technology	Impella® 5.5 with SmartAssist(R) System
COVID-19 Vaccine COVID-19 Vaccine Booster COVID-19 Vaccine Dose 1 COVID-19 Vaccine Dose 2 COVID-19 Vaccine Dose 3	COMIRNATY® SPIKEVAX™
Cytarabine and Daunorubicin Liposome Antineoplastic	VYXEOS™
Defibrotide Sodium Anticoagulant	Defitelio
Donislecel-jujn Allogeneic Pancreatic Islet Cellular Suspension	Lantidra™
Durvalumab Antineoplastic	IMFINZI®
Eculizumab	Soliris®
Elranatamab Antineoplastic	ELREXFIO™
Endothelial Damage Inhibitor	DuraGraft® Endothelial Damage Inhibitor
Epcoritamab Monoclonal Antibody	EPKINLY™
~~Esketamine Hydrochloride~~	~~SPRAVATO™~~
Exagamglogene Autotemcel	CASGEVY™
Facet Joint Fusion Device, Paired Titanium Cages in New Technology	Facet FiXation implant FFX® (Facet FiXation) implant
~~Fosfomycin Anti-infective~~	~~CONTEPO™~~ ~~Fosfomycin injection~~
~~Gilteritinib Antineoplastic~~	~~XOSPATA®~~
Glofitamab Antineoplastic	Columvi™
High-Dose Intravenous Immune Globulin	GAMUNEX-C, for COVID-19 treatment hdIVIG (high-dose intravenous immunoglobulin), for COVID-19 treatment High-dose intravenous immunoglobulin for COVID-19 treatment Octagam 10%, for COVID-19 treatment
Hyperimmune Globulin	Anti-SARS-CoV-2 hyperimmune globulin HIG (hyperimmune globulin), for COVID-19 treatment hIVIG (hyperimmune intravenous immunoglobulin), for COVID-19 treatment Hyperimmune intravenous immunoglobulin (hIVIG), for COVID-19 treatment IGIV-C, for COVID-19 treatment
Idecabtagene Vicleucel Immunotherapy	ABECMA® Ide-cel Idecabtagene Vicleucel

New/Revised Text in Green ~~deleted~~ Deleted

SECTION X - NEW TECHNOLOGY
CHARACTER 6 - DEVICE / SUBSTANCE / TECHNOLOGY

~~Imipenem-cilastatin-relebactam Anti-infective~~	~~IMI/REL~~
Interbody Fusion Device, Custom-Made Anatomically Designed in New Technology	aprevo™
Interbody Fusion Device, Nanotextured Surface in New Technology	nanoLOCK™ interbody fusion device
Interbody Fusion Device, Radiolucent Porous in New Technology	COALESCE® radiolucent interbody fusion device COHERE® radiolucent interbody fusion device
Internal Fixation Device, Gyroid-Sheet Lattice Design in New Technology	restor3d TIDAL™ Fusion Cage
Internal Fixation Device, Open-truss Design in New Technology	Ankle Truss System™ (ATS)
Intracardiac Pacemaker, Dual-Chamber in New Technology	Aveir™ AR, as dual chamber Aveir™ DR, dual chamber
Intraluminal Device, Bioprosthetic Valve in New Technology	TricValve® Transcatheter Bicaval Valve System VenoValve®
~~Intraluminal Device, Sustained Release Drug-eluting in New Technology~~	~~Eluvia™ Drug-Eluting Vascular Stent System~~ ~~SAVAL below-the-knee (BTK) drug-eluting~~
~~Intraluminal Device, Sustained Release Drug-eluting, Four or More in New Technology~~	~~Eluvia™ Drug-Eluting Vascular Stent System~~ ~~SAVAL below-the-knee (BTK) drug-eluting~~
~~Intraluminal Device, Sustained Release Drug-eluting, Three in New Technology~~	~~Eluvia™ Drug-Eluting Vascular Stent System~~ ~~SAVAL below-the-knee (BTK) drug-eluting~~
~~Intraluminal Device, Sustained Release Drug-eluting, Two in New Technology~~	~~Eluvia™ Drug-Eluting Vascular Stent System~~ ~~SAVAL below-the-knee (BTK) drug-eluting~~
Intraluminal Device, Everolimus-eluting Resorbable Scaffold(s) in New Technology	Drug-eluting resorbable scaffold intraluminal device Esprit™ BTK (scaffold) (stent) Everolimus Eluting Resorbable Scaffold System
Iobenguane I-131 Antineoplastic	AZEDRA® Iobenguane I-131, High Specific Activity (HSA)
Lefamulin Anti-infective	XENLETA™
Lifileucel Immunotherapy	AMTAGVI™ Lifileucel
Lisocabatagene Maraleucel Immunotherapy	Lisocabtagene Maraleucel
Lovotibeglogene Autotemcel	LYFGENIA™

Lurbinectedin	ZEPZELCA™
Magnetically Controlled Growth Rod(s) in New Technology	MAGEC® Spinal Bracing and Distraction System Spinal growth rods, magnetically controlled
Marnetegragene Autotemcel	RP-L201
Melphalan Hydrochloride Antineoplastic	HEPZATO™ KIT (melphalan hydrochloride Hepatic Delivery System)
~~Meropenem-vaborbactam Anti-infective~~	~~Vabomere™~~
Mineral-based Topcal Hemostatic Agent	Hemospray® Endoscopic Hemostat
Mosunetuzumab Antineoplastic	LUNSUMIO™
Multi-plane Flex Technology Bioprosthetic Valve in New Technology	Edwards EVOQUE tricuspid valve replacement system
Nafamostat Anticoagulant	LTX Regional Anticoagulant Niyad™
Nerinitide	NA-1 (Nerinitide)
Non-Chimeric Antigen Receptor T-cell Immune Effector Cell Therapy	T-cell Antigen Coupler T-cell (TAC-T) Therapy T-cell Receptor-Engineered T-cell Receptor-Engineered T-cell (TCR-T) Therapy Tumor-Infiltrating Lymphocyte (TIL) Therapy
Obecabtagene Autoleucel	obe-cel
Omadacycline Anti-infective	NUZYRA™
Omidubicel	Omisirge®
Other New Technology Therapeutic Substance	STELARA® Ustekinumab
Posterior (Dynamic) Distraction Device in New Technology	ApiFix® Minimally Invasive Deformity Correction (MID-C) System
Prademagene Zamikeracel, Genetically Engineered Autologous Cell Therapy in New Technology	EB-101 gene-corrected autologous cell therapy EB-101 gene-corrected keratinocyte sheets LZRSE-COL7A1 engineered autologous epidermal sheets pz-cel
Reduction Device in New Technology	Neovasc Reducer™ Reducer™ System
~~Ruxolitinib~~	~~Jakafi®~~
Satralizumab-mwge	ENSPRYNG™
SER-109	VOWST™
Skin Substitute, Porcine Liver Derived in New Technology	MIRODERM™ Biologic Wound Matrix
Spesolimab Monoclonal Antibody	SPEVIGO®

New/Revised Text in Green ~~deleted~~ Deleted

APPENDIX A

SECTION X - NEW TECHNOLOGY
CHARACTER 6 - DEVICE / SUBSTANCE / TECHNOLOGY

Sulbactam-Durlobactam	SUL-DUR Xacduro®
Synthetic Substitute,Extraluminal Support Device in New Technology	VasQ™ External Support device
Synthetic Substitute, Talar Prosthesis in New Technology	Total Ankle Talar Replacement™ (TATR)
Synthetic Substitute,Ultrasound Penetrable in New Technology	Longeviti ClearFit® Cranial Implant Longeviti ClearFit® OTS Cranial Implant
Synthetic Substitute, Mechanically Expandable (Paired) in New Technology	SpineJack® system
Tabelecleucel Immunotherapy	EBVALLO™
Tagraxofusp-erzs Antineoplastic	ELZONRIS™
Talquetamab Antineoplastic	TALVEY™
Teclistamab Antineoplastic	TECVAYLI™
Terlipressin	TERLIVAZ®
Tibial Extension with Motion Sensors in New Technology	Canturio™ te (Tibial Extension)
Tisagenlecleucel Immunotherapy	KYMRIAH® Tisagenlecleucel
Trilaciclib	COSELA™
Uridine Triacetate	Vistogard®
Vancomycin Hydrochloride and Tobramycin Sulfate Anti-Infective, Temporary Irrigation Spacer System	VT-X7 (Irrigation System) (Spacer)
Vein Graft Extraluminal Support Device(s) in New Technology	VEST™ Venous External Support device
~~Venetoclax Antineoplastic~~	~~Venclexta®~~
Zooplastic Tissue, Rapid Deployment Technique in New Technology	EDWARDS INTUITY Elite valve system INTUITY Elite valve system, EDWARDS Perceval sutureless valve Sutureless valve, Perceval

SECTION X, CHARACTER 6

New/Revised Text in Green ~~deleted~~ Deleted

BODY PART KEY

Abdominal aortic plexus	**Use:** Abdominal Sympathetic Nerve
Abdominal esophagus	**Use:** Esophagus, Lower
Abductor hallucis muscle	**Use:** Foot Muscle, Right Foot Muscle, Left
Accessory cephalic vein	**Use:** Cephalic Vein, Right Cephalic Vein, Left
Accessory obturator nerve	**Use:** Lumbar Plexus
Accessory phrenic nerve	**Use:** Phrenic Nerve
Accessory spleen	**Use:** Spleen
Acetabulofemoral joint	**Use:** Hip Joint, Right Hip Joint, Left
Achilles tendon	**Use:** Lower Leg Tendon, Right Lower Leg Tendon, Left
Acromioclavicular ligament	**Use:** Shoulder Bursa and Ligament, Right Shoulder Bursa and Ligament, Left
Acromion (process)	**Use:** Scapula, Right Scapula, Left
Adductor brevis muscle	**Use:** Upper Leg Muscle, Right Upper Leg Muscle, Left
Adductor hallucis muscle	**Use:** Foot Muscle, Right Foot Muscle, Left
Adductor longus muscle Adductor magnus muscle	**Use:** Upper Leg Muscle, Right Upper Leg Muscle, Left
Adenohypophysis	**Use:** Pituitary Gland
Alar ligament of axis	**Use:** Head and Neck Bursa and Ligament
Alveolar process of mandible	**Use:** Mandible, Right Mandible, Left
Alveolar process of maxilla	**Use:** Maxilla
Anal orifice	**Use:** Anus
Anatomical snuffbox	**Use:** Lower Arm and Wrist Muscle, Right Lower Arm and Wrist Muscle, Left
Angular artery	**Use:** Face Artery
Angular vein	**Use:** Face Vein, Right Face Vein, Left
Annular ligament	**Use:** Elbow Bursa and Ligament, Right Elbow Bursa and Ligament, Left
Anorectal junction	**Use:** Rectum
Ansa cervicalis	**Use:** Cervical Plexus
Antebrachial fascia	**Use:** Subcutaneous Tissue and Fascia, Right Lower Arm Subcutaneous Tissue and Fascia, Left Lower Arm
Anterior (pectoral) lymph node	**Use:** Lymphatic, Right Axillary Lymphatic, Left Axillary
Anterior cerebral artery	**Use:** Intracranial Artery
Anterior cerebral vein	**Use:** Intracranial Vein
Anterior choroidal artery	**Use:** Intracranial Artery
Anterior circumflex humeral artery	**Use:** Axillary Artery, Right Axillary Artery, Left
Anterior communicating artery	**Use:** Intracranial Artery
Anterior cruciate ligament (ACL)	**Use:** Knee Bursa and Ligament, Right Knee Bursa and Ligament, Left
Anterior crural nerve	**Use:** Femoral Nerve
Anterior facial vein	**Use:** Face Vein, Right Face Vein, Left

APPENDIX B

BODY PART KEY

Anterior intercostal artery	**Use:** Internal Mammary Artery, Right Internal Mammary Artery, Left
Anterior interosseous nerve	**Use:** Median Nerve
Anterior lateral malleolar artery	**Use:** Anterior Tibial Artery, Right Anterior Tibial Artery, Left
Anterior lingual gland	**Use:** Minor Salivary Gland
Anterior medial malleolar artery	**Use:** Anterior Tibial Artery, Right Anterior Tibial Artery, Left
Anterior spinal artery	**Use:** Vertebral Artery, Right Vertebral Artery, Left
Anterior tibial recurrent artery	**Use:** Anterior Tibial Artery, Right Anterior Tibial Artery, Left
Anterior ulnar recurrent artery	**Use:** Ulnar Artery, Right Ulnar Artery, Left
Anterior vagal trunk	**Use:** Vagus Nerve
Anterior vertebral muscle	**Use:** Neck Muscle, Right Neck Muscle, Left
Antihelix Antitragus	**Use:** External Ear, Right External Ear, Left External Ear, Bilateral
Antrum of Highmore	**Use:** Maxillary Sinus, Right Maxillary Sinus, Left
Aortic annulus	**Use:** Aortic Valve
Aortic arch	**Use:** Thoracic Aorta, Ascending/Arch
Aortic intercostal artery	**Use:** Upper Artery
Apical (subclavicular) lymph node	**Use:** Lymphatic, Right Axillary Lymphatic, Left Axillary
Apneustic center	**Use:** Pons
Aqueduct of Sylvius	**Use:** Cerebral Ventricle

Aqueous humour	**Use:** Anterior Chamber, Right Anterior Chamber, Left
Arachnoid mater	**Use:** Cerebral Meninges Spinal Meninges
Arcuate artery	**Use:** Foot Artery, Right Foot Artery, Left
Areola	**Use:** Nipple, Right Nipple, Left
Arterial canal (duct)	**Use:** Pulmonary Artery, Left
Aryepiglottic fold Arytenoid cartilage	**Use:** Larynx
Arytenoid muscle	**Use:** Neck Muscle, Right Neck Muscle, Left
Ascending aorta	**Use:** Thoracic Aorta, Ascending/Arch
Ascending palatine artery	**Use:** Face Artery
Ascending pharyngeal artery	**Use:** External Carotid Artery, Right External Carotid Artery, Left
Atlantoaxial joint	**Use:** Cervical Vertebral Joint
Atrioventricular node	**Use:** Conduction Mechanism
Atrium dextrum cordis	**Use:** Atrium, Right
Atrium pulmonale	**Use:** Atrium, Left
Auditory tube	**Use:** Eustachian Tube, Right Eustachian Tube, Left
Auerbach's (myenteric) plexus	**Use:** Abdominal Sympathetic Nerve
Auricle	**Use:** External Ear, Right External Ear, Left External Ear, Bilateral
Auricularis muscle	**Use:** Head Muscle

BODY PART KEY

New/Revised Text in Green ~~deleted~~ Deleted

BODY PART KEY

Axillary fascia	**Use:** Subcutaneous Tissue and Fascia, Right Upper Arm Subcutaneous Tissue and Fascia, Left Upper Arm
Axillary nerve	**Use:** Brachial Plexus
Bartholin's (greater vestibular) gland	**Use:** Vestibular Gland
Basal (internal) cerebral vein	**Use:** Intracranial Vein
Basal nuclei	**Use:** Basal Ganglia
Base of Tongue	**Use:** Pharynx
Basilar artery	**Use:** Intracranial Artery
Basis pontis	**Use:** Pons
Biceps brachii muscle	**Use:** Upper Arm Muscle, Right Upper Arm Muscle, Left
Biceps femoris muscle	**Use:** Upper Leg Muscle, Right Upper Leg Muscle, Left
Bicipital aponeurosis	**Use:** Subcutaneous Tissue and Fascia, Right Lower Arm Subcutaneous Tissue and Fascia, Left Lower Arm
Bicuspid valve	**Use:** Mitral Valve
Body of femur	**Use:** Femoral Shaft, Right Femoral Shaft, Left
Body of fibula	**Use:** Fibula, Right Fibula, Left
Bony labyrinth	**Use:** Inner Ear, Right Inner Ear, Left
Bony orbit	**Use:** Orbit, Right Orbit, Left
Bony vestibule	**Use:** Inner Ear, Right Inner Ear, Left
Botallo's duct	**Use:** Pulmonary Artery, Left
Brachial (lateral) lymph node	**Use:** Lymphatic, Right Axillary Lymphatic, Left Axillary
Brachialis muscle	**Use:** Upper Arm Muscle, Right Upper Arm Muscle, Left
Brachiocephalic artery Brachiocephalic trunk	**Use:** Innominate Artery
Brachiocephalic vein	**Use:** Innominate Vein, Right Innominate Vein, Left
Brachioradialis muscle	**Use:** Lower Arm and Wrist Muscle, Right Lower Arm and Wrist Muscle, Left
Broad ligament	**Use:** Uterine Supporting Structure
Bronchial artery	**Use:** Upper Artery
Bronchus Intermedius	**Use:** Main Bronchus, Right
Buccal gland	**Use:** Buccal Mucosa
Buccinator lymph node	**Use:** Lymphatic, Head
Buccinator muscle	**Use:** Facial Muscle
Bulbospongiosus muscle	**Use:** Perineum Muscle
Bulbourethral (Cowper's) gland	**Use:** Urethra
Bundle of His Bundle of Kent	**Use:** Conduction Mechanism
Calcaneocuboid joint	**Use:** Tarsal Joint, Right Tarsal Joint, Left
Calcaneocuboid ligament	**Use:** Foot Bursa and Ligament, Right Foot Bursa and Ligament, Left
Calcaneofibular ligament	**Use:** Ankle Bursa and Ligament, Right Ankle Bursa and Ligament, Left
Calcaneus	**Use:** Tarsal, Right Tarsal, Left

BODY PART KEY

Capitate bone	**Use:** Carpal, Right Carpal, Left
Cardia	**Use:** Esophagogastric Junction
Cardiac plexus	**Use:** Thoracic Sympathetic Nerve
Cardioesophageal junction	**Use:** Esophagogastric Junction
Caroticotympanic artery	**Use:** Internal Carotid Artery, Right Internal Carotid Artery, Left
Carotid glomus	**Use:** Carotid Body, Left Carotid Body, Right Carotid Bodies, Bilateral
Carotid sinus	**Use:** Internal Carotid Artery, Right Internal Carotid Artery, Left
Carotid sinus nerve	**Use:** Glossopharyngeal Nerve
Carpometacarpal ligament	**Use:** Hand Bursa and Ligament, Right Hand Bursa and Ligament, Left
Cauda equina	**Use:** Lumbar Spinal Cord
Cavernous plexus	**Use:** Head and Neck Sympathetic Nerve
Celiac (solar) plexus Celiac ganglion	**Use:** Abdominal Sympathetic Nerve
Celiac lymph node	**Use:** Lymphatic, Aortic
Celiac trunk	**Use:** Celiac Artery
Central axillary lymph node	**Use:** Lymphatic, Right Axillary Lymphatic, Left Axillary
Cerebral aqueduct (Sylvius)	**Use:** Cerebral Ventricle
Cerebrum	**Use:** Brain
Cervical esophagus	**Use:** Esophagus, Upper
Cervical facet joint	**Use:** Cervical Vertebral Joint Cervical Vertebral Joints, 2 or more
Cervical ganglion	**Use:** Head and Neck Sympathetic Nerve
Cervical interspinous ligament Cervical intertransverse ligament Cervical ligamentum flavum	**Use:** Head and Neck Bursa and Ligament
Cervical lymph node	**Use:** Lymphatic, Right Neck Lymphatic, Left Neck
Cervicothoracic facet joint	**Use:** Cervicothoracic Vertebral Joint
Choana	**Use:** Nasopharynx
Chondroglossus muscle	**Use:** Tongue, Palate, Pharynx Muscle
Chorda tympani	**Use:** Facial Nerve
Choroid plexus	**Use:** Cerebral Ventricle
Ciliary body	**Use:** Eye, Right Eye, Left
Ciliary ganglion	**Use:** Head and Neck Sympathetic Nerve
Circle of Willis	**Use:** Intracranial Artery
Circumflex iliac artery	**Use:** Femoral Artery, Right Femoral Artery, Left
Claustrum	**Use:** Basal Ganglia
Coccygeal body	**Use:** Coccygeal Glomus
Coccygeus muscle	**Use:** Trunk Muscle, Right Trunk Muscle, Left
Cochlea	**Use:** Inner Ear, Right Inner Ear, Left
Cochlear nerve	**Use:** Acoustic Nerve
Columella	**Use:** Nasal Mucosa and Soft Tissue

BODY PART KEY

New/Revised Text in Green ~~deleted~~ Deleted

BODY PART KEY

Common digital vein	**Use:** Foot Vein, Right Foot Vein, Left
Common facial vein	**Use:** Face Vein, Right Face Vein, Left
Common fibular nerve	**Use:** Peroneal Nerve
Common hepatic artery	**Use:** Hepatic Artery
Common iliac (subaortic) lymph node	**Use:** Lymphatic, Pelvis
Common interosseous artery	**Use:** Ulnar Artery, Right Ulnar Artery, Left
Common peroneal nerve	**Use:** Peroneal Nerve
Condyloid process	**Use:** Mandible, Right Mandible, Left
Conus arteriosus	**Use:** Ventricle, Right
Conus medullaris	**Use:** Lumbar Spinal Cord
Coracoacromial ligament	**Use:** Shoulder Bursa and Ligament, Right Shoulder Bursa and Ligament, Left
Coracobrachialis muscle	**Use:** Upper Arm Muscle, Right Upper Arm Muscle, Left
Coracoclavicular ligament Coracohumeral ligament	**Use:** Shoulder Bursa and Ligament, Right Shoulder Bursa and Ligament, Left
Coracoid process	**Use:** Scapula, Right Scapula, Left
Corniculate cartilage	**Use:** Larynx
Corpus callosum	**Use:** Brain
Corpus cavernosum Corpus spongiosum	**Use:** Penis
Corpus striatum	**Use:** Basal Ganglia
Corrugator supercilii muscle	**Use:** Facial Muscle
Costocervical trunk	**Use:** Subclavian Artery, Right Subclavian Artery, Left
Costoclavicular ligament	**Use:** Shoulder Bursa and Ligament, Right Shoulder Bursa and Ligament, Left
Costotransverse joint	**Use:** Thoracic Vertebral Joint Thoracic Vertebral Joints, 2 to 7 Thoracic Vertebral Joints, 8 or more
Costotransverse ligament	**Use:** Sternum Bursa and Ligament Rib(s) Bursa and Ligament
Costovertebral joint	**Use:** Thoracic Vertebral Joint Thoracic Vertebral Joints, 2 to 7 Thoracic Vertebral Joints, 8 or more
Costoxiphoid ligament	**Use:** Sternum Bursa and Ligament Rib(s) Bursa and Ligament
Cowper's (bulbourethral) gland	**Use:** Urethra
Cremaster muscle	**Use:** Perineum Muscle
Cribriform plate	**Use:** Ethmoid Bone, Right Ethmoid Bone, Left
Cricoid cartilage	**Use:** Trachea
Cricothyroid artery	**Use:** Thyroid Artery, Right Thyroid Artery, Left
Cricothyroid muscle	**Use:** Neck Muscle, Right Neck Muscle, Left
Crural fascia	**Use:** Subcutaneous Tissue and Fascia, Right Upper Leg Subcutaneous Tissue and Fascia, Left Upper Leg
Cubital lymph node	**Use:** Lymphatic, Right Upper Extremity Lymphatic, Left Upper Extremity
Cubital nerve	**Use:** Ulnar Nerve

BODY PART KEY

Cuboid bone	**Use:** Tarsal, Right Tarsal, Left
Cuboideonavicular joint	**Use:** Tarsal Joint, Right Tarsal Joint, Left
Culmen	**Use:** Cerebellum
Cuneiform cartilage	**Use:** Larynx
Cuneonavicular joint	**Use:** Tarsal Joint, Right Tarsal Joint, Left
Cuneonavicular ligament	**Use:** Foot Bursa and Ligament, Right Foot Bursa and Ligament, Left
Cutaneous (transverse) cervical nerve	**Use:** Cervical Plexus
Deep cervical fascia	**Use:** Subcutaneous Tissue and Fascia, Right Neck Subcutaneous Tissue and Fascia, Left Neck
Deep cervical vein	**Use:** Vertebral Vein, Right Vertebral Vein, Left
Deep circumflex iliac artery	**Use:** External Iliac Artery, Right External Iliac Artery, Left
Deep facial vein	**Use:** Face Vein, Right Face Vein, Left
Deep femoral (profunda femoris) vein	**Use:** Femoral Vein, Right Femoral Vein, Left
Deep femoral artery	**Use:** Femoral Artery, Right Femoral Artery, Left
Deep palmar arch	**Use:** Hand Artery, Right Hand Artery, Left
Deep transverse perineal muscle	**Use:** Perineum Muscle
Deferential artery	**Use:** Internal Iliac Artery, Right Internal Iliac Artery, Left
Deltoid fascia	**Use:** Subcutaneous Tissue and Fascia, Right Upper Arm Subcutaneous Tissue and Fascia, Left Upper Arm
Deltoid ligament	**Use:** Ankle Bursa and Ligament, Right Ankle Bursa and Ligament, Left
Deltoid muscle	**Use:** Shoulder Muscle, Right Shoulder Muscle, Left
Deltopectoral (infraclavicular) lymph node	**Use:** Lymphatic, Right Upper Extremity Lymphatic, Left Upper Extremity
Dens	**Use:** Cervical Vertebra
Denticulate (dentate) ligament	**Use:** Spinal Cord
Depressor anguli oris muscle Depressor labii inferioris muscle Depressor septi nasi muscle Depressor supercilii muscle	**Use:** Facial Muscle
Dermis	**Use:** Skin
Descending genicular artery	**Use:** Femoral Artery, Right Femoral Artery, Left
Diaphragma sellae	**Use:** Dura Mater
Distal humerus	**Use:** Humeral Shaft, Right Humeral Shaft, Left
Distal humerus, involving joint	**Use:** Elbow Joint, Right Elbow Joint, Left
Distal radioulnar joint	**Use:** Wrist Joint, Right Wrist Joint, Left
Dorsal digital nerve	**Use:** Radial Nerve
Dorsal metacarpal vein	**Use:** Hand Vein, Right Hand Vein, Left
Dorsal metatarsal artery	**Use:** Foot Artery, Right Foot Artery, Left

BODY PART KEY

Dorsal metatarsal vein	**Use:** Foot Vein, Right Foot Vein, Left
Dorsal scapular artery	**Use:** Subclavian Artery, Right Subclavian Artery, Left
Dorsal scapular nerve	**Use:** Brachial Plexus
Dorsal venous arch	**Use:** Foot Vein, Right Foot Vein, Left
Dorsalis pedis artery	**Use:** Anterior Tibial Artery, Right Anterior Tibial Artery, Left
Duct of Santorini	**Use:** Pancreatic Duct, Accessory
Duct of Wirsung	**Use:** Pancreatic Duct
Ductus deferens	**Use:** Vas Deferens, Right Vas Deferens, Left Vas Deferens, Bilateral Vas Deferens
Duodenal ampulla	**Use:** Ampulla of Vater
Duodenojejunal flexure	**Use:** Jejunum
Dura mater, intracranial	**Use:** Dura Mater
Dura mater, spinal	**Use:** Spinal Meninges
Dural venous sinus	**Use:** Intracranial Vein
Earlobe	**Use:** External Ear, Right External Ear, Left External Ear, Bilateral
Eighth cranial nerve	**Use:** Acoustic Nerve
Ejaculatory duct	**Use:** Vas Deferens, Right Vas Deferens, Left Vas Deferens, Bilateral Vas Deferens
Eleventh cranial nerve	**Use:** Accessory Nerve
Encephalon	**Use:** Brain
Ependyma	**Use:** Cerebral Ventricle
Epidermis	**Use:** Skin
Epidural space, spinal	**Use:** Spinal Canal
Epiploic foramen	**Use:** Peritoneum
Epithalamus	**Use:** Thalamus
Epitrochlear lymph node	**Use:** Lymphatic, Right Upper Extremity Lymphatic, Left Upper Extremity
Erector spinae muscle	**Use:** Trunk Muscle, Right Trunk Muscle, Left
Esophageal artery	**Use:** Upper Artery
Esophageal plexus	**Use:** Thoracic Sympathetic Nerve
Ethmoidal air cell	**Use:** Ethmoid Sinus, Right Ethmoid Sinus, Left
Extensor carpi radialis muscle Extensor carpi ulnaris muscle	**Use:** Lower Arm and Wrist Muscle, Right Lower Arm and Wrist Muscle, Left
Extensor digitorum brevis muscle	**Use:** Foot Muscle, Right Foot Muscle, Left
Extensor digitorum longus muscle	**Use:** Lower Leg Muscle, Right Lower Leg Muscle, Left
Extensor hallucis brevis muscle	**Use:** Foot Muscle, Right Foot Muscle, Left
Extensor hallucis longus muscle	**Use:** Lower Leg Muscle, Right Lower Leg Muscle, Left
External anal sphincter	**Use:** Anal Sphincter

APPENDIX B

BODY PART KEY

External auditory meatus	**Use:** External Auditory Canal, Right External Auditory Canal, Left
External maxillary artery	**Use:** Face Artery
External naris	**Use:** Nasal Mucosa and Soft Tissue
External oblique aponeurosis	**Use:** Subcutaneous Tissue and Fascia, Trunk
External oblique muscle	**Use:** Abdomen Muscle, Right Abdomen Muscle, Left
External popliteal nerve	**Use:** Peroneal Nerve
External pudendal artery	**Use:** Femoral Artery, Right Femoral Artery, Left
External pudendal vein	**Use:** Saphenous Vein, Right Saphenous Vein, Left
External urethral sphincter	**Use:** Urethra
Extradural space, intracranial	**Use:** Epidural Space, Intracranial
Extradural space, spinal	**Use:** Spinal Canal
Facial artery	**Use:** Face Artery
False vocal cord	**Use:** Larynx
Falx cerebri	**Use:** Dura Mater
Fascia lata	**Use:** Subcutaneous Tissue and Fascia, Right Upper Leg Subcutaneous Tissue and Fascia, Left Upper Leg
Femoral head	**Use:** Upper Femur, Right Upper Femur, Left
Femoral lymph node	**Use:** Lymphatic, Right Lower Extremity Lymphatic, Left Lower Extremity
Femoropatellar joint Femorotibial joint	**Use:** Knee Joint, Right Knee Joint, Left
Fibular artery	**Use:** Peroneal Artery, Right Peroneal Artery, Left
Fibularis brevis muscle Fibularis longus muscle	**Use:** Lower Leg Muscle, Right Lower Leg Muscle, Left
Fifth cranial nerve	**Use:** Trigeminal Nerve
Filum terminale	**Use:** Spinal Meninges
First cranial nerve	**Use:** Olfactory Nerve
First intercostal nerve	**Use:** Brachial Plexus
Flexor carpi radialis muscle Flexor carpi ulnaris muscle	**Use:** Lower Arm and Wrist Muscle, Right Lower Arm and Wrist Muscle, Left
Flexor digitorum brevis muscle	**Use:** Foot Muscle, Right Foot Muscle, Left
Flexor digitorum longus muscle	**Use:** Lower Leg Muscle, Right Lower Leg Muscle, Left
Flexor hallucis brevis muscle	**Use:** Foot Muscle, Right Foot Muscle, Left
Flexor hallucis longus muscle	**Use:** Lower Leg Muscle, Right Lower Leg Muscle, Left
Flexor pollicis longus muscle	**Use:** Lower Arm and Wrist Muscle, Right Lower Arm and Wrist Muscle, Left
Foramen magnum	**Use:** Occipital Bone
Foramen of Monro (intraventricular)	**Use:** Cerebral Ventricle
Foreskin	**Use:** Prepuce
Fossa of Rosenmuller	**Use:** Nasopharynx

BODY PART KEY

Fourth cranial nerve	**Use:** Trochlear Nerve
Fourth ventricle	**Use:** Cerebral Ventricle
Fovea	**Use:** Retina, Right Retina, Left
Frenulum labii inferioris	**Use:** Lower Lip
Frenulum labii superioris	**Use:** Upper Lip
Frenulum linguae	**Use:** Tongue
Frontal lobe	**Use:** Cerebral Hemisphere
Frontal vein	**Use:** Face Vein, Right Face Vein, Left
Fundus uteri	**Use:** Uterus
Galea aponeurotica	**Use:** Subcutaneous Tissue and Fascia, Scalp
Ganglion impar (ganglion of Walther)	**Use:** Sacral Sympathetic Nerve
Gasserian ganglion	**Use:** Trigeminal Nerve
Gastric lymph node	**Use:** Lymphatic, Aortic
Gastric plexus	**Use:** Abdominal Sympathetic Nerve
Gastrocnemius muscle	**Use:** Lower Leg Muscle, Right Lower Leg Muscle, Left
Gastrocolic ligament Gastrocolic omentum	**Use:** Omentum
Gastroduodenal artery	**Use:** Hepatic Artery
Gastroesophageal (GE) junction	**Use:** Esophagogastric Junction
Gastrohepatic omentum Gastrophrenic ligament Gastrosplenic ligament	**Use:** Omentum
Gemellus muscle	**Use:** Hip Muscle, Right Hip Muscle, Left
Geniculate ganglion	**Use:** Facial Nerve
Geniculate nucleus	**Use:** Thalamus
Genioglossus muscle	**Use:** Tongue, Palate, Pharynx Muscle
Genitofemoral nerve	**Use:** Lumbar Plexus
Glans penis	**Use:** Prepuce
Glenohumeral joint	**Use:** Shoulder Joint, Right Shoulder Joint, Left
Glenohumeral ligament	**Use:** Shoulder Bursa and Ligament, Right Shoulder Bursa and Ligament, Left
Glenoid fossa (of scapula)	**Use:** Glenoid Cavity, Right Glenoid Cavity, Left
Glenoid ligament (labrum)	**Use:** Shoulder Bursa and Ligament, Right Shoulder Bursa and Ligament, Left
Globus pallidus	**Use:** Basal Ganglia
Glossoepiglottic fold	**Use:** Epiglottis
Glottis	**Use:** Larynx
Gluteal lymph node	**Use:** Lymphatic, Pelvis
Gluteal vein	**Use:** Hypogastric Vein, Right Hypogastric Vein, Left
Gluteus maximus muscle Gluteus medius muscle Gluteus minimus muscle	**Use:** Hip Muscle, Right Hip Muscle, Left
Gracilis muscle	**Use:** Upper Leg Muscle, Right Upper Leg Muscle, Left

APPENDIX B

BODY PART KEY

Great auricular nerve	**Use:** Cervical Plexus
Great cerebral vein	**Use:** Intracranial Vein
Greater saphenous vein	**Use:** Saphenous Vein, Right Saphenous Vein, Left
Greater alar cartilage	**Use:** Nasal Mucosa and Soft Tissue
Greater occipital nerve	**Use:** Cervical Nerve
Greater Omentum	**Use:** Omentum
Greater splanchnic nerve	**Use:** Thoracic Sympathetic Nerve
Greater superficial petrosal nerve	**Use:** Facial Nerve
Greater trochanter	**Use:** Upper Femur, Right Upper Femur, Left
Greater tuberosity	**Use:** Humeral Head, Right Humeral Head, Left
Greater vestibular (Bartholin's) gland	**Use:** Vestibular Gland
Greater wing	**Use:** Sphenoid Bone
Hallux	**Use:** 1st Toe, Right 1st Toe, Left
Hamate bone	**Use:** Carpal, Right Carpal, Left
Head of fibula	**Use:** Fibula, Right Fibula, Left
Helix	**Use:** External Ear, Right External Ear, Left External Ear, Bilateral
Hepatic artery proper	**Use:** Hepatic Artery
Hepatic flexure	**Use:** Transverse Colon
Hepatic lymph node	**Use:** Lymphatic, Aortic
Hepatic plexus	**Use:** Abdominal Sympathetic Nerve
Hepatic portal vein	**Use:** Portal Vein
Hepatogastric ligament	**Use:** Omentum
Hepatopancreatic ampulla	**Use:** Ampulla of Vater
Humeroradial joint Humeroulnar joint	**Use:** Elbow Joint, Right Elbow Joint, Left
Humerus, distal	**Use:** Humeral Shaft, Right Humeral Shaft, Left
Hyoglossus muscle	**Use:** Tongue, Palate, Pharynx Muscle
Hyoid artery	**Use:** Thyroid Artery, Right Thyroid Artery, Left
Hypogastric artery	**Use:** Internal Iliac Artery, Right Internal Iliac Artery, Left
Hypopharynx	**Use:** Pharynx
Hypophysis	**Use:** Pituitary Gland
Hypothenar muscle	**Use:** Hand Muscle, Right Hand Muscle, Left
Ileal artery Ileocolic artery	**Use:** Superior Mesenteric Artery
Ileocolic vein	**Use:** Colic Vein
Iliac crest	**Use:** Pelvic Bone, Right Pelvic Bone, Left
Iliac fascia	**Use:** Subcutaneous Tissue and Fascia, Right Upper Leg Subcutaneous Tissue and Fascia, Left Upper Leg

BODY PART KEY

Iliac lymph node	**Use:** Lymphatic, Pelvis
Iliacus muscle	**Use:** Hip Muscle, Right Hip Muscle, Left
Iliofemoral ligament	**Use:** Hip Bursa and Ligament, Right Hip Bursa and Ligament, Left
Iliohypogastric nerve Ilioinguinal nerve	**Use:** Lumbar Plexus
Iliolumbar artery	**Use:** Internal Iliac Artery, Right Internal Iliac Artery, Left
Iliolumbar ligament	**Use:** Lower Spine Bursa and Ligament
Iliotibial tract (band)	**Use:** Subcutaneous Tissue and Fascia, Right Upper Leg Subcutaneous Tissue and Fascia, Left Upper Leg
Ilium	**Use:** Pelvic Bone, Right Pelvic Bone, Left
Incus	**Use:** Auditory Ossicle, Right Auditory Ossicle, Left
Inferior cardiac nerve	**Use:** Thoracic Sympathetic Nerve
Inferior cerebellar vein Inferior cerebral vein	**Use:** Intracranial Vein
Inferior epigastric artery	**Use:** External Iliac Artery, Right External Iliac Artery, Left
Inferior epigastric lymph node	**Use:** Lymphatic, Pelvis
Inferior genicular artery	**Use:** Popliteal Artery, Right Popliteal Artery, Left
Inferior gluteal artery	**Use:** Internal Iliac Artery, Right Internal Iliac Artery, Left
Inferior gluteal nerve	**Use:** Sacral Plexus
Inferior hypogastric plexus	**Use:** Abdominal Sympathetic Nerve
Inferior labial artery	**Use:** Face Artery
Inferior longitudinal muscle	**Use:** Tongue, Palate, Pharynx Muscle
Inferior mesenteric ganglion	**Use:** Abdominal Sympathetic Nerve
Inferior mesenteric lymph node	**Use:** Lymphatic, Mesenteric
Inferior mesenteric plexus	**Use:** Abdominal Sympathetic Nerve
Inferior oblique muscle	**Use:** Extraocular Muscle, Right Extraocular Muscle, Left
Inferior pancreaticoduodenal artery	**Use:** Superior Mesenteric Artery
Inferior phrenic artery	**Use:** Abdominal Aorta
Inferior rectus muscle	**Use:** Extraocular Muscle, Right Extraocular Muscle, Left
Inferior suprarenal artery	**Use:** Renal Artery, Right Renal Artery, Left
Inferior tarsal plate	**Use:** Lower Eyelid, Right Lower Eyelid, Left
Inferior thyroid vein	**Use:** Innominate Vein, Right Innominate Vein, Left
Inferior tibiofibular joint	**Use:** Ankle Joint, Right Ankle Joint, Left
Inferior turbinate	**Use:** Nasal Turbinate
Inferior ulnar collateral artery	**Use:** Brachial Artery, Right Brachial Artery, Left
Inferior vesical artery	**Use:** Internal Iliac Artery, Right Internal Iliac Artery, Left
Infraauricular lymph node	**Use:** Lymphatic, Head
Infraclavicular (deltopectoral) lymph node	**Use:** Lymphatic, Right Upper Extremity Lymphatic, Left Upper Extremity

APPENDIX B

BODY PART KEY

Infrahyoid muscle	**Use:** Neck Muscle, Right Neck Muscle, Left
Infraparotid lymph node	**Use:** Lymphatic, Head
Infraspinatus fascia	**Use:** Subcutaneous Tissue and Fascia, Right Upper Arm Subcutaneous Tissue and Fascia, Left Upper Arm
Infraspinatus muscle	**Use:** Shoulder Muscle, Right Shoulder Muscle, Left
Infundibulopelvic ligament	**Use:** Uterine Supporting Structure
Inguinal canal Inguinal triangle	**Use:** Inguinal Region, Right Inguinal Region, Left Inguinal Region, Bilateral
Interatrial septum	**Use:** Atrial Septum
Intercarpal joint	**Use:** Carpal Joint, Right Carpal Joint, Left
Intercarpal ligament	**Use:** Hand Bursa and Ligament, Right Hand Bursa and Ligament, Left
Interclavicular ligament	**Use:** Shoulder Bursa and Ligament, Right Shoulder Bursa and Ligament, Left
Intercostal lymph node	**Use:** Lymphatic, Thorax
Intercostal muscle	**Use:** Thorax Muscle, Right Thorax Muscle, Left
Intercostal nerve Intercostobrachial nerve	**Use:** Thoracic Nerve
Intercuneiform joint	**Use:** Tarsal Joint, Right Tarsal Joint, Left
Intercuneiform ligament	**Use:** Foot Bursa and Ligament, Right Foot Bursa and Ligament, Left
Intermediate bronchus	**Use:** Main Bronchus, Right
Intermediate cuneiform bone	**Use:** Tarsal, Right Tarsal, Left
Internal (basal) cerebral vein	**Use:** Intracranial Vein
Internal anal sphincter	**Use:** Anal Sphincter
Internal carotid artery, intracranial portion	**Use:** Intracranial Artery
Internal carotid plexus	**Use:** Head and Neck Sympathetic Nerve
Internal iliac vein	**Use:** Hypogastric Vein, Right Hypogastric Vein, Left
Internal maxillary artery	**Use:** External Carotid Artery, Right External Carotid Artery, Left
Internal naris	**Use:** Nasal Mucosa and Soft Tissue
Internal oblique muscle	**Use:** Abdomen Muscle, Right Abdomen Muscle, Left
Internal pudendal artery	**Use:** Internal Iliac Artery, Right Internal Iliac Artery, Left
Internal pudendal vein	**Use:** Hypogastric Vein, Right Hypogastric Vein, Left
Internal thoracic artery	**Use:** Internal Mammary Artery, Right Internal Mammary Artery, Left Subclavian Artery, Right Subclavian Artery, Left
Internal urethral sphincter	**Use:** Urethra
Interphalangeal (IP) joint	**Use:** Finger Phalangeal Joint, Right Finger Phalangeal Joint, Left Toe Phalangeal Joint, Right Toe Phalangeal Joint, Left
Interphalangeal ligament	**Use:** Hand Bursa and Ligament, Right Hand Bursa and Ligament, Left Foot Bursa and Ligament, Right Foot Bursa and Ligament, Left
Interspinalis muscle	**Use:** Trunk Muscle, Right Trunk Muscle, Left

BODY PART KEY

Interspinous ligament	**Use:** Head and Neck Bursa and Ligament Upper Spine Bursa and Ligament Lower Spine Bursa and Ligament
Intertransversarius muscle	**Use:** Trunk Muscle, Right Trunk Muscle, Left
Intertransverse ligament	**Use:** Upper Spine Bursa and Ligament Lower Spine Bursa and Ligament
Interventricular foramen (Monro)	**Use:** Cerebral Ventricle
Interventricular septum	**Use:** Ventricular Septum
Intestinal lymphatic trunk	**Use:** Cisterna Chyli
Ischiatic nerve	**Use:** Sciatic Nerve
Ischiocavernosus muscle	**Use:** Perineum Muscle
Ischiofemoral ligament	**Use:** Hip Bursa and Ligament, Right Hip Bursa and Ligament, Left
Ischium	**Use:** Pelvic Bone, Right Pelvic Bone, Left
Jejunal artery	**Use:** Superior Mesenteric Artery
Jugular body	**Use:** Glomus Jugulare
Jugular lymph node	**Use:** Lymphatic, Right Neck Lymphatic, Left Neck
Labia majora Labia minora	**Use:** Vulva
Labial gland	**Use:** Upper Lip Lower Lip
Lacrimal canaliculus Lacrimal punctum Lacrimal sac	**Use:** Lacrimal Duct, Right Lacrimal Duct, Left
Laryngopharynx	**Use:** Pharynx
Lateral (brachial) lymph node	**Use:** Lymphatic, Right Axillary Lymphatic, Left Axillary
Lateral canthus	**Use:** Upper Eyelid, Right Upper Eyelid, Left
Lateral collateral ligament (LCL)	**Use:** Knee Bursa and Ligament, Right Knee Bursa and Ligament, Left
Lateral condyle of femur	**Use:** Lower Femur, Right Lower Femur, Left
Lateral condyle of tibia	**Use:** Tibia, Right Tibia, Left
Lateral cuneiform bone	**Use:** Tarsal, Right Tarsal, Left
Lateral epicondyle of femur	**Use:** Lower Femur, Right Lower Femur, Left
Lateral epicondyle of humerus	**Use:** Humeral Shaft, Right Humeral Shaft, Left
Lateral femoral cutaneous nerve	**Use:** Lumbar Plexus
Lateral malleolus	**Use:** Fibula, Right Fibula, Left
Lateral meniscus	**Use:** Knee Joint, Right Knee Joint, Left
Lateral nasal cartilage	**Use:** Nasal Mucosa and Soft Tissue
Lateral plantar artery	**Use:** Foot Artery, Right Foot Artery, Left
Lateral plantar nerve	**Use:** Tibial Nerve
Lateral rectus muscle	**Use:** Extraocular Muscle, Right Extraocular Muscle, Left
Lateral sacral artery	**Use:** Internal Iliac Artery, Right Internal Iliac Artery, Left

APPENDIX B

BODY PART KEY

Lateral sacral vein	**Use:** Hypogastric Vein, Right Hypogastric Vein, Left
Lateral sural cutaneous nerve	**Use:** Peroneal Nerve
Lateral tarsal artery	**Use:** Foot Artery, Right Foot Artery, Left
Lateral temporomandibular ligament	**Use:** Head and Neck Bursa and Ligament
Lateral thoracic artery	**Use:** Axillary Artery, Right Axillary Artery, Left
Latissimus dorsi muscle	**Use:** Trunk Muscle, Right Trunk Muscle, Left
Least splanchnic nerve	**Use:** Thoracic Sympathetic Nerve
Left ascending lumbar vein	**Use:** Hemiazygos Vein
Left atrioventricular valve	**Use:** Mitral Valve
Left auricular appendix	**Use:** Atrium, Left
Left colic vein	**Use:** Colic Vein
Left coronary sulcus	**Use:** Heart, Left
Left gastric artery	**Use:** Gastric Artery
Left gastroepiploic artery	**Use:** Splenic Artery
Left gastroepiploic vein	**Use:** Splenic Vein
Left inferior phrenic vein	**Use:** Renal Vein, Left
Left inferior pulmonary vein	**Use:** Pulmonary Vein, Left
Left jugular trunk	**Use:** Thoracic Duct
Left lateral ventricle	**Use:** Cerebral Ventricle
Left ovarian vein Left second lumbar vein	**Use:** Renal Vein, Left
Left subclavian trunk	**Use:** Thoracic Duct
Left subcostal vein	**Use:** Hemiazygos Vein
Left superior pulmonary vein	**Use:** Pulmonary Vein, Left
Left suprarenal vein Left testicular vein	**Use:** Renal Vein, Left
Leptomeninges, intracranial	**Use:** Cerebral Meninges
Leptomeninges, spinal	**Use:** Spinal Meninges
Lesser alar cartilage	**Use:** Nasal Mucosa and Soft Tissue
Lesser occipital nerve	**Use:** Cervical Plexus
Lesser Omentum	**Use:** Omentum
Lesser saphenous vein	**Use:** Saphenous Vein, Right Saphenous Vein, Left
Lesser splanchnic nerve	**Use:** Thoracic Sympathetic Nerve
Lesser trochanter	**Use:** Upper Femur, Right Upper Femur, Left
Lesser tuberosity	**Use:** Humeral Head, Right Humeral Head, Left
Lesser wing	**Use:** Sphenoid Bone
Levator anguli oris muscle	**Use:** Facial Muscle
Levator ani muscle	**Use:** Perineum Muscle
Levator labii superioris alaeque nasi muscle Levator labii superioris muscle	**Use:** Facial Muscle
Levator palpebrae superioris muscle	**Use:** Upper Eyelid, Right Upper Eyelid, Left
Levator scapulae muscle	**Use:** Neck Muscle, Right Neck Muscle, Left
Levator veli palatini muscle	**Use:** Tongue, Palate, Pharynx Muscle

BODY PART KEY

Levatores costarum muscle	**Use:** Thorax Muscle, Right Thorax Muscle, Left
Ligament of head of fibula	**Use:** Knee Bursa and Ligament, Right Knee Bursa and Ligament, Left
Ligament of the lateral malleolus	**Use:** Ankle Bursa and Ligament, Right Ankle Bursa and Ligament, Left
Ligamentum flavum	**Use:** Upper Spine Bursa and Ligament Lower Spine Bursa and Ligament
Lingual artery	**Use:** External Carotid Artery, Right External Carotid Artery, Left
Lingual tonsil	**Use:** Pharynx
Locus ceruleus	**Use:** Pons
Long thoracic nerve	**Use:** Brachial Plexus
Lumbar artery	**Use:** Abdominal Aorta
Lumbar facet joint	**Use:** Lumbar Vertebral Joint Lumbar Vertebral Joints, 2 or more
Lumbar ganglion	**Use:** Lumbar Sympathetic Nerve
Lumbar lymph node	**Use:** Lymphatic, Aortic
Lumbar lymphatic trunk	**Use:** Cisterna Chyli
Lumbar splanchnic nerve	**Use:** Lumbar Sympathetic Nerve
Lumbosacral facet joint	**Use:** Lumbosacral Joint
Lumbosacral trunk	**Use:** Lumbar Nerve
Lunate bone	**Use:** Carpal, Right Carpal, Left
Lunotriquetral ligament	**Use:** Hand Bursa and Ligament, Right Hand Bursa and Ligament, Left
Macula	**Use:** Retina, Right Retina, Left
Malleus	**Use:** Auditory Ossicle, Right Auditory Ossicle, Left
Mammary duct Mammary gland	**Use:** Breast, Right Breast, Left Breast, Bilateral
Mammillary body	**Use:** Hypothalamus
Mandibular nerve	**Use:** Trigeminal Nerve
Mandibular notch	**Use:** Mandible, Right Mandible, Left
Manubrium	**Use:** Sternum
Masseter muscle	**Use:** Head Muscle
Masseteric fascia	**Use:** Subcutaneous Tissue and Fascia, Face
Mastoid (postauricular) lymph node	**Use:** Lymphatic, Right Neck Lymphatic, Left Neck
Mastoid air cells	**Use:** Mastoid Sinus, Right Mastoid Sinus, Left
Mastoid process	**Use:** Temporal Bone, Right Temporal Bone, Left
Maxillary artery	**Use:** External Carotid Artery, Right External Carotid Artery, Left
Maxillary nerve	**Use:** Trigeminal Nerve
Medial canthus	**Use:** Lower Eyelid, Right Lower Eyelid, Left
Medial collateral ligament (MCL)	**Use:** Knee Bursa and Ligament, Right Knee Bursa and Ligament, Left
Medial condyle of femur	**Use:** Lower Femur, Right Lower Femur, Left
Medial condyle of tibia	**Use:** Tibia, Right Tibia, Left

APPENDIX B

New/Revised Text in Green ~~deleted~~ Deleted

BODY PART KEY

Medial cuneiform bone	**Use:** Tarsal, Right Tarsal, Left
Medial epicondyle of femur	**Use:** Lower Femur, Right Lower Femur, Left
Medial epicondyle of humerus	**Use:** Humeral Shaft, Right Humeral Shaft, Left
Medial malleolus	**Use:** Tibia, Right Tibia, Left
Medial meniscus	**Use:** Knee Joint, Right Knee Joint, Left
Medial plantar artery	**Use:** Foot Artery, Right Foot Artery, Left
Medial plantar nerve Medial popliteal nerve	**Use:** Tibial Nerve
Medial rectus muscle	**Use:** Extraocular Muscle, Right Extraocular Muscle, Left
Medial sural cutaneous nerve	**Use:** Tibial Nerve
Median antebrachial vein Median cubital vein	**Use:** Basilic Vein, Right Basilic Vein, Left
Median sacral artery	**Use:** Abdominal Aorta
Mediastinal lymph node	**Use:** Lymphatic, Thorax
Meissner's (submucous) plexus	**Use:** Abdominal Sympathetic Nerve
Membranous urethra	**Use:** Urethra
Mental foramen	**Use:** Mandible, Right Mandible, Left
Mentalis muscle	**Use:** Facial Muscle
Mesoappendix Mesocolon	**Use:** Mesentery
Metacarpal ligament Metacarpophalangeal ligament	**Use:** Hand Bursa and Ligament, Right Hand Bursa and Ligament, Left
Metatarsal ligament	**Use:** Foot Bursa and Ligament, Right Foot Bursa and Ligament, Left
Metatarsophalangeal (MTP) joint	**Use:** Metatarsal-Phalangeal Joint, Right Metatarsal-Phalangeal Joint, Left
Metatarsophalangeal ligament	**Use:** Foot Bursa and Ligament, Right Foot Bursa and Ligament, Left
Metathalamus	**Use:** Thalamus
Midcarpal joint	**Use:** Carpal Joint, Right Carpal Joint, Left
Middle cardiac nerve	**Use:** Thoracic Sympathetic Nerve
Middle cerebral artery	**Use:** Intracranial Artery
Middle cerebral vein	**Use:** Intracranial Vein
Middle colic vein	**Use:** Colic Vein
Middle genicular artery	**Use:** Popliteal Artery, Right Popliteal Artery, Left
Middle hemorrhoidal vein	**Use:** Hypogastric Vein, Right Hypogastric Vein, Left
Middle rectal artery	**Use:** Internal Iliac Artery, Right Internal Iliac Artery, Left
Middle suprarenal artery	**Use:** Abdominal Aorta
Middle temporal artery	**Use:** Temporal Artery, Right Temporal Artery, Left
Middle turbinate	**Use:** Nasal Turbinate
Mitral annulus	**Use:** Mitral Valve
Molar gland	**Use:** Buccal Mucosa
Musculocutaneous nerve	**Use:** Brachial Plexus
Musculophrenic artery	**Use:** Internal Mammary Artery, Right Internal Mammary Artery, Left

New/Revised Text in Green ~~deleted~~ Deleted

BODY PART KEY

Musculospiral nerve	**Use:** Radial Nerve
Myelencephalon	**Use:** Medulla Oblongata
Myenteric (Auerbach's) plexus	**Use:** Abdominal Sympathetic Nerve
Myometrium	**Use:** Uterus
Nail bed Nail plate	**Use:** Finger Nail Toe Nail
Nasal cavity	**Use:** Nasal Mucosa and Soft Tissue
Nasal concha	**Use:** Nasal Turbinate
Nasalis muscle	**Use:** Facial Muscle
Nasolacrimal duct	**Use:** Lacrimal Duct, Right Lacrimal Duct, Left
Navicular bone	**Use:** Tarsal, Right Tarsal, Left
Neck of femur	**Use:** Upper Femur, Right Upper Femur, Left
Neck of humerus (anatomical) (surgical)	**Use:** Humeral Head, Right Humeral Head, Left
Nerve to the stapedius	**Use:** Facial Nerve
Neurohypophysis	**Use:** Pituitary Gland
Ninth cranial nerve	**Use:** Glossopharyngeal Nerve
Nostril	**Use:** Nasal Mucosa and Soft Tissue
Obturator artery	**Use:** Internal Iliac Artery, Right Internal Iliac Artery, Left
Obturator lymph node	**Use:** Lymphatic, Pelvis
Obturator muscle	**Use:** Hip Muscle, Right Hip Muscle, Left
Obturator nerve	**Use:** Lumbar Plexus
Obturator vein	**Use:** Hypogastric Vein, Right Hypogastric Vein, Left
Obtuse margin	**Use:** Heart, Left
Occipital artery	**Use:** External Carotid Artery, Right External Carotid Artery, Left
Occipital lobe	**Use:** Cerebral Hemisphere
Occipital lymph node	**Use:** Lymphatic, Right Neck Lymphatic, Left Neck
Occipitofrontalis muscle	**Use:** Facial Muscle
Odontoid process	**Use:** Cervical Vertebra
Olecranon bursa	**Use:** Elbow Bursa and Ligament, Right Elbow Bursa and Ligament, Left
Olecranon process	**Use:** Ulna, Right Ulna, Left
Olfactory bulb	**Use:** Olfactory Nerve
Ophthalmic artery	**Use:** Intracranial Artery
Ophthalmic nerve	**Use:** Trigeminal Nerve
Ophthalmic vein	**Use:** Intracranial Vein
Optic chiasma	**Use:** Optic Nerve
Optic disc	**Use:** Retina, Right Retina, Left
Optic foramen	**Use:** Sphenoid Bone
Orbicularis oculi muscle	**Use:** Upper Eyelid, Right Upper Eyelid, Left
Orbicularis oris muscle	**Use:** Facial Muscle
Orbital fascia	**Use:** Subcutaneous Tissue and Fascia, Face

APPENDIX B

BODY PART KEY

Orbital portion of ethmoid bone Orbital portion of frontal bone Orbital portion of lacrimal bone Orbital portion of maxilla Orbital portion of palatine bone Orbital portion of sphenoid bone Orbital portion of zygomatic bone	**Use:** Orbit, Right Orbit, Left
Oropharynx	**Use:** Pharynx
Otic ganglion	**Use:** Head and Neck Sympathetic Nerve
Oval window	**Use:** Middle Ear, Right Middle Ear, Left
Ovarian artery	**Use:** Abdominal Aorta
Ovarian ligament	**Use:** Uterine Supporting Structure
Oviduct	**Use:** Fallopian Tube, Right Fallopian Tube, Left
Palatine gland	**Use:** Buccal Mucosa
Palatine tonsil	**Use:** Tonsils
Palatine uvula	**Use:** Uvula
Palatoglossal muscle Palatopharyngeal muscle	**Use:** Tongue, Palate, Pharynx Muscle
Palmar (volar) digital vein Palmar (volar) metacarpal vein	**Use:** Hand Vein, Right Hand Vein, Left
Palmar cutaneous nerve	**Use:** Median Nerve Radial Nerve
Palmar fascia (aponeurosis)	**Use:** Subcutaneous Tissue and Fascia, Right Hand Subcutaneous Tissue and Fascia, Left Hand
Palmar interosseous muscle	**Use:** Hand Muscle, Right Hand Muscle, Left
Palmar ulnocarpal ligament	**Use:** Wrist Bursa and Ligament, Right Wrist Bursa and Ligament, Left
Palmaris longus muscle	**Use:** Lower Arm and Wrist Muscle, Right Lower Arm and Wrist Muscle, Left
Pancreatic artery	**Use:** Splenic Artery
Pancreatic plexus	**Use:** Abdominal Sympathetic Nerve
Pancreatic vein	**Use:** Splenic Vein
Pancreaticosplenic lymph node Paraaortic lymph node	**Use:** Lymphatic, Aortic
Pararectal lymph node	**Use:** Lymphatic, Mesenteric
Parasternal lymph node Paratracheal lymph node	**Use:** Lymphatic, Thorax
Paraurethral (Skene's) gland	**Use:** Vestibular Gland
Parietal lobe	**Use:** Cerebral Hemisphere
Parotid lymph node	**Use:** Lymphatic, Head
Parotid plexus	**Use:** Facial Nerve
Pars flaccida	**Use:** Tympanic Membrane, Right Tympanic Membrane, Left
Patellar ligament	**Use:** Knee Bursa and Ligament, Right Knee Bursa and Ligament, Left
Patellar tendon	**Use:** Knee Tendon, Right Knee Tendon, Left
Pectineus muscle	**Use:** Upper Leg Muscle, Right Upper Leg Muscle, Left
Pectoral (anterior) lymph node	**Use:** Lymphatic, Right Axillary Lymphatic, Left Axillary
Pectoral fascia	**Use:** Subcutaneous Tissue and Fascia, Chest
Pectoralis major muscle Pectoralis minor muscle	**Use:** Thorax Muscle, Right Thorax Muscle, Left
Pelvic splanchnic nerve	**Use:** Abdominal Sympathetic Nerve Sacral Sympathetic Nerve
Penile urethra	**Use:** Urethra

BODY PART KEY

Pericardiophrenic artery	**Use:** Internal Mammary Artery, Right Internal Mammary Artery, Left
Perimetrium	**Use:** Uterus
Peroneus brevis muscle Peroneus longus muscle	**Use:** Lower Leg Muscle, Right Lower Leg Muscle, Left
Petrous part of temporal bone	**Use:** Temporal Bone, Right Temporal Bone, Left
Pharyngeal constrictor muscle	**Use:** Tongue, Palate, Pharynx Muscle
Pharyngeal plexus	**Use:** Vagus Nerve
Pharyngeal recess	**Use:** Nasopharynx
Pharyngeal tonsil	**Use:** Adenoids
Pharyngotympanic tube	**Use:** Eustachian Tube, Right Eustachian Tube, Left
Pia mater, intracranial	**Use:** Cerebral Meninges
Pia mater, spinal	**Use:** Spinal Meninges
Pinna	**Use:** External Ear, Right External Ear, Left External Ear, Bilateral
Piriform recess (sinus)	**Use:** Pharynx
Piriformis muscle	**Use:** Hip Muscle, Right Hip Muscle, Left
Pisiform bone	**Use:** Carpal, Right Carpal, Left
Pisohamate ligament Pisometacarpal ligament	**Use:** Hand Bursa and Ligament, Right Hand Bursa and Ligament, Left
Plantar digital vein	**Use:** Foot Vein, Right Foot Vein, Left
Plantar fascia (aponeurosis)	**Use:** Subcutaneous Tissue and Fascia, Right Foot Subcutaneous Tissue and Fascia, Left Foot
Plantar metatarsal vein Plantar venous arch	**Use:** Foot Vein, Right Foot Vein, Left
Platysma muscle	**Use:** Neck Muscle, Right Neck Muscle, Left
Plica semilunaris	**Use:** Conjunctiva, Right Conjunctiva, Left
Pneumogastric nerve	**Use:** Vagus Nerve
Pneumotaxic center Pontine tegmentum	**Use:** Pons
Popliteal ligament	**Use:** Knee Bursa and Ligament, Right Knee Bursa and Ligament, Left
Popliteal lymph node	**Use:** Lymphatic, Right Lower Extremity Lymphatic, Left Lower Extremity
Popliteal vein	**Use:** Femoral Vein, Right Femoral Vein, Left
Popliteus muscle	**Use:** Lower Leg Muscle, Right Lower Leg Muscle, Left
Postauricular (mastoid) lymph node	**Use:** Lymphatic, Right Neck Lymphatic, Left Neck
Postcava	**Use:** Inferior Vena Cava
Posterior (subscapular) lymph node	**Use:** Lymphatic, Right Axillary Lymphatic, Left Axillary
Posterior auricular artery	**Use:** External Carotid Artery, Right External Carotid Artery, Left
Posterior auricular nerve	**Use:** Facial Nerve
Posterior auricular vein	**Use:** External Jugular Vein, Right External Jugular Vein, Left
Posterior cerebral artery	**Use:** Intracranial Artery

APPENDIX B

BODY PART KEY

Posterior chamber	**Use:** Eye, Right Eye, Left
Posterior circumflex humeral artery	**Use:** Axillary Artery, Right Axillary Artery, Left
Posterior communicating artery	**Use:** Intracranial Artery
Posterior cruciate ligament (PCL)	**Use:** Knee Bursa and Ligament, Right Knee Bursa and Ligament, Left
Posterior facial (retromandibular) vein	**Use:** Face Vein, Right Face Vein, Left
Posterior femoral cutaneous nerve	**Use:** Sacral Plexus
Posterior inferior cerebellar artery (PICA)	**Use:** Intracranial Artery
Posterior interosseous nerve	**Use:** Radial Nerve
Posterior labial nerve Posterior scrotal nerve	**Use:** Pudendal Nerve
Posterior spinal artery	**Use:** Vertebral Artery, Right Vertebral Artery, Left
Posterior tibial recurrent artery	**Use:** Anterior Tibial Artery, Right Anterior Tibial Artery, Left
Posterior ulnar recurrent artery	**Use:** Ulnar Artery, Right Ulnar Artery, Left
Posterior vagal trunk	**Use:** Vagus Nerve
Preauricular lymph node	**Use:** Lymphatic, Head
Precava	**Use:** Superior Vena Cava
Prepatellar bursa	**Use:** Knee Bursa and Ligament, Right Knee Bursa and Ligament, Left
Pretracheal fascia Prevertebral fascia	**Use:** Subcutaneous Tissue and Fascia, Right Neck Subcutaneous Tissue and Fascia, Left Neck
Princeps pollicis artery	**Use:** Hand Artery, Right Hand Artery, Left
Procerus muscle	**Use:** Facial Muscle
Profunda brachii	**Use:** Brachial Artery, Right Brachial Artery, Left
Profunda femoris (deep femoral) vein	**Use:** Femoral Vein, Right Femoral Vein, Left
Pronator quadratus muscle Pronator teres muscle	**Use:** Lower Arm and Wrist Muscle, Right Lower Arm and Wrist Muscle, Left
Prostatic urethra	**Use:** Urethra
Proximal radioulnar joint	**Use:** Elbow Joint, Right Elbow Joint, Left
Psoas muscle	**Use:** Hip Muscle, Right Hip Muscle, Left
Pterygoid muscle	**Use:** Head Muscle
Pterygoid process	**Use:** Sphenoid Bone
Pterygopalatine (sphenopalatine) ganglion	**Use:** Head and Neck Sympathetic Nerve
Pubis	**Use:** Pelvic Bone, Right Pelvic Bone, Left
Pubofemoral ligament	**Use:** Hip Bursa and Ligament, Right Hip Bursa and Ligament, Left
Pudendal nerve	**Use:** Sacral Plexus
Pulmoaortic canal	**Use:** Pulmonary Artery, Left
Pulmonary annulus	**Use:** Pulmonary Valve
Pulmonary plexus	**Use:** Vagus Nerve Thoracic Sympathetic Nerve
Pulmonic valve	**Use:** Pulmonary Valve
Pulvinar	**Use:** Thalamus
Pyloric antrum Pyloric canal Pyloric sphincter	**Use:** Stomach, Pylorus

BODY PART KEY

Pyramidalis muscle	**Use:** Abdomen Muscle, Right Abdomen Muscle, Left
Quadrangular cartilage	**Use:** Nasal Septum
Quadrate lobe	**Use:** Liver
Quadratus femoris muscle	**Use:** Hip Muscle, Right Hip Muscle, Left
Quadratus lumborum muscle	**Use:** Trunk Muscle, Right Trunk Muscle, Left
Quadratus plantae muscle	**Use:** Foot Muscle, Right Foot Muscle, Left
Quadriceps (femoris)	**Use:** Upper Leg Muscle, Right Upper Leg Muscle, Left
Radial collateral carpal ligament	**Use:** Wrist Bursa and Ligament, Right Wrist Bursa and Ligament, Left
Radial collateral ligament	**Use:** Elbow Bursa and Ligament, Right Elbow Bursa and Ligament, Left
Radial notch	**Use:** Ulna, Right Ulna, Left
Radial recurrent artery	**Use:** Radial Artery, Right Radial Artery, Left
Radial vein	**Use:** Brachial Vein, Right Brachial Vein, Left
Radialis indicis	**Use:** Hand Artery, Right Hand Artery, Left
Radiocarpal joint	**Use:** Wrist Joint, Right Wrist Joint, Left
Radiocarpal ligament Radioulnar ligament	**Use:** Wrist Bursa and Ligament, Right Wrist Bursa and Ligament, Left
Rectosigmoid junction	**Use:** Sigmoid Colon
Rectus abdominis muscle	**Use:** Abdomen Muscle, Right Abdomen Muscle, Left
Rectus femoris muscle	**Use:** Upper Leg Muscle, Right Upper Leg Muscle, Left
Recurrent laryngeal nerve	**Use:** Vagus Nerve
Renal calyx Renal capsule Renal cortex	**Use:** Kidney, Right Kidney, Left Kidneys, Bilateral Kidney
Renal plexus	**Use:** Abdominal Sympathetic Nerve
Renal segment	**Use:** Kidney, Right Kidney, Left Kidneys, Bilateral Kidney
Renal segmental artery	**Use:** Renal Artery, Right Renal Artery, Left
Retroperitoneal lymph node	**Use:** Lymphatic, Aortic
Retroperitoneal space	**Use:** Retroperitoneum
Retropharyngeal lymph node	**Use:** Lymphatic, Right Neck Lymphatic, Left Neck
Retropubic space	**Use:** Pelvic Cavity
Rhinopharynx	**Use:** Nasopharynx
Rhomboid major muscle Rhomboid minor muscle	**Use:** Trunk Muscle, Right Trunk Muscle, Left
Right ascending lumbar vein	**Use:** Azygos Vein
Right atrioventricular valve	**Use:** Tricuspid Valve
Right auricular appendix	**Use:** Atrium, Right
Right colic vein	**Use:** Colic Vein
Right coronary sulcus	**Use:** Heart, Right

APPENDIX B

BODY PART KEY

Right gastric artery	**Use:** Gastric Artery
Right gastroepiploic vein	**Use:** Superior Mesenteric Vein
Right inferior phrenic vein	**Use:** Inferior Vena Cava
Right inferior pulmonary vein	**Use:** Pulmonary Vein, Right
Right jugular trunk	**Use:** Lymphatic, Right Neck
Right lateral ventricle	**Use:** Cerebral Ventricle
Right lymphatic duct	**Use:** Lymphatic, Right Neck
Right ovarian vein Right second lumbar vein	**Use:** Inferior Vena Cava
Right subclavian trunk	**Use:** Lymphatic, Right Neck
Right subcostal vein	**Use:** Azygos Vein
Right superior pulmonary vein	**Use:** Pulmonary Vein, Right
Right suprarenal vein Right testicular vein	**Use:** Inferior Vena Cava
Rima glottidis	**Use:** Larynx
Risorius muscle	**Use:** Facial Muscle
Round ligament of uterus	**Use:** Uterine Supporting Structure
Round window	**Use:** Inner Ear, Right Inner Ear, Left
Sacral ganglion	**Use:** Sacral Sympathetic Nerve
Sacral lymph node	**Use:** Lymphatic, Pelvis
Sacral splanchnic nerve	**Use:** Sacral Sympathetic Nerve
Sacrococcygeal ligament	**Use:** Lower Spine Bursa and Ligament
Sacrococcygeal symphysis	**Use:** Sacrococcygeal Joint
Sacroiliac ligament Sacrospinous ligament Sacrotuberous ligament	**Use:** Lower Spine Bursa and Ligament
Salpingopharyngeus muscle	**Use:** Tongue, Palate, Pharynx Muscle
Salpinx	**Use:** Fallopian Tube, Right Fallopian Tube, Left
Saphenous nerve	**Use:** Femoral Nerve
Sartorius muscle	**Use:** Upper Leg Muscle, Right Upper Leg Muscle, Left
Scalene muscle	**Use:** Neck Muscle, Right Neck Muscle, Left
Scaphoid bone	**Use:** Carpal, Right Carpal, Left
Scapholunate ligament Scaphotrapezium ligament	**Use:** Hand Bursa and Ligament, Right Hand Bursa and Ligament, Left
Scarpa's (vestibular) ganglion	**Use:** Acoustic Nerve
Sebaceous gland	**Use:** Skin
Second cranial nerve	**Use:** Optic Nerve
Sella turcica	**Use:** Sphenoid Bone
Semicircular canal	**Use:** Inner Ear, Right Inner Ear, Left
Semimembranosus muscle Semitendinosus muscle	**Use:** Upper Leg Muscle, Right Upper Leg Muscle, Left
Septal cartilage	**Use:** Nasal Septum
Serratus anterior muscle	**Use:** Thorax Muscle, Right Thorax Muscle, Left
Serratus posterior muscle	**Use:** Trunk Muscle, Right Trunk Muscle, Left

BODY PART KEY

Seventh cranial nerve	**Use:** Facial Nerve
Short gastric artery	**Use:** Splenic Artery
Sigmoid artery	**Use:** Inferior Mesenteric Artery
Sigmoid flexure	**Use:** Sigmoid Colon
Sigmoid vein	**Use:** Inferior Mesenteric Vein
Sinoatrial node	**Use:** Conduction Mechanism
Sinus venosus	**Use:** Atrium, Right
Sixth cranial nerve	**Use:** Abducens Nerve
Skene's (paraurethral) gland	**Use:** Vestibular Gland
Small saphenous vein	**Use:** Saphenous Vein, Right Saphenous Vein, Left
Solar (celiac) plexus	**Use:** Abdominal Sympathetic Nerve
Soleus muscle	**Use:** Lower Leg Muscle, Right Lower Leg Muscle, Left
Sphenomandibular ligament	**Use:** Head and Neck Bursa and Ligament
Sphenopalatine (pterygopalatine) ganglion	**Use:** Head and Neck Sympathetic Nerve
Spinal nerve, cervical	**Use:** Cervical Nerve
Spinal nerve, lumbar	**Use:** Lumbar Nerve
Spinal nerve, sacral	**Use:** Sacral Nerve
Spinal nerve, thoracic	**Use:** Thoracic Nerve
Spinous process	**Use:** Cervical Vertebra Thoracic Vertebra Lumbar Vertebra
Spiral ganglion	**Use:** Acoustic Nerve
Splenic flexure	**Use:** Transverse Colon
Splenic plexus	**Use:** Abdominal Sympathetic Nerve
Splenius capitis muscle	**Use:** Head Muscle
Splenius cervicis muscle	**Use:** Neck Muscle, Right Neck Muscle, Left
Stapes	**Use:** Auditory Ossicle, Right Auditory Ossicle, Left
Stellate ganglion	**Use:** Head and Neck Sympathetic Nerve
Stensen's duct	**Use:** Parotid Duct, Right Parotid Duct, Left
Sternoclavicular ligament	**Use:** Shoulder Bursa and Ligament, Right Shoulder Bursa and Ligament, Left
Sternocleidomastoid artery	**Use:** Thyroid Artery, Right Thyroid Artery, Left
Sternocleidomastoid muscle	**Use:** Neck Muscle, Right Neck Muscle, Left
Sternocostal ligament	**Use:** Sternum Bursa and Ligament Rib(s) Bursa and Ligament
Styloglossus muscle	**Use:** Tongue, Palate, Pharynx Muscle
Stylomandibular ligament	**Use:** Head and Neck Bursa and Ligament
Stylopharyngeus muscle	**Use:** Tongue, Palate, Pharynx Muscle
Subacromial bursa	**Use:** Shoulder Bursa and Ligament, Right Shoulder Bursa and Ligament, Left
Subaortic (common iliac) lymph node	**Use:** Lymphatic, Pelvis
Subarachnoid space, spinal	**Use:** Spinal Canal
Subclavicular (apical) lymph node	**Use:** Lymphatic, Right Axillary Lymphatic, Left Axillary

APPENDIX B

BODY PART KEY

Subclavius muscle	**Use:** Thorax Muscle, Right Thorax Muscle, Left
Subclavius nerve	**Use:** Brachial Plexus
Subcostal artery	**Use:** Upper Artery
Subcostal muscle	**Use:** Thorax Muscle, Right Thorax Muscle, Left
Subcostal nerve	**Use:** Thoracic Nerve
Subdural space, spinal	**Use:** Spinal Canal
Submandibular ganglion	**Use:** Facial Nerve Head and Neck Sympathetic Nerve
Submandibular gland	**Use:** Submaxillary Gland, Right Submaxillary Gland, Left
Submandibular lymph node	**Use:** Lymphatic, Head
Submaxillary ganglion	**Use:** Head and Neck Sympathetic Nerve
Submaxillary lymph node	**Use:** Lymphatic, Head
Submental artery	**Use:** Face Artery
Submental lymph node	**Use:** Lymphatic, Head
Submucous (Meissner's) plexus	**Use:** Abdominal Sympathetic Nerve
Suboccipital nerve	**Use:** Cervical Nerve
Suboccipital venous plexus	**Use:** Vertebral Vein, Right Vertebral Vein, Left
Subparotid lymph node	**Use:** Lymphatic, Head
Subscapular (posterior) lymph node	**Use:** Lymphatic, Right Axillary Lymphatic, Left Axillary

Subscapular aponeurosis	**Use:** Subcutaneous Tissue and Fascia, Right Upper Arm Subcutaneous Tissue and Fascia, Left Upper Arm
Subscapular artery	**Use:** Axillary Artery, Right Axillary Artery, Left
Subscapularis muscle	**Use:** Shoulder Muscle, Right Shoulder Muscle, Left
Substantia nigra	**Use:** Basal Ganglia
Subtalar (talocalcaneal) joint	**Use:** Tarsal Joint, Right Tarsal Joint, Left
Subtalar ligament	**Use:** Foot Bursa and Ligament, Right Foot Bursa and Ligament, Left
Subthalamic nucleus	**Use:** Basal Ganglia
Superficial circumflex iliac vein	**Use:** Saphenous Vein, Right Saphenous Vein, Left
Superficial epigastric artery	**Use:** Femoral Artery, Right Femoral Artery, Left
Superficial epigastric vein	**Use:** Saphenous Vein, Right Saphenous Vein, Left
Superficial palmar arch	**Use:** Hand Artery, Right Hand Artery, Left
Superficial palmar venous arch	**Use:** Hand Vein, Right Hand Vein, Left
Superficial temporal artery	**Use:** Temporal Artery, Right Temporal Artery, Left
Superficial transverse perineal muscle	**Use:** Perineum Muscle
Superior cardiac nerve	**Use:** Thoracic Sympathetic Nerve
Superior cerebellar vein Superior cerebral vein	**Use:** Intracranial Vein
Superior clunic (cluneal) nerve	**Use:** Lumbar Nerve

BODY PART KEY

Superior epigastric artery	**Use:** Internal Mammary Artery, Right Internal Mammary Artery, Left
Superior genicular artery	**Use:** Popliteal Artery, Right Popliteal Artery, Left
Superior gluteal artery	**Use:** Internal Iliac Artery, Right Internal Iliac Artery, Left
Superior gluteal nerve	**Use:** Lumbar Plexus
Superior hypogastric plexus	**Use:** Abdominal Sympathetic Nerve
Superior labial artery	**Use:** Face Artery
Superior laryngeal artery	**Use:** Thyroid Artery, Right Thyroid Artery, Left
Superior laryngeal nerve	**Use:** Vagus Nerve
Superior longitudinal muscle	**Use:** Tongue, Palate, Pharynx Muscle
Superior mesenteric ganglion	**Use:** Abdominal Sympathetic Nerve
Superior mesenteric lymph node	**Use:** Lymphatic, Mesenteric
Superior mesenteric plexus	**Use:** Abdominal Sympathetic Nerve
Superior oblique muscle	**Use:** Extraocular Muscle, Right Extraocular Muscle, Left
Superior olivary nucleus	**Use:** Pons
Superior rectal artery	**Use:** Inferior Mesenteric Artery
Superior rectal vein	**Use:** Inferior Mesenteric Vein
Superior rectus muscle	**Use:** Extraocular Muscle, Right Extraocular Muscle, Left
Superior tarsal plate	**Use:** Upper Eyelid, Right Upper Eyelid, Left
Superior thoracic artery	**Use:** Axillary Artery, Right Axillary Artery, Left
Superior thyroid artery	**Use:** External Carotid Artery, Right External Carotid Artery, Left Thyroid Artery, Right Thyroid Artery, Left
Superior turbinate	**Use:** Nasal Turbinate
Superior ulnar collateral artery	**Use:** Brachial Artery, Right Brachial Artery, Left
Supraclavicular (Virchow's) lymph node	**Use:** Lymphatic, Right Neck Lymphatic, Left Neck
Supraclavicular nerve	**Use:** Cervical Plexus
Suprahyoid lymph node	**Use:** Lymphatic, Head
Suprahyoid muscle	**Use:** Neck Muscle, Right Neck Muscle, Left
Suprainguinal lymph node	**Use:** Lymphatic, Pelvis
Supraorbital vein	**Use:** Face Vein, Right Face Vein, Left
Suprarenal gland	**Use:** Adrenal Gland, Left Adrenal Gland, Right Adrenal Glands, Bilateral Adrenal Gland
Suprarenal plexus	**Use:** Abdominal Sympathetic Nerve
Suprascapular nerve	**Use:** Brachial Plexus
Supraspinatus fascia	**Use:** Subcutaneous Tissue and Fascia, Right Upper Arm Subcutaneous Tissue and Fascia, Left Upper Arm
Supraspinatus muscle	**Use:** Shoulder Muscle, Right Shoulder Muscle, Left
Supraspinous ligament	**Use:** Upper Spine Bursa and Ligament Lower Spine Bursa and Ligament
Suprasternal notch	**Use:** Sternum

APPENDIX B

BODY PART KEY

Supratrochlear lymph node	**Use:** Lymphatic, Right Upper Extremity Lymphatic, Left Upper Extremity
Sural artery	**Use:** Popliteal Artery, Right Popliteal Artery, Left
Sweat gland	**Use:** Skin
Talocalcaneal (subtalar) joint	**Use:** Tarsal Joint, Right Tarsal Joint, Left
Talocalcaneal ligament	**Use:** Foot Bursa and Ligament, Right Foot Bursa and Ligament, Left
Talocalcaneonavicular joint	**Use:** Tarsal Joint, Right Tarsal Joint, Left
Talocalcaneonavicular ligament	**Use:** Foot Bursa and Ligament, Right Foot Bursa and Ligament, Left
Talocrural joint	**Use:** Ankle Joint, Right Ankle Joint, Left
Talofibular ligament	**Use:** Ankle Bursa and Ligament, Right Ankle Bursa and Ligament, Left
Talus bone	**Use:** Tarsal, Right Tarsal, Left
Tarsometatarsal ligament	**Use:** Foot Bursa and Ligament, Right Foot Bursa and Ligament, Left
Temporal lobe	**Use:** Cerebral Hemisphere
Temporalis muscle Temporoparietalis muscle	**Use:** Head Muscle
Tensor fasciae latae muscle	**Use:** Hip Muscle, Right Hip Muscle, Left
Tensor veli palatini muscle	**Use:** Tongue, Palate, Pharynx Muscle
Tenth cranial nerve	**Use:** Vagus Nerve
Tentorium cerebelli	**Use:** Dura Mater
Teres major muscle Teres minor muscle	**Use:** Shoulder Muscle, Right Shoulder Muscle, Left
Testicular artery	**Use:** Abdominal Aorta
Thenar muscle	**Use:** Hand Muscle, Right Hand Muscle, Left
Third cranial nerve	**Use:** Oculomotor Nerve
Third occipital nerve	**Use:** Cervical Nerve
Third ventricle	**Use:** Cerebral Ventricle
Thoracic aortic plexus	**Use:** Thoracic Sympathetic Nerve
Thoracic esophagus	**Use:** Esophagus, Middle
Thoracic facet joint	**Use:** Thoracic Vertebral Joint Thoracic Vertebral Joints, 2 to 7 Thoracic Vertebral Joints, 8 or more
Thoracic ganglion	**Use:** Thoracic Sympathetic Nerve
Thoracoacromial artery	**Use:** Axillary Artery, Right Axillary Artery, Left
Thoracolumbar facet joint	**Use:** Thoracolumbar Vertebral Joint
Thymus gland	**Use:** Thymus
Thyroarytenoid muscle	**Use:** Neck Muscle, Right Neck Muscle, Left
Thyrocervical trunk	**Use:** Thyroid Artery, Right Thyroid Artery, Left
Thyroid cartilage	**Use:** Larynx
Tibialis anterior muscle Tibialis posterior muscle	**Use:** Lower Leg Muscle, Right Lower Leg Muscle, Left
Tibiofemoral joint	**Use:** Knee Joint, Right Knee Joint, Left Knee Joint, Tibial Surface, Right Knee Joint, Tibial Surface, Left
Tongue, base of	**Use:** Pharynx

BODY PART KEY

Tracheobronchial lymph node	**Use:** Lymphatic, Thorax
Tragus	**Use:** External Ear, Right External Ear, Left External Ear, Bilateral
Transversalis fascia	**Use:** Subcutaneous Tissue and Fascia, Trunk
Transverse (cutaneous) cervical nerve	**Use:** Cervical Plexus
Transverse acetabular ligament	**Use:** Hip Bursa and Ligament, Right Hip Bursa and Ligament, Left
Transverse facial artery	**Use:** Temporal Artery, Right Temporal Artery, Left
Transverse foramen	**Use:** Cervical Vertebra
Transverse humeral ligament	**Use:** Shoulder Bursa and Ligament, Right Shoulder Bursa and Ligament, Left
Transverse ligament of atlas	**Use:** Head and Neck Bursa and Ligament
Transverse process	**Use:** Cervical Vertebra Thoracic Vertebra Lumbar Vertebra
Transverse scapular ligament	**Use:** Shoulder Bursa and Ligament, Right Shoulder Bursa and Ligament, Left
Transverse thoracis muscle	**Use:** Thorax Muscle, Right Thorax Muscle, Left
Transversospinalis muscle	**Use:** Trunk Muscle, Right Trunk Muscle, Left
Transversus abdominis muscle	**Use:** Abdomen Muscle, Right Abdomen Muscle, Left
Trapezium bone	**Use:** Carpal, Right Carpal, Left
Trapezius muscle	**Use:** Trunk Muscle, Right Trunk Muscle, Left
Trapezoid bone	**Use:** Carpal, Right Carpal, Left
Triceps brachii muscle	**Use:** Upper Arm Muscle, Right Upper Arm Muscle, Left
Tricuspid annulus	**Use:** Tricuspid Valve
Trifacial nerve	**Use:** Trigeminal Nerve
Trigone of bladder	**Use:** Bladder
Triquetral bone	**Use:** Carpal, Right Carpal, Left
Trochanteric bursa	**Use:** Hip Bursa and Ligament, Right Hip Bursa and Ligament, Left
Twelfth cranial nerve	**Use:** Hypoglossal Nerve
Tympanic cavity	**Use:** Middle Ear, Right Middle Ear, Left
Tympanic nerve	**Use:** Glossopharyngeal Nerve
Tympanic part of temporal bone	**Use:** Temporal Bone, Right Temporal Bone, Left
Ulnar collateral carpal ligament	**Use:** Wrist Bursa and Ligament, Right Wrist Bursa and Ligament, Left
Ulnar collateral ligament	**Use:** Elbow Bursa and Ligament, Right Elbow Bursa and Ligament, Left
Ulnar notch	**Use:** Radius, Right Radius, Left
Ulnar vein	**Use:** Brachial Vein, Right Brachial Vein, Left
Umbilical artery	**Use:** Internal Iliac Artery, Right Internal Iliac Artery, Left Lower Artery
Ureteral orifice	**Use:** Ureter, Right Ureter, Left Ureters, Bilateral Ureter

BODY PART KEY

Ureteropelvic junction (UPJ)	**Use:** Kidney Pelvis, Right Kidney Pelvis, Left
Ureterovesical orifice	**Use:** Ureter, Right Ureter, Left Ureters, Bilateral Ureter
Uterine artery	**Use:** Internal Iliac Artery, Right Internal Iliac Artery, Left
Uterine cornu	**Use:** Uterus
Uterine tube	**Use:** Fallopian Tube, Right Fallopian Tube, Left
Uterine vein	**Use:** Hypogastric Vein, Right Hypogastric Vein, Left
Vaginal artery	**Use:** Internal Iliac Artery, Right Internal Iliac Artery, Left
Vaginal vein	**Use:** Hypogastric Vein, Right Hypogastric Vein, Left
Vastus intermedius muscle Vastus lateralis muscle Vastus medialis muscle	**Use:** Upper Leg Muscle, Right Upper Leg Muscle, Left
Ventricular fold	**Use:** Larynx
Vermiform appendix	**Use:** Appendix
Vermilion border	**Use:** Upper Lip Lower Lip
Vertebral arch Vertebral body	**Use:** Cervical Vertebra Thoracic Vertebra Lumbar Vertebra
Vertebral canal	**Use:** Spinal Canal
Vertebral foramen Vertebral lamina Vertebral pedicle	**Use:** Cervical Vertebra Thoracic Vertebra Lumbar Vertebra
Vesical vein	**Use:** Hypogastric Vein, Right Hypogastric Vein, Left
Vestibular (Scarpa's) ganglion Vestibular nerve Vestibulocochlear nerve	**Use:** Acoustic Nerve
Virchow's (supraclavicular) lymph node	**Use:** Lymphatic, Right Neck Lymphatic, Left Neck
Vitreous body	**Use:** Vitreous, Right Vitreous, Left
Vocal fold	**Use:** Vocal Cord, Right Vocal Cord, Left
Volar (palmar) digital vein Volar (palmar) metacarpal vein	**Use:** Hand Vein, Right Hand Vein, Left
Vomer bone	**Use:** Nasal Septum
Vomer of nasal septum	**Use:** Nasal Bone
Xiphoid process	**Use:** Sternum
Zonule of Zinn	**Use:** Lens, Right Lens, Left
Zygomatic process of frontal bone	**Use:** Frontal Bone
Zygomatic process of temporal bone	**Use:** Temporal Bone, Right Temporal Bone, Left
Zygomaticus muscle	**Use:** Facial Muscle

BODY PART KEY

New/Revised Text in Green ~~deleted~~ Deleted

DEVICE KEY

3f (Aortic) Bioprosthesis valve	**Use:** Zooplastic Tissue in Heart and Great Vessels
AbioCor® Total Replacement Heart	**Use:** Synthetic Substitute
Acellular Hydrated Dermis	**Use:** Nonautologous Tissue Substitute
Acetabular cup	**Use:** Liner in Lower Joints
Activa PC neurostimulator	**Use:** Stimulator Generator, Multiple Array for Insertion in Subcutaneous Tissue and Fascia
Activa RC neurostimulator	**Use:** Stimulator Generator, Multiple Array Rechargeable for Insertion in Subcutaneous Tissue and Fascia
Activa SC neurostimulator	**Use:** Stimulator Generator, Single Array for Insertion in Subcutaneous Tissue and Fascia
ACUITY™ Steerable Lead	**Use:** Cardiac Lead, Pacemaker for Insertion in Heart and Great Vessels Cardiac Lead, Defibrillator for Insertion in Heart and Great Vessels
Advisa (MRI)	**Use:** Pacemaker, Dual Chamber for Insertion in Subcutaneous Tissue and Fascia
AFX® Endovascular AAA System	**Use:** Intraluminal Device
AMPLATZER® Muscular VSD Occluder	**Use:** Synthetic Substitute
AMS 800® Urinary Control System	**Use:** Artificial Sphincter in Urinary System
AneuRx® AAA Advantage®	**Use:** Intraluminal Device
Annuloplasty ring	**Use:** Synthetic Substitute
Artificial anal sphincter (AAS)	**Use:** Artificial Sphincter in Gastrointestinal System
Artificial bowel sphincter (neosphincter)	**Use:** Artificial Sphincter in Gastrointestinal System
Artificial urinary sphincter (AUS)	**Use:** Artificial Sphincter in Urinary System
Assurant (Cobalt) stent	**Use:** Intraluminal Device
AtriClip LAA Exclusion System	**Use:** Extraluminal Device
Attain Ability® lead	**Use:** Cardiac Lead, Pacemaker for Insertion in Heart and Great Vessels Cardiac Lead, Defibrillator for Insertion in Heart and Great Vessels
Attain StarFix® (OTW) lead	**Use:** Cardiac Lead, Pacemaker for Insertion in Heart and Great Vessels Cardiac Lead, Defibrillator for Insertion in Heart and Great Vessels
Autograft	**Use:** Autologous Tissue Substitute
Autologous artery graft	**Use:** Autologous Arterial Tissue in Heart and Great Vessels Autologous Arterial Tissue in Upper Arteries Autologous Arterial Tissue in Lower Arteries Autologous Arterial Tissue in Upper Veins Autologous Arterial Tissue in Lower Veins
Autologous vein graft	**Use:** Autologous Venous Tissue in Heart and Great Vessels Autologous Venous Tissue in Upper Arteries Autologous Venous Tissue in Lower Arteries Autologous Venous Tissue in Upper Veins Autologous Venous Tissue in Lower Veins
Axial Lumbar Interbody Fusion System	**Use:** Interbody Fusion Device in Lower Joints

DEVICE KEY

AxiaLIF® System	**Use:** Interbody Fusion Device in Lower Joints
BAK/C® Interbody Cervical Fusion System	**Use:** Interbody Fusion Device in Upper Joints
Bard® Composix® (E/X) (LP) mesh	**Use:** Synthetic Substitute
Bard® Composix® Kugel® patch	**Use:** Synthetic Substitute
Bard® Dulex™ mesh	**Use:** Synthetic Substitute
Bard® Ventralex™ hernia patch	**Use:** Synthetic Substitute
Baroreflex Activation Therapy® (BAT®)	**Use:** Stimulator Lead in Upper Arteries Cardiac Rhythm Related Device in Subcutaneous Tissue and Fascia
Berlin Heart Ventricular Assist Device	**Use:** Implantable Heart Assist System in Heart and Great Vessels
Bioactive embolization coil(s)	**Use:** Intraluminal Device, Bioactive in Upper Arteries
Biventricular external heart assist system	**Use:** Short-term External Heart Assist System in Heart and Great Vessels
Blood glucose monitoring system	**Use:** Monitoring Device
Bone anchored hearing device	**Use:** Hearing Device, Bone Conduction for Insertion in Ear, Nose, Sinus Hearing Device in Head and Facial Bones
Bone bank bone graft	**Use:** Nonautologous Tissue Substitute
Bone screw (interlocking) (lag) (pedicle) (recessed)	**Use:** Internal Fixation Device in Head and Facial Bones Internal Fixation Device in Upper Bones Internal Fixation Device in Lower Bones
Bovine pericardial valve	**Use:** Zooplastic Tissue in Heart and Great Vessels
Bovine pericardium graft	**Use:** Zooplastic Tissue in Heart and Great Vessels
Brachytherapy seeds	**Use:** Radioactive Element
BRYAN® Cervical Disc System	**Use:** Synthetic Substitute
BVS 5000 Ventricular Assist Device	**Use:** Short-term External Heart Assist System in Heart and Great Vessels
Cardiac contractility modulation lead	**Use:** Cardiac Lead in Heart and Great Vessels
Cardiac event recorder	**Use:** Monitoring Device
Cardiac resynchronization therapy (CRT) lead	**Use:** Cardiac Lead, Pacemaker for Insertion in Heart and Great Vessels Cardiac Lead, Defibrillator for Insertion in Heart and Great Vessels
CardioMEMS® pressure sensor	**Use:** Monitoring Device, Pressure Sensor for Insertion in Heart and Great Vessels
Carotid (artery) sinus (baroreceptor) lead	**Use:** Stimulator Lead in Upper Arteries
Carotid WALLSTENT® Monorail® Endoprosthesis	**Use:** Intraluminal Device
Centrimag® Blood Pump	**Use:** Short-term External Heart Assist System in Heart and Great Vessels
Ceramic on ceramic bearing surface	**Use:** Synthetic Substitute, Ceramic for Replacement in Lower Joints
Cesium-131 Collagen Implant	**Use:** Radioactive Element, Cesium-131 Collagen Implant for Insertion in Central Nervous System and Cranial Nerves
Clamp and rod internal fixation system (CRIF)	**Use:** Internal Fixation Device in Upper Bones Internal Fixation Device in Lower Bones

DEVICE KEY

COALESCE® radiolucent interbody fusion device	**Use:** Interbody Fusion Device, Radiolucent Porous in New Technology
CoAxia NeuroFlo catheter	**Use:** Intraluminal Device
Cobalt/chromium head and polyethylene socket	**Use:** Synthetic Substitute, Metal on Polyethylene for Replacement in Lower Joints
Cobalt/chromium head and socket	**Use:** Synthetic Substitute, Metal for Replacement in Lower Joints
Cochlear implant (CI), multiple channel (electrode)	**Use:** Hearing Device, Multiple Channel Cochlear Prosthesis for Insertion in Ear, Nose, Sinus
Cochlear implant (CI), single channel (electrode)	**Use:** Hearing Device, Single Channel Cochlear Prosthesis for Insertion in Ear, Nose, Sinus
COGNIS® CRT-D	**Use:** Cardiac Resynchronization Defibrillator Pulse Generator for Insertion in Subcutaneous Tissue and Fascia
COHERE® radiolucent interbody fusion device	**Use:** Interbody Fusion Device, Radiolucent Porous in New Technology
Colonic Z-Stent®	**Use:** Intraluminal Device
Complete (SE) stent	**Use:** Intraluminal Device
Concerto II CRT-D	**Use:** Cardiac Resynchronization Defibrillator Pulse Generator for Insertion in Subcutaneous Tissue and Fascia
CONSERVE® PLUS Total Resurfacing Hip System	**Use:** Resurfacing Device in Lower Joints
Consulta CRT-D	**Use:** Cardiac Resynchronization Defibrillator Pulse Generator for Insertion in Subcutaneous Tissue and Fascia
Consulta CRT-P	**Use:** Cardiac Resynchronization Pacemaker Pulse Generator for Insertion in Subcutaneous Tissue and Fascia
CONTAK RENEWAL® 3 RF (HE) CRT-D	**Use:** Cardiac Resynchronization Defibrillator Pulse Generator for Insertion in Subcutaneous Tissue and Fascia
Contegra Pulmonary Valved Conduit	**Use:** Zooplastic Tissue in Heart and Great Vessels
Continuous Glucose Monitoring (CGM) device	**Use:** Monitoring Device
Cook Biodesign® Fistula Plug(s)	**Use:** Nonautologous Tissue Substitute
Cook Biodesign® Hernia Graft(s)	**Use:** Nonautologous Tissue Substitute
Cook Biodesign® Layered Graft(s)	**Use:** Nonautologous Tissue Substitute
Cook Zenapro™ Layered Graft(s)	**Use:** Nonautologous Tissue Substitute
Cook Zenith AAA Endovascular Graft	**Use:** Intraluminal Device, Branched or Fenestrated, One or Two Arteries for Restriction in Lower Arteries Intraluminal Device, Branched or Fenestrated, Three or More Arteries for Restriction in Lower Arteries Intraluminal Device
CoreValve transcatheter aortic valve	**Use:** Zooplastic Tissue in Heart and Great Vessels
Cormet Hip Resurfacing System	**Use:** Resurfacing Device in Lower Joints
CoRoent® XL	**Use:** Interbody Fusion Device in Lower Joints
Corox (OTW) Bipolar Lead	**Use:** Cardiac Lead, Pacemaker for Insertion in Heart and Great Vessels Cardiac Lead, Defibrillator for Insertion in Heart and Great Vessels

APPENDIX C

DEVICE KEY

Cortical strip neurostimulator lead	**Use:** Neurostimulator Lead in Central Nervous System and Cranial Nerves
Cultured epidermal cell autograft	**Use:** Autologous Tissue Substitute
CYPHER® Stent	**Use:** Intraluminal Device, Drug-eluting in Heart and Great Vessels
Cystostomy tube	**Use:** Drainage Device
DBS lead	**Use:** Neurostimulator Lead in Central Nervous System and Cranial Nerves
DeBakey Left Ventricular Assist Device	**Use:** Implantable Heart Assist System in Heart and Great Vessels
Deep brain neurostimulator lead	**Use:** Neurostimulator Lead in Central Nervous System and Cranial Nerves
Delta frame external fixator	**Use:** External Fixation Device, Hybrid for Insertion in Upper Bones External Fixation Device, Hybrid for Reposition in Upper Bones External Fixation Device, Hybrid for Insertion in Lower Bones External Fixation Device, Hybrid for Reposition in Lower Bones
Delta III Reverse shoulder prosthesis	**Use:** Synthetic Substitute, Reverse Ball and Socket for Replacement in Upper Joints
Diaphragmatic pacemaker generator	**Use:** Stimulator Generator in Subcutaneous Tissue and Fascia
Direct Lateral Interbody Fusion (DLIF) device	**Use:** Interbody Fusion Device in Lower Joints
Driver stent (RX) (OTW)	**Use:** Intraluminal Device
DuraHeart Left Ventricular Assist System	**Use:** Implantable Heart Assist System in Heart and Great Vessels
Durata® Defibrillation Lead	**Use:** Cardiac Lead, Defibrillator for Insertion in Heart and Great Vessels
Dynesys® Dynamic Stabilization System	**Use:** Spinal Stabilization Device, Pedicle-Based for Insertion in Upper Joints Spinal Stabilization Device, Pedicle-Based for Insertion in Lower Joints
E-Luminexx™ (Biliary) (Vascular) Stent	**Use:** Intraluminal Device
EDWARDS INTUITY Elite valve system	**Use:** Zooplastic Tissue, Rapid Deployment Technique in New Technology
Electrical bone growth stimulator (EBGS)	**Use:** Bone Growth Stimulator in Head and Facial Bones Bone Growth Stimulator in Upper Bones Bone Growth Stimulator in Lower Bones
Electrical muscle stimulation (EMS) lead	**Use:** Stimulator Lead in Muscles
Electronic muscle stimulator lead	**Use:** Stimulator Lead in Muscles
Embolization coil(s)	**Use:** Intraluminal Device
Endeavor® (III) (IV) (Sprint) Zotarolimus-eluting Coronary Stent System	**Use:** Intraluminal Device, Drug-eluting in Heart and Great Vessels
Endologix AFX® Endovascular AAA System	**Use:** Intraluminal Device
EndoSure® sensor	**Use:** Monitoring Device, Pressure Sensor for Insertion in Heart and Great Vessels
ENDOTAK RELIANCE® (G) Defibrillation Lead	**Use:** Cardiac Lead, Defibrillator for Insertion in Heart and Great Vessels
Endotracheal tube (cuffed) (double-lumen)	**Use:** Intraluminal Device, Endotracheal Airway in Respiratory System
Endurant® Endovascular Stent Graft	**Use:** Intraluminal Device

DEVICE KEY

Endurant® II AAA stent graft system	**Use:** Intraluminal Device
EnRhythm	**Use:** Pacemaker, Dual Chamber for Insertion in Subcutaneous Tissue and Fascia
Enterra gastric neurostimulator	**Use:** Stimulator Generator, Multiple Array for Insertion in Subcutaneous Tissue and Fascia
Epic™ Stented Tissue Valve (aortic)	**Use:** Zooplastic Tissue in Heart and Great Vessels
Epicel® cultured epidermal autograft	**Use:** Autologous Tissue Substitute
Esophageal obturator airway (EOA)	**Use:** Intraluminal Device, Airway in Gastrointestinal System
Esteem® implantable hearing system	**Use:** Hearing Device in Ear, Nose, Sinus
Everolimus-eluting coronary stent	**Use:** Intraluminal Device, Drug-eluting in Heart and Great Vessels
Ex-PRESS™ mini glaucoma shunt	**Use:** Synthetic Substitute
EXCLUDER® AAA Endoprosthesis	**Use:** Intraluminal Device, Branched or Fenestrated, One or Two Arteries for Restriction in Lower Arteries Intraluminal Device, Branched or Fenestrated, Three or More Arteries for Restriction in Lower Arteries
EXCLUDER® IBE Endoprosthesis	**Use:** Intraluminal Device, Branched or Fenestrated, One or Two Arteries for Restriction in Lower Arteries
Express® (LD) Premounted Stent System	**Use:** Intraluminal Device
Express® Biliary SD Monorail® Premounted Stent System	**Use:** Intraluminal Device
Express® SD Renal Monorail® Premounted Stent System	**Use:** Intraluminal Device
External fixator	**Use:** External Fixation Device in Head and Facial Bones External Fixation Device in Upper Bones External Fixation Device in Lower Bones External Fixation Device in Upper Joints External Fixation Device in Lower Joints
EXtreme Lateral Interbody Fusion (XLIF) device	**Use:** Interbody Fusion Device in Lower Joints
Facet replacement spinal stabilization device	**Use:** Spinal Stabilization Device, Facet Replacement for Insertion in Upper Joints Spinal Stabilization Device, Facet Replacement for Insertion in Lower Joints
FLAIR® Endovascular Stent Graft	**Use:** Intraluminal Device
Flexible Composite Mesh	**Use:** Synthetic Substitute
Foley catheter	**Use:** Drainage Device
Formula™ Balloon-Expandable Renal Stent System	**Use:** Intraluminal Device
Freestyle (Stentless) Aortic Root Bioprosthesis	**Use:** Zooplastic Tissue in Heart and Great Vessels
Fusion screw (compression) (lag) (locking)	**Use:** Internal Fixation Device in Upper Joints Internal Fixation Device in Lower Joints
GammaTile™	**Use:** Radioactive Element, Cesium-131 Collagen Implant for Insertion in Central Nervous System and Cranial Nerves
Gastric electrical stimulation (GES) lead	**Use:** Stimulator Lead in Gastrointestinal System
Gastric pacemaker lead	**Use:** Stimulator Lead in Gastrointestinal System

APPENDIX C

DEVICE KEY

GORE EXCLUDER® AAA Endoprosthesis	**Use:** Intraluminal Device, Branched or Fenestrated, One or Two Arteries for Restriction in Lower Arteries
GORE EXCLUDER® IBE Endoprosthesis	**Use:** Intraluminal Device, Branched or Fenestrated, One or Two Arteries for Restriction in Lower Arteries
GORE TAG® Thoracic Endoprosthesis	**Use:** Intraluminal Device
GORE® DUALMESH®	**Use:** Synthetic Substitute
Guedel airway	**Use:** Intraluminal Device, Airway in Mouth and Throat
Hancock Bioprosthesis (aortic) (mitral) valve	**Use:** Zooplastic Tissue in Heart and Great Vessels
Hancock Bioprosthetic Valved Conduit	**Use:** Zooplastic Tissue in Heart and Great Vessels
HeartMate 3™ LVAS	**Use:** Implantable Heart Assist System in Heart and Great Vessels
HeartMate II® Left Ventricular Assist Device (LVAD)	**Use:** Implantable Heart Assist System in Heart and Great Vessels
HeartMate XVE® Left Ventricular Assist Device (LVAD)	**Use:** Implantable Heart Assist System in Heart and Great Vessels
Hip (joint) liner	**Use:** Liner in Lower Joints
Holter valve ventricular shunt	**Use:** Synthetic Substitute
Ilizarov external fixator	**Use:** External Fixation Device, Ring for Insertion in Upper Bones External Fixation Device, Ring for Reposition in Upper Bones External Fixation Device, Ring for Insertion in Lower Bones External Fixation Device, Ring for Reposition in Lower Bones
Ilizarov-Vecklich device	**Use:** External Fixation Device, Limb Lengthening for Insertion in Upper Bones External Fixation Device, Limb Lengthening for Insertion in Lower Bones
Impella® heart pump	**Use:** Short-term External Heart Assist System in Heart and Great Vessels
Implantable cardioverter-defibrillator (ICD)	**Use:** Defibrillator Generator for Insertion in Subcutaneous Tissue and Fascia
Implantable drug infusion pump (anti-spasmodic) (chemotherapy) (pain)	**Use:** Infusion Device, Pump in Subcutaneous Tissue and Fascia
Implantable glucose monitoring device	**Use:** Monitoring Device
Implantable hemodynamic monitor (IHM)	**Use:** Monitoring Device, Hemodynamic for Insertion in Subcutaneous Tissue and Fascia
Implantable hemodynamic monitoring system (IHMS)	**Use:** Monitoring Device, Hemodynamic for Insertion in Subcutaneous Tissue and Fascia
Implantable Miniature Telescope™ (IMT)	**Use:** Synthetic Substitute, Intraocular Telescope for Replacement in Eye
Implanted (venous) (access) port	**Use:** Vascular Access Device, Totally Implantable in Subcutaneous Tissue and Fascia
InDura, intrathecal catheter (1P) (spinal)	**Use:** Infusion Device
Injection reservoir, port	**Use:** Vascular Access Device, Totally Implantable in Subcutaneous Tissue and Fascia
Injection reservoir, pump	**Use:** Infusion Device, Pump in Subcutaneous Tissue and Fascia

DEVICE KEY

Interbody fusion (spine) cage	**Use:** Interbody Fusion Device in Upper Joints Interbody Fusion Device in Lower Joints
Interspinous process spinal stabilization device	**Use:** Spinal Stabilization Device, Interspinous Process for Insertion in Upper Joints Spinal Stabilization Device, Interspinous Process for Insertion in Lower Joints
InterStim® Therapy lead	**Use:** Neurostimulator Lead in Peripheral Nervous System
InterStim® Therapy neurostimulator	**Use:** Stimulator Generator, Single Array for Insertion in Subcutaneous Tissue and Fascia
Intramedullary (IM) rod (nail)	**Use:** Internal Fixation Device, Intramedullary in Upper Bones Internal Fixation Device, Intramedullary in Lower Bones
Intramedullary skeletal kinetic distractor (ISKD)	**Use:** Internal Fixation Device, Intramedullary in Upper Bones Internal Fixation Device, Intramedullary in Lower Bones
Intrauterine device (IUD)	**Use:** Contraceptive Device in Female Reproductive System
INTUITY Elite valve system, EDWARDS	**Use:** Zooplastic Tissue, Rapid Deployment Technique in New Technology
Itrel (3) (4) neurostimulator	**Use:** Stimulator Generator, Single Array for Insertion in Subcutaneous Tissue and Fascia
Joint fixation plate	**Use:** Internal Fixation Device in Upper Joints Internal Fixation Device in Lower Joints
Joint liner (insert)	**Use:** Liner in Lower Joints
Joint spacer (antibiotic)	**Use:** Spacer in Upper Joints Spacer in Lower Joints
Kappa	**Use:** Pacemaker, Dual Chamber for Insertion in Subcutaneous Tissue and Fascia
Kinetra® neurostimulator	**Use:** Stimulator Generator, Multiple Array for Insertion in Subcutaneous Tissue and Fascia
Kirschner wire (K-wire)	**Use:** Internal Fixation Device in Head and Facial Bones Internal Fixation Device in Upper Bones Internal Fixation Device in Lower Bones Internal Fixation Device in Upper Joints Internal Fixation Device in Lower Joints
Knee (implant) insert	**Use:** Liner in Lower Joints
Kuntscher nail	**Use:** Internal Fixation Device, Intramedullary in Upper Bones Internal Fixation Device, Intramedullary in Lower Bones
LAP-BAND® adjustable gastric banding system	**Use:** Extraluminal Device
LifeStent® (Flexstar) (XL) Vascular Stent System	**Use:** Intraluminal Device
LIVIAN™ CRT-D	**Use:** Cardiac Resynchronization Defibrillator Pulse Generator for Insertion in Subcutaneous Tissue and Fascia
Loop recorder, implantable	**Use:** Monitoring Device
MAGEC® Spinal Bracing and Distraction System	**Use:** Magnetically Controlled Growth Rod(s) in New Technology
Mark IV Breathing Pacemaker System	Stimulator Generator in Subcutaneous Tissue and Fascia
Maximo II DR (VR)	**Use:** Defibrillator Generator for Insertion in Subcutaneous Tissue and Fascia
Maximo II DR CRT-D	**Use:** Cardiac Resynchronization Defibrillator Pulse Generator for Insertion in Subcutaneous Tissue and Fascia

APPENDIX C

DEVICE KEY

Medtronic Endurant® II AAA stent graft system	**Use:** Intraluminal Device
Melody® transcatheter pulmonary valve	**Use:** Zooplastic Tissue in Heart and Great Vessels
Metal on metal bearing surface	**Use:** Synthetic Substitute, Metal for Replacement in Lower Joints
Micro-Driver stent (RX) (OTW)	**Use:** Intraluminal Device
Micrus CERECYTE microcoil	**Use:** Intraluminal Device, Bioactive in Upper Arteries
MIRODERM™ Biologic Wound Matrix	**Use:** Skin Substitute, Porcine Liver Derived in New Technology
MitraClip valve repair system	**Use:** Synthetic Substitute
Mitroflow® Aortic Pericardial Heart Valve	**Use:** Zooplastic Tissue in Heart and Great Vessels
Mosaic Bioprosthesis (aortic) (mitral) valve	**Use:** Zooplastic Tissue in Heart and Great Vessels
MULTI-LINK (VISION)(MINIVISION) (ULTRA) Coronary Stent System	**Use:** Intraluminal Device
nanoLOCK™ interbody fusion device	**Use:** Interbody Fusion Device, Nanotextured Surface in New Technology
Nasopharyngeal airway (NPA)	**Use:** Intraluminal Device, Airway in Ear, Nose, Sinus
Neuromuscular electrical stimulation (NEMS) lead	**Use:** Stimulator Lead in Muscles
Neurostimulator generator, multiple channel	**Use:** Stimulator Generator, Multiple Array for Insertion in Subcutaneous Tissue and Fascia
Neurostimulator generator, multiple channel rechargeable	**Use:** Stimulator Generator, Multiple Array Rechargeable for Insertion in Subcutaneous Tissue and Fascia
Neurostimulator generator, single channel	**Use:** Stimulator Generator, Single Array for Insertion in Subcutaneous Tissue and Fascia
Neurostimulator generator, single channel rechargeable	**Use:** Stimulator Generator, Single Array Rechargeable for Insertion in Subcutaneous Tissue and Fascia
Neutralization plate	**Use:** Internal Fixation Device in Head and Facial Bones Internal Fixation Device in Upper Bones Internal Fixation Device in Lower Bones
Nitinol framed polymer mesh	**Use:** Synthetic Substitute
Non-tunneled central venous catheter	**Use:** Infusion Device
Novacor Left Ventricular Assist Device	**Use:** Implantable Heart Assist System in Heart and Great Vessels
Novation® Ceramic AHS® (Articulation Hip System)	**Use:** Synthetic Substitute, Ceramic for Replacement in Lower Joints
Optimizer™ III implantable pulse generator	**Use:** Contractility Modulation Device for Insertion in Subcutaneous Tissue and Fascia
Oropharyngeal airway (OPA)	**Use:** Intraluminal Device, Airway in Mouth and Throat
Ovatio™ CRT-D	**Use:** Cardiac Resynchronization Defibrillator Pulse Generator for Insertion in Subcutaneous Tissue and Fascia
OXINIUM	**Use:** Synthetic Substitute, Oxidized Zirconium on Polyethylene for Replacement in Lower Joints
Paclitaxel-eluting coronary stent	**Use:** Intraluminal Device, Drug-eluting in Heart and Great Vessels
Paclitaxel-eluting peripheral stent	**Use:** Intraluminal Device, Drug-eluting in Upper Arteries Intraluminal Device, Drug-eluting in Lower Arteries

DEVICE KEY

Partially absorbable mesh	**Use:** Synthetic Substitute
Pedicle-based dynamic stabilization device	**Use:** Spinal Stabilization Device, Pedicle-Based for Insertion in Upper Joints Spinal Stabilization Device, Pedicle-Based for Insertion in Lower Joints
Perceval sutureless valve	**Use:** Zooplastic Tissue, Rapid Deployment Technique in New Technology
Percutaneous endoscopic gastrojejunostomy (PEG/J) tube	**Use:** Feeding Device in Gastrointestinal System
Percutaneous endoscopic gastrostomy (PEG) tube	**Use:** Feeding Device in Gastrointestinal System
Percutaneous nephrostomy catheter	**Use:** Drainage Device
Peripherally inserted central catheter (PICC)	**Use:** Infusion Device
Pessary ring	**Use:** Intraluminal Device, Pessary in Female Reproductive System
Phrenic nerve stimulator generator	**Use:** Stimulator Generator in Subcutaneous Tissue and Fascia
Phrenic nerve stimulator lead	**Use:** Diaphragmatic Pacemaker Lead in Respiratory System
PHYSIOMESH™ Flexible Composite Mesh	**Use:** Synthetic Substitute
Pipeline™ Embolization device (PED)	**Use:** Intraluminal Device
Polyethylene socket	**Use:** Synthetic Substitute, Polyethylene for Replacement in Lower Joints
Polymethylmethacrylate (PMMA)	**Use:** Synthetic Substitute
Polypropylene mesh	**Use:** Synthetic Substitute
Porcine (bioprosthetic) valve	**Use:** Zooplastic Tissue in Heart and Great Vessels
PRESTIGE® Cervical Disc	**Use:** Synthetic Substitute
PrimeAdvanced neurostimulator	**Use:** Stimulator Generator, Multiple Array for Insertion in Subcutaneous Tissue and Fascia
PROCEED™ Ventral Patch	**Use:** Synthetic Substitute
Prodisc-C	**Use:** Synthetic Substitute
Prodisc-L	**Use:** Synthetic Substitute
PROLENE Polypropylene Hernia System (PHS)	**Use:** Synthetic Substitute
Protecta XT CRT-D	**Use:** Cardiac Resynchronization Defibrillator Pulse Generator for Insertion in Subcutaneous Tissue and Fascia
Protecta XT DR (XT VR)	**Use:** Defibrillator Generator for Insertion in Subcutaneous Tissue and Fascia
Protégé® RX Carotid Stent System	**Use:** Intraluminal Device
Pump reservoir	**Use:** Infusion Device, Pump in Subcutaneous Tissue and Fascia
PVAD™ Ventricular Assist Device	**Use:** External Heart Assist System in Heart and Great Vessels
REALIZE® Adjustable Gastric Band	**Use:** Extraluminal Device
Rebound HRD® (Hernia Repair Device)	**Use:** Synthetic Substitute
RestoreAdvanced neurostimulator	**Use:** Stimulator Generator, Multiple Array Rechargeable for Insertion in Subcutaneous Tissue and Fascia
RestoreSensor neurostimulator	**Use:** Stimulator Generator, Multiple Array Rechargeable for Insertion in Subcutaneous Tissue and Fascia

APPENDIX C

DEVICE KEY

RestoreUltra neurostimulator	**Use:** Stimulator Generator, Multiple Array Rechargeable for Insertion in Subcutaneous Tissue and Fascia
Reveal (DX) (XT)	**Use:** Monitoring Device
Reverse® Shoulder Prosthesis	**Use:** Synthetic Substitute, Reverse Ball and Socket for Replacement in Upper Joints
Revo MRI™ SureScan® pacemaker	**Use:** Pacemaker, Dual Chamber for Insertion in Subcutaneous Tissue and Fascia
Rheos® System device	**Use:** Cardiac Rhythm Related Device in Subcutaneous Tissue and Fascia
Rheos® System lead	**Use:** Stimulator Lead in Upper Arteries
RNS System lead	**Use:** Neurostimulator Lead in Central Nervous System and Cranial Nerves
RNS system neurostimulator generator	**Use:** Neurostimulator Generator in Head and Facial Bones
Sacral nerve modulation (SNM) lead	**Use:** Stimulator Lead in Urinary System
Sacral neuromodulation lead	**Use:** Stimulator Lead in Urinary System
SAPIEN transcatheter aortic valve	**Use:** Zooplastic Tissue in Heart and Great Vessels
Secura (DR) (VR)	**Use:** Defibrillator Generator for Insertion in Subcutaneous Tissue and Fascia
Sheffield hybrid external fixator	**Use:** External Fixation Device, Hybrid for Insertion in Upper Bones External Fixation Device, Hybrid for Reposition in Upper Bones External Fixation Device, Hybrid for Insertion in Lower Bones External Fixation Device, Hybrid for Reposition in Lower Bones
Sheffield ring external fixator	**Use:** External Fixation Device, Ring for Insertion in Upper Bones External Fixation Device, Ring for Reposition in Upper Bones External Fixation Device, Ring for Insertion in Lower Bones External Fixation Device, Ring for Reposition in Lower Bones
Single lead pacemaker (atrium) (ventricle)	**Use:** Pacemaker, Single Chamber for Insertion in Subcutaneous Tissue and Fascia
Single lead rate responsive pacemaker (atrium) (ventricle)	**Use:** Pacemaker, Single Chamber Rate Responsive for Insertion in Subcutaneous Tissue and Fascia
Sirolimus-eluting coronary stent	**Use:** Intraluminal Device, Drug-eluting in Heart and Great Vessels
SJM Biocor® Stented Valve System	**Use:** Zooplastic Tissue in Heart and Great Vessels
Soletra® neurostimulator	**Use:** Stimulator Generator, Single Array for Insertion in Subcutaneous Tissue and Fascia
Spinal cord neurostimulator lead	**Use:** Neurostimulator Lead in Central Nervous System and Cranial Nerves
Spinal growth rods, magnetically controlled	**Use:** Magnetically Controlled Growth Rod(s) in New Technology
Spiration IBV™ Valve System	**Use:** Intraluminal Device, Endobronchial Valve in Respiratory System
Stent (angioplasty) (embolization)	**Use:** Intraluminal Device
Stented tissue valve	**Use:** Zooplastic Tissue in Heart and Great Vessels
Stratos LV	**Use:** Cardiac Resynchronization Pacemaker Pulse Generator for Insertion in Subcutaneous Tissue and Fascia

DEVICE KEY

Subcutaneous injection reservoir, port	**Use:** Vascular Access Device, Totally Implantable in Subcutaneous Tissue and Fascia
Subcutaneous injection reservoir, pump	**Use:** Infusion Device, Pump in Subcutaneous Tissue and Fascia
Subdermal progesterone implant	**Use:** Contraceptive Device in Subcutaneous Tissue and Fascia
Sutureless valve, Perceval	**Use:** Zooplastic Tissue, Rapid Deployment Technique in New Technology
SynCardia Total Artificial Heart	**Use:** Synthetic Substitute
Synchra CRT-P	**Use:** Cardiac Resynchronization Pacemaker Pulse Generator for Insertion in Subcutaneous Tissue and Fascia
Talent® Converter	**Use:** Intraluminal Device
Talent® Occluder	**Use:** Intraluminal Device
Talent® Stent Graft (abdominal) (thoracic)	**Use:** Intraluminal Device
TandemHeart® System	**Use:** Short-term External Heart Assist System in Heart and Great Vessels
TAXUS® Liberté® Paclitaxel-eluting Coronary Stent System	**Use:** Intraluminal Device, Drug-eluting in Heart and Great Vessels
Therapeutic occlusion coil(s)	**Use:** Intraluminal Device
Thoracostomy tube	**Use:** Drainage Device
Thoratec IVAD (Implantable Ventricular Assist Device)	**Use:** Implantable Heart Assist System in Heart and Great Vessels
Thoratec Paracorporeal Ventricular Assist Device	**Use:** Short-term External Heart Assist System in Heart and Great Vessels
Tibial insert	**Use:** Liner in Lower Joints
Tissue bank graft	**Use:** Nonautologous Tissue Substitute
Tissue expander (inflatable) (injectable)	**Use:** Tissue Expander in Skin and Breast Tissue Expander in Subcutaneous Tissue and Fascia
Titanium Sternal Fixation System (TSFS)	**Use:** Internal Fixation Device, Rigid Plate for Insertion in Upper Bones Internal Fixation Device, Rigid Plate for Reposition in Upper Bones
Total artificial (replacement) heart	**Use:** Synthetic Substitute
Tracheostomy tube	**Use:** Tracheostomy Device in Respiratory System
Trifecta™ Valve (aortic)	**Use:** Zooplastic Tissue in Heart and Great Vessels
Tunneled central venous catheter	**Use:** Vascular Access Device, Tunneled in Subcutaneous Tissue and Fascia
Tunneled spinal (intrathecal) catheter	**Use:** Infusion Device
Two lead pacemaker	**Use:** Pacemaker, Dual Chamber for Insertion in Subcutaneous Tissue and Fascia
Ultraflex™ Precision Colonic Stent System	**Use:** Intraluminal Device
ULTRAPRO Hernia System (UHS)	**Use:** Synthetic Substitute
ULTRAPRO Partially Absorbable Lightweight Mesh	**Use:** Synthetic Substitute
ULTRAPRO Plug	**Use:** Synthetic Substitute
Ultrasonic osteogenic stimulator	**Use:** Bone Growth Stimulator in Head and Facial Bones Bone Growth Stimulator in Upper Bones Bone Growth Stimulator in Lower Bones

APPENDIX C

DEVICE KEY

Ultrasound bone healing system	**Use:** Bone Growth Stimulator in Head and Facial Bones Bone Growth Stimulator in Upper Bones Bone Growth Stimulator in Lower Bones
Uniplanar external fixator	**Use:** External Fixation Device, Monoplanar for Insertion in Upper Bones External Fixation Device, Monoplanar for Reposition in Upper Bones External Fixation Device, Monoplanar for Insertion in Lower Bones External Fixation Device, Monoplanar for Reposition in Lower Bones
Urinary incontinence stimulator lead	**Use:** Stimulator Lead in Urinary System
Vaginal pessary	**Use:** Intraluminal Device, Pessary in Female Reproductive System
Valiant Thoracic Stent Graft	**Use:** Intraluminal Device
Vectra® Vascular Access Graft	**Use:** Vascular Access Device, Tunneled in Subcutaneous Tissue and Fascia
Ventrio™ Hernia Patch	**Use:** Synthetic Substitute
Versa	**Use:** Pacemaker, Dual Chamber for Insertion in Subcutaneous Tissue and Fascia
Virtuoso (II) (DR) (VR)	**Use:** Defibrillator Generator for Insertion in Subcutaneous Tissue and Fascia
WALLSTENT® Endoprosthesis	**Use:** Intraluminal Device
X-STOP® Spacer	**Use:** Spinal Stabilization Device, Interspinous Process for Insertion in Upper Joints Spinal Stabilization Device, Interspinous Process for Insertion in Lower Joints
Xenograft	**Use:** Zooplastic Tissue in Heart and Great Vessels
XIENCE V Everolimus Eluting Coronary Stent System	**Use:** Intraluminal Device, Drug-eluting in Heart and Great Vessels
XLIF® System	**Use:** Interbody Fusion Device in Lower Joints
Zenith Flex® AAA Endovascular Graft	**Use:** Intraluminal Device
Zenith TX2® TAA Endovascular Graft	**Use:** Intraluminal Device
Zenith® Renu™ AAA Ancillary Graft	**Use:** Intraluminal Device
Zilver® PTX® (paclitaxel) Drug-Eluting Peripheral Stent	**Use:** Intraluminal Device, Drug-eluting in Upper Arteries Intraluminal Device, Drug-eluting in Lower Arteries
Zimmer® NexGen® LPS Mobile Bearing Knee	**Use:** Synthetic Substitute
Zimmer® NexGen® LPS-Flex Mobile Knee	**Use:** Synthetic Substitute
Zotarolimus-eluting coronary stent	**Use:** Intraluminal Device, Drug-eluting in Heart and Great Vessels

SUBSTANCE KEY

Term	ICD-10-PCS Value
AIGISRx Antibacterial Envelope Antimicrobial envelope	**Use:** Anti-Infective Envelope
Axicabtagene Ciloeucel	**Use:** Engineered Autologous Chimeric Antigen Receptor T-cell Immunotherapy
Bone morphogenetic protein 2 (BMP 2)	**Use:** Recombinant Bone Morphogenetic Protein
CBMA (Concentrated Bone Marrow Aspirate)	**Use:** Concentrated Bone Marrow Aspirate
Clolar	**Use:** Clofarabine
Defitelio	**Use:** Defibrotide Sodium Anticoagulant
DuraGraft® Endothelial Damage Inhibitor	**Use:** Endothelial Damage Inhibitor
Factor Xa Inhibitor Reversal Agent, Andexanet Alfa	**Use:** Andexanet Alfa, Factor Xa Inhibitor Reversal Agent
Kcentra	**Use:** 4-Factor Prothrombin Complex Concentrate
Nesiritide	**Use:** Human B-type Natriuretic Peptide
rhBMP-2	**Use:** Recombinant Bone Morphogenetic Protein
Seprafilm	**Use:** Adhesion Barrier
STELARA®	**Use:** Other New Technology Therapeutic Substance
Tissue Plasminogen Activator (tPA) (rtPA)	**Use:** Other Thrombolytic
Ustekinumab	**Use:** Other New Technology Therapeutic Substance
Vistogard®	**Use:** Uridine Triacetate
Voraxaze	**Use:** Glucarpidase
VYXEOS™	**Use:** Cytarabine and Daunorubicin Liposome Antineoplastic
ZINPLAVA™	**Use:** Bezlotoxumab Monoclonal Antibody
Zyvox	**Use:** Oxazolidinones

DEVICE AGGREGATION TABLE

Specific Device	for Operation	in Body System	General Device
Autologous Arterial Tissue	All applicable	Heart and Great Vessels Lower Arteries Lower Veins Upper Arteries Upper Veins	**7** Autologous Tissue Substitute
Autologous Venous Tissue	All applicable	Heart and Great Vessels Lower Arteries Lower Veins Upper Arteries Upper Veins	**7** Autologous Tissue Substitute
Cardiac Lead, Defibrillator	Insertion	Heart and Great Vessels	**M** Cardiac Lead
Cardiac Lead, Pacemaker	Insertion	Heart and Great Vessels	**M** Cardiac Lead
Cardiac Resynchronization Defibrillator Pulse Generator	Insertion	Subcutaneous Tissue and Fascia	**P** Cardiac Rhythm Related Device
Cardiac Resynchronization Pacemaker Pulse Generator	Insertion	Subcutaneous Tissue and Fascia	**P** Cardiac Rhythm Related Device
Contractility Modulation Device	Insertion	Subcutaneous Tissue and Fascia	**P** Cardiac Rhythm Related Device
Defibrillator Generator	Insertion	Subcutaneous Tissue and Fascia	**P** Cardiac Rhythm Related Device
Epiretinal Visual Prosthesis	All applicable	Eye	**J** Synthetic Substitute
External Fixation Device, Hybrid	Insertion	Lower Bones Upper Bones	**5** External Fixation Device
External Fixation Device, Hybrid	Reposition	Lower Bones Upper Bones	**5** External Fixation Device
External Fixation Device, Limb Lengthening	Insertion	Lower Bones Upper Bones	**5** External Fixation Device
External Fixation Device, Monoplanar	Insertion	Lower Bones Upper Bones	**5** External Fixation Device
External Fixation Device, Monoplanar	Reposition	Lower Bones Upper Bones	**5** External Fixation Device
External Fixation Device, Ring	Insertion	Lower Bones Upper Bones	**5** External Fixation Device
External Fixation Device, Ring	Reposition	Lower Bones Upper Bones	**5** External Fixation Device
Hearing Device, Bone Conduction	Insertion	Ear, Nose, Sinus	**S** Hearing Device
Hearing Device, Multiple Channel Cochlear Prosthesis	Insertion	Ear, Nose, Sinus	**S** Hearing Device
Hearing Device, Single Channel Cochlear Prosthesis	Insertion	Ear, Nose, Sinus	**S** Hearing Device
Internal Fixation Device, Intramedullary	All applicable	Lower Bones Upper Bones	**4** Internal Fixation Device
Internal Fixation Device, Intramedullary Limb Lengthening	Insertion	Lower Bones Upper Bones	**6** Internal Fixation Device, Intramedullary
Internal Fixation Device, Rigid Plate	Insertion	Upper Bones	**4** Internal Fixation Device
Internal Fixation Device, Rigid Plate	Reposition	Upper Bones	**4** Internal Fixation Device
Intraluminal Device, Flow Diverter	Restriction	Upper Arteries	**D** Intraluminal Device

DEVICE AGGREGATION TABLE

Specific Device	for Operation	in Body System	General Device
Intraluminal Device, Pessary	All applicable	Female Reproductive System	**D** Intraluminal Device
Intraluminal Device, Airway	All applicable	Ear, Nose, Sinus Gastrointestinal System Mouth and Throat	**D** Intraluminal Device
Intraluminal Device, Bioactive	All applicable	Upper Arteries	**D** Intraluminal Device
Intraluminal Device, Branched or Fenestrated, One or Two Arteries	Restriction	Heart and Great Vessels Lower Arteries	**D** Intraluminal Device
Intraluminal Device, Branched or Fenestrated, Three or More Arteries	Restriction	Heart and Great Vessels Lower Arteries	**D** Intraluminal Device
Intraluminal Device, Drug-eluting	All applicable	Heart and Great Vessels Lower Arteries Upper Arteries	**D** Intraluminal Device
Intraluminal Device, Drug-eluting, Four or More	All applicable	Heart and Great Vessels Lower Arteries Upper Arteries	**D** Intraluminal Device
Intraluminal Device, Drug-eluting, Three	All applicable	Heart and Great Vessels Lower Arteries Upper Arteries	**D** Intraluminal Device
Intraluminal Device, Drug-eluting, Two	All applicable	Heart and Great Vessels Lower Arteries Upper Arteries	**D** Intraluminal Device
Intraluminal Device, Endobronchial Valve	All applicable	Respiratory System	**D** Intraluminal Device
Intraluminal Device, Endotracheal Airway	All applicable	Respiratory System	**D** Intraluminal Device
Intraluminal Device, Four or More	All applicable	Heart and Great Vessels Lower Arteries Upper Arteries	**D** Intraluminal Device
Intraluminal Device, Radioactive	All applicable	Heart and Great Vessels	**D** Intraluminal Device
Intraluminal Device, Three	All applicable	Heart and Great Vessels Lower Arteries Upper Arteries	**D** Intraluminal Device
Intraluminal Device, Two	All applicable	Heart and Great Vessels Lower Arteries Upper Arteries	**D** Intraluminal Device
Monitoring Device, Hemodynamic	Insertion	Subcutaneous Tissue and Fascia	**2** Monitoring Device
Monitoring Device, Pressure Sensor	Insertion	Heart and Great Vessels	**2** Monitoring Device
Pacemaker, Dual Chamber	Insertion	Subcutaneous Tissue and Fascia	**P** Cardiac Rhythm Related Device
Pacemaker, Single Chamber	Insertion	Subcutaneous Tissue and Fascia	**P** Cardiac Rhythm Related Device
Pacemaker, Single Chamber Rate Responsive	Insertion	Subcutaneous Tissue and Fascia	**P** Cardiac Rhythm Related Device
Spinal Stabilization Device, Facet Replacement	Insertion	Lower Joints Upper Joints	**4** Internal Fixation Device
Spinal Stabilization Device, Interspinous Process	Insertion	Lower Joints Upper Joints	**4** Internal Fixation Device
Spinal Stabilization Device, Pedicle-Based	Insertion	Lower Joints Upper Joints	**4** Internal Fixation Device

DEVICE AGGREGATION TABLE

Specific Device	for Operation	in Body System	General Device
Spinal Stabilization Device,Vertebral Body Tether	Reposition	Lower Bones Upper Bones	**4** Internal Fixation Device
Stimulator Generator, Multiple Array	Insertion	Subcutaneous Tissue and Fascia	**M** Stimulator Generator
Stimulator Generator, Multiple Array Rechargeable	Insertion	Subcutaneous Tissue and Fascia	**M** Stimulator Generator
Stimulator Generator, Single Array	Insertion	Subcutaneous Tissue and Fascia	**M** Stimulator Generator
Stimulator Generator, Single Array Rechargeable	Insertion	Subcutaneous Tissue and Fascia	**M** Stimulator Generator
Synthetic Substitute, Ceramic	Replacement	Lower Joints	**J** Synthetic Substitute
Synthetic Substitute, Ceramic on Polyethylene	Replacement	Lower Joints	**J** Synthetic Substitute
Synthetic Substitute, Intraocular Telescope	Replacement	Eye	**J** Synthetic Substitute
Synthetic Substitute, Metal	Replacement	Lower Joints	**J** Synthetic Substitute
Synthetic Substitute, Metal on Polyethylene	Replacement	Lower Joints	**J** Synthetic Substitute
Synthetic Substitute, Oxidized Zirconium on Polyethylene	Replacement	Lower Joints	**J** Synthetic Substitute
Synthetic Substitute, Polyethylene	Replacement	Lower Joints	**J** Synthetic Substitute
Synthetic Substitute, Reverse Ball and Socket	Replacement	Upper Joints	**J** Synthetic Substitute

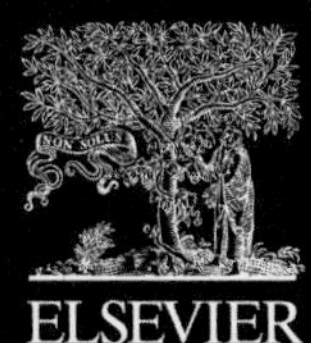
ELSEVIER

Trust Elsevier to support you every step of your coding career!

From beginning to advanced, from the classroom to the workplace, from application to certification, Elsevier coding solutions are your guide to greater opportunities and successful career advancement.

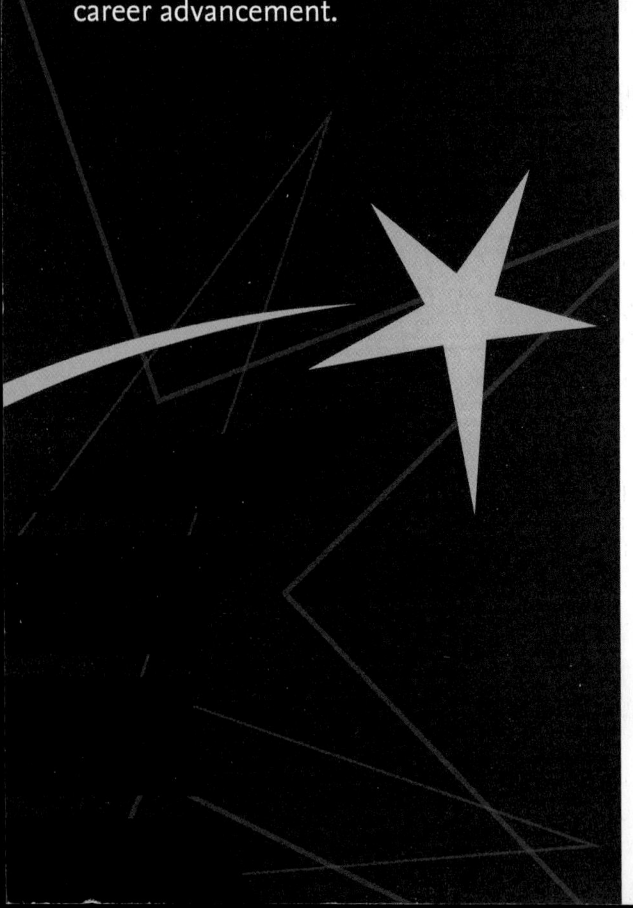

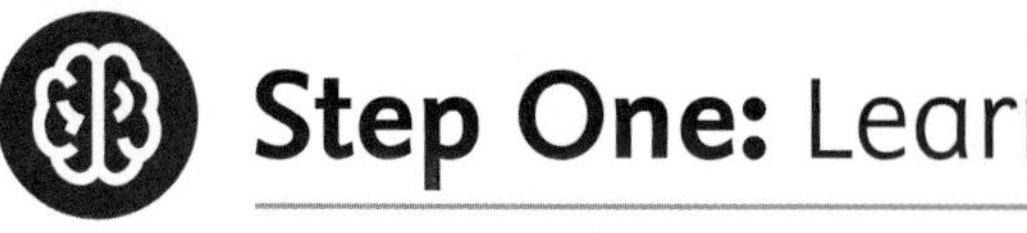

Step One: Lear

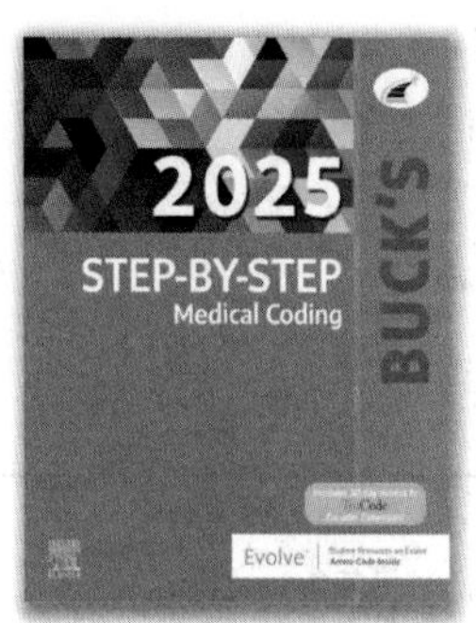
2025
STEP-BY-STEP
Medical Coding
BUCK'S
Evolve

Buck's Step-by-Step Medical Coding, 2025 Editio
ISBN: 978-0-443-24878-8

Also available:
Buck's Workbook for Step-by-Step Medical Coding, 2025 Edition
ISBN: 978-0-443-24879-5

Buck's Medical Coding Online for Step-by-Step Medical Coding, 2025 Edition
ISBN: 978-0-443-26462-7

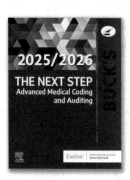

Step Two: Practic

2025/2026
THE NEXT STEP
Advanced Medical Coding and Auditing
BUCK'S
Evolve

Buck's The Next Step: Advanced Medical Coding and Auditing, 2025/2026 Edition
ISBN: 978-0-443-24880-1

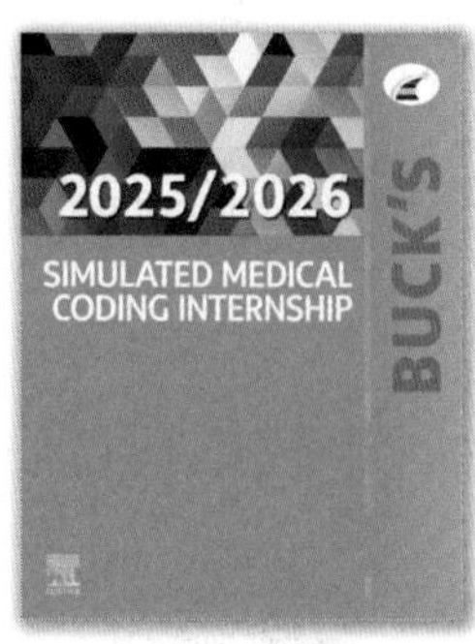
2025/2026
SIMULATED MEDICAL CODING INTERNSHIP
BUCK'S

Buck's Simulated Medical Coding Internship, 2025/2026 Edition
ISBN: 978-0-443-26464-1

Practice Management with Auditing for Coders
POWERED BY
SimChart® for the medical office
ELSEVIER

Practice Management with Auditing for Coders Powered by SimChart for the Medical Office
ISBN: 978-0-323-43011-1

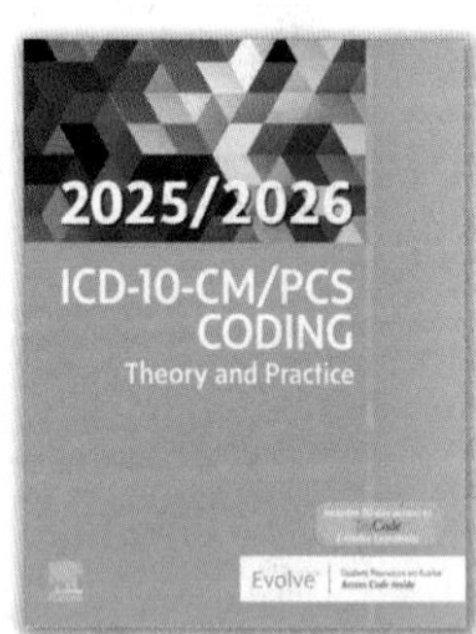

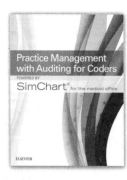
2025/2026
ICD-10-CM/PCS CODING
Theory and Practice
Evolve

ICD-10-CM/PCS Coding Theory and Practice, 2025/2026 Edition
ISBN: 978-0-443-24893-1